PHARMACOTHERAPY
HANDBOOK

PHARMACOTHERAPY HANDBOOK

Barbara G. Wells, PharmD, FASHP, FCCP
Professor and Dean
Idaho State University College of Pharmacy
Pocatello, Idaho

Joseph T. DiPiro, PharmD, FCCP
Professor, College of Pharmacy
Head, Department of Pharmacy Practice
University of Georgia

Clinical Professor of Surgery
Medical College of Georgia
Augusta, Georgia

Terry L. Schwinghammer, PharmD, FCCP, BCPS
Associate Professor
Department of Pharmaceutical Sciences
School of Pharmacy, University of Pittsburgh
Pittsburgh, Pennsylvania

Cindy W. Hamilton, PharmD
Principal, Hamilton House
Virginia Beach, Virginia

Clinical Instructor
Virginia Commonwealth University School of Pharmacy
Richmond, Virginia

APPLETON & LANGE
Stamford, Connecticut

Copyright © 1998 by Appleton & Lange
A Simon & Schuster Company

98 99 00 01 02 / 10 9 8 7 6 5 4 3 2 1

Prentice Hall International (UK) Limited, *London*
Prentice Hall of Australia Pty. Limited, *Sydney*
Prentice Hall Canada, Inc., *Toronto*
Prentice Hall Hispanoamericana, S.A., *Mexico*
Prentice Hall of India Private Limited, *New Delhi*
Prentice Hall of Japan, Inc., *Tokyo*
Simon & Schuster Asia Pte. Ltd., *Singapore*
Editora Prentice Hall do Brasil Ltda., *Rio de Janeiro*
Prentice Hall, *Upper Saddle River, New Jersey*

Editor-in-Chief: Cheryl L. Mehalik
Managing Editor, Development: Kathleen McCullough
Production Editor: Elizabeth C. Ryan
Designer: Mary Skudlarek

ISBN 0-8385-8140-4

9 780838 581407

90000

PRINTED IN THE UNITED STATES OF AMERICA

CONTENTS

Contents

Contents

NEUROLOGIC DISORDERS
Edited by Barbara G. Wells, PharmD, FASHP, FCCP

NUTRITIONAL DISORDERS
Edited by Cindy W. Hamilton, PharmD

ONCOLOGIC DISORDERS
Edited by Terry L. Schwinghammer, PharmD, FCCP, BCPS

OPHTHALMIC DISORDERS
Edited by Cindy W. Hamilton, PharmD

Contents

PREFACE

This pocket companion to *Pharmacotherapy: A Pathophysiologic Approach,* Third Edition, was created to provide practitioners and students with critical information that can be easily used to guide drug therapy decision-making in the clinical setting. To ensure brevity and portability, the bulleted format provides the user with *essential textual information, key tables* and *figures,* and *treatment algorithms.*

Corresponding to the major sections in the main text, disorders are alphabetized within the following sections which appear as a tabbing guide on the back of the book: Bone and Joint Disorders; Cardiovascular Disorders; Dermatologic Disorders; Endocrinologic Disorders; Gastrointestinal Disorders; Gynecologic and Obstetric Disorders; Hematologic Disorders; Infectious Diseases; Neurologic Disorders; Nutritional Disorders; Oncologic Disorders; Ophthalmic Disorders; Psychiatric Disorders; Renal Disorders; and Respiratory Disorders. Drug-induced conditions associated with skin disorders, renal diseases, and pulmonary diseases appear in three tabular appendices.

Carrying over a popular feature from *Pharmacotherapy,* each chapter is organized in a consistent format:

- Disease state definition
- Concise review of relevant pathophysiology
- Clinical presentation
- Diagnosis
- Desired outcome
- Treatment and monitoring

The treatment section may include non-pharmacologic therapy, drug selection guidelines, dosing recommendations, major adverse effects, pharmacokinetic considerations, and important drug–drug interactions. Treatment algorithms are included when available. If more in-depth information is required, the reader is encouraged to refer to the primary text, *Pharmacotherapy: A Pathophysiologic Approach,* Third Edition.

It is our sincere hope that students and practitioners find this book helpful as they continuously strive to deliver the highest quality care to patients. We invite your comments on how we may improve subsequent editions of this work.

Barbara G. Wells
Joseph T. DiPiro
Terry L. Schwinghammer
Cindy W. Hamilton

ACKNOWLEDGMENTS

The editors wish to express our sincere appreciation to the authors whose chapters in the third edition of *Pharmacotherapy: A Pathophysiologic Approach* served as the basis for this book. The dedication and professionalism of these outstanding practitioners, teachers, and clinical scientists are evident on every page of this work. The authors of the chapters from the third edition are acknowledged at the end of each respective *Handbook* chapter. We also thank Gary R. Matzke and Courtney V. Fletcher for their assistance with selected chapters. Cheryl Mehalik, our Executive Editor at Appleton & Lange, deserves special recognition for her creativity, her unique ideas, and for shepherding the book through all stages of the production process. We also wish to thank our spouses, Richard Wells, Cecily DiPiro, Donna Schwinghammer, and Raleigh Hamilton for their love, encouragement, and patience.

TO THE READER

Basic and clinical research provide a continuous flow of biomedical information that enables practitioners to use medications more effectively and safely. The editors, authors, and publisher of this book have made every effort to ensure accuracy of information provided. *However, it is the responsibility of all practitioners to assess the appropriateness of published drug therapy information, especially in light of the specific clinical situation and new developments in the field.* The editors and authors have taken care to recommend dosages that are consistent with current published guidelines and other responsible literature. However, when dealing with new and unfamiliar drug therapies, students and practitioners should consult several appropriate information sources.

Bone and Joint Disorders
Edited by Terry L. Schwinghammer, PharmD, FCCP, BCPS

Chapter 1

▶ GOUT AND HYPERURICEMIA

▶ DEFINITIONS

- The term gout describes a disease spectrum including hyperuricemia, recurrent attacks of acute arthritis associated with monosodium urate crystals in leukocytes found in synovial fluid, deposits of monosodium urate crystals in tissues (tophi), interstitial renal disease, and uric acid nephrolithiasis.
- Hyperuricemia may be an asymptomatic condition, with an increased serum uric acid as the only apparent abnormality. A urate concentration greater than 7.0 mg/dL is abnormal and is associated with an increased risk for gout.

▶ PATHOPHYSIOLOGY

- In humans, uric acid is the product of the degradation of purines. It serves no known physiologic purpose and therefore is regarded as a waste product. The size of the urate pool is increased several-fold in individuals with gout. This excess accumulation may result from either overproduction or underexcretion.
- The purines from which uric acid is produced originate from three sources: dietary purine, conversion of tissue nucleic acid to purine nucleotides, and *de novo* synthesis of purine bases.
- Abnormalities in the enzyme systems that regulate purine metabolism may result in overproduction of uric acid. An increase in the activity of phosphoribosyl pyrophosphate (PRPP) synthetase leads to an increased concentration of PRPP, a key determinant of purine synthesis and thus uric acid production. A deficiency of hypoxanthine–guanine phosphoribosyl transferase (HGPRT) may also result in overproduction of uric acid. HGPRT is responsible for the conversion of guanine to guanylic acid and hypoxanthine to inosinic acid. These two conversions require PRPP as the cosubstrate and are important reutilization reactions involved in the synthesis of nucleic acids. A deficiency in the HGPRT enzyme leads to increased metabolism of guanine and hypoxanthine to uric acid and more PRPP to interact with glutamine in the first step of the purine pathway. Complete absence of HGPRT results in the childhood Lesch–Nyhan syndrome, characterized by choreoathetosis, spasticity, mental retardation, and markedly excessive production of uric acid.

- Uric acid may also be overproduced as a consequence of increased breakdown of tissue nucleic acids such as occurs with myeloproliferative and lymphoproliferative disorders.
- Dietary purines play an unimportant role in the generation of hyperuricemia in the absence of some derangement in purine metabolism or elimination.
- About two-thirds of the uric acid produced each day is excreted in the urine. The rest is eliminated through the gastrointestinal tract, after enzymatic degradation by colonic bacteria. A decline in the urinary excretion of uric acid to a level below the rate of production leads to hyperuricemia and an increased miscible pool of sodium urate.
- Drugs that decrease renal clearance of uric acid through modification of filtered load or one of the tubular transport processes include diuretics, salicylates (<2 g/day), pyrazinamide, ethambutol, nicotinic acid, ethanol, levodopa, and cytotoxic drugs.
- Normal individuals produce 600–800 mg of uric acid daily and excrete less than 600 mg in urine. Individuals who excrete more than 600 mg on a purine-free diet may be considered overproducers. Hyperuricemic individuals who excrete less than 600 mg of uric acid per 24 hours on a purine-free diet may be defined as underexcretors of uric acid. On a regular diet, excretion of greater than 1000 mg per 24 hours reflects overproduction; less than this is probably normal.
- Deposition of urate crystals in synovial fluid results in an inflammatory process involving chemical mediators that cause vasodilation, increased vascular permeability, and chemotactic activity for polymorphonuclear leukocytes. Phagocytosis of urate crystals by the leukocytes results in rapid lysis of cells and a discharge of proteolytic enzymes into the cytoplasm. The inflammatory reaction that ensues is associated with intense joint pain, erythema, warmth, and swelling.
- Uric acid nephrolithiasis occurs in 10–25% of patients with gout. Factors that predispose individuals to uric acid nephrolithiasis include excessive urinary excretion of uric acid, an acidic urine, and a highly concentrated urine.
- In acute uric acid nephropathy, acute renal failure occurs as a result of blockage of urine flow secondary to massive precipitation of uric acid crystals in the collecting ducts and ureters. This syndrome is a well-recognized complication in patients with myeloproliferative or lymphoproliferative disorders and is a result of massive malignant cell turnover, particularly after initiation of chemotherapy. Chronic urate nephropathy is caused by the long-term deposition of urate crystals in the renal parenchyma.
- Tophi (urate deposits) are uncommon in the general population of gouty subjects and are a late complication of hyperuricemia. The most common sites of tophaceous deposits in patients with recurrent acute gouty arthritis are the base of the great toe, the helix of the ear, olecranon bursae, Achilles tendon, knees, wrists, and hands.

▶ CLINICAL PRESENTATION

- Acute attacks of gouty arthritis are characterized by rapid onset of excruciating pain, swelling, and inflammation. The attack is typically monoarticular at first, most often affecting the first metatarsophalangeal joint (podagra), and then, in order of frequency, the insteps, ankles, heels, knees, wrists, fingers, and elbows. Attacks commonly begin at night with the patient awakening from sleep with excruciating pain. The affected joints are erythematous, warm, and swollen. Fever and leukocytosis are common. Untreated attacks may last from 3–14 days before spontaneous recovery.
- Although acute attacks of gouty arthritis may occur without apparent provocation, attacks may be precipitated by stress, trauma, alcohol ingestion, infection, surgery, rapid lowering of serum uric acid by ingestion of uric acid–lowering agents, and ingestion of certain drugs known to elevate serum uric acid concentrations.

▶ DIAGNOSIS

- When joint aspiration is not a viable option, a presumptive diagnosis of acute gouty arthritis may be made on the basis of the presence of the characteristic signs and symptoms as well as the response to treatment. The definitive diagnosis is accomplished by aspiration of synovial fluid from the affected joint and identification of intracellular crystals of monosodium urate monohydrate in synovial fluid leukocytes.

▶ DESIRED OUTCOME

The goals in the treatment of gout are to terminate the acute attack, prevent recurrent attacks of gouty arthritis, and prevent complications associated with chronic deposition of urate crystals in tissues.

▶ TREATMENT

ACUTE GOUTY ARTHRITIS

Colchicine
- The usual oral dose of colchicine is 0.5 or 0.6 mg at hourly intervals until the joint symptoms subside; the patient develops nausea, vomiting, or diarrhea; or the patient has taken a maximum of 12 tablets. About 75–95% of patients with acute gouty arthritis respond favorably to colchicine when ingestion of the drug is begun within 12 hours of the onset of joint symptoms. Gastrointestinal (GI) toxicity occurs in 50–80% of patients before the relief of the attack. Elderly patients may become severely dehydrated and incur serious electrolyte losses.
- This high incidence of GI toxicity may be circumvented by administering colchicine intravenously. The initial intravenous (IV) dose of col-

chicine is 2 mg. If relief is not obtained, an additional 1-mg dose may be given at 6 and at 12 hours to a total dose of 4 mg for a specific attack. The colchicine should be diluted with 20 mL of normal saline before administration to minimize sclerosis of the vein. IV colchicine subjects patients to the risk of local extravasation, which can cause inflammation in and necrosis of the surrounding tissue. Very small, difficult-to-inject veins and renal impairment are relative contraindications to IV colchicine therapy. Colchicine should not be used intravenously in individuals who are neutropenic, have severe renal impairment (creatinine clearance <10 mL/min), or have combined renal and hepatic insufficiency.

Indomethacin

- Indomethacin is as effective as colchicine in the treatment of acute gouty arthritis and is preferred because acute GI toxicity occurs far less frequently than with colchicine. It is customary to start with a relatively large dose for the first 24–48 hours and then taper the therapy over 3–4 days to minimize the risk of recurrent attacks. For example, 75 mg of indomethacin may be given initially, followed by 50 mg every 6 hours for 2 days, then 50 mg every 8 hours for 1 or 2 days.
- Side effects unique to indomethacin include headache and dizziness. All nonsteroidal anti-inflammatory drugs (NSAIDs) have been implicated in causing gastric ulceration and bleeding, but this is unlikely with short-term therapy.

Other NSAIDs

- Other NSAIDs are also effective in relieving the inflammation of acute gout (Table 1.1). NSAIDs should be used with caution in individuals with a history of acid peptic disease, congestive heart failure, chronic renal failure, or coronary artery disease.

TABLE 1.1. Dosage Regimens of Nonsteroidal Anti-inflammatory Drugs (NSAIDs) for Treatment of Acute Gouty Arthritis

Generic (Brand) Name	Dosage and Frequency
Fenoprofen (Nalfon)	800 mg Q6H
Flurbiprofen (Ansaid)	100 mg QID for 1 day, then 50 mg QID
Ibuprofen (Motrin)	600–800 mg QID
Ketoprofen (Orudis)	50 mg QID or 75 mg TID
Meclofenamate (Meclomen)	100 mg TID-QID
Naproxen (Naprosyn)	750 mg initially, then 250 mg Q8H
Piroxicam (Feldene)	40 mg QD
Sulindac (Clinoril)	200 mg BID
Tolmetin (Tolectin)	400 mg TID-QID

Corticosteroids
- Corticosteroids may be used to treat acute attacks of gouty arthritis, but they are reserved primarily for resistant cases. Prednisone may be administered orally in doses of 30–60 mg daily in patients with multiple-joint involvement. Because rebound attacks may occur upon steroid withdrawal, colchicine 0.6 mg should be given two or three times daily during and for several days after steroid therapy.
- Doses of 40–80 USP units of ACTH gel are given intramuscularly (IM) every 6–8 hours for 2–3 days and then the doses are reduced in stepwise fashion and discontinued.
- Intra-articular administration of triamcinolone hexacetonide in a dose of 20–40 mg may be useful in treating acute gout limited to a single joint.

PROPHYLACTIC THERAPY

General Principles
- If the first episode of acute gouty arthritis was mild and responded promptly to treatment, the patient's serum urate concentration was only minimally elevated, and the 24-hour urinary uric acid excretion was not excessive (<1000 mg/24 hours on a regular diet), then prophylactic treatment can be withheld.
- If the patient had a severe attack of gouty arthritis, a complicated course of uric acid lithiasis, a substantially elevated serum uric acid (>10.0 mg/dL), or a 24-hour urinary excretion of uric acid of more than 1000 mg, then prophylactic treatment should be instituted immediately after resolution of the acute episode.
- Prophylactic therapy is also appropriate for patients with frequent (i.e., more than two or three per year) attacks of gouty arthritis even if the serum uric acid concentration is normal or only minimally elevated.

Colchicine
- Prophylactic therapy with low-dose oral colchicine, 0.5–0.6 mg twice daily, may be effective in preventing recurrent arthritis in patients with no evidence of visible tophi and a normal or slightly elevated serum urate concentration. Patients do not become resistant to or tolerant of daily colchicine, and if they sense the beginning of an acute attack, they should increase the dose to 1 mg every 2 hours; in most instances the attack aborts after 1 or 2 mg of colchicine.

Uric Acid Lowering Therapy
- Patients with a history of recurrent acute gouty arthritis and a significantly elevated serum uric acid concentration are probably best managed with uric acid lowering therapy.
- Colchicine at a dose of 0.5 mg twice daily should be administered during the first 6–12 months of antihyperuricemic therapy to minimize the risk of acute attacks that may occur during initiation of uric acid lowering therapy.

- The therapeutic objective of antihyperuricemic therapy is to reduce the serum urate concentration below 6 mg/dL, well below the saturation point.

Uricosuric Drugs

- Uricosuric drugs (probenecid, sulfinpyrazone) increase the renal clearance of uric acid by inhibiting the renal tubular reabsorption of uric acid. Therapy with uricosuric drugs should be started at a low dose to avoid marked uricosuria and possible stone formation. The maintenance of adequate urine flow and alkalinization of the urine with sodium bicarbonate or Shohl's solution during the first several days of uricosuric therapy further diminish the possibility of uric acid stone formation.
- Probenecid is given initially at a dose of 250 mg twice a day for 1–2 weeks, then 500 mg twice a day for 2 weeks. Thereafter, the daily dose is increased by 500-mg increments every 1–2 weeks until satisfactory control is achieved or a maximum dose of 3.0 g is reached.
- The initial dose of sulfinpyrazone is 50 mg twice a day for 3–4 days, then 100 mg twice a day, increasing the daily dose by 100-mg increments each week until the serum urate concentration is in the desired range.
- The major side effects associated with uricosuric therapy are GI irritation, rash and hypersensitivity, precipitation of acute gouty arthritis, and stone formation. These drugs are contraindicated in patients who are allergic to them and in patients with impaired renal function (i.e., creatinine clearance <50 mL/min).

Xanthine Oxidase Inhibitor

- Both allopurinol and its major metabolite, oxypurinol, are xanthine oxidase inhibitors and thus impair the conversion of hypoxanthine to xanthine and xanthine to uric acid. Allopurinol also lowers the intracellular concentration of PRPP. Because of the long half-life of its metabolite, allopurinol can be given once daily. An oral daily dose of 300 mg is usually sufficient. Occasionally, as much as 600–800 mg/d may be necessary.
- Allopurinol is the antihyperuricemic drug of choice in patients with a history of urinary stones or impaired renal function, in patients who have lymphoproliferative or myeloproliferative disorders and need pretreatment with a xanthine oxidase inhibitor before initiation of cytotoxic therapy to protect against acute uric acid nephropathy, and in patients with gout who are overproducers of uric acid.
- The major side effects of allopurinol are skin rash, leukopenia, occasional GI toxicity, and increased frequency of acute gouty attacks with the initiation of therapy.

EVALUATION OF THERAPEUTIC OUTCOMES

- Patients should be monitored for symptomatic relief of joint pain as well as potential adverse effects and drug interactions related to drug therapy. The acute pain of an initial attack of gouty arthritis should begin to ease within about eight hours of treatment initiation. Complete resolution of pain, erythema, and inflammation usually occurs within 48 to 72 hours.

- Asymptomatic hyperuricemia need not be treated, especially if the serum urate concentration remains below 10 mg/dL.

See Chapter 86, Gout and Hyperuricemia, authored by David W. Hawkins, PharmD, and Daniel W. Rahn for a more detailed discussion of this topic.

Chapter 2

▶ OSTEOARTHRITIS

▶ DEFINITION

Osteoarthritis (OA) is a common, slowly progressive disorder affecting primarily the weight-bearing diarthrodial joints of the peripheral and axial skeleton. It is characterized by progressive deterioration and loss of articular cartilage resulting in osteophyte formation, pain, limitation of motion, deformity, and progressive disability. Inflammation may or may not be present in the affected joints.

▶ PATHOPHYSIOLOGY

- An initial biochemical change in cartilage appears to be an increase in water content of the cartilage matrix despite a reduction in hydrophilic proteoglycans. This initial change results in a thickened articular cartilage but one less able to withstand mechanical forces.
- Soon after these changes in water content occur, the glycosaminoglycan composition changes, reflecting changes in keratan sulfate and the ratio of chondroitin 4-sulfate to chondroitin 6-sulfate. These changes may result in decreased proteoglycan–collagen interaction in the cartilage. The collagen content does not appear to change until severe disease is present. Increases in collagen synthesis and in the distribution and diameter of the fibers have been noted.
- The net effect of these biochemical changes is the failure of the cartilage to repair itself, resulting in loss of cartilage, eburnation of bone, and pain.
- Pathologic changes in the cartilage and bone also occur. There is an initial thickening of the articular cartilage, reflecting the damage to the collagen network and increase of water content. Joint synovial lining may show moderate degrees of inflammation. Fibrillation, a splitting of the noncalcified cartilage, exposes the underlying bone, which may ultimately lead to microfractures of the subchondral bone. Horizontal splitting of cartilage between the calcified and uncalcified layers occurs secondary to shearing damage. Cartilage thinning and erosions progress to focal exposure of the calcified cartilage and underlying bone as a result of grinding damage or abrasive wear.
- Microfractures result in the production of callus and increased amounts of osteoid. New bone (osteophytes) forms at the joint margins, away from the area of cartilage destruction. Osteophytes may be an attempt to stabilize the joints and may not be part of the destructive aspects of osteoarthritis.
- Inflammation, such as synovitis, is seen and may result from the release of inflammatory mediators such as prostaglandins secreted by the chondrocytes.

▶ CLINICAL PRESENTATION

- In the United States, both sexes tend to be affected equally; potential risk factors include obesity, repetitive use through work or leisure activities, and heredity.
- The clinical presentation depends on the duration of disease, the joints affected, and the severity of joint involvement (Table 2.1). The predominant symptom is a localized deep, aching pain associated with the affected joint. Early in the course of the disease, pain occurs when the joint is first used and becomes relieved by rest or removal of weight from the affected joint. Later, the pain occurs with minimal motion or activity and may be present even during rest.
- In addition to pain in the affected joint, limitation of motion, stiffness, crepitus, and deformities may be present. A sense of weakness or instability may be associated with this limitation of motion in patients with lower extremity involvement.
- The joint stiffness lasts less than 30 minutes and often occurs after sitting or resting for some time. Joint enlargement typically is related to bony proliferation or, in some cases, thickening of the synovium and joint capsule. The presence of a warm, red, tender joint may suggest an inflammatory synovitis.
- Joint deformity may be present in the later stages and is the result of subluxation, collapse of subchondral bone, formation of bone cysts, or bony overgrowths.
- Physical examination of the affected joint or joints reveals pain, tenderness, crepitus, and possible joint enlargement. Heberden's nodes are bony enlargements (osteophytes) of the distal interphalangeal (DIP) and Bouchard's nodes are osteophytes of the proximal interphalangeal (PIP) joints.

▶ DIAGNOSIS

- The diagnosis of osteoarthritis is strongly dependent on an evaluation of the patient's history, clinical examination of the affected joint(s), and radiologic findings.
- Radiologic evaluation is necessary for the accurate diagnosis of OA. In early, mild OA, radiographic changes may be normal. With the progression of degenerative changes in cartilage, the joint space may begin to narrow, subchondral bony sclerosis occurs, and marginal osteophyte and cyst formation may develop. Late in the disease process, subluxation and deformity may be apparent. Osteoporosis and joint erosions are not usually seen but may occur in some patients with erosive OA.
- Joint arthroscopic examination also can confirm the diagnosis or extent of OA present in a particular joint, but few clinical situations require this procedure to establish the diagnosis.
- No specific clinical laboratory abnormalities occur in primary OA. The erythrocyte sedimentation rate (ESR) may be slightly elevated in

TABLE 2.1. Clinical Presentation of Osteoarthritis

Age
Usually elderly

Sex
Age <45 more common in men
>45 more common in women (hands)

Symptoms
Deep, aching pain
Pain on motion
Early in disease—pain with use
Late in disease—pain at rest
Stiffness
Rarely exceeds 15 min; related to weather
Localized to involved joints
Limited joint motion
Instability of weight-bearing joints
Crepitus, crackling

Signs/Physical Examination
Monoarticular or oligoarticular; asymmetrical involvement
Joints frequently involved
Hands—DIP, PIP, first carpometacarpal joint
Foot—first metatarsophalangeal
Hips, knees, cervical spine, lumbar spine
Observations on joint examination
Bony proliferation or occasional synovitis
Local tenderness
Crepitus
Muscle atrophy
Limited motion with passive/active movement
Effusions
Characteristics of synovial fluid
High viscosity
Mild leukocytosis (<2000 WBC/mm^3)

Laboratory Values
No specific test
ESR, hematologic survey, chemistry survey are normal
No systemic manifestations

Key: DIP, distal interphalangeal; PIP, proximal interphalangeal; WBC, white blood cell count; ESR, erythrocyte sedimentation rate.

patients with generalized or erosive inflammatory OA. The rheumatoid factor test is negative. Analysis of the synovial fluid reveals fluid with high viscosity. This fluid demonstrates a mild leukocytosis (<2000 WBC/mm^3) with predominantly mononuclear cells.

▶ DESIRED OUTCOME

The major goals for the management of osteoarthritis are: (1) to educate the patient, caregivers, and relatives; (2) to relieve symptoms such as pain and stiffness; (3) to preserve the joint motion and function by limiting disease progression; and (4) to minimize the disability.

▶ TREATMENT

NONPHARMACOLOGIC TREATMENT

- The first step is to educate the patient about the extent, degree of involvement, prognosis, and management approach. For the patient who is overweight, dietary counseling is an important recommendation.
- Physical therapy—with heat or cold treatments and an exercise program—helps to maintain and regain joint range of motion, relieve pain, and reduce muscle spasms. Transcutaneous electrical nerve stimulation (TENS) may provide some relief of acute pain, but it is cumbersome and expensive. Exercise programs using isometric techniques are designed to strengthen the muscles and improve joint function and motion.
- Various assistive devices—including splints, canes, walkers, and braces—can be used during exercise or daily activities. Other orthotic devices such as heel cups or insoles may also be tried to help relieve pain and improve the patient's ability to walk.
- Surgical procedures (e.g., osteotomy, joint debridement, osteophyte removal, partial or total arthroplasty, joint fusion) are indicated for patients who have severe disease or who have substantial pain or marked functional disabilities and in whom conservative therapy has not been effective.

DRUG THERAPY

General Principles

- Drug therapy in OA is directed at the symptomatic relief of pain and inflammation when present.
- Because OA often occurs in older individuals who may also have other preexisting medical conditions, a conservative approach to the use of medications is warranted.
- An individualized approach to treatment is necessary (Fig. 2.1). Some patients with mild symptoms may require simple topical or oral analgesics; patients who receive no relief from the analgesics or who have signs of active inflammation may benefit from the use of an anti-inflammatory medication.

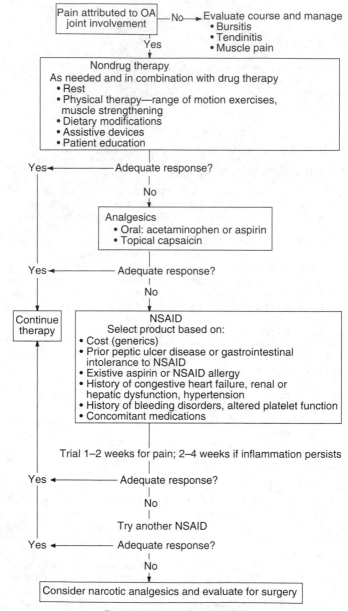

Figure 2.1. Treatment for osteoarthritis.

Analgesics

Acetaminophen

- For patients who need only analgesic therapy, acetaminophen 650 mg four times daily provides analgesia comparable to that provided by aspirin 650 mg four times daily without the associated GI toxicity. Several recent reports have demonstrated the comparable efficacy of acetaminophen (2.6–4 g/d) to either ibuprofen at doses of 1200 or 2400 mg/d or naproxen 750 mg/d in relieving the pain symptoms associated with OA of the knee. This has led some clinicians to recommend the use of acetaminophen in doses less than 4 g/d as first-line therapy for the short-term symptomatic relief of OA pain.
- Acetaminophen is usually well tolerated by patients, but hepatic and renal toxicity have been reported when it has been taken in excess, for prolonged periods of time, or by at-risk populations.

Salicylates

- Aspirin in doses of 325–650 mg four times daily also provides analgesia; doses greater than 3.6 g/d are necessary to achieve anti-inflammatory activity.
- Salicylates can cause adverse gastrointestinal (GI) effects ranging from mild discomfort to gastric ulcers. To minimize these effects, the salicylates should be taken with food or milk. Enteric-coated products cause less gastric mucosal injury compared with buffered or plain aspirin. The nonacetylated salicylate products also produce less GI irritation and bleeding than plain aspirin but are considerably more expensive. Aspirin products may cause impaired renal function and increases in serum transaminases.

Capsaicin

- Topical administration of capsaicin, an extract of red peppers that produces release of and ultimately depletion of substance P, has been beneficial in providing pain relief in OA.
- When used alone or as an adjunct to oral analgesics or nonsteroidal anti-inflammatory drugs (NSAIDs), capsaicin may help to avoid or minimize the systemic effects associated with those medications.
- Capsaicin is administered two to four times a day by gently rubbing the cream around the affected joint. Several weeks of consistent application may be required before maximal pain relief is achieved.
- Capsaicin is generally well tolerated, but some patients report a burning or stinging sensation when it is first applied.

Other Analgesics

- Tramadol, propoxyphene, or stronger opioids such as codeine are usually reserved for patients who have failed single- or multiple-agent therapy with simple analgesics, topical agents, or NSAIDs.
- Patients should be instructed to use these products primarily for severe pain and for the shortest duration possible. Ideally, prescriptions should

be written for a limited quantity with only one or two refills to minimize the potential for abuse and assist with assessing the degree of pain
relief obtained.

Nonsteroidal Anti-Inflammatory Drugs

- In general, the NSAIDs are indicated after simple analgesics have failed
  to relieve pain, toxic effects have developed, or inflammation is present.
- As a class, the NSAIDs are comparably effective in reducing pain and
  modifying the inflammatory process (Table 2.2). NSAIDs are as effective as aspirin and cause fewer GI complaints.
- The choice of a particular NSAID is frequently a matter of prescriber
  preference based on past treatment, cost, patient preference, toxic
  effects, and compliance.
- A patient may respond well to one drug in a particular chemical class
  but experience little or no benefit from another NSAID in the same
  class. Therefore, other NSAIDs may be used in a selective manner after
  an adequate trial (2–3 weeks) at an adequate dose (either anti-inflammatory or analgesic) of other NSAIDs in a chemical class.
- Combination of NSAIDs with other NSAIDs or aspirin increases toxic
  effects while providing no added benefit.
- Gastrointestinal complaints are the most common adverse effects
  observed with NSAIDs, and administration with food or milk should be
  encouraged, except for the enteric-coated products (milk or antacids
  may destroy the enteric coating and cause increased GI symptoms in
  some patients). Diarrhea can occur but is more commonly observed
  with meclofenamate than the other NSAIDs.
- All NSAIDs have the potential to cause GI bleeding through a variety
  of mechanisms related to direct topical or systemic effects of the
  NSAIDs. Several factors increase the risk of ulcers and ulcer complications related to NSAIDs. These include patient age greater than age 65;
  prior ulcer disease or complications; therapy with high-dose or multiple
  NSAIDs; concomitant corticosteroid therapy; and NSAID therapy duration of less than 3 months. Concomitant therapy with a mucosal protective agent (e.g., misoprostol) should be considered in patients who are
  considered to be at high risk.
- NSAIDs may also cause renal complications, hepatitis, platelet dysfunction, hypersensitivity reactions, rash, or central nervous system
  (CNS) complaints such as drowsiness, dizziness, headaches, depression, confusion, and tinnitus.
- The most potentially serious drug interactions include the concomitant
  use of NSAIDs with lithium, warfarin, oral hypoglycemics, methotrexate, antihypertensives, angiotensin-converting enzyme (ACE) inhibitors, beta blockers, and diuretics.

Corticosteroids

- Systemic corticosteroid therapy is not recommended in the treatment of
  OA, as side effects associated with prolonged use outweigh any potential benefits of therapy.

TABLE 2.2. Medications Commonly Used in the Treatment of Osteoarthritis

Medication	Dosage and Frequency	Maximum Dosage (mg/d)
Oral analgesics		
Acetaminophen	325–650 mg every 4–6 hours or 1 g 3–4 times per day	4000
Tramadol	50–100 mg every 4–6 hours	400
Topical analgesics		
Capsaicin 0.025% or 0.075%	Apply to affected joint 3–4 times per day	—
Nonsteroidal anti-inflammatory drugs (NSAIDs)		
Carboxylic acids		
Acetylated salicylates		
Aspirin, plain, buffered or enteric coated	325–650 mg every 4–6 hours for pain. Anti-inflammatory doses start at 3600 mg/d in divided doses	3600[a]
Nonacetylated salicylates		
Salsalate	500–1000 mg 2–3 times per day	3000[a]
Diflunisal	500–1000 mg 2 times per day	
Choline salicylate[b]	500–1000 mg 2–3 times per day	3000[a]
Choline magnesium salicylate	500–1000 mg 2–3 times per day	3000[a]
Acetic acids		
Etodolac	800–1200 mg/d in divided doses	120–1200
Diclofenac	100–150 mg/d in divided doses	200
Indomethacin	25 mg 2–3 times a day; 75 mg SR once daily	200; 150
Ketorolac[c]	10 mg every 4–6 hours	40
Nabumetono[d]	500–1000 mg 1–2 times a day	2000
Propionic acids		
Fenoprofen	300–600 mg 3–4 times per day	3200
Flurbiprofen	200–300 mg/d in 2–4 divided doses	300
Ibuprofen	1200–3200 mg/d in 3–4 divided doses	3200
Ketoprofen	150–300 mg/d in 3–4 divided doses	300
Naproxen	250–500 mg twice per day	1500
Naproxen sodium	275–550 mg twice per day	1375
Oxaprozin	1200 mg daily	1800
Fenamates		
Meclofenamate	200–400 mg/d in 3–4 divided doses	400
Mefenamic acid[e]	250 mg every 6 hours	1000
Oxicams		
Piroxicam	20 mg daily	20

[a]Monitor serum salicylate levels over 3–3.6 g/d.
[b]Only available as a liquid; 870 mg salicylate/5 mL.
[c]Not FDA approved for treatment of OA for more than 5 days.
[d]Nonorganic acid but metabolite is an acetic acid.
[e]Not FDA approved for treatment of OA.

- The use of intra-articular corticosteroids (IAC) may temporarily be helpful, but their long-term benefit remains controversial. If used, IAC should be administered infrequently at intervals of 4–6 months for any given joint. If no improvement occurs from one or two injections, then further treatment is not likely to succeed. After injection, the patient should be instructed to minimize joint activity and the joint stress load for several days. Injection into the ligaments or pericapsular areas can be beneficial and is associated with reduced risks relative to IAC administration.

▶ EVALUATION OF THERAPEUTIC OUTCOMES

- The monitoring plan for assessing therapeutic efficacy consists of establishing the patient's baseline pain through the use of a pain visual analogue scale (VAS) and identifying the range of motion for the affected joint (flexion, extension, abduction, or adduction).
- Depending on the joint affected, measurement of grip strength may aid in the measurement of hand OA; measuring the time needed to walk 50 feet may aid in the assessment of hip and knee OA.
- Baseline radiographs of the respective joint are often performed to assist with establishing the degree and/or extent of joint involvement; these may be repeated when the clinical course indicates a worsening of symptoms.
- Other measures include the clinician's global assessment based on the patient's history of activities and limitations caused by the OA as well as documentation of analgesic or NSAID use.
- The use of disease-specific quality of life (QOL) questionnaires for arthritis provides another valuable tool in assessing a patient's clinical response to various therapeutic interventions.
- Patients should be questioned directly to determine if they are having adverse effects from their medications. They should also be monitored for any signs of drug-related effects, such as skin rash, headaches, drowsiness, weight gain, or alterations in blood pressure from NSAIDs. Baseline serum creatinine determinations, hematology profiles, and ␣um transaminases with repeat levels as needed are useful in identifying ␣cific toxicities to the kidney, liver, GI tract, or bone marrow.

See Ch.
a more a⹁5, Osteoarthritis, authored by Larry E. Boh, MS, RPh, for
⹁iscussion of this topic.

Chapter 3

▶ OSTEOPOROSIS

▶ DEFINITION

Osteoporosis is a gradual reduction in bone mass (osteopenia) such that the skeleton is compromised, resulting in fractures with minimal trauma. Type I (postmenopausal osteoporosis) affects primarily trabecular bone in women within 15–20 years following menopause. Type II (senile osteoporosis) affects men and women older than age 70. Type III is secondary to other diseases or medications and occurs in either sex at any age (Table 3.1).

▶ PATHOPHYSIOLOGY

- Estrogen deficiency is associated with an increase in bone resorption without an increase in bone formation.

TABLE 3.1. Classification of Osteoporotic Types

	Type I Post-menopausal	Type II Senile	Type III Secondary
Age	55–70	75–90	Any age
Years past menopause	5–15	25–40	Any age
Sex ratio F:M	20:1	2:1	1:1
Fracture site	Spine	Hip, spine, pelvis, humerus	Spine, hip, peripheral
Bone loss			
Trabecular	+++	++	+++
Cortical	+	++	+++
Contributing factor			
Menopause	+++	++	++
Age	+	+++	++
Biochemistry			
PTH	↓	↑	↓↑
1,25(OH)$_2$D$_3$	↓	↓	↓↑
Calcium absorption	↓	↓	↓
1 α hydroxylase response to PTH	↓	→	?

- In women, cortical bone loss proceeds at a rate of 3% per decade until menopause, at which time it accelerates to about 9% per decade. The rate returns to normal 10–20 years after menopause.
- Four factors contribute to the onset of age-related bone loss: (1) decreased osteoblast function; (2) decreased calcium and vitamin D absorption; (3) biochemical imbalances; and (4) sex hormone deficiencies.
- The lower osteoporosis incidence in men may result from higher peak bone mass at skeletal maturity, shorter life expectancy, lower bone loss rate during aging, fewer falls, and/or a gradual (versus a distinct) cessation of hormone production.

▶ CLINICAL PRESENTATION

- The usual presentation of osteoporosis is shortened stature, kyphosis, lordosis, or a fracture, most commonly of a vertebra, hip, or forearm. Recurrent fractures are common and the time frame is unpredictable. Vertebral body collapse is the most frequently seen fracture, especially in early postmenopausal women.
- The acute phase may be followed by chronic back pain.
- Chest wall changes can lead to pulmonary and cardiovascular complications.
- Collapsed vertebrae rarely lead to spinal cord compression.

▶ DIAGNOSIS

- History and physical exam should identify osteoporotic risk factors (Table 3.2).
- Bone can be quantified using several noninvasive techniques (Table 3.3).
- The quality and quantity of bone, as well as the rate of turnover, can be studied by obtaining an intact core of cortical and trabecular bone from the iliac crest.
- The preferred tests to determine if bone formation is ongoing are the presence or rise in osteocalcin and total alkaline phosphatase. Rises in alkaline phosphatase are not sensitive and specific to bone formation.
- The preferred tests to determine if bone resorption is ongoing are fasting urinary hydroxyproline and calcium corrected for creatine production and pyridinoline and deoxypyridinoline cross-links.
- Other tests that may be helpful to detect other causes of bone disease are serum calcium, phosphorus, vitamin D, vitamin D metabolites, and parathyroid hormone (PTH) concentrations.

▶ DESIRED OUTCOMES

- Prevention of osteoporosis should be undertaken by increasing peak bone mass in women and men younger than age 35–40 years and elim-

TABLE 3.2. Factors Commonly Associated with Osteoporosis

Genetic
White or Asiatic ethnicity
Positive family history
Small body frame (less than 58 kg)

Lifestyle
Smoking
Inactivity
Nulliparity
Excessive exercise (producing amenorrhoea)
Early natural menopause
Late menarche

Nutritional Factors
Milk intolerance
Lifelong low dietary calcium intake
Excessive alcohol intake
Consistently high animal protein intake

Medical Disorders
Anorexia nervosa
Thyrotoxicosis
Cushing's syndrome
Type I diabetes
Alterations in gastrointestinal and hepatobiliary function
Occult osteogenesis imperfecta
Mastocytosis
Rheumatoid arthritis
Long-term parenteral nutrition
Prolactinoma
Hemolytic anemia, hemochromatosis, and thalassaemia
Ankylosing spondylitis

Drugs
Thyroid replacement drugs
Glucocorticoid drugs
Anticoagulants (heparin)
Chronic lithium therapy
Chemotherapy
GnRH agonist or antagonist therapy
Anticonvulsant drugs
Extended tetracycline use[a]
Diuretics producing calciuria[a]
Phenothiazine derivatives[a]
Cyclosporine[a]
Aluminum-containing antacids[a]

[a]Not yet associated with decreased bone mass although identified as either toxic to bone in animals or inducing calciuria and/or calcium malabsorption in human beings.
Key: GnRH, gonadotropin releasing hormone.

TABLE 3.3. Noninvasive Measurements of Bone Mineral Density

Technique	Site	Precision[a] (%)	Accuracy[b] (%)	Examination Time (min)	Absorbed Dose of Radiation[c] (mrem)
Single-photon absorptiometry	Proximal and distal radius, calcaneus	1–3	5	15	10–20
Dual-energy photon absorptiometry	Spine, hip, total body	2–4	4–10	20–40	5
Dual-energy x-ray absorptiometry	Spine, hip, total body	0.5–2	3–5	3–7	1–3
Quantitative computed tomography	Spine	2–5	5–20	10–15	100–1000

[a]Precision is the coefficient of variation (standard deviation divided by the mean) for repeated measurements over a short period of time in young, healthy persons.
[b]Accuracy is the coefficient of variation for measurements in a specimen whose mineral content has been determined by other means (e.g., measurement of ashed weight).
[c]To convert millirems to millijoules per kilogram of body weight, multiply by 0.01.

inating or decreasing the bone loss in postmenopausal women and older men.
• There are two goals for existing osteoporosis: prevent further bone loss and prevent subsequent fractures. Pain control may also be an important issue.

▶ PREVENTION AND TREATMENT

NONPHARMACOLOGIC APPROACHES

• As caffeine increases urinary calcium excretion, caffeine ingestion should be decreased to less than 2–5 cups of coffee daily in both genders.
• Women and men should stop smoking, as smoking is associated with lower bone mass, increased fracture rates, and earlier menopause.
• Aerobic and strengthening exercises prevent bone loss and falls.
• Prevention of falls in the elderly is critical. Home environments may need to be redesigned. Sedatives should be discontinued or switched to short-acting agents, diuretics should be given during the day, and orthostatic blood pressure problems should be resolved.

ANTIRESORPTIVE APPROACHES

Calcium

- Most studies support supplemental calcium to decrease bone loss. Comparison studies find calcium to be less beneficial than hormone-replacement therapy, especially for women in whom therapy is initiated within 5 years of menopause. Estrogen users require only 1 g of daily calcium versus 1.5 g in nonusers of estrogen.
- All patients should meet the National Institutes of Health (NIH) consensus conference recommendations for calcium intake (Table 3.4). More than 75% of women older than 35 years have calcium intakes of less than the recommended daily allowance (RDA). Table 3.5 lists foods with high calcium content. Calcium absorption from milk is about 25–35%.
- Table 3.6 lists common forms of calcium supplementation and their calcium content. Calcium carbonate contains the most elemental calcium by weight (40%).
- Calcium tablets should be ingested between meals in 500 mg doses or less to enhance absorption. Calcium carbonate has acid-dependent absorption, whereas calcium citrate has acid-independent absorption. The citrate salt may therefore have particular usefulness in elderly patients who have decreased acid secretion.

TABLE 3.4. Optimal Calcium Requirements Recommended by the National Institutes of Health Consensus Panel

Age Group	Optimal Daily Intake of Calcium (mg)
Infants	
Birth–6 mo	400
6 mo–1 yr	600
Children	
1–5 yr	800
6–10 yr	800–1200
Adolescents/young adults	
11–24 yr	1200–1500
Men	
25–65 yr	1000
Over 65 yr	1500
Women	
25–50 yr	1000
Over 50 yr (postmenopausal)	
On estrogens	1000
Not on estrogens	1500
Over 65 yr	1500
Pregnant and nursing	1200–1500

TABLE 3.5. Calcium Content of Various Foods

Food	Serving Size	Calcium Content (mg)
Milk (skim)	1 qt	1212
Milk (whole)	1 qt	1152
Sardines	8 medium	354
Yogurt (low-fat)	1 cup	345
Swiss cheese	1 oz	250
Red salmon	½ cup	250
Turnip greens, cooked	½ cup	245
Creamed cottage cheese	1 cup	211
Cheddar cheese	1 oz	211
Ice cream	1 cup	200
American processed cheese	1 oz	150
Spinach (frozen, chopped, cooked)	½ cup	113
Chocolate fudge	3½ oz	100

TABLE 3.6. Oral Calcium Supplementation Products

Preparation	Tablet Size		To Supply 1 g Elemental Calcium (tablets/d)
	mg	*mg Elemental Calcium/Tablet*	
Calcium carbonate (40% elemental calcium)			
Generic	650	260	4
Cal-Sup (Riker Laboratories)	750	300	4
Caltrate (Lederle Laboratories)	1500	600	2
Os-Cal 500 (Marion Laboratories)	1250	500	2
Tums (Norcliff-Thayer)	500	200	5
Titralac (3M Company)	420	168	6
Generic calcium gluconate (9% elemental calcium)	650	58.5	17
Generic calcium lactate (13% elemental calcium)	650	84.5	12
Generic dibasic calcium phosphate (23% elemental calcium)	500	115	9

- The most common side effect is constipation. Calcium should not be administered with fiber laxatives. Calcium can decrease iron, tetracycline, ciprofloxacin, etidronate, phenytoin, and fluoride absorption if given concomitantly. The activity of calcium channel blockers may be decreased if the serum calcium concentration is higher than normal.

Diuretics
- Thiazide diuretics promote a decrease in renal calcium excretion, whereas loop diuretics increase renal calcium excretion. Concurrent thiazides and estrogens result in greater bone mineral density than do estrogens alone.

Vitamin D and Its Metabolites
- Vitamin D is obtained by dietary intake and created by ultraviolet light's effect on 7-dehydrocholesterol. Vitamin D is metabolized in the liver to 25-hydroxyvitamin D and then to the active metabolite 1,25-dihydroxyvitamin D in the kidney.
- 1,25-dihydroxyvitamin D increases calcium absorption and stimulates osteoblasts and osteoclasts. The increased calcium concentration decreases PTH release, thereby decreasing bone resorption.
- Pharmacologic doses of vitamin D or its metabolites are not yet considered standard therapy for preventing osteoporosis, but are sometimes used for treating patients with serious osteoporosis or low 1,25-dihydroxyvitamin D concentrations.
- Vitamin D products can cause hypercalcemia and hypercalciuria.
- Determination of 1,25-dihydroxyvitamin D concentration may be desired to establish if liver and kidney metabolism of vitamin D has occurred, especially in patients with advanced osteoporosis.

Hormone Therapy
- Estrogens produce a decrease in bone resorption, an increase in calcitriol concentrations, and an increase in intestinal calcium absorption and retention.
- In 1993, the Osteoporosis Consensus Development Conference stated that estrogen replacement therapy (ERT) is the medication of choice for preventing osteoporosis in postmenopausal women.
- A significant increase in bone mass (2–3% per year) may occur if estrogen therapy has been initiated within the first 3–6 years following menopause.
- Continuous hormone replacement therapy (HRT) (estrogens and progesterones), appears to be similar to cyclic HRT in preserving bone mass at cortical and trabecular bone sites.
- ERT decreases osteoporotic fracture incidence. Greater effects are seen with decreasing hip and spine fractures versus radius fractures.
- Because transdermal ERT bypasses the liver, less positive lipid effects, which occur after about 6 months of therapy, are achieved compared with oral ERT. Combination therapy with progesterones and androgens can minimize or eliminate the positive lipid effect.

- A dose–response relationship exists between bone mass and conjugated estrogens in daily doses of 0.3–2.5 mg, estradiol 0.5–2.0 mg, and transdermal estradiol 0.05–0.1 mg. The suggested doses of ERT for osteoporosis prevention are conjugated estrogens 0.625 mg, ethinyl estradiol 0.02 mg, estropipate 0.625 mg, esterified estrogens 0.625 mg, estradiol 0.5 mg, and transdermal estradiol 0.05 mg/day.
- For continuous therapy, conjugated estrogen 0.625 mg or equivalent is administered daily, and medroxyprogesterone 10 mg is administered for 10–14 days at the beginning of the month or 2.5–5.0 mg is administered daily. For the cyclic regimen, conjugated estrogen 0.625 mg or equivalent is administered for 3 weeks, with medroxyprogesterone 10 mg administered for the last 10–14 days.
- The optimal duration of therapy is not known. Currently, lifetime use of estrogens is being considered. The positive lipid effect with ERT is maintained for at least 20 years.
- Unopposed ERT for more than 6 months causes up to a tenfold increased risk for endometrial cancer. Concomitant progesterone therapy for at least 10–14 days a month usually eliminates or reduces this risk even to lower than that of nonusers. Progesterone therapy is not needed for women who have had a hysterectomy.
- Common adverse reactions of HRT include vaginal spotting and bleeding; breast tenderness and breast enlargement, especially in older women; pedal edema; and weight gain. Uncommon adverse reactions are facial hair growth, bloating, nausea, vomiting, leg pain, headache, increase or decrease in sexual desire, dizziness, and mood changes. A 2.5-fold increase in cholelithiasis exists with HRT.
- Current thromboembolic disease is considered a relative contraindication by some, whereas some consider thromboembolic disease during pregnancy or with past oral contraceptive use an absolute contraindication.

Tamoxifen
- Tamoxifen is both an estrogen antagonist and an estrogen agonist.
- Tamoxifen 10 mg twice daily for 5 years was associated with an increase in lumbar bone density. It has been associated with an increase in endometrial cancer. It may be an option for prevention of osteoporosis in breast cancer patients.

Progesterones
- The addition of progesterone to estrogen therapy does not seem to have any additional beneficial effects on bone when compared with estrogen alone.

Testosterone
- In men who are deficient in testosterone, 10–115 months of replacement therapy resulted in increased distal bone density or spinal bone density. It is contraindicated in men with prostatic cancer and should be used with caution in men with prostatic hypertrophy.

Calcitonin

- Salmon calcitonin is approved by the Food and Drug Administration (FDA) for prevention of postmenopausal osteoporosis and Paget's disease. Salmon calcitonin is 50 times more potent than human calcitonin. Calcitonin decreases osteoclast bone attachment, motility, life span, and numbers along with altering the cellular structure. Bone density is preserved.
- Patients with high bone turnover respond best to calcitonin; however, elderly women also benefit. Calcitonin also has a beneficial effect for steroid-induced osteoporosis. Calcitonin, given intranasally or subcutaneously, also causes pain relief within 1–12 weeks. Daily administration is used initially, then decreased to 50–100 IU two to three times weekly.
- Calcitonin's effect on bone density may plateau or decrease after 12–18 months.
- If calcitonin is used, calcium and, when needed, vitamin D should also be used.
- Nasal administration produces fewer side effects than subcutaneous administration.

Bisphosphonates

- Bisphosphonates adsorb to bone hydroxyapatite, become a permanent part of bone structure, and are resistant to enzymatic hydrolysis. The estimated half-life of bisphosphonates is similar to the half-life of bone (1–10 years).
- The effect of bisphosphonates is greater for lumbar bone than for cortical bone; however, unlike fluoride therapy, cortical bone is not weakened as a result of increased lumbar bone density.
- Etidronate disodium 400 mg/day 2 hours before or after a meal for 14 days, given every 3–3.5 months, can increase bone mass and offers an effective alternative for patients unable to take estrogens.
- Alendronate is another alternative to estrogen therapy. It is approved for prevention and treatment of osteoporosis.
- Alendronate 10 mg/day orally has increased bone mass and reduced vertebral fractures and loss of height. A trend toward reduction in nonvertebral fractures also occurs. It is taken 30 minutes before the first food, beverage, or medication in the morning with a full glass of water only. Patients should be instructed to remain upright after taking the tablet because erosive esophagitis has been reported.
- Nausea and diarrhea are the most common side effects.
- Calcium and, when needed, vitamin D should also be given, but at different times from the biphosphonates.

BONE FORMATION APPROACHES

Fluoride

- Fluoride increases bone formation in trabecular bone and may increase osteoblasts. It serves as a hydroxy radical in the hydroxyapatite crystals, forming fluorapatite, which is a mineral system more resistant to resorption. New bone formed may be somewhat disorganized and more resistant to compression fractures but less resistant to torsional strain, which is believed to be responsible for hip fractures.

- Twenty to 40% of fluoride users are nonresponders. Hip and peripheral fractures have been increased in some studies.
- Slow-release fluoride appears to be useful in a dose of 25 mg/day for less than 5 years. At least 1–1.5 g/day of calcium and, when needed, vitamin D should also be prescribed. Calcium and fluoride should be given at different times to prevent chemical binding. Antacids can also decrease fluoride absorption.
- Dosage adjustments are necessary for patients with creatinine clearances of less than 50 mL/min.
- The most common side effects (e.g., gastrointestinal, osteoarticular) are less frequent with slow-release products. These disappear within 1–8 weeks of discontinuation of treatment and generally reappear when treatment is reinstituted, even at lower doses.

Androgens and Anabolic Steroids
- Androgens may enhance osteoblast activity. Results have been mixed for the various androgens (e.g., nandrolone decanoate, stanozolol, methandrostenolone). Most women develop adverse reactions such as liver function alterations, negative lipid effects, hirsutism, hoarseness, and acne.

▶ GLUCOCORTICOID–INDUCED OSTEOPOROSIS

- Bone loss begins within the first 6–12 months on glucocorticoid therapy, and trabecular bone has the greatest loss. Daily doses of 7.5 mg or more of prednisone cause substantial loss of bone in most patients. Men and women are equally affected.
- Long-term effects of inhaled steroids are still unknown but probably minimal with standard therapy.
- Glucocorticoids decrease bone formation and increase bone resorption. Decreased calcium gastrointestinal absorption and increased renal excretion leads to a negative calcium balance and secondary hyperparathyroidism.
- Osteonecrosis, also called aseptic necrosis, and muscle wasting are serious complications of steroid therapy. This usually involves the femoral and humeral heads and causes intense pain and decreased mobility.
- Glucocorticoids should be used in the lowest possible doses and for the shortest period of time. Alternate day therapy does not appear to lessen bone loss.
- Some of the medications used to prevent and treat Type I osteoporosis (e.g., supplemental calcium, thiazides, vitamin D, ERT, calcitonin, alendronate, nandrolone decanoate) may be of some benefit.

▶ EVALUATION OF THERAPEUTIC OUTCOMES

- The indications for radiologic quantification of bone mass have not been definitively established, but suggested indications include characterizing bone loss as fast or slow, establishing fracture risk, determining the efficacy of preventive or treatment regimens, and assisting patients in prevention and treatment decisions.
- It is critical to involve the patient in treatment decisions whenever possible and to monitor regularly for efficacy, side effects, and compliance with prescribed regimens.
- It is also advisable to monitor for compliance with prescribed diets and exercise regimens, and to assess propensity for falling.

See Chapter 83, Osteoporosis and Osteomalacia, authored by Mary Beth O'Connell, PharmD, FASHP, FCCP, and Steven F. Bauwens, PharmD, FASCP, for a more detailed discussion of this topic.

Chapter 4

▶ RHEUMATOID ARTHRITIS

▶ DEFINITION

Rheumatoid arthritis (RA) is a chronic and usually progressive inflammatory disorder of unknown etiology characterized by polyarticular symmetrical joint involvement and systemic manifestations.

▶ PATHOPHYSIOLOGY

- Although the precise etiology is unknown, RA results from a dysregulation of the humoral and cell-mediated components of the immune system.
- Most patients produce antibodies called rheumatoid factors; these seropositive patients tend to have a more aggressive course than do patients who are seronegative.
- In the initial cell-mediated process, macrophages engulf and process antigens and present them to T-lymphocytes. The processed antigen is recognized by the major histocompatibility complex (MHC) proteins on the lymphocyte surface, resulting in T-cell activation and production of cytotoxins and cytokines that result in joint damage.
- Activated B-lymphocytes produce plasma cells that form antibodies that, in combination with complement, result in accumulation of polymorphonuclear leukocytes (PMNs). PMNs release cytotoxins, free oxygen radicals, and hydroxyl radicals that promote cellular damage to synovium and bone.
- Vasoactive substances (histamine, kinins, prostaglandins) are released at the site of inflammation, increasing blood flow and vascular permeability; this causes edema, warmth, and pain.
- Chronic inflammatory changes may result in loss of joint space, loss of joint motion, bony fusion (ankylosis), joint subluxation, tendon contractures, and chronic deformity.

▶ CLINICAL PRESENTATION

- Nonspecific prodromal symptoms may include fatigue, weakness, low-grade fever, loss of appetite, and joint pain. Stiffness and myalgias may precede development of synovitis.
- Joint involvement tends to be symmetric and involve the small joints of the hands, wrists, and feet; the elbows, shoulders, hips, knees, and ankles may also be affected.
- Joint stiffness typically is worse in the morning and usually lasts at least 1 hour before maximal improvement is seen for the day.
- Chronic joint deformities commonly involve subluxations of the wrists, metacarpophalangeal (MCP) joints, and proximal interphalan-

geal (PIP) joints (swan-neck deformity, boutonniere deformity, ulnar deviation).
- Extra-articular involvement may include subcutaneous nodules, vasculitis, pleural effusions, pulmonary fibrosis, ocular manifestations, pericarditis, cardiac conduction abnormalities, and bone marrow suppression.

▶ DIAGNOSIS

- The American Rheumatism Association criteria for the classification of RA are included in Table 4.1.

TABLE 4.1. American Rheumatism Association Criteria for Classification of Rheumatoid Arthritis–1987 Revision

Criteria[a]	Definition
1. Morning stiffness	Morning stiffness in and around the joints lasting at least 1 hour before maximal improvement
2. Arthritis of three or more joint areas	At least three joint areas have simultaneously had soft tissue swelling or fluid (not bony overgrowth alone) observed by a physician. The 14 possible joint areas are (right or left): PIP,[b] MCP,[b] wrist, elbow, knee, ankle, and MTP[b] joints
3. Arthritis of hand joints	At least one joint area swollen as above in wrist, MCP, or PIP joint
4. Symmetric arthritis	Simultaneous involvement of the same joint areas (as in No. 2) on both sides of the body (bilateral involvement of PIP, MCP, or MTP joints is acceptable without absolute symmetry)
5. Rheumatoid nodules	Nodules may be subcutaneous, over bony prominences, or extensor surfaces, or in juxta-articular regions, observed by a physician
6. Serum rheumatoid factor	Demonstration of abnormal amounts of serum "rheumatoid factor" by any method that has been positive in less than 5% of normal control subjects
7. Radiographic changes	Radiographic changes typical of RA on posterior–anterior hand and wrist x-rays, which must include erosions or unequivocal bony decalcification localized to or most marked adjacent to the involved joints (osteoarthritis changes alone do not qualify)

[a]For classification purposes, a patient is said to have rheumatoid arthritis (RA) if he or she has satisfied at least four of the above seven criteria. Criteria 1 through 4 must be present for at least 6 weeks. Patients with two clinical diagnoses are not excluded. Designation as classic, definite, or probable rheumatoid arthritis is *not* to be made.
[b]PIP, proximal interphalangeal; MCP, metacarpophalangeal; MTP, metatarsophalangeal.

- Additional laboratory abnormalities that may be seen include normo-cytic, normochromic anemia; thrombocytosis or thrombocytopenia; leukopenia; elevated erythrocyte sedimentation rate (ESR); and positive antinuclear antibodies (ANA) (25% of patients).
- Examination of aspirated synovial fluid may reveal turbidity, leukocy-tosis, reduced viscosity, and normal or low glucose relative to serum concentrations.

▶ DESIRED OUTCOME

- The ultimate goal of RA treatment is to induce a complete remission, which is only rarely achievable.
- Other reasonable goals are to reduce symptoms of joint stiffness and pain, decrease joint swelling, preserve range of motion and joint func-tion for essential activities of daily living, maximize quality of life, pre-vent systemic complications, and slow the rate of joint damage.

▶ TREATMENT

GENERAL MANAGEMENT PRINCIPLES

- There is no known cure for RA and no known method to prevent it.
- Early diagnosis and prompt therapeutic intervention are necessary to reduce the likelihood and severity of irreversible joint damage.
- Aggressive treatment early in the disease course may slow progression and delay development of joint damage and erosions.
- Combination drug therapy is frequently beneficial but results in increased cost and toxicity.
- Regular follow-up is essential to assess disease activity and detect adverse drug effects.
- Patient education about the nature of the disease and the potential ben-efits and limitations of drug therapy is critical to the success of phar-macotherapy for RA.
- An algorithm for the treatment of RA is included in Fig. 4.1.

NONPHARMACOLOGIC TREATMENT

- Adequate rest, weight reduction if obese, occupational therapy, physical therapy, and use of assistive devices may improve symptoms and help maintain joint function.
- Patients with severe disease may benefit from surgical procedures such as tenosynovectomy, tendon repair, and joint replacements.

NONSTEROIDAL ANTI-INFLAMMATORY DRUGS

- Nonsteroidal anti-inflammatory drugs (NSAIDs) act by inhibiting syn-thesis of prostaglandins involved in the inflammatory cascade; other mechanisms may also be operative. These drugs possess both analgesic and anti-inflammatory properties and are first-line therapy for treatment

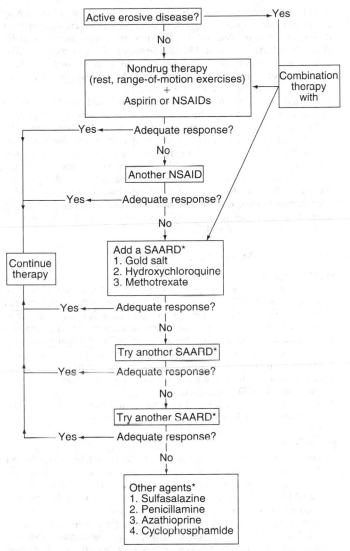

Figure 4.1. Algorithm for treatment of rheumatoid arthritis. *Corticosteroids may be necessary for patients with severe inflammatory disease in any of these phases to enable the patient to be more functional while awaiting the beneficial effects of therapy or in patients with partial responses to therapy. SAARD, slow-acting antirhumatic drug.

of mild RA symptoms. NSAIDs are effective for symptom relief only and do not slow disease progression or prevent bony erosions or joint deformity. At equivalent doses, NSAIDs are approximately equally effective in the treatment of RA. Combinations of two or more NSAIDs should be avoided because they are no more effective and may have additive adverse effects. NSAIDs are generally continued when disease-modifying antirheumatic drugs (DMARDs) are added.

- In general, NSAIDs are well absorbed orally and highly bound to plasma proteins (causing some drug interactions); most are hepatically metabolized with renal excretion of metabolites. Gastrointestinal (GI) toxicity (GI distress, nausea, vomiting, ulceration, bleeding) is common and results from direct GI irritation as well as prostaglandin inhibition; preventive measures should be considered in patients at greatest risk. Renal insufficiency may occur, especially in older patients, patients with comorbidities (e.g., hypertension, diabetes, congestive heart failure (CHF), renal impairment, cirrhosis), and patients taking other drugs that may reduce renal blood flow. Common dosage regimens are shown in Table 4.2.

DISEASE-MODIFYING ANTIRHEUMATIC DRUGS

General Principles
- Patients with active RA despite adequate NSAID treatment should be considered for DMARD therapy because these drugs have the potential to reduce or prevent joint damage, preserve joint function, and potentially reduce health care costs and improve the economic productivity of patients. Early initiation of therapy is crucial for optimal benefit.
- All DMARDs are relatively slow-acting (onset delay of 1–6 months), but the majority of patients ultimately achieve benefit from these drugs.
- Effective contraception is required for women of childbearing potential when most DMARDs are prescribed.
- Common dosage regimens and monitoring parameters for DMARDs are contained in Table 4.3.

Methotrexate
- Methotrexate is often selected as the initial DMARD, especially for patients with more severe disease. It may have the best long-term outcome because it is less toxic and less likely to be discontinued than other DMARDs. Its onset is relatively rapid (as early as 2–3 weeks), and more than 50% of patients continue it beyond 3 years.
- Toxicities are gastrointestinal (stomatitis, diarrhea, nausea, vomiting), hematologic (thrombocytopenia, leukopenia), pulmonary (fibrosis, pneumonitis), and hepatic (elevated enzymes, rare cirrhosis). Concomitant folic or folinic acid may reduce some adverse effects without loss of efficacy. Liver function must be monitored periodically, but a liver biopsy is recommended only in patients with persistently elevated hepatic enzymes.

TABLE 4.2. Dosage Regimens for Nonsteroidal Anti-Inflammatory Drugs

| Drug | Recommended Anti-Inflammatory Total Daily Dosage | | |
	Adult	*Children*	*Dosing Schedule*
Aspirin	2.6–5.2 g	60–100 mg/kg	qid
Diclofenac	150–200 mg	—	tid to qid
Diflunisal	0.5–1.5 g	—	bid
Etodolac	0.2–1.2 g (max 20 mg/kg)	—	tid to qid
Fenoprofen	0.9–3.0 g	—	qid
Flurbiprofen	200–300 mg	—	bid to qid
Ibuprofen	1.2–3.2 g	20–40 mg/kg	tid to qid
Indomethacin	50–200 mg	2–4 mg/kg (max 200 mg)	bid to qid
Ketoprofen	150–300 mg	—	tid to qid
Meclofenamate	200–400 mg	—	tid to qid
Nabumetone	1–2 g	—	daily to bid
Naproxen	0.5–1.0 g	10 mg/kg	bid
Naproxen sodium	0.55–1.1 g	—	bid
Nonacetylated salicylates[a]	1.2–4.8 g	—	bid to 6×/day
Oxaprozin	0.6–1.8 g (max 26 mg/kg)	—	daily to tid
Piroxicam	10–20 mg	—	daily
Sulindac	300–400 mg	—	bid
Tolmetin	0.6–1.8 g	15–30 mg/kg	tid to qid

[a]Choline salicylate, magnesium salicylate, salsalate, sodium salicylate, and sodium thiosalicylate

Gold Preparations

- Intramuscular or oral gold preparations are effective but the onset may be delayed for 3 to 6 months. Aurothioglucose (suspension in oil) and gold sodium thiomalate (aqueous solution) require weekly injections for about 22 weeks before a less frequent maintenance regimen may be initiated. Oral gold (auranofin) is more convenient than IM gold, but it is less effective.
- Adverse effects are gastrointestinal (nausea, vomiting, diarrhea), dermatologic (rash, stomatitis), renal (proteinuria, hematuria), and hematologic (anemia, leukopenia, thrombocytopenia). Gold sodium thiomalate is associated with nitritoid reactions (flushing, palpitations, hypotension, tachycardia, headache, blurred vision). Patients receiving IM gold may experience a postinjection disease flare for 1 to 2 days after an injection.

TABLE 4.3. Usual Doses and Monitoring Parameters for Antirheumatic Drugs

Drug	Usual Dose	Monitoring Parameters	
		Initial	*Maintenance*
NSAIDs	See Table 4.2	Scr or BUN, CBC q 2–4 weeks after starting therapy for 1–2 months salicylates: serum salicylate levels if therapeutic dose and no response	Same as initial plus stool guaiac q 6–12 months
Methotrexate	Oral or IM: 7.5–15 mg q week	Baseline: AST, ALT, alk phos, alb, t. bili, hep B & C studies, CBC w/plt, Scr	CBC w/plt, AST, alb q 1–2 months
Gold			
Auranofin	Oral: 3 mg daily to bid	Baseline: UA, CBC w/plt	Same as initial q 1–2 months
Gold sodium thiomalate or aurothioglucose	IM: 10-mg test dose, then weekly dosing 25–50 mg, after response may increase dosing interval	Baseline and until stable: UA, CBC w/plt preinjection	Same as initial every other dose
Hydroxychloroquine	Oral: 200–300 mg bid, after 1–2 months may decrease to 200 mg bid or daily	Baseline: color fundus photography and automated central perimetric analysis	Ophthalmoscopy q 9–12 months and Amsler grid at home q 2 weeks
Sulfasalazine	Oral: 500 mg bid, then increase to 1 g bid max	Baseline: CBC w/plt, then q week for 1 month	Same as initial q 1–2 months
Azathioprine	Oral: 50–150 mg daily	CBC w/plt, AST q 2 weeks for 1–2 months	Same as initial q 1–2 months
D-Penicillamine	Oral: 125–250 mg daily, may increase by 125–250 mg q 1–2 months, max: 750 mg daily	Baseline: UA, CBC w/plt, then q week for 1 month	Same as initial q 1–2 months, but q 2 weeks if dose change
Cyclophosphamide	Oral: 1–2 mg/kg/d	UA, CBC w/plt q week for 1 month	Same as initial q 2–4 weeks
Cyclosporine	Oral: 2.5 mg/kg/d	Scr, blood pressure q month	Same as initial

Key: alb, albumin; alk phos, alkaline phosphatase; ALT, alanine aminotransferase; AST, aspartate aminotransferase; BUN, blood urea nitrogen; CBC, complete blood count; hep, hepatitis; IA, intra-articular; IM, intramuscular; IV, intravenous; plt, platelet; q, every; Scr, serum creatinine; t. bili, total bilirubin; UA, urinalysis.

Hydroxychloroquine

- The antimalarial hydroxychloroquine is a good initial choice for patients with mild disease because of its safety, convenience, and low cost. It lacks the myelosuppressive, hepatic, and renal toxicities seen with some other DMARDs, simplifying its monitoring. Its onset may be as early as 6 weeks, but it may take as long as 6 months in some cases.
- Short-term toxicities include gastrointestinal (nausea, vomiting, diarrhea), ocular (accommodation defects, benign corneal deposits, blurred vision scotomas, night blindness, rare retinopathy), dermatologic (rash, alopecia, skin pigmentation), and neurologic (headache, vertigo, insomnia) effects. Periodic ophthalmologic examinations are necessary for early detection of reversible retinal toxicity.

Sulfasalazine

- This sulfonamide derivative is also effective for mild disease and is relatively safe and inexpensive. Its onset of action may occur in 1–2 months.
- Adverse effects include gastrointestinal (anorexia, nausea, vomiting, diarrhea), dermatologic (rash, urticaria), hematologic (leukopenia, rare agranulocytosis), and hepatic (elevated enzymes) effects. GI symptoms may be minimized by starting with low doses and taking the medication with food. Complete blood counts should be monitored periodically.

Penicillamine

- This chelating agent is effective and its effects may be seen in 1–3 months. Its use is limited by its infrequent but potentially serious induction of autoimmune diseases (e.g., Goodpasture's syndrome, myasthenia gravis).
- Other adverse effects include skin rash, metallic taste, hypogeusia, stomatitis, anorexia, nausea, vomiting, dyspepsia. Glomerular nephritis, manifested as proteinuria and hematuria, may also occur.

Azathioprine and Cyclophosphamide

- These potent immunosuppressives are reserved for patients unresponsive to or intolerant of other DMARDs.
- Azathioprine is a purine analog with immunosuppressive properties. Its effects may be seen in 3–4 weeks, but may take as long as 12 weeks at maximal dosages. Its major adverse effects are bone marrow suppression (leukopenia, macrocytic anemia, thrombocytopenia, pancytopenia), stomatitis, GI intolerance, infections, hepatoxicity, and oncogenic potential.
- Cyclophosphamide has similar or more severe adverse effects and is usually reserved for life-threatening RA complications.

Cyclosporine

- This drug is an effective immunosuppressive agent with an onset in 1–3 months. Its use is limited by drug cost and the occurrence of frequent toxicities (hypertension, hyperglycemia, nephrotoxicity, tremor, GI intolerance, hirsutism, gingival hyperplasia). Hypertension and nephrotoxicity are usually reversible after drug discontinuation. For these reasons, it is usually reserved for patients who are refractory to or intolerant of other DMARDs.

GLUCOCORTICOIDS

- Glucocorticoids have anti-inflammatory and immunosuppressive properties, and some evidence suggests that low oral doses may slow the rate of joint damage.
- In low oral doses (<10 mg/day of prednisone equivalent), they may be used as "bridging therapy" during the period before a DMARD has gained its full effect or for continuous therapy in patients whose disease is difficult to control with an NSAID and one or more DMARDs.
- High-dose oral bursts may be used to suppress disease flares. The adverse effects of systemic glucocorticoids limit their long-term use. Dosage tapering and eventual discontinuation should be considered at some point in patients receiving chronic therapy.
- Intra-articular injections may be useful when only a few joints are involved. The same joint should not be injected more frequently than once every 3 months.

▶ EVALUATION OF THERAPEUTIC OUTCOMES

- Patients with quiescent disease may be seen twice yearly, with the frequency of laboratory and clinical monitoring determined by the particular drug regimen; patients with active disease should be seen more frequently until disease control is achieved.
- Clinical signs of improvement include reduction in joint swelling, decreased warmth over actively involved joints, and decreased tenderness to joint palpation.
- Symptom improvement includes reduction in joint pain and morning stiffness, longer time to onset of afternoon fatigue, and improvement in ability to perform daily activities.
- Laboratory monitoring is of little value in monitoring individual patient response to therapy but is essential for detecting and preventing adverse drug effects (Table 4.3).
- Functional status may be assessed with the Arthritis Impact Measurement Scale or the Health Assessment Questionnaire.
- Patients should be questioned about the presence of symptoms that may be related to adverse effects of their particular regimen.
- Joint radiographs may be of some value in assessing disease progression.

See Chapter 84, Rheumatoid Arthritis and the Seronegative Spondy-loarthropathies, authored by Arthur A. Schuna, PharmD, Michael J. Schmidt, PharmD, and Denise Walbrandt Pigarelli, PharmD, for a detailed discussion of this topic.

Cardiovascular Disorders

Edited by Terry L. Schwinghammer, PharmD, FCCP, BCPS,
and Cindy W. Hamilton, PharmD

Chapter 5

► ARRHYTHMIAS

► DEFINITION

Arrhythmia is defined as loss of cardiac rhythm, especially irregularity of heartbeat. This chapter covers the group of conditions caused by any abnormality in the rate, regularity, or sequence of cardiac activation.

► PATHOPHYSIOLOGY

SUPRAVENTRICULAR TACHYCARDIA

- Common supraventricular tachycardias requiring drug treatment are atrial fibrillation or atrial flutter, paroxysmal supraventricular tachycardia, and automatic atrial tachycardias. Other common supraventricular arrhythmias that usually do not require drug therapy (e.g., premature atrial complexes, wandering atrial pacemaker, sinus arrhythmia, sinus tachycardia) are not included in this chapter.

Atrial Fibrillation and Atrial Flutter

- Atrial fibrillation is characterized as an extremely rapid (400–600 atrial beats/min) and disorganized atrial activation. There is a loss of atrial contraction (atrial kick), and supraventricular impulses penetrate the atrioventricular (AV) conduction system in variable degrees, resulting in irregular ventricular activation and irregularly irregular pulse (120–180 beats/min).
- Atrial flutter is characterized by rapid (270–330 atrial beats/min) but regular atrial activation. The ventricular response usually has a regular pattern. This arrhythmia occurs less frequently than atrial fibrillation, but it has similar precipitating factors, consequences, and drug therapy.
- The predominant mechanism of atrial fibrillation and atrial flutter is reentry, which is usually associated with organic heart disease that causes atrial distention (e.g., ischemia or infarction, hypertensive heart disease, valvular disorders). Additional associated disorders include acute pulmonary embolus and chronic lung disease, resulting in pulmonary hypertension and cor pulmonale; and states of high adrenergic tone such as thyrotoxicosis, alcohol withdrawal, sepsis, or excess physical exertion.

Paroxysmal Supraventricular Tachycardia

- Paroxysmal supraventricular tachycardia (PSVT) arising by reentrant mechanisms includes arrhythmias caused by AV nodal reentry and AV reentry incorporating an anomalous AV pathway, and, less commonly, sinoatrial (SA) nodal reentry, and intra-atrial reentry.

Automatic Atrial Tachycardias

- Automatic atrial tachycardias such as multifocal atrial tachycardia appear to arise from multifocal or unifocal supraventricular foci with enhanced automatic properties. Severe pulmonary disease is the underlying precipitating disorder present in 60–80% of patients.

VENTRICULAR ARRHYTHMIAS

- Common ventricular arrhythmias include ventricular premature beats (VPBs), ventricular tachycardia (VT), and ventricular fibrillation (VF). Less common ventricular arrhythmias include proarrhythmia and torsade de pointes (TdP).

Ventricular Premature Beats

- VPBs are very common ventricular rhythm disturbances that occur in patients with or without heart disease and may be elicited experimentally by abnormal automaticity, triggered activity, or reentrant mechanisms.

Ventricular Tachycardia

- VT is defined by three or more repetitive VPBs occurring at >100 beats/min. The most common precipitating factor for an acute episode is acute myocardial infarction; other causes are severe electrolyte abnormalities (e.g., hypokalemia), hypoxemia, and digitalis toxicity. The chronic recurrent form is almost always associated with underlying organic heart disease (e.g., idiopathic dilated congestive cardiomyopathy or remote myocardial infarction with left ventricular aneurysm).
- Sustained VT requires therapeutic intervention to restore a stable rhythm or it lasts a relatively long time (usually >30 seconds). Nonsustained VT (NSVT) self-terminates after a brief duration (usually <30 seconds). Incessant VT refers to VT occurring more frequently than sinus rhythm so that VT becomes the dominant rhythm. Exercise-induced VT occurs during high sympathetic tone (e.g., physical exertion). Monomorphic VT has a consistent QRS configuration, whereas polymorphic VT has varying QRS complexes.

Proarrhythmia

- Proarrhythmia refers to development of a significant new arrhythmia (such as VT, VF, or TdP) or worsening of an existing arrhythmia. Proarrhythmia results from the same mechanisms that cause other arrhythmias or an alteration in the underlying substrate due to the antiarrhythmic agent (e.g., development of an accelerated tachycardia due to flecainide, which decreases conduction velocity without significantly altering the refractory period). Antiarrhythmic drugs cause proarrhythmia in 5–20% of patients. Although initially thought to occur within several days of drug initiation, risk may persist throughout treatment.

Definite patient risk factors are underlying ventricular arrhythmias, ischemic heart disease, and poor left ventricular function; less well-defined risk factors are elevated antiarrhythmic serum concentrations (and rapid dosage escalation), recent therapy with a type Ia antiarrhythmic, and underlying ventricular conduction delays.

II

Torsades de Pointes

- TdP is a rapid form of polymorphic VT that is associated with evidence of delayed ventricular repolarization due to blockade or abnormal potassium conductance. TdP may be hereditary or acquired. Acquired forms are associated with many clinical conditions and drugs, especially type Ia antiarrhythmics. Quinidine-induced TdP or quinidine syncope occurs in 4–8% of patients treated with this agent.

Ventricular Fibrillation

- VF is electrical anarchy of the ventricle resulting in no cardiac output and cardiovascular collapse. VF, often preceded by VT, is the most frequently documented rhythm in patients who die suddenly during electrocardiographic (ECG) monitoring. Sudden cardiac death occurs most commonly in patients with ischemic heart disease and primary myocardial disease.

BRADYARRHYTHMIAS

- Sinus bradyarrhythmias (heart rate <60 beats/min) are common especially in young athletes. However, some patients have sinus node dysfunction or sick sinus syndrome because of underlying organic heart disease and normal aging process, which results in symptomatic sinus bradycardia, periods of sinus arrest, or both. Sinus node dysfunction is usually representative of diffuse conduction disease, which may be accompanied by AV block and by paroxysmal tachycardias such as atrial fibrillation. Alternating bradyarrhythmias and tachyarrhythmias are referred to as tachy–brady syndrome.
- AV block is caused by conduction delay or block, which may occur in any area of AV conduction. AV block may be found in patients without underlying heart disease, such as trained athletes, or it may occur during sleep when vagal tone is high. AV block may be transient where the underlying etiology is reversible (e.g., myocarditis, myocardial ischemia, after cardiovascular surgery, during drug therapy) or irreversible. Beta blockers, digitalis, or calcium antagonists may cause AV block, primarily in the AV nodal area. Type I antiarrhythmic agents may exacerbate conduction delays below the level of the AV node.

▶ CLINICAL PRESENTATION

- Supraventricular tachycardias may cause a variety of clinical manifestations ranging from no symptoms to minor palpitations and/or irregular pulse to severe and even life-threatening symptoms. Patients may experience dizziness or acute syncopal episodes; symptoms of congestive heart failure; anginal chest pain; or, more often, choking or pressure sensation during the tachycardia episode. Symptoms such as palpitations and even syncope correlate poorly with documented recurrences of tachycardia.

- Atrial fibrillation or flutter may be manifested by the entire range of symptoms associated with other supraventricular tachycardias, but syncope is not a common presenting symptom. An additional complication of atrial fibrillation is arterial embolization resulting from atrial stasis and poorly adherent mural thrombi, which accounts for the most devastating complication, embolic stroke. In patients with atrial fibrillation, risk factors for cerebral embolism are concurrent mitral stenosis or severe systolic heart failure.
- Ventricular arrhythmias may yield manifestations ranging from no symptoms or only mild palpitations to a life-threatening situation associated with hemodynamic collapse. Consequences of proarrhythmia range from no symptoms to worsening of symptoms to sudden death. VF, by definition, is an acute medical emergency resulting in no cardiac output, cardiovascular collapse, and death if effective treatment measures are not taken.
- Patients with bradyarrhythmias experience symptoms associated with hypotension such as dizziness, syncope, fatigue, and confusion. If left ventricular dysfunction exists, symptoms of congestive heart failure may be exacerbated. Except for recurrent syncope, these symptoms are often subtle and nonspecific.

▶ DIAGNOSIS

- Surface electrocardiogram (ECG) is the cornerstone of diagnostic tools for cardiac rhythm disturbances.
- Less sophisticated methods are often the initial tools for detecting qualitative and quantitative alterations of heartbeat. For example, direct auscultation can reveal the irregularly irregular pulse that is characteristic of atrial fibrillation.
- Proarrhythmia can be difficult to diagnose because of the variable nature of underlying arrhythmias. Flecainide and encainide have been known to cause a rapid, sustained, monomorphic VT with a characteristic sinusoidal QRS pattern.
- TdP is characterized by long QT interval or prominent U waves on surface ECG.
- Specific maneuvers may be required to delineate the etiology of syncope associated with bradyarrhythmias. Diagnosis of carotid sinus hypersensitivity can be confirmed by performing carotid sinus massage with ECG and blood pressure monitoring. Vasovagal syncope can be diagnosed using the upright body tilt test. β blockers may be administered IV to predict response to oral therapy.
- AV block is usually categorized into three different types based on surface ECG findings (Table 5.1).

TABLE 5.1. Forms of Atrioventricular Block

Type	Criteria
First-degree block	Prolonged PR interval (>0.2 s), 1:1 AV conduction
Second-degree block	
Mobitz I	Progressive PR prolongation until QRS is dropped, <1:1 AV conduction
Mobitz II	Random nonconducted beats (absence of QRS), <1:1 AV conduction
Third-degree block	AV dissociation, absence of AV conduction

▶ DESIRED OUTCOME

The desired outcome depends on the underlying arrhythmia. For example, the ultimate treatment goals of treating atrial fibrillation or flutter are restoring sinus rhythm, preventing thromboembolic complications, and preventing further recurrences.

▶ TREATMENT

GENERAL PRINCIPLES

- Treatment approach is determined by the underlying arrhythmia. Before addressing specific arrhythmias, it is appropriate to consider general principles of therapy.
- The Cardiac Arrhythmias Suppression Trial (CAST) is perhaps the most important study on treating rhythm disorders. CAST revealed that patients with VPBs postmyocardial infarction do not benefit from chronic antiarrhythmic drug therapy (beyond general β-blocker use). In fact, this type of therapy is detrimental, presumably because of proarrhythmia. The results have colored long-term use of all antiarrhythmics, causing broad skepticism regarding risk–benefit ratios. Pharmaceutical companies have shifted investigative efforts away from potent sodium channel blockers and removed encainide from the market. These findings also provide incentive for pursuing nondrug therapies.
  - The antiarrhythmic agent should be discontinued if proarrhythmia is detected or suspected.
  - Internal cardioverter/defibrillators are becoming first-line treatment for many serious, recurrent ventricular arrhythmias because of technologic advances combined with the now known hazards of drugs.

MECHANISMS OF ANTIARRHYTHMIC DRUGS

- Drugs may have antiarrhythmic activity by directly altering conduction in several ways. Drugs may depress the automatic properties of abnormal pacemaker cells by decreasing the slope of phase 4 depolarization and/or by elevating threshold potential. Drugs may alter the conduction characteristics of the pathways of a reentrant loop.

- Although often criticized, the most frequently used classification system was first proposed by Vaughan Williams (Table 5.2). Type Ia drugs slow conduction velocity, prolong refractoriness, and decrease the automatic properties of sodium-dependent (normal and diseased) conduction tissue. Clinically, type Ia drugs are broad-spectrum antiarrhythmics, being effective for both supraventricular and ventricular arrhythmias.

- Although categorized separately, type Ib drugs probably act similarly to type Ia drugs (i.e., accentuated effects in diseased tissues leading to bidirectional block in a reentrant circuit), except that type Ib agents are considerably more effective in ventricular than supraventricular arrhythmias.

- Type Ic drugs profoundly slow conduction velocity while leaving refractoriness relatively unaltered. Although effective for both ventricular and supraventricular arrhythmias, their use for ventricular arrhythmias has been limited by the risk of proarrhythmia.

- Collectively, type I drugs can be referred to as sodium channel blockers. Antiarrhythmic sodium channel receptor theories account for additive (e.g., quinidine and mexiletine) and antagonistic (e.g., flecainide

TABLE 5.2. Classification of Antiarrhythmic Drugs

Type	Drug	Conduction Velocity[a]	Refractory Period	Automaticity	Ion Block
Ia	Quinidine Procainamide Disopyramide	↓	↑	↓	Sodium (intermediate)
Ib	Lidocaine Mexiletine Tocainide	0/↓	↓	↓	Sodium (fast on–off)
Ic	Flecainide Propafenone[b] Moricizine[c]	↓↓	0	↓	Sodium (slow on–off)
II[d]	β blockers	↓	↑	↓	Calcium (indirect)
III	Amiodarone[b,e] Bretylium[b] Sotalol[b]	0	↑↑	0	Potassium
IV[d]	Verapamil Diltiazem	↓	↑	↓	Calcium

Key: ↑, increase; ↓, decrease.
[a]Variables for normal tissue models in ventricular tissue.
[b]Also has type II β-blocking actions.
[c]Classification controversial.
[d]Variables for SA and AV nodal tissue only.
[e]Amiodarone also blocks calcium and sodium channels (fast on–off).

and lidocaine) drug combinations, as well as potential antidotes to excess sodium-channel blockade (e.g., sodium bicarbonate, propranolol).

- Type II drugs include β-adrenergic antagonists; clinically relevant mechanisms result from their antiadrenergic actions. β blockers are most useful in tachycardias in which nodal tissues are abnormally automatic or are a portion of a reentrant loop. These agents are also helpful in slowing ventricular response in atrial tachycardias (e.g., atrial fibrillation) by their effects on the AV node.

- Type III drugs specifically prolong refractoriness in atrial and ventricular fibers and include three very different drugs that share the common effect of delaying repolarization by blocking potassium channels.

  - Bretylium prolongs repolarization by blocking potassium conductance independent of the sympathetic nervous system, increases the VF threshold, and seems to have selective antifibrillatory but not antitachycardic effects. Bretylium can be effective in VF but is rarely effective in ventricular tachycardia.

  - In contrast, amiodarone and sotalol are effective in many tachycardias. Amiodarone displays electrophysiologic characteristics consistent with each type of antiarrhythmic drug. It is a sodium-channel blocker with relatively fast on–off kinetics, has β-blocking actions, blocks potassium channels, and has slight calcium antagonist activity. Amiodarone seems to be the most effective antiarrhythmic agent, but it also has the most impressive side-effect profile. Sotalol is a potent inhibitor of outward potassium movement during repolarization and also possesses β-blocking actions. Sotalol and similar drugs also appear to be more effective in preventing VF (in dog models) than traditional sodium blockers. They also decrease defibrillation threshold in contrast with type I agents.

- Type IV drugs inhibit calcium entry into the cell, which slows conduction, prolongs refractoriness, and decreases SA and AV nodal automaticity. Calcium channel antagonists are effective for automatic or reentrant tachycardias, which arise from or use the SA or AV nodes.

- In addition to exhibiting different mechanisms, antiarrhythmic agents are distinguished by their pharmacokinetic (Table 5.3) and safety profiles (Table 5.4).

ATRIAL FIBRILLATION OR ATRIAL FLUTTER

- Many methods are available for restoring sinus rhythm, preventing thromboembolic complications, and preventing further recurrences (Fig. 5.1); however, treatment selection is widely debated depending, in part, on onset and severity of symptoms.

- If symptoms are severe and of recent onset, patients may require direct-current cardioversion (DCC) to restore sinus rhythm immediately.

- If symptoms are tolerable, drugs that slow conduction and increase refractoriness in the AV node should be used as initial therapy. Type Ia

Cardiovascular Disorders

TABLE 5.3. Pharmacokinetics of Antiarrhythmic Drugs

Drug	Bioavail-ability (%)	Primary Route of Elimination[a]	$V_{D,ss}$ (L/kg)	Protein Binding (%)	$t_{1/2}$	Therapeutic Range (mg/L)
Quinidine	70–80	H	2.0–3.5	80–90	5–9 h	2–6
Procainamide	75–95	H/R	1.5–3.0	10–20	2.5–5.0 h	4–15
Disopyramide	70–95	H/R	0.8–2.0	50–80	4–8 h	2–6
Lidocaine	20–40	H	1–2	65–75	60–180 min	1.5–5.0
Mexiletine	80–95	H	5–12	60–75	6–12 h	0.8–2.0
Tocainide	90–95	H	1.5–3.0	10–30	12–15 h	4–10
Moricizine	34–38	H	6–11	92–95	1–6 h	—
Flecainide	90–95	H/R	8–10	35–45	13–20 h	0.3–2.5
Propafenone[b]						
Poor	11–39	H	2.5–4.0	85–95	12–32 h	—
Extensive					2–10 h	
Amiodarone	22–88	H	70–150	95–99	15–100 d	1.0–2.5
Sotalol	90–95	R	1.2–2.4	30–40	12–20 h	—
Bretylium	15–20	R	4–8	Negligible	5–10 h	0.5–2.0
Verapamil	20–40	H	1.5–5.0	95–99	4–12 h	>0.05
Diltiazem	35–50	H	3–5	70–85	4–10 h	>0.05

[a]H, hepatic; R, renal.
[b]Variables for parent compound (not 5–OH propafenone).

antiarrhythmic agents should not be administered initially because they may paradoxically increase ventricular response in the absence of drugs that slow AV nodal conduction. Digoxin's place in therapy has been questioned because it is sometimes ineffective and often slow in onset. Many clinicians prefer calcium antagonists (e.g., IV verapamil, diltiazem). If a high adrenergic state is the precipitating factor, IV β blockers (e.g., propranolol, esmolol) can be highly effective.

- After treatment with AV nodal blocking agents and a subsequent decrease in ventricular response, the patient should be evaluated for the possibility of restoring sinus rhythm.
- If sinus rhythm is restored, anticoagulation should be initiated because return of atrial contraction increases risk of thromboembolism. Current recommendations are warfarin treatment (INR 2.0–3.0) for at least 3 weeks prior to cardioversion and continuing for about 1 month after effective cardioversion. Exceptions in which anticoagulation may not be necessary are atrial flutter (unless concurrent risks for thrombosis are present); lone atrial fibrillation; atrial fibrillation of less than 48 hours'

TABLE 5.4. Side Effects of Antiarrhythmic Drugs

Quinidine	Cinchonism, diarrhea, GI,[a] hypotension, torsades de pointes, aggravation of underlying heart failure, conduction disturbances or ventricular arrhythmias, hepatitis, thrombocytopenia, hemolytic anemia
Procainamide	Systemic lupus erythematosus, GI, torsades de pointes, aggravation of underlying heart failure, conduction disturbances or ventricular arrhythmias, agranulocytosis
Disopyramide	Anticholinergic symptoms, GI, torsades de pointes, heart failure, aggravation of underlying conduction disturbances and/or ventricular arrhythmias, hypoglycemia, hepatic cholestasis
Lidocaine	CNS,[b] seizures, psychosis, sinus arrest, aggravation of underlying conduction disturbances
Mexiletine	CNS, psychosis, GI, aggravation of underlying conduction disturbances or ventricular arrhythmias
Tocainide	CNS, psychosis, GI, aggravation of underlying conduction disturbances or ventricular arrhythmias, rash/arthralgias, pulmonary infiltrates, agranulocytosis, thrombocytopenia
Moricizine	Dizziness, headache, GI, aggravation of underlying conduction disturbances or ventricular arrhythmias
Flecainide, propafenone	Blurred vision, dizziness, headache, GI, bronchospasm,[c] aggravation of underlying heart failure, conduction disturbances or ventricular arrhythmias
Amiodarone	CNS, corneal microdeposits/blurred vision, GI, aggravation of underlying ventricular arrhythmias, torsades de pointes, bradycardia or AV block, bruising without thrombocytopenia, pulmonary fibrosis, hepatitis, hypothyroidism, hyperthyroidism, photosensitivity, blue-gray skin discoloration, myopathy
Sotalol	Fatigue, GI, depression, torsades de pointes, bronchospasm, aggravation of underlying heart failure, conduction disturbances or ventricular arrhythmias
Bretylium	Hypotension, GI

[a]GI = nausea, anorexia.
[b]CNS = confusion, paresthesias, tremor, ataxia, etc.
[c]Propafenone only.

duration; and absence of atrial thrombus or severe stasis on transesophageal echocardiography (TEE).
- After prior anticoagulation, methods for restoring sinus rhythm in patients with atrial fibrillation or flutter are pharmacologic cardioversion and DCC. The time-honored method for pharmacologic cardioversion is oral quinidine therapy beginning with maintenance dosages; IV procainamide, oral flecainide, and sotalol are suitable alternatives. Advantages of initial drug therapy are that an effective agent may be

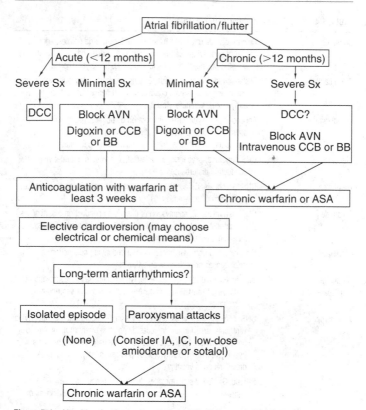

Figure 5.1. Algorithm for the treatment of atrial fibrillation and atrial flutter. Sx, symptoms; AVN, AV node; DCC, direct-current cardioversion; CCB, calcium channel antagonist (verapamil or diltiazem); BB, β blocker; ASA, aspirin. *(From Bauman JL et al. Tachycardias, in Carter B, Angaran D, Lake K, Raebel M [eds]: Pharmacotherapy Self-Assessment Program, 2nd ed. Kansas City, MO, ACCP, 1995, with permission.)*

determined in case long-term therapy is required and there is little to lose with a 2- to 3-day trial; disadvantages are significant side effects such as drug-induced TdP, drug–drug interactions, and lower cardioversion rate for drugs compared with DCC. Disadvantages of DCC are need for prior sedation/anesthesia and a risk of serious complications, although the latter is small.

- Maintenance medications after sinus rhythm is restored may consist of digoxin, antithrombotic therapy, and antiarrhythmic drugs.

- Digoxin is often continued because of underlying ventricular dysfunction, but this practice has been questioned because digoxin may occasionally be profibrillatory.
- Warfarin significantly reduces the incidence of stroke in patients with atrial fibrillation (not associated with prior thromboembolic episodes or mitral valve disease) with an acceptable risk of bleeding complications. The American College of Chest Physicians Consensus Conference on antithrombotic therapy recommends chronic warfarin treatment (INR 2.0–3.0) for all patients with atrial fibrillation except for young (<60 years of age) patients with "lone" atrial fibrillation, patients with only atrial flutter, and patients who are unreliable or whose compliance is poor. There is evidence that aspirin (325 mg/day) should be used instead of warfarin in the absence of risk factors (i.e., hypertension, recent heart failure, and prior thromboembolism).
- Atrial fibrillation usually recurs after initial cardioversion because most patients have irreversible underlying heart disease. A meta-analysis confirmed that quinidine maintained sinus rhythm better than placebo; however, 50% of patients had recurrent atrial fibrillation within a year, and more importantly, quinidine increased mortality, presumably due to proarrhythmia. Newer type Ic (e.g., flecainide, propafenone) and type III (e.g., amiodarone, sotalol) antiarrhythmic agents may provide alternatives to quinidine; however, these agents are also associated with proarrhythmia. Consequently, chronic antiarrhythmic drugs should be reserved for patients with symptomatic recurrences or symptomatic paroxysmal atrial fibrillation.

PAROXYSMAL SUPRAVENTRICULAR TACHYCARDIA DUE TO REENTRY

- The choice between pharmacologic and nonpharmacologic methods for treating PSVT depends on symptom severity (Fig. 5.2). Synchronized DCC is the treatment of choice if symptoms are severe (e.g., syncope, near syncope, anginal chest pain, severe heart failure). Non-drug measures (e.g., carotid massage, valsalva maneuver) can be used for mild to moderate symptoms. If these methods fail, drug therapy is the next option.
- The choice among drugs is based on the QRS complex (Fig. 5.2). Drugs can be divided into three broad categories: those that directly or indirectly increase vagal tone to the AV node (e.g., edrophonium, vasopressors, and digoxin); those that depress conduction through slow, calcium-dependent tissue (e.g., adenosine, β blockers, calcium channel blockers); and those that depress conduction through fast, sodium-dependent tissue (e.g., quinidine, procainamide, disopyramide, flecainide).
- Adenosine has been recommended as the drug of first choice in patients with PSVT because its short duration of action will not cause prolonged

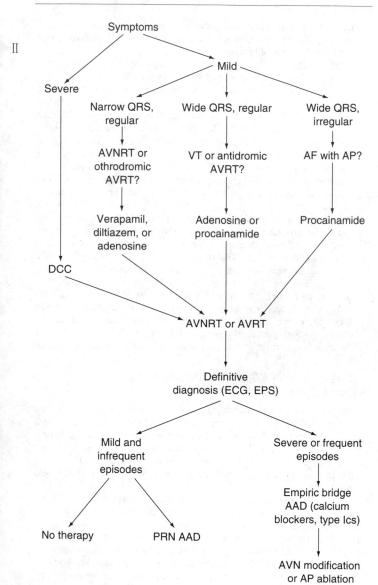

hemodynamic compromise in patients with wide QRS complexes who actually have VT rather than PSVT.

- After acute PSVT is terminated, long-term preventive treatment is indicated if frequent episodes necessitate therapeutic intervention, or episodes are infrequent but severely symptomatic. Serial testing of antiarrhythmic agents can be evaluated in the ambulatory setting via ambulatory ECG recordings (Holter) or telephonic transmissions of cardiac rhythm (event monitors), during hospitalization with Holter monitoring or telemetry, or by invasive electrophysiologic techniques in the laboratory.
- Chronic antiarrhythmic drug treatment in young, otherwise healthy patients is problematic because of possible necessity of life-long daily medication, poor tolerability, occasionally severe side effects, and frequent lack of efficacy.
- Transcutaneous catheter ablation using radio frequency (rf) current of the PSVT substrate is being considered as a nondrug alternative to chronic antiarrhythmic drug treatment because it is highly effective and curative, rarely results in complications, and obviates the need for chronic antiarrhythmic drug therapy.

AUTOMATIC ATRIAL TACHYCARDIAS

- Underlying precipitating factors should be corrected by ensuring proper oxygenation and ventilation, and by correcting acid–base or electrolyte disturbances.
- If tachycardia persists, the need for additional treatment is determined by symptoms. Patients with asymptomatic atrial tachycardia and relatively slow ventricular response usually require no drug therapy.
- If patients are symptomatic, medical therapy can be tailored either to control ventricular response or to restore sinus rhythm. Calcium antagonists (e.g., verapamil) are considered first-line drug therapy. Intravenous magnesium (independent of serum magnesium) can also be effective. Both probably act by suppressing calcium-mediated triggered activity.

Figure 5.2. Algorithm for the treatment of acute (top) PSVT and chronic prevention of recurrences (bottom). DCC, direct current cardioversion; AVN, atrioventricular node; AVRT, AV reentrant tachycardia; AVNRT, AV nodal reentrant tachycardia; VT, ventricular tachycardia; AF, atrial fibrillation; AP, accessory pathway; ECG, electrocardiographic monitoring; EPS, electrophysiologic studies; PRN, as needed; AAD, antiarrhythmic drugs. Note that for empiric bridge therapy prior to radiofrequency ablation procedures, calcium antagonists (or other AV nodal blockers) should not be used if the patient has AV reentry with preexcitation. (*From Bauman JL et al. Tachycardias, in Carter B, Angaran D, Lake K, Raebel M [eds]: Pharmacotherapy Self-Assessment Program, 2nd ed. Kansas City, MO, ACCP, 1995, with permission.*)

VENTRICULAR PREMATURE BEATS

II
- In apparently healthy individuals, drug therapy is unnecessary because VPBs without associated heart disease carry little or no risk. If drug therapy is necessary, β blockers are the drugs of choice because they are generally better tolerated than type I agents and decrease mortality, particularly after myocardial infarction. The endpoint of drug therapy is symptomatic relief, not quantitative reduction in VPB frequency.
- Chronic antiarrhythmic drug treatment of VPBs in patients with associated heart disease (usually postmyocardial infarction) is controversial. Aggressive antiarrhythmic drug therapy is recommended to suppress a high percentage of VPBs, thereby eliminating a risk factor for cardiac death in patients with coronary disease. However, the frequency of VPBs is sporadic and extremely variable, which makes it difficult to determine effective drug therapy; antiarrhythmic agents are associated with impressive side effects (Table 5.4). A more conservative approach, withholding drug therapy in the absence of significant symptoms, is supported by CAST results.

VENTRICULAR TACHYCARDIA

Acute Ventricular Tachycardia
- Initial management of an acute episode of VT requires a quick assessment of the patient's status and symptoms. If severe symptoms are present, then DCC should be instituted to restore sinus rhythm immediately. Precipitating factors should be corrected. If VT is an isolated electrical event associated with a transient initiating factor (e.g., acute myocardial ischemia, digitalis toxicity), then lidocaine should be administered and continued for 24–48 hours or until the patient is stable. There is no need for long-term antiarrhythmic therapy after precipitating factors are corrected.
- Patients with mild or no symptoms can be treated initially with antiarrhythmic drugs. Lidocaine (loading dose and infusion) is usually the drug of choice because of effectiveness, quick onset, and ease of administration. If lidocaine fails to terminate tachycardia, IV procainamide (loading dose and infusion) can be tried. DCC should be instituted or a transvenous pacing wire should be inserted if the patient's status deteriorates, VT degenerates to VF, or drug therapy fails.

Sustained Ventricular Tachycardia
- Chronic recurrent sustained VT deserves attention because of the high risk of death; trial-and-error attempts are unwarranted. Neither electrophysiologic studies nor Holter monitoring is ideal. These findings and the side-effect profiles of antiarrhythmic agents have led to nondrug approaches.
- Electrophysiologic studies can be used for serial testing of antiarrhythmic drugs. Drawbacks are invasiveness; low yield for finding an effec-

tive drug, which necessitates use of alternate treatment endpoints; and lack of predictive value for selected drugs (e.g., amiodarone).

- Holter monitoring can also be performed with serial drug testing; the II surrogate endpoint is suppression of ventricular ectopy (>83%) and total abolition of NSVT compared to control (drug-free) recordings. In a large comparative study, Holter testing successfully identified more effective agents than electrophysiologic monitoring; there were no differences in VT recurrence or sudden death. Sotalol was the most effective drug in the trial.

- Implantable automatic cardioverter defibrillator (ICD) is becoming popular because it is highly effective in preventing sudden death due to recurrent VT or VF and because technologic advances have been introduced that, for example, obviate the need for thoracotomy. Limitations include high cost of the device and of implantation, ultimate need for antiarrhythmic drugs (usually amiodarone) in up to 50% of patients, and lack of evidence of decrease in overall mortality.

- Patients with complex ventricular ectopy should not be treated with traditional (type I) antiarrhythmic drugs.

Nonsustained Ventricular Tachycardia

- The approach to NSVT is controversial (Fig. 5.3). Obviously, patients with long symptomatic episodes require drug therapy, but most are asymptomatic. Epidemiologic data indicate that patients with NSVT and coronary disease are at risk for sudden death, particularly if they have inducible sustained tachycardias on invasive electrophysiologic studies. Serial drug testing can be used, but electrophysiologic-guided drug therapy has not been shown to decrease long-term mortality. Noninvasive tools are an alternate approach to risk stratification; abnormal signal-averaged ECG is a significant risk factor for subsequent arrhythmia (sustained VT) or sudden death. Large prospective trials are necessary and ongoing to discern the proper approach to NSVT.

PROARRHYTHMIA

- Proarrhythmia is resistant to resuscitation with cardioversion or overdrive pacing. Some clinicians have had success with IV lidocaine or sodium bicarbonate.

TORSADES DE POINTES

- For an acute episode, most patients will require and respond to DCC. However, TdP tends to be paroxysmal and often recurs rapidly after countershock.

- Preventive therapy should increase heart rate and thereby shorten ventricular repolarization. Initial treatment after DCC includes either temporary transvenous pacing (105–120 beats/min) or pharmacologic pacing (e.g., isoproterenol or epinephrine infusion). IV magnesium sulfate, independent of serum magnesium concentration, also provides valuable adjunctive therapy. Agents that prolong QT interval should be

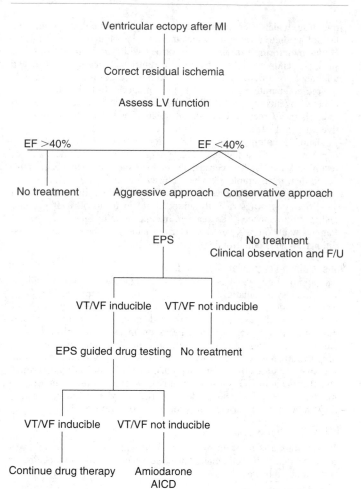

Figure 5.3. An algorithm for management of patients with ventricular ectopy after myocardial infarction. Correction of residual ischemia may include treatment with antianginal drug therapy, percutaneous transluminal coronary angioplasty, or bypass surgery. No treatment indicates that antiarrhythmic therapy (either pharmacologic or nonpharmacologic therapy) is not indicated. MI, myocardial infarction; LV, left ventricular; EF, ejection fraction; EPS, electrophysiologic studies; VT/VF, ventricular tachycardia/ventricular fibrillation; AICD, automatic implantable cardioverter–defibrillator; F/U, follow-up. (*From Bauman JL et al. Tachycardias, in Carter B, Angaran D, Lake K, Raebel M [eds]: Pharmacotherapy Self-Assessment Program, 2nd ed. Kansas City, MO, ACCP, 1995, with permission.*)

discontinued and exacerbating factors corrected. Drugs that further prolong repolarization (e.g., procainamide) are contraindicated. Lidocaine
is usually ineffective. II
- In heritable TdP, propranolol has been shown to prevent recurrences
and sudden death. In refractory patients, phenytoin or ICD placement
have been used.
- In acquired long-QT syndromes, correction of underlying cause is crucial for successful preventive therapy. In quinidine syncope, type Ia
agents should be avoided as future treatment. No drugs need be used
chronically.

VENTRICULAR FIBRILLATION

- VF should be managed according to the American Heart Association's
recommendations for advanced cardiac life support; additional details
can be found in Chapter 6, Cardiopulmonary Resuscitation.

BRADYARRHYTHMIA DUE TO SINUS NODE DYSFUNCTION

- Treatment of sinus node dysfunction involves elimination of symptomatic bradycardia and possibly managing alternating tachycardias such
as atrial fibrillation. Asymptomatic sinus bradyarrhythmias usually do
not require therapeutic intervention.
- In general, long-term therapy of choice for patients with significant
symptoms is a permanent ventricular pacemaker.
- Drugs commonly employed to treat supraventricular tachycardias
should be used with caution, if at all, in the absence of a functioning
pacemaker.
- Carotid-sinus hypersensitivity can also be treated with permanent pacemaker therapy. Patients who remain symptomatic may benefit from
adding α-adrenergic stimulants (e.g., ephedrine), sometimes with β
blockers to maximize α-sympathetic stimulation.
- Vasovagal syncope can usually be treated successfully with oral β
blockers to inhibit the sympathetic surge that causes forceful ventricular contraction and precedes the onset of hypotension and bradycardia.
Other drugs that have been used successfully (with or without β blockers) include scopolamine patches, α-adrenergic agonists, theophylline,
dipyridamole, and disopyramide.

ATRIOVENTRICULAR BLOCK

- Temporary transvenous pacing is the cornerstone for acute treatment of
symptomatic bradycardia or AV block. Until the right ventricular lead
can be inserted, bridge therapy may include transcutaneous pacing
devices or drugs that improve sinus and AV nodal conduction (e.g.,
atropine, epinephrine infusion). Pharmacologic therapies such as
atropine or sympathomimetics may improve symptoms and conduction
in sinus bradycardia/arrest and AV nodal block, but they will not help if
AV block is below the AV node (e.g., Mobitz II or trifascicular AV
block).

II

- Chronic symptomatic AV block should be treated by inserting a permanent pacemaker.
- Patients without symptoms usually can be followed closely without a pacemaker.

▶ EVALUATION OF THERAPEUTIC OUTCOMES

- The most important monitoring parameters fall into the following categories: (1) mortality (total and arrhythmic), (2) arrhythmia recurrence (duration, frequency, and symptoms), (3) hemodynamic consequences (rate, blood pressure, and symptoms), and (4) treatment complications (need for alternative or additional drugs, devices, or surgery).
- Presence or recurrence of any arrhythmia can be documented by ECG means (e.g., surface ECG, Holter monitor, event monitor).
- Some therapeutic outcomes are unique to certain arrhythmias. For instance, patients with atrial fibrillation or flutter need to be monitored for thromboembolism and for complications of anticoagulation therapy (bleeding or drug interactions).

See Chapter 16, The Arrhythmias, authored by Jerry L. Bauman, PharmD, FCCP, FACC and Marieke Dekker Schoen, PharmD, for a more detailed discussion of this topic.

Chapter 6

► CARDIOPULMONARY RESUSCITATION

► DEFINITION

Cardiopulmonary arrest occurs when spontaneous and effective ventilation and circulation abruptly terminate following a cardiac or respiratory event.

► PATHOPHYSIOLOGY

- Cardiac arrhythmias, such as ventricular tachycardia (VT) and ventricular fibrillation (VF), are the usual cause of sudden cardiac death. Other presenting arrhythmias include bradyarrhythmias, asystole, and pulseless electrical activity (PEA).
- Respiratory arrests can occur subsequent to sudden infant death syndrome, drowning, drug overdose, stroke, chronic obstructive pulmonary disease, infection, foreign-body aspiration, and electrocution. Primary respiratory arrests occur most commonly in children.
- Although approximately 80–90% of nontraumatic cardiac arrests are initiated by either VT or VF, only 35-55% of patients with out-of-hospital cardiac arrests are actually found to be in VF or VT. These statistics are relevant because the survival rate to hospital discharge is higher for patients found initially in VF or VT versus that of patients in asystole or PEA activity (20% versus 1-7%).
- Two theories exist regarding the mechanism of blood flow in cardiopulmonary resuscitation (CPR). The initial theory, known as the cardiac pump theory, explains forward blood flow based on active compression of the heart between the sternum and vertebrae. After the discovery of cough CPR, the thoracic pump theory was founded on the belief that blood flow during CPR results from intrathoracic pressure alterations induced by chest compressions. In reality, components of both theories may operate during CPR.
- Acid–base imbalances result from decreased perfusion and ineffective ventilation. Despite CPR, which raises cardiac output to approximately 30% of baseline, anaerobic metabolism predominates and raises Pco_2 concentrations. Elimination of Pco_2 is hampered by diminished blood flow.

► CLINICAL MANIFESTATIONS

- Termination of spontaneous and effective ventilation and circulation may be preceded by cardiac symptoms, easy fatigability, or nonspecific complaints lasting days to months.

- The onset of cardiac arrest may be characterized by typical symptoms of an acute cardiac event (e.g., prolonged angina or pain of myocardial infarction), acute dyspnea or orthopnea, palpitations, or light-headedness. Alternatively, the onset may occur without warning. Loss of consciousness and pulse are sine qua nons in cardiac arrest.

▶ DIAGNOSIS

- Rapid diagnosis is vital to the success of CPR. Patients must receive early intervention to prevent cardiac rhythms from degenerating into less treatable arrhythmias.
- Cardiac arrest is diagnosed initially by observation of clinical manifestations consistent with cardiac arrest. The diagnosis is confirmed by evaluating vital signs, especially heart rate and respirations.
- Electrocardiography (ECG) is useful for determining the cardiac rhythm, which in turn determines drug therapy.

▶ DESIRED OUTCOME

Successful CPR comprises restoration of stable heart rate, cardiac rhythm, and blood pressure [systolic blood pressure (SBP) >70 mm Hg]. To truly be successful, patients should remain neurologically intact with minimal morbidity. After successful resuscitation, the primary goals include optimizing tissue oxygenation, identifying the precipitating cause(s) of arrest, and preventing subsequent episodes.

▶ TREATMENT

GENERAL PRINCIPLES

- The philosophies for providing CPR and emergency cardiac care have been organized and updated by the American Heart Association. The following guidelines are taken primarily from the 1992 update.
- Although controversial, factors proven to enhance prehospital survival include occurrence of a witnessed arrest, presence of VT or VF, rapid implementation of bystander CPR, early administration of defibrillation therapy for VF, and early application of prehospital advanced cardiac life support (ACLS). In-hospital cardiac resuscitation teams were developed to address these factors.
- Basic life support is based on the assessment and application of the ABCs: airway, breathing, and circulation. If spontaneous breathing is absent, the airway should be opened and rescue breathing attempted. If the victim is pulseless, closed-chest compressions should be combined with rescue breathing. Basic life support should be continued until spontaneous circulation returns, advanced ACLS is obtained, or exhaustion prohibits continued efforts.

- ACLS incorporates CPR, electrical defibrillation, airway management, ECG monitoring, and drug administration.
- Patients found in either pulseless VT or VF should receive immediate electrical defibrillation using up to three countershocks using 200 J, 200–300 J, and 360 J, respectively.
- Pharmacists should participate in cardiac resuscitation teams by preparing medications for administration; providing drug information; documenting medication administration including name, dose, route, and time; and assisting with chest compressions.
- Drug therapy may consist of sympathomimetics, antiarrhythmics, atropine, and electrolytes, which are described later in this chapter. The preferred intravenous (IV) solution is normal saline or lactated Ringer's. Dextrose solutions should be reserved for patients with documented or suspected hypoglycemia.
- The ideal route of drug administration is easily accessible during CPR and provides rapid entry into the central circulation. Although central venous administration results in earlier and higher peak drug concentrations than peripheral venous administration, the former route may not be available early in the cardiac arrest event. Additionally, attempts to obtain central access may interrupt CPR.
- Peripheral venous access, using the antecubital vein, is acceptable if central access is not available. Peripheral IV injections should be followed with a 20-mL fluid bolus; the extremity should be elevated to speed drug entry into the central circulation.
- If neither central nor peripheral access is available, endotracheal administration of epinephrine, lidocaine, and atropine may be used. Although recommendations vary, endotracheal doses should be 2–2.5 times corresponding IV doses. Increased drug effects may occur when spontaneous circulation returns because endotracheal administration is associated with delayed onset and prolonged duration of action. The recommended method for endotracheal administration is as follows: (1) dilution of the dose in 10 mL of distilled water or normal saline, (2) interruption of CPR, (3) rapid drug administration beyond the tip of the endotracheal tube, (4) three to five quick insufflations using a bag-valve device to aerosolize the drug, and (5) resumption of CPR.
- In pediatric patients, the intraosseous route may be used temporarily if no other routes of drug administration are available.
- Intracardiac drug administration is not recommended during closed-chest CPR.

▶ PHARMACOTHERAPY FOR VF AND PULSELESS VT

SYMPATHOMIMETICS

- The goal of adrenergic agonist therapy is to augment both coronary and cerebral blood flow present during the low flow state associated with CPR.

- Although the optimal adrenergic agent has not been identified, epinephrine (an α_1, α_2, β_1, and β_2 agonist) is recommended as first-line pharmacologic therapy in the treatment of VF, pulseless VT, asystole, and PEA.
- The standard dose of epinephrine is 1 mg (10 mL of 1:10,000 solution) administered by intravenous push (IVP) every 3–5 minutes. If the initial 1-mg dose is unsuccessful, alternative doses are 2–5 mg IVP every 3–5 minutes; 1 mg, 3 mg, 5 mg IVP given 3 minutes apart; or 0.1 mg/kg IVP every 3–5 minutes.
- Although higher doses may increase the initial resuscitation success rate, they do not improve survival to hospital discharge or neurologic outcome.
- Norepinephrine (an α_1, α_2, β_1 agonist) improves myocardial oxygen balance and regional cerebral blood flow compared with epinephrine in animals, but human studies have not confirmed this benefit.

ANTIARRHYTHMICS

- Antiarrhythmic agents are administered in the treatment of persistent pulseless VT or VF following unsuccessful defibrillation with initial epinephrine administration. The first-line antiarrhythmic agent is lidocaine, followed by bretylium. The selection of lidocaine over bretylium is based on the increased familiarity and preferred adverse effect profile of lidocaine, not on clinical trial evidence. Procainamide remains a third-line agent due to the length of time necessary for drug administration.
- Successive doses of antiarrhythmic agents should be administered at more frequent intervals during cardiac arrest to increase circulating blood concentrations and subsequently improve their efficacy.

Lidocaine

- The initial dose of lidocaine is 1.5 mg/kg by IVP. If defibrillation is unsuccessful, an additional 1.5-mg/kg bolus can be administered in 3–5 minutes for a total dose of 3 mg/kg. A continuous lidocaine infusion of 2–4 mg/min should be started after the arrhythmia is suppressed.
- Lidocaine may reduce arrhythmia recurrence following successful defibrillation. Plasma concentrations >6 µg/mL were necessary for antifibrillatory effects in an animal model.

Bretylium

- The antiarrhythmic actions of bretylium result from a complex combination of direct myocardial and indirect adrenergic effects. Initially, bretylium administration potentiates norepinephrine release, which can be manifested clinically by increases in blood pressure, heart rate, and cardiac output, which may facilitate return of spontaneous circulation. Approximately 15–20 minutes after administration, bretylium blocks further release of norepinephrine, which may lead to hypotension and the need for fluids and vasopressors.

- The initial dose of bretylium is 5 mg/kg by IVP. The drug should be allowed to circulate for 1 or 2 minutes before defibrillation. If defibrillation is unsuccessful, subsequent bolus doses of 10 mg/kg may be administered at 5-minute intervals up to a total dose of 30–35 mg/kg. After the arrhythmia is suppressed, a continuous infusion may be initiated at 1–2 mg/min. If VT persists, 5–10 mg/kg should be diluted in 50 mL of fluid and infused over 8–10 minutes. Intravenous infusions should be used in conscious patients to avoid peak serum concentrations, which may induce nausea and vomiting.

Procainamide

- To decrease the risk of hypotension, procainamide infusions should not exceed 20 mg/min in nonemergency situations. However, current guidelines suggest that procainamide infusion rates up to 30 mg/min may be used. Procainamide should be continued until the arrhythmia is suppressed, the patient becomes hypotensive, QRS widens 50% above baseline, or total dose reaches 17 mg/kg. After the arrhythmia is suppressed, procainamide may be infused at a continuous rate of 1–4 mg/min.
- In patients with severe renal or cardiac dysfunction, the initial procainamide loading dose should be decreased to 12 mg/kg. The normal maintenance infusion, 2.8 mg/kg/hour, should also be reduced by one-third if organ impairment is moderate or by two-thirds if it is severe.

ALTERNATIVES FOR REFRACTORY VF OR VT

- Refractory ventricular arrhythmias may be associated with electrolyte abnormalities, primarily hyperkalemia, hypokalemia, and hypomagnesemia.
- Calcium chloride solution 10% should be administered IV at 4 mg/kg for known or suspected hyperkalemia (K^+ >6.0 mEq/L). Sodium bicarbonate 1 mEq/kg may also be given to drive potassium into the cell.
- Potassium 10 mEq should be administered IV over 30 minutes for refractory VF and known or suspected hypokalemia.
- Magnesium sulfate 1–2 g should be diluted in 10 mL of fluid and administered IV over 1–2 minutes for refractory VF and known or suspected hypomagnesemia (Mg^{+2} <1.4 mEq/L). Caution should be used because rapid magnesium supplementation may produce significant hypotension or asystole.

► PHARMACOTHERAPY FOR ASYSTOLE AND PEA

- Patients with asystole should receive CPR, intubation, and IV access. Isoproterenol is contraindicated as a means of pharmacologic pacing because this β_1, β_2 agonist greatly increases myocardial oxygen demand. Defibrillation should also be avoided because it may increase parasympathetic tone, which, in turn, may shorten survival in patients

II

with asystole. The primary pharmacologic agents are epinephrine and atropine.

- Epinephrine doses are identical to those for VF and pulseless VT, including higher doses if the initial 1-mg dose fails.
- Atropine should be initiated at a dose of 1 mg, which can be repeated at 3- to 5-minute intervals up to a total dose of 0.04 mg/kg (approximately 3 mg in a 70-kg adult). This recommendation differs from that for bradycardia, which begins with 0.5–1 mg up to a total dose of 0.04 mg/kg. In either case, doses <0.5 mg should be avoided because of a potential paradoxical vagotonic effect.
- Calcium is only recommended for hyperkalemia, hypocalcemia, and calcium antagonist toxicity.

ACID–BASE MANAGEMENT

- Sodium bicarbonate has a limited role during CPR because it did not improve survival in clinical trials and may worsen acidosis. Selected patients, however, may benefit from bicarbonate therapy if the following conditions are present: (1) known bicarbonate-responsive acidosis, (2) hyperkalemia, or (3) tricyclic antidepressant or phenobarbital overdose. Sodium bicarbonate may also be useful in cases with prolonged arrest times (i.e., >10 minutes); these patients should first receive adequate CPR, intubation, ventilation, and multiple epinephrine doses before sodium bicarbonate.
- The initial recommended dose of sodium bicarbonate is 1 mEq/kg. Subsequent doses of 0.5 mEq/kg can be administered at 10-minute intervals.

▶ LONG-TERM STRATEGIES

- Education plays a pivotal role in long-term strategies to optimize CPR. All health care professionals should be proficient in current CPR procedures. Public awareness of the prevention of cardiovascular and cerebrovascular disease should be increased. Patients should be educated to identify early warning signs and symptoms so that medical care could be accessed earlier.

▶ EVALUATION OF THERAPEUTIC OUTCOMES

- To gauge the success of CPR, therapeutic outcome should be monitored throughout the attempt, after each intervention, and during the postresuscitation phase. Respiratory rate, heart rate, cardiac rhythm, and blood pressure should be assessed.
- The pharmacokinetic disposition of lidocaine may be altered because the primary determinant of clearance, hepatic blood flow, declines during cardiac arrest. In addition, the percentage of unbound lidocaine (free fraction) may be reduced. Toxicity may occur because of the aggressive lidocaine loading recommended by the American Heart

Association. Dosage reductions are suggested for maintenance infusions in patients with reduced cardiac output, hepatic dysfunction, or >70 years of age. Plasma lidocaine concentrations should be monitored during prolonged maintenance infusions. Patients should be assessed for adverse effects such as slurred speech, altered consciousness, muscle twitching, and seizures.

- Serum concentration monitoring is not useful with bretylium therapy because antifibrillatory activity correlates better with myocardial concentrations.
- In patients receiving procainamide, blood pressure and ECG changes should be monitored throughout the infusion. If infusions are continued for more than 24 hours, plasma procainamide and *N*-acetylprocainamide (NAPA) concentrations should be monitored.
- Patients with persistent or recurrent VT or VF following antiarrhythmic administration should be assessed for electrolyte abnormalities.
- Blood gas analysis should be performed to guide administration of sodium bicarbonate.
- During the postresuscitation period, patients should receive a 12-lead ECG, chest x-ray, arterial blood gas, blood chemistry determinations, frequent vital signs, continuous ECG monitoring, and ventilatory support if necessary.

See Chapter 11, Pharmacotherapy of Cardiopulmonary Resuscitation, authored by Lori A. Jones, PharmD, for a more detailed discussion of this topic.

Chapter 7

▶ CONGESTIVE HEART FAILURE

▶ DEFINITION

Congestive heart failure (CHF) is a pathophysiologic state in which the heart is unable to pump blood at a rate sufficient to meet the metabolic needs of the body.

▶ PATHOPHYSIOLOGY

- CHF can result from many cardiac diseases or disorders that alter systolic function, diastolic function, or both.
  - Causes of systolic dysfunction (i.e., decreased contractility) are dilated cardiomyopathies, ventricular hypertrophy, and reduction in muscle mass (e.g., myocardial infarction). Ventricular hypertrophy can be caused by pressure overload (e.g., systemic or pulmonary hypertension, aortic or pulmonic valve stenosis) or volume overload (e.g., valvular regurgitation, shunts, high-output states).
  - Causes of diastolic dysfunction (i.e., restricted ventricular filling) are increased ventricular stiffness, mitral or tricuspid valve stenosis, and pericardial disease (e.g., pericarditis, pericardial tamponade). Ventricular stiffness can be caused by ventricular hypertrophy, infiltrative diseases, and myocardial ischemia and infarction.
- The most common underlying etiologies are ischemic heart disease, which occurs in 47% of women and 59% of men with CHF, followed by hypertension in 37% and 30%, respectively.
- Cardiac output (CO) is defined as the volume of blood ejected per unit time (L/min) according to the following formula: $CO = HR \times SV$. HR is heart rate, which is controlled by the autonomic nervous system. SV is stroke volume, which depends on preload, afterload, and contractility.
  - Preload can be estimated by the left ventricular end diastolic pressure (LVEDP), which in turn is estimated by pulmonary capillary wedge pressure (PCWP).
  - Systemic vascular resistance (SVR) is used to approximate left ventricular afterload.
  - Contractility is difficult to measure accurately in the clinical setting.
- Mean arterial pressure (MAP) is defined by the following equation: $MAP = CO \times SVR$.
- As cardiac function decreases, the heart relies on the following compensatory mechanisms: (1) increased sympathetic nervous system activity; (2) the Frank–Starling mechanism, whereby increased preload increases stroke volume; and (3) ventricular hypertrophy. Although these compensatory mechanisms initially maintain cardiac function, they initiate vicious cycles that lead to continued worsening of CHF (Table 7.1).

TABLE 7.1. Beneficial and Detrimental Effects of the Compensatory Mechanisms in CHF

Compensatory Response	Mechanism(s) of Compensation	Beneficial Effects of Compensation	Detrimental Effects of Compensation
Na+ and water retention	Decreased renal perfusion Aldosterone release	Optimize stroke volume through Frank–Starling mechanism	Pulmonary and systemic congestion and edema
Vasoconstriction	Increased SNS activity Angiotensin II Arginine vasopressin (?)	Maintain BP in face of reduced CO	Increased MVO_2 Increased afterload, which decreases stroke volume and further activates the compensatory mechanisms
Tachycardia	Increased SNS activity Baroreceptor-mediated response to decreased BP	Help maintain CO	Increased MVO_2 Precipitation of ventricular arrhythmias (?) Shortened diastolic filling time β_1-receptor down-regulation, decreased receptor sensitivity
Ventricular hypertrophy	Increased afterload Decreased cardiac output Increased preload	Help maintain CO Reduced myocardial wall stress Decreased MVO_2	Diastolic dysfunction Hypertrophied ventricle does not have normal function Risk of myocardial cell death

Key: SNS, sympathetic nervous system; BP, blood pressure; MVO_2, myocardial oxygen demand; CO, cardiac output.

- Common precipitating factors that may cause a previously compensated patient to decompensate include noncompliance with diet or drug therapy, uncontrolled hypertension, and arrhythmia.
- Drugs may precipitate or exacerbate CHF because of negative inotropic or cardiotoxic effects, or because of sodium and water retention (Table 7.2).

▶ CLINICAL PRESENTATION

- Manifestations of CHF result from congestion developing behind the failing ventricle and therefore depend on whether failure is left or right sided (Table 7.3). Most patients initially have left ventricular failure, but both ventricles eventually fail because ventricles share a sep-

TABLE 7.2. Drugs That May Precipitate or Exacerbate CHF

Negative Inotropic Effect
Antiarrhythmics (e.g., disopyramide, flecainide, others)
β Blockers (e.g., propranolol, metoprolol, atenolol, others)
Calcium channel blockers (e.g., verapamil, others)

Cardiotoxic
Doxorubicin
Daunomycin
Cyclophosphamide

Sodium and Water Retention
Glucocorticoids
Androgens
Estrogens
Nonsteroidal anti-inflammatory agents
Salicylates (high dose)
Sodium-containing drugs (e.g., carbenicillin disodium, ticarcillin disodium)

TABLE 7.3. Signs and Symptoms of CHF

Symptoms	Signs
Right Ventricular Dysfunction	
Abdominal pain	Peripheral edema
Anorexia	Jugular venous distension
Nausea	Hepatojugular reflux
Bloating	Hepatomegaly
Constipation	
Ascites	
Left Ventricular Dysfunction	
Dyspnea on exertion	Bibasilar rales
Paroxysmal nocturnal dyspnea	Pulmonary edema
Orthopnea	S3 gallop
Tachypnea	Pleural effusion
Cough	Cheyne–Stokes respiration
Hemoptysis	
Nonspecific Findings	
Exercise intolerance	Tachycardia
Fatigue	Pallor
Weakness	Cyanosis of digits
Nocturia	Cardiomegaly
CNS symptoms	

tal wall and because left ventricular failure increases right ventricular workload.
- Left ventricular failure causes signs and symptoms of pulmonary congestion. Associated signs and symptoms include dyspnea on exertion, orthopnea, paroxysmal nocturnal dyspnea, dyspnea at rest, and pulmonary edema.
- Right ventricular failure causes signs and symptoms consistent with systemic congestion. Peripheral edema is a cardinal finding in right-sided heart failure.

▶ DIAGNOSIS

- A diagnosis of CHF should be considered in patients exhibiting characteristic signs and symptoms (Table 7.3).
- Ventricular hypertrophy can be demonstrated on chest x-ray or electrocardiogram (ECG).
- The chest x-ray also provides a relatively specific but insensitive measure of the degree of pulmonary congestion.
- The most widely used classification system is the New York Heart Association (NYHA) Functional Classification System. Functional class (FC)-I patients have no limitation of physical activity, FC-II patients have slight limitation of physical activity, FC-III patients have marked limitation of physical activity, and FC-IV patients are unable to carry on physical activity without discomfort.

▶ DESIRED OUTCOME

Goals for the pharmacologic management of CHF include improved symptoms and quality of life, reduced mortality, altered natural history of CHF after symptoms are present, and prevention of progression to severe heart failure and cardiogenic shock. The treatment approach depends on the severity of CHF and whether it is acute or chronic.

▶ TREATMENT OF ACUTE OR SEVERE CHF

GENERAL PRINCIPLES

- Drug therapy for acute or severe CHF consists of positive inotropes, arterial vasodilators, diuretics, or a combination thereof. Individual agents are discussed in more detail in the following sections (see also Chapter 12, Shock: Hypovolemic and Cardiogenic).
- The choice between positive inotropes and arterial vasodilators depends on patient factors. Arterial vasodilators are useful for significantly elevated SVR, but they should be avoided if there is significant hypotension. Inotropes with pressor activity (i.e., dopamine) are usually recommended when the systolic arterial pressure is <90–100 mm Hg or MAP is <70–75 mm Hg, but they are hazardous if cardiac arrhythmias,

myocardial ischemia, or both are present. In severe ventricular dysfunction, combination therapy may be necessary to raise cardiac index above 2.2 L/min/m2.

- IV agents used to treat acute or severe CHF can be distinguished by their hemodynamic effects (Table 7.4) and pharmacokinetic profiles. Short half-lives are advantageous because of the ability to titrate the dose rapidly according to individual response, but drugs with short half-lives must be administered by continuous infusion.

- Positive inotropes include adrenergic agents, phosphodiesterase inhibitors, and digitalis.
  - Adrenergic agents (e.g., dopamine, dobutamine) have half-lives of only a few minutes, quick onset of action, and short duration of action. Although potentially useful in special circumstances, isoproterenol, epinephrine, and norepinephrine are less commonly used in the treatment of severe CHF and have largely been replaced by dopamine and dobutamine.
  - Phosphodiesterase inhibitors (e.g., amrinone, milrinone) suitable for IV administration exhibit hemodynamic effects that are generally similar to those of dobutamine, but they have longer half-lives.
  - Digoxin is rarely used in patients with acute CHF who are hemodynamically unstable and is therefore discussed in the section on chronic CHF.

- Patients with acute or severe heart failure can be divided into four subsets based on their cardiac index and PCWP. This hemodynamic classification is useful for guiding selection of drug therapy (Fig. 7.1).

TABLE 7.4. Usual Hemodynamic Effects of Intravenous Agents Commonly Used for the Treatment of Acute/Severe Heart Failure[a]

Drug	Dose	HR	MAP	PCWP	CO	SVR
Dopamine	1–3 μg/kg/min	0	0	0	0/+	−
Dopamine	3–10 μg/kg/min	+	+	0	+	0
Dopamine	>10 μg/kg/min	+	+	+	+	+
Dobutamine	2.5–15 μg/kg/min	0/+	0	−	+	−
Amrinone	5–10 μg/kg/min	0/+	0/−	−	+	−
Milrinone	0.375–0.75 μg/kg/min	0/+	0/−	−	+	−
Nitroprusside	0.25–3 μg/kg/min	0/+	0/−	−	+	−
Nitroglycerin	5–200 μg/min	0/+	0/−	−	0/+	0/−
Furosemide	20–80 mg, repeated as needed up to 4–6 times/d	0	0	−	0	0

[a]See text for a more detailed description of the interpatient variability in response. *Key:* +, increase; −, decrease; 0, no change; HR, heart rate; MAP, mean arterial pressure; PCWP, pulmonary capillary wedge pressure; CO, cardiac output; SVR, systemic vascular resistance.

- Subset I (i.e., acceptable cardiac index and PCWP) does not need immediate specific intervention.
- Subset II (i.e., acceptable cardiac index and PCWP >18 mm Hg) has pulmonary congestion. Although the normal range of PCWP is 5–12 mm Hg for individuals without cardiac dysfunction, pressures of 15–18 mm Hg are preferred for patients with CHF to optimize cardiac index and avoid pulmonary congestion. PCWP can be reduced by IV administration of preload reducing agents such as loop diuretics or nitroglycerin.
- Subset III (i.e., cardiac index <2.2 L/min/m^2 and acceptable PCWP) has peripheral hypoperfusion. If PCWP is significantly <15 mm Hg, IV fluids should be administered initially to improve ventricular filling pressure and, consequently, cardiac index. If patients have significant left ventricular dysfunction and a depressed Starling relationship, positive inotropes, arterial vasodilators, or both may be necessary to further increase cardiac index.
- Subset IV (i.e., cardiac index <2.2 L/min/m^2 and PCWP >18 mm Hg) has both pulmonary congestion and peripheral hypoperfusion, and the worst prognosis. Therapy involves a combination of agents used for subsets II and III.
- The intraaortic balloon pump is the most widely used form of mechanical circulatory assistance and is typically used in patients with acute/severe heart failure who do not respond adequately to positive inotropic agents and vasodilators.

ADRENERGIC AGENTS: DOPAMINE AND DOBUTAMINE

- Dopamine produces dose-dependent hemodynamic effects because of its relative affinity for α_1, β_1, and β_2 receptors as well as D_1 (dopaminergic) receptors. Low doses increase renal blood flow, glomerular filtration, urine output, natriuresis, and kaliuresis. Positive inotropic effects mediated primarily by β_1 receptors become more prominent with doses of 3–10 µg/kg/min (Table 7.4). As the dose is increased to more than 10 µg/kg/min, chronotropic and α_1 mediated vasoconstricting effects become more prominent. Dopamine, particularly at higher doses, alters several parameters that increase myocardial oxygen demand and potentially decrease myocardial blood flow.
- Dobutamine is a potent inotropic agent with vasodilating action (Table 7.4). Its combined effects on myocardial contractility, heart rate, blood pressure, PCWP, and coronary blood flow suggest that it produces its desired hemodynamic effects while not adversely affecting the balance between myocardial oxygen demand and supply. Initial doses are usually 2.5–5 µg/kg/min and can be progressively increased to 15 µg/kg/min or higher based on clinical and hemodynamic responses.
- There are hemodynamic differences between dopamine and dobutamine because of differences in their binding affinities for adrenergic receptors. Dobutamine increases cardiac index because of an increase in stroke volume and a variable increase in heart rate. Dobutamine

67

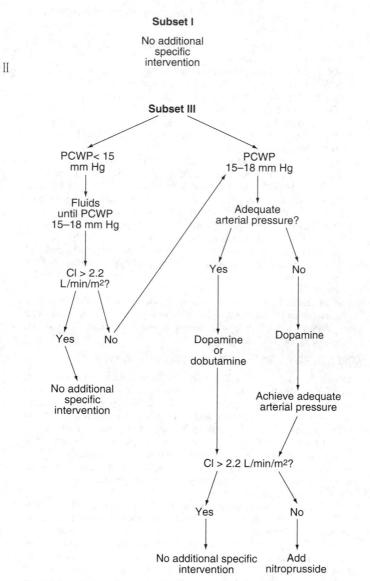

Subset I

No additional
specific
intervention

II

Subset III

PCWP< 15
mm Hg

Fluids
until PCWP
15–18 mm Hg

CI > 2.2
L/min/m²?

Yes   No

No additional
specific
intervention

PCWP
15–18 mm Hg

Adequate
arterial pressure?

Yes   No

Dopamine
or
dobutamine

Dopamine

Achieve adequate
arterial pressure

CI > 2.2 L/min/m²?

Yes   No

No additional specific
intervention

Add
nitroprusside

Figure 7.1. General treatment algorithm for acute/severe heart failure based on hemody-namic subsets. This is a suggested approach which may need to be modified for certain patients (see text).

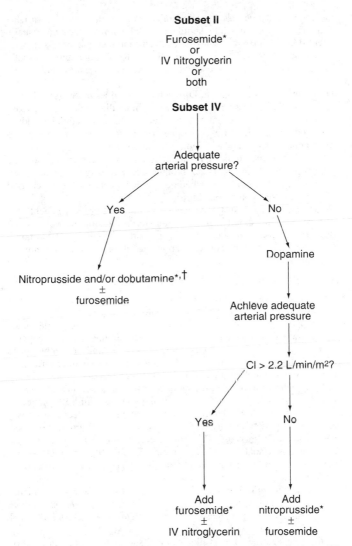

Figure 7.1. (continued). *Usual goals for hemodynamic parameters: cardiac index (CI) > 2.2 L/min/m², PCWP 15–18 mm Hg while maintaining adequate blood pressure and perfusion to essential organs. †Amrinone or milrinone are alternative agents.

increases heart rate less than dopamine, but the difference is variable and may not be clinically significant. Dobutamine does not usually alter MAP compared to the more consistent increase observed with dopamine. Because of its vasodilating effects, dobutamine usually decreases PCWP, as opposed to the increase observed with dopamine.

- Dobutamine does not bind to D_1 receptors and does not cause selective renal vasodilation; however, the increase in cardiac index can increase renal blood flow, urine output, and natriuresis. Some clinicians advocate combining low-dose dopamine for its renovascular effects and dobutamine for its inotropic and systemic effects.
- Although one study indicated that dobutamine was less arrhythmogenic than dopamine, both agents can produce cardiac arrhythmias.
- Attenuation of dobutamine's hemodynamic effects has been reported after 72 hours of continuous infusion.
- Some patients have sustained hemodynamic and clinical benefits for several days or months after a short-term infusion of dobutamine despite its 2.5-minute half-life. The potential for increased mortality, however, raises serious concerns about the chronic use of intermittent dobutamine infusions.

PHOSPHODIESTERASE INHIBITORS: AMRINONE AND MILRINONE

- Phosphodiesterase inhibitors have positive inotropic and vasodilating effects and are sometimes called inodilators.
- The bipyridine derivatives, amrinone and milrinone, have similar pharmacologic and hemodynamic effects after IV administration. In patients with heart failure, their hemodynamic effects generally resemble those of dobutamine or nitroprusside. The most consistent difference is a greater increase in heart rate with dobutamine.
- After IV administration, amrinone or milrinone increases cardiac index primarily because of an increase in stroke volume with little change in heart rate (Table 7.4). Amrinone and milrinone also decrease PCWP and thus are particularly useful in patients with a low cardiac index and an elevated PCWP (subset IV). This decrease in preload, however, can be hazardous for patients without an elevated PCWP (subset III). Amrinone and milrinone produce relatively little change in myocardial oxygen demand.
- Amrinone and milrinone should not be used as single agents in patients with heart failure who have moderate or severe hypotension because these drugs will not increase, and may even decrease, arterial blood pressure.
- Until more data become available, the issue of tolerance during prolonged continuous infusions of phosphodiesterase inhibitors must be considered an unresolved issue.
- The mean terminal half-life of milrinone in patients with heart failure is 2.3 hours, whereas that of amrinone ranges from 2–4 hours in healthy subjects and up to 12 hours in patients with severe heart failure.

- The usual loading dose of amrinone is 0.75 mg/kg over 2–3 minutes, followed by a continuous infusion of 5–10 µg/kg/min. If the therapeutic response is inadequate, an additional loading dose of 0.75 mg/kg may be repeated after 30 minutes. Maintenance doses >20 µg/kg/min may not produce additional hemodynamic benefits.
- The recommended loading dose of milrinone is 50 µg/kg over 10 minutes, followed by a continuous infusion of 0.5 µg/kg/min (range: 0.375–0.75 µg/kg/min).
- IV formulations of milrinone and amrinone are usually well tolerated, unlike the relatively high incidence of adverse effects associated with chronic oral amrinone.
- Generally, milrinone or amrinone should be considered only in patients who have not responded adequately to dobutamine, dopamine, IV vasodilators, or a combination of these agents.
- A combination of amrinone or milrinone with dopamine or dobutamine may be helpful in patients with dose-limiting adverse effects.

VASODILATORS: NITROPRUSSIDE, NITROGLYCERIN, AND HYDRALAZINE

- Arterial vasodilators (e.g., hydralazine) act as afterload-reducing agents and typically increase cardiac output. Venous vasodilators (e.g., nitroglycerin) act as preload reducers by affecting venous capacitance—they reduce pulmonary congestion in patients with high cardiac filling pressures. Mixed vasodilators (e.g., nitroprusside, angiotensin-converting enzyme inhibitors) act on both arterial resistance and venous capacitance vessels, and can therefore reduce congestive symptoms and increase cardiac output.

Nitroprusside

- Sodium nitroprusside is a mixed arterial–venous vasodilator that acts directly on vascular smooth muscle to increase cardiac index and decrease PCWP. Despite its lack of direct inotropic activity, nitroprusside exerts hemodynamic effects that are qualitatively similar to those of dobutamine, amrinone, and milrinone (Table 7.4); however, nitroprusside generally decreases PCWP and SVR more than dobutamine.
- Decreased blood pressure is an important dose-limiting adverse effect of nitroprusside and other vasodilators. Therefore, nitroprusside is particularly useful for patients who are in subset IV and have a significantly elevated SVR but who are not hypotensive.
- The combination of nitroprusside and dopamine or dobutamine is useful for patients in subset IV who fail to respond to nitroprusside or positive inotropic agents alone.
- Generally, nitroprusside will not adversely affect, and may improve, the balance between myocardial oxygen demand and supply. However, an excessive decrease in systemic arterial pressure can decrease coronary perfusion and worsen ischemia.

II

- Nitroprusside has a rapid onset and a duration of action of <10 minutes. Nitroprusside should be initiated at a low dose (i.e., 0.1–0.25 μg/kg/min) to avoid an excessive drop in arterial pressure, and then increased by small increments (i.e., 0.1–0.2 μg/kg/min) every 5–10 minutes as needed and tolerated. Usually effective doses range from 0.5–3.0 μg/kg/min. Because of a rebound phenomenon after abrupt withdrawal of nitroprusside in patients with heart failure, doses should be tapered slowly when stopping nitroprusside therapy. Nitroprusside-induced cyanide and thiocyanate toxicity is unlikely when doses <3 μg/kg/min are administered for <3 days.

Nitroglycerin

- The major hemodynamic effects of nitroglycerin are decreased preload and PCWP due to its venous vasodilation. Nitroglycerin also has mild arterial vasodilating effects, which generally lead to a relatively small increase in cardiac index compared to that of inotropic agents. Combination therapy with nitroglycerin and dobutamine or dopamine is appealing because of complementary effects to increase cardiac index and decrease PCWP.
- Nitroglycerin should be initiated at 5–10 μg/min (0.1 μg/kg/min) and increased progressively every 5–10 minutes as necessary and tolerated. Maintenance doses usually vary from 35–200 μg/min (0.5–3.0 μg/kg/min). Some tolerance develops in most patients over 12–72 hours.

LOOP DIURETICS

- Diuretics decrease intravascular volume and preload, thereby improving pulmonary congestion. They are particularly useful for patients in subset II and in combination with vasodilators/inotropes for patients in subset IV.
- Furosemide is the most widely used and studied IV loop diuretic for acute or severe CHF. Others are ethacrynic acid, bumetanide, and torsemide.
- Despite the controversy over the short-term (i.e., 5–20 minutes) effects of IV furosemide on PCWP and SVR, the diuretic effects predominate after 20 minutes and lead to a consistent decrease in PCWP and an improvement in pulmonary congestion.

▶ TREATMENT OF CHRONIC CHF

GENERAL PRINCIPLES

- The first step in management of chronic CHF is to determine the etiology or precipitating factors so that underlying disorders can be treated.
- Important nonpharmacologic interventions include cardiac rehabilitation and restriction of dietary sodium.
- Drugs available for the management of chronic CHF are shown in Table 7.5.

TABLE 7.5. Comparative Hemodynamic Effects of Drugs Used Routinely in the Management of Chronic Heart Failure

Drug	Daily Dose (mg)[a]	Usual Frequency	HR	MBP	PCWP	CO	SVR
Diuretics							
Furosemide	20–120	qd or bid	0	0	↓	0	0
Bumetanide	0.5–10	qd or bid	0	0	↓	0	0
ACE Inhibitors							
Captopril	37.5–300	tid	↓	↓	↓	↑	↓
Enalapril	5–40	bid	↓	↓	↓	↑	↓
Lisinopril	5–40	qd	↓	↓	↓	↑	↓
Hydralazine	100–400	qid	0/↑	0/↓	0	↑	↓
Isosorbide dinitrate	80–240	qid	0/↑	0/↓	↓	0/↑	0/↓
Digoxin	0.125–0.5	qd	↓	0	0/↓	↑	0/↓

[a]For many of the drugs, the low end of the dosage range represents appropriate starting doses with upward titration to the target dose. *Key:* HR, heart rate; MBP, mean blood pressure; PCWP, pulmonary capillary wedge pressure; CO, cardiac output; SVR, systemic vascular resistance; 0, no change; ↑, increase; ↓, decrease.

DIURETICS

- Diuretics decrease edema and pulmonary congestion by reducing preload (Table 7.5). Although diuretics are widely used because they control symptoms of CHF, especially when combined with vasodilator therapy, diuretics have not been shown to reduce mortality.
- Thiazide diuretics are relatively weak diuretics and may be effective in the early stages of CHF, but more potent diuretics are commonly needed.
- Loop diuretics (e.g., furosemide, bumetanide) are the most widely used diuretics for CHF. In addition to acting in the thick ascending limb of the loop of Henle, loop diuretics induce a prostaglandin-mediated increase in renal blood flow. Coadministration of nonsteroidal anti-inflammatory drugs (NSAIDs) blocks this effect and can diminish diuretic response.
- Diuretic dosages are titrated according to symptoms and body weight. Typical daily doses of furosemide range from 40 to 240 mg given in one or two doses. Unlike thiazide diuretics, loop diuretics maintain their effectiveness in the presence of impaired renal function, although higher doses may be necessary.
- Hypokalemia, the most common metabolic disturbance associated with both thiazide and loop diuretics, may be exacerbated by hyperaldosteronism. Hypokalemia is especially worrisome because it can precipitate ventricular arrhythmias in CHF patients, especially if they are also taking digoxin.

- Hypomagnesemia is also common with diuretic therapy; it also increases the risk of arrhythmias.
- Resistance to diuretic therapy may be mediated by pharmacokinetic or pharmacodynamic mechanisms, or both.
  - Absorption of furosemide from the gut may be reduced or delayed, which can be overcome by giving the diuretic orally in larger doses or intravenously.
  - Although the pharmacodynamic mechanism is not clear, suppressed responses may be related to increased proximal and distal tubular sodium reabsorption. Maneuvers to overcome this resistance include treating the primary disease by other strategies (i.e., afterload reduction), giving low-dose dopamine to enhance diuresis, using larger IV bolus or continuous IV doses of furosemide, and adding a second diuretic with a different mechanism of action. Although the loop diuretic–thiazide combination is synergistic, this approach is generally reserved for the inpatient setting where the patient can be monitored closely because of the risk of profound diuresis and severe sodium, potassium, and volume depletion. Very low doses or only occasional doses of the thiazide-type diuretic should be used in the outpatient setting.

VASODILATORS: NITRATES AND HYDRALAZINE

- The predominant hemodynamic effect of nitrates is to reduce preload (Table 7.5), although a slight reduction in SVR may be seen.
- Isosorbide dinitrate (ISDN) is the most extensively studied nitrate product for CHF. The usual dose of ISDN is 40 mg (range: 20–80 mg) every 6 hours. Oral nitroglycerin products are probably equally effective.
- The best alternative for minimizing nitrate tolerance appears to be 8- to 12-hour nitrate-free intervals.
- Hydralazine is a direct-acting vasodilator that acts predominantly on arterial smooth muscle and reduces SVR with resultant increases in stroke volume index and cardiac index (Table 7.5); effects on preload are minimal. Average doses range from 200 to 300 mg/d, but doses as high as 3000 mg have been used.
- To achieve both preload and afterload reduction, the two vasodilators are frequently combined. Hydralazine 300 mg/d plus ISDN 160 mg/d significantly reduced mortality in NYHA FC-II and FC-III patients in the Veterans Administration Cooperative Study (Vasodilators in Heart Failure Trial, VHeFT-I).
- Adverse effects to both nitrates and hydralazine are common, which limits use of this combination in many patients.

VASODILATORS: ANGIOTENSIN-CONVERTING ENZYME INHIBITORS

- ACE inhibitors cause arterial and venous dilatation, thus reducing both preload and afterload (Table 7.5). Hemodynamic effects observed with long-term therapy include significant increases in cardiac index, stroke work index, and stroke volume index, as well as significant reductions in left ventricular filling pressure, SVR, MAP, and heart rate.

- In clinical studies, ACE inhibitors significantly improved clinical status, functional class, exercise tolerance, left ventricular size, and mortality. In fact, enalapril reduced mortality more than hydralazine-ISDN in VHeFT-II.
- ACE inhibitors may also prevent the development of CHF in properly selected, high-risk patients. Decreased mortality has been shown in patients who had a left ventricular ejection fraction of $\leq 40\%$ after myocardial infarction. Although ACE inhibitor therapy should be initiated in the immediate postinfarction period, significant benefit may still be derived from starting therapy at any time in patients with asymptomatic left ventricular dysfunction.
- All patients with symptomatic heart failure should receive chronic ACE inhibitor therapy; patients who do not tolerate or have contraindications to ACE inhibitors should receive hydralazine and a nitrate. Although not all ACE inhibitors are approved for use in CHF, their benefits probably represent a drug class effect. The major differences among ACE inhibitors are with their pharmacokinetic properties, not their pharmacologic properties.
- Although the exact mechanism is not clear, ACE inhibitors may reduce mortality by preventing the progression of CHF. Cardiac tissue angiotensin II may be a proto-oncogene that contributes to the hypertrophy and ventricular dilatation associated with progressive heart failure.
- The primary adverse effects of ACE inhibitor therapy in CHF are hypotension and functional renal insufficiency.
  - Risk factors for hypotension are hyponatremia (serum sodium <130 mEq/L) and recent increases in diuretic dose; the risk may be minimized by initiating therapy with lower doses.
  - The most important risk factor for functional renal insufficiency is hyponatremia usually secondary to diuretic therapy; severe heart failure and dehydration are also risk factors. The risk of renal insufficiency can be minimized by reducing diuretic dosage or liberalizing sodium intake.
- Retention of potassium with ACE inhibitor therapy is common. Although hyperkalemia rarely develops, caution is necessary if patients have renal insufficiency or receive concomitant potassium supplementation, potassium-containing salt substitutes, or potassium-sparing diuretic therapy.
- Troublesome but less common side effects are rash, dysgeusia, and dry hacking cough.

DIGITALIS

- Digitalis glycosides exert positive inotropic effects by binding to sodium-activated and potassium-activated adenosine triphosphatase (NaK ATPase or sodium pump). The overall response is usually increased cardiac index, decreased SVR and PCWP, and relatively little change in arterial blood pressure.

- Questions about the role of digitalis in heart failure have been raised by flaws in and inconsistent results of controlled trials of digoxin, the controversy over the long-term use of positive inotropes, and the documented benefits of vasodilators. Digoxin appears to reduce hospitalizations and symptoms, but there is no evidence that it reduces mortality. Digoxin, like several other inotropic agents, could have an adverse effect on the natural progression of the disease and/or the risk of sudden death and could increase mortality.
  - Efficacy in patients with CHF and supraventricular tachyarrhythmias such as atrial fibrillation is relatively well established and widely accepted.
  - Patients who remain symptomatic on optimal doses of vasodilators and diuretics and who have systolic dysfunction are candidates for digoxin. Patients most likely to benefit from digoxin have significant left ventricular systolic dysfunction and supraventricular tachyarrhythmias, or symptoms of moderate-to-severe heart failure (NYHA FC-III and FC-IV) and dilated left ventricles with systolic dysfunction (often with a third heart sound). If patients remain symptomatic after adding digoxin, clinicians may consider adding another vasodilator or a trial of low-dose β-blocker therapy.
- The pharmacokinetics of digoxin are highly variable and depend on patient characteristics, concomitant drugs and disease states, and dosage forms employed. Blood samples for serum digoxin determinations should be collected at least 6 hours and preferably 12 hours or more after the last dose. The desired range of serum digoxin concentrations is generally quoted as 0.8–2.0 ng/mL. A more conservative target of 1.0–1.5 ng/mL has also been advocated.
- There are many drug interactions with digoxin, which can be clinically important.
- Usual maintenance doses with digoxin tablets range from 0.125 to 0.5 mg/day. Lower doses are usually necessary in patients with significant renal impairment. Although loading doses are not generally required by patients in normal sinus rhythm, 15 μg/kg of lean body weight (range: 10–20 μg/kg) is usually appropriate. Lower IV loading doses should be used (e.g., 10 μg/kg of lean body weight) to compensate for the difference in bioavailability.
- Digoxin and other digitalis glycosides produce many cardiac and noncardiac adverse effects (Table 7.6). Despite the general perception that digoxin is often poorly tolerated, some multicenter randomized double-blind trials indicate that digoxin is relatively well tolerated compared to milrinone, captopril, and even placebo.

ANTIARRHYTHMIC THERAPY

- Antiarrhythmic therapy is appealing because sudden cardiac death, presumably due to ventricular arrhythmias, is the mode of death in up to 50% of CHF patients.

TABLE 7.6. Signs and Symptoms of Digitalis Toxicity

Noncardiac (Mostly CNS) Adverse Effects[a]

Anorexia, nausea, vomiting, abdominal pain

Visual disturbances: halos, photophobia, problems with color perception (i.e., red-green or yellow-green vision), scotomata

Fatigue, weakness, dizziness, headache, neuralgia, confusion, delirium, psychosis

Cardiac Adverse Effects[a,b]

Ventricular arrhythmias

Premature ventricular depolarizations, bigeminy, trigeminy, ventricular tachycardia, ventricular fibrillation

Atrioventricular (AV) block

First degree, second degree (Mobitz type I), third degree

AV junctional escape rhythms, junctional tachycardia

Atrial arrhythmias with slowed AV conduction or AV block

Particularly paroxysmal atrial tachycardia with AV block

Sinus bradycardia

[a]Some adverse effects may be difficult to distinguish from the signs/symptoms of heart failure.
[b]Digitalis toxicity has been associated with almost every known rhythm abnormality (only the more common manifestations are listed).

- No antiarrhythmic regimen can be recommended routinely for patients with CHF until the results from large ongoing clinical trials are published.
  - Class I antiarrhythmics should probably be avoided in all patients with left ventricular dysfunction.
  - The role of amiodarone therapy for patients with CHF remains unclear because of conflicting data regarding its effect on mortality.

POTENTIALLY USEFUL DRUGS: β BLOCKERS

- Although normal doses of β blockers worsen CHF, stable patients may benefit from properly titrated doses. Many clinical trials document sustained improvement in symptoms and hemodynamic parameters. Although β blockers cannot be recommended as routine therapy, they may be considered if a patient remains symptomatic on conventional therapy.
- Metoprolol should be initiated at a low dosage of approximately 6.25 mg twice daily and titrated upward over 4–6 weeks to a target dose of 100–150 mg per day.
- Carvedilol has been shown to reduce mortality by 67% in patients with FC-II to -IV heart failure. It is not clear whether this benefit is related exclusively to β-blocking properties, or whether α_1-receptor blocking properties and anti-oxidant effects contribute to its mortality-reducing effects. This provocative finding underscores the need for additional studies to define the role of β blockers in CHF.

▶ EVALUATION OF THERAPEUTIC OUTCOMES

II

- Patients should be monitored for signs and symptoms of CHF caused by excess fluid retention (Table 7.3).
- Body weight should be monitored, especially in patients with chronic CHF who receive diuretic therapy, because change in body weight is a sensitive marker of fluid status that reflects excess fluid retention or fluid loss.
- Invasive hemodynamic monitoring using a balloon-tipped, flow-directed pulmonary artery catheter has become a critically important tool in the management of patients with severe heart failure because the results can be used to guide selection of appropriate medical therapy. Typical goals are cardiac index >2.2 L/min/m^2, PCWP of 15–18 mm Hg, SVR of 800–1200 dyne•sec/cm^3, and systolic blood pressure >90 mm Hg or MAP >70 mm Hg.
- Improved peripheral perfusion can be evaluated by increased urine output, decreased peripheral vasoconstriction, and stronger peripheral pulses.
- Clinicians should monitor potassium closely in CHF patients; caution patients about the use of salt substitutes, which are commonly potassium chloride; and add potassium supplementation only when necessary.

See Chapter 13, Congestive Heart Failure, authored by Julie A. Johnson, PharmD, FCCP, and Richard L. Lalonde, PharmD, for a more detailed discussion of this topic.

Chapter 8

► HYPERLIPIDEMIA

► DEFINITION

Hyperlipidemia is defined as an elevation of one or more of the following: cholesterol, cholesterol esters, phospholipids, or triglycerides. Cholesterol and triglycerides, as the major plasma lipids, are essential substrates for cell membrane formation and hormone synthesis, and they provide a source of free fatty acids.

► PATHOPHYSIOLOGY

- Cholesterol, triglycerides, and phospholipids are transported as complexes of lipid and specialized proteins (apolipoproteins) known as lipoproteins. Abnormalities of plasma lipoproteins can result in a predisposition to coronary artery disease, pancreatitis, xanthomas, or neurologic disease. Elevated total and low density lipoprotein cholesterol (LDL-C) and reduced high density lipoprotein cholesterol (HDL-C) are associated with the development of coronary heart disease (CHD).
- The response-to-injury hypothesis states that risk factors such as oxidized LDL, mechanical injury to the endothelium, excessive homocysteine, immunologic attack, or viral-induced changes in endothelial and intimal function lead to endothelial dysfunction and a series of cellular interactions that culminate in atherosclerosis and eventually angina and myocardial infarction. Atherosclerotic lesions are thought to arise from transport and retention of plasma LDL-C through the endothelial cell layer into the extracellular matrix of the subendothelial space. Once in the artery wall, LDL is oxidized by various oxidative products produced locally. Mildly oxidized LDL then recruits monocytes into the artery wall. These monocytes then become transformed into macrophages that accelerate LDL oxidation.
- Oxidized LDL provokes an inflammatory response mediated by a number of chemoattractants and cytokines (e.g., monocyte colony-stimulating factor, intercellular adhesion molecule, platelet-derived growth factor, transforming growth factors, interleukin-1, interleukin-6).
- The extent of oxidation and the inflammatory response are under genetic control, and primary or genetic lipoprotein disorders have been classified into six categories commonly used for the phenotypical description of hyperlipidemia (Table 8.1). Secondary forms of hyperlipidemia also exist, and several drugs may elevate lipid levels (Table 8.2).
- The primary defect in familial hypercholesterolemia is the inability to bind LDL to the LDL receptor (LDL-R) or, rarely, a defect of internalizing the LDL-R complex into the cell after normal binding. This leads

TABLE 8.1. Fredrickson–Levy–Lees Classification of Hyperlipoproteinemia

| | | Approximate Mean Lipid Elevation | |
| | | *Cholesterol* | *Triglycerides* |
Type	Lipoprotein Elevation	*(mg/dL)*	*(mg/dL)*
I	Chylomicrons	324	3316
IIa	LDL[a]	368	148
IIb	LDL + VLDL	354	135
III	IDL (LDL$_1$)	441	694
IV	VLDL	251	438
V	VLDL + chylomicrons	373	2071

[a]Heterozygotes for familial hypercholesterolemia.
Modified from Schafer EJ, Levy RI. N Engl J Med 1985;312:1302.

TABLE 8.2. Secondary Forms of Hyperlipoproteinemia

Disease-Induced	Drug-Induced
Endocrine/Metabolic	Alcohol
Diabetes mellitus	Progestins
von Gierke's disease	Thiazide diuretics
Lipodystrophies	β Blockers
Cushing's syndrome	Glucocorticoids
Sexual ateliotic dwarfism	
Acromegaly	
Hypothyroidism	
Anorexia nervosa	
Werner's syndrome	
Acute intermittent porphyria	
Renal	
Uremia	
Nephrotic syndrome	
Hepatic	
Primary biliary cirrhosis	
Acute hepatitis	
Hepatoma	
Immunologic	
Systemic lupus erythematosis	
Monoclonal gammapathies	
Stress-Induced	

to lack of LDL degradation by cells and unregulated biosynthesis of cholesterol, with total cholesterol and LDL-C being inversely proportional to the deficit in LDL receptors.

II

▶ CLINICAL PRESENTATION

- Familial hypercholesterolemia is characterized by a selective elevation in plasma LDL and deposition of LDL-derived cholesterol in tendons (xanthomas) and arteries (atheromas).
- Familial lipoprotein lipase deficiency is characterized by a massive accumulation of chylomicrons and a corresponding increase in plasma triglycerides or a type I lipoprotein pattern. VLDL concentration is normal. Presenting manifestations include repeated attacks of pancreatitis and abdominal pain, eruptive cutaneous xanthomatosis, and hepatosplenomegaly beginning in childhood. Symptom severity is proportional to dietary fat intake, and consequently to the elevation of chylomicrons. Accelerated atherosclerosis is not associated with this disease.
- Patients with familial type III hyperlipoproteinemia develop the following clinical features after age 20: xanthoma striata palmaris (yellow discolorations of the palmar and digital creases); tuberous or tuberocruptive xanthomas (bulbous cutaneous xanthomas); and severe atherosclerosis involving the coronary arteries, internal carotids, and abdominal aorta.
- Type IV hyperlipoproteinemia is common and occurs primarily in adult patients who are obese, diabetic, and hyperuricemic and do not have xanthomas. It may be secondary to alcohol ingestion and can be aggravated by stress, progestins, oral contraceptives, thiazides, or β-blockers.
- Type V (VLDL + chylomicrons) is characterized by abdominal pain, pancreatitis, eruptive xanthomas, and peripheral polyneuropathy. These patients are commonly obese, hyperuricemic, and diabetic; alcohol intake, exogenous estrogens, and renal insufficiency tend to be exacerbating factors. The risk of atherosclerosis is increased with this disorder.

▶ DIAGNOSIS

- Total cholesterol and HDL should be measured in all adults 20 years of age or older at least once every 5 years.
- Once hyperlipidemia is suspected, two major components of the evaluation are the history (including age, gender, and, if female, menstrual and estrogen replacement status) and physical examination and laboratory investigations.
- A complete history and physical exam should assess the following: (1) presence or absence of cardiovascular risk factors or definite cardiovascular disease in the individual; (2) family history of premature cardio-

vascular disease or lipid disorders; (3) presence or absence of secondary causes of hyperlipidemia, including concurrent medications (Table 8.2); and (4) presence or absence of xanthomas, abdominal pain, or history of pancreatitis, renal or liver disease, peripheral vascular disease, or cerebral vascular disease (carotid bruits, stroke, or transient ischemic attack).

- Measurement of plasma cholesterol (which is about 3% lower than serum determinations), triglyceride, and HDL-C levels after a 12-hour or longer fast is important, because triglycerides may be elevated in nonfasted individuals; total cholesterol is only modestly affected by fasting.

- Two determinations, 1–8 weeks apart, with the patient on a stable diet and weight, and in the absence of acute illness, are recommended to minimize variability and to obtain a reliable baseline. If the total cholesterol is greater than 200 mg/dL, a second determination is recommended and, if the values are more than 30 mg/dL apart, the average of three values should be used.

- If the physical examination and history are insufficient to diagnose a familial disorder, then agarose-gel lipoprotein electrophoresis is useful to determine which class of lipoproteins is affected. If the triglyceride levels are below 400 mg/dL and neither type III hyperlipidemia nor chylomicrons are detected by electrophoresis, then one can calculate VLDL-C and LDL-C concentrations: VLDL-C = triglyceride/5; LDL-C = total cholesterol − (VLDL-C + HDL-C). Initial testing uses total cholesterol for case finding but subsequent management decisions should be based on LDL-C.

- Because total cholesterol is comprised of cholesterol derived from LDL, VLDL, and HDL, determination of HDL-C is useful when total plasma cholesterol is elevated. HDL-C may be elevated by moderate alcohol ingestion (less than 2 drinks per day), physical exercise, smoking cessation, weight loss, oral contraceptives, phenytoin, and terbutaline. HDL may be lowered by smoking, obesity, a sedentary lifestyle and drugs such as β blockers.

- Diagnosis of lipoprotein lipase deficiency is based on low or absent enzyme activity with normal human plasma or apolipoprotein C-II, a cofactor of the enzyme.

▶ DESIRED OUTCOME

- The goals of treatment are to reduce total and LDL cholesterol in order to prevent the development of new atherosclerotic plaques in coronary arteries, to halt progression of established lesions, and to induce the regression of existing lesions. Data from secondary and primary intervention trials also provide evidence that CHD morbidity and mortality as well as total mortality can be reduced with diet and drug therapy.

▶ TREATMENT

GENERAL GUIDELINES

- The Adult Treatment Panel II of the National Cholesterol Education Panel (NCEP) has recommended that total cholesterol determinations and risk factor assessment be used in the initial classification of adults (Table 8.3).
- If the total cholesterol is below 200 mg/dL and the HDL is higher than 35 mg/dL, no further follow-up is recommended for patients without known CHD and less than two risk factors (Table 8.4).
- In patients with borderline high blood cholesterol, assessment of risk factors is needed to more clearly define disease risk.
- When the serum total cholesterol is 200 mg/dL or higher, or when the HDL cholesterol is less than 35 mg/dL or at borderline high levels with two or more risk factors, a lipoprotein analysis (two measurements 1–8 weeks apart) to measure total and HDL cholesterol and triglycerides so that LDL-C may be estimated is recommended.
- In patients with evidence of CHD or other clinical atherosclerotic disease, the LDL goal is lower than 100 mg/dL, and most patients require diet and/or drug intervention.
- Decisions regarding management are based on the LDL-C levels. The goals of therapy expressed as LDL-C levels and the level of initiation of diet and drug therapy are provided in Table 8.5. The extent of lipid reduction is related to CHD risk reduction, and the goals outlined in the tables should be considered as *minimal* goals. If possible, dietary means should be used to attain even lower LDL-C to achieve further reductions in CHD risk.
- Secondary forms of hyperlipidemia should be managed initially by correcting the underlying abnormality, including modification of drug therapy when appropriate.

TABLE 8.3. Initial Classification of Total, LDL, and HDL Cholesterol and Triglycerides

Classification	Total Cholesterol	LDL Cholesterol	HDL Cholesterol	Triglycerides
Desirable/ normal	<200 mg/dL	<130 mg/dL	—	<200 mg/dL
Borderline high	200–239 mg/dL	130–159 mg/dL	—	200–400 mg/dL
High	≥240 mg/dL	>160 mg/dL	>60 mg/dL	400–1000 mg/dL
Very high	—	—	—	>1000 mg/dL
Low	—	—	<35 mg/dL	—

Key: HDL, high-density lipoproteins; LDL, low-density lipoproteins.

TABLE 8.4. Risk Status Based on Presence of CHD Risk Factors Other Than LDL Cholesterol

Positive Risk Factors

Men: ≥45 years

Women: ≥55 years or premature menopause without estrogen replacement therapy

Family history of premature CHD (definite myocardial infarction or sudden death before 55 years of age in father or other male first-degree relative, or before 65 years of age in mother or other female first-degree relative)

Current cigarette smoking

Hypertension (≥140/90 mm Hg or on antihypertensive medication)

Low HDL cholesterol (<35 mg/dL)

Diabetes mellitus

Negative Risk Factor[a]

High HDL cholesterol (≥60 mg/dL)

Key: CHD, coronary heart disease; LDL, low-density lipoproteins; HDL, high-density lipoproteins.
Note: High risk is defined as a net of two or more CHD risk factors or the presence of coronary or peripheral atherosclerosis.
[a]If the HDL cholesterol level is ≥60 mg/dL, subtract one risk factor because high HDL cholesterol levels decrease CHD risk.

TABLE 8.5. Treatment Decisions Based on LDL Cholesterol

	Initiation Level	LDL Goal
Dietary therapy		
Without CHD and <2 risk factors	≥160 mg/dL	<160 mg/dL
Without CHD and ≥2 risk factors	≥130 mg/dL	<130 mg/dL
With CHD	>100 mg/dL	≤100 mg/dL
	Consideration Level	LDL Goal
Drug treatment		
Without CHD and <2 risk factors	≥190 mg/dL[a]	<160 mg/dL
Without CHD and ≥2 risk factors	≥160 mg/dL	<130 mg/dL
With CHD	≥130 mg/dL[b]	≤100 mg/dL

Key: LDL, low-density lipoproteins; CHD, coronary heart disease.
[a]In men less than 35 years old and premenopausal women with LDL cholesterol levels of 190–219 mg/dL, drug therapy should be delayed except in high-risk patients such as those with diabetes.
[b]In patients with CHD and LDL cholesterol levels of 100–129 mg/dL, the clinician should exercise clinical judgment in deciding whether to initiate drug treatment.

DIETARY THERAPY

- The objectives of dietary therapy are to decrease progressively the intake of total fat, saturated fatty acids (i.e., saturated fat), and cholesterol and to achieve a desirable body weight.
- Dietary modification, weight control, and increased physical activity are essential first steps in the treatment of most lipid disorders. The recommended dietary approach is outlined in Table 8.6.
- The basic rationale for reducing dietary cholesterol, saturated fat, and excessive calories is based on the overproduction of VLDL and, subsequently, LDL. Excessive dietary intake of cholesterol and saturated fatty acids leads to decreased hepatic clearance of LDL and deposition of LDL and oxidized LDL in peripheral tissues.
- The predicted reduction in total serum cholesterol following institution of the step I diet would be reduction of 3–14%, with average reductions of about 5–7% in men consuming 13–14% of their calories as saturated fat. Progressing to step II diet therapy should provide an additional reduction of about 3–7%.
- Each phase of the diet should be maintained for a minimum of 4–6 weeks for the minimal goal; however, the optimal response may not be seen for 3–6 months or more. In general, drug therapy should not be instituted until the trial of diet has continued for 6 months in primary prevention except in patients with severe forms of hyperlipidemia, those with two or more risk factors, or definite CHD.

TABLE 8.6. Dietary Therapy of High Blood Cholesterol

Nutrient[a]	Step I Diet	Recommended intake	Step II Diet
Total fat		≤30% of total calories	
Saturated fatty acids	8–10% of total calories		<7% of total calories
Polyunsaturated fatty acids		Up to 10% of total calories	
Monounsaturated fatty acids		Up to 15% of total calories	
Carbohydrates		≥55% of total calories	
Cholesterol	<300 mg/d		<200 mg/d
Total calories		To achieve and maintain desirable body weight	

[a]Calories from alcohol not included.

- Reduction of cholesterol and saturated fat intake provides a reduction of CHD risk regardless of the time of intervention (primary versus secondary). Diet modification works adjunctively with other risk factor interventions, such as cessation of smoking and treating hypertension. Continuation of diet therapy is imperative if drug therapy is to be optimal.
- Increased intake of soluble fiber in the form of oat bran, pectins, certain gums, and psyllium products can result in useful adjunctive reductions in total and LDL cholesterol (5–20%), but these dietary alterations or supplements should not be substituted for more active forms of treatment. They have little or no effect on HDL-C or triglyceride concentrations. These products may also be useful in managing constipation associated with the bile acid sequestrants.
- Fish oil supplementation has a fairly large effect in reducing triglycerides and VLDL-C, but it either has no effect on total and LDL cholesterol or may cause elevations in these fractions.

DRUG THERAPY

- The effect of drug therapy on lipids and lipoproteins is shown in Table 8.7.
- Recommended drugs of choice for each lipoprotein phenotype and alternate agents are given in Table 8.8.
- Available products and their doses are provided in Table 8.9.

Bile Acid Sequestrants (Cholestyramine and Colestipol)

- The primary action of both agents is to bind bile acids in the intestinal lumen, with a concurrent interruption of enterohepatic circulation of bile acids, which decreases the bile acid pool size and stimulates hepatic synthesis of bile acids from cholesterol. Depletion of the hepatic pool of cholesterol results in an increase in cholesterol biosynthesis and an increase in the number of LDL-R on the hepatocyte membrane, which stimulates an enhanced rate of catabolism from plasma and lowers LDL levels. The increase in hepatic cholesterol biosynthesis may be paralleled by increased hepatic VLDL production and, consequently, bile acid resins may aggravate hypertriglyceridemia in patients with combined hyperlipidemia.
- Bile acid sequestrants are useful in treating primary hypercholesterolemia (familial hypercholesterolemia, familial combined hyperlipidemia, type IIa hyperlipoproteinemia).
- Gastrointestinal complaints of constipation, bloating, epigastric fullness, nausea, and flatulence are most commonly reported. These adverse effects can be managed by increasing the fluid intake, modifying the diet to increase bulk, and by use of stool softeners.
- The gritty texture and bulk may be minimized by mixing the powder with orange drink or juice. Colestipol may have better palatability because it is odorless and tasteless. Tablet forms of bile acid sequestrants should help in improving compliance with this form of therapy.

TABLE 8.7. Effects of Drug Therapy on Lipids and Lipoproteins

Drug	Mechanism of Action	Effects on Lipids	Effects on Lipoproteins	Comment
Cholestyramine and colestipol	↑ LDL catabolism ↓ Cholesterol absorption	↓ Cholesterol	↓ LDL ↑ VLDL	Problem with compliance; binds many coadministered drugs
Niacin	↓ LDL and VLDL synthesis	↓ Triglyceride and cholesterol	↓ VLDL, ↓ LDL, ↑ HDL	Problems with patient acceptance; good in combination with bile acid resins
Dextrothyroxine sodium	↑ LDL catabolism	↓ Cholesterol	↓ LDL	Caution in patients with heart disease
Clofibrate	↑ VLDL clearance	↓ Triglyceride and cholesterol	↓ VLDL and LDL; ↑ HDL	Possible long-term toxicity; only modest effects on cholesterol
Neomycin sulfate	↑ LDL catabolism ↓ Cholesterol absorption	↓ Cholesterol	↓ LDL	Potentially ototoxic and nephrotixic
Probucol[a]	↑ LDL clearance	↓ Cholesterol	↓ LDL and HDL	Lowers HDL; modest efficacy but inhibits LDL oxidation and facilitates reverse cholesterol transport
Gemfibrozil	↑ VLDL clearance ↓ VLDL synthesis	↓ Triglyceride and cholesterol	↓ VLDL, ↑ ↓ LDL, ↑ HDL	Similar to clofibrate; long-term toxicity may be less than clofibrate; raises HDL
Atorvastatin, fluvastatin, lovastatin, pravastatin, simvastatin	↑ LDL catabolism; inhibit LDL synthesis	↓ Cholesterol	↓ LDL	Highly effective in heterozygotous familial hypercholesterolemia and in combination with other agents

[a] *Withdrawn from the US market in 1995.*

TABLE 8.8. Lipoprotein Phenotype and Recommended Drug Treatment

Lipoprotein Type	Drug of Choice	Combination Therapy	Alternative Agents
I	Not indicated	—	—
IIa	Cholestyramine or colestipol HMG Co-ARI[a]	Niacin Neomycin	HMG Co-ARI Neomycin
IIb	Gemfibrozil Niacin	Cholestyramine or colestipol	Cholestyramine or colestipol HMG Co-ARI Clofibrate
III	Gemfibrozil Niacin	HMG Co-ARI	HMG Co-ARI Clofibrate Estrogen
IV	Gemfibrozil Niacin	Niacin Gemfibrozil	Clofibrate
V	Gemfibrozil Niacin		Clofibrate Oxandrolone Norethisterone Fish oils

[a]Not presently recommended as a first-line drug by the National Cholesterol Education Program. HMG Co-ARI, hydroxymethylglutaryl coenzyme-A reductase inhibitors.

- Other potential adverse effects include impaired absorption of fat-soluble vitamins A, D, E, and K with high doses; hypernatremia and hyperchloremia; gastrointestinal obstruction; and reduced bioavailability of acidic drugs such as coumarin anticoagulants, digitoxin, nicotinic acid, thyroxine, acetaminophen, hydrocortisone, hydrochlorothiazide, loperamide, and possibly iron. Drug interactions may be avoided by alternating administration times with an interval of 6 hours or greater between the bile acid resin and other drugs.

Niacin
- Niacin reduces the hepatic synthesis of VLDL, which in turn leads to a reduction in the synthesis of LDL. Niacin also increases HDL by reducing its catabolism.
- The principal use of niacin is for mixed hyperlipemia or as a second-line agent in combination therapy for hypercholesterolemia. It is also considered to be the first-line agent or an alternative for the treatment of hypertriglyceridemia.

TABLE 8.9. Comparison of Drugs Used in the Treatment of Hyperlipidemia

Drug	Manufacturer	Dosage Forms	Usual Daily Dose	Maximum Daily Dose
Cholestyramine (Questran, Questran Light)	Bristol-Myers Squibb	Bulk powder/ 4-g packets	8 g tid	32 g
Cholestyramine (Cholybar)	Parke-Davis	4-g resin per bar		
Colestipol hydrochloride (Colestid)	Upjohn	Bulk powder/ 5-g packets	10 g bid	30 g
Niacin	Various	50-, 100-, 250-, and 500-mg tablets; 125-, 250-, and 500-mg capsules	2 g tid	9 g
Dextrothyroxine sodium (Choloxin)	Boots	1-, 2-, and 4-mg tablets	6 mg qd	8 mg
Neomycin sulfate	Various	500-mg tablets	1 g bid	2 g
Clofibrate (Atromid-S)	Ayerst	500-mg capsules	1 g bid	2 g
Gemfibrozil (Lopid)	Parke-Davis	300-mg capsules	600 mg bid	1.5 g
Lovastatin (Mevacor)	Merck	20- and 40-mg tablets	20–40 mg	80 mg
Pravastatin (Pravachol)	Bristol-Myers Squibb	10- and 20-mg tablets	20–40 mg	40 mg
Simvastatin (Zocor)	Merck	5-, 10-, 20-, and 40-mg tablets	10–20 mg	40 mg
Fluvastatin (Lescol)	Sandoz	20- and 40-mg tablets	20–40 mg	40 mg
Atorvastatin (Lipitor)	Parke-Davis	10-, 20-, and 40-mg tablets	10–40 mg	80 mg

II

- Niacin has many common adverse drug reactions; fortunately, most of the symptoms and biochemical abnormalities seen do not require discontinuation of therapy.
- Cutaneous flushing and itching appear to be prostaglandin mediated and can be reduced by aspirin 325 mg given shortly before niacin ingestion. Taking the dose with meals and slowly titrating the dose upward may minimize these effects. Concomitant alcohol and hot drinks may magnify flushing and pruritus with niacin, and they should be avoided at the time of ingestion. Gastrointestinal intolerance is also a common problem.
- Potentially important laboratory abnormalities occurring with niacin therapy include elevated liver function tests, hyperuricemia, and hyperglycemia. Niacin-associated hepatitis is more common with sustained-release preparations, and their use should be restricted to patients intolerant of regular-release products. Niacin is contraindicated in patients with active liver disease, and it may exacerbate preexisting gout and diabetes.
- Nicotinamide should not be used in the treatment of hyperlipidemia, because it does not effectively lower cholesterol or triglyceride levels.

HMG-CoA Reductase Inhibitors (Atorvastatin, Fluvastatin, Lovastatin, Pravastatin, Simvastatin)

- Reductase inhibitors interrupt the conversion of HMG-CoA to mevalonate, the rate-limiting step in *de novo* cholesterol biosynthesis, by inhibiting HMG-CoA reductase. Reduced synthesis of LDL-C and enhanced catabolism of LDL mediated through LDL receptors appear to be the principal mechanisms for lipid-lowering effects.
- When used as monotherapy, the HMG-CoA reductase inhibitors are the most potent total and LDL cholesterol lowering agents and among the best tolerated.
- Total and LDL cholesterol are reduced in a dose-related fashion by 30% or more on average when added to dietary therapy, with the effects being more pronounced in nonfamilial hypercholesterolemia than in the familial form. Simvastatin and atorvastatin are more potent than lovastatin, pravastatin, and fluvastatin.
- Combination therapy with bile acid sequestrants and lovastatin is rational as LDL receptor numbers are increased, leading to greater degradation of LDL-C; intracellular synthesis of cholesterol is inhibited; and enterohepatic recycling of bile acids is interrupted.
- Constipation occurs in less than 10% of patients taking reductase inhibitors.
- In the EXCEL study of more than 8000 patients, elevation of serum transaminase levels (primarily alanine aminotransferase) to more than three times the upper limit of normal and associated muscle symptoms (myopathy) were seen in 1.5% of patients taking lovastatin 40 mg given twice a day (vs. 0.1% in patients taking placebo).

- Also in the EXCEL study, creatine kinase (CK) greater than 10 times the upper limit of normal and muscle symptoms occurred in 0.2% of the lovastatin group, and any elevation of CK was highest at 40 mg given twice a day, 3.5% versus 1.6% for placebo.

II

Gemfibrozil

- Gemfibrozil, a fibric acid derivative of clofibrate, reduces the synthesis of VLDL and, to a lesser extent, apolipoprotein B with a concurrent increase in the rate of removal of triglyceride-rich lipoproteins from plasma.
- As a single agent, it is effective in reducing VLDL but a reciprocal rise in LDL may occur, and total cholesterol values may remain relatively unchanged. Plasma HDL concentrations may rise 10–15% or more with gemfibrozil.
- Gastrointestinal complaints occur in 3–5% of patients, rash in 2%, dizziness in 2.4%, and transient elevations in transaminase levels and alkaline phosphatase in 4.5% and 1.3%, respectively.
- Similar to clofibrate, gemfibrozil may enhance the formation of gallstones associated with an increase in the lithogenic index; however, the rate is low (0.6%) and similar to that seen with placebo in the Helsinki Heart Study.
- Gemfibrozil may potentiate the effects of oral anticoagulants as seen with clofibrate, but this is not well documented.

Clofibrate

- Clofibrate increases the activity of lipoprotein lipase and reduces to a lesser extent the synthesis or secretion of VLDL from the liver into the plasma. Clofibrate is less effective than gemfibrozil or niacin in reducing VLDL production.
- Although clofibrate has been suggested as the drug of choice for type III hyperlipoproteinemia, it has not been shown to reduce cardiovascular mortality and it has numerous well-documented and serious adverse effects, relegating it to third-line therapy after niacin or gemfibrozil.
- Clofibrate may induce gallstones (4.7%, clofibrate; 0.54%, placebo), promote ventricular ectopy, and potentially cause gastrointestinal malignancy causing a greater overall mortality than placebo alone.
- A myositis syndrome of myalgia, weakness, stiffness, malaise, and elevations in creatinine phosphokinase and aspartate aminotransferase may occur and seems to be more common in patients with renal insufficiency.
- Enhanced hypoprothrombinemic and hypoglycemic effects are reported to occur when clofibrate is given to patients on coumarin anticoagulants and sulfonylurea compounds, but the mechanisms for these interactions are not well understood.

Neomycin

- Neomycin is a second-line drug for use in patients with primary hypercholesterolemia who are unable to take bile acid sequestrants. It reduces

the absorption of cholesterol from the small intestine, but its utility is limited by detrimental changes in lipoproteins, adverse effects, and lack of efficacy.
* Early in therapy 38–80% of patients experience increased stool frequency or diarrhea, but this usually resolves after 1–3 weeks of therapy.
* Although small amounts are absorbed (3–5%), no ototoxicity has been reported at doses of 2 g/d or less for up to 3 years.
* Neomycin may increase the absorption of digoxin, enhance the hypoprothrombinemic effects of warfarin, and interact synergistically with other nephrotoxic drugs and neuromuscular blocking agents.

Dextrothyroxine
* Dextrothyroxine can no longer be recommended for the treatment of hyperlipemia based on the Coronary Drug Project experience in which dextrothyroxine-treated patients experienced a higher mortality rate if ventricular ectopy was present at the initiation of therapy.

Fish Oil Supplementation
* Diets high in omega-3 polyunsaturated fatty acids (from fish oil), most commonly eicosapentaenoic acid (EPA), reduce cholesterol, triglycerides, LDL-C, VLDL-C, and may elevate HDL-C.
* Fish oil supplementation may be most useful in patients with hypertriglyceridemia, but its role in treatment is not well defined.
* Potential complications of fish oil supplementation such as thrombocytopenia and bleeding disorders have been noted, especially with high doses (EPA, 15–30 g/d).

Treatment Recommendations
* Treatment of type I hyperlipoproteinemia is directed toward reduction of chylomicrons derived from dietary fat with the subsequent reduction in plasma triglycerides. Total daily fat intake should be no more than 10–25 g/d, or approximately 15% of total calories. Secondary causes of hypertriglyceridemia (Table 8.2) should be excluded or, if present, the underlying disorder should be treated appropriately.
* Primary hypercholesterolemia (familial hypercholesterolemia, familial combined hyperlipidemia, type IIa hyperlipoproteinemia) is treated with the bile acid sequestrants cholestyramine and colestipol.
* Combined hyperlipoproteinemia (type IIb) may be treated with niacin or gemfibrozil to lower LDL cholesterol without elevating VLDL and triglycerides. Niacin is the most effective agent and may be combined with a bile acid sequestrant. Cholestyramine or colestipol alone in this disorder may elevate VLDL and triglycerides and their use as single agents for treating combined hyperlipoproteinemia should be avoided.
* Type III hyperlipoproteinemia may be treated with niacin, gemfibrozil, or (rarely) clofibrate. Fish oil supplementation may be an alternative therapy.

- Type V hyperlipoproteinemia requires a stringent restriction of the fat component of dietary intake. In addition, drug therapy is indicated, as outlined in Table 8.8, if the response to diet alone is inadequate. Medium-chain triglycerides, which are absorbed without chylomicron formation, may be used as a dietary supplement for caloric intake if needed for both types I and V.

Combination Drug Therapy

- Combination therapy may be considered after adequate trials of monotherapy and in patients documented as being compliant to the prescribed regimen. Two to three monthly lipoprotein determinations should confirm lack of response prior to initiation of combination therapy.
- Contraindications to and drug interactions with combined therapy should be screened carefully, as well as consideration of the extra cost of drug product and monitoring that may be required.
- An HMG-CoA reductase inhibitor and a bile acid sequestrant or niacin with a bile acid sequestrant provide the greatest reduction in total and LDL cholesterol.
- Regimens intended to increase HDL levels should include either gemfibrozil or niacin, and it should be remembered that reductase inhibitors combined with either of these drugs may result in a greater incidence of hepatotoxicity or myositis.
- Familial combined hyperlipidemia may respond better to gemfibrozil and lovastatin than gemfibrozil and colestipol.

Treatment of Hypertriglyceridemia

- Lipoprotein pattern types I, III, IV, and V are associated with hypertriglyceridemia, and these primary lipoprotein disorders should be excluded prior to implementing therapy.
- A positive family history of CHD is important in identifying patients at risk for premature atherosclerosis, and if a patient with CHD has elevated triglycerides, the associated abnormality is probably a contributing factor to CHD and should be treated.
- The goal of therapy is to lower triglycerides and VLDL particles that may be atherogenic, increase HDL, and reduce LDL. Success in treatment is defined as a reduction in triglycerides below 500 mg/dL.
- High serum triglycerides (Table 8.3) should be treated by achieving desirable body weight, consumption of a low saturated and cholesterol diet, regular exercise, smoking cessation, and restriction of alcohol (in selected patients).
- In patients with borderline-high triglycerides but with accompanying CHD, risk factors and genetic forms of hypertriglyceridemia associated with CHD drug therapy with niacin should be considered.
- Niacin should not be used in diabetics because of the risk of worsening glycemic control. Alternative therapies include gemfibrozil and reductase inhibitors.

▶ EVALUATION OF THERAPEUTIC OUTCOMES

II

- Short-term evaluation of therapy for hyperlipidemia is based on response to diet and drug treatment as measured in the clinical laboratory by total cholesterol, LDL-C, HDL-C, and triglycerides.
- Patients treated for primary prevention may have no symptoms or clinical manifestations of a genetic lipid disorder (e.g., xanthomas), so monitoring is solely laboratory based. The goals for LDL and HDL cholesterol are provided in Table 8.5.
- In patients treated for secondary intervention, symptoms of atherosclerotic cardiovascular disease, such as angina or intermittent claudication, may improve over months to years. Xanthomas or other external manifestations of hyperlipidemia should regress with therapy.
- Lipid measurements should be obtained in the fasted state to minimize interference from chylomicrons and, once the patient is stable, monitoring is needed at intervals of 6 months to 1 year.
- Patients with multiple risk factors and established CHD should also be monitored and evaluated for progress in managing their other risk factors such as hypertension, smoking cessation, exercise and weight control, and glycemic control (if diabetic).
- Evaluation of dietary therapy with diet diaries and recall survey instruments allows information about diet to be collected in a systemic fashion and may improve patient adherence to dietary recommendations.

See Chapter 21, Hyperlipidemia, authored by Robert L. Talbert, PharmD, FCCP, for a more detailed discussion of this topic.

Chapter 9

► HYPERTENSION

► DEFINITION

- Based on the impact on risk for cardiovascular morbidity and mortality, the Fifth Joint National Committee on the Detection, Evaluation, and Treatment of High Blood Pressure (JNC-V) classified adult blood pressure as follows:

Category	Systolic (mm Hg)	Diastolic (mm Hg)
Normal	<130	<85
High normal	130–139	85–89
Hypertension		
Stage 1 (mild)	140–159	90–99
Stage 2 (moderate)	160–179	100–109
Stage 3 (severe)	180–209	110–119
Stage 4 (very severe)	>209	>119

- If the diastolic blood pressure (DBP) is less than 90 mm Hg and the systolic blood pressure (SBP) is 140 mm Hg or higher, then the term *isolated systolic hypertension* is applicable. Isolated systolic hypertension is believed to result from the pathophysiology of aging and portends an increased risk of cardiovascular morbidity and mortality.
- A marked or sharp increase in DBP is considered a hypertensive crisis, which may represent either a hypertensive emergency—an elevation of diastolic blood pressure accompanied by acute target organ injury—or a hypertensive urgency—severe hypertension without signs or symptoms of acute target organ complications.

► PATHOPHYSIOLOGY

- Hypertension is a heterogeneous disorder that may result either from a specific cause (secondary hypertension) or from some underlying pathophysiologic mechanism stemming from an unknown etiology (primary or essential hypertension). Secondary hypertension accounts for fewer than 5% of cases, and most of these are caused by chronic renal disease or renovascular disease. Other conditions causing secondary hypertension include pheochromocytoma, Cushing's syndrome, primary aldosteronism, coarctation of the aorta, and exogenous substances such as estrogens, glucocorticoids, licorice, sympathomimetic amines, nonsteroidal anti-inflammatory drugs (NSAIDs), chronic alcohol

II
- use, and tyramine-containing foods in combination with monoamine oxidase (MAO) inhibitors.
- Multiple factors may contribute to the development of primary hypertension. Postulated mechanisms include:
  - A pathologic disturbance in the central nervous system (CNS), autonomic nerve fibers, adrenergic receptors, or baroreceptors.
  - Abnormalities in either the renal or tissue autoregulatory processes for sodium excretion, plasma volume, and arteriolar constriction.
  - Humoral abnormalities involving the renin–angiotensin–aldosterone system (RAS), natriuretic hormone, or hyperinsulinemia.
  - A deficiency in the local synthesis of vasodilating substances in the vascular endothelium, such as prostacyclin, bradykinin, and nitric oxide, or an increase in the production of vasoconstricting substances such as angiotensin II and endothelin I.
  - Increased sodium intake together with an inherited defect in the kidney's ability to excrete sodium, leading to an increase in circulating natriuretic hormone, which inhibits intracellular sodium transport resulting in increased vascular reactivity.
  - Increased intracellular concentration of calcium, leading to altered vascular smooth muscle function and increased peripheral vascular resistance.
- Early in the course of primary hypertension, the blood pressure may fluctuate between abnormal and normal levels. As the disease progresses, peripheral vascular resistance increases and patients develop a sustained increase in blood pressure. In most cases the DBP does not exceed 115 mm Hg. Individuals with secondary hypertension are more likely to experience severe elevations in blood pressure. Only a small proportion of patients suffering from primary hypertension develops accelerated or severe hypertension.
- The target organ damage secondary to chronic hypertension principally involves the brain, the eye, the heart, and the kidney. The main causes of death in hypertensive subjects are cerebrovascular accidents, cardiovascular events, and renal failure. The probability of premature death from any of these causes increases with increasing SBP or DBP.

▶ CLINICAL PRESENTATION

- Patients with uncomplicated, primary hypertension are usually asymptomatic initially. As the hypertension progresses, however, symptoms characteristic of cardiovascular, cerebrovascular, or renal disease may occur as the patient develops target organ damage.
- Patients with secondary hypertension usually complain of symptoms suggestive of the underlying disorder. For example, patients with pheochromocytoma may have a history of paroxysmal headaches, sweating, tachycardia, palpitations, orthostatic dizziness, or syncope. In primary aldosteronism, hypokalemic symptoms of muscle cramps and

weakness may be present. Patients with hypertension secondary to Cushing's syndrome may complain of weight gain, polyuria, edema, menstrual irregularities, recurrent acne, or muscular weakness.

▶ DIAGNOSIS

- Frequently, the only sign of primary hypertension on physical examination is an elevated blood pressure. As the disease progresses, signs of end-organ damage begin to appear, chiefly related to pathologic changes in the eye, brain, heart, kidneys, and peripheral blood vessels.
- The funduscopic exam may reveal arteriolar narrowing, arteriovenous nicking, retinal hemorrhages, and infarcts. Papilledema suggests a malignant stage of high blood pressure requiring rapid treatment.
- Auscultation of the heart may identify an accentuated second heart sound (S_2), a systolic ejection murmur, an S_4 gallop, or an S_3 gallop sound associated with congestive heart failure (CHF).
- The physical examination may provide clues for diagnosing secondary hypertension. For example, patients with renal artery stenosis may have an abdominal systolic–diastolic bruit; patients with Cushing's syndrome may have the classic physical features of moon face, buffalo hump, hirsutism, and abdominal striae.
- A low serum potassium before antihypertensive therapy is begun may suggest mineralocorticoid-induced hypertension. The presence of protein, blood cells, and casts in the urine may indicate an underlying parenchymal kidney disease as the cause of hypertension.
- Routine laboratory tests that should be obtained in all patients prior to initiating drug therapy include hemoglobin and hematocrit, urinalysis, serum potassium and creatinine, liver function tests, and electrocardiogram (ECG). Total and high density lipoprotein (HDL) cholesterol, plasma glucose, and serum uric acid are indicated to assess other risk factors and to develop baseline data for monitoring drug-induced metabolic changes.
- More specific laboratory tests are used to diagnose secondary hypertension. These include plasma norepinephrine and urinary metanephrine for pheochromocytoma, plasma and urinary aldosterone levels for primary aldosteronism, and plasma renin activity, captopril stimulation test, renal vein renins, and renal artery angiography for renovascular disease.
- A single reading of blood pressure elevation does not constitute a diagnosis of hypertension. If the blood pressure taken on two or more subsequent days is 140/90 mm Hg or higher, then a diagnosis of hypertension is confirmed.

▶ DESIRED OUTCOME

The long-term goal for the treatment of hypertension is to reduce blood pressure to the desired goal with minimal adverse effects in order to reduce target organ damage and prevent the development of the cerebrovascular, cardiovascular, ophthalmic, and renal complications of the disease.

▶ TREATMENT

GENERAL PRINCIPLES

- The treatment plan for hypertension should include measures to minimize contributing factors and to reduce or prevent other known risk factors. Obesity, hyperlipidemia, glucose intolerance, excessive salt intake, cigarette smoking, and alcohol consumption are important risk factors that should be addressed.
- Initial treatment steps should include lifestyle modifications, including: (1) a sensible dietary program designed for gradual weight reduction, if appropriate, and for reducing the saturated fat and salt content of the diet; (2) restriction of alcohol intake, which may worsen hypertension; (3) cessation of smoking; and (4) aerobic exercise, if medically feasible.
- Pharmacologic therapy should be individualized based on a patient's age, race, known pathophysiologic variables, and concurrent conditions. Treatment should be designed not only to lower blood pressure safely and effectively, but also to avoid or reverse hyperlipidemia, glucose intolerance, and left ventricular hypertrophy.
- Individual drug selection should also be based on safety, efficacy, cost, and the presence of concomitant diseases and other risk factors. Table 9.1 provides a list of agents currently available for the treatment of hypertension in the United States.

DIURETICS

- Thiazides are generally the diuretics of choice for the treatment of hypertension, and all are equally effective in lowering blood pressure. In patients with adequate renal function [i.e., glomerular filtration rate (GFR) >30 mL/min], thiazides are more effective hypotensive agents than loop diuretics. As renal function declines, however, sodium and fluid accumulate, and the use of a more potent diuretic is necessary to counter the effects that volume and sodium expansion have on arterial blood pressure.
- The potassium-sparing diuretics are weak antihypertensive agents when used alone, but provide an additive hypotensive effect when used in combination with thiazide or loop diuretics. Moreover, they counteract the potassium- and magnesium-losing properties of other diuretic agents.
- Acutely, diuretics lower blood pressure by causing a diuresis. The reduction in plasma volume and stroke volume associated with a diuresis decreases cardiac output and, consequently, blood pressure. The initial drop in cardiac output produced by the diuresis causes a compen-

satory increase in peripheral vascular resistance. With continuing diuretic therapy, the extracellular fluid volume and plasma volume return almost to pretreatment levels, and peripheral vascular resistance falls below its pretreatment baseline. The reduction in peripheral vascular resistance is responsible for the long-term hypotensive effectiveness. It has been postulated that thiazides lower blood pressure by mobilizing sodium and water from arteriolar walls.

- When diuretics are used in combination with other antihypertensive agents, an additive hypotensive effect is usually observed because of independent mechanisms of action. Furthermore, many nondiuretic antihypertensive agents induce salt and water retention, which is counteracted by concurrent use of a diuretic.

- Side effects of thiazides include hypokalemia, hypomagnesemia, hypercalcemia, hyperuricemia, hyperglycemia, hyperlipidemia, and sexual dysfunction. Loop diuretics cause a lesser effect on serum lipids and glucose, but hypocalcemia may occur. Short-term studies indicate that indapamide does not adversely effect lipids or glucose tolerance or cause sexual dysfunction.

- The hypokalemia and hypomagnesemia caused by diuretics may lead to cardiac arrhythmias, especially in patients receiving digitalis therapy, patients with left ventricular hypertrophy, and patients with ischemic heart disease.

- Hypokalemia may be prevented by using low daily doses (e.g., 12.5–25 mg of hydrochlorothiazide or 25 mg of chlorthalidone) and reducing sodium and increasing potassium in the diet. Salt substitutes containing potassium should be used with caution in patients who are on potassium-sparing diuretics, angiotensin converting enzyme (ACE) inhibitors, or NSAIDs. If hypokalemia occurs despite these preventive measures, the use of a potassium chloride supplement or a potassium-sparing diuretic is indicated.

- Diuretic-induced hyperuricemia may produce gouty arthritis or uric acid stones, especially in individuals who are predisposed to gout. If this occurs in patients requiring diuretic therapy, allopurinol or a uricosuric agent can be given to prevent recurrent gouty attacks without compromising the antihypertensive effects of the diuretic.

- Chronic use of thiazide diuretic therapy may alter glucose metabolism by reducing postprandial insulin secretion and by causing insulin resistance, which may contribute to the production of diabetes in prediabetic individuals or worsen metabolic control in diabetic patients.

- The effect thiazide diuretics have on serum lipid concentrations is debatable. Some studies show only a transient increase in total cholesterol and triglycerides, whereas others show a persistent adverse effect.

- Potassium-sparing diuretics may cause hyperkalemia, especially in patients with renal insufficiency or diabetes, and in patients receiving concurrent treatment with an ACE inhibitor, NSAIDs, or potassium supplements. Spironolactone may cause gynecomastia.

TABLE 9.1. The Antihypertensive Agents

Drug	Dose Range (mg/d)	
	Initial	*Maximum*
Diuretics		
Thiazides and related sulfonamide diuretics		
Bendroflumethiazide	2.5	5
Benzthiazide	25	50
Chlorothiazide sodium	250	500
Chlorthalidone	25	50
Cyclothiazide	1	2
Hydrochlorothiazide	25	50
Hydroflumethiazide	25	50
Indapamide	2.5	5
Methyclothiazide	2.5	5
Metolazone	2.5	5
Polythiazide	2	4
Quinethazone	50	100
Trichlormethiazide	2	4
Loop diuretics		
Bumetanide	0.5	10
Ethacrynic acid	50	200
Furosemide	80	480
Torsemide	5	10
Potassium-sparing agents		
Amiloride hydrochloride	5	10
Spironolactone	50	100
Triamterene	50	100
Adrenergic Inhibitors		
β-Adrenergic blockers		
Acebutolol	400	1200
Atenolol	25	100
Betaxolol	10	40
Bisoprolol	5	20
Carteolol	2.5	10
Labetolol	200	2400
Metoprolol tartrate	50	300
Nadolol	20	120
Penbutolol	20	80
Pindolol	20	60
Propranolol hydrochloride	40	480
Propranolol, long-acting (LA)	80	480
Timolol maleate	20	60
Central-acting adrenergic inhibitors		
Clonidine hydrochloride	0.2	1.2

TABLE 9.1. continued

Drug	Dose Range (mg/d)	
	Initial	*Maximum*
Adrenergic Inhibitors (cont.)		
Guanabenz acetate	8	32
Guanfacine	1	3.0
Methyldopa	500	2000
Peripheral-acting adrenergic antagonists		
Guanadrel sulfate	10	150
Guanethidine monosulfate	10	300
Rauwolfia alkaloids		
Rauwolfia (whole root)	50	100
Reserpine	0.05	0.25
α_1-Adrenergic blocker		
Doxazosin	1	16
Prazosin hydrochloride	2	20
Terazosin	1	5.0
Combined α- and β-adrenergic blockers		
Labetolol	200	1200
Vasodilators		
Hydralazine hydrochloride	50	300
Minoxidil	5	100
Angiotensin-converting enzyme inhibitors		
Benazepril	10	20
Captopril	25	150
Enalapril maleate	10	40
Fosinopril	10	80
Lisinopril	10	80
Moexipril	7.5	30
Quinapril	10	80
Ramipril	1.25	20
Trandolapril	1	6
Angiotensin II Receptor Antagonists		
Losartan	50	100
Valsartan	80	320
Calcium channel antagonists		
Amlodipine	5	10
Diltiazem hydrochloride	120	240
Felodipine	5	10
Isradipine	5	20
Nicardipine	60	120
Nifedipine	30	180
Nisoldipine	20	60
Nitrendipine	10	40
Verapamil hydrochloride	240	480

II

CENTRAL α_2-RECEPTOR AGONISTS

II

- Clonidine, guanabenz, guanfacine, and methyldopa all lower blood pressure primarily by stimulating α_2-adrenergic receptors in the brain, which reduces sympathetic outflow from the vasomotor center in the brain and increases vagal tone. Stimulation of presynaptic α_2 receptors peripherally may contribute to the reduction in sympathetic tone. Consequently, heart rate is decreased, cardiac output decreases slightly, total peripheral resistance is lowered, plasma renin activity is reduced, and baroreceptor reflexes are blunted.

- Chronic use results in sodium and fluid retention, which appear to be most prominent with methyldopa. Low doses of either clonidine, guanfacine, or guanabenz can be used to treat mild hypertension without the addition of a diuretic.

- Sedation and dry mouth are common side effects of these antihypertensive agents. These symptoms may diminish or completely abate with chronic use of low doses. As with other centrally acting antihypertensive drugs, these agents may cause depression.

- Rebound hypertension may rarely occur when a central α-receptor agonist is stopped. This is thought to occur secondary to a compensatory increase in norepinephrine release that follows a discontinuation of presynaptic α-receptor stimulation.

- Methyldopa rarely may cause hepatitis or hemolytic anemia. A transient elevation in liver function tests is occasionally associated with methyldopa therapy and is clinically unimportant. A persistent increase in serum transaminases or alkaline phosphatase may herald the onset of a fulminant hepatitis, which can be fatal. A Coombs'-positive hemolytic anemia occurs in less than 1% of patients receiving methyldopa, although 20% exhibit a positive direct Coombs' test without anemia.

- The transdermal delivery system for clonidine is applied to the skin and left in place one week before being replaced. It reduces blood pressure while facilitating compliance and avoiding the high peak serum drug concentrations that are thought to contribute to adverse effects. The disadvantages of this system are its cost, a 20% incidence of local skin rash or irritation, and a 2- or 3-day delay of onset of effect.

PERIPHERAL α_1-RECEPTOR BLOCKERS

- Prazosin, terazosin, and doxazosin are selective α_1-receptor blockers that do not alter α_2-receptor activity and therefore do not usually cause reflex tachycardia.

- At low doses, selective α blockers may be used as monotherapy in the treatment of mild hypertension. At higher doses, fluid and sodium accumulation necessitate concurrent diuretic therapy to maintain hypotensive efficacy.

- CNS side effects include lassitude, vivid dreams, and depression. The so-called "first-dose phenomenon" is characterized by orthostatic hypotension, transient dizziness or faintness, palpitations, and even syncope occurring within 1–3 hours of the first dose, or subsequently after the first increased dose. These episodes can be obviated by having the patient take the first dose, and first increased dose, at bedtime. Occasionally, orthostatic dizziness persists with chronic administration.

β-Adrenoceptor Blockers

- The exact hypotensive mechanism of β-adrenoceptor blockers (β blockers) is not known. Postulated mechanisms include reduction in cardiac output through negative chronotropic and inotropic effects on the heart, a central action on β receptors in the brain, reduction in renin release from the kidney, and possibly blockade of peripheral β receptors on the surface of presynaptic sympathetic neuronal endings.
- Even though there are important pharmacodynamic and pharmacokinetic differences among the various β blockers (Table 9.2), there is no difference in their clinical antihypertensive efficacy.
- At low doses, bisoprolol, metoprolol, atenolol, and acebutolol are cardioselective and bind more avidly to β_1 receptors than to β_2 receptors. As a result, they are less likely to provoke bronchospasm and vasoconstriction and may be safer than nonselective β blockers to use in patients with asthma, chronic obstructive pulmonary disease (COPD), and peripheral vascular disease. Selective β blockers may be safer in diabetes mellitus as well, because both insulin secretion and glycogenolysis are adrenergically mediated; blockade of β_2 receptors may reduce either process and cause hyperglycemia or blunt recovery from hypoglycemia, respectively. Because cardioselectivity is a dose-

TABLE 9.2. Pharmacodynamic and Pharmacokinetic Properties of the β-Adrenoceptor Blocking Agents

	α_1 Blockade	β_1 Selectivity	MSA[a]	ISA[a]	Lipid Solubility	Bioavail-ability (%)	Half-Life (hours)
Acebutolol	0	+	+	+	Low	20–60	3–4
Atenolol	0	+	0	0	Low	50	6–9
Betaxolol	0	+	±	0	Low	100	14–24
Bisoprololol	0	+++	0	0	Low	85	10–12
Carteolol	0	0	0	+	Low	50	6
Labetalol	+	0	+	0	Moderate	40	3–5
Metoprolol	0	+	0	0	Moderate	50	3–4
Nadolol	0	0	0	0	Low	30	14–24
Penbutolol	0	0	0	+	High	100	5
Pindolol	0	0	+	+++	Moderate	100	3–4
Propranolol	0	0	+	0	High	35	4–6
Timolol	0	0	0	0	Low	75	3–4

[a]MSA, membrane stabilizing activity; ISA, intrinsic sympathomimetic activity.

II

dependent phenomenon and the effect is lost at higher doses, even β_1 selective blockers should be avoided if at all possible in hypertensive patients with those concomitant diseases.

- Pindolol, penbutolol, carteolol, and acebutolol possess intrinsic sympathomimetic activity (ISA) or partial β-receptor agonist activity and are therefore capable of maintaining normal basal sympathetic tone while blocking the effects of excessive adrenergic stimulation. When sympathetic tone is low, as it is during resting states, β receptors are partially stimulated, so resting heart rate, cardiac output, and peripheral blood flow are not reduced when receptors are blocked. Theoretically, these drugs may be less hazardous in patients with borderline CHF, sinus bradycardia, or perhaps even peripheral vascular disease.

- All β blockers are capable of exerting a membrane-stabilizing action on cardiac cells if large enough doses are given, but the dose required usually greatly exceeds that used in treating hypertension or cardiac arrhythmias.

- Pharmacokinetic differences among β blockers can be found in first-pass metabolism, serum half-lives, degree of lipophilicity, and route of elimination. Propranolol and metoprolol undergo extensive first-pass metabolism. Atenolol and nadolol, which have relatively long half-lives, are excreted renally, and the dosage of each may need to be adjusted in patients with renal insufficiency. Even though the half-lives of the other β blockers are much shorter, once-daily administration may still be effective. Beta blockers vary in terms of their lipophilic properties and CNS penetration, but the more water-soluble β blockers are not reliably less likely to cause CNS side effects.

- Side effects from β blockade in the myocardium include bradycardia, atrioventricular conduction abnormalities, and CHF. Pulmonary β blockade may lead to acute exacerbations of bronchospasm in patients with asthma or COPD. Blocking β_2 receptors in arteriolar smooth muscle may aggravate intermittent claudication or Raynaud's phenomenon and may cause cold extremities as a result of decreased peripheral blood flow.

- Abrupt cessation of β-blocker therapy may produce unstable angina, myocardial infarction, or even death in patients predisposed to ischemic myocardial events. In patients without coronary artery disease, abrupt discontinuation of β-blocker therapy may be associated with sinus tachycardia, increased sweating, and generalized malaise. For these reasons, it is always prudent to taper the dose gradually over 14 days before discontinuation.

- Adverse effects on serum lipids and glucose tolerance may offset some of the beneficial effects on cardiovascular morbidity and mortality. β blockers increase serum triglyceride levels and decrease HDL cholesterol levels. β blockers with α-blocking properties produce no appreciable change in serum lipid concentration. Also, β blockers with ISA do not affect serum lipids adversely and may even increase HDL cholesterol.

- β blockers may induce glucose intolerance by inhibiting insulin secretion and by generating insulin resistance. These adverse effects are not usually associated with the use of β blockers that possess ISA or α-receptor blocking properties.

ANGIOTENSIN-CONVERTING ENZYME INHIBITORS

- ACE is widely distributed in many tissues. It is present in several different cell types, but its principal location is in endothelial cells. Because the vascular endothelium covers a large surface area, the major site for angiotensin II production in the body is the blood vessels, not the kidney. ACE inhibitors block the conversion of angiotensin I to angiotensin II, a potent vasoconstrictor and stimulator of aldosterone secretion. Blockade of angiotensin II also increases the compliance of large arteries, which may effectively prevent or reverse left ventricular hypertrophy. ACE inhibitors may also help prevent or slow the rate of arteriosclerosis in these large vessels, which is the major cause of cardiovascular complications. ACE inhibitors also block the degradation of bradykinin and stimulate the synthesis of other vasodilating substances including prostaglandin E_2 and prostacyclin. The observation that ACE inhibitors lower blood pressure in patients with normal plasma renin and ACE activity clearly indicates the importance of tissue production of ACE as a cause of increased vascular resistance.
- Captopril has a relatively short half-life and is usually administered two to three times daily. Recent studies indicate that once-daily administration of captopril may be adequate for the treatment of hypertension in salt-restricted patients. The remaining ACE inhibitors have long half-lives and are given once daily in the treatment of hypertension. The absorption of captopril is reduced 30–40% by the presence of food in the stomach.
- The most serious adverse effects of the ACE inhibitors are neutropenia and agranulocytosis, proteinuria, glomerulonephritis, and angioedema; these effects occur in less than 1% of patients. Patients with preexisting renal or connective tissue diseases appear to be most vulnerable to the renal and hematologic side effects. Patients with bilateral renal artery stenosis or unilateral stenosis of a solitary functioning kidney and patients dependent on the vasoconstrictive effect of angiotensin II on the efferent arteriole are particularly susceptible to developing acute renal failure on ACE inhibitors.
- Approximately 10% of patients who receive captopril develop a skin rash, which is usually transient and disappears despite continued treatment. A reversible loss of taste or taste disturbance (dysgeusia) has been reported in about 6% of patients receiving captopril. The higher incidence of skin rash, dysgeusia, and proteinuria with captopril has been attributed to its sulfhydryl group, which is not present on enalapril or lisinopril. Approximately 10–20% of patients develop a persistent cough, and some may develop acute bronchospasm.

- Acute hypotension may occur at the onset on ACE inhibitor therapy, especially in patients who are severely sodium or volume depleted. It may be necessary to discontinue diuretics and reduce the dosage of other antihypertensive agents before initiating therapy. Initiating therapy at the lowest dose possible and administering the first dose at bedtime may also minimize acute hypotension.
- ACE inhibitors are absolutely contraindicated in pregnancy because serious neonatal problems, including renal failure and death, have been reported when mothers took these agents during the second and third trimesters of pregnancy.
- Hyperkalemia is seen primarily in patients with renal disease or diabetes mellitus (especially with type IV renal tubular acidosis) or patients on concomitant NSAIDs, potassium supplements, or potassium-sparing diuretics.

ANGIOTENSIN II RECEPTOR ANTAGONISTS

- Losartan and valsartan are angiotensin analogues that inhibit the renin system by competing directly with angiotensin II for tissue binding sites. Therefore, they block the effects of angiotensin II generated by either ACE or the enzyme chymase.
- These drugs appear to have effects on blood pressure and systemic and renal hemodynamics that are comparable to the ACE inhibitors. They are less likely than ACE inhibitors to cause a nonproductive cough or hyperkalemia.

VASODILATORS

- Hydralazine and minoxidil cause direct arteriolar smooth muscle relaxation through mechanisms that increase the intracellular concentration of cyclic guanosine monophosphate (GMP).
- A compensatory activation of the baroreceptor reflexes results in an increase in sympathetic outflow from the vasomotor center, producing an increase in heart rate, cardiac output, and renin release. Consequently, the hypotensive effectiveness of direct vasodilators diminishes in time unless the patient is also taking a sympathetic inhibitor and a diuretic. In older patients, baroreceptor mechanisms may be blunted enough that blood pressure may be lowered with vasodilatory therapy without causing sympathetic overactivity.
- Direct vasodilator use can precipitate angina in patients with underlying coronary artery disease unless the baroreceptor reflex mechanism is completely blocked with a sympathetic inhibitor; the β-adrenergic blocking agents are most effective.
- Hydralazine may cause a dose-related, reversible lupus-like syndrome, which is more common in slow acetylators of the drug. Lupus-like reactions can usually be avoided by using total daily doses of less than 200 mg. Other hydralazine side effects include dermatitis, drug fever, peripheral neuropathy, hepatitis, and vascular headaches.

- Minoxidil causes a reversible hypertrichosis on the face, arms, back, and chest. Other side effects include pericardial effusion and a nonspecific T-wave change on the ECG.

II

CALCIUM CHANNEL ANTAGONISTS

- Calcium channel antagonists cause relaxation of cardiac and smooth muscle by blocking voltage-sensitive calcium channels, thereby reducing the entry of extracellular calcium into the cells. Vascular smooth muscle relaxation leads to vasodilation and a corresponding reduction in blood pressure.
- Verapamil decreases heart rate, slows atrioventricular (AV) nodal conduction, and produces a negative inotropic effect that may precipitate heart failure in subjects with borderline cardiac reserve. Diltiazem decreases atrioventricular conduction and heart rate to a lesser extent than verapamil.
- Nifedipine has potent peripheral vasodilating effects, causing a baroreceptor-mediated reflex increase in heart rate. It does not usually alter conduction through the AV node. Nifedipine rarely may cause an increase in the frequency, intensity, and duration of angina in association with acute hypotension. However, this effect may be obviated by using sustained-released formulations. Other side effects of nifedipine include dizziness, flushing, headache, peripheral edema, mood changes, and various gastrointestinal complaints.
- Diltiazem and verapamil rarely cause cardiac conduction abnormalities such as bradycardia, AV block, and CHF. Both can cause anorexia, nausea, peripheral edema, and hypotension. Verapamil causes constipation in about 7% of patients.

POSTGANGLIONIC SYMPATHETIC INHIBITORS

- Guanethidine and guanadrel deplete norepinephrine from postganglionic sympathetic nerve terminals and inhibit the release of norepinephrine in response to sympathetic nerve stimulation. This results in a reduction in cardiac output and peripheral vascular resistance.
- Postural hypotension is common because reflex-mediated vasoconstriction is blocked by these drugs. Other undesired side effects include impotence, explosive diarrhea (due to unopposed parasympathetic activity), and weight gain. These drugs are usually reserved for patients with refractory hypertension because of their side effect profiles.

RESERPINE

- Reserpine depletes norepinephrine from sympathetic nerve endings and blocks the transport of norepinephrine into its storage granules. When the nerve is stimulated, less than the usual amount of norepinephrine is released into the synapse. This reduces sympathetic tone, decreasing peripheral vascular resistance and blood pressure.

- Its use is associated with significant sodium and fluid retention, and it should be administered in combination with a diuretic.
- Reserpine's strong inhibition of sympathetic activity allows increased parasympathetic activity to occur, which is responsible for side effects of nasal stuffiness, increased gastric acid secretion, diarrhea, and bradycardia.
- The most important side effect is a dose-related mental depression, which is a consequence of CNS depletion of catecholamines and serotonin. The problem can be minimized by not exceeding 0.25 mg daily.

DIFFERENTIAL APPROACH TO THE MANAGEMENT OF HYPERTENSION

- Hypertension is a heterogeneous disorder that poses special therapeutic problems in several specific clinical situations, as shown in Table 9.3.

TABLE 9.3. Differential Antihypertensive Therapy in Specific Clinical Situations

	Advantageous	Disadvantageous
CHF[a]	ACE inhibitor, diuretic, hydralazine	β Blocker, reserpine, Ca channel antagonist
Angina	β Blocker, Ca channel antagonist	Hydralazine, minoxidil
Elderly	Diuretic, α agonist, Ca channel antagonist	
Black	Diuretic, Ca channel antagonist	β blocker as initial therapy
Young	β Blocker, α agonist, ACE inhibitor	Diuretic
Diabetes	α Agonist, ACE inhibitor, Ca channel antagonist	β Blocker, diuretic
Asthma, COPD	Ca channel antagonist	β Blocker, ACE inhibitor
Pregnancy	Methyldopa, hydralazine, labetolol	Diuretic, β blocker
Renal insufficiency	α Agonist, Ca channel antagonist, minoxidil, hydralazine, loop diuretic	Thiazide diuretic
Tachycardia	β Blocker, α agonist, reserpine, verapamil, diltiazem	Nifedipine, hydralazine, minoxidil
Hyperlipidemia	α Blocker, ACE inhibitor, Ca channel antagonist	Diuretic, β blocker
Gout/hyperuricemia	α Agonist, α blocker, Ca channel antagonist, ACE inhibitor[b]	Diuretic, β blocker, ACE inhibitor[b]

[a]CHF, congestive heart failure; ACE, angiotensin-converting enzyme; COPD, chronic obstructive pulmonary disease.
[b]ACE inhibitors may increase urinary clearance of uric acid thereby reducing hyperuricemia but increasing the risk of uric acid deposition in the urine or kidneys.

Hypertension in Childhood

- In most cases, the factors associated with hypertension in children are identical to those in adults. However, secondary hypertension is much more common in children than in adults.
- Renal disease (e.g., pyelonephritis, glomerulonephritis, renal artery stenosis, renal cysts) is the most common cause of secondary hypertension in children. Medical or surgical management of the underlying renal disorder usually restores normal blood pressure.
- In many young people, primary hypertension is associated with an increased cardiac output and a normal plasma volume and total peripheral vascular resistance. This hyperdynamic or hyperkinetic circulatory state might best be treated with a β blocker. Alternative agents include clonidine, guanfacine, or guanabenz, which are known to lower serum norepinephrine levels and thus reduce hyperadrenergic activity.

Hypertension in Pregnancy

- Pre-eclampsia can lead rapidly to life-threatening complications for both the mother and fetus; it usually presents after 20 weeks' gestation in primigravid women. The diagnosis is based on the appearance of hypertension or a significant increase in blood pressure with proteinuria, edema, or both. The hypertension and other signs of pre eclampsia are thought to reflect pathophysiologic changes that induce vasospasm and may cause hematologic, renal, hepatic, brain, and uteroplacental damage. The underlying pathology, not simply the blood pressure elevation, is responsible for the complications; it is uncertain whether blood pressure reduction is of any benefit in reducing the complications of pre-eclampsia.
- Definitive treatment of pre-eclampsia is delivery or abortion, and this is clearly indicated if pending or frank eclampsia (pre-eclampsia plus convulsions) is present. Otherwise, measures such as restriction of activity, bed rest, and close monitoring are in order. If drug treatment of hypertension is indicated (DBP >100 mm Hg), methyldopa (or perhaps another α-agonist) is the recommended drug of choice.
- β blockers appear safe and effective in simple hypertension of pregnancy even though there is some concern about effects on fetal heart rate, glucose intolerance, and growth retardation.

Hypertension in Elderly Patients

- Elderly patients may present with either isolated systolic hypertension or an elevation in both systolic and diastolic blood pressure. In the double-blind placebo-controlled trial called the Systolic Hypertension in the Elderly Program (SHEP), active treatment of isolated systolic hypertension resulted in a 36% reduction in the incidence of total stroke and a 27% reduction in the total number of cardiovascular events.
- The JNC-V recommends a reduction in the SBP to less than 160 mm Hg for patients with a SBP greater than 180 mm Hg and a reduction in

II

blood pressure by 20 mm Hg for those with SBP between 160 and 179 mm Hg.
- Elderly patients are usually more sensitive to volume depletion and sympathetic inhibition, and treatment generally should be initiated with a small dose of a diuretic (e.g., 12.5 mg of hydrochlorothiazide) and increased gradually. If diuretic therapy alone does not achieve the desired reduction in SBP, a sympathetic inhibitor can be added at low doses with gradual increases. Calcium channel blockers or β blockers should be considered in elderly patients with hypertension and angina, and ACE inhibitors might be preferred for hypertensive patients with CHF. The pharmacologic management of diastolic hypertension in the elderly should be similar to that outlined for isolated systolic hypertension.

Hypertension in African Americans
- Hypertension is more common and more severe in black persons than other races. Differences in electrolyte homeostasis, glomerular filtration rate, sodium excretion and transport mechanisms, plasma renin activity, and blood pressure response to plasma volume expansion have been noted.
- Supplemental potassium and calcium have both been shown to cause a modest reduction in blood pressure in some studies.
- The lower plasma renin activity and increased blood pressure response to sodium and fluid loading observed suggest a more sodium- and volume-dependent hypertension. Black individuals are hyperresponsive to diuretic therapy; therefore, diuretics are usually recommended as initial treatment.
- If diuretic therapy alone does not provide adequate control, addition of a sympathetic inhibitor is appropriate. Diuretic therapy combined with β blockers or ACE inhibitors is equally efficacious in hypertensive blacks and whites.
- Calcium channel antagonists are as effective as diuretics for initial treatment and provide an alternative that may be preferable under certain conditions.

Hypertension with Diabetes Mellitus
- Diuretics and β blockers generally should be avoided in diabetic hypertensive patients because they cause insulin resistance and glucose intolerance. β blockers also mask most of the signs and symptoms of hypoglycemia (tremor, tachycardia, palpitations), delay recovery from hypoglycemia, and may produce elevations in blood pressure due to vasoconstriction caused by unopposed α-receptor stimulation during the hypoglycemic recovery phase.
- The α_1 antagonists may increase the risk of orthostatic hypotension, and the α_2 agonists may cause a paradoxical increase in blood pressure. These effects appear to be due to a more sensitive autonomic nervous system in patients with diabetic neuropathy.

- ACE inhibitors may increase insulin sensitivity and provide renal protective effects. Thus these agents may be considered the preferred pharmacologic treatment of hypertension in the diabetic subject. However, hyperkalemia may occur in diabetic patients with type 4 renal tubular acidosis or in any diabetic on potassium supplements or potassium-sparing diuretics.

II

Hypertension with Hyperlipidemia

- Because hyperlipidemia compounds the risk of coronary artery disease, it should be effectively managed or prevented in hypertensive patients.
- Thiazide diuretics and β blockers without ISA or α-blocking properties may affect serum lipids adversely, although it is controversial whether the effect persists over time. It may be prudent to avoid diuretics and β blockers in hypertensive patients with hyperlipidemia and to consider alternative agents in patients who develop lipid abnormalities while on diuretics or β blockers.

Hypertension and Coronary Artery Disease

- For hypertensive patients with ischemic heart disease, β blockers and calcium channel antagonists lower blood pressure and reduce myocardial oxygen demand. The cardiac stimulation that may occur with nifedipine or β blockers with ISA, however, may make these agents less desirable in this clinical setting.
- Reducing the DBP excessively may compromise coronary perfusion, especially in patients with fixed coronary artery stenosis, and lead to myocardial infarction (MI).
- For secondary prevention of infarction in hypertensive patients, calcium channel blockers do not afford the same degree of benefit as β blockers. Diltiazem has been shown to reduce reinfarction in patients with non–Q-wave infarcts and may reduce cardiac events in post-MI patients who do not have CHF.

Hypertension and Congestive Heart Failure

- In patients with CHF, captopril, enalapril, and ramipril have been shown to improve symptomatology and reduce mortality. Because of the high renin and angiotensin II status of patients with CHF, therapy should be initiated at low doses to avoid a profound drop in blood pressure.
- A β-blocker or nondihydropyridine calcium channel antagonist may improve left ventricular filling and cardiac output in patients with reduced cardiac output due to diastolic dysfunction. However, these agents may worsen CHF in patients with systolic decompensation.

Hypertensive Urgencies and Emergencies

- Hypertensive urgencies may be treated effectively with oral loading with:
  - Clonidine, with 0.2 mg given initially followed by 0.1 mg hourly until the DBP falls below 110 mm Hg or a total of 0.7 mg has been administered; a single dose may be sufficient.

II

- Nifedipine, by having the patient swallow a perforated capsule.
- Captopril, with doses of 25–50 mg given at 1- to 2-hour intervals.
- Hypertensive emergencies must be treated aggressively immediately to salvage viable tissue. DBP should not be lowered below 100–110 mm Hg over several minutes to several hours depending on the clinical situation. Precipitous drops in blood pressure to the normotensive range or lower may lead to end-organ ischemia or infarction. After the goal DBP is reached, treatment should be designed to hold that level of pressure for several days to allow physiologic adjustments in autoregulatory function. Then the blood pressure can be further reduced to normotensive levels.
- Nitroprusside is usually given as a continuous IV infusion at a rate of 0.5–8.0 μg/kg/min. Its onset of hypotensive action is immediate and its effect disappears within 2–5 minutes of discontinuation of the infusion. When the infusion must be continued longer than 72 hours, serum thiocyanate levels should be measured, and the infusion should be discontinued if the level exceeds 12 mg/dL. The risk of thiocyanate toxicity is increased in patients with impaired renal function. Other side effects of nitroprusside include fatigue, nausea, anorexia, disorientation, psychotic behavior, muscle spasms, and, rarely, hypothyroidism. Nitroprusside administration requires constant intra-arterial pressure monitoring.
- IV nitroglycerin may be given at a rate of 5–100 μg/min. As with oral nitrates, IV nitroglycerin is associated with tolerance over 24–48 hours.
- Diazoxide given in small IV bolus doses (50–100 mg every 5–10 minutes) or by slow IV infusion over 15–30 minutes avoids the precipitous fall in pressure that occurs when given as a 300-mg rapid IV bolus. Because diazoxide increases plasma volume, it is common practice to give a diuretic concurrently unless the patient is volume depleted. Diazoxide has quick onset and a duration of action ranging from 4–12 hours. It occasionally causes overshoot hypotension, which can be reversed by pressor agents. Other side effects include nausea, vomiting, tachycardia, hyperglycemia, and hyperuricemia.
- Trimethaphan camsylate is a ganglionic blocking agent that is particularly useful for treating hypertension in patients with acute aortic dissection. It is administered by continuous IV infusion with constant or frequent intra-arterial pressure monitoring at an initial infusion rate of 1 mg/min; the dose can be adjusted up to 10 mg/min. Its onset of action is immediate and its effects disappear within 10 minutes of discontinuation. Trimethaphan may cause profound orthostatic hypotension, ileus, urinary retention, dry mouth, and visual impairment. Respiratory arrest has been reported at infusion rates greater than 5 mg/min.
- Labetolol may be given at an initial dose of 20 mg by slow IV injection over a 2-minute period, followed by repeated injections of 40–80 mg at 10-minute intervals, up to a total dose of 300 mg. It can also be

administered by continuous infusion at an initial rate of 2 mg/min and adjusted according to blood pressure response. Because of its α-blocking effects, labetolol can cause orthostatic hypotension. Other side effects include nausea, vomiting, paresthesias, sweating, dizziness, flushing, and headaches.

- Hydralazine may be given intravenously by diluting 10–20 mg in 20 mL of 5% dextrose in water (D$_5$W) and administering it at a rate of 0.5–1.0 mL/min. Its onset of action ranges from 10–30 minutes and its effects last 2–4 hours. Because the hypotensive response is less predictable than with other parenteral agents, its major role is in the treatment of eclampsia or hypertensive encephalopathy associated with renal insufficiency.
- Nicardipine IV may be administered for short-term treatment of hypertension using doses of 5–15 mg/h, which is adjusted by 1–2.5 mg/h after 15 minutes. Headaches, nausea, and vomiting are common side effects, and the use of the agent increases heart rate by 8–18 beats per minute.

See Chapter 12, Hypertension, authored by David W. Hawkins, PharmD, Henry I. Bussey, PharmD, and L. Michael Prisant, MD, for a more detailed discussion of this topic.

Chapter 10

► ISCHEMIC HEART DISEASE

► DEFINITION

Ischemic heart disease (IHD) is defined as a lack of oxygen and decreased or no blood flow in the myocardium. The disease results from coronary artery narrowing or obstruction and is manifested as the clinical syndrome of angina pectoris. IHD has many clinical expressions including stable exertional angina; unstable (rest, preinfarction, crescendo) angina; silent myocardial ischemia; acute coronary insufficiency; coronary vasomotion or vasospasm associated with atypical, variant, or Prinzmetal's angina; and myocardial infarction (MI).

► PATHOPHYSIOLOGY

- The major determinants of myocardial oxygen demand (MVo_2) are heart rate, contractility, and intramyocardial wall tension. Wall tension is thought to be the most important factor. Because the consequences of IHD usually result from increased demand in the face of a fixed oxygen supply, alterations in MVo_2 are important as a cause of and as an intervention intended to alleviate it.
- A clinically useful indirect estimate of MVo_2 is the double product (DP), which is heart rate (HR) multiplied by systolic blood pressure (SBP) (DP = HR × SBP). The DP does not consider changes in contractility (an independent variable), and because only changes in pressure are considered, volume loading of the left ventricle and increased MVo_2 related to ventricular dilation are underestimated.
- MVo_2 and the caliber of the resistance vessels delivering blood to the myocardium are the prime determinants in the occurrence of ischemia.
- The normal coronary system consists of large epicardial or surface vessels (R_1) that offer little resistance to myocardial flow and intramyocardial arteries and arterioles (R_2), which branch into a dense capillary network to supply basal blood. Under normal circumstances, the resistance in R_2 is much greater than that in R_1. Myocardial blood flow is inversely related to arteriolar resistance and directly related to the coronary driving pressure.
- Atherosclerotic lesions occluding R_1 increase arteriolar resistance, and R_2 can vasodilate to maintain coronary blood flow. With greater degrees of obstruction, this response is inadequate, and the coronary flow reserve afforded by R_2 vasodilation is insufficient to meet oxygen demand. Relatively severe stenosis (80–85%) may provoke ischemia and symptoms at rest while less severe stenosis may allow a reserve of coronary blood flow for exertion.
- The diameter and length of obstructing lesions and the influence of pressure drop across an area of stenosis affect coronary blood flow and

function of the collateral circulation. Dynamic coronary obstruction can occur in normal vessels and vessels with stenosis in which vasomotion or spasm may be superimposed on a fixed stenosis. Persisting ischemia may promote growth of developed collateral blood flow.

- Critical stenosis occurs when the obstructing lesion encroaches on the luminal diameter and exceeds 70–80%. Lesions creating obstruction of 50–70% may reduce blood flow, but these obstructions are not consistent, and vasospasm and thrombosis superimposed on a "noncritical" lesion may lead to clinical events such as MI. If the lesion enlarges from 80 to 90%, resistance in that vessel is tripled. Coronary reserve is diminished at about 85% obstruction due to vasoconstriction.

- Abnormalities of ventricular contraction can occur, and regional loss of contractility may impose a burden on the remaining myocardial tissue, resulting in heart failure, increased MV_{O_2}, and rapid depletion of oxygen stores. Zones of tissue with marginal blood flow may develop that are at risk for more severe damage, if the ischemic episode persists or becomes more severe. Nonischemic areas of myocardium may compensate for the severely ischemic and border zones of ischemia by developing more tension than usual in an attempt to maintain cardiac output. Changes at the cellular level may impair the association of actin and myosin. The left or right ventricular dysfunction that ensues may be associated with clinical findings of an S_3, dyspnea, orthopnea, tachycardia, fluctuating blood pressure, transient murmurs, and mitral or tricuspid regurgitation.

▶ CLINICAL PRESENTATION

- The classic symptoms associated with typical chest pain and angina due to IHD appear in Table 10.1. For some patients, the presenting symptoms due to ischemia differ from the classical symptoms, and these are referred to as anginal equivalents.

- Patients suffering from variant or Prinzmetal's angina secondary to coronary spasm are more likely to experience pain at rest and in the early morning hours. Pain is not usually brought on by exertion or emotional stress nor relieved by rest; the electrocardiogram (ECG) pattern is that of current of injury with ST elevation rather than depression.

- Unstable angina is generally defined as the presence of one or more of the following: (1) new onset (<2 months) exertional angina resulting in marked limitations of ordinary physical activity; (2) recent (<2 months) acceleration of angina as reflected by an increase in severity; or (3) pain at rest which lasts for >20 minutes.

- Ischemia may also be painless or "silent" in many patients. Silent ischemia is more common in diabetic patients, perhaps due to neuropathy and inability to sense pain.

TABLE 10.1. Characteristics of Angina Pectoris

II

Quality

Sensation of pressure or heavy weight on the chest
Burning sensation
Feeling of tightness
Shortness of breath with feeling of constriction about the larynx or upper trachea
Visceral quality (deep, heavy, squeezing, aching)
Gradual increase in intensity followed by gradual fading away

Location

Over the sternum or very near to it
Anywhere between epigastrium and pharynx
Occasionally limited to left shoulder and left arm
Rarely limited to right arm
Limited to lower jaw
Lower cervical or upper thoracic spine
Left interscapular or suprascapular area

Duration

0.5–30 minutes

Precipitating Factors

Relationship to exercise
Effort that involves use of arms above the head
Cold environment
Walking against the wind
Walking after a large meal
Emotional factors involved with physical exercise
Fright, anger
Coitus

Nitroglycerin Relief

Relief of pain occurring within 45 seconds to 5 minutes of taking nitroglycerin

Radiation

Medial aspect of left arm
Left shoulder
Jaw
Occasionally right arm

From Helfant RH, Banka VS. A Clinical and Angiographic Approach to Coronary Heart Disease. Philadelphia, FA Davis, 1978:47, with permission.

▶ DIAGNOSIS

- Important aspects of the clinical history include the nature or quality of the chest pain, precipitating factors, duration, pain radiation, and the response to nitroglycerin or rest. There appears to be little relationship between the historical features of angina and the severity or extent of coronary artery vessel involvement. Ischemic chest pain may resemble pain arising from a variety of noncardiac sources, and the differential diagnosis of anginal pain from other etiologies may be difficult based on history alone.

II

- The patient should be asked about major risk factors for coronary disease, including smoking and a family history of coronary artery disease (CAD), familial lipid disorders, and diabetes mellitus.

- There are few signs on physical examination to indicate the presence of CAD. Findings on the cardiac examination may include abnormal precordial systolic bulge, decreased intensity of S_1, paradoxical splitting of S_2, S_3 (ventricular gallop), S_4 (atrial gallop), apical systolic murmur, and diastolic murmur. Elevated heart rate or blood pressure can yield an increased DP and may be associated with angina. Other noncardiac physical findings suggesting that significant cardiovascular disease may be present include abdominal aortic aneurysms or peripheral vascular disease.

- Other than risk-factor screening (lipid profiling, fasting glucose to exclude diabetes), there are no specific laboratory tests that are useful in diagnosing CAD. Cardiac enzymes should be normal in the angina patient.

- The ECG is normal in about one-half of patients with angina who are not experiencing an acute attack. Typical ST-T wave changes include depression, T-wave inversion, and ST-segment elevation. Variant angina is associated with ST-segment elevation, whereas silent ischemia may produce elevation or depression. Significant ischemia is associated with ST-segment depression of >2 mm, exertional hypotension, and reduced exercise tolerance.

- Exercise tolerance (stress) testing (ETT) is useful for a history of chest pain that is equivocal, for risk stratification, implementation of medical versus surgical therapy, and to assess the efficacy of treatment. Ischemic ST depression that occurs during ETT is an independent risk factor for cardiac events and cardiovascular mortality. Thallium (^{201}Tl) myocardial perfusion scintigraphy may be used in conjunction with ETT to detect reversible and irreversible defects in blood flow to the myocardium.

- Radionuclide angiocardiography (performed with technetium-99m, a radioisotope) is used to measure ejection fraction (EF), regional ventricular performance, cardiac output, ventricular volumes, valvular regurgitation, asynchrony or wall motion abnormalities, and intracardiac shunts.

- Echocardiography is useful for direct visualization of lesions in the left main coronary artery and in detecting the presence of ventricular aneurysms, assessing EF, and detecting regional or global left ventricular (LV) function abnormalities that occur during ischemia episodes.

- Ambulatory ECG (Holter) monitoring is useful in detecting ischemia during symptomatic and asymptomatic episodes and provides information for an extended period of time.

- Cardiac catheterization and angiography in patients with suspected CAD are used diagnostically to document the presence and severity of disease as well as for prognostic purposes.

▶ DESIRED OUTCOME

The goals of treatment are to relieve the patient's symptoms, maintain functional capacity, minimize adverse effects of treatment, and prevent progression to MI.

▶ TREATMENT

MODIFICATION OF RISK FACTORS

- Primary prevention through the identification and modification of risk factors should result in a significant impact on the prevalence of IHD. Secondary intervention is effective in reducing subsequent morbidity and mortality.
- Risk factors are additive and can be classified as alterable or unalterable. Unalterable risk factors include gender, age, family history or genetic composition, environmental influences, and, to some extent, diabetes mellitus. Risk factors that can be altered include smoking, hypertension, hyperlipidemia, obesity, sedentary lifestyle, hyperuricemia, psychosocial factors such as stress and type A behavior patterns, and the use of certain drugs that may be detrimental including progestins, corticosteroids, cyclosporine, thiazide diuretics, and β blockers. Although thiazide diuretics and β blockers (nonselective without intrinsic sympathomimetic activity) may elevate both cholesterol and triglycerides by 10–20%, and these effects may be detrimental, no objective evidence exists from prospective well-controlled studies to support avoiding these drugs.
- Alcohol ingestion in small to moderate amounts (<40 g/d of pure ethanol) reduces the risk of CAD; however, consumption of large amounts (>50 g/d) or binge drinking of alcohol are associated with increased mortality from stroke, malignant neoplasms, and cirrhosis.

DRUG THERAPY

Nitrates

- The major mechanism of action of nitrates appears to be mediated indirectly through a reduction of myocardial oxygen demand secondary to venodilation and arterial–arteriolar dilation, leading to a reduction in wall stress from reduced ventricular volume and pressure (Table 10.2). Direct actions on the coronary circulation include dilation of large and small intramural coronary arteries, collateral dilation, coronary artery stenosis dilation, abolition of normal tone in narrowed vessels, and relief of spasm.

TABLE 10.2. Effect of Drug Therapy on Myocardial Oxygen Demand[a]

| | Heart Rate | Myocardial Contractility | LV Wall Tension | |
			Systolic Pressure	*LV Volume*
Nitrates	↑	0	↓	↓↓
β Blockers	↓↓	↓	↓	↑
Nifedipine	↑	0 or ↓	↓↓	0 or ↓
Verapamil	↓	↓	↓	0 or ↓
Diltiazem	↓↓	0 or ↓	↓	0 or ↓

Key: LV, left ventricular.
[a]Calcium channel antagonists and nitrates may also increase myocardial oxygen supply through coronary vasodilation. Diastolic function may also be improved with verapamil, nifedipine, and, perhaps, diltiazem. These effects may vary from those indicated in the table depending on individual patient baseline hemodynamics.

- Nitrate therapy may be used to terminate an acute anginal attack, prevent effort- or stress-induced attacks, or for long-term prophylaxis. Sublingual, buccal, or spray nitroglycerin products are the treatment of choice for the alleviation of anginal attacks because of rapid absorption (Table 10.3). Prevention of symptoms may be accomplished by the prophylactic use of oral or transdermal products, but the development of tolerance may be problematic.

TABLE 10.3. Nitrate Products

Product	Onset (min)	Duration	Initial Dose
Nitroglycerin			
IV	1–2	3–5 min	5 μg
SL/lingual	1–3	30–60 min	0.3 mg
PO	40	3–6 h	2.5–9 mg TID
Ointment	20–60	2–8 h	0.5–1 inch
Patch	40–60	>8 h	1 patch
Erythritol tetranitrate	5–30	4–6 h	5–10 mg TID
Penterythritol tetranitrate	30	4–8 h	10–20 mg TID
Isosorbide dinitrate			
SL/chewable	2–5	1–2 h	2.5–5 mg TID
PO	20–40	4–6 h	5–20 mg TID
Isosorbide mononitrate	30–60	6–8 h	20 mg QD, BID[a]

[a]Product dependent.

- Sublingual nitroglycerin 0.3–0.4 mg relieves pain in about 75% of patients within 3 minutes, with another 15% becoming pain free in 5–15 minutes. Pain persisting beyond about 20–30 minutes after the use of two or three nitroglycerin tablets is suggestive of evolving MI or unstable angina, and the patient should be instructed to seek emergency aid.

- Chewable, oral, and transdermal products are acceptable for the long-term prophylaxis of angina; dosing of the longer acting preparations should be adjusted to provide a hemodynamic response. This may require doses of oral isosorbide dinatrate (ISDN) ranging from 10–60 mg as often as every 3–4 hours due to tolerance or first-pass metabolism. Intermittent (12 hours on, 12 hours off) transdermal nitroglycerin therapy has been shown to produce modest but significant improvement in exercise time in chronic stable angina. Because nitrates work primarily through a reduction in MVo_2, the DP can be used to optimize the dose of sublingual and oral nitrate products.

- Nitrates may be combined with other drugs with complementary mechanisms of action for chronic prophylactic therapy. Combination therapy is generally used in patients with more severe symptoms that do not respond to nitrates alone (nitrates plus β blockers or calcium channel blockers) and in patients having an element of vasospasm leading to decreased supply (nitrates plus calcium channel blockers).

- Pharmacokinetic characteristics common to nitrates include a large first-pass effect of hepatic metabolism, short to very short half-lives (except for isosorbide mononitrate [ISMN]), large volumes of distribution, high clearance rates, and large interindividual variations in plasma or blood concentrations. The half-life of nitroglycerin is 1–5 minutes regardless of route, hence the potential advantage of sustained-release and transdermal products. ISDN is metabolized to isosorbide 2 mono- and 5-mononitrate (ISMN). ISMN has a half-life of about 5 hours and may be given once or twice daily depending on the product chosen.

- Patients should be instructed to keep nitroglycerin in the original, tightly closed glass container and to avoid mixing with other medication. Patients should also be aware that enhanced venous pooling in the sitting or standing positions may improve the effect as well as the symptoms of postural hypotension.

- Adverse reactions include postural hypotension, reflex tachycardia, headaches and flushing, and occasional nausea. Excessive hypotension may result in MI or stroke. Noncardiovascular adverse effects include rash (especially with transdermal nitroglycerin) and methemoglobinemia with high doses given for extended periods.

- Because both the onset and offset of tolerance to nitrates occurs quickly, one dosing strategy to circumvent it is to provide a daily nitrate-free interval of 8 to 12 hours. ISDN, for example, should not be used more often than three times per day if tolerance is to be avoided.

β-Adrenergic Blocking Agents

- Decreased heart rate, decreased contractility, and a slight to moderate decrease in blood pressure with β-adrenergic receptor antagonism reduce MVo_2. The overall effect in patients with effort-induced angina is a reduction in oxygen demand. β blockers do not improve oxygen supply and, in certain instances, unopposed α-adrenergic stimulation may lead to coronary vasoconstriction.

- β blockers improve symptoms in about 80% of patients with chronic exertional stable angina, and objective measures of efficacy demonstrate improved exercise duration and delay in the time at which ST-segment changes and initial or limiting symptoms occur. β blockade may allow angina patients previously limited by symptoms to perform more exercise and ultimately improve overall cardiovascular performance through a training effect.

- Postacute MI patients with angina are particularly good candidates for β blockade because of a reduced risk of reinfarction. A beneficial effect on mortality has been demonstrated with timolol, propranolol, and metoprolol. Patients with preexisting LV dysfunction may receive digitalis glycosides to maintain cardiac output if β blockade is necessary for IHD.

- β blockade is effective in chronic exertional angina as monotherapy and in combination with nitrates and/or calcium channel antagonists. β blockers are frequently added to nitrate therapy in patients with inadequate control of symptoms because of their complementary mechanism of action, relatively low cost, and general tolerability. β-blockers also blunt the reflex tachycardia from nitrate therapy. Patients with severe angina, rest angina, or variant angina may be better treated with nitrates or calcium channel antagonists.

- Initial doses of β blockers should be at the lower end of the usual dosing range and titrated to response. General guidelines include the objective of lowering resting heart rate to 50 to 60 beats per minute and limiting maximal exercise heart rate to about 100 beats per minute or less. Heart rate with modest exercise should be no more than about 20 beats per minute above resting heart rate (or a 10% increment over resting heart rate).

- There is little evidence to suggest superiority of any particular β blocker. Those with longer half-lives may be dosed less frequently, but even propranolol may be dosed twice a day in most patients with angina. The ancillary property of intrinsic sympathomimetic activity appears to be detrimental in patients with rest or severe angina because the reduction in heart rate would be minimized, therefore limiting a reduction in MVo_2. Cardioselective β blockers may be used in some patients to minimize adverse effects such as bronchospasm. Combined nonselective β and α blockade with labetolol may be useful in some patients with marginal LV reserve.

- Adverse effects associated with β blockade include hypotension, heart failure, bradycardia and heart block, bronchospasm, peripheral vasoconstriction and intermittent claudication, and altered glucose metabolism. Central nervous system adverse effects include fatigue, malaise, and depression. Abrupt withdrawal of therapy in patients with angina has been associated with increased severity and number of pain episodes and MI. Tapering of therapy in the course of 2 days should minimize the risk of withdrawal reactions if therapy is to be discontinued.

Calcium Channel Antagonists

- Direct actions of the calcium antagonists include vasodilation of systemic arterioles and coronary arteries leading to a reduction of arterial pressure and coronary vascular resistance as well as depression of the myocardial contractility and conduction velocity of the SA and AV nodes (Table 10.2). Reflex β-adrenergic stimulation overcomes much of the negative inotropic effect, and depression of contractility becomes clinically apparent only in the presence of LV dysfunction and when other negative inotropic drugs are used concurrently.

- Verapamil and diltiazem cause less peripheral vasodilation than nifedipine and, consequently, the risk of myocardial depression is greater with these two agents. Conduction through the AV node is predictably depressed with verapamil and to some extent with diltiazem, and they must be used with caution in patients with preexisting conduction abnormalities or in the presence of other drugs with negative chronotropic properties.

- MV_{O_2} is reduced with use of all the calcium channel antagonists primarily because of reduced wall tension secondary to reduced arterial pressure. Overall, the benefit provided by calcium channel antagonists is related to reduced MV_{O_2} rather than improved oxygen supply.

- In contrast to the β blockers, calcium channel antagonists have the potential to improve coronary blood flow through areas of fixed coronary obstruction by inhibiting coronary artery vasomotion and vasospasm.

- Additional product information on calcium channel antagonists is provided in Chapter 9.

Management of Stable Exertional Angina Pectoris

- After assessing and manipulating alterable risk factors, a regular exercise program should be undertaken in a graduated fashion and with adequate supervision to improve cardiovascular and muscular fitness.

- Nitrate therapy should be the first step in managing acute attacks for patients with chronic stable angina. If angina occurs no more often than once every few days, then sublingual nitroglycerin or the spray or buccal products may be sufficient.

- For episodes of "first-effort" angina occurring in a predictable fashion, nitroglycerin may be used in a prophylactic manner with the patient taking 0.3–0.4 mg sublingually about 5 minutes prior to the anticipated time of activity. Nitroglycerin spray may be useful when inadequate saliva is produced to rapidly dissolve sublingual nitroglycerin or if a patient has difficulty opening the container. The response usually lasts about 30 minutes.

- When angina occurs more than once a day, a chronic prophylactic regimen using nitrates or β blockers should be considered. Long-acting forms of nitroglycerin (oral or transdermal), ISDN, ISMN, and pentaerythritol trinitrate may be effective. A nitrate-free interval of 8 hours per day or longer should be provided to maintain efficacy. Dose titration should be based on changes in the DP. The choice among nitrate products should be based on familiarity with the preparation, cost, and patient acceptance.

- Chronic prophylactic therapy may also be instituted with β-adrenergic blocking agents; they may be preferable in some situations because of less frequent dosing and other desirable pharmacologic properties (e.g., potential cardioprotective effects, antiarrhythmic effects, lack of tolerance, antihypertensive efficacy). The appropriate dose should be determined by the goals outlined for heart rate and DP. An agent should be selected that is well tolerated by individual patients at a reasonable cost. Patients most likely to respond well to β blockade are those with a high resting heart rate and those with a relatively fixed anginal threshold (i.e., their symptoms appear at the same level of exercise or workload on a consistent basis).

- Calcium channel antagonists have the potential advantage of improving coronary blood flow through coronary artery vasodilation as well as decreasing MVo_2 and may be used instead of β blockers for chronic prophylactic therapy. They are as effective as β blockers and are most useful in patients who have a variable threshold for exertional angina, which suggests fluctuations in myocardial oxygen supply that may be due to coronary artery vasomotion. Calcium antagonists may provide better skeletal muscle oxygenation, resulting in decreased fatigue and better exercise tolerance. They can be used safely in many patients with contraindications to β blocker therapy. Nifedipine, verapamil, and diltiazem have similar efficacy in the management of chronic stable angina. Patients with conduction abnormalities and moderate to severe LV dysfunction (EF <35%) should be treated cautiously with verapamil. Diltiazem has significant effects on the AV node and can produce heart block in patients with preexisting conduction disease or when other drugs with effects on conduction (e.g., digoxin, β blockers) are used concurrently. Nifedipine may cause excessive heart rate elevation, especially if the patient is not receiving a β blocker, and this may offset its beneficial effect on MVo_2. The hemodynamic effect of calcium antagonists is complementary to β blockade and, consequently, combination therapy is rational. Because both β blockers and calcium antagonists have the potential for depressing contractility, this combination should be used with care in patients with poor ventricular function.

MANAGEMENT OF UNSTABLE ANGINA PECTORIS (Figure 10.1)

- Precipitation of the acute ischemic syndromes of unstable angina and MI are thought to be due to progression of atherosclerosis, acute coronary thrombosis, coronary artery spasm, and platelet aggregation. Patients at high risk of death or nonfatal MI are those presenting with prolonged ongoing (>20 minutes) rest pain, pulmonary edema related to ischemia, angina at rest with dynamic ST changes of ≥1 mm, angina with new or worsening mitral regurgitation, S_3 or rales, and angina with hypotension. Unstable angina differs from stable angina in that the primary event is thought to be a reduction in coronary blood flow rather than an increase in MV_{O_2}.
- Initial patient management should include history, physical examination, ECG (within 20 minutes), bed rest with continuous monitoring for ischemia and arrhythmia detection, supplemental oxygen if cyanotic or hypoxemic, and immediate consideration of the use of aspirin, heparin, β blockers, and narcotics (if pain is not relieved by nitrates and β blockers).
- Aspirin should be dosed at 160–325 mg, and heparin is given as an IV bolus of 80 units/kg followed by a continuous IV infusion of 18 units/kg/h to maintain the activated partial thromboplastin time at 1.5–2.5 times control and continued for 2–5 days or until revascularization is performed.
- Thrombolysis is not indicated in patients who do not have evidence of acute ST-segment elevation or left bundle branch block on ECG.
- Long-term antiplatelet therapy with aspirin in doses ranging from 324–1300 mg/day has been shown to reduce the occurrence of mortality and nonfatal infarction in unstable angina by about 50%. Ticlopidine (250 mg two times per day) may be considered in patients with aspirin hypersensitivity or recent major gastrointestinal bleeding.
- If three doses of sublingual nitroglycerin do not relieve the patient's pain, then IV nitroglycerin may be initiated at low doses (5–10 μg/kg/min) and titrated upward by 10 μg/min every 5–10 minutes until symptoms are relieved or limiting adverse effects occur. A reduction in SBP is expected and should be about 15 mm Hg or to a systolic pressure of 100–110 mm Hg. After 24 hours free of symptoms, patients may be switched over to oral or topical nitrates.
- IV β blockers are recommended for high-risk patients (oral for intermediate- and low-risk patients) in the absence of contraindications. β blockers in unstable angina reduce the risk of progression to MI by 13% but have not been shown to reduce mortality. Regimens are similar to those used in acute MI.
- Unstable patients with persisting or recurring pain while on nitrates and β blockers should receive a calcium channel antagonist. Calcium antagonists may be added to nitrates and β blockers, and some authors suggest that they are most useful in combination with pretreatment β blockade. Nifedipine should not be used in the absence of concurrent β blockade. Diltiazem may be more useful than other agents in the setting

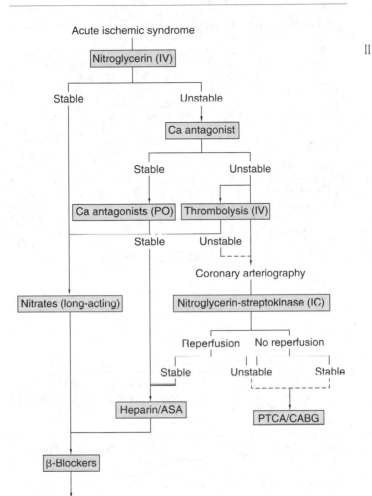

Figure 10.1. Therapeutic guidelines for managing patients who present with acute ischemic syndromes. ASA, acetylsalicylic acid; CABG, coronary artery bypass graft; IC, intracoronary; IV, intravenous; PO, orally; PTCA, percutaneous transluminal coronary angioplasty. *(From Epstein SE, Palmeri ST. Am J Cardiol 1984;54:1250, with permission.)*

II

of unstable angina and non–Q-wave MI because it has been shown to reduce reinfarction and refractory angina.

- Cardiac catheterization should be considered in the following groups of patients: (1) patients with prior angioplasty, bypass surgery, or MI; (2) patients who fail to stabilize on medical therapy; (3) patients opting for early invasive strategy (coronary artery bypass graft [CABG] or percutaneous transluminal coronary angioplasty [PTCA]); (4) patients with high-risk clinical findings or noninvasive test results; or (5) patients with significant congestive heart failure (CHF) or LV dysfunction.

- CABG is recommended for patients found to have ≥50% occlusion of the left main artery or ≥70% three-vessel disease with depressed LV function (EF <0.50). Patients with two-vessel disease with proximal LAD stenosis ≥95% and depressed LV function should be referred promptly for CABG or PTCA. Patients with significant CAD who fail to stabilize on medical therapy or have symptoms with low levels of exertion or have ischemia accompanied by CHF should have prompt revascularization.

- If cardiac catheterization is not indicated, noninvasive exercise or pharmacologic stress testing should be performed in low- and intermediate-risk patients who have been free of angina and CHF for 48 hours.

- In the event of prolonged chest pain and ischemic ECG changes unrelieved by nitrate therapy or calcium channel antagonists, one may assume total occlusion of a coronary vessel and steps should be taken to restore blood flow (e.g., thrombolytic therapy either alone or preceding PTCA).

CORONARY ARTERY SPASM AND VARIANT ANGINA PECTORIS

- All patients should be treated for acute attacks and maintained on prophylactic treatment for 6–12 months following the initial episode. Aggravating factors such as alcohol and cigarette smoking should be eliminated.

- Nitrates are the mainstay of therapy, and most patients respond rapidly to sublingual nitroglycerin or ISDN. IV and intracoronary nitroglycerin may be very useful for patients not responding to sublingual preparations.

- Chronic nitrate therapy has not been investigated extensively in variant angina; however, ISDN in doses of 40–120 (mean 65 mg/d) has been shown to decrease anginal frequency.

- Because calcium channel antagonists may be more effective, have few serious adverse effects in effective doses, and can be given less frequently than nitrates, some consider them the agents of choice for variant angina. Nifedipine, verapamil, and diltiazem are all equally effective as single agents for the initial management of variant angina and coronary artery spasm. In patients unresponsive to calcium channel antagonists alone, nitrates may be added. Combination therapy with nifedipine plus diltiazem or nifedipine plus verapamil has been reported to be useful in patients unresponsive to single-drug regimens.

- β blockers have little or no role in the management of variant angina, as they may induce coronary vasoconstriction and prolong ischemia as documented by continuous ECG monitoring.
- The effects of aspirin in variant angina have not been as successful as in unstable angina, perhaps reflecting differences in the underlying pathophysiology.

▶ EVALUATION OF THERAPEUTIC OUTCOMES

- Subjective measures of drug response include the number of painful episodes, amount of rapid-acting nitroglycerin consumed, and patient-reported alterations in activities of daily living (e.g., time to walk two blocks, number of stairs climbed without pain).
- Objective clinical measures of response include HR, blood pressure, and the DP as a measure of MVO_2. Nitrates may increase HR but lower SBP, whereas calcium channel blockers and β blockers reduce the DP.
- Objective assessment also includes the resolution of ECG changes at rest, during exercise, or with ambulatory ECG monitoring.
- Monitoring for major adverse effects includes headache and dizziness with nitrates; fatigue and lassitude with β blockers; and peripheral edema, constipation, and dizziness with the calcium channel blockers.
- The ECG is very useful, particularly if the patient is experiencing chest pain or other symptoms thought to be of ischemic origin. ST-segment deviations are very important, and the extent of their deviation is related to the severity of ischemia.
- ETT may also be used to evaluate the response to therapy, but the expense and time needed to perform this test precludes routine use.
- Cardiac catheterization, radionuclide scans, and echocardiography are used primarily for risk stratification and selecting patients for more invasive procedures rather than for monitoring therapy.
- A comprehensive plan includes ancillary monitoring of lipid profiles, fasting plasma glucose, thyroid function tests, hemoglobin/hematocrit, and electrolytes.
- For variant angina, reduction in symptoms and nitroglycerin consumption as documented by a patient diary can assist the interpretation of objective data obtained from ambulatory ECG recordings. Evidence of efficacy includes the reduction of ischemic events, both ST-segment depression and elevation. Additional evidence is a reduced number of attacks of angina requiring hospitalization, and the absence of MI and sudden death.

See Chapter 14, Ischemic Heart Disease, authored by Robert L. Talbert, PharmD, FCCP, for a more detailed discussion of this topic.

Chapter 11

▶ MYOCARDIAL INFARCTION

▶ DEFINITION

Acute myocardial infarction (MI) results from a sudden interruption of blood supply to an area of myocardium resulting from complete, or near complete, occlusion of a coronary artery. The occlusion persists long enough that myocardial function is compromised and myocardium becomes necrotic (nonviable).

▶ PATHOPHYSIOLOGY

- In many cases, coronary artery disease (CAD) is the primary underlying process that leads to MI. Fatty streaks are deposited on coronary artery endothelium and may progress to form atherosclerotic plaques, depending on the absence or presence of specific risk factors (hypertension, diabetes mellitus, smoking, and hyperlipidemia).
- If progression occurs, plaques develop, proliferate, and eventually disrupt the integrity and function of the endothelium. Myocardial ischemia may occur owing to the narrowing of one or more coronary arteries. However, thrombus formation, not coronary artery narrowing, is believed to be the cause of >85% of acute MIs. The precipitating event is disruption of a coronary plaque, which initiates a thrombotic process.
- The thrombotic process involves activation of platelets, thrombin, and fibrin and subsequently formation of a thrombus, which completely occludes the coronary vessel.
- Infarction is characterized by a "wavefront" of ischemia that progresses from the endocardium to the epicardium. If coronary blood flow is not restored, myocardium dies within approximately 3 hours, based on animal models. Despite this rapid time course, a significant percentage of myocardium is salvageable after as long as 12–24 hours of ischemia, perhaps because of the presence of collateral blood flow within the infarcted area.
- Coronary vasospasm may play a role in and can cause an acute MI, but it is not the primary etiology. Circumstances that may contribute to vasospasm include excessive physical exertion, abrupt exposure to extreme cold, and drugs, specifically catecholamines and cocaine.
- Anterior wall MI (AWMI) involves the anterior wall of the left ventricle and most often represents occlusion of the left anterior descending (LAD) artery (Figure 11.1). AWMI involves a much larger area of myocardium than inferior wall MI (IWMI) and, consequently, there is a risk of a greater loss of myocardium and myocardial function.
- Although isolated right ventricular infarction accounts for <3% of all acute MIs, infarction of the right ventricle occurs in nearly 50% of the

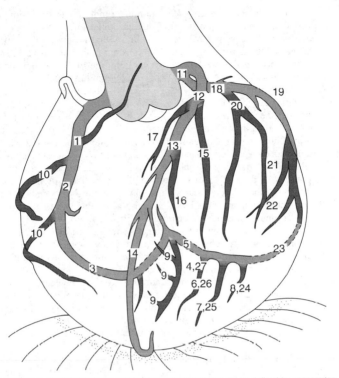

Figure 11.1. Coronary artery anatomy visualized at angiography, as defined by cooperating centers in the Coronary Artery Surgery Study. (1) Proximal right, (2) midright, (3) distal right, (4) right posterior descending, (5) right posterior lateral segment, (6) first right posterior lateral, (7) second right posterior lateral, (8) third right posterior lateral, (9) inferior septal, (10) acute marginal, (11) left main, (12) proximal left anterior descending, (13) mid left anterior descending, (14) distal left anterior descending, (15) first diagonal, (16) second diagonal, (17) first septal, (18) proximal circumflex, (19) distal circumflex, (20) first obtuse marginal, (21) second obtuse marginal, (22) third obtuse marginal, (23) left atrioventricular, (24) first left posterior lateral, (25) second left posterior lateral, (26) third left posterior lateral, (27) left posterior descending. *(From the Principal Investigators of CASS and their associates. The National Heart, Lung, and Blood Institute coronary artery surgery study (CASS). Circulation 1981;62(suppl I):I-1, with permission.)*

patients with IWMI. In many patients, the right coronary artery (RCA) is a large, dominant vessel that not only supplies the right ventricle but also supplies a significant portion of inferior wall of the left ventricle. Therefore, occlusion of the RCA may result in an IWMI or the combination of an IWMI and right ventricular MI, depending on where the

II

occlusion in the RCA occurs. In left dominant individuals, occlusion of the circumflex artery can result in right ventricular infarction.

- A transmural, or Q-wave, MI results in injury that penetrates the entire thickness of the myocardial wall. Nontransmural, or non–Q-wave, MI involves only the subendocardial myocardium; the ECG may not show ST-segment elevation but may only have subtle findings such as T wave inversion, nonspecific ST-T–wave changes, or ST-segment depression.

- Enlargement of the left ventricle plays a critical role in the development of post-MI heart failure and subsequent mortality. The response of the left ventricle to injury (called *ventricular remodeling*) involves activation of neurohumoral and renin–angiotensin systems and the release of vasopressin once a decrease in cardiac output occurs. Sinus tachycardia, mediated by activation of the adrenergic system, occurs first as a response to a drop in cardiac output and, within hours of infarction, expansion of the infarcted area occurs due to thinning and stretching of the infarcted segment. This is followed by acute dilatation and hypertrophy of the noninfarcted myocardium. This initial process precipitates chronic changes in ventricular volume leading to further ventricular dilatation and hypertrophy and eventually the development of left ventricular failure and ultimately, death. Scar formation and healing follow these early events with the entire process taking up to several months.

- Outcome after acute MI depends upon the extent of myocardial damage, left ventricular function, infarct location, the presence or absence of congestive heart failure (CHF), and patient age. Anterior wall infarction tends to be larger and therefore associated with a poorer outcome than inferior wall infarction or right ventricular infarction.

▶ CLINICAL PRESENTATION

- The predominant symptom is chest pain that is frequently described as chest pressure or a squeezing sensation rather than pain. As many as 15–25% of patients with acute MI have no pain, particularly those with diabetes mellitus who may have autonomic dysfunction.

- Physical findings may include diaphoresis, nausea and vomiting, arm tingling/numbness, and shortness of breath.

- Hypotension, clear lung fields, and elevated jugular venous pressure in a patient with an IWMI are indications of right ventricular involvement. Patients with right ventricular MI may present with or quickly develop hemodynamic compromise or cardiogenic shock. Because of right ventricular dysfunction, there is inadequate filling of the left ventricle.

▶ DIAGNOSIS

- Because the clinical presentation cannot differentiate acute MI from other cardiac and noncardiac causes of chest pain, objective criteria (ECG, cardiac enzymes) are needed to confirm the diagnosis.

- The diagnostic ECG feature of acute MI is the Q wave associated with a pattern of prolonged, peaked, or inverted ST-segments. The earliest change in the ECG is associated with the T wave; it may be prolonged, peaked, or inverted. T wave alterations are soon followed by ST-segment elevation. A Q wave may or may not be present on the initial ECG or may appear hours or sometimes days after MI.
- Serial blood samples for the determination of cardiac enzyme concentrations should be obtained every 6–8 hours for 24 hours if MI is suspected. Creatine kinase (CK) concentration peaks within 24 hours after acute MI, followed by a decline and return to baseline by the third or fourth day. There must be an elevation of the total CK with at least a 4% CK-MB isoenzyme fraction to confirm the diagnosis of Q wave MI. The higher the total CK and percent MB, the larger the infarct. Peak lactate dehydrogenase (LDH) concentrations usually occur between 3 and 4 days after MI and return to normal by day 14. The utility of serial LDH determinations is limited; if the patient presents late (beyond 24 hours) from the onset of symptoms, determination of serial LDH concentrations every 6–8 hours may be useful in confirming the diagnosis. Peak concentrations should be at least two times above normal with an increase in the LDH-1 fraction that ultimately exceeds the concentration of the LDH-2 fraction (referred to as the LDH "flip").
- The diagnosis of Q wave acute MI is made if the following criteria are met: the presence of ischemic chest pain for at least 30 minutes and/or ST-segment elevation on the ECG with the subsequent development of significant Q waves. The diagnosis is then confirmed by a rise in cardiac enzymes as described above.

▶ DESIRED OUTCOME

The primary goals of therapy for patients with acute MI are to relieve pain and anxiety, minimize infarct size, salvage ischemic myocardium, prevent or minimize complications, and reduce mortality and improve quality of life.

GENERAL PRINCIPLES

- Admission to an intensive care or coronary care unit is mandatory for close observation and acute care.
- Close monitoring of vital signs, symptoms, and the ECG is recommended for the first 48–72 hours after MI in uncomplicated patients. Continued intensive monitoring is recommended beyond 72 hours if the patient is hemodynamically unstable and has persistent ischemia and/or hemodynamically significant cardiac arrhythmias.
- Activity should be restricted for the first 3–4 days and gradually increased as tolerated by the patient.
- The diet should include use of multiple small meals, sodium restriction, and reduced content of saturated fats and cholesterol.

- A stool softener, either docusate sodium 100 mg or docusate calcium 240 mg once or twice a day, is recommended to avoid the stress associated with defecation.
- If possible, patients with presumed acute MI should have three large-bore (18-gauge) peripheral intravenous (IV) lines placed upon admission to the emergency department to permit prompt drug therapy and facilitate collection of blood for diagnostic tests.
- Pertinent laboratory tests on admission should include CBC with platelet count, activated partial thromboplastin time (aPTT), and prothrombin time (PT). If the patient receives thrombolytic therapy, regular assessment of hemoglobin, hematocrit, and platelets should be obtained.
- For the first few hours of acute MI, supplemental oxygen (2–4 L/min by nasal cannula) should be administered because even uncomplicated patients may be moderately hypoxic.

DRUG THERAPY

Analgesics

- IV morphine sulfate is the drug of choice for acute pain associated with MI. It results in peripheral arteriolar dilation which decreases systemic vascular resistance and reduces myocardial oxygen demand (MVo_2). It also reduces afterload and decreases circulating concentrations of catecholamines, which may reduce the likelihood of ventricular arrhythmias.
- Meperidine and hydromorphone may also be useful for pain relief, but neither has been shown to be superior to morphine.
- IV morphine should be administered slowly in small doses of 2–5 mg every 5–15 minutes, as needed. Some patients with persistent pain may require maintenance doses of 4–8 mg every 4–6 hours.
- Therapy should be continued until pain relief is achieved or an unacceptable endpoint, such as hypotension (systolic blood pressure <90 mm Hg), is reached. Patients should be monitored closely for hypotension, respiratory depression, and allergic reactions.

Nitroglycerin

- Nitroglycerin (NTG) causes peripheral venodilation and coronary dilation, which relieves chest discomfort and helps to salvage ischemic myocardium. NTG reduces susceptibility to ventricular arrhythmias (specifically ventricular fibrillation), limits infarct size, and may reduce mortality by 10–30% in patients with large acute MI. Pain relief results from improvement in myocardial oxygen supply owing to the dilation of epicardial and collateral vessels that improve blood supply to ischemic myocardium. In addition, NTG reduces MVo_2 by decreasing myocardial wall tension. Nitroprusside is generally not used because it has been associated with coronary "steal."
- Long-term NTG use (beyond the peri-infarction period) may be necessary only in patients with persistent angina.

- NTG should be avoided in patients with right ventricular MI and should be used with caution in patients with hypotension, tachycardia, or bradycardia.
- Sublingual (SL) NTG (0.4 mg) is frequently used to determine whether chest pain is due to MI or ischemia. Typically, 0.4 mg SL NTG is administered, and chest pain intensity and the ECG are assessed. This dose may be repeated three times, once every 5 minutes, as long as heart rate and blood pressure are stable. If the ECG changes persist despite relief of chest pain, the diagnosis is MI.
- IV NTG is preferred in the management of MI because it is easily titrated. Therapy may be initiated with or without a 15-µg bolus followed by a initial infusion rate of 5–10 µg/min via an infusion pump. The infusion may be increased every 5–10 minutes by 5–10 µg/min increments for chest pain relief, resolution of ECG abnormalities, or until the systolic blood pressure is between 90 and 100 mm Hg. Patients with an uncomplicated MI may require only 24–48 hours of therapy before switching to an oral or transdermal dosage form.
- Heart rate and blood pressure must be monitored during IV NTG administration. If hypotension develops, the rate of infusion should be reduced or gradually discontinued. IV fluids should be administered if the patient remains hypotensive upon discontinuation. If the patient becomes either symptomatically tachycardic or bradycardic, the NTG infusion rate should be decreased. The ECG should also be closely monitored for reemergence of ischemia, even if the patient does not have recurrent chest pain.
- Headache is common with NTG (>50%); decreasing the infusion rate and use of acetaminophen may be effective and should be given consideration prior to discontinuation of the NTG infusion.

Thrombolytic Therapy
- Agents approved for use by the FDA in patients with acute MI in the United States include:
  - Alteplase (recombinant tissue-type plasminogen activator [Activase])
  - Anistreplase (anisoylated plasminogen streptokinase activator complex or APSAC [Eminase])
  - Reteplase (recombinant plasminogen activator [Retavase])
  - Streptokinase (Streptase/Kabikinase)
- These agents improve myocardial oxygen supply by dissolving the thrombus associated with acute MI, reestablishing blood flow to ischemic myocardium. Consequently, the extent of myocardial necrosis and infarct size are limited and the likelihood of survival is significantly improved if thrombolysis is achieved in a timely fashion.
- Patients treated within 4 hours from the onset of their chest pain have a better outcome in regard to infarct artery patency and preservation of left ventricular function. However, patients who present within the first 12 hours should be evaluated as candidates for thrombolytic therapy. Patients who present between 12 and 24 hours may be considered if

they have signs and symptoms of ongoing ischemia such as persistent ST-segment elevation and chest pain. Patients who present after 24 hours should not be considered eligible.

- Absolute and relative contraindications to thrombolytic therapy are outlined in Table 11.1. The presence of more than one relative contraindication is considered an *absolute* contraindication to therapy. Age is neither an absolute nor relative contraindication.
- Although there may be a slight mortality benefit in favor of alteplase, it is more expensive than streptokinase. The choice of thrombolytic agent is less important than ensuring that a thrombolytic drug is given in a timely manner to eligible patients.
- Current recommendations call for the administration of thrombolytic therapy to patients with ECG evidence of Q wave MI who present within 12 hours of the onset of chest pain without contraindications to therapy. Eligible patients should be treated as soon as possible, but preferably within 70 minutes from the time they present to the emergency department, with one of the following regimens:
  - Alteplase: 15 mg IV bolus followed by 0.75 mg/kg infusion (not to exceed 50 mg) over 30 minutes followed by 0.5 mg/kg infusion (not to exceed 35 mg) over the next 60 minutes
  - Anistreplase: 30 units IV over 2–5 minutes
  - Reteplase: 10-unit IV bolus followed by a second 10-unit bolus 30 minutes later

TABLE 11.1. Relative and Absolute Contraindications to Thrombolytic Therapy

Relative
Recent trauma or surgery (i.e., <2 weeks)
History of cerebrovascular accident
History of GI or GU surgery or stroke within last 6 months
Active peptic ulcer
History of chronic severe HTN with or without drug therapy
Significant liver dysfunction
Prior exposure to streptokinase or anistreplase
Known bleeding diathesis

Absolute
Possible aortic dissection
Acute pericarditis
Active internal bleeding
Severe uncontrolled hypertension (BP >220/110 mm Hg)
Recent head trauma or known intracranial neoplasm
History of hemorrhagic cerebrovascular accident
Diabetic hemorrhagic retinopathy or other hemorrhagic ophthalmic condition
Previous allergic reaction to streptokinase or anistreplase; use alteplase
Prolonged cardiopulmonary resuscitation with evidence of chest trauma
Pregnancy

GI, gastrointestinal; GU, genitourinary; HTN, hypertension.

- Streptokinase: 1.5 million units in 50 mL of normal saline or D_5W IV over 60 minutes
- A lytic state characterized by a fall in fibrinogen concentration, an increase in fibrin degradation products, and prolongation of the aPTT increases the risk of bleeding. Hemorrhagic stroke is the most serious adverse effect; others include hypotension and allergic reactions (primarily with streptokinase).
- Successful reperfusion with thrombolytic therapy can be assessed by normalization of the ECG, relief of chest pain, and onset of reperfusion arrhythmias, which are usually ventricular in nature.
- Patients in whom symptoms of MI persist beyond 1 to 2 hours from the start of thrombolytic therapy may benefit from rescue percutaneous transluminal coronary angioplasty (PTCA).

Lidocaine

- Although ventricular tachycardia (VT) and ventricular fibrillation (VF), are the most common consequences of MI, prophylactic lidocaine is not recommended because it has not been shown to reduce mortality and is associated with potentially serious risks.
- IV lidocaine is the drug of choice in patients who manifest ventricular arrhythmias. It should be reserved for patients who have either sustained or symptomatic ventricular arrhythmias or patients who have received thrombolytic therapy and develop the following symptoms since the incidence of reperfusion arrhythmias is high:
  - PVCs occurring >6/min
  - Closely coupled (R on T) PVCs
  - Multiform PVCs
  - Short bursts of ≥ 3 in succession
  - VT/VF in association with CPR and electrical cardioversion
- The duration of lidocaine therapy should not exceed 48 hours since the incidence of ventricular arrhythmias declines to nearly zero by 24–36 hours after MI.
- Therapy should be initiated with an IV bolus dose of 1 mg/kg (maximum 100 mg). Additional bolus doses may be given every 8–10 minutes up to a total loading dose of 4 mg/kg. Simultaneously, a constant IV infusion of 22–50 mg/kg/min should be started. Doses of lidocaine may need to be reduced in patients with CHF and/or liver disease.
- The ECG should be closely observed for PVCs and VT/VF. Recurrent arrhythmias may indicate the need for additional lidocaine or alternative therapy.
- Adverse effects include nausea, drowsiness, perioral numbness, dizziness, confusion, hypotension, bradycardia, asystole, and seizures. Determination of serum lidocaine concentrations may not be useful because of the short duration of therapy and alteration of lidocaine pharmacokinetics in acute MI.
- Patients whose ventricular arrhythmias do not respond to lidocaine should be switched to IV procainamide.

Early Administration of β-Adrenergic Blockers

- Administration of β blockers within 12 hours of the onset of chest pain reduces the incidence of ventricular arrhythmias, recurrent ischemia, and reinfarction, and, most important, mortality in patients with acute MI.
- If there are no contraindications, β blocker therapy is recommended for hemodynamically stable patients with tachycardia or hypertension whether or not they receive thrombolytic therapy and patients with continuing ischemia or postinfarction angina.
- The choice of agent does not appear to be an issue except that those with intrinsic sympathomimetic activity (ISA) should be avoided since they have not been shown to be of benefit. Examples of IV dosing regimens include:
  - Propranolol 0.1 mg/kg in two to three divided doses every 10 minutes
  - Metoprolol 15 mg in three divided doses every 5 minutes
  - Atenolol 5–10 mg in two divided doses every 5–10 minutes
- An oral regimen can be initiated 6–12 hours after the last IV dose depending on the β blocker used. An algorithm outlining the decision-making process for acute β-blocker therapy with metoprolol is outlined in Fig. 11.2.

Late Administration of β-Adrenergic Blockers

- The goal of late (at least 24 hours after MI) oral administration of β-blocker therapy is secondary prevention of recurrent ischemia and reinfarction. Studies have demonstrated an improvement in survival and a reduction in reinfarction when therapy is initiated between 24 and 72 hours after MI.
- Examples of dosing regimens include:
  - Propranolol 180–240 mg/d in three or four divided doses
  - Metoprolol 100 mg twice daily
  - Atenolol 100 mg once daily
  - Timolol 10 mg twice daily
- The medication should be dosed such that the exercising heart rate of the patient does not exceed 75 beats/min or to the maximum dose.
- For secondary prevention, β-blocker therapy should be continued for at least 2 years.

Calcium Channel Antagonists

- Diltiazem is recommended for patients with non–Q-wave MI for the prevention of post-MI angina and reinfarction. Calcium channel antagonists are not routinely recommended in patients with Q-wave MI.
- In patients with non–Q-wave MI who have no contraindications, diltiazem 90 mg every 6 hours should be initiated between 24 and 72 hours after the onset of MI and continued for 2 years. Diltiazem should be avoided in patients with heart block and/or hypotension.
- Heart rate, blood pressure, and the frequency of anginal episodes should be monitored closely. Other side effects of diltiazem include constipation, nausea, and dizziness.

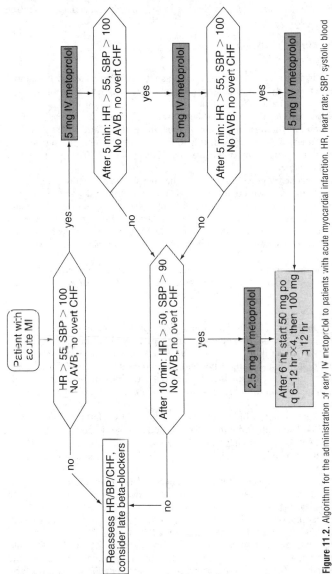

Figure 11.2. Algorithm for the administration of early IV metoprolol to patients with acute myocardial infarction. HR, heart rate; SBP, systolic blood pressure; AVB, atrioventricular block; CHF, congestive heart failure.

137

- Because of equivocal results from clinical trials, calcium channel blockers are not recommended for routine use for secondary prevention of acute MI.

Antithrombotic Therapy

Aspirin

- Aspirin is a potent inhibitor of platelet cyclooxygenase with a rapid onset, usually before aspirin concentrations are detectable in the systemic circulation.
- Aspirin 160–325 mg should be chewed and swallowed as soon as possible after the onset of symptoms or immediately after presentation to the emergency department whether or not the patient is considered a candidate for thrombolytic therapy. Exceptions include aspirin allergy or GI intolerance.
- For secondary prevention, aspirin has been shown to reduce the risk of recurrent cardiovascular events when started within days or even years of acute MI. A single loading dose of 300–325 mg followed by long-term therapy with 160–325 mg/d may be started in patients not already receiving aspirin as part of their acute MI care. Enteric-coated aspirin reduces the incidence of GI side effects (stomach pain, heartburn, nausea).
- Patients should be evaluated regularly for signs and symptoms of recurrent ischemia, as up to 30–40% of patients experience recurrent ischemia or reinfarction despite aspirin therapy.

Heparin

- When combined with thrombolytic therapy, IV heparin may have a beneficial effect on maintaining artery patency, but this comes at the expense of an increased risk of bleeding. Ongoing trials are evaluating use of a weight-based dosing regimen and established guidelines for the adjustment of heparin based on the aPTT. Until more information is acquired, the current recommendations for concomitant heparin therapy are as follows:
  - Alteplase: Heparin 75 U/kg bolus followed by continuous infusion of 1000 U/h at the time the alteplase infusion is initiated.
  - Streptokinase: No heparin bolus; a maintenance infusion of 1000 U/h should be initiated 1–3 hours after the start of the streptokinase infusion.
  - Anistreplase: Same heparin regimen as for streptokinase.
  - Reteplase: Heparin 5000 unit bolus followed by continuous infusion of 1000 U/h.
- Heparin should be titrated to maintain the aPTT at 1.5 to 2 times control and continued for approximately 24–48 hours. The patient can then be switched to low-dose subcutaneous heparin (5000 U BID) until ambulatory. Patients at high risk for systemic embolism then should remain on full-dose IV heparin while oral anticoagulation with warfarin is initiated.

- In patients with AWMI, either full-dose IV or high-dose SQ heparin (12,500 units SQ every 12 hours) is recommended for short-term prevention of mural thrombus. Heparin should be followed by warfarin therapy titrated to prolong the INR to 2.0 to 3.0.
- In patients not receiving full-dose IV or SQ heparin, low-dose heparin (5000 units SQ every 8–12 hours) should be started within 12–18 hours after onset of chest pain to prevent systemic thromboembolic complications of MI. This regimen should be continued for 24–72 hours or until the patient is ambulatory.

Warfarin

- Secondary prevention of recurrent ischemia or reinfarction with long-term warfarin is controversial. Until more data are available, routine use of warfarin is not considered standard practice.

Angiotensin-Converting Enzyme (ACE) Inhibitors

- The primary goal of an ACE inhibitor after acute MI is to limit postinfarction left ventricular dilatation and hypertrophy so that pump function is preserved or improved and CHF is prevented.
- Based on present information, it is difficult to make definitive recommendations about the use of ACE inhibitors in patients after acute MI. Patients with a first acute MI who have a left ventricular ejection fraction of <40% and who are not hypotensive (systolic blood pressure <100 mm Hg) may derive the greatest benefit from either lisinopril or long-term oral captopril therapy.
- Captopril should be initiated no sooner than 72 hours after MI with a test dose of 6.25 mg followed by 12.5 mg. If tolerated, the dose should be titrated up to 50 mg three times a day.
- Lisinopril may be initiated within 24 hours of the onset of symptoms at 5 mg/d, then increased to 10 mg/d.

▶ EVALUATION OF THERAPEUTIC OUTCOMES

- At the time of or near the time of hospital discharge, patients should be carefully evaluated to ensure the appropriate plan for rehabilitation.
- Patients should understand important aspects of their medications, particularly secondary prevention; modification of risk factors such as smoking, cholesterol, and hypertension; exercise program; and diet.
- An objective assessment of a patient's prognosis and stratification for risk of recurrent cardiovascular events should be made, usually by exercise tolerance testing (ETT) and determination of left ventricular function. ETT with continuous ECG and blood pressure monitoring will determine the overall exercise capacity of the patient, blood pressure response to exercise, and if angina occurs, at what point during exercise it occurs, as well as if activity precipitates arrhythmias. Submaximal exercise testing can usually be performed just prior to hospital discharge and can then be followed by a full exercise test 1 month after infarction.

II

- High-risk patients are easily identified by their low exercise capability, failure of the systolic blood pressure to rise above the resting value during exercise (frequently referred to as an inadequate blood pressure response to exercise), and chest pain associated with ischemic changes on the ECG.
- Current guidelines recommend that post-MI patients undergo exercise testing annually following acute MI.
- Left ventricular function may be evaluated by echocardiography, coronary angiography, or radionuclear ventriculograms.

See Chapter 15, Acute Myocardial Infarction, authored by Kathleen A. Stringer, PharmD, FCCP, and Larry M. Lopez, PharmD, FCCP, for a more detailed discussion of this topic.

Chapter 12

▶ SHOCK

▶ DEFINITION

Shock refers to conditions manifested by hemodynamic alterations (e.g., hypotension, tachycardia, low cardiac output [CO], and oliguria) caused by intravascular volume deficit (hypovolemic shock), myocardial pump failure (cardiogenic shock), or peripheral vasodilation (septic, anaphylactic, or neurogenic shock). Cardiogenic shock will be only briefly considered in this chapter (see Chapter 7, Congestive Heart Failure and Chapter 11, Myocardial Infarction).

▶ PATHOPHYSIOLOGY

- General pathophysiologic mechanisms of different forms of shock are similar, except for initiating events.
- Hypovolemic shock is characterized by acute intravascular volume deficiency owing to external losses or internal redistribution of extracellular water. This type of shock can be precipitated by hemorrhage, burns, trauma, intestinal obstruction, and dehydration from considerable insensible fluid loss, over-aggressive loop-diuretic administration, and severe vomiting or diarrhea. Relative hypovolemia leading to hypovolemic shock occurs during significant vasodilation, which accompanies anaphylaxis, sepsis, and neurogenic shock.
- Cardiogenic shock results from direct insult to heart muscle (e.g., acute myocardial infarction), other mechanical heart problem (e.g., valvular dysfunction), restricted muscle function (e.g., tamponade, pericardotomy syndrome), or exacerbation of congestive heart failure due to drug or nondrug factors.
- Regardless of the etiology, fall in blood pressure (BP) is compensated by an increase in sympathetic outflow, activation of the renin–angiotensin system, and other humoral factors that stimulate peripheral vasoconstriction. Compensatory vasoconstriction redistributes blood away from extremities and kidneys toward vital organs (e.g., heart, brain) in an attempt to maintain oxygenation, nutrition, and organ function.
- Severe metabolic lactic acidosis often develops secondary to tissue ischemia and causes localized vasodilation, which further exacerbates the impaired cardiovascular state. Death follows from multisystem organ failure.
- Extent of damage and reversibility depend primarily on severity and duration of insult.
- Shock results in failure of the circulatory system to deliver sufficient oxygen (O_2) to body tissues despite normal or reduced O_2 consumption.

II

Rate of oxygen delivery (Do_2) to tissues is estimated from the following formula: Do_2 mL/min = CO × (Hgb × 1.39 × Sao_2) × 10.

- Oxygen-carrying capacity (Cao_2) is essentially the product of hemoglobin (Hgb), volume of oxygen (O_2) carried per gram of hemoglobin (1.39), and arterial O_2 saturation (Sao_2). Ten is a conversion factor for correcting units of measure.

- Critical Do_2 levels, about 600 mL/min or 8 mL/kg/min in normal patients, may increase to 15 mL/kg/min in patients with septic shock.

- Oxygen consumption (Vo_2) can be thought of as the amount of O_2 extracted by cells from the circulation, which is related to cellular metabolism. Vo_2 is expressed by the following relationship: Vo_2 mL/min = CO × [Hgb × 1.39] × ($Sao_2 - Svo_2$)] × 10, which is similar to the equation for calculating oxygen delivery.

- Normally, Vo_2 is *independent* of Do_2. Once Do_2 falls below the critical value, Vo_2 becomes *dependent* on Do_2. Venous oxygen saturation (Svo_2) of <40% usually indicates inability to compensate and maintain sufficient Do_2.

► CLINICAL PRESENTATION

- Shock presents with a diversity of signs and symptoms. Hypotension, tachycardia, confusion, and oliguria are key symptoms. Myocardial and cerebral ischemia, pulmonary edema (cardiogenic shock), and multisystem organ failure often follow.

- Significant hypotension (sytolic blood pressure [SBP] <90 mm Hg) with reflex sinus tachycardia (>120–130 beats/min) is often observed in the hypovolemic patient. Clinically, the patient presents with extremities cool to the touch and a "thready" pulse. If coronary hypoxia persists, cardiac arrhythmias may occur, which eventually lead to irreversible myocardial pump failure, pulmonary edema, and cardiovascular collapse.

- In the patient with extensive myocardial damage, chest auscultation may reveal heart sounds consistent with valvular heart disease (regurgitation, outflow obstruction) or significant ventricular dysfunction (S_3). Chest roentgenogram may detect dissecting ascending aortic aneurysm (widened mediastinum) or cardiomegaly (large heart shadow).

- Altered sensorium (confusion or combativeness) may be one of the first symptoms of shock.

- Respiratory alkalosis secondary to hyperventilation is usually observed secondary to CNS stimulation of ventilatory centers as a result of trauma, sepsis, or shock. Lung auscultation may reveal rales (pulmonary edema) or absence of breath sounds (pneumothorax, hemothorax). Chest roentgenogram can confirm early suspicions or disclose an undetected abnormality such as pneumonia (pulmonary infiltrates). Continued insult to the lungs may result in adult respiratory distress syndrome (ARDS).

- Kidneys are exquisitely sensitive to changes in perfusion pressures. Moderate alterations can lead to significant changes in glomerular filtration rate (GFR). Oliguria, progressing to anuria, occurs because of vasoconstriction of afferent arterioles.

- Skin is often cool, pale, or cyanotic (bluish) due to hypoxemia. Sweating results in a moist, clammy feel. Digits will have severely slowed capillary refill.
- Redistribution of blood flow away from the gastrointestinal (GI) tract may cause stress gastritis, gut ischemia, and in some cases, infarction, resulting in GI bleeding.
- Reduced hepatic blood flow, especially in vasodilatory forms of shock, can alter metabolism of endogenous compounds and drugs. Progressive liver damage (shock liver) manifests as elevated serum hepatic transaminases and unconjugated bilirubin. Impaired synthesis of clotting factors may increase prothrombin time (PT), international normalized ratio (INR), and activated partial thromboplastin time (aPTT).

▶ DIAGNOSIS

- Information from noninvasive and invasive monitoring (Table 12.1) and evaluation of past medical history, clinical presentation, and laboratory findings are key components in establishing the diagnosis as well as in assessing general mechanisms responsible for shock (Table 12.2) and thus guiding therapy. Regardless of the etiology, consistent findings include hypotension (SBP <90 mm Hg), depressed cardiac index (CI <2.2 L/min/m^2), tachycardia (heart rate [HR] >100 beats/min), and low urine output (<20 mL/h).
- Trends must be considered rather than isolated numbers because misinterpretation can yield an incorrect diagnosis, which may delay appropriate therapy. In addition, instrumentation must be calibrated to ensure accurate results.
- Noninvasive assessment of BP using the sphygmomanometer and stethoscope may be inaccurate in the shock state.
- Swan–Ganz catheter is the preferred instrument for invasive monitoring of central cardiovascular pressures. This flow-directed balloon-tipped catheter is inserted via the subclavian or internal jugular vein through the superior vena cava, right atrium, and ventricle, into the pulmonary artery. Depending on the location of its tip, Swan–Ganz catheter can be used to determine central venous pressure (CVP), which is essentially the same as right atrial pressure (RAP) and therefore an estimate of intravascular volume and right ventricular preload; pulmonary artery systolic and diastolic pressures (PAS and PAD); and pulmonary capillary wedge pressure (PCWP), which affords an estimate of the left ventricular end diastolic pressure (LVEDP) and an indication of pulmonary congestion.
- Cardiac output (2.5–3 L/min) and Svo$_2$ (70–75%) may be very low in the patient with extensive myocardial damage. These values are determined by Swan–Ganz catheterization.

Cardiovascular Disorders

II

- CO and CI are estimated using the thermodilution method. Systemic vascular resistance (SVR), an indication of peripheral vascular impedance to blood flow (afterload), is calculated from CO, mean arterial pressure (MAP), and RAP.
- Svo_2 is obtained by venipuncture or monitored directly by a Swan–Ganz oximeter.
- Metabolic changes associated with progression of shock include increased Vo_2, shift from aerobic to anaerobic metabolism, elevated serum lactate, and metabolic acidosis.

TABLE 12.1. Key Cardiovascular and Respiratory Parameters

Parameter	Abbreviation	Formula	Normal
Noninvasive			
Heart rate	HR	Direct measure	72–88 beats/min
Blood pressure (systolic/diastolic)	SBP/DBP	Direct measure cuff or arterial line	100–140/60–100 mm Hg
Mean arterial pressure	MAP	DBP + 1/3 (SBP − DBP) or arterial line	82–102 mm Hg
Pulse pressure	PP	SBP − DBP	40–80 mm Hg
Invasive: Swan–Ganz Determinations			
Central venous pressure (right atrial pressure)	CVP (RAP)	Direct measure	1–10 mm Hg
Pulmonary artery pressure (systolic/diastolic)	PAS/PAD	Direct measure	25–35 mm Hg/ 10–20 mm Hg
Mean pulmonary artery pressure	MPAP	Direct measure	11–15 mm Hg
Pulmonary capillary wedge pressure	PCWP	Direct measure	8–12 mm Hg
Cardiac output	CO	Thermodilution measure	4.5–6.5 L/min
Cardiac index	CI	CO/BSA	2.8–3.6 L/min/m^2
Calculated Parameters			
Rate pressure product	RPP	HR × SBP	12,000
Stroke volume	SV	CO/HR × 1000	60–90 mL
Stroke index	SI	CI/HR × 1000	30–50 mL/m^2
Left ventricular stroke work index	LVSWI	SI × MAP × 0.0136	44–68 g/m^2
Left cardiac work index	LCWI	CI × MAP × 0.0136	3–4.6 kg-m/m^2
Right ventricular stroke work index	RVSWI	SI × MPAP × 0.0136	4–8 g/m^2

TABLE 12.1. continued

Parameter	Abbreviation	Formula	Normal
Calculated Parameters (cont.)			
Right cardiac work index	RCWI	CI × MPAP × 0.0136	0.4–0.6 kg-m/m^2
Systemic vascular resistance	SVR	[(MAP − CVP) /CO] × 79.9	900–1200 dynes- s/cm^5
Systemic vascular resistance index	SVRI	[(MAP − CVP)/CI] × 79.9	1760–2600 dynes- s/cm^5 × m^2
Pulmonary vascular resistance	PVR	[(MPAP − PCWP) /CO] × 79.9	75–400 dynes- s/cm^5 × m^2
Pulmonary vascular resistance index	PVRI	[(MPAP − PCWP) /CI] × 79.9	45–225 dynes- s/cm^5
Oxygen Transport			
Arterial pH	pH	Direct measure	7.36–7.44
Arterial oxygen tension	Pao_2	Direct measure	80–100 mm Hg
Arterial carbon dioxide tension	$Paco_2$	Direct measure	36–44 mm Hg (torr)
Arterial oxygen hemoglobin saturation	Sao_2	Direct measure	95–99%
Mixed venous oxygen tension	Pvo_2	Direct measure	33–53 mm Hg
Mixed venous oxygen saturation	Svo_2	Direct measure	60–80 mm Hg
Arterial oxygen content	Cao_2	Hb × Sao_2 × 1.39	20.1 vol%
Venous oxygen content	Cvo_2	Hb × Svo_2 × 1.39	15.5 vol%
Arterial–mixed venous content difference	$o_2C(a-v)o_2$	Cao_2 − Cvo_2	4–5.5 mL/dL
Oxygen delivery	Do_2	CO × Cao_2 × 10	900–1100 mL/min
Oxygen consumption	Vo_2	CO × Cvo_2 × 10	225–235 mL/min
Oxygen extraction	o_2 ext	$(Cao_2 − Cvo_2)/Cao_2$	22–30%

Reprinted with modifications from Shoemaker WC. In Shoemaker WC, Ayers S, Grenvik A, et al. (eds): Textbook of Critical Care, 2nd ed. Philadelphia, WB Saunders, 1989:979, with permission.

- Respiratory alkalosis is associated with low partial pressure of O_2 (Pao_2) (25–35 mm Hg) and alkaline pH, but normal bicarbonate. The first two values are measured by arterial blood gas, which also yields partial pressure of carbon dioxide ($Paco_2$) and Sao_2. Circulating Sao_2 can also be measured by an oximeter, which is a noninvasive method that is fairly accurate and useful at the patient's bedside.
- Renal function can be grossly assessed by hourly measurements of urine output, but estimation of creatinine clearance based on isolated serum creatinine values in critically ill patients may yield erroneous

Cardiovascular Disorders

TABLE 12.2. Comparative Hemodynamic Profiles of Hypovolemic and Cardiogenic Shock

	MAP	RAP (CVP)	PCWP	HR	CO	SVR
Hypovolemic shock	↓↓	↓↓	↓↓	↑↑	↓–↓↓↓	↑–↑↑
Cardiogenic shock						
Left ventricular/ biventricular failure	↔↓	↑–↑↑	↑↑	↓↔↑	↓↓	↑–↑↑
Right ventricular failure	↔↓	↑↑–↑↑↑	↓–↓↓	↓↔↑	↓↓	↑–↑↑

Key: MAP, mean arterial pressure; RAP, right atrial pressure; CVP, central venous pressure; PCWP, pulmonary capillary wedge pressure, HR, heart rate; CO, cardiac output; SVR, systemic vascular resistance; ↓, decrease; ↔, no change; ↑, increase.

Compiled from Sypniewski E, Ornato JP. In Ornato JP, Gonzalez ER (eds): Drug Therapy in Emergency Medicine. New York, Churchill Livingstone, 1990, p 55; and Kirby RR, Taylor RW, Civetta JM (eds). Shock in Handbook of Critical Care. Philadelphia, JB Lippincott, 1994:19, with permission.

results. Decreased renal perfusion and aldosterone release result in sodium retention, and thus, low urinary sodium (U_{Na} <30 mEq/L).

▶ DESIRED OUTCOME

The initial goal is to support oxygen delivery through the circulatory system by assuring effective intravascular plasma volume, optimal oxygen-carrying capacity, and adequate BP while definitive diagnosis and therapeutic strategies are being determined. The goal is not to normalize each parameter because compensatory mechanisms such as sinus tachycardia are clearly necessary.

▶ GENERAL TREATMENT PRINCIPLES

- Supplemental oxygen should be initiated at the earliest signs of shock, beginning with 4–6 L/min via nasal cannula or 6–10 L/min by face mask.
- Fluid resuscitation is essential. Different therapeutic options are discussed below.
- If fluid challenge does not achieve desired endpoints, pharmacologic support is necessary (Figure 12.1). Dose titration will depend on desired and observed clinical outcomes, as well as type of shock (Table 12.3). Because dose recommendations for inotropic and vasoactive drugs are primarily based on ideal body weight, careful dose selection is required to avoid overdose in obese individuals. Vasoactive and inotropic medications must be administered by infusion pump.
  - If the hypotension has a primary vascular component (secondary to vasodilation causing a relative hypovolemia such as in septic, neurogenic, or anaphylactic shock), vasopressors such as dopamine or norepinephrine should be administered through a central intravenous (IV) line. Catecholamines, in general, have very short half-lives (2 min-

utes), which affords quick onset and short duration of action, thus facilitating titration.

- If the patient experiences significant myocardial dysfunction *without* signs or symptoms of shock, yet presents with mild to severe hypotension (SBP = 70–100 mm Hg), a β_1-adrenergic inotrope such as dobutamine may be beneficial. If the patient presents *with* signs and symptoms of shock, dopamine may be preferred. Dopamine exerts dose-dependent hemodynamic effects (Table 12.3). Alternatively, if the patient with myocardial pump problems has an SBP of >100 mm Hg, a vasodilator such as nitroglycerin should be initiated before or soon after inotropic therapy. Nitroglycerin also has dose-dependent effects, causing venous dilation at lower doses (<100–150 µg/min) and both venous and arterial dilation at higher doses (>100–150 µg/min).
- If the patient has myocardial dysfunction because of calcium-channel blocker administration, hypocalcemia, or severe hyperkalemia, calcium 1 g can be administered by slow IV push to improve myocardial contractility.
- Phosphodiesterase III inhibitors have hemodynamic effects resembling those of dobutamine. Amrinone, for example, is less likely to induce arrhythmia, but its long half-life (3–5 hours) limits titration during acute management.
- Normalization of pH to at least 7.3 is essential because metabolic acidosis interferes with the hemodynamic response to endogenous and exogenous catecholamines. Although metabolic acidosis can be avoided by optimizing ventilation and preventing maldistribution of blood flow, sodium bicarbonate may be required if the patient has ventilation–perfusion mismatch (e.g., pulmonary embolus or edema, mucous plug, alveolar damage) or persistent source of acid load (e.g., continued hypoperfusion, ischemic limb, severe trauma). Additional information can be found in Chapter 74, Acid–Base Disorders.

▶ FLUID RESUSCITATION FOR HYPOVOLEMIC SHOCK

GENERAL PRINCIPLES

- Initial fluid resuscitation consists of isotonic crystalloid (0.9% sodium chloride or lactated Ringer's solution), colloid (5% plasmanate or albumin, 6% hetastarch), or whole blood (Tables 12.4 and 12.5). Choice of solution is based on oxygen-carrying capacity (e.g., hemoglobin, hematocrit), cause of hypovolemic shock, accompanying disease states, degree of fluid loss, and required speed of fluid delivery.
- Degree of blood loss can be estimated by evaluating signs and symptoms (Table 12.6). Patients with class I or II blood loss can usually be managed by crystalloid alone. Patients with class III or IV blood loss require both crystalloid and colloid because of significant fluid loss, and hence oxygen-carrying capacity.

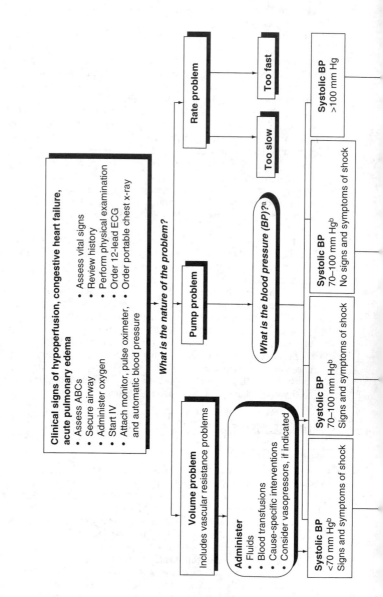

Clinical signs of hypoperfusion, congestive heart failure, acute pulmonary edema

- Assess ABCs
- Secure airway
- Administer oxygen
- Start IV
- Attach monitor, pulse oximeter, and automatic blood pressure

- Assess vital signs
- Review history
- Perform physical examination
- Order 12-lead ECG
- Order portable chest x-ray

What is the nature of the problem?

Rate problem

Too slow

Too fast

Pump problem

What is the blood pressure (BP)?[a]

Systolic BP >100 mm Hg

Systolic BP 70–100 mm Hg[b] No signs and symptoms of shock

Systolic BP 70–100 mm Hg[b] Signs and symptoms of shock

Volume problem

Includes vascular resistance problems

Administer
- Fluids
- Blood transfusions
- Cause-specific interventions
- Consider vasopressors, if indicated

Systolic BP <70 mm Hg[b] Signs and symptoms of shock

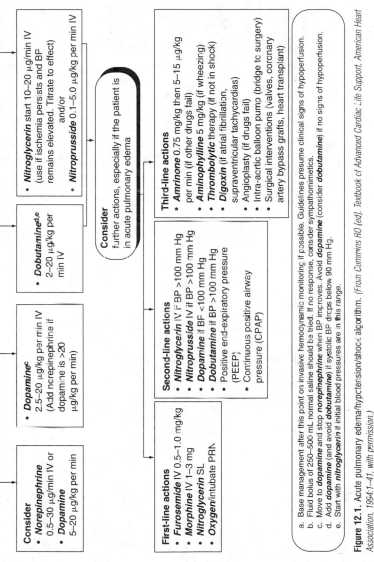

Figure 12.1. Acute pulmonary edema/hypotension/shock algorithm. *(From Cummins RO [ed]. Textbook of Advanced Cardiac Life Support, American Heart Association, 1994:1–41, with permission.)*

Consider
- *Norepinephrine*
  0.5–30 µg/min IV or
- *Dopamine*
  5–20 µg/kg per min

- *Dopamine*[c]
  2.5–20 µg/kg per min IV
  (Add norepinephrine if
  dopamine is >20
  µg/kg per min)

- *Dobutamine*[d,e]
  2–20 µg/kg per
  min IV

- *Nitroglycerin* start 10–20 µg/min IV
  (use if ischemia persists and BP
  remains elevated. Titrate to effect)
  and/or
- *Nitroprusside* 0.1–5.0 µg/kg per min IV

Consider
further actions, especially if the patient is
in acute pulmonary edema

First-line actions
- *Furosemide* IV 0.5–1.0 mg/kg
- *Morphine* IV 1–3 mg
- *Nitroglycerin* SL
- *Oxygen*/intubate PRN

Second-line actions
- *Nitroglycerin* IV if BP >100 mm Hg
- *Nitroprusside* IV if BP >100 mm Hg
- *Dopamine* if BP <100 mm Hg
- *Dobutamine* if BP >100 mm Hg
- Positive end-expiratory pressure
  (PEEP)
- Continuous positive airway
  pressure (CPAP)

Third-line actions
- *Amrinone* 0.75 mg/kg then 5–15 µg/kg
  per min (if other drugs fail)
- *Aminophylline* 5 mg/kg (if wheezing)
- *Thrombolytic* therapy (if not in shock)
- *Digoxin* (if atrial fibrillation,
  supraventricular tachycardias)
- Angioplasty (if drugs fail)
- Intra-aortic balloon pump (bridge to surgery)
- Surgical interventions (valves, coronary
  artery bypass grafts, heart transplant)

a. Base management after this point on invasive hemodynamic monitoring if possible. Guidelines presume clinical signs of hypoperfusion.
b. Fluid bolus of 250–500 mL normal saline should be tried. If no response, consider sympathomimetics.
c. Move to *dopamine* and stop *norepinephrine* when BP improves. Avoid *dopamine* (consider *dobutamine*) if no signs of hypoperfusion.
d. Add *dopamine* (and avoid *dobutamine*) if systolic BP drops below 90 mm Hg.
e. Start with *nitroglycerin* if initial blood pressures are in this range.

TABLE 12.3. Pharmacologic Properties and Clinical Effects of Selected Vasoactive Drugs

Drug/Usual Dose	Receptor Specificity					Pharmacologic Effect				Hemodynamic Effect							Adverse Effects/Comments
	α	β₁	β₂	Dop	Sm Msc	VD	VC	INT	CHT	AP	RBF	MAP	PCWP	CO	SVR	UO	
Amrinone (Inocor) (750 mg/250 mL NS) (P,C) LD = 0.75 – 1.0 mg/kg MD = 5 – 15 μg/kg/min	—	—	—	—	++	++	—	+++	+++	++		↔↑↓	↓	↑	↓↓	↑	Thrombocytopenia, nausea, flulike syndrome, hypotension, arrhythmias, dilute in saline only
Dobutamine (Dobutrex) (500 mg/250 mL D₅W or NS) (P,C) 2–10 μg/kg/min >10–20 μg/kg/min	+ ++	+++ ++++	++ +++	— —	— —	+ ++	+ +	+++ ++++	+ ++	+ ++	↑ ↑	↑ ↔↑↓	→ →	↔↑ ↑	↔↓ →	↑ ↑	Hypotension, tachycardia, headache
Dopamine (Intropin) (800 mg/250 mL D₅W or NS) (C) 1–3 μg/kg/min 3–10 μg/kg/min >10–20 μg/kg/min	— — +++	+ ++++ ++++	— ++ +	++++ ++++ —	— — —	+ + —	— — +++	++ ++++ +++	+ ++ ++	+ ++ +++	↑↑ ↑↑ ↓↑	↔ ↔ ↑	↔↑ ↔↑ ↑	↔ ↑ ↑	↔ ↔↓ ↑	↑↑ ↑↑ ↓↑	Tachyarrhythmias, painful extravasation, hypertension, decreased peripheral perfusion, angina, headache
Epinephrine (Adrenalin) (2 mg/250 mL D₅W or NS) (C) 0.01–0.05 μg/kg/min >0.05 μg/kg/min	+ +++	++++ +++	++ +	— —	— —	+ —	+ +++	+++ +++	++ +++	++ +++	↑ ↓↑	↑ ↑↑	↔↓ ↑	↑↑ ↑↑	↔↓ ↑↑	↑ ↓↑	Hypertension, arrhythmias, decreased peripheral perfusion, angina, painful extravasation

TABLE 12.3. continued

Drug/Usual Dose	Receptor Specificity					Pharmacologic Effect					Hemodynamic Effect						Adverse Effects/Comments
	α	β₁	β₂	Dop	Sm Msc	VD	VC	INT	CHT	AP	RBF	MAP	PCWP	CO	SVR	UO	
Milrinone (Primacor) (50 mg/250 mL D₅W or NS) (P,C) LD = 50 µg/kg MD = 0.375–0.75 µg/kg/min	—	—	—	—	++	++	—	+++	+++	++	↑	↔↑↓	↓	↑	↓↓	↑	Hypotension, possible increased incidence of tachyarrhythmias vs. amrinone, decreased incidence of thrombocytopenia vs. amrinone
Norepinephrine (Levophed) (4 mg/250 mL D₅W or NS) (C) >2–20 µg/min (0.02–1.0 µg/kg/min)	++++	++	—	—	—	—	++++	+	++	++	↑↓	↑↑↑	↑↑	↔↑↓	↑↑↑	↑↓	Arrhythmias, angina, hypertension, decreased peripheral perfusion, painful extravasation
Isoproterenol (Isuprel) (2 mg/250 mL D₅W or NS) (P,C) 2–10 µg/min	—	++++	+++	—	—	+++	—	+++	+++	++++	↑	↓↓	↓↓	↑↑	↓↓↓	↑	Hypotension, arrhythmias, tachycardia
Phenylephrine (Neosynephrine) (50 mg/250 mL D₅W or NS) (C) 0.5–5 µg/min	++++	—	—	—	—	—	+++	—	—	—	↑	↑	↑	↔↑↓	↑	↑	Reflex bradycardia, hypertension, painful extravasation

II

151

TABLE 12.3. continued

Drug/Usual Dose	Receptor Specificity					Pharmacologic Effect				Hemodynamic Effect							Adverse Effects/Comments
	α	β₁	β₂	Dop	Sm Msc	VD	VC	INT	CHT	AP	RBF	MAP	PCWP	CO	SVR	UO	
Nitroglycerin (Nitrol, Tridil) (50 mg/250 mL D₅W or NS) (P,C) 5–300 µg/min	—	—	—	—	++++	++++ A<V	—	—	+	—	↑	↓	↓	↔↑↓	↔↓	↑	Headache, hypotension, reflex tachycardia, nausea
Nitroprusside (Nipride) (50 mg/250 mL D₅W or NS) (P,C) 0.5–10 µg/kg/min	—	—	—	—	++++	++++ A=V	—	—	+	—	↑	↓↓	↓↓	↑	↓↓	↑	Headache, hypotension, nausea, tremor, confusion, reflex tachycardia, cyanide and thiocynate toxicity

Key: α, alpha-adrenergic; β₁, beta-one adrenergic; β₂, beta-two adrenergic; Dop, dopaminergic; Sm Msc, smooth muscle; VD, vasodilation; VC, vasoconstriction; INT, inotropic; CHT, chronotropic; AP, arrhythmogenic potential; RBF, renal blood flow; MAP, mean arterial pressure; PCWP, pulmonary capillary wedge pressure; CO, cardiac output; SVR, systemic vascular resistance; UO, urine output; C, central administration; LD, loading dose; MD, maintenance dose; A, arterial; V, venous; +, mild; ++, moderate; +++ high; ++++, maximal; —, no effect; ↑, increase; ↓, decrease; ↑↓, increase or decrease; ↔ no change.

Reprinted with modification from Gonzalez ER and Meyers DG. In Ornato JC (ed): Clinics in Emergency Medicine: Cardiovascular Emergencies. New York, Churchill Livingstone, 1986:125, with permission.

TABLE 12.4. Crystalloid and Colloid Preparations

	0.9% NaCl (NS)	Lactated Ringer's	Plasma Protein Fraction 5%	Albumin 5%	Albumin 25%	Hetastarch 6% in NS
Sodium (mEq/L)	154	130	130–160	130–160	130–160	154
Chloride (mEq/L)	154	109	130–160	130–160	130–160	154
Other	—	Lactate 28 mEq/L, potassium 4 mEq, calcium 3 mEq/L	—	—	—	Hydroxyethyl starch average MW 450,000
Osmolality (mOsm)	308	273	290	300	1500	310
Albumin	—	—	≈44 g/L	≈50 g/L	≈250 g/L	—
Globulin	—	—	≈6 g/L	—	—	—
Colloid oncotic pressure (mm Hg)	—	—	20	20	100	30
Plasma volume expansion (per amount infused)	250 mL (per 1000 mL)	250 mL (per 1000 mL)	250–500 mL (per 250 mL)	250–500 mL (per 250 mL)	250 mL (per 50 mL)	500–750 mL (per 500 mL)
Distribution	ECW[a]	ECW[a]	Intravascular[b]	Intravascular[b]	Intravascular[b]	Intravascular[b]
Half-life of effect	Minutes	Minutes	5–6 hours	5–6 hours	5–6 hours	6–8 hours
Metabolism	—	Liver (lactate to bicarbonate)	Liver (amino acids)	Liver (amino acids)	Liver (amino acids)	40% urine unchanged, enzymatic degradation to smaller particles and glucose

TABLE 12.4. continued

	0.9% NaCl (NS)	Lactated Ringer's	Plasma Protein Fraction 5%	Albumin 5%	Albumin 25%	Hetastarch 6% in NS
Anaphylactoid reactions	—	—	0.019%[c]	0.019%	0.019%	0.085%
Life-threatening reactions	—	—	0.003%[c]	0.003%	0.003%	0.006%
Precautions	—	—	Dilutional effect on coagulation factors. Relatively contraindicated during coagulopathy			Dilutional effect on coagulation factors, lowers factor VIII, do not exceed 1500 mL per 24 hours, do not administer to patients with history of coagulation or bleeding problems

[a]Will distribute into ICW if intracellular osmolarity > normal from dehydration.

[b]Will distribute into interstitial space if presence of "leaky capillary syndrome" associated with septic shock.

[c]Incidence slightly higher than 5% and 25% albumin due to presence of globulins.

Adapted from Ross AD, Angaran DM. Drug Intell Clin Pharm 1984;18, 108; and Gould SA, Sehgal LR, Sehgal HL, Moss GS. Crit Care Clin 1993;9:240, with permission.

TABLE 12.5. Blood and Blood Products

Blood Product	Usual Package	Content	Complications
Whole blood	Unit	450 mL of blood; plasma (some clotting factors) RBCs, WBCs, platelets	Hepatitis, fever, chills, hemolytic/allergic reactions, hyperkalemia, hypocalcemia, intra-vascular overload, rare hemolytic reactions, CMV, HIV
Packed red blood cells (PRBCs)	Unit	220–300 mL of RBCs, includes WBCs and platelets	Same as with whole blood, except decreased risk, of intravascular overload
Platelets	Unit	$5.5-10 \times 10^{10}$ platelets in 30–50 mL plasma	Hepatitis, fever, chills, allergic reactions, development of antiplatelet antibodies, graft-versus-host disease, HIV
Fresh frozen plasma (FFP)	Unit	200–250 mL plasma; 200 units of all coagulation factors, 400 mg of fibrinogen, complement	Hepatitis, fever, chills, allergic reactions, HIV
Cryoprecipitate	Unit	80–120 units of factor VIII, 250 mg of fibrinogen 15–25 mL of plasma	Hepatitis, fever, chills, allergic reactions, hemolysis from anti-A or anti-B, HIV

Adapted from Bojar RM. Manual of Perioperative Care in Cardiac and Thoracic Surgery, 2nd ed. Boston, Blackwell Scientific Publications, 1994:93–97; and Kirby RR, Taylor IIW, Civetta JM (eds). Handbook of Critical Care. Philadelphia, JB Lippincott, 1994:32, with permission.

- Most clinicians agree that crystalloids should be initial therapy. If volume resuscitation is suboptimal following several liters of crystalloid, colloids should be considered. Some patients may require blood products to assure maintenance of oxygen-carrying capacity, as well as clotting factors and platelets for blood hemostasis.

CRYSTALLOIDS

- Crystalloids consist of electrolytes (e.g., Na^+, Cl^-, K^+) in water solutions, with or without dextrose. There is little clinical evidence to support the superiority of lactated Ringer's solution compared to normal saline in fluid resuscitation of patients.

TABLE 12.6. Hypovolemic Classes

Blood Loss	Blood Pressure	Vascular Response	Temperature	Color	Circulation (Blanching)	Endocrine Response	Metabolic Response	Signs and Symptoms
Class I (<15%) (750 mL)	Normal to 20%, ↓ BP	Contraction of great veins, ECF shift intravascularly	Cool	Pale	Normal, slight slowing	Slight	Slight	Mild thirst UO > 30 mL/h
Class II (20–25%) (1000–1250 mL)	↓ SBP, ↑ DBP, narrow pulse pressure	All of the above, mild tachycardia (>100 beats/min), ↓ CO, ↓ blood flow to all organs, shunting of blood flow to heart and brain	Cool	Pale	Definite slowing	↑ aldosterone, ADH, growth hormone and interleukin-1-β; some ↑ cortisol, catecholamines, clotting factors, no ↑ in insulin	↑ glycolysis, mild ↑ glucose, ↑ lipolysis/ FFA, small ↑ lactate, respiratory alkalosis, ↑ O_2 consumption, ↓ U_{Na}	Thirst, orthostasis, hyperventilation, apprehension, weakness UO = 20–30 mL/h
Class III (30–35%) (1500–1750 mL)	Frank hypotension, ↓ BP 20–40%	As above, tachycardia (>120 beats/min), ↓↓ CO, ↓↓ blood flow to organs	Cold	Pale	Definite slowing	As above	As above	As above, confusion UO = 5–15 mL/h

TABLE 12.6. continued

Blood Loss	Blood Pressure	Vascular Response	Temperature	Color	Circulation (Blanching)	Endocrine Response	Metabolic Response	Signs and Symptoms
Class IV (40–45%; (2000–2500 mL)	Very narrow pulse pressure, ↓↓ BP or nonrecordable	As above, CO < 50% tachycardia (>140 beats/min), increased shunting to heart and brain; bradycardia, asystole or ventricular fibrillation	Cold	Ashen, cyanotic (mottling)	Definite slowing	As above, marked ↑ in catecholamines	As above, ↑↑ lactic acidosis, mVo$_2$ 20 mm Hg or less	As above, lethargic, comatose, anuria

Key: ↑, increase; ↓, decrease; BP, blood pressure; SBP, systolic blood pressure; DBP, diastolic blood pressure; ADH, antidiuretic hormone; FFA, free fatty acids; U$_{Na}$, urine sodium concentration; mVo$_2$, mixed venous oxygen; UO, urine output.
Compiled from Packman MI, Rackow EC. Crit Care Med 1983;11:165–169; and Advanced Trauma Life Support Student Manual. American College of Surgeons Committee on Trauma, 1993:86, with permission.

II

- Crystalloids are administered at a rate of 500–2000 mL/h, depending on the severity of the deficit, degree of ongoing fluid loss, and tolerance to infusion volume. Usually 2–4 L of crystalloid normalizes intravascular volume.
- Advantages of crystalloids include rapidity and ease of administration, compatibility with most drugs, absence of serum sickness, and low cost. Isotonic solutions may be safer for patients who may not tolerate fluid challenges (e.g., myocardial dysfunction) or who have "leaky capillary syndrome."
- The primary disadvantage is the large volume necessary to replace or augment intravascular volume. Approximately 4 L of normal saline must be infused to replace 1 L of blood loss. In addition, dilution of colloid oncotic pressure leading to pulmonary edema is more likely to follow crystalloid than colloid resuscitation.

COLLOIDS

- Colloids consist of natural protein solutions (e.g., albumin, plasmanate), synthetic complex sugars (e.g., dextran, hetastarch), and blood products. (Blood products are discussed separately in the following section). All exert oncotic pressure within the vascular tree. No colloid is ideal because none has all of the following properties: osmotic pressure similar to plasma; oxygen carrying and distribution properties; reasonable duration of action; multiple routes of metabolism and elimination; lack of antigenicity, allergenicity, and pyrogenicity; easy production and sterilization; pharmacologic inertness; and low cost.
- Albumin and hetastarch are considered equivalent for treatment of hypovolemic shock.
  - Albumin is more widely used than plasmanate. Plasmanate contains approximately 88% albumin and 12% globulins; globulins are responsible for a higher incidence of serum sickness.
  - Hetastarch, a complex sugar (starch), has essentially replaced dextran as a synthetic plasma volume expander. Patients with coagulation disorders should probably avoid hetastarch because of reported coagulation effects.
- Colloids must be administered through large-bore central lines because of their viscosity.
- Colloids expand intravascular volume in at least a 1:1 ratio, depending on dose and rate of administration, and on patient factors. It is not uncommon for 250 mL of albumin 5% or hetastarch to increase relative intravascular volume by 400- to 500-mL. Four-to-one volume expansion may occur after 25% albumin.
- Advantages of colloids include long dwell time in vasculature ranging from several hours to days, lower volume requirement compared with crystalloids, and lower incidence of pulmonary edema.
- Disadvantages mirror the advantages. Fluid overload is a more serious complication because diuretics do not affect circulating colloids. Colloids may precipitate congestive heart failure if cardiovascular function

is compromised. Colloids may be detrimental in patients with increased capillary permeability because leakage into the interstitium exerts oncotic pressure that increases risk of pulmonary edema. Finally, colloids cost more than crystalloids.

BLOOD

- Blood transfusion is indicated if hemoglobin is <10 g/dL because of its central role in Do_2.
- Banked whole blood is often used; however, it lacks labile clotting factors (V, VIII, IX) and platelets. Fresh whole blood (<6 hours old) has intact clotting factors and platelets; however, it is not as available as banked whole blood.
- Blood administration is associated with some potentially serious risks.
  - Blood should be cross-matched for ABO and Rh antigens. Acute hemolytic transfusion reactions necessitate stopping blood transfusion, and administering crystalloid to treat hypotension and maintain urine output at >100 mL/h to prevent hemoglobinuria-induced renal failure. A vasopressor may be required to reverse hypotension. Loop diuretics or mannitol (25 g) can be added to maintain renal blood flow and urine output. Delayed hemolytic reactions occur 7–10 days after the transfusion and are rarely dangerous.
  - Potential for viral transmission (e.g., hepatitis, cytomegalovirus, and human immunodeficiency virus) must be considered.
  - Transfusion of >2 units can be problematic because blood is stored in acid citrate dextrose or citrate phosphate dextrose. Calcium 4 mEq should be administered per unit of blood to prevent hypocalcemia caused by citrate phosphate dextrose sequestration of calcium ion. Hyperkalemia, which may be caused by hemolysis of stored blood, does not usually require therapy. Metabolism of citrate to bicarbonate may induce metabolic alkalosis. Urticarial reactions may be treated with IV H_1 antihistamines (diphenhydramine) without interrupting transfusion.
  - Multiple transfusions can aggravate hypothermia because blood is stored in the refrigerator.
- Blood is usually administered through a 170-μm filter to remove microaggregates. Blood is compatible with normal saline, but not with dextrose or lactated Ringer's solution. Usual administration time is 1 unit per 1 hour, which can be shortened but should not be prolonged beyond 4 hours.
- Each unit of whole blood raises hemoglobin by approximately 1 g/dL.
- Packed red blood cells are used in fluid-restricted patients.
- Platelets and fresh-frozen plasma are cornerstones of hemorrhage management. One unit of platelets usually increases the platelet count by about 7000–10,000/mm^3. Fresh-frozen plasma contains clotting factors and fibrinogen, and is therefore added to platelets for severe bleeding. Cryoprecipitate provides the best source of factors I, VIII, and XIII as well as fibrinogen for severe coagulopathy.

▶ EVALUATION OF THERAPEUTIC OUTCOMES

II
- Cardiovascular and respiratory parameters should be monitored continuously (Table 12.1). Trends, rather than specific CVP or PCWP numbers, should be attempted because of interpatient variability in response.
- Successful fluid resuscitation should increase SBP (>90 mm Hg), CI (>2.2 L/min/m^2), and urine output (0.5–1 mL/kg/h) while decreasing SVR to the normal range (900–1200 dynes-s/cm^5). MAP of >60 mm Hg should be achieved to ensure adequate cerebral and coronary perfusion pressure.
- Intravascular volume overload is characterized by high filling pressures (CVP > 12–15 mm Hg, PCWP > 20–24 mm Hg) and decreased CO (<3.5 L/min). If volume overload occurs, furosemide 20–40 mg should be administered by slow IV push to produce rapid diuresis of intravascular volume and "unload" the heart through venous dilation.
- Coagulation problems are primarily associated with low levels of clotting factors in stored blood as well as dilution of endogenous clotting factors and platelets following administration of the blood. As a result, a coagulation panel (PT, INR, aPTT) should be checked in patients undergoing replacement of 50–100% or more of blood volume in 12–24 hours.

See Chapter 23, Hypovolemic and Cardiogenic Shock, authored by Edward Sypniewski, Jr., PharmD, for a more detailed discussion of this topic.

Chapter 13

▶ STROKE

▶ DEFINITION

Stroke is the syndrome caused by disruption in blood flow to the brain resulting in sudden onset of a focal neurologic deficit that persists for at least 24 hours. Stroke is a major manifestation of cerebrovascular disease, which in turn refers to any type of pathophysiologic vascular disease of the brain.

▶ PATHOPHYSIOLOGY

- Vascular pathology leading to stroke can include any abnormality of the vessel, blood flow, or blood quality. Vessel abnormalities include many processes such as developmental defects, arteritis, aneurysm, hypertensive disease, vasoconstriction, and atherosclerosis. Blood flow can be affected by vessel disease and also by thrombotic or embolic processes. Decreased blood flow in the brain (i.e., ischemia) or cerebral bleeding can produce these abnormalities.
- Of the many potential causes of stroke, infarction accounts for 85% and hemorrhage accounts for only 15% (Fig. 13.1). Atherothrombotic infarction is the most common type of stroke, representing almost 66% of reported cases.

TREATABLE RISK FACTORS

- Hypertension is the major predisposing treatable risk factor for stroke and is strongly related to atherothrombotic brain infarction as well as cerebral hemorrhage.
- Individuals with cardiac diseases [e.g., coronary heart disease, congestive heart failure, left ventricular hypertrophy, and arrhythmias (i.e., atrial fibrillation)] have more than twice the stroke risk compared with those with normal cardiac function.
- Transient ischemic attacks (TIAs) are focal ischemic neurologic deficits lasting <24 hours. TIAs precede an ischemic stroke in about 60% of cases; 35% of untreated patients develop a stroke within 5 years of a TIA.
- Multiple factors identified in the Framingham study [i.e., elevated systolic blood pressure, elevated serum cholesterol, glucose intolerance, cigarette smoking, and left ventricular hypertrophy by electrocardiogram (ECG)] can be used to identify the 10% of the population who will have one-third of the strokes.

CEREBROVASCULAR DISEASE

Atherothrombotic Disease

- Atherosclerosis of brain arteries is a process similar to that found in extracranial vessels. Atherosclerosis and subsequent plaque formation

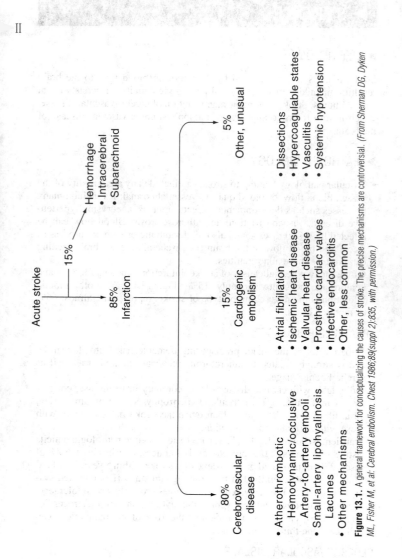

Figure 13.1. A general framework for conceptualizing the causes of stroke. The precise mechanisms are controversial. *(From Sherman DG, Dyken ML, Fisher M, et al: Cerebral embolism. Chest 1986;89(suppl 2):835, with permission.)*

result in arterial narrowing or occlusion and constitute the most common cause of aortacranial stenosis. Thrombosis is most likely to occur where plaque causes the most vessel narrowing. Embolism can produce a stroke when a clot, plaque, or platelet aggregate breaks off into the circulation and blocks an artery. Platelets contribute to thrombosis. Platelet activation, whether by plaque formation or trauma, initiates a series of events including release of adenine diphosphate (ADP) from platelets, which enhances platelet aggregation. Aggregation is consolidated by coagulation factors, red blood cells, and formation of a fibrin network. Thromboxane A_2 promotes platelet aggregation and vasoconstriction, which is balanced by prostacyclin (PGI_2). The atherosclerotic process is variable; resultant ischemic consequences depend on adequacy of blood flow and collateral circulation and embolism.

Cerebral Ischemia

- Cerebral ischemia can be global or focal. Global ischemia is associated with lack of collateral blood flow, and irreversible brain damage occurs in 4–8 minutes. In focal ischemia, collateral circulation may allow for survival of brain cells and reversal of neuronal damage after ischemia.
- Cell function can be preserved for up to 4 hours provided reductions in cerebral blood flow (CBF) are between ranges associated with electrical (i.e., 15–18 mL/100 g/min) and ionic failure (10 mL/100 g/min).
- When CBF is 10 mL/100 g/min, metabolic derangements (e.g., accumulation of lactic acid, adenosine triphosphate (ATP) depletion, and increased intracellular calcium) ultimately decrease cell integrity, increase membrane permeability, perpetuate intracellular acidosis, and impair cell function.
- Swelling is one of the primary responses of brain tissue to acute injury. Movement of plasma into the extracellular space results in increased intracranial pressure, which can result in brain herniation.

Lacunar Infarcts

- Lacuna refers to the small cavity left after necrotic tissue has been removed. Occlusion of small arterial branches of the circle of Willis and of anterior, middle, and posterior cerebral and basilar arteries can result in infarcts deep in the cerebral hemispheres and brain stem. The associated pathophysiology is somewhat different compared with that of infarcts located closer to the brain surface. The pathophysiology has been described as being a degenerative process in the media of the artery (lipohyalinosis), leading to vessel occlusion.

Transient Ischemic Attacks

- TIA pathophysiology involves atherosclerotic process, thrombus formation, and low CBF. Small microemboli break off from the cerebral thrombus and lodge in distal areas, producing temporary focal cerebral dysfunction.

CEREBRAL EMBOLISM

II
- Any region of the brain can be affected by embolism; however, the middle cerebral artery is commonly involved. Embolism has been associated with many types of heart disease.
- Chronic atrial fibrillation is the most common cause of cardiogenic embolism and is the most common sustained arrhythmia (see Chapter 5).
- Factors that further increase the risk of embolism in patients with valvular heart disease include mitral stenosis with or without incompetence (versus mitral incompetence alone), atrial fibrillation, increased left atrial size, increased age, and previous embolic event.
- Thrombus formation on prosthetic cardiac valves is related to valve-induced turbulence in blood flow and thrombogenic potential of valve material. Early Starr–Edwards valve and original Bjork–Shiley valve have higher embolic rates than newer valves. Bioprosthetic valves (e.g., Hancock, Carpentier–Edwards, Lonescu–Shiley) have a central flow design, which produces less turbulence, and a biologic material (i.e., porcine valve), which is less thrombogenic. Other risk factors include atrial fibrillation, large left atrium, inadequate anticoagulation, and previous embolic event.
- The highest frequency of emboli induced by infective endocarditis is associated with infections on the left side of the heart that produce large, mobile vegetations from *Haemophilus parainfluenzae,* or slow-growing, fastidious, gram-negative bacilli, fungi *(Aspergillus* spp.), and *Streptococcus viridans.*

INTRACRANIAL HEMORRHAGE

- Frequent causes of hemorrhagic stroke are hypertensive intracerebral hemorrhage, ruptured saccular aneurysms, hemorrhage associated with bleeding disorders, and arteriovenous malformations. Bleeding from a ruptured artery allows for an extravasation of blood into brain tissue and mass formation. Brain tissue is pushed, displaced, and compressed; brain functions may be impaired.

▶ CLINICAL PRESENTATION

- Neurologic manifestations differ depending on stroke type; location of insult; and extent of ischemia, infarct, or hemorrhage. Stroke may show varied manifestations, which are reversible or irreversible and which range from hemiplegia to sensory deficits. Hemiplegia may or may not be accompanied by other manifestations.
- Thrombosis of cerebral vessels produces variable clinical manifestations compared with other stroke types. Stroke is preceded by TIA(s) in >50% of cases. If thrombosis involves internal carotid and middle cerebral arteries, focal symptoms may include mono- or hemiplegia, mono- or hemiparesthesia, blindness in one eye, and speech disturbance. If the vertebrobasilar system is involved, symptoms may include dizziness,

diplopia, numbness, impaired vision, and dysarthria. Usually these attacks are short lived and resolve in <10 minutes. Stroke itself most often develops suddenly as a single attack. Stroke in evolution or progressing stroke evolves over hours, days, or weeks. Most cerebral thrombotic strokes occur at rest while sleeping or after arising. Headache may precede other symptoms, but it is often absent.

- Clinical presentation of lacunar infarcts varies depending on their location. The most frequently occurring lacunar syndrome is pure motor hemiparesis (e.g., hemiparesis or hemiplegia of arm, leg, face, and trunk) due to infarction in the posterior portion of the internal capsule. Mild dysarthria occurs without sensory or consciousness alterations or visual field defects. Affected body parts display the same degree of weakness. In contrast, stroke in the cortical region usually leads to unequal distribution of weakness.
- Most TIAs last 5–10 minutes; those lasting ≥1 hours may result from embolism. Symptoms are determined by lesion location (Table 13.1).

TABLE 13.1. Symptoms of Transient Ischemic Attacks

Carotid system TIAs
Unilateral weakness—usually hemiparesis
Unilateral sensory complaints—numbness, paresthesia
Aphasia—language comprehension, output, or both
Monocular visual loss (amaurosis fugax)

Vertebrobasilar system TIAs
Motor deficit—especially if bilateral
Sensory complaints—especially if bilateral
Simultaneous, bilateral visual complaints
Diplopia ⎫
Vertigo ⎪
Dysarthria[a] ⎬ Only in combination, not as
Ataxia without weakness ⎪ isolated symptoms
Dysphagia ⎭

Either carotid or vertebral TIAs
Severe dysarthria[a]
Homonymous visual complaints

Isolated symptoms rarely resulting from TIAs
Vertigo, dizziness
Diplopia
Loss of consciousness
Confusion
Bilateral leg weakness, falling spells

[a]Often difficult to distinguish from nonfluent dysphasia on the basis of history.
From Easton JD, Hart RG, Sherman DG, et al: Diagnosis and management of ischemic stroke. Part 1. Threatened stroke and its management. Curr Prob Cardiol 1983;8:13, with permission.

- Onset of cerebral embolism is characteristically abrupt, often occurring in an awake patient. Cardiogenic embolism is associated with multifocal neurologic findings.
- Clinical manifestations of intracranial hemorrhage have an abrupt onset; changes generally occur over minutes to hours (up to 24 hours). Most patients lose consciousness, which is often preceded by head pain and dizziness. Headache is more likely to occur at the onset than with thromboembolism (50% versus <25% of cases). Neck rigidity, convulsions, and vomiting are common. Hypertension-related external capsule (putaminal) hemorrhage is manifested by rapid onset of hemiplegia, loss of consciousness, and conjugate deviation of eyes to contralateral side. As the lesion enlarges, compression of upper brain stem produces deepening coma, dilated and fixed pupils, Babinski signs, bilateral motor hypertonus, and irregular respirations. Internal capsule (thalamic) hemorrhage is also characterized by rapid onset; however, loss of vision occurs on the same side as optic nerve involvement in the internal capsule. Gaze disturbances include defective vertical and lateral gaze, fixed downward deviation of eyes, and unequal pupils.

▶ DIAGNOSIS

- It is challenging to diagnose accurately a particular lesion because of variations in presentation; however, good clinical examination can help to locate a lesion and to delineate between ischemic and hemorrhagic stroke. Imaging studies [e.g, computed tomography (CT) scan and magnetic resonance imaging (MRI)] are important diagnostic tools. CT scan results must be known before therapy of stroke with anticoagulants or platelet antiaggregating agents.
- Diagnosis of atherothrombotic stroke requires evaluation of clinical presentation and laboratory findings. Tests may include cerebral arteriography, CT and MRI scans, radioactive brain scan study (e.g., technetium scan), head x-rays, electroencephalogram (EEC), ECG, transcranial Doppler studies, and lumbar puncture (LP). Arteriogram is the definitive test for arterial occlusion or narrowing; however, because of associated neurologic risk, arteriogram should be reserved for unclear diagnosis or pending vascular surgery. Hydration may reduce risks of arteriogram. Because of these risks, brain imaging is most important. CT scan is often normal during the first 48 hours after thrombotic infarct. In contrast, MRI can adequately detect small infarcts in the cortical surface and elsewhere usually within 1 hour of occurrence. Promising new techniques include digital subtraction angiography, transesophageal echocardiography, xenon blood flow, and positron emission tomography (PET) scan.
- CT or MRI scan can provide evidence of lacunar infarction if performed within 7–10 days; however, infarcts <2 mm may be missed.
- Diagnosis of TIA is confounded by short duration, which necessitates reliance on the patient's recollection of symptoms (Table 13.1). Labo-

ratory studies are performed to rule out blood or other disorders that may decrease CBF. Embolism of cardiac origin should be considered by performing ECG, chest x-ray, and echocardiography, especially with two-dimensional technique.

II

- Cardiogenic embolism should be considered when the following are present: patient older than age 60, sudden onset of maximal neurologic deficit, prior cortical infarct, history of valvular heart disease or left ventricular myocardial infarct, and atrial fibrillation or congestive heart failure. Two-dimensional, M-mode, and transesophogeal echocardiography are all useful for demonstrating thrombi, valve dysfunction, and cardiac dysfunction. ECG may indicate arrhythmia (e.g., atrial fibrillation). MRI and CT are being evaluated for their ability to detect cardiogenic emboli.
- In hypertensive intracerebral hemorrhage, important diagnostic clues are sudden onset and quick evolution of physical findings, and history of hypertension. Ocular signs are helpful in localizing hemorrhages of putaminal and thalamic origin; funduscopic examination may reveal periarteriolar hemorrhages and decreased arteriolar size. CT is the diagnostic procedure of choice because it can detect small amounts of blood and distinguish between hemorrhage and infarction.

▶ DESIRED OUTCOME

The desired outcome depends on the etiology of stroke. For example, a comprehensive approach to cerebrovascular disease consists of general prophylaxis against stroke and vascular disease, supportive and medical management during the acute phase of stroke, mitigation of the pathologic or atherothrombotic process, and appropriate rehabilitative and physical therapy programs during the poststroke period.

▶ TREATMENT

GENERAL PRINCIPLES

- Control of hypertension, hyperlipidemia, obesity, tobacco use, and other risk factors (Table 13.2) is essential to overall care of the patient with cerebrovascular disease.

ISCHEMIC CEREBROVASCULAR DISEASE

Anticoagulants

- Anticoagulation should not be used routinely for TIAs and should not be used at all for completed stroke. Anticoagulation is still controversial for progressing stroke; however, individual judgment must be used when intracerebral hemorrhage has been ruled out by CT scan.
- If indicated, heparin should be administered acutely by continuous IV infusion to a target activated partial thromboplastin time (aPTT) of 1.5 times control value.

TABLE 13.2. Risk Factors in Stroke

Single risk factors
  Well-documented risk factors
    Treatment not feasible or value not established
      Age and gender
      Familial factors
      Race
      Diabetes mellitus
      Prior stroke
      Asymptomatic carotid bruits
    Treatable
      Hypertension
      Cardiac disease
      Transient ischemic attacks
      Elevated hematocrit
      Sickle cell disease
  Less well-documented risk factors
    Treatment not feasible or value not established
      Geographic location
      Season and climate
      Socioeconomic factors
    Treatable but value not established
      Elevated blood cholesterol and lipids
      Cigarette smoking
      Alcohol consumption
      Oral contraceptive use
      Physical inactivity
      Obesity
Multiple risk factors
  Framingham profile
    Systolic blood pressure
    Serum cholesterol
    Glucose tolerance
    Cigarette smoking
    Electrocardiogram
    Left ventricular hypertrophy
  Paffenbarger and Williams criteria
    Cigarette smoking
    Systolic blood pressure
    Low ponderal index
    Body height
    A parent dead
    Not a varsity athlete

From Dyken ML, Wolf PA, Barnett HJM, et al: Risk factors in stroke—a statement for physicians by the Subcommittee on Risk Factors and Stroke of the Stroke Council. Stroke 1984;15:1106, with permission.

- If indicated, warfarin should overlap with heparin for approximately 5 days. A slightly less intensive anticoagulation regimen [i.e., international normalized ratio (INR) of 2.0–3.0] reduces the incidence of bleeding without decreasing efficacy.

Thrombolytic Agents

- Alteplase carries FDA approval for use in acute ischemic stroke, but several other thrombolytics have also been investigated.
- Alteplase must be initiated within 3 hours of onset, and diagnosis of ischemic stroke (including CT scan) must be made by a physician with expertise in verifying stroke. Alteplase is not recommended when the time of stroke onset cannot be ascertained reliably (e.g., strokes recognized on awakening).
- The recommended dose of alteplase is 0.9 mg/kg (maximum 90 mg) infused over 60 minutes, with 10% of the total dose administered as an initial IV bolus over 1 minute.
- Hemorrhage is the most common and potentially severe complication of thrombolytic therapy for acute ischemic stroke. Treatment should only be administered if bleeding complications can be managed promptly. Patients taking heparin or warfarin should not be given alteplase.

Antiplatelet Agents

- Of the many antiplatelet agents that have been studied for use in ischemic cerebrovascular disease, aspirin and ticlopidine are the only commercially available agents with convincing clinical effects.
- Aspirin inhibits platelet aggregation by irreversible inactivation of cyclooxygenase, which prevents conversion of arachidonic acid to thromboxane A_2. Optimal dose should inhibit thromboxane A_2, but not prostacyclin. Recent studies indicate the lowest effective dose may be 20–40 mg/day; however, effectiveness of doses less than 300 mg/day for TIA or minor strokes of arterial origin is not resolved. A dose of 325–975 mg/d is recommended for preventing TIAs and stroke. Enteric-coated products may be better tolerated.
- Ticlopidine has unique platelet antiaggregatory effects and is superior to aspirin in patients with TIAs; however, it is less tolerable and more costly. Side effects occur in >50% of patients (e.g., gastrointestinal complaints); some side effects are significant (e.g., bone marrow suppression, rash, diarrhea, elevated serum cholesterol, reversible neutropenia). Ticlopidine may interact with digoxin, theophylline, and antacids. Although its place in therapy requires further evaluation, ticlopidine 250 mg twice daily is an alternative if aspirin is not tolerated or not effective.

Surgery

- Surgery is performed to prevent cerebral infarctions and TIAs by removing the source of occlusion and/or embolus, which should increase CBF to an ischemic area. Carotid endarterectomy is the most common surgical procedure for occlusive cerebrovascular disease. Indications are TIAs and mild completed stroke in the presence of ulcerated or highly stenotic (>75%) plaque. Carotid endarterectomy was superior to medical treatment alone in symptomatic patients with stenosis of ≥70%, but it was not beneficial in patients with <70% stenosis.

CEREBRAL EMBOLISM OF CARDIAC ORIGIN

- Immediate anticoagulation with heparin should be considered to reduce the risk of recurrent embolic events if CT scan documents absence of hemorrhagic transformation. Heparin is usually given 24 hours after stroke onset without a loading dose; aPTT should be maintained no greater than 1.5 times control. Warfarin (INR 2.0–3.0) should follow heparin therapy.
- Patients at high risk of embolic events because of atrial fibrillation should receive prophylactic chronic anticoagulation with warfarin. Because of the potential of intracerebral hemorrhage in elderly patients and the probability of lifetime treatment, subgroups with high and low rates of stroke have been identified (see Chapter 5, Arrhythmias).
  - Younger low-risk patients (<75 years) and patients with lone atrial fibrillation can be treated with aspirin 325 mg/day.
  - High-risk patients in whom anticoagulation is judged to be safe can be treated with warfarin to an INR of 2.0–3.0.
  - High-risk patients >75 years may be treated with lower intensity warfarin at an INR of 2.0. Aspirin is the alternative.
  - Anticoagulation is necessary for most patients with atrial fibrillation who have had an ischemic stroke.
- Patients who have had prosthetic cardiac valve replacement should begin anticoagulation immediately after surgery to reduce risk of thromboembolism. The regimen depends on valve type.
  - Mechanical prosthetic cardiac valve: Six hours after implantation, therapy should begin with IV heparin to maintain aPTT at 1.5–2 times control, followed by subcutaneous heparin 10,000 U every 12 hours after chest tube removal until discharge. Warfarin should be started as soon as possible after the operation and dosed to maintain INR of 2.5–3.5. Aspirin 160 mg/day or dipyridamole 5–6 mg/kg/day may be added to warfarin for additional protection. For patients who cannot take oral anticoagulants, dipyridamole plus sulfinpyrazone 800 mg/d may be tried empirically.
  - Bioprosthetic cardiac valve: Initial heparin therapy is similar to that given to patients with a mechanical prosthetic cardiac valve. For mitral valve, warfarin therapy should be initiated soon after operation and continued for 3 months at a less intense INR of 2.0–3.0. Warfarin (INR of 2.0–3.0) should be continued indefinitely in patients who have atrial fibrillation, enlarged left atrium, or previous thromboembolism. For aortic valve and sinus rhythm, anticoagulation is optional. Aspirin 325 mg/day can be used empirically in patients with bioprosthetic cardiac valves.

INTRACRANIAL HEMORRHAGE

- Surgery can be performed in the acute or early stage to remove the clot by aspiration or evacuation in patients whose hemorrhage is near the brain surface and who are not comatose.
- To reduce edema around the hemorrhage, mannitol 0.25–2 g/kg can be administered intravenously every 4–8 hours until the serum osmolality is raised between 300 and 310 mOsm/L. This regimen is also suitable for ischemic stroke; however, cerebral edema is rarely present unless there is a large infarction in the middle cerebral artery. Corticosteroids (e.g., dexamethasone) are no longer recommended.
- Cerebral vasospasm in subarachnoid hemorrhage can be severe; reserpine, kanamycin, isoproterenol, aminophylline, and nitroprusside have all failed. Dopamine, 3–6 µg/kg/min, has been used, but there is a risk of rebleeding. Barbiturate coma has been used to reduce intracranial pressure when dopamine or mannitol has not been successful.

▶ EVALUATION OF THERAPEUTIC OUTCOMES

- Treatable single risk factors should be vigorously addressed. When risk factors occur in combination, therapy is initiated aggressively, with particular emphasis on hypertension and lifestyle changes. Blood pressure is monitored to ensure effective management of hypertension; drug-induced hypotension must be avoided. Lipid profiles, body weight, tobacco use, and other risk factors should also be monitored.
- Patients receiving anticoagulant therapy are carefully monitored for maintenance of appropriate coagulation parameters and for minor and major bleeding.
- Patients receiving aspirin are monitored for gastrointestinal bleeding because risk of bleeding is slightly increased.
- Patients receiving ticlopidine are monitored for side effects and potential drug interactions. Complete blood count with differential should be performed every 2 weeks for 3 months.

See Chapter 20, Stroke, authored by J. Chris Bradberry, PharmD, for a more detailed discussion of this topic.

Chapter 14 _____

▶ THROMBOEMBOLIC DISORDERS

▶ DEFINITION

Venous thromboembolism includes both venous thrombosis and pulmonary embolism. A deep vein thrombosis (DVT) is a thrombus composed of cellular material (red and white blood cells, platelets) bound together with fibrin strands, which form in the venous portion of the vasculature. A pulmonary embolism (PE) is a thrombus or foreign substance that arises from the systemic circulation and lodges in the pulmonary artery or one of its branches, causing complete or partial obstruction of pulmonary blood flow.

▶ PATHOPHYSIOLOGY

• Three primary components—venous stasis, vascular injury, and hypercoagulability (Virchow's triad)—play a role in the development of a thrombus.

• Venous stasis is characterized by altered or decreased blood flow in the deep veins of the lower limbs resulting from immobility, prolonged bed rest, massive obesity, venous obstruction, congestive heart failure, hypovolemia, varicose veins, late-stage pregnancy, shock, or severe myocardial infarction.

• Vascular wall injury or endothelial damage occurs from mechanical (e.g., venipuncture, fractures) or chemical (e.g., potassium, hypertonic glucose) trauma that evokes an inflammatory response (phlebitis), in addition to locally activating the coagulation cascade to form an intraluminal thrombus.

• Hypercoagulability and excessive activation of the coagulation cascade can occur in activated protein C resistance; deficiencies of protein C, protein S, or antithrombin III; and certain types of malignancy.

• The coagulation cascade can be triggered through either the intrinsic or extrinsic pathways (Fig. 14.1). The intrinsic pathway is activated by the contact of factor XII with exposed collagen from damaged subendothelial vessels. The extrinsic pathway is activated by the exposure of blood to tissue thromboplastin, a tissue factor released after vascular wall damage.

• Most venous thrombi involve the veins of the lower extremities where they develop behind venous valve cusps or at bifurcations in the intramuscular veins of the calf. Consequences of DVT include the postphlebitic syndrome, compromise of venous blood flow to the lower extremity, chronic venous insufficiency, and embolization of the thrombus to the lungs or elsewhere.

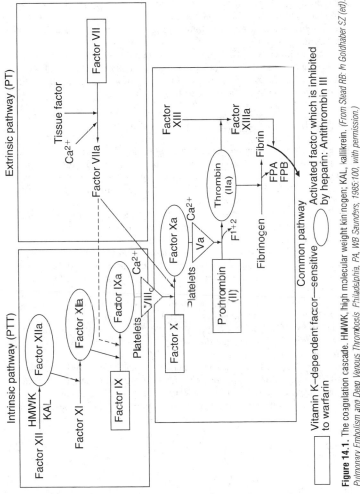

Figure 14.1. The coagulation cascade. HMWK, high molecular weight kininogen; KAL, kallikrein. *(From Stead RB: In Goldhaber SZ (ed). Pulmonary Embolism and Deep Venous Thrombosis. Philadelphia, PA, WB Saunders, 1985:100, with permission.)*

II

- In most patients, venous thrombi and PE are broken up by the endogenous lytic system, with complete clot resolution occurring over several weeks.
- The pulmonary effects of a PE may include the formation of an alveolar dead space, pneumoconstriction, arterial hypoxemia, loss of pulmonary surfactant (which occurs after 24 hours) leading to atelectasis and transudation of alveolar fluid into alveolar spaces, and pulmonary infarction (<10%).
- Hemodynamically, a PE increases pulmonary vascular resistance and subsequently right ventricular afterload. If these changes become marked, they may lead to tricuspid regurgitation, pulmonary hypertension, right ventricular failure, and low cardiac output.

▶ CLINICAL PRESENTATION

- Venous thrombi frequently are clinically silent. The most common clinical symptoms include pain, tenderness, swelling, and discoloration. The pain and tenderness are usually localized to the calf in patients with calf vein thrombosis and tend to be more diffuse and intense in patients with proximal vein thrombosis.
- Edema secondary to proximal vein obstruction or vascular inflammation is most often responsible for the swelling and ranges in severity. The swelling typically is localized or unilateral and can occur with or without pain. Patients with DVT may exhibit a discolored lower extremity from cyanosis because of a large venous obstruction; it may also be pale secondary to reflex arterial vasospasm or reddish from perivascular inflammation.
- Physical signs that may be present include a palpable cord and a positive Homan's sign (a nonspecific and insensitive test).
- Symptoms of postphlebitic syndrome may range from chronic pain and swelling in the lower extremities to the formation of stasis ulcers and the development of infection.
- Although many PE are clinically silent, signs and symptoms may include a sudden onset of unexplained dyspnea, cough, tachypnea, tachycardia, pleuritic chest pain, and anxiety or a feeling of impending doom. Diaphoresis, substernal chest pain, and hemoptysis (which may indicate pulmonary infarction or congestive atelectasis) are sometimes seen.
- Patients with massive PE often present with signs of circulatory collapse, such as syncope or shock due to a reduced cardiac output, or with evidence of acute cor pulmonale or right ventricular failure.

▶ DIAGNOSIS

- The diagnosis of DVT or PE should be suspected in any patient with suggestive clinical signs and symptoms. Because none are specific, objective testing methods are necessary.

- A medical history, medication history, and thorough physical examination are important in identifying underlying risk factors that may have led to the development of the thrombus.

II

DIAGNOSTIC TECHNIQUES FOR DVT

- Diagnostic techniques may visualize the thrombus (contrast venography, ultrasound, magnetic resonance imaging); measure obstructions to venous outflow (impedance plethysmography, Doppler ultrasound); or detect the incorporation of radiolabeled proteins into the developing thrombus (^{125}I-fibrinogen scan).
- Impedance plethysmography (IPG) is a noninvasive test that is sensitive and specific for thrombosis of the proximal veins; it is less sensitive for thrombosis of the calf veins and cannot distinguish between thrombotic and nonthrombotic obstruction to venous outflow. A normal result essentially excludes the diagnosis of proximal vein thrombosis, but not calf vein thrombosis.
- Doppler ultrasonography is a noninvasive diagnostic test used for the evaluation of patients with suspected DVT that is highly sensitive in detecting thrombi in proximal veins but less sensitive to thrombi that are nonocclusive or located in the calf veins. Advantages of the Doppler are that it is almost as sensitive as IPG in detecting symptomatic DVT, it is convenient and inexpensive, and it has better sensitivity to calf vein thrombosis. It also has applicability to patients with arterial insufficiency or plaster casts.
- Real-time ultrasonography may be useful in detecting acute and chronic thrombi in the lower extremities. It is very accurate and sensitive in the diagnosis of proximal vein thrombosis but less accurate in detecting calf vein thrombi.
- Serial Doppler ultrasonography, IPG, and real-time ultrasonography tests are often obtained the day after the initial test, on day 5 to 7, and again between days 10 and 14. If the test becomes positive during the serial testing, the patient is diagnosed with DVT and anticoagulant therapy is initiated.
- ^{125}I-fibrinogen leg scanning can be used as a screening tool in high-risk patients or as an adjunctive test to IPG in patients with suspected DVT. This technique detects more than 90% of calf vein thrombi, but only 60–80% of proximal vein thrombi. It should never be used as the only diagnostic tool because it fails to detect many high proximal vein thrombi.
- Venography may be used in patients in whom noninvasive techniques are inconclusive, or in whom ultrasonic techniques are not useful (morbidly obese, edema).
- New plasma markers, such as D-dimer, are currently being evaluated as negative predictors of DVT and PE.

DIAGNOSTIC TECHNIQUES FOR PE

- An electrocardiogram (ECG), chest roentgenogram, and arterial blood gas should be obtained in any patient with suspected PE. ECG patterns may include nonspecific ST-segment elevations or depression, T wave inversion, right axis deviation, new incomplete right bundle-branch block, or evidence of right ventricular hypertrophy. The radiographic patterns may include effusions, infiltrates, enlargement of right descending pulmonary artery, Westermark's sign (avascular lung zones), and elevation of the diaphragm.

- An arterial blood gas may be useful in assessing the degree of ventilation; however, approximately 10–20% of patients with PE have Po_2 values of >80 mm Hg.
- A ventilation–perfusion (V/Q) radionuclide scan estimates the probability of PE based on the anatomic patterns of injected and inhaled radioactive materials. Pulmonary perfusion defects are nonspecific, so assessment of ventilation is necessary. Because an embolus obstructs arterial blood flow in one of the pulmonary arteries but does not affect ventilation, this scan can detect areas that are being ventilated but not perfused (a V/Q mismatch). If results are inconclusive, further objective testing is necessary to confirm the diagnosis of PE.
- Pulmonary angiography may be indicated when there is a nondiagnostic V/Q scan with or without a normal IPG in a patient with a picture suggestive of PE; disagreement between V/Q scan interpretation and clinical impression; a contraindication to anticoagulation; and anticipation of thrombolytic therapy, inferior vena cava interruption, or embolectomy.

▶ DESIRED OUTCOME

The main objectives of treating venous thrombosis are to prevent the development of pulmonary embolism and the postphlebitic syndrome, to reduce morbidity from the acute event, and to achieve these objectives with a minimum of adverse effects and cost. Successful treatment of DVT should prevent extension of the thrombus, prevent embolism to the lungs, and restore patency to the venous circulation while maintaining normal venous valve function.

▶ TREATMENT

GENERAL PRINCIPLES

- In any patient suspected of having a DVT or PE, empiric therapy (e.g., heparin) is started to decrease the risk of further embolic events while waiting for the results of diagnostic tests.
- General management of DVT includes bed rest, with the heels elevated above the heart to enhance venous return, and administration of nonaspirin analgesics for pain.
- For PE, oxygen should be given and, if necessary, patients should be mechanically ventilated.
- Coagulation tests (aPTT, PT, INR) should be performed prior to the initiation of therapy to establish the patient's baseline values, which assists

in determining the endpoint for heparin therapy and guides later oral anticoagulation with warfarin.

HEPARIN

- The anticoagulant function of heparin is thought to depend on its ability to bind to and catalyze antithrombin III (ATIII) or heparin cofactor, a circulating anticoagulant that neutralizes the proteolytic activities of several clotting factors that have a serine residue at their enzymatically active site (XII, XI, X, and IX, kallikrein, and thrombin).
- Heparin halts further growth and propagation of the thrombus, allowing the endogenous thrombolytic system to eradicate the existing clot. In addition, heparin may also promote thrombus resolution.
- Heparin is indicated in patients with a thrombus extending above the popliteal vein because of the high risk of PE and postphlebitic syndrome in these patients. Patients with symptomatic calf vein thrombosis should also receive heparin. Patients with superficial thrombophlebitis should not receive anticoagulation. Heparin is clearly indicated for patients with documented PE and is also used for the prevention of venous thromboembolism.
- Contraindications include hypersensitivity to the drug, active bleeding, hemophilia, thrombocytopenia, intracranial hemorrhage, bacterial endocarditis, active tuberculosis, ulcerative lesions of the GI tract, severe hypertension, threatened abortion, or visceral carcinoma.
- Figure 14.2 is an algorithm for the acute management of DVT or PE with heparin therapy and management of excessive anticoagulation. Doses should be based on total body weight with a loading dose of 70–100 U/kg followed by an initial IV infusion rate of 15–25 U/kg/h. One popular regimen is an initial dose of 80 U/kg followed by 18 U/kg/h. Continuous intravenous (IV) infusion is the recommended method of administration because it produces a more consistent degree of anticoagulation and may be associated with lower risk for bleeding than intermittent bolus dosing.
  - The activated partial thromboplastin time (aPTT) should be checked no sooner than 6 hours after beginning the heparin infusion or after any dosage change (target aPTT: 1.5–2.0 times control).
  - Once the target aPTT is achieved, daily monitoring is indicated for minor dosing adjustments.
  - In uncomplicated patients or less extensive disease, a short course of heparin therapy may be appropriate (4–5 days of continuous IV heparin with warfarin started on day 1). Patients with massive pulmonary embolism or ileofemoral thrombosis may require a more traditional duration of heparin therapy (i.e., 10 days), with warfarin being started on day 5.
- If continuous infusion is not feasible, intermittent IV injections may be given every 4 hours in most patients, with aPTT performed 3.5–4 hours after the heparin injection.

II

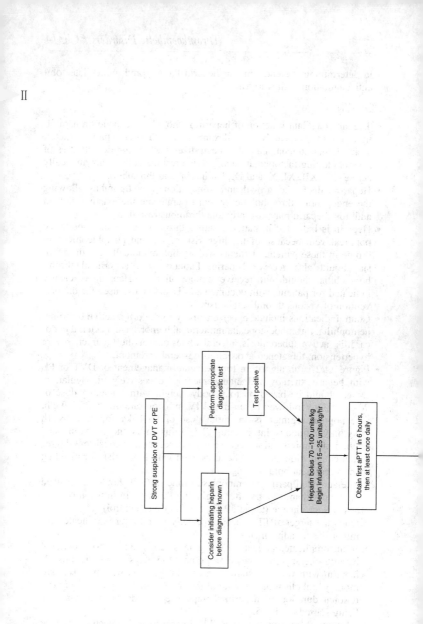

Strong suspicion of DVT or PE

Consider initiating heparin before diagnosis known

Perform appropriate diagnostic test

Test positive

Heparin bolus 70–100 units/kg
Begin infusion 15–25 units/kg/hr

Obtain first aPTT in 6 hours, then at least once daily

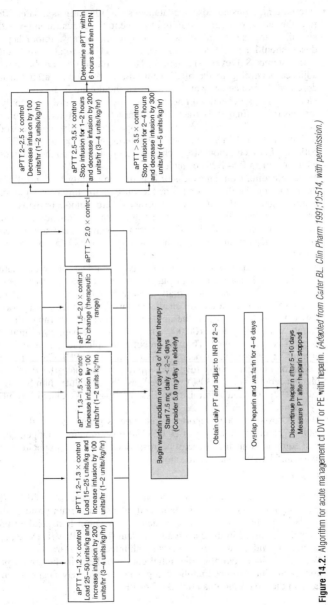

Figure 14.2. Algorithm for acute management of DVT or PE with heparin. (Adapted from Carter BL. Clin Pharm 1991;10:514, with permission.)

The algorithm contains the following text boxes:

aPTT 1–1.2 × control
Load 25–50 units/kg and increase infusion by 200 units/hr (3–4 units/kg/hr)

aPTT 1.2–1.3 × control
Load 15–25 units/kg and increase infusion by 100 units/hr (1–2 units/kg/hr)

aPTT 1.3–1.5 × control
Increase infusion by 100 units/hr (1–2 units/kg/hr)

aPTT 1.5–2.0 × control
No change (therapeutic range)

aPTT > 2.0 × control

aPTT 2–2.5 × control
Decrease infusion by 100 units/hr (1–2 units/kg/hr)

aPTT 2.5–3.5 × control
Stop infusion for 1–2 hours and decrease infusion by 200 units/hr (3–4 units/kg/hr)

aPTT > 3.5 × control
Stop infusion for 2–4 hours and decrease infusion by 300 units/hr (4–5 units/kg/hr)

Determine aPTT within 6 hours and then PRN

Begin warfarin sodium on day 1–3 of heparin therapy
Start 7.5 mg daily × 2–3 days
(Consider 5.0 mg/day in elderly)

Obtain daily PT and adjust to INR of 2–3

Overlap heparin and warfarin for 4–6 days

Discontinue heparin after 5–10 days
Measure PT after heparin stopped

II

179

- Intermittent, adjusted-dose subcutaneous (SQ) heparin is a safe, effective alternative route for the initial treatment of venous thrombosis that simplifies treatment and allows for outpatient therapy. Initial heparin doses should be 15,000–17,500 U or 250 U/kg total body weight administered SQ every 12 hours. The initial dose can be rapidly adjusted according to the aPTT value drawn 4–6 hours after the first dose and then once daily at the middle of the dosing interval.

- Hemorrhage associated with heparin therapy occurs most commonly in the gastrointestinal (GI) tract, the urinary tract, soft tissues, and the oropharynx. The most frequently encountered bleeding episodes include melena, hematomas, and hematuria, which occur in 2–3% of patients. Less common are ecchymosis, epistaxis, and hematemesis, which occur in 0.5–1.2% of patients.

- Minor bleeding from an excess of heparin can usually be controlled by discontinuing the drug. For major bleeding or the threat of significant hemorrhage, specific therapy is warranted (e.g., blood transfusion or protamine sulfate) For patients receiving continuous infusion heparin, 1 mg of protamine should be administered by slow IV infusion for each 100 U of heparin delivered during the past 4 hours ($\leq$50 mg over 10 minutes).

- Thrombocytopenia may occur as an early, slight decrease in circulating platelets that is transient, with platelet counts seldom dropping below 100,000/mm^3; this does not usually require drug discontinuation. A rare but severe immunologically mediated thrombocytopenia may occur between 5–14 days after the initiation of heparin therapy. Platelet counts may fall below 100,000/mm^3 and will remain low until the heparin is discontinued. Thromboembolic complications may occur in arteries or veins (i.e., myocardial infarction, DVT, PE). Careful monitoring of platelet counts (every 2–3 days) to evaluate the decline of platelet count (i.e., >30%) as well as the absolute number (i.e., <100,000/mm^3) can minimize the risk of heparin-associated thrombocytopenia.

- Osteoporosis has been reported rarely and is generally found only in patients receiving in excess of 20,000 U/d for 6 months or longer. Other rare complications include skin necrosis, local urticaria, hypoaldosteronism, and hypersensitivity reactions.

WARFARIN

- Warfarin prevents formation of γ-carboxyglutamic acid residues (by blocking the carboxylation system) and release of certain proteins that are deficient in γ-carboxyglutamic acid. Six vitamin K-dependent proteins are involved in the coagulation system (factors II, VII, IX, X, and proteins C and S), whose synthesis is inhibited by warfarin.

- Warfarin is indicated after the initial course of heparin therapy to prevent recurrent thromboembolic complications that may occur particularly in the first 3 months after DVT or PE.

- Although inhibition of coagulation factors occurs 12–24 hours after oral administration, the antithrombotic effects may not occur until 2–7 days after the initiation of therapy.

II

- Warfarin is indicated for at least 3 months after an initial episode of DVT and indefinitely for long-term anticoagulation in patients with recurrent venous thromboembolism.
- All of the contraindications listed for heparin also apply to warfarin. Relative contraindications for warfarin include severe hepatic or renal disease, vitamin K deficiency, chronic alcoholism, a requirement for intensive salicylate or NSAID therapy, and the inability of the patient to comply with the regimen.
- Warfarin can be initiated at any time during heparin treatment and should be initiated as soon as it becomes apparent that oral anticoagulation will be used. Initiation of warfarin should occur before IV heparin is discontinued to prevent a break in the level of anticoagulation. The overlapping period of heparin and warfarin should be 4–5 days because of the delayed onset of the effect of warfarin and the hypercoagulable state occurring after heparin is discontinued. Heparin can usually be discontinued once the INR is within the desired range for 2 consecutive days.
- Warfarin should be initiated with small doses (5–10 mg/d for 2–4 days); elderly patients (i.e., age >65 years) may need even lower initial doses (i.e., 1–3 mg/d).
- Warfarin therapy is monitored by the INR (target: 2.0–3.0 for DVT or PE) every 24–48 hours after therapy is initiated and until the INR results have stabilized (i.e., INRs that are similar for 2 or 3 consecutive days with the same warfarin dosage) or until a maintenance dose is determined.
- The frequency of fatal, major, and major plus minor bleeding during warfarin therapy has been estimated to be 0.6, 3.0, and 9.6%, respectively. Table 14.1 outlines guidelines for reversing the anticoagulant effect of warfarin according to the INR and the clinical situation (i.e., presence of bleeding). Vitamin K given orally, SQ, or by slow IV infusion will usually reverse the effects of warfarin in 6–12 hours. Patients who will be resumed on warfarin therapy should receive lower doses of vitamin K to avoid full normalization of the INR and subsequent warfarin resistance.
- Warfarin-induced skin necrosis and purple toe syndrome are rare non-dose-related side effects of warfarin.
- Heparin is currently the anticoagulant of choice in pregnant females because it does not cross the placenta and does not cause fetal complications; warfarin should be avoided because it crosses the placenta and causes fetal malformation at *any* time during pregnancy. During lactation, heparin is not secreted in breast milk and can be safely administered to nursing mothers.
- Because of the large number of food and drug–drug interactions with warfarin, close monitoring and additional INR determinations may be

TABLE 14.1. Reversing the Anticoagulant Effect of Warfarin

Clinical Situation	Recommended Treatment Action
INR >3 but <6, patient is not bleeding, and rapid reversal is not indicated for reasons of surgical intervention	Omit the next few warfarin doses and resume warfarin therapy at a lower dose when the patient's INR is between 2 and 3.
INR ≥6 but <10 and the patient is not bleeding, or more rapid reversal is required because the patient requires elective surgery	Administer vitamin K 0.5–1 mg, oral or SQ; reduction in INR will occur within 8 hours and many patients' INRs may be in the range of 2–3 in 24 hours. If the INR at 24 hours is still high, a second dose of vitamin K 0.5 mg SQ can be repeated. Warfarin can then be restarted at a lower dose.
INR ≥10 but <20 and the patient is not bleeding	Vitamin K 3–4 mg, oral or SQ, should be given with the INR reduced substantially at 6 hours. The INR should be checked every 6–12 hours, and vitamin K can be repeated as necessary.
Major warfarin overdose (e.g., INR >20) or a rapid reversal of an anticoagulant effect is required because of serious bleeding	Vitamin K 10 mg slow IV infusion (e.g., over 20–30 minutes) and the INR checked every 6 hours. Vitamin K may be repeated every 12 hours and supplemented with plasma transfusion or factor concentrate depending on the urgency of the situation.
Life-threatening bleeding or serious warfarin overdose	Replacement with factor concentrates as indicated supplemented with vitamin K 10 mg slow IV infusion (e.g., over 20–30 minutes). Vitamin K may be repeated as necessary depending on the INR.

Adapted from Hirsh J, Poller L. Arch Intern Med 1994;154:282–288, with permission.

indicated whenever other medications are initiated or discontinued, or an alteration in consumption of vitamin K–containing foods is noted.

- Patient education information is outlined in Table 14.2.

THROMBOLYTIC THERAPY

- Thrombolytic agents are not generally accepted as a standard form of therapy for DVT or PE because of potential bleeding complications, lack of mortality differences and adequate long-term follow-up among studies performed, the amount of patient monitoring required once therapy is initiated, and the substantial cost of these agents.
- All thrombolytics are plasminogen activators and act either directly (urokinase, alteplase) or indirectly (streptokinase). Plasminogen, an inactive proteolytic enzyme, is converted to plasmin, which has the ability to lyse fibrin, as well as to hydrolyze fibrinogen and other coagulation factors, leading to a systemic lytic state.

TABLE 14.2. Information for the Patient on Warfarin

1. *Need for strict compliance:* The importance of taking warfarin and other medications as directed and of following instructions regarding prothrombin times and follow-up office visits must be stressed.

2. *Side effects:* The sites and signs of bleeding as well as instructions on when and where to call if bleeding occurs should be reviewed.

3. *Dietary instruction.* The patient should be told that no major dietary restrictions are necessary; however, no abrupt changes in dietary habits should be made. Rarely, diets with excessive quantities of vitamin K have interfered with warfarin therapy.

4. *Frequent prothrombin times:* The patient needs to be aware of the required monitoring of prothrombin times and why this is necessary. Some patients question the need for continued monitoring of warfarin, and this issue is best addressed early in the course of treatment.

5. *Drug interactions:* The patient should be informed that other drugs can greatly influence the effect of warfarin and should be told not to start or stop medications without first asking the physician. It may be useful to make specific recommendations regarding the use of common nonprescription drugs, e.g., antacids, analgesics, and cold products.

Adapted from Carter BL, Jones ME, Waickman LA. Clin Pharm 1985;4:292–293, with permission.

- Proposed indications for thrombolytic therapy of thromboembolic disease include massive/submassive PE with hemodynamic compromise, massive PE without hemodynamic compromise, submassive PE in patients who cannot tolerate further cardiopulmonary compromise, heparin treatment failures, and extensive proximal DVT. Thrombolytic agents offer the greatest benefit to PE patients with acute decompensation (hypotension and low cardiac output); their role in patients with less severe episodes remains to be defined.
- Patients receiving thrombolytics should have a documented diagnosis of thromboembolism and evidence that the thrombus is of recent origin (within the last 7 days).
- Three thrombolytic agents and regimens are available for treatment of DVT and PE (Table 14.3):
  - Streptokinase: Loading dose of 250,000 units in normal saline or 5% dextrose in water IV over 30 minutes followed by a continuous IV infusion of 100,000 U/h for 24 (PE) to 72 (DVT) hours.
  - Urokinase: Loading dose of 4400 U/kg in normal saline or 5% dextrose in water IV over 10 minutes followed by 4400 U/kg/h IV for a total of 12 hours (PE).
  - Alteplase: 100 mg by IV infusion over 2 hours (PE).
- Laboratory monitoring is used to determine whether some degree of systemic fibrinolysis has been achieved (Table 14.4). Once thrombolytic therapy is discontinued and the thrombin time or aPTT has fallen to less than twice the normal values (usually in 2–4 hours), continuous IV heparin should be given for 7–14 days.
- Laboratory monitoring guidelines to minimize local and major hemorrhage of patients receiving thrombolytic therapy are summarized in

Table 14.3. Thrombolytic therapy is associated with a 6–30% frequency of major bleeding complications in patients treated for DVT and approximately 20% for patients being treated for PE. Minor bleeding or oozing at cutaneous puncture sites can be controlled locally with pressure dressings. In cases of serious bleeding, thrombolytic therapy should be discontinued quickly. If blood replacement is indicated, whole blood or blood products (packed red blood cells, fresh-frozen plasma, or cryoprecipitate) may be given. In situations where bleeding unresponsive to blood replacement therapy must be rapidly corrected, e-aminocaproic acid (EACA) may be given in 5-g doses.

- Allergic or hypersensitivity reactions associated with streptokinase include urticaria, itching, flushing, nausea, headache, and transient elevation or decrease of systolic blood pressure. Anaphylaxis (1.3–2.5%) has ranged in severity from minor breathing difficulties to bronchospasm, periorbital swelling, or angioneurotic edema. Mild allergic reactions have been reported with urokinase and alteplase.
- Fever is more common with streptokinase therapy but can also occur with urokinase and alteplase. Allergic and febrile reactions may be treated with antihistamines, and acetaminophen is effective for fever. Corticosteroids have also been used for the prophylaxis of these adverse reactions.
- Hypotension can occur with rapid infusions of streptokinase and has also been reported with urokinase and alteplase. The hypotension can often be prevented by slowing the rate of administration.

TABLE 14.3. Laboratory Monitoring for Thrombolytic Therapy

Tests
　Whole-blood euglobulin lysis time, or
　Thrombin time, or
　PTT and PT, or
　Fibrin(ogen) degradation products

Time of Testing
　Before therapy
　　Detect and correct coagulation defects (by means of thrombin time, PTT and PT)
　　Determine baseline or control for fibrinolysis (any of the above tests; euglobulin lysis time or
　　　fibrin[ogen] degradation products if patient has been receiving heparin)
　During therapy (3–4 h after start)
　　Use same test(s) used for establishing baseline or control
　After therapy
　　Use PTT if heparin therapy is to begin

From Sharma CVRK, Cella G, Parisi AF, Sasahara AA. N Engl J Med 1982;306:1271, with permission.

SURGICAL THERAPY

- Thrombectomy for DVT is reserved for patients with severe limb ischemia.
- Pulmonary embolectomy and venous interruption are the most common procedures considered for PE. The placement of percutaneous transvenous filters (i.e., Greenfield filter) and umbrellas (Mobin–Uddin) may prevent recurrence of thromboembolism from the lower extremities.

PREVENTION OF VENOUS THROMBOEMBOLISM

- General guidelines for identifying patients at risk for thromboembolism are contained in Table 14.4.
- Nonpharmacologic prophylactic techniques include early ambulation, leg elevation, leg exercises, elastic compression or thromboembolic deterrent stockings, intermittent calf compression, electrical stimulation of calf muscles during surgery, and inferior vena cava interruption.
- Low-dose heparin therapy involves the administration of 5000 U SQ every 8–12 hours. Dosing every 8 hours (15,000 U/d) is no more effec-

TABLE 14.4. Guidelines for Prophylaxis of Thromboembolism

Type of Surgery/Indication	Recommended Prophylaxis
General surgery	
Low-risk (minor surgery, <40 years old, no risk factors)	Early ambulation
Moderate-risk (major surgery, >40 years old, no risk factors)	GCS, LDH (every 12 hours), or IPC
High-risk (major surgery, >40 years old some risk factors)	LDH (every 8 hours), or LMWH
Above characteristics but prone to wound complications (hematoma)	Above or IPC or dextran
Very high-risk (above with multiple risk factors)	LDH (every 8 hours), LMWH, or dextran with IPC, perioperative warfarin in some
Total hip replacement	Warfarin, LMWH, or dose-adjusted heparin
Hip fracture surgery	Warfarin or LMWH
Knee surgery	IPC (? LMWH)
Multiple trauma patients	IPC, warfarin, or LMWH
High-risk orthopedic and multiple trauma patients, other prophylaxis contraindicated	IVC filter
Neurosurgery, intracranial	IPC and/or GCS
Acute spinal cord injury	Dose-adjusted heparin, LMWH, IPC, or warfarin
Immobile general medicine patients	GCS, IPC, or LDH

Key: GCS, graduated compression stockings; IPC, intermittent pneumatic compression; LDH, low-dose subcutaneous heparin; LMWH, low molecular weight heparin; IVC, inferior vena cava.

tive and may be associated with a slightly higher rate of bleeding episodes. In surgery patients, heparin should be started 2 hours before the surgical procedure and then given every 12 hours thereafter.

- Dose-adjusted heparin (given subcutaneously every 12 hours) has also been used in high-risk patients in whom low-dose heparin is not effective or has limited effectiveness (i.e., hip surgery patients). The aPTT is drawn 4–6 hours after the first dose and at the midpoint of the dosing interval thereafter to maintain the aPTT in the high-normal range (i.e., 31.5–36 seconds).

- Warfarin has been used in high-risk patients in either a fixed low dose (1–2 mg daily) or a dose adjusted to slightly prolong the prothrombin time (INR of 2–2.5; for hip surgery, INR of 2–3).

- Low molecular weight heparins (LMWHs), when compared with unfractionated heparin, possess greater bioavailability after SQ administration, a longer duration of anti-factor Xa activity, linear pharmacokinetics, possibly fewer adverse effects, and lack of required routine laboratory monitoring (i.e., aPTT). Prophylactic regimens and FDA-approved indications for the LMWHs currently available are as follows:

  - Enoxaparin (Lovenox) 30 mg SQ twice daily (hip or knee replacement surgery); 40 mg once daily (abdominal surgery)

  - Dalteparin (Fragmin) 2500 units SQ once daily (abdominal surgery)

  - Danaparoid sodium (Orgaron) 750 units SQ twice daily (hip replacement surgery)

  - Ardeparin sodium (Normiflo) 50 units/kg twice daily (knee replacement surgery)

▶ EVALUATION OF THERAPEUTIC OUTCOMES

- Patients should be monitored for the resolution of symptoms, the development of recurrent thrombosis, and symptoms of the postphlebitic syndrome, as well as for adverse effects from treatment.

- Patients treated for DVT should be initially monitored twice daily and then daily for changes in pain, limb circumference, swelling, and tenderness.

- Patients treated for DVT or PE should be monitored for signs and symptoms of PE every shift for 1–2 days, followed by daily monitoring for the incidence or changes in dyspnea, apprehension, cough, pleuritic chest pain, and hemoptysis.

- Repeat arterial blood gases and/or V/Q studies may be indicated to assess progress of antithrombotic therapy in patients being treated for PE.

- Patients should be examined twice daily during hospitalization for signs of bleeding including IV catheter sites, hematomas, and ecchymosis. Intramuscular injections should be avoided in patients receiving therapeutic heparin.

- A platelet count should be obtained prior to heparinization, every 2 or 3 days during therapy, and after the discontinuation of therapy to monitor for heparin-associated thrombocytopenia.

II

- Hemoglobin and hematocrit are indicated prior to heparinization and every 1–2 days during therapy to identify the presence of bleeding. The stool should be examined daily for the presence of blood.
- Alterations in warfarin dosage should be made in small increments to prevent excessive changes in the INR.
- Careful follow-up and weekly monitoring of the INR is required during the first 4 weeks of therapy after discharge from the hospital. Changes in diet, exercise, clinical state, social habits, and compliance frequently alter maintenance dose requirements. Once a stable therapeutic warfarin dose has been attained, the INR can be monitored less frequently (i.e., once monthly).

See Chapter 19, Thromboembolic Disorders, authored by Sharon M. Erdman, PharmD, Keith A. Rodvold, PharmD, and William R. Friedenberg, MD, for a more detailed discussion of this topic.

Dermatologic Disorders
Edited by Barbara G. Wells, PharmD, FASHP, FCCP

Chapter 15

▶ ACNE

▶ DEFINITION

Acne is a common, self-limiting, multifactorial disease involving inflammation of the sebaceous follicles of the face and upper trunk.

▶ PATHOPHYSIOLOGY

- Acne is believed to be caused by a derangement in the structure or function of the sebaceous follicle (Fig. 15.1).
- A widening of the follicular canal with an increase in cell production occurs. Sebaceous glands atrophy, and sebum mixes with excess loose cells in the follicular canal to form a keratinous plug. This appears as a "blackhead," or open comedo. Trauma or inflammatory changes may lead to formation of a "whitehead," or closed comedo. If the follicular wall is damaged or ruptured, the contents of the follicle may extrude into the dermis and initiate an inflammatory reaction clinically seen as a pustule.
- Androgens stimulate growth of sebaceous follicles and enhance production of sebum.
- The glyceride component of sebum is converted to free fatty acids and glycerol by lipases, products of *Propionibacterium acnes* (*P. acnes*). Free fatty acids may irritate the follicular wall and cause increased cell turnover and inflammation.
- The increased production of loosely adherent keratin cells has been correlated with obstruction of the follicles seen in comedo formation.
- *P. acnes* is part of the normal flora in the sebaceous follicle and plays an important role in the initial development and maintenance of the inflammatory response. *P. acnes* is antigenic and causes increased antibody formation, leading to an inflammatory response. Immune complex–mediated complement activation may lead to vascular leakage, mast cell degranulation, and leukocyte chemotaxis. Hydrolytic enzymes released by complement activation may damage the follicle wall and lead to more severe acne. *P. acnes* may also evoke a cell-mediated immune response.

▶ CLINICAL PRESENTATION

- Acne ranges from mild (few open comedones) to severe (multiple inflamed papules, pustules, and nodule-sized lesions).
- Fibrosis associated with healing may lead to permanent scarring.

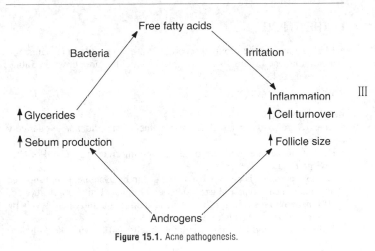

Figure 15.1. Acne pathogenesis.

▶ DIAGNOSIS

- Diagnosis is based on the presence of characteristic lesions. A drug and medical history should be obtained to determine what, if any, exacerbating factors can be eliminated and to assist in drug selection (Table 15.1).

▶ DESIRED OUTCOME

The goal of treatment is to heal lesions and to prevent or minimize scarring.

TABLE 15.1. Examples of Components to Patient History for Acne

Onset and duration of acne

Family history

Exacerbating factors

Previous history of antiacne agents with efficacy and adverse effect data

All current and recent topical and systemic medications

All topical products such as soaps, moisturizers, astringents, and cosmetics

Environmental and occupational exposures to chemicals and toxins

Allergies (food, drug, environmental)

▶ TREATMENT

- Medications may be grouped according to their proposed mechanism of action on acne (Table 15.2). Treatment guidelines are shown in Tables 15.3 and 15.4.

III TOPICAL TREATMENTS

Benzoyl Peroxide

- Benzoyl peroxide is an effective treatment for mild and moderately severe acne.
- Further studies are required to assess the tumorigenic potential of benzoyl peroxide.
- Benzoyl peroxide is decomposed on the skin by cysteine, liberating free oxygen radicals that oxidize bacterial proteins. Daily application of 10% benzoyl peroxide for 2 weeks can reduce free fatty acid levels by 50% and *P. acnes* levels by 98%.
- It increases sloughing rate of epithelial cells and loosens the follicular plug.
- Side effects include dryness, irritation, and contact dermatitis. To limit irritation, therapy may be initiated with a low potency product (2.5%), and then the strength may be increased (5–10%) or application frequency slowly increased (every other day, then each day, then twice daily).
- Gel formations are usually most potent, whereas the lotions and soaps are of weaker potency. The alcohol-based preparations generally cause more dryness and irritation. Fair or moist skin is more sensitive, thus, patients should be advised to apply medication to dry skin at least 30 minutes after washing.

TABLE 15.2. Agents that Decrease Pathogenic Mechanisms in Acne

Cell Turnover	*P. acnes*	Inflammation	Sebum Production/Secretion
Benzoyl peroxide	Benzoyl peroxide	Sulfur	Corticosteroids
Tretinoin	Tetracycline	Resorcinol	Estrogens
Salicylic acid	Erythromycin	Nonsteroidal anti-inflammatory	Isotretinoin
Abrasives	Clindamycin	drugs	
Isotretinoin	Co-trimoxazole	Isotretinoin	
	Minocycline		
	Isotretinoin		
	Azelaic acid		

TABLE 15.3. Topical Treatment Guidelines

Active Ingredient	Formulation	Strength	Regimen	Potential Side Effects
Benzoyl peroxide	Soaps, lotions, creams, gels	2.5–10%	Initially every other day or daily, then twice daily	Irritation based on form and strength
Tretinoin	Cream, gel, solution	0.025–0.05%	Initially every other day or daily	Excessive drying, erythema Concomitant use of other irritants increases adverse effects
Sulfur/resorcinol/ salicylic acid	Creams, lotions, gels, soaps	0.5–10% in various combinations	Daily	
Clindamycin	Solution, gel, lotion	1%	Twice daily	Drying, gastrointestinal effects
Tetracycline	Solution	2.2%	Twice daily	Burning and stinging following application, skin discoloration
Erythromycin	Solution, powder; gel as a combination product	1.5–2%	Twice daily	Drying, erythema

TABLE 15.4. Oral Treatment Guidelines

Active Ingredient	Formulation	Strength	Regimen	Potential Side Effects
Tetracycline	Tablets, capsules	250–500 mg	1 g/d initial; if no response in 2–3 weeks or severe acne, 2–3 g/d Maintenance 125–500 mg/d	Gastrointestinal upset, hypersensitivity syndromes Photosensitivity Drug and food interactions
Erythromycin	Tablets as various salts	250–500 mg	1 g/d as base; if no response in 2–3 weeks or severe acne, 2–3 g/d Maintenance 250–500 mg/d	Gastrointestinal upset, rashes Drug interactions
Clindamycin	Capsules	75–150–300 mg	300–450 mg/d	Diarrhea, pseudomembranous colitis
Isotretinoin	Capsules	10–20–40 mg	0.5–1 mg/kg/d in two divided doses Maximum of 2 mg/kg/d	Cheilitis, erythema, dryness Gastrointestinal effects Teratogenicity

Azelaic Acid

- Topical azelaic acid apparently interferes with DNA synthesis in some of the bacteria associated with acne vulgaris. It significantly reduced inflamed lesions after 1 month and noninflamed lesions after 2 months.
- Azelaic acid cream 20% is effective therapy chiefly for papulopustular acne.

Tretinoin

- Tretinoin (topical vitamin A acid) increases cell turnover in the follicular wall and decreases cohesiveness of cells, leading to extrusion of existing comedones and inhibition of the formation of new comedones. It also decreases the number of cell layers in the stratum corneum from 14 to 5. A "flare" of acne may suddenly appear after 3–6 weeks of treatment, followed by clinical clearing in 8–12 weeks.
- Side effects include irritation, erythema, peeling, allergic contact dermatitis, and increased sensitivity to sun exposure, wind, cold, and other irritants.
- Irritation may be managed by titrating strength and frequency of application. Treatment can be initiated with 0.025% cream for mild acne in people with fair complexions, 0.01% gel for moderate acne in fair skin with oily complexions, and 0.025% gel for severe acne with oily skin. Irritation is also minimized by applying to dry skin approximately 30 minutes after washing and by slowly increasing application frequency from every other day to daily, then twice daily.
- A combination of benzoyl peroxide each morning and tretinoin at bedtime may enhance efficacy and be less irritating than either agent used alone.

Adapalene

- Adapalene is a retinoid with potent anti-inflammatory and comedolytic properties. When applied once daily for 12 weeks, it is effective in reducing acne lesions and is better tolerated than tretinoin gel.
- Hypopigmentation is not a problem, but exposure to sunlight should be limited. It is not recommended to be taken during pregnancy or lactation.

Sulfur/Resorcinol/Salicylic Acid

- These agents are keratolytic and mildly antibacterial. Keratolytic refers to the effect of solubilization of the intracellular cement of keratin cells in the stratum corneum.
- Combinations of these agents are often considered synergistic.
- They are not considered to be as effective comedolytic agents as are benzoyl peroxide and tretinoin.
- Disadvantages include odor created by a hydrogen sulfide reaction of sulfur with the skin, the brown scale from resorcinol, and salicylism from long-term use of high concentrations of salicylic acid on permeable skin.

III

Topical Antibacterial Products

- Topical clindamycin, erythromycin, and tetracycline have been used effectively.
- Clindamycin is considered the most effective topical antibacterial agent for acne.
- A topical preparation of erythromycin plus zinc is reported to be significantly better than 500 mg/d oral tetracycline in reducing overall acne severity and papule lesion counts.
- Disadvantages of topical antibiotic agents include occasional irritation and stinging. On the skin, tetracycline photooxidizes to produce a visible yellow tinting with a relative lack of efficacy. Diarrhea and pseudomembranous colitis may occur with the use of topical clindamycin.

ORAL TREATMENTS

Oral Antibacterial Agents

- Oral antibiotics are effective and relatively safe for inflammatory types of acne.
- Tetracycline (and derivatives), erythromycin, clindamycin, and trimethoprim/sulfamethoxazole decreases the percentage of free fatty acids in skin surface lipids and also decreases numbers of *P. acnes.* Tetracycline also reduces the amount of keratin in sebaceous follicles and inhibits chemotaxis, phagocytosis, complement activation, and cell-mediated immunity. Tetracycline also achieves higher drug concentrations in areas of inflamed than normal skin. Minocycline and doxycycline have enhanced penetration into tissue and sebaceous follicles compared to tetracycline.
- Drawbacks to use of tetracycline include drug–food interactions with dairy products, photosensitivity, gastrointestinal disturbances, and predisposition to superinfections (i.e., vaginal candidiasis). Disadvantages of minocycline include vestibular toxicity and discoloration of skin and teeth.
- Side effects of clindamycin include diarrhea and a risk for pseudomembranous colitis.
- Trimethoprim/sulfamethoxazole should perhaps be reserved for refractory cases to minimize the risk of resistance.
- Ampicillin and tetracycline apparently decrease the intestinal flora needed to hydrolyze conjugated ethinyl estradiol excreted into bile; thus, enterohepatic recirculation is interrupted and the amount of active estrogen is reduced. Several pregnancies have been reported, and women taking oral contraceptives given ampicillin or tetracycline should be informed of the potential for this interaction.

Isotretinoin

- Isotretinoin is indicated for patients with severe recalcitrant comedonal acne unresponsive to conventional therapies.

- It decreases sebum production and changes sebum composition, inhibits *P. acnes,* inhibits inflammation, and alters patterns of keratinization within follicles.
- After 16 weeks of therapy, isotretinoin produced a greater than 70% success rate followed by a prolonged remission of more than 20 months.

III

- Adverse effects are often dose-related and include dry lips (90% of patients), dryness and desquamation of the face (30%), hypertriglyceridemia (25%), conjunctivitis and eye irritation, muscle and joint pain, skeletal hyperostosis, increased creatinine phosphokinas, increased blood glucose, photosensitivity, pseudotumor cerebri, excess granulation tissue, and teratogenicity.
- Incidence of teratogenicity is high. Nine spontaneous abortions and 7 major birth defects (hydrocephalus, small or partially occluded external auditory canals, and cardiac abnormalities) have been reported.

▶ EVALUATION OF THERAPEUTIC OUTCOMES

- Information regarding pathogenic factors and the importance of medication compliance should be conveyed to patients.
- Patients should understand that effectiveness of any therapeutic regimen may require 6–8 weeks and that they may also notice an "exacerbation" of acne after initiation of therapy. Inflammatory acne lesions may take approximately 4 weeks to surface.

See Chapter 90, Common Skin Disorders: Acne and Psoriasis, authored by Phillip A. Nowakowski, PharmD, Jean A. Rumsfield, PharmD, and Dennis P. West, PhD, FCCP, for a more detailed discussion of this topic.

Chapter 16

▶ PSORIASIS

▶ DEFINITION

Psoriasis is a common chronic disease characterized by recurrent exacerbations and remissions of thickened, erythematous, and scaling lesions.

▶ PATHOPHYSIOLOGY

- The cause of psoriasis is unknown. Hypotheses of etiology are shown in Table 16.1.
- Psoriatic epidermal cells proliferate at a rate sevenfold faster than normal epidermal cells. Duration of the cell cycle is 37.5 hours, versus 300 hours in normal skin.
- Psoriatic skin shows evidence of increased metabolic activity and increased cGMP, DNA, RNA, IgG, and C3. Arachidonic acid levels are 30 times normal, and prostaglandin E_2 levels are 50% higher than normal.
- Thirty-six percent of patients with psoriasis have at least one immediate relative with the disorder.
- Climate, stress, infection, trauma, and drugs may aggravate psoriasis. Warm seasons and sunlight improved psoriasis in 80% of patients, whereas 90% of patients worsen in cold weather.
- Infection (e.g., streptococcal, upper respiratory) may be a precipitating factor.
- Injury (e.g., rubbing, venipuncture, bites, surgery) to normal appearing skin may precipiate psoriasis (Koebner response).
- Lithium carbonate and β-adrenergic blocking agents exacerbate psoriasis.

▶ CLINICAL PRESENTATION

- Lesions are characterized by sharply demarcated, erythematous papules and plaques often covered with silver-white fine scales. Lesions start small and enlarge over time.
- Scalp psoriasis ranges from diffuse scaling on an erythematous scalp to thickened plaques with exudation, microabscesses, and fissures. Trunk, back, arm, and leg lesions may be generalized, scattered, discrete, droplike lesions or large plaques. Palms, soles, face, and genitalia may be involved, as well. Usually pustular psoriasis affects the palms and soles symmetrically, but more severe forms may occur with coalescent pustules, fever, malaise, and leukocytosis.
- Psoriatic arthritis is a distinct clinical entity in which both psoriatic lesions and inflammatory "arthritis" occur.

TABLE 16.1. Possible Etiologic Factors of Psoriasis

Defects in epidermal cell cycle
Disruption in arachidonic acid metabolism
Genetics
Exogenous trigger factors
  Climate
  Stress
  Infection
  Trauma
  Drugs
Immunologic mechanisms

▶ DIAGNOSIS

- The diagnosis is made based on history and physical exam, which reveals characteristic lesions as described previously. Patient assessment is summarized in Table 16.2.

▶ DESIRED OUTCOME

The goal of therapy is to achieve complete clearing of lesions, but partial clearing is acceptable at times, using regimens with decreased toxicity and increased patient acceptability.

▶ TREATMENT

- Drug treatments are listed in Table 16.3, and treatment guidelines are shown in Tables 16.4 and 16.5.

EMOLLIENTS–KERATOLYTICS

- Emollients hydrate the stratum corneum and minimize water evaporation. They may enhance desquamation, eliminate scaling, and decrease itching.

TABLE 16.2. Psoriatic Patient Assessment

Onset and duration of psoriasis
Family history
Exacerbating factors
Previous history of antipsoriasis agents with efficacy and side effect data
All current and recent topical and systemic medications
Environmental and occupational exposure to chemicals and toxins
Allergies (food, drug, environmental)

TABLE 16.3. Examples of Drug Treatments for Psoriasis

Topical	Systemic
Emollients and keratolytics	Ultraviolet-A and oral psoralens (systemic PUVA)
Coal tar	
Anthralin	Methotrexate
Calcipotriene	Retinoids
Methotrexate (under investigation)	Sulfasalazine
UVA and topical psoralens (topical PUVA)	Cyclosporine
	Tacrolimus

TABLE 16.4. Topical Treatment Guidelines

Active Ingredient	Formulation	Strength	Regimen	Potential Side Effects
Emollients	Lotions, creams, ointments	N/A	Three to four times daily	Folliculitis Contact dermatitis
Salicylic acid (keratolytic)	Gels, lotions	2–10%	Two to three times daily	Can be irritating Has resulted in salicylism
Coal tar	Creams, gels, lotions, ointments, solutions	1–48.5%	Apply in the evening, allowing to remain through the night	Messy and burdensome Can be irritating, photoreactions
Anthralin	Creams, ointments	0.1–1%	Usually in the evening, allowing to remain through the night. Short contact regimens also have been used	Stains skin and clothing Can be irritating
Calcipotriene	Ointment	50 µg/g	Twice daily, no more than 100 g/week, for up to 8 days	Burning and stinging in 10% of patients
Corticosteroids	Creams, lotions, ointments, solutions	Variable potency	Two to four times daily for maintenance; may use occlusion at night	Local tissue atrophy, striae, epidermal thinning, glucocorticoid systematic effects
Methoxsalen	Lotion	1%	Apply to area prior to UVA therapy	Photoreaction, exaggerated burning

TABLE 16.5. Oral Treatment Guidelines

Active Ingredient	Formulation	Strength	Regimen	Potential Side Effects
Sulfasalazine	Suspension, tablets	250 mg/5 mL, 500 mg	3–4 g/d	Gastrointestinal upset
Methoxsalen	Capsules	10 mg	Dosed on a mg/kg basis, 2 hours before UVA exposure	Burns, erythema, gastrointestinal upset, CNS effects, ocular damage, skin cancer
Methotrexate	Tablets, injection	2.5 mg, 20–25 mg/mL	2.5–5 mg every 12 hours for three doses every week	Anemia, leukopenia, thrombocytopenia, gastro-intestinal upset
Etretinate	Capsules	10 mg, 25 mg	0.75–1 mg/kg/d in divided doses	Dry mouth and lips, eye irritation, gastrointestinal upset, hematologic and hepatic effects
Cyclosporine	Capsules, solution	25 mg, 100 mg, 100 mg/mL	3–4 mg/kg/d in two divided doses; may increase to 5 mg/kg/d (ideal body weight), in 1 month if no response.	Nephrotoxicity, gastrointestinal upset, hypertension, tremor, monitor liver function tests
Tacrolimus	Capsules	1 mg, 5 mg	0.15 mg/kg twice daily; titrate based on side effects	Nephrotoxicity, gastrointestinal upset, hypertension, tremor, monitor liver function tests

III

- Moisturizers often need to be applied three times daily.
- Side effects of moisturizers include folliculitis and allergic contact dermatitis.
- Keratolytics are used to remove scales and decrease hyperkeratosis. Salicylic acid is the most frequently used agent, usually used in 2–20% strengths. Lower concentrations have a keratin-dispersing effect, whereas concentrations of 5% or higher have a corneolytic (exfoliative) action.
- Side effects of salicylic acid include local irritation and salicylism with nausea, vomiting, tinnitus, or hyperventilation.

COAL TAR

- Coal tar contains thousands of hydrocarbon compounds formed from distillation of bituminous coal.
- Coal tar can cross-link with DNA and, in combination with ultraviolet (UV) light, may increase prostaglandin synthesis.
- Disadvantages include unpleasant odor, staining of skin and clothing, ability to reversibly darken or alter light hair colors, and ability to tarnish silver jewelry.
- It may be applied directly to skin and may also be used in bath water and as a shampoo.

- Although many of its polynuclear aromatic hydrocarbons are known carcinogens, no increase in cancer risk has been identified. However, there are cases indicating a higher rate of cutaneous carcinoma in patients exposed to coal tar and UV light.

ANTHRALIN

III

- Anthralin appears to inhibit DNA synthesis by intercalation between DNA strands. It may also decrease epidermal proliferation by mitochondrial inhibition.
- Irritation, inflammation, and staining of skin and clothing are common.
- Application for 20 minutes has been found effective with decreased side effects. Titrating the strength of anthralin slowly from 0.1–0.25% to a concentration of 0.5–1% may minimize irritation. It should be applied only to affected areas of skin.

CALCIPOTRIENE

- Calcipotriene is a synthetic vitamin D analogue. It inhibits cell proliferation and induction of cell differentiation.
- Improvement usually requires 2 weeks of treatment, and approximately 70% of patients demonstrate marked improvement after 8 weeks. Maintenance therapy may be required.
- Side effects include burning, stinging, dry skin, peeling, rash, and worsening of psoriasis. Hypercalcemia is rare.

TOPICAL CORTICOSTEROIDS

- Topical steroids may play an important adjunctive role in treatment.
- They may halt synthesis and mitosis of DNA in epidermal cells and appear to inhibit phospholipase A, lowering the amounts of arachidonic acid, prostaglandins, and leukotrienes in the skin.
- Low-potency products have a modest anti-inflammatory effect and are safest for long-term application, for application on the face and intertriginous areas, for use with occlusion and in infants and young children.
- High-potency preparations are used for more severe inflammatory dermatoses. They may be used for an intermediate duration, or for longer periods on thickened skin. They may also be used on the face and intertriginous areas, but only for a short treatment duration.
- Very high potency products are used for short durations and on small surface areas. Occlusive dressings should not be used with these products.
- Ointments are considered the most clinically effective preparation for psoriasis. They are not suited for use in areas such as the axilla, groin, or other intertriginous areas where maceration and folliculitis may develop secondary to the occlusive effect. Creams are often preferred by patients and may be used in intertriginous areas.
- For severe acute forms of psoriasis, a patient may be instructed to apply a high-potency topical steroid every 2 hours for 24–48 hours, followed by application three to four times daily. For maintenance application two to four times daily is adequate.

III

- Adverse effects include tissue atrophy, degeneration, and striae. If detected early, these effects may be reversible with discontinuation. Thinning of epidermis and purpura may occur. Acneform eruptions and masking of symptoms of bacterial or fungal skin infections have been reported. Systemic side effects include risk of suppression of the hypothalamic–pituitary–adrenal axis, hyperglycemia, and development of cushinoid features. Tachyphylaxis and rebound psoriasis after abrupt cessation of topical corticosteroid therapy can also occur.

SULFASALAZINE

- Oral sulfasalazine (3–4 g/d for 8 weeks) has been reported to be effective for plaque-type psoriasis in some patients. When used alone, it is not as effective as methotrexate, psoralen plus ultraviolet A (UVA) light, or etretinate, but it has a lowered incidence of severe side effects.

SYSTEMIC THERAPY–PHOTOCHEMOTHERAPY: ORAL AND TOPICAL PSORALEN AND LONG-WAVE ULTRAVIOLET A LIGHT

- Use of psoralens with UVA (PUVA) controls psoriasis in nearly 90% of patients.
- Psoralens react with nucleic acids and intercalate between base pairs. When DNA is irradiated with long-wave ultraviolet light (320–400 nm, UVA) the psoralens covalently bind to pyrimidine bases, forming a cross-link.
- Candidates for PUVA therapy usually have severe incapacitating psoriasis unresponsive to topical therapies without history of photosensitivity, skin cancers, cataracts, or x-ray therapy of the skin. Methoxsalen (8-methoxypsoralen or 8-MOP) is usually dosed at 0.6–0.8 mg/kg and is given 2 hours before exposure to UVA. Serum methoxsalen concentrations usually peak within 0.5–2 hours of ingestion. Dosing of UVA is determined by patient skin type and history of previous response to UV radiation.

TOPICAL PSORALENS

- Trioxsalen baths and UV light have proved to be beneficial for psoriasis.

METHOTREXATE

- Oral methotrexate is indicated in the treatment of severe forms of psoriasis (e.g., psoriatic arthritis, erythrodermic psoriasis, pustular psoriasis, extensive psoriasis) refractory to other therapy.
- It inhibits synthesis of thymidylate, thus cell division is halted. Methotrexate is somewhat specific for cells in the S phase of the cell cycle.
- The "triple dose" regimen is probably the most common, and involves oral methotrexate administration at 12-hour intervals for three doses to provide inhibition for the 36-hour cell cycle period in psoriasis. The patient can be given a single weekly oral dose or 1/3 of the weekly dose every 12 hours for 3 doses.

- A liver biopsy is recommended at baseline and at intervals of 1.0–1.5 g cumulative dose of methotrexate. Leukocyte and platelet counts should be monitored every 4 weeks with hemoglobin, serum creatinine, aspartate and alanine transaminases, alkaline phosphatase, and urinalysis performed every 3–4 months. A yearly chest x-ray is recommended.
- Potentially interacting drugs are salicylates, many nonsteroidal anti-inflammatory drugs (NSAIDs), ethanol, sulfonamides, barbiturates, and retinoids.

III

ETRETINATE

- Etretinate is a vitamin A derivative (retinol) effective in treating severe pustular and erythrodermic forms of psoriasis. Fifteen percent of patients had clearing, 37% of patients had greater than 75% clearing, 31% of patients had 50–75% clearing, and 17% of patients had unsatisfactory response.
- Doses of 1 mg/kg/d are used and are titrated to the lowest effective dose.
- Monotherapy does not achieve total clearing in all patients, but may be a useful adjuvant therapy for PUVA by reducing the carcinogenic risks of that modality.
- Side effects include peeling of palms and soles, softening of the nails, diffuse hair loss, and dryness of mucous membranes. Additionally, it may cause an increase in serum triglycerides and cholesterol, with a lowering of high density lipoprotein. Transient increases in aspartate and alanine transaminases and lactate dehydrogenase and a few cases of hepatitis have been reported.

ACITRETIN

- Acitretin is an aromatic retinoid. Acitretin plus ultraviolet B (UVB) combination treatment represents a possible therapeutic regimen in severe psoriasis.
- It metabolizes to etretinate in some degree.

CYCLOSPORINE

- Systemically administered cyclosporine is increasingly used in treatment of severe psoriasis. It is not used with PUVA or intensive UVB.
- Side effects include renal dysfunction, hypertension, paresthesias, hypertrichosis, gingival hyperplasia, and gastrointestinal disorders.
- Intralesional cyclosporine has been clinically effective. A topical preparation can serve as monotherapy or as a dose-sparing modality in conjunction with systemically administered cyclosporine.

▶ EVALUATION OF THERAPEUTIC OUTCOMES

- Monitoring for disease resolution and side effects is critical to successful therapy. Positive response to therapy is noted as normalization of involved areas of skin as measured by reduced erythema and scaling as well as flattening of plaques.

III

- Patients should understand general concepts of therapy, and the importance of compliance should be emphasized.
- Achievement of efficacy by any therapeutic regimen requires days to weeks. Initial dramatic response may be achieved with some agents such as corticosteroids; however, sustained benefit with pharmacologically specific antipsoriatic therapy usually requires a range of about 2–4 weeks for noticeable response.

See Chapter 90, Common Skin Disorders: Acne and Psoriasis, authored by Phillip A. Nowakowski, PharmD, Jean A. Rumsfield, PharmD, and Dennis P. West, PhD, FCCP, for a more detailed discussion of this topic.

Endocrinologic Disorders

Edited by Terry L. Schwinghammer, PharmD, FCCP, BCPS

Chapter 17

▶ DIABETES MELLITUS

▶ DEFINITION

The term diabetes mellitus describes a series of complex and chronic metabolic disorders characterized by symptomatic glucose intolerance. All diabetics eventually show abnormalities of insulin secretion and complications of the disease, such as vascular and neurologic abnormalities; most manifest some degree of cellular resistance to insulin in type 2 diabetes mellitus.

▶ PATHOPHYSIOLOGY

DIABETES CLASSIFICATION

- In 1979, the National Diabetes Data Group reclassified diabetes into two main types: insulin-dependent diabetes mellitus (IDDM or type I) and non-insulin dependent diabetes mellitus (NIDDM or type II). In 1997, an international expert committee proposed changing the classification to type 1 and type 2 diabetes.
  - Type 1 diabetes (previously termed IDDM or juvenile-onset diabetes) is primarily due to pancreatic islet β-cell destruction, usually leading to absolute insulin deficiency. These patients are prone to developing diabetic ketoacidosis (DKA) if insulin is withheld. This form may be related to an autoimmune process or may be idiopathic.
  - Type 2 diabetes (previously termed NIDDM or adult-onset diabetes) is the more prevalent form and results from insulin resistance with a relative (rather than absolute) defect in the secretion of insulin.
  - Diabetes can also develop as a result of preexisting pancreatic disease or a hormone excess (e.g., ACTH, cortisol) from the use of certain medications (e.g., thiazide diuretics), or from insulin receptor abnormalities.

CARBOHYDRATE METABOLISM

- Carbohydrates are metabolized in the body to glucose, which is absorbed from the gastrointestinal (GI) tract into the bloodstream and oxidized in skeletal muscle to produce energy. Glucose is also stored in the liver in the form of glycogen and is converted in adipose tissue to fats and triglycerides.
- Insulin is produced and stored in the ß cells of the pancreas; its release increases uptake of glucose by the tissues, increases liver glycogen levels, decreases glycogen breakdown (glycogenolysis) by the liver,

increases synthesis of fatty acids, decreases breakdown of fatty acids into ketone bodies, and promotes incorporation of amino acids into proteins.

- Glucose can diffuse into the brain without the aid of insulin, but muscle and fat require the presence of insulin to receive glucose for energy. If glucose is not available, these tissues convert amino acids and fatty acids to carbohydrates (called gluconeogenesis). If deprivation continues, the tissue will eventually metabolize stored fats, resulting in the production of free fatty acids that are eventually oxidized to ketone bodies.

IV

- Plasma glucose concentrations are usually maintained between 40 and 160 mg/dL. Symptoms of hypoglycemia are usually present at concentrations <40 mg/dL. Plasma concentrations in excess of 180 mg/dL usually exceed the renal tubular maximal threshold for reabsorption, and glucose will spill into the urine. Higher concentrations may cause an osmotic diuresis.

- Counterregulatory hormones that increase blood glucose levels include glucagon, growth hormone, epinephrine, glucocorticoids, and thyroid hormone; somatostatin reduces blood glucose levels because it suppresses glucagon secretion and inhibits absorption of glucose from the GI tract.

▶ CLINICAL PRESENTATION

TYPE 1 DIABETES

- The classic symptoms of diabetes include polyuria, polydipsia, and polyphagia (increased appetite with increased calorie intake).
- Osmotic diuresis from urinary glucose produces polyuria, which can lead to dehydration with accompanying polydipsia.
- Because glucose cannot be adequately transported into cells, the hunger sensation is triggered, resulting in polyphagia.
- Other common symptoms in type 1 patients include weight loss, weakness, and dry skin. The onset of these symptoms is rapid, and secondary ketoacidosis is common.

TYPE 2 DIABETES

- Type 2 diabetes presents gradually and may be present without symptoms.
- Because obesity is common, weight loss and/or polyphagia may be absent or go unnoticed.
- Polyuria may be a presenting complaint, but most type 2 diabetics are discovered because of an abnormal blood or urine glucose on routine physical examination or screening.

DIABETIC KETOACIDOSIS (DKA)

- Patients in DKA often present with:
  - Lethargy (from hyperglycemia, hyperosmolality, ketonemia, and acidosis).

- Hyperventilation with possible Kussmaul's respirations (from compensatory respiratory alkalosis).
- Fruity odor to the breath (from acetonemia).
- Changes in mental status (from hyperosmolality).
- Nausea and vomiting (from metabolic acidosis).
- Abdominal pain (from gastric distention).
- Thirst and polyuria (from osmotic diuresis), or decreased urine output (from progressive DKA causing decreased glomerular filtration rate [GFR]).
- Dry mucous membranes.
- Poor skin turgor (from dehydration).
- Tachycardia.

IV

▶ DIAGNOSIS

- The 1997 international expert committee recommended that all persons over the age of 45 be tested for diabetes and that the test be repeated every three years if blood glucose is normal. Persons at risk for developing diabetes (e.g., those with a diabetic family member) should be tested at younger ages.
- Preganant women do not need to be screened for gestational diabetes if they meet the following criteria: <25 years old, normal body weight, no family history of diabetes, *and* not a member of an ethnic group with a high incidence of diabetes.
- The 1997 revised diagnostic criteria for diabetes mellitus are contained in Table 17.1.
- Impaired fasting glucose (IFG) is defined as a fasting plasma glucose (FPG) >110 mg/dL but <126 mg/dL.

TABLE 17.1. Criteria for the Diagnosis of Diabetes Mellitus

Diabetes can be diagnosed by any of three ways, confirmed on a different day by any one of the following three methods:

1. Symptoms of diabetes plus a casual plasma glucose concentration ≥200 mg/dl. Casual is defined as any time of day without regard to time since last meal. The classic symptoms of diabetes include polyuria, polydipsia, and unexplained weight loss.
2. Fasting plasma glucose (FPG) ≥200 mg/dL. Fasting is defined as no caloric intake for at least 8 hours.
3. Oral glucose tolerance test (OGTT) with the two-hour postload value >200 mg/dL. The test should be performed as described by the World Health Organization, using a glucose load containing the equivalent of 75-g anhydrous glucose dissolved in water.

The FPG is the preferred test because it is simple, convenient, widely available, acceptable to patients, and inexpensive compared to the OGTT.

- Impaired glucose tolerance (IGT) is diagnosed when the two-hour post-load sample of the oral glucose tolerance test (OGTT) is >140 mg/dL but <200 mg/dL.
- Diagnosis of DKA is established by testing for the presence of signs and symptoms and one or more of the following: (1) urine ketones, (2) serum ketones, (3) lowered serum bicarbonate level, and (4) lowered arterial pH. Patients usually have an increased anion gap. More than three-fourths of patients exhibit an increased serum amylase, but its cause and significance are unclear.

IV

▶ DESIRED OUTCOME

The goals of diabetes treatment are to maintain the blood glucose level in an acceptable range throughout the day to prevent symptoms of hyperglycemia, prevent the long-term microvascular and neurologic complications of the disease, and minimize the likelihood of hypoglycemia. Desirable plasma glucose and glycosylated hemoglobin (HbA_{1c}) levels are listed in Table 17.2.

▶ TREATMENT

GENERAL PRINCIPLES

- Patient education about the causes, symptoms, complications, and treatment of diabetes is essential for proper management.
- A diet plan for type 1 patients should be based on healthy daily nutrition to allow flexibility in insulin therapy and home monitoring. Dietary therapy for type 2 patients should be directed toward achieving blood glucose, lipid, and blood pressure goals and weight loss, if appropriate. Less than 10% of the total daily intake should come from saturated fats, and up to 10% from polyunsaturated fats, leaving 60–70% of the total calories from carbohydrates and monounsaturated fats. Home glucose monitoring is helpful in determining which foods adversely affect blood glucose control.

TABLE 17.2. Goals of Therapy

Parameter	Normal	Acceptable	Fair	Poor
Fasting plasma glucose (mg/dL)	115	140	200	>200
Postprandial plasma glucose (mg/dL)	140	175	235	>235
Glycosylated hemoglobin[a] (%)	6	<8	8–9.5	>10

[a] Increase limits 10% for elderly patients

- Appropriate physical activity should be recommended (unless contraindicated) to improve insulin sensitivity and possibly improve glucose tolerance. Exercise can also help promote weight loss and maintain ideal body weight when combined with restricted caloric intake.

ORAL AGENTS

- Oral agents are indicated for type 2 diabetics who have failed to control blood glucose adequately despite weight loss, proper diet, and exercise. A treatment algorithm for implementing therapy of type 2 diabetes is shown in Figure 17.1. IV

Sulfonylureas (Table 17.3)

- Sulfonylureas increase ß-cell insulin secretion; extrapancreatic effects may include reducing the rate of hepatic glucose production, increasing the insulin receptor sensitivity, and increasing the number of insulin receptors.
- There are few therapeutic differences among these agents; except for hypoglycemia, the second-generation oral hypoglycemics appear to produce fewer side effects than do the older drugs.
- The best candidates for sulfonylurea therapy are patients who are at least 40 years of age at the onset of the disease, have been diabetic for <5 years prior to the initiation of therapy, and have a fasting plasma glucose concentration of less than 300 mg/dL.
- Approximately 60–70% of patients have an initial response; about 5–20% of patients experience secondary failure. If a patient fails to respond to sulfonylureas because of disease progression, the dose of the present drug may be increased, therapy may be changed to another oral agent, another oral agent from a different class may be added, the patient may be switched to insulin, or combined insulin–oral hypoglycemic therapy may be prescribed. Only about 10% of patients respond when changed from one sulfonylurea to another because of the patient's failure to follow a dietary plan or because of an underlying stressful condition or disease.
- If the patient fails to respond to sulfonylurea therapy because of underlying stress or disease, he or she should receive insulin at least until termination of the stressful period, at which time oral therapy can usually be successfully reinitiated.
- These drugs should be administered 30 minutes before breakfast for maximum absorption.
- The dosage should be increased every 1–2 weeks until satisfactory control has been achieved or until the maximum dose has been reached.
- The major adverse effect is hypoglycemia, which is more problematic with long half-life drugs (e.g., chlorpropamide). Elderly patients are more susceptible, especially when they skip meals or when there is some degree of renal or liver impairment. Other side effects include hematologic reactions such as leukopenia, thrombocytopenia, and hemolytic anemia; skin reactions, particularly rashes, purpura, and pruritus; antithyroid activity; and diffuse pulmonary reactions. Renal side

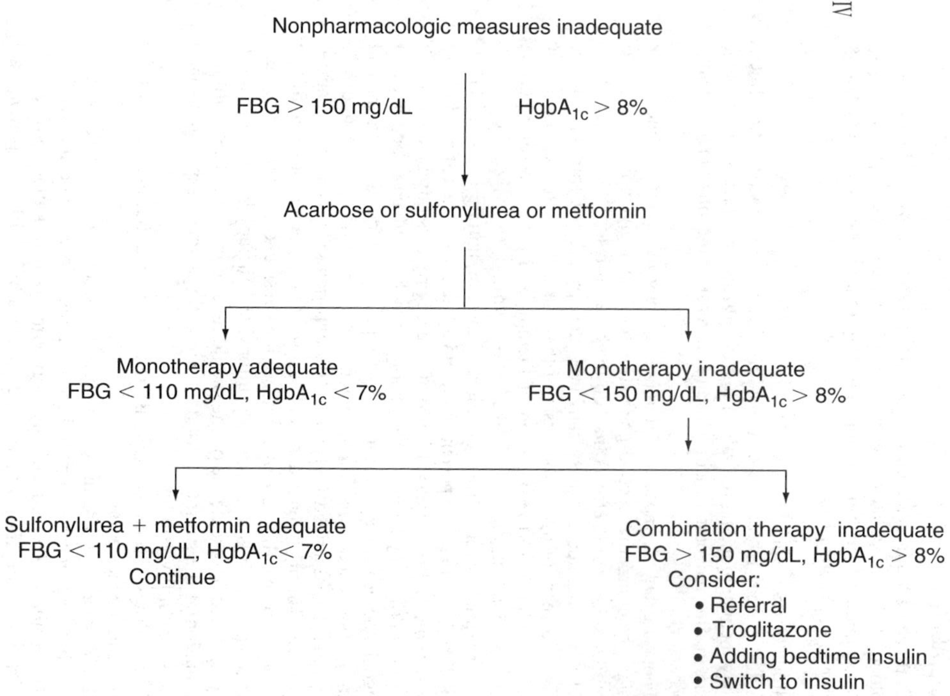

Figure 17.1. Proposed treatment algorithm for type 2 diabetes. (FBG, fasting blood glucose; Hgb A_{1c} glycosylated hemoglobin.)

IV

Nonpharmacologic measures inadequate

FBG > 150 mg/dL   HgbA$_{1c}$ > 8%

Acarbose or sulfonylurea or metformin

Monotherapy adequate
FBG < 110 mg/dL, HgbA$_{1c}$ < 7%

Sulfonylurea + metformin adequate
FBG < 110 mg/dL, HgbA$_{1c}$ < 7%
Continue

Monotherapy inadequate
FBG < 150 mg/dL, HgbA$_{1c}$ > 8%

Combination therapy inadequate
FBG > 150 mg/dL, HgbA$_{1c}$ > 8%
Consider:
• Referral
• Troglitazone
• Adding bedtime insulin
• Switch to insulin

effects include mild diuresis (especially with tolazamide and aceto-hexamide), and fluid retention and hyponatremia (chlorpropamide). Gastrointestinal side effects include nausea, vomiting, and cholestasis (with or without jaundice).

Metformin

- Metformin (Glucophage) is a biguanide that enhances peripheral mus-cle glucose uptake and inhibits glucose release from the liver. It also increases insulin sensitivity more consistently in obese than in lean patients, resulting in modest weight loss in some patients. It does not induce hypoglycemia when used alone.
- Metformin is as effective as a sulfonylurea in controlling blood glucose levels.
- The most frequent side effects are gastrointestinal (diarrhea up to 30%). Lactic acidosis occurs rarely, and is more likely in patients with renal disease (SCr >1.5 for males, >1.4 for females), liver disease, history of alcohol abuse, acute/chronic metabolic acidosis, and patients with con-ditions that predispose them to renal insufficiency or hypoxia.

Acarbose

- Acarbose (Precose) inhibits the enzyme α-glucosidase in the brush bor-der of the intestine which facilitates absorption of starch and disaccha-rides such as sucrose. This decreases the absorption rate of carbohy-drate, slowing or lowering the peak postprandial blood glucose concentration without causing hypoglycemia.
- Studies have demonstrated a decrease in postprandial blood glucose with some improvement of HbA_{1c} but less than that observed with sul-fonylureas or metformin.
- The usual recommended dose is 50–100 mg with each large meal; this drug is most effective when given with a starchy high-fiber meal.
- The most common side effects are increased flatulence and abdominal bloating. When used in combination with a hypoglycemic agent (sul-fonylurea or insulin), patients must be taught the importance of treating hypoglycemia with glucose- (dextrose-) based products since acarbose will block absorption of more complex disaccharide sugars (e.g., sucrose).

Troglitazone

- Troglitazone (Rezulin) is a thiazolidinedione derivative that decreases gluconeogenesis, increases glucose uptake and utilization in skeletal muscle, and increases glucose uptake and decreases fatty acid output in adipose tissue. It does not affect insulin secretion.
- The drug is FDA-approved for use in type 2 patients currently taking insulin but inadequately controlled (HbA_{1c} >8.5% and insulin >30 units/d in multiple injections). It decreases insulin resistance and lowers fasting plasma glucose and HbA_{1c} concentrations. It is also indicated for use as monotherapy or in combination with sulfonylurea.

IV

IV

TABLE 17.3. Oral Agents for Diabetes

Generic (trade)	Onset (h)	Half-Life (h)	Duration (h)	Recommended Starting Dose		Maximum Dose per Day	Metabolism/ Elimination
				Nonelderly	Elderly		
Sulfonylureas							
First-generation agents							
Tolbutamide (orinase)	1	5.6	6–12	1–2 g/d	500 mg/d to 500 mg twice daily	2–3 g	Metabolized in liver to inactive metabolites that are excreted renally
Acetohexamide (Dymelor)	1	5	10–14	250 mg– 1.5 g/d	125–250 mg/d	1.5 g	Metabolized in liver; metabolite's potency is equal to or greater than that of parent compound; renally eliminated
Tolazamide (Tolinase)	4–6	7	10–14	100– 250 mg/d	100 mg/d	750 mg– 1 g	Metabolized in liver; metabolite less active than parent compound; renally eliminated
Chlorpropamide (Diabinese)	1	35	72	250 mg/d	100 mg/d	500 mg	Metabolized in liver; also excreted unchanged in the urine
Second-generation agents							
Glyburide (DiaBeta, Micronase)	1.5	2–4	18–24	2.5 mg/d	1.25–2.5 mg/d	20 mg	Metabolized in liver; 50% of metabolites eliminated in urine, 50% in feces

TABLE 17.3. continued

Generic (trade)	Onset (h)	Half-Life (h)	Duration (h)	Recommended Starting Dose Nonelderly	Recommended Starting Dose Elderly	Maximum Dose per Day	Metabolism/ Elimination
Glyburide, micronized (Glynase)	1.5	2–4	18–24	1.5 mg	1.5–3 mg	12 mg	Metabolized in liver; 50% metabolites eliminated in urine, 50% in feces
Glipizide (Glucotrol)	1	3–7	16–24	5 mg/d	2.5–5 mg/d	40 mg	Metabolized in liver to inactive metabolites; renally eliminated
Glimepiride (Amaryl)	1	9	24	1–2 mg/d	1 mg/d	8 mg/d	Hepatic metabolism
Biguanides							
Metformin (Glucophage)	1.5	1.5–4.9	16–20	500 mg	500–1000 mg	2550 mg	Urinary excretion
Other							
Acarbose (Precose)	<1	2	~3	25 mg TID	25 mg TID	100 mg TID	Metabolized within the GI tract
Troglitazone (Rezulin)	—	16–34	—	200 mg/d	200 mg/d	600 mg/d	Hepatic metabolism

IV

- The initial dose is 200 mg once daily with a meal; the dose may be increased to 400 mg once daily after 2–4 weeks (maximum 600 mg/d).
- Adverse effects include mild, reversible increases in hepatic transaminases (1–2%). The drug lowers serum concentrations of oral contraceptives. Cholestyramine reduces absorption of troglitazone; they should be taken at different times of the day.
- The drug is substantially more expensive than sulfonylureas.

Oral Hypoglycemic Combinations

IV
- The combination of a sulfonylurea and metformin or troglitazone may lower blood glucose by a greater amount than one of the agents alone.
- Oral agents and insulin have also been used in combination. The proposed mechanism is the ability of the oral agent to increase endogenous insulin secretion rather than to improve the insulin sensitivity of tissues. Nighttime insulin is administered to suppress hepatic glucose production.

INSULINS

- Table 17.4 compares the onset, peak, and duration of various insulin preparations.
- Regular insulin is a solution, and it can be administered by the intravenous (IV), intramuscular (IM), or subcutaneous (SQ) route. All other types of insulin are suspensions and can be administered subcutaneously only.
- NPH and Lente insulins differ in their ability to be mixed with other types of insulin. NPH and regular insulins can be combined in the same syringe and refrigerated for up to 21 days without changes in potency. Lente insulin has an excess of zinc that binds with regular insulin and delays its absorption. The interaction also produces more Lente insulin, possibly causing hypoglycemia when the absorption of Lente reaches its peak. Since the interaction occurs within 15 minutes after mixing and lasts for 24 hours, patients should be instructed either to inject the mixture immediately or to consistently wait 24 hours before administration.
- NPH insulin should not be combined with Lente insulins. Human NPH and human regular preparations can be mixed with no consequences.

TABLE 17.4. Onset, Peak, and Duration of Various Insulin Preparations

Type of Insulin	Onset (h)	Peak (h)	Duration (h)
Short acting			
Regular	0.5–1	2–4	5–7
Intermediate acting			
NPH	1–2	6–14	18–24
Lente	1–2	6–14	18–24
Long acting			
Ultralente	4–6	18–26	36+

- Type 2 patients can be started on a single injection of 15–20 U/d of an intermediate-acting (NPH or Lente) insulin with dosage adjustments made according to plasma glucose levels. Patients receiving insulin for the first time should be started on human insulin.
- Since many type 1 and type 2 patients do not exhibit 24-hour control on a single daily injection, twice daily injections of NPH and regular insulin are often used; premixed NPH/regular insulins are available. The first injection (NPH-to-regular ratio of 2:1) is given 30 minutes before breakfast. The second injection (NPH-to-regular ratio of 1:1) is given 30 minutes before the evening meal.
- If regular insulin only is used, the patient's total daily insulin requirement is divided into four equal doses, each given 30 minutes before meals and at bedtime.
- Continuous subcutaneous insulin infusion (CSII) by pump is administered continuously and as bolus doses before meals. Because of a high incidence of complications, pump use should be restricted to those patients who are knowledgeable, stable, and well motivated.
- Guidelines for dose adjustments based on clinical response are given in Table 17.5.

TREATMENT OF HYPOGLYCEMIA

- In a conscious patient, immediate treatment involves the administration of food, preferably sugar. Eight Lifesavers, 4–6 ounces of a sugar-containing soft drink, a piece of fruit, one-half cup fruit juice, 2–3 glucose tablets (5 g each), a tube of glucose gel, or 1 cup skim milk usually reverses the symptoms in 10–20 minutes.
- In the unconscious patient, 1 mg of glucagon injected subcutaneously should provide relief within 10–15 minutes. Patients who weigh less than 20 kg should receive 0.5 mg. Common side effects are nausea and vomiting. Once the patient regains consciousness, oral liquids containing sugar should be administered. In the hospitalized hypoglycemic patient, 50 mL of $D_{50}W$ provides rapid reversal of symptoms.

TREATMENT OF DKA

- Therapy should be targeted toward correcting dehydration, reducing the plasma glucose concentration to normal, reversing the acidosis and ketosis, replenishing electrolyte and volume losses, and identifying the underlying cause.
- Normal saline should be administered at a rate of 1 L/h for 2–3 hours. After the patient's heart rate rhythm and blood pressure have normalized, IV fluids can be changed to 0.45% sodium chloride.
- Low-dose IV regular insulin may be initiated with a bolus of 0.1 U/kg before starting a continuous infusion (e.g., dilute 100 units of regular insulin in 100 mL of 0.9% sodium chloride and infuse at an initial rate of 0.1 U/kg/h.) Plasma glucose determinations should be made hourly. If there has been less than a 10% drop in 2 hours, then the insulin drip rate should be doubled.

TABLE 17.5. Adjusting Insulin Dosages Based on Clinical Response

Problem	Time Problem Experienced	Possible Solutions
Hyperglycemia	Fasting	If the patient is receiving a single dose of an intermediate-acting insulin, split into 2 doses—2/3 of total dose before breakfast, 1/3 of dose before supper
		If the patient is receiving split-dose intermediate insulin, increase presupper dose or move present dose to a later time in the evening
	Midmorning	Add Regular to morning dose
	Midafternoon	Increase morning NPH or Lente dose *or* add Regular at lunch time
	Bedtime	Add Regular with presupper dose if not currently receiving *or* increase Regular at presupper dose
	Early morning (2:00–3:00 AM)	If using Regular/intermediate dose before the evening meal, split the dose and give the Regular dose before the meal and the intermediate dose at bedtime (consider the dawn effect)
Hypoglycemia	Fasting	Decrease evening insulin dose, but first check timing of AM test and dose
	Midmorning	Decrease or omit prebreakfast dose of Regular insulin
	Midafternoon	Decrease morning NPH or Lente dose
		Be sure patient is withdrawing correct dosage into syringe in the correct order if he/she is receiving more than one type of insulin
	Bedtime	Instruct patient to eat a bedtime snack and/or check dose of PM NPH/Lente (again, "fall back")
		Decrease presupper dose of Regular insulin
		Decrease presupper dose of intermediate-acting insulin if it is being administered earlier in the afternoon
	Early morning (2:00–3:00 AM)	Consider Somogyi effect—decrease the evening dose of intermediate-acting insulin

Note: If more than one monitoring time throughout the day is abnormal, try to adjust only one insulin dose at a time. Adequately titrating more than one dose adjustment and gauging the effects is quite difficult and often creates more adjustment problems.

- When the plasma glucose concentration declines to approximately 250 mg/dL, the primary IV fluid should be changed from 0.45% sodium chloride to 5% dextrose in 0.45% sodium chloride and the infusion rate of the insulin drip should be cut in half to avoid hyperchloremic acidosis and to prevent hypoglycemia.
- The endpoint of insulin therapy is not euglycemia but correction of acidosis and ketonemia. The insulin infusion should be continued until the acidosis has been corrected (arterial pH, >7.30; plasma glucose concentration, <250 mg/dL; anion gap, 13–17; serum bicarbonate, >15 mEq/L; no ketonemia).
- Electrolytes depleted from osmotic diuresis and acidosis should be replaced as quickly as possible. Sodium is generally replaced by administering 2–4 L of normal saline during the initial management of DKA. Potassium can be replaced by adding 40–60 mEq to each liter of IV fluid and administering it at a rate of 10–20 mEq/h.
- Phosphate replacement should be instituted if the serum level approaches the lower end of the normal range.
- Bicarbonate is generally administered only to patients whose arterial pH is below 7.0. When indicated, bicarbonate should be administered via infusion of 50 mEq (or 1 mEq/Kg) during 1 hour. The goal of therapy is to raise the arterial pH to 7.10–7.15.

IV

TREATMENT OF NEUROPATHY

- Symptoms may begin as tingling, or burning sensations, particularly in the distal tissues with a definite loss in vibratory sensation. The patient may eventually lose all sensation in a particular area, becoming unable to detect hot, cold, or pain. Circulation is usually impaired to these areas because of diabetes related vascular changes.
- Narcotic analgesics and nonsteroidal anti-inflammatory drugs (NSAIDs) may provide some relief for painful neuropathy.
- Anticonvulsants (phenytoin and carbamazepine) should be reserved for severe cases that have been resistant to other treatments.
- Psychotropic drugs, such as tricyclic antidepressants, trazodone, fluoxetine, and phenothiazines, have mixed favorable responses but seem to provide greater pain relief than anticonvulsants. Doses for the treatment of painful neuropathies should be low initially and titrated to effect.
- Neurogenic bladder, with loss of autonomic mediated urinary continence, may benefit from treatment with bethanechol and/or anticholinergics.
- Symptoms of gastroparesis (nausea, vomiting, abdominal distension) may be reduced with the prokinetic agents metoclopramide and cisapride. Cisapride may induce fewer side effects, such as extrapyramidal reactions, but is more costly.
- Treatment for diabetic diarrhea has included anticholinergic agents, dietary change, antibiotics, bulk and bile salt resins, kaolin/pectin, and diphenoxylate/atropine. Somatostatin analogues have shown some promise in this disorder.

TREATMENT OF RETINOPATHY

- Nonproliferative retinopathy can be treated with laser photocoagulation therapy that may help to arrest progression and decrease the loss of vision associated with macular edema.
- Because hypertension and smoking lead to more rapid progression of ocular damage, it is very important to halt or to eliminate these risk factors.
- Aldose reductase inhibitors (e.g., sorbinil) are investigational agents that have not yet been proven to be beneficial in progressive retinopathy.

IV

TREATMENT OF NEPHROPATHY

- ACE inhibitors are most useful during the early stages of diabetic nephropathy. They seem to normalize systemic and glomerular capillary pressures, resulting in reduced proteinuria and glomerulosclerosis. When the ACE inhibitors are started the patient may have a transient rise in serum creatinine, which usually returns to baseline within a few days. Caution must be advised, however, when using these agents in severe renal disease, since ACE inhibitors can worsen or cause renal impairment.
- Other agents that may play a role in preventing and reversing kidney disease include aspirin, dipyridamole, somatostatin analogues, certain antihypertensive medications, and aldose reductase inhibitors.

▶ EVALUATION OF THERAPEUTIC OUTCOMES

- Blood glucose determination is the standard for diabetes monitoring. Most patients use whole-blood glucose determinations as a means of monitoring diabetic control in the ambulatory setting. In the laboratory, serum or plasma is utilized. Chemically impregnated strips or hand-held electronic glucose monitoring machines that utilize strips are available that can monitor whole-blood glucose from several drops of blood obtained by a fingerstick. The goals of therapy are included in Table 17.2.
- The HbA_{1c} is useful for monitoring long-term control of diabetes (see Table 17.2). Bringing the blood glucose under control for 4–6 weeks will result in a fall in the percentage of HbA_{1c}. However, a patient must have experienced hyperglycemia for 1–4 weeks before the HbA_{1c} concentration rises substantially.
- Urine glucose testing is the least expensive monitoring device but has several limitations. Urine testing may lack correlation between urine and blood glucose values. The tests are technique dependent, and the patient must read the results at the appropriate time. Urine ketone determination is commonly recommended to patients with type 1 diabetes or who are ketosis prone (e.g., Ketostix).
- For monitoring therapy of DKA, plasma or whole-blood glucose concentrations should be monitored hourly until they have stabilized below

250 mg/dL. Electrolytes, especially potassium, should be monitored every hour until stabilized within the normal range, then every 2–4 hours until the acidosis has been corrected. Heart rhythm should be monitored, especially in comatose patients.

See Chapter 72, Diabetes Mellitus, authored by Condit F. Steil, PharmD, CDE, for a more detailed discussion of this topic.

IV

Chapter 18

► THYROID DISORDERS

► DEFINITION

Thyroid disorders encompass a variety of disease states affecting thyroid hormone production or secretion that result in alterations in metabolic stability. Hyperthyroidism and hypothyroidism are defined as the clinical and biochemical syndromes resulting from increased and decreased thyroid hormone production, respectively.

► THYROID HORMONE PHYSIOLOGY

- The thyroid hormones thyroxine (T_4) and triiodothyronine (T_3) are formed on thyroglobulin, a large glycoprotein synthesized within the thyroid cell. Inorganic iodide enters the thyroid follicular cell and is oxidized by thyroid peroxidase and is covalently bound (organified) to tyrosine residues of thyroglobulin.
- The iodinated tyrosine residues monoiodotyrosine (MIT) and diiodotyrosine (DIT) combine (couple) to form iodothyronines in reactions catalyzed by thyroid peroxidase. Thus, DIT and DIT combine to form T_4, while MIT and DIT form T_3.
- Thyroid hormone is liberated into the bloodstream by the process of proteolysis within thyroid cells. T_4 and T_3 are transported in the bloodstream by three proteins: thyroid-binding globulin (TBG), thyroid-binding prealbumin (TBPA), and albumin. Only the unbound (free) thyroid hormone is able to diffuse into the cell, elicit a biologic effect, and regulate thyroid-stimulating hormone (TSH) secretion from the pituitary.
- T_4 is secreted solely from the thyroid gland, but <20% of T_3 is produced there; the majority of T_3 is formed from the breakdown of T_4 catalyzed by the enzyme 5′-monodeiodinase found in peripheral tissues. T_3 is about five times more active than T_4.
- T_4 may also be acted on by the enzyme 5′-monodeiodinase to form reverse T_3, which has no significant biologic activity.
- Thyroid hormone production is regulated by TSH secreted by the anterior pituitary, which in turn is under negative feedback control by the level of free thyroid hormone and the positive influence of hypothalamic thyrotropin-releasing hormone (TRH). Thyroid hormone production is also regulated by extrathyroidal deiodination of T_4 to T_3, which can be affected by nutrition, nonthyroidal hormones, drugs, and illness.

► THYROTOXICOSIS (HYPERTHYROIDISM)

PATHOPHYSIOLOGY

- Thyrotoxicosis results when tissues are exposed to excessive levels of T_4, T_3, or both. In Graves' disease, hyperthyroidism results from the action of thyroid-stimulating antibodies (TSAb) directed against the thyrotropin receptor on the surface of the thyroid cell. These immunoglobulin G (IgG) antibodies bind to the receptor and activate the enzyme adenylate cyclase in the same manner as TSH.

CLINICAL PRESENTATION

- Symptoms include nervousness, emotional lability, easy fatigability, heat intolerance, loss of weight concurrent with an increased appetite, increased frequency of bowel movements, palpitations, proximal muscle weakness (noted on climbing stairs or in arising from a sitting position), and scanty or irregular menses in women.
- Physical signs may include warm, smooth, moist skin and unusually fine hair; separation of the end of the fingernails from the nail beds (onycholysis); retraction of the eyelids and lagging of the upper lid behind the globe upon downward gaze (lid lag); tachycardia at rest, a widened pulse pressure, and a systolic ejection murmur; occasional gynecomastia in men; a fine tremor of the protruded tongue and outstretched hands; and hyperactive deep tendon reflexes.
- Graves' disease is manifested by hyperthyroidism, diffuse thyroid enlargement, and the extrathyroidal findings of exophthalmos, pretibial myxedema, and thyroid acropachy. The thyroid gland is usually diffusely enlarged, with a smooth surface and consistency varying from soft to firm. In severe disease, a thrill may be felt and a systolic bruit may be heard over the gland.
- In painful subacute (viral, or DeQuervain's) thyroiditis, patients complain of severe pain in the thyroid region, which often extends to the ear on the affected side. Low-grade fever is common, and systemic signs and symptoms of thyrotoxicosis are present. The thyroid gland is firm and exquisitely tender on physical examination.
- Painless (silent, lymphocytic, postpartum) thyroiditis has a triphasic course that mimics that of painful thyroiditis. Most patients present with mild thyrotoxic symptoms; lid retraction and lid lag are present but exophthalmos is absent. The thyroid gland may be diffusely enlarged but thyroid tenderness is absent.
- Thyroid storm is a life-threatening medical emergency characterized by severe thyrotoxicosis, high fever (often >103°F), tachycardia, tachypnea, dehydration, delirium, coma, nausea, vomiting, and diarrhea. Precipitating factors include infection, trauma, surgery, radioactive iodine treatment, and withdrawal from antithyroid drugs.

DIAGNOSIS

- An elevated 24-hour radioactive iodine uptake (RAIU) indicates *true hyperthyroidism,* i.e., the patient's thyroid gland is actively overproducing T_4, T_3, or both (normal RAIU 10–30%).
  - TSH-induced hyperthyroidism is diagnosed by evidence of peripheral hypermetabolism, diffuse thyroid gland enlargement, elevated free thyroid hormone levels, and elevated serum immunoreactive TSH

IV

IV

concentrations. Because the pituitary gland is extremely sensitive to even minimal elevations of free T_4, a detectable TSH level in any thyrotoxic patient indicates the inappropriate production of TSH.

- TSH-secreting pituitary adenomas are diagnosed by demonstrating lack of response to TRH stimulation, elevated TSH α-subunit levels, and radiologic imaging.
- An autonomous thyroid nodule (toxic adenoma) usually occurs with larger nodules, i.e., those more than 4 cm in diameter. If the T_4 level is normal, a T_3 level is measured to rule out T_3 toxicosis. Once a radioiodine scan has demonstrated that the toxic thyroid adenoma would collect more radioiodine than the surrounding tissue, independent function is documented by a failure of the autonomous nodule to decrease its iodine uptake during exogenous T_3 administration.
- In multinodular goiters, a thyroid scan will show patchy areas of autonomously functioning thyroid tissue.
- A low RAIU indicates the excess thyroid hormone is not a consequence of thyroid gland hyperfunction.
  - This may be seen in subacute thyroiditis, painless thyroiditis, struma ovarii, follicular cancer, and factitious ingestion of exogenous thyroid hormone.
- In thyrotoxic Graves' disease, there is an increase in the overall hormone production rate with a disproportionate increase in T_3 relative to T_4 (Table 18.1). Saturation of TBG is increased owing to the elevated levels of serum T_4 and T_3, which is reflected in an elevated T_3 resin uptake. As a result, the concentrations of free T_4, free T_3, and the free T_4 and T_3 indices are increased to an even greater extent than are the measured serum total T_4 and T_3 concentrations. The TSH level is undetectable owing to negative feedback by elevated levels of thyroid hormone at the pituitary. The diagnosis of thyrotoxicosis is confirmed by measurement of the serum T_4 concentration, T_3 resin uptake (or free T_4), and TSH. An increased 24-hour RAIU (obtained in nonpregnant individuals) documents that the thyroid gland is inappropriately utiliz-

TABLE 18.1. Thyroid Function Test Results in Different Thyroid Conditions

	Total T_4	Free T_4	Total T_3	T_3 Resin Uptake	Free Thyroxine Index	TSH
Normal	4.5–12.5 µg/dL	0.8–2.8 ng/dL	80–220 ng/dL	22–34%	1.0–4.3 U	0.25–6.7 µU/mL
Hyperthyroid	↑↑	↑↑	↑↑↑	↑	↑↑↑	↓↓
Hypothyroid	↓↓	↓↓	↓	↓↓	↓↓↓	↑↑
Increased TBG	↑	Normal	↑	↓	Normal	Normal

Key: TSH, thyroid-stimulating hormone; TBG, thyroid-binding globulin.

ing the iodine to produce more thyroid hormone at a time when the patient is thyrotoxic.

- In subacute thyroiditis, thyroid function tests typically run a triphasic course in this self-limited disease. Initially, serum thyroxine levels are elevated due to release of preformed thyroid hormone from disrupted follicles. The 24-hour RAIU during this time is <2% owing to thyroid inflammation and TSH suppression by the elevated thyroxine level. As the disease progresses, intrathyroidal hormone stores are depleted, and the patient may become mildly hypothyroid with an appropriately elevated TSH level. During the recovery phase thyroid hormone stores are replenished and serum TSH elevation gradually returns to normal.

IV

DESIRED OUTCOME

The therapeutic objectives for hyperthyroidism are to normalize the production of thyroid hormone; minimize the symptoms and long-term consequences of the disorder; and provide individualized therapy based on the type and severity of disease, patient age and gender, existence of nonthyroidal conditions, and response to previous therapy.

TREATMENT

Antithyroid Medications (Table 18.2)

Thiourea Drugs

- The thioureas propylthiouracil (PTU) and methimazole block thyroid hormone synthesis by inhibiting the peroxidase enzyme system of the thyroid gland, thus preventing oxidation of trapped iodide and subsequent incorporation into iodotyrosines and ultimately iodothyronine ("organification"), and by inhibiting coupling of monoiodotyrosine and diiodotyrosine to form T_4 and T_3. PTU (but not methimazole) also inhibits the peripheral conversion of T_4 to T_3.
- The thioureas are the preferred treatment for children and pregnant women. The increased risk of hypothyroidism following RAI or surgery makes thioureas a reasonable treatment alternative in young adults.
- Usual initial doses include PTU 300–600 mg daily (usually in 3 divided doses) or methimazole 30–60 mg/d (usually in 3 divided doses). Some evidence suggest single daily doses of either drug may be effective.
- Improvement in symptoms and laboratory abnormalities should ensue within 4–8 weeks, at which time a tapering regimen to maintenance doses can be started. Dosage changes should be made on a monthly basis, since the endogenously produced T_4 will reach a new steady-state concentration in this interval. Typical daily maintenance doses are PTU 50–300 mg and methimazole 5–30 mg.
- If clinical improvement is not observed, consider noncompliance, insufficient dosage to block hormone synthesis, and inadequate dosing interval if a single daily dose has been used.
- Antithyroid drug therapy should continue for 12–24 months to induce a long-term remission. The presence of TSAb is predictive for relapse.

IV

TABLE 18.2. Management of Hyperthyroidism

Modality	Maintenance Dose (mg/d)	Maximal Dose (mg/d)	Actions	Indications
Thiourea drugs				
Propylthiouracil (PTU) 50 mg tablets	200–600	1200	Inhibit thyroid hormone synthesis (PTU also inhibits peripheral conversion of T_4 to T_3); may exert immunosuppressive actions	First-line therapy for Graves' hyperthyroidism; short-term therapy before ^{131}I or surgery
Methimazole (Tapazole) 5 and 10 mg tablets	10–60	120		
β-Adrenergic antagonists[a]			Ameliorate action of thyroid hormone in tissues	Adjunctive therapy, often therapy required for thyroiditis
Propranolol	80–160	480		
Nadolol	80–160	320		
Iodine-containing compounds			Inhibit T_4 and T_3 release	Preparation for surgery; thyrotoxic crisis
Lugol's solution	750	750		
Potassium iodide (SSKI)	10–300	400		
Miscellaneous				
Potassium perchlorate	NA	NA	Inhibits iodine transport	No routine indications
Lithium carbonate	NA	NA	Inhibits thyroid hormone synthesis and release	No routine indications
Glucocorticoids			Ameliorates actions of thyroid hormones in tissues; exerts immunosuppressive action (Graves' disease)	Severe subacute thyroiditis; thyrotoxic crisis
Radioactive iodine (RAI,[131]I)	NA	2–10 mCi	Ablation of thyroid gland	First-line therapy for Graves' hyperthyroidism, treatment of choice for recurrent thyrotoxicosis; young adults to elderly; contraindicated in pregnancy, children, and active ophthalmopathy
Surgery	NA	NA	Removal of thyroid gland	Patients should be euthyroid prior to surgery; caution in elderly; cold iodine given prior to surgery

Key: SSKI, Saturated solution of potassium iodide; NA, not applicable.
[a]Not approved in the United States by the FDA for the treatment of thyrotoxicosis.

- Patient characteristics for a favorable outcome include a small goiter (less than 50 g), short duration of disease (<6 months), no previous history of relapse with antithyroid drugs, and low maintenance dosage requirements of antithyroid drug therapy.
- Patients should be monitored every 6–12 months after remission. If a relapse occurs, alternate therapy with RAI is preferred to a second course of antithyroid drugs, as subsequent courses of therapy are less likely to induce remission.
- In one study, concurrent therapy of Graves' disease with methimazole and thyroxine for 1 year, followed by thyroxine alone for 3 years resulted in lower relapse rates than methimazole alone. It is theorized that thyroxine induced suppression of thyroid antigens.
- Minor adverse reactions include pruritic maculopapular rashes, fever, and a benign transient leukopenia (WBC <4000/mm^3). The alternate thiourea may be tried in these situations, but cross-sensitivity occurs in about 50% of patients.
- Major adverse effects include agranulocytosis (with fever, malaise, gingivitis, oropharyngeal infection, and a granulocyte count of <250/mm^3), aplastic anemia, arthralgias, a lupus-like syndrome, polymyositis, gastrointestinal intolerance, hepatotoxicity, and hypoprothrombinemia. Agranulocytosis, if it occurs, almost always develops in the first 3 months of therapy; routine monitoring is not recommended because of its sudden onset. Patients should be counseled to discontinue therapy and contact their physician if flu-like symptoms such as fever, malaise, or sore throat develop. Patients who have experienced a *major* adverse reaction to one thiourea drug should not be converted to the alternate drug because of cross-sensitivity.

Iodides

- Iodide acutely blocks thyroid hormone release, inhibits thyroid hormone biosynthesis by interfering with intrathyroidal iodide utilization, and decreases the size and vascularity of the gland.
- Symptom improvement occurs within 2–7 days of initiating therapy, and serum T$_4$ and T$_3$ concentrations may be reduced for a few weeks.
- Iodides are often used as adjunctive therapy to prepare a patient with Graves' disease for surgery, to acutely inhibit thyroid hormone release and quickly attain the euthyroid state in severely thyrotoxic patients with cardiac decompensation, or to inhibit thyroid hormone release following radioactive iodine therapy.
- Potassium iodide is available as a saturated solution (SSKI, 40 mg iodide per drop), or as Lugol's solution, containing 8 mg of iodide per drop (Table 18.2).
- The typical starting dose of SSKI is 3–10 drops daily (120–400 mg) in water or juice.
- When used to prepare a patient for surgery, it should be administered 7–14 days preoperatively.

IV

- As an adjunct to radioactive iodine (RAI), SSKI should not be used before, but rather 3–7 days after RAI treatment so that the radioactive iodide can concentrate in the thyroid.
- Adverse effects include hypersensitivity reactions (skin rashes, drug fever, rhinitis, conjunctivitis); salivary gland swelling; "iodism" (metallic taste, burning mouth and throat, sore teeth and gums, symptoms of a head cold, and sometimes stomach upset and diarrhea); and gynecomastia.

IV *Adrenergic Blockers*

- β blockers (especially propranolol) have been used widely to ameliorate thyrotoxic symptoms such as palpitations, anxiety, tremor, and heat intolerance. They have no effect on peripheral thyrotoxicosis and protein metabolism and do not reduce TSAb or prevent thyroid storm. Propranolol and nadolol partially block the conversion of T_4 to T_3 but this contribution to the overall therapeutic effect is small.
- β blockers are usually used as adjunctive therapy with antithyroid drugs, RAI, or iodides when treating Graves' disease or toxic nodules; in preparation for surgery; or in thyroid storm. β blockers are primary therapy only for thyroiditis and iodine-induced hyperthyroidism.
- Propranolol doses required to relieve adrenergic symptoms are variable but an initial dose of 20–40 mg four times daily is effective (heart rate <90 beats/min) for most patients. A comparable nadolol dose is 80 mg daily.
- β blockers are contraindicated in patients with congestive heart failure unless it is due solely to tachycardia (high output) and in patients who have developed cardiomyopathy and heart failure. Other side effects include nausea, vomiting, anxiety, insomnia, lightheadedness, bradycardia, and hematologic disturbances.
- Centrally acting sympatholytics (e.g., clonidine) and calcium channel antagonists (e.g., diltiazem) may be useful for symptom control when contraindications to β blockade exist.

Radioactive Iodine

- Sodium iodide 131 (^{131}I) is an oral liquid that concentrates in the thyroid and initially disrupts hormone synthesis by incorporating into thyroid hormones and thyroglobulin. Over a period of weeks, follicles that have taken up RAI and surrounding follicles develop evidence of cellular necrosis and fibrosis of the interstitial tissue.
- RAI is the preferred treatment of debilitated, cardiac, and elderly patients and patients who have had a failure or toxic reaction on drug therapy. RAI is also used in patients who relapse after surgery. Pregnancy is an absolute contraindication to the use of RAI.
- β blockers are the primary adjunctive therapy to RAI, since they may be given anytime without compromising RAI therapy.
- In patients whose symptoms are not controlled with β blockers alone, symptomatic control with adjunctive thioureas to attain a euthyroid

state up until 1 week prior to RAI is warranted because of the slow onset of effect with RAI. Patients with cardiac disease and elderly patients are often treated with thioureas prior to RAI ablation because thyroid hormone levels will transiently increase following RAI treatment, owing to release of performed thyroid hormone.

- Thioureas should not routinely be administered after RAI, because their use is associated with a higher incidence of early post-treatment recurrence or persistence of hyperthyroidism.
- If iodides are administered, they should be given 3–7 days *after* RAI to prevent interference with the uptake of RAI in the thyroid gland.
- The goal of therapy is to destroy overactive thyroid cells, and a single dose of 4000–8000 rads results in a euthyroid state in 60% of patients at 6 months or less. A second dose of RAI should be given 6 months after the first RAI treatment if the patient remains hyperthyroid.
- Hypothyroidism commonly occurs months to years following RAI. The acute, short-term side effects include mild thyroidal tenderness and dysphagia. Long-term follow-up has not revealed an increased risk for development of thyroid carcinoma, leukemia, or congenital defects.

Surgery

- Surgical removal of the thyroid gland is the treatment of choice for coexisting cold nodules, extremely large goiters (over 80 g), and patients with contraindications to thioureas (i.e., allergy or adverse effects) and RAI (i.e., pregnancy).
- If thyroidectomy is planned, PTU or methimazole is usually given until the patient is biochemically euthyroid (usually 6–8 weeks), followed by the addition of iodides (500 mg/d) for 10–14 days before surgery to decrease the vascularity of the gland. Levothyroxine may be added to maintain the euthyroid state while the thioureas are continued.
- Use of levothyroxine to prevent postoperative recurrence of goiter is controversial.
- Propranolol has been used for several weeks preoperatively and 7–10 days after surgery to maintain a heart rate <90 beats/min. Combined pretreatment with propranolol and 10–14 days of potassium iodide also has been advocated.
- Complications of surgery include persistent or recurrent hyperthyroidism (up to 18%), hypothyroidism (up to about 49%), hypoparathyroidism (up to 4%), and vocal cord abnormalities (up to 5%). The frequent occurrence of hypothyroidism requires periodic follow-up for identification and treatment.

Treatment of Thyroid Storm

- The following therapeutic measures should be instituted promptly: suppression of thyroid hormone formation and secretion, antiadrenergic therapy, administration of corticosteroids, and treatment of associated complications or coexisting factors that may have precipitated the storm (Table 18.3).

TABLE 18.3. Drug Dosages Used in the Management of Thyroid Storm

Drug	Regimen
Propythiouracil	900–1200 mg/d PO in four or six divided doses
Methimazole	90–120 mg/d PO in four or six divided doses
Sodium iodide	Up to 2 g/d IV in single or divided doses
Lugol's solution	5–10 drops TID in water or juice
Saturated solution of potassium iodide	1–2 drops TID in water or juice
Propranolol	40–80 mg every 6 h
Lithium	600–1500 mg/d PO in three or four divided doses
Dexamethasone	5–20 mg/d PO or IV in divided doses
Prednisone	25–100 mg/d PO in divided doses
Methylprednisolone	20–80 mg/d IV in divided doses
Hydrocortisone	100–400 mg/d IV in divided doses

- PTU in large doses is the preferred thiourea because it interferes with the production of thyroid hormones and blocks the peripheral conversion of T_4 to T_3.
- Iodides, which rapidly block the release of preformed thyroid hormone, should be administered *after* PTU is initiated to inhibit iodide use by the overactive gland.
- General supportive measures, including acetaminophen as an antipyretic (aspirin or other nonsteroidal anti-inflammatory drugs [NSAIDs] may displace bound thyroid hormone), fluid and electrolyte replacement, sedatives, digitalis, antiarrhythmics, insulin, and antibiotics should be given as indicated. Plasmapheresis and peritoneal dialysis have been used to remove excess hormone when the patient has not responded to more conservative measures.

EVALUATION OF THERAPEUTIC OUTCOMES

- After therapy (thioureas, RAI, or surgery) for hyperthyroidism has been initiated, patients should be evaluated on a monthly basis until they reach a euthyroid condition.
- Clinical signs of continuing thyrotoxicosis or the development of hypothyroidism should be noted.
- If hypothyroidism develops after RAI treatment or surgery, thyroxine replacement may be given when the free T_4 level is below normal and the TSH concentration is above 10 μU/mL. The goal is to maintain both the free thyroxine level and the TSH concentration in the normal range. Once a stable dose of thyroxine is identified, the patient may be followed every 6–12 months.

▶ HYPOTHYROIDISM

PATHOPHYSIOLOGY

- The vast majority of hypothyroid patients have thyroid gland failure (primary hypothyroidism). Causes include chronic autoimmune thyroiditis (Hashimoto's disease), iatrogenic hypothyroidism, iodine deficiency, enzyme defects, thyroid hypoplasia, and goitrogens.
- Pituitary failure (secondary hypothyroidism) is an uncommon cause resulting from pituitary tumors, surgical therapy, external pituitary radiation, postpartum pituitary necrosis, metastatic tumors, tuberculosis, histiocytosis, and autoimmune mechanisms.

IV

CLINICAL PRESENTATION

- Adult manifestations of hypothyroidism include dry skin, cold intolerance, weight gain, constipation, weakness, lethargy, fatigue, loss of ambition or energy, depression, and slowed and hoarse speech. In children, thyroid hormone deficiency may manifest as growth retardation.
- Physical signs include coarse skin and hair, cold skin, periorbital puffiness, bradycardia, muscle cramps, myalgia, and stiffness. Reversible neurologic syndromes such as carpal tunnel syndrome, polyneuropathy, and cerebellar dysfunction may also occur. Objective weakness (with proximal muscles being affected more than distal muscles) and slow relaxation of deep tendon reflexes are common.
- Most patients with pituitary failure (secondary hypothyroidism) have clinical signs of generalized pituitary insufficiency such as abnormal menses and decreased libido, or evidence of a pituitary adenoma such as visual field defects, galactorrhea, or acromegaloid features.
- Myxedema coma is the end stage of long-standing uncorrected hypothyroidism and is manifested by hypothermia, advanced stages of hypothyroid symptoms, and altered sensorium ranging from delirium to coma. Untreated disease is associated with a high mortality rate.

DIAGNOSIS

- A rise in the TSH level is the first evidence of primary hypothyroidism.
  - Many patients have a T_4 level within the normal range (compensated hypothyroidism) and few, if any, symptoms of hypothyroidism. As the disease progresses the T_4 concentration drops below the normal level.
  - The T_3 concentration is often maintained in the normal range despite a low T_4.
  - The RAIU is not a useful test in the evaluation of a hypothyroid patient.
- Pituitary failure (secondary hypothyroidism) should be suspected in a patient with decreased levels of thyroxine and inappropriately normal or low TSH levels.

DESIRED OUTCOME

The treatment goals for hypothyroidism are to normalize the amount of thyroid hormone in the body, minimize the symptoms and long-term consequences of the disorder, and provide individualized therapy based on the type and severity of disease, patient age and gender, existence of non-thyroidal conditions, and response to previous therapy.

TREATMENT OF HYPOTHYROIDISM

IV

- Levothyroxine (L-thyroxine) is the drug of choice for thyroid hormone replacement and suppressive therapy, because it is chemically stable, relatively inexpensive, free of antigenicity, and has uniform potency; however, any of the commercially available thyroid preparations can be used (Table 18.4).
- Although T_3 (and not T_4) is the biologically active form, levothyroxine administration results in a pool of thyroid hormone that is readily and consistently converted to T_3.
- Cholestyramine, sucralfate, aluminum hydroxide, ferrous sulfate, soybean formula, and possibly lovastatin may impair the absorption of levothyroxine from the gastrointestinal tract. Drugs that increase non-deiodinative T_4 clearance include rifampin, carbamazepine, and possibly phenytoin. Amiodarone may block the conversion of T_4 to T_3.
- Substitution of generic levothyroxine preparations should be undertaken with caution, as products may not be bioequivalent.
- The average maintenance dose for most adults is about 110–120 µg/d, but there is a wide range of replacement doses, necessitating individualized therapy and appropriate monitoring to determine an appropriate dose.
- Young patients with long-standing disease and patients over age 45 without known cardiac disease can be started on 50 µg daily of levothyroxine and increased to 100 µg daily after 1 month.
- The recommended initial daily dose for older patients or those with known cardiac disease is 25 µg/d titrated upward in increments of 25 µg at monthly intervals to prevent stress on the cardiovascular system.
- Patients with subclinical hypothyroidism and marked elevations in TSH (>10 µU/mL) and high titers of TSAb or prior treatment with ^{131}I may benefit from treatment with levothyroxine of 50–75 µg per day.
- Serum TSH concentration is the most sensitive and specific monitoring parameter for adjustment of levothyroxine dose. Concentrations begin to fall within hours and are usually normalized within 2 to 6 weeks. An elevated level indicates insufficient replacement.
- TSH and T_4 concentrations should both be checked monthly until a euthyroid state is achieved. Serum T_4 concentrations can be useful in detecting noncompliance, malabsorption, or changes in levothyroxine product bioequivalence. TSH may also be used to check for noncompliance.
- In patients with hypothyroidism caused by hypothalamic or pituitary failure, alleviation of the clinical syndrome and restoration of serum T_4

TABLE 18.4. Thyroid Preparations Used in the Treatment of Hypothyroidism

Drug/Dosage Form	Content	Relative	Comments/Equivalency
Thyroid, USP ¼-, ½-, 1-, 1½-, 2-, 3-, 4-, and 5-grain tablets	Desiccated hog, beef, or sheep thyroid gland	1 grain (equivalent to 60 µg of T_4)	Unpredictable hormonal stability, inexpensive generic brands may not be bioequivalent
Thyroglobulin 32 mg (½ grain), 65 mg (1 grain), 100 mg (1½ grain), 130 mg (2 grain), and 200 mg (3 grain)	Partially purified hog thyroglobulin	1 grain	Standardized biologically to give T_4:T_3 ratio of 2.5:1; more expensive than thyroid extract; no clinical advantage
L-Thyroxine 25, 50, 75, 88, 100, 112, 125, 137, 150, 175, 200, and 300 µg tablets; 200, 500 µg per vial powder for injection	Synthetic T_4	100 µg	Stable; predictable potency; generics may be bioequivalent; when switching from natural thyroid to L-thyroxine, lower dose by ½ grain; variable absorption between products; $t_{1/2}$ = 7 days so daily dosing
Liothyronine 5-, 25-, and 50-µg tablets	Synthetic T_3	25 µg	Uniform absorption; rapid onset; $t_{1/2}$ = 1.5 days, multiple daily dosing; monitor response with TSH assays
Liotrix ¼, ½, 1, 2, and 3 strength tablets	Synthetic T_4:T_3 in 4:1 ratio		Stable, predictable, expensive; lacks therapeutic rationale because T_4 is converted to T_3 peripherally

IV

229

to the normal range are the only criteria available for estimating the appropriate replacement dose of levothyroxine.

- TSH suppressive levothyroxine therapy may also be given to patients with nodular thyroid disease and diffuse goiter, to patients with a history of thyroid irradiation, and to patients with thyroid cancer.
- Excessive doses of thyroid hormone may lead to congestive heart failure, angina pectoris, and myocardial infarction. Allergic or idiosyncratic reactions can occur with the natural animal-derived products such as desiccated thyroid and thyroglobulin but they are extremely rare with the synthetic products used today. Excess exogenous thyroid hormone may reduce bone density and increase the risk of fracture.

IV

TREATMENT OF MYXEDEMA COMA

- Immediate and aggressive therapy with IV bolus thyroxine 300–500 µg is needed to prevent mortality.
- Glucocorticoid therapy with IV hydrocortisone 100 mg every 8 hours should be given until coexisting adrenal suppression is ruled out.
- Consciousness, lowered TSH concentrations, and normal vital signs are expected within 24 hours.
- Maintenance doses of tyroxine are typically 75–100 µg IV until the patient stabilizes and oral therapy is begun.
- Supportive therapy must be instituted to maintain adequate ventilation, euglycemia, blood pressure, and body temperature. Underlying disorders such as sepsis and myocardial infarction must be diagnosed and treated.

EVALUATION OF THERAPEUTIC OUTCOMES

- Patients with uncomplicated hypothyroidism receiving typical doses of levothyroxine will have an increase in metabolic activity and be out of the myxedematous zone within 1 week of initiating therapy.
- An impressive diuresis usually occurs within 2–3 days, with an improvement in the puffy facial appearance and with weight loss. Speech, skin temperature, mental alertness, and physical activity show improvement within 72 hours.
- Levothyroxine is the drug of choice in pregnant women, and the objective of treatment is to decrease TSH to <6 µU/mL and to maintain T_4 concentrations in the range of ~2–4 µg/dL.
- In children with hypothyroidism developing beyond 2–3 years of age, normal CNS and physiologic development are expected with thyroid replacement therapy.

See Chapter 73, Thyroid Disorders, authored by Charles A. Reasner, MD, FACE and Robert L. Talbert, PharmD, FCCP, for a more detailed discussion of this topic.

Chapter 19

▶ ALCOHOLIC LIVER DISEASE

▶ DEFINITION

Alcoholic liver disease (ALD) is defined as chronic insufficiency of the liver as a result of alcohol abuse.

▶ EPIDEMIOLOGY

- Alcohol is one of the most common causes of liver disease worldwide. In the United States, mortality and rate of hospitalization from chronic liver diseases have been declining.
- Up to 90% of deaths due to cirrhosis may be prevented by elimination of alcohol use.
- ALD is associated with chronic ingestion of 60–80 g of ethanol daily for long periods of time (e.g., >10 years).
- With chronic ethanol abuse there is a 1 in 12 risk of developing cirrhosis.
- Other factors related to increased risk of developing ALD include poor nutritional status and female sex.

▶ PATHOPHYSIOLOGY

- ALD can be viewed as a progressive, chronic condition with four basic stages.
- The initial lesion, steatosis or fatty metamorphosis, may begin as early as the first drink. If the pattern of heavy alcohol use is continued, these lesions become necrotic, inducing a mild inflammatory reaction called alcoholic hepatitis or steatonecrosis. In some cases, these lesions lead to a third stage involving fibrotic changes of cirrhosis. The endpoint of the disease is hepatic failure and death.
- Genetic make-up, gender, nutrition, and other hepatotoxins may predispose individuals to alcoholic hepatitis.
- Continued use of alcohol appears to induce the mixed-function oxidase system that increases lipid synthesis and decreases oxidation of fatty acids perhaps caused by acetaldehyde. This leads directly to steatosis, which is the first lesion of ALD.
- Steatosis is a lesion characteristic of, although not exclusive to, ALD. When seen at biopsy, the hepatocytes are filled with large lipid-containing vesicles. This pathologic change is easily reversed by abstinence from alcohol, and little functional impairment is usually encountered.

- The next major pathologic event in the progression of ALD is steatonecrosis or alcoholic hepatitis. Lysis and necrosis of the fat-filled hepatocytes provoke an immune response. Alcohol may lead to cell necrosis by increasing the metabolic rate of cells that are already relatively hypoxic. The fibrosis that occurs in alcoholic hepatitis often obliterates the central veins, leading to portal vein hypertension even before the patient has progressed to cirrhosis. If there is no continued insult to the liver, a resolution of symptoms can be anticipated in 3 to 8 months.
- The 7-year survival rate for abstainers is 80%, whereas for those continuing to drink the rate is only 50%.
- Cirrhosis leading to hepatic failure and its complications is the terminal event in ALD. The fibrosis may compress the hepatic veins, decreasing hepatic outflow, and thus leading to portal hypertension.

V

▶ CLINICAL PRESENTATION

- Patients with ALD typically present with scleral icterus, spider angiomata (star-shaped vascular defects observed on the skin) generally observed on the trunk, and palmar erythema.
- Icterus, also called jaundice, is characterized by a yellow tinge to the skin or eyes that is noticeable when total bilirubin levels exceed 3 to 5 mg %.
- The liver is usually distended. Typically the spleen is palpable because of increased pressures from the portal hypertension.
- Gynecomastia is common in males because of the testicular atrophy induced by alcohol.

LABORATORY

- With advancing liver disease, less bilirubin (a breakdown product of hemoglobin) is conjugated by the liver, leading to increases in indirect bilirubin (insoluble form which is bound to plasma proteins) in blood. Liver cell death leads to release of conjugated bilirubin (or direct bilirubin) from the liver into the systemic circulation. Excess conjugated bilirubin may be filtered by the kidneys, giving urine the characteristic "cola" color and leads to accumulation in the epidermis and sclera.
- Alkaline phosphatase, an enzyme made in the cells lining the biliary tract and in bone tissue, increases in the blood with processes that disrupt bile flow.
- With alcoholic hepatitis, values of alanine aminotransferase (ALT) and aspartate aminotransferase (AST) may reach into the hundreds (normal range for these is generally 5–40 IU/dL). As liver disease progresses into cirrhosis, the transaminases may actually fall, despite decreasing liver function.
- With ALD, a disproportionate increase in γ-glutamyltranspeptidase (GGTP, a biliary excretory enzyme that is more specific for liver disease) can be expected and is a useful diagnostic clue.

- As liver damage progresses, protein synthesis decreases. Prolongation of clotting tests such as prothrombin time and activated partial thromboplastin time can be expected. The serum albumin may fall as low as 2 g/dL (normal 4.5–5.5 g/dL).
- The Child–Pugh classification is frequently used to stratify patients into categories for selection of various therapies (Table 19.1).

PORTAL HYPERTENSION

- Portal hypertension in ALD is the direct result of increased mechanical resistance to blood flow through the liver. Thus, the manifestations of portal hypertension are primarily the result of low-pressure vessels handling high-pressure loads. Esophageal and abdominal varices often develop; these can rupture and sometimes lead to life-threatening hemorrhage.
- Another significant complication of portal hypertension is ascites.

DECREASED LIVER FUNCTION

- With cirrhosis there is a progressive loss of basic hepatocyte function because of an overall loss of parenchymal mass that results in a decrease in protein synthesis and utilization of available substrates.
- A loss of enzymes leads to a decrease in the ability of the liver to handle both drugs and endogenous toxins, which then begin to accumulate.
- A decrease in serum albumin leads to a decrease in the protein binding of certain drugs and a decrease in the serum oncotic pressure.
- Vitamin K–dependent coagulation factors (II, VII, IX, X) synthesized by the liver slowly diminish, resulting in an increased frequency of bleeding problems
- The ability of the hepatic transaminases to detoxify ammonia is decreased. Ammonia, octopamine, mercaptans, phenols, methanethiols, and other by-products of metabolism begin to accumulate. Along with this decrease in transamination there is an apparent increase in ammonia production in the gut.

TABLE 19.1. Child–Pugh Grading of Liver Disease

Clinical and Biochemical Measurements	Points Scored for Increasing Abnormality		
	1	*2*	*3*
Encephalopathy (grade)	None	1 and 2	3 and 4
Ascites	Absent	Slight	Moderate
Bilirubin (mg/dL)	1–2	2–3	>3
Albumin (g/dL)	3.5	2.8–3.5	<2.8
Prothrombin time (increased seconds)	1–4	4–6	>6

TABLE 19.2. Scale for Assessing the Depth of Hepatic Encephalopathy

Grade	Cognitive/Motor	Behavior
1	Mild tremor, altered handwriting	Anxiety, insomnia, mild confusion
2	Dysarthria, ataxia asterixis	Lethargy, disorientation
3	Seizures, muscle twitching	Delirium, bizarre behavior
4	Posturing	Coma

From Barber JR, Teasley KM. Clin Pharm 1984;3:245–253, with permission.

V

- There is some evidence that benzodiazepine-receptor reactivity is increased and that an endogenous benzodiazepine-receptor ligand accumulates in liver disease. This ligand is known to be produced in very small amounts by plants.
- There is an increase in aromatic amino acids (AAAs) at a rate 24 times the production of branched-chain amino acids (BCAAs).

HEPATIC ENCEPHALOPATHY

- Hepatic encephalopathy (HE) is a syndrome of altered mental status associated with liver impairment and is characterized by impaired cognitive skills, worsened motor abilities, and steadily depressed levels of consciousness, beginning with somnolence and ending with coma.
- The spectrum of impairment is broad and may be classified in stages as the syndrome progresses (Table 19.2).
- The cause of HE is not known; several factors, such as increased blood levels of ammonia and aromatic amino acids, have been associated with the development of HE (Table 19.3).

TABLE 19.3. Theories for the Development of Hepatic Encephalopathy

Toxin	Description
Ammonia	Direct neurotoxin
Multiple synergistic neurotoxins	Mercaptans (produced by dietary methionine), elevated free fatty acids
False neurotransmitters	Elevated aromatic amino acids lead to increased serotonin, octopamine, and phenylethylamine (depressants) while decreasing dopamine and noradrenaline (stimulants)
γ-Aminobutyric acid neurotransmission	Endogenous and/or exogenous benzodiazepine-like compounds

- There are a variety of precipitating causes for hepatic encephalopathy (Table 19.4).
- There is also a tremendous increase in the relative levels of aromatic amino acids in the encephalopathic patient. The abnormal ratio of BCAAs to AAAs in liver disease allows for enhanced CNS entry of tryptophan, tyrosine, and phenylalanine.

PHARMACOKINETIC/PHARMACODYNAMIC CHANGES ASSOCIATED WITH LIVER FAILURE

- Table 19.5 lists a few drugs and the known pharmacokinetic changes associated with liver impairment.
- Highly extracted drugs tend to be affected more by changes in hepatic blood flow than by changes in metabolic rate. The opposite is true of low-extraction ratio drugs. V

TABLE 19.4. Precipitating Causes of Hepatic Encephalopathy

Cause	Mechanism	Management
Infection	Increased tissue catabolism leads to more nitrogen load; hypotension-induced azotemia	Treat infection
Constipation	Increased production and absorption of ammonia from longer contact time for bacteria and substrates	Prophylactic use of stool softeners or laxatives
Metabolic alkalosis	Leads to diffusion of un-ionized ammonia across blood–brain barrier	KCl treatment in moderate cases; 0.1 N HCl infusion in severe cases
Excess dietary protein	Substrate for bacterial production of ammonia or other nitrogenous toxins	Limit total protein intake or restrict red meat protein
Gastrointestinal bleeding	Hypovolemia may decrease perfusion to liver/brain/kidneys; blood provides 15–20 g protein/100 mL as ammonia substrate	Evacuate bowel
Drugs: sedative/hypnotics; opiates	Direct CNS depression	Avoid use; otherwise select short-acting nonliver metabolized or adjust dose
Azotemia	Sedative effect of uremia	Use diuretics gently

V

TABLE 19.5. Selected Examples of Pharmacokinetic Changes During Liver Failure

Drug	Extraction	Disease	Plasma Clearance	Volume of Distribution	Terminal Half-Life
Diazepam	Low	Cirrhosis	Decreases 30–50%	May increase slightly	Increases 40–50%
Diazepam	Low	Acute hepatitis	Decreases	May increase slightly	Increases 20–40%
Oxazepam	Low	Cirrhosis	Increases slightly	Increases 10–20%	Increases slightly
Phenobarbital	Low	Cirrhosis			Increases 10–30%
Phenobarbital	Low	Acute hepatitis			Increases 10–40%
Propranolol	High	Cirrhosis	Decreases 33–50%	Increases 50%	Increases 100–200%
Labetolol	High	Cirrhosis	Decreases 25–60%	Decreases 20–40%	Increases slightly
Lidocaine	High	Cirrhosis	Decreases 35–40%		
Clindamycin	Low	Cirrhosis	Decreases 60%	Decreases 40%	Increases slightly
Theophylline	High	Cirrhosis	Decreases 33–50%	Increases 30–40%	Increases 100–300%

Some pharmacokinetic/pharmacodynamic changes with liver disease include:

- Highly protein-bound drugs have increased unbound (or free) fractions owing to reduced albumin concentrations.
- An increased free fraction also means that there is more drug available to be metabolized by the still-functioning hepatic enzymes. Thus, until these enzymes become saturated, the clearance of a highly protein-bound drug during liver impairment can increase and the half-life can shorten.
- Patients with high GGTP and alkaline phosphatase levels may experience a decrease in biliary excretion. Drugs that are excreted through the bile will accumulate in these patients.
- Dramatic shifts in fluid can be expected in ALD, thus increasing the distribution volume of drugs with low protein binding.
- The clinical components of liver disease also can change the dose-response relationships of drugs. Encephalopathic patients will be much more sensitive to central nervous system (CNS) depressants.
- Bleeding varices may increase the absorption of drugs that would normally exhibit poor absorption.
- Diarrhea associated with hepatitis will decrease the absorption of many drugs.

▶ DESIRED OUTCOME

The ideal goal for treatment of ALD is that the patient stops drinking alcohol before irreversible hepatic damage has occurred. This would reduce long-term complications. When there is chronic liver dysfunction, the goals are restoration of liver function and avoidance of life-threatening complications.

▶ TREATMENT

GENERAL PRINCIPLES

- The most important treatment for ALD is the discontinuance of alcohol exposure. With discontinuation of alcohol exposure, many patients improve dramatically.
- After the discontinuation of alcohol, the therapy for ALD is primarily symptomatic.

ALCOHOLIC HEPATITIS

- A treatment algorithm for alcoholic hepatitis is shown in Figure 19.1.
- In alcoholic hepatitis, glucocorticoids are sometimes used during the acute phase to decrease the inflammatory response to the alcoholic hyaline and other antigenic substances present. Dramatic improvement in short-term mortality has been demonstrated with methylprednisolone in very sick patients.

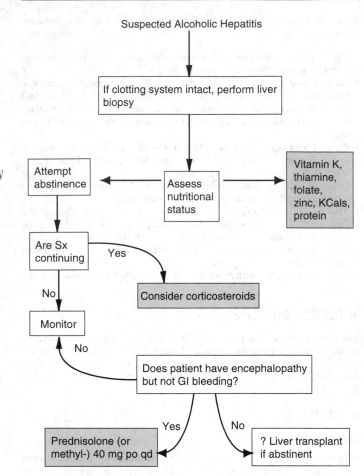

Figure 19.1. Treatment algorithm for a patient with alcoholic hepatitis.

- Encephalopathy was a predictor for success and additionally, that the presence of GI bleeding would reverse the positive effects of glucocorticoids.
- Generally, prednisolone or methylprednisolone are the preferred steroids since they do not require liver metabolism to an active compound as prednisone does.

CIRRHOSIS

- The treatment of cirrhosis is also symptomatic, directed at the manifestations in the particular patient.
- If the patient shows signs of nutritional deficiency, it should be corrected. Deficiencies in folate, thiamine, and vitamin C are very common and often severe. In addition, potassium, phosphorus, magnesium, and iron can be quite low in these patients.
- Replacement of iron should be done with particular caution in cirrhotic patients, because liver iron stores are often higher than normal despite low serum concentrations, and hemochromatosis can develop.
- Vitamin K injections can sometimes help regenerate clotting factors, but as cirrhosis worsens the response to vitamin K lessens. Treatment of the coagulopathy may require fresh whole blood or fresh frozen plasma transfusions.
- Replenishment of serum protein can be very difficult in cirrhotic patients who often require protein restriction, but adequate calories should be given.
- Liver transplantation is a consideration for end-stage liver disease.

V

ASCITES

- Ascites is primarily an accumulation of fluid; therefore, the objective in treating ascites should be removal of fluid. In practice, this is often not an easy task.
- Table 19.6 summarizes the stepwise treatment of ascites.
- Sodium restriction is the first step in treating ascites. Most patients with ascites can tolerate 1 g of sodium per day, which essentially means no

TABLE 19.6. Treatment Algorithm for Ascites

Therapy	Goal
Sodium and water restriction	Loss = 1–2 L/d (weight loss = 1–2 kg)
If inadequate response after 3–5 d, add	
Mild diuretic (spironolactone 100–400 mg/d)	As above
If inadequate response after 4–7 d, add	
Loop diuretic (furosemide 40–120 mg/d)	As above
If inadequate response after 30–60 d, add	
Peritoneal dialysis with reinfusion	As above
or	
Peritoneovenous shunt	As above

added salt and no salted foods. The diuresis observed from this approach, however, is very slow, often taking as long as 30 days for obvious loss of ascites volume.

- Salt restriction is generally accompanied by a concurrent restriction of fluid intake to a few hundred mL per day. As the ascites begins to resolve, the amount of sodium can sometimes be increased to a more tolerable 2 to 3 g, and the amount of fluid intake increased upward to a liter per day.

- The overall fluid loss per day should not exceed 1–2 L. Non-edematous patients should not be diuresed beyond a weight loss of about 0.5 kg/d. Diuresis that is too brisk can lead to problems of relative dehydration and a potentially fatal hepatorenal syndrome.

- Paracentesis or diuretic therapy can be used to deplete the volume of ascites when sodium and fluid restriction fail to produce adequate diuresis. Paracentesis of large volumes of fluid usually results in immediate resorption of water from the vascular space into the peritoneal space that may lead to vascular volume depletion. To avoid these shifts, simultaneous administration of parenteral albumin has been used.

- Many patients who continue to develop ascites and those who do not respond to diuretics or paracentesis may be eligible to receive a LeVeen or peritoneovenous shunt.

- Diuretic therapy for ascites is effective in most patients; however, the process is slow (35–40 days of continuous therapy may be required before the ascites resolves).

- The drugs most frequently used are the potassium-sparing diuretics, in particular, spironolactone, because of its ability to inhibit the action of aldosterone in the kidney tubule. The dose of spironolactone required ranges from 100–800 mg/d and is usually not effective without concurrent sodium and water restriction. The onset of the diuretic effect with spironolactone is slow, 3–5 days in some cases, and loop diuretics such as furosemide are sometimes added to increase the rate of weight loss.

PORTAL HYPERTENSION

- The therapy for portal hypertension is directed at reducing flow to the portal bed.

- Operative procedures such as splenectomy or portacaval shunts attempt to do this mechanically.

- Drug therapy with propranolol is also used with some success at a dose sufficient to decrease the blood pressure by 25 mm Hg or to reduce the heart rate by 20–25%.

- Propranolol reduces the incidence of first rebleeding and lowers the mortality rate relative to placebo. However, it produces desirable (decreased portal vein pressure) and undesirable effects (decreased liver blood flow).

- Sclerotherapy is the direct application of a chemical with necroinflammatory or thrombotic properties (ethanolamine, sodium tetradecyl sulfate, and sodium morrhuate) to manage the acute bleeding episode and, when used prophylactically, to prevent relapse. There is no consensus regarding the sclerosant of choice.

- An intravenous infusion of vasopressin at 0.2–0.6 unit per minute can be used to treat acutely bleeding varices.
- Coronary and venous thrombosis can occur along with arrhythmias secondary to ischemia as a result of the use of vasopressin. Increases in blood pressure are possible as are severe vascular headaches and angina. It is prudent to have any patient treated with vasopressin monitored by electrocardiogram.
- Nitroglycerin has been advocated as an adjunct to vasopressin to limit the coronary vasospasm.

HEPATIC ENCEPHALOPATHY

V

- Most patients with HE respond to some type of protein restriction. Care must be exercised since nearly all patients with ALD have varying degrees of protein malnutrition and would require at least 60 g of protein daily to maintain positive nitrogen balance.
- The source and types of amino acids in the diet may also be important, because AAAs, already higher than normal in cirrhotics, can be utilized in the CNS to produce false neurotransmitters. This ratio of AAAs to BCAAs can be reversed by the use of feedings high in BCAAs.
- The classic management has been to restrict intake to about 20 g of protein per day; this is increased as the patient's symptoms improve. This approach is refuted by the false neurotransmitter theory for HE that suggests quality of protein rather than quantity is important, especially in light of protein malnutrition and anorexia present in this population.
- In latent (i.e., subclinical) HE, oral BCAA improves psychomotor disturbances and automobile driving capacity compared to placebo.
- The status of BCAA in *acute* HE is more uncertain. In contrast, oral BCAA has improved some measures in *chronic* HE including liver function tests (increased serum albumin), nutritional measures (amino-acid profile, nitrogen balance), and mortality, in some studies. To prevent negative nitrogen balance, stable cirrhotic patients may require 0.5–1 g/kg of protein. However, catabolic states such as alcoholic hepatitis require intakes of 1.0 g/kg of protein.
- Therapies that reduce the blood ammonia level appear to be effective in the management of HE that does not respond to protein restriction alone (Figure 19.2).
- Lactulose, a nonabsorbed disaccharide, decreases this rate of urea breakdown and thus decreases the ammonia in the blood derived from the gut. Optimally, the lactulose dose should be titrated to produce two to three stools per day. Lactulose should be started at 50 mL every hour until catharsis occurs.
- Neomycin given orally is also used to change colonic flora and decrease blood ammonia. The optimal dosing regimen is not known; however, a starting dose of 0.5 g four times daily may be used up to 4–6 g/d.

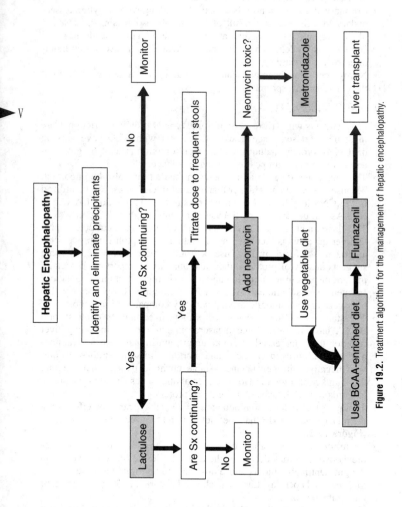

Figure 19.2. Treatment algorithm for the management of hepatic encephalopathy.

V

242

- The benzodiazepine antagonist flumazenil is an alternative when conventional treatment of HE has failed. Rapid and startling clinical response has been reported with doses of 0.2–15 mg IV in uncontrolled studies. Studies show improvement in 40–70% of patients treated with flumazenil and no response to placebo.

See Chapter 37, Alcoholic Liver Disease, authored by Mark A. Gill, PharmD and William R. Kirchain, PharmD, for a more detailed discussion of this topic.

V

Chapter 20

▶ CONSTIPATION

▶ DEFINITION

A number of different definitions of constipation have been used in clinical studies. Some of the definitions used include: less than three stools per week for women and five for men despite a high residue diet, or a period of >3 days without a bowel movement; straining at stool >25% of the time and/or two or fewer stools per week; or straining at defecation and less than one stool daily with minimal effort. These varying definitions demonstrate the difficulty in characterizing this problem.

▶ PATHOPHYSIOLOGY

- Constipation is not a disease but a symptom of an underlying disease or problem.
- Approaches to treatment of constipation should begin with attempts to determine its cause. Disorders of the gastrointestinal (GI) tract (e.g., irritable bowel syndrome or diverticulitis), metabolic disorders (e.g., diabetes), or endocrine disorders (e.g., hypothyroidism) may be involved.
- Constipation commonly results from a diet low in fiber or from use of constipating drugs such as opiates.
- Finally, it is believed that constipation may sometimes be psychogenic in origin. Diseases or conditions that may cause constipation are:
  - Gastrointestinal Disorders
    Gastroduodenal obstruction from ulceration or cancer
    Irritable bowel syndrome
    Diverticulitis
    Hemorrhoids, anal fissures
    Ulcerative proctitis
    Tumors
  - Metabolic and Endocrine Disorders
    Diabetes mellitus
    Hypothyroidism
    Panhypopituitarism
    Pheochromocytoma
    Hypercalcemia
  - Pregnancy
  - Neurogenic Constipation
    Head trauma
    Central nervous system tumors
    Stroke
    Parkinson's disease
  - Psychogenic Constipation

Psychiatric disorders
Innapropriate bowel habits
- Drug-Induced Constipation
Analgesics
Inhibitors of prostaglandin synthesis
Opiates
Anticholinergics
Antihistamines
Antiparkinsonian agents (e.g., benztropine or trihexyphenidyl)
Phenothiazines
Tricyclic antidepressants
Antacids containing calcium carbonate or aluminum hydroxide
Barium sulfate
Clonidine
Diuretics (non-potassium sparing)
Ganglionic blockers
Iron preparations
Muscle blockers (d-tubocurarine, succinylcholine)
Polystyrene sodium sulfonate
- All opiate derivatives are associated with constipation, but the degree of intestinal inhibitory effects seems to differ between agents. Orally administered opiates appear to have greater inhibitory effect than parenterally administered agents; oral codeine is well known as a potent antimotility agent.
- Agents with anticholinergic properties inhibit bowel function by parasympatholytic actions on innervation to many regions of the GI tract, particularly the colon and rectum. Many types of drugs possess anticholinergic action, and these agents are used commonly in hospitalized and nonhospitalized patients.

▶ CLINICAL PRESENTATION

- The patient presenting with constipation usually complains of abdominal discomfort and distention.
- Constipation may vary in implication from a minor discomfort in the otherwise healthy adult to a symptom of colon cancer or other serious diseases.
- A basis for evaluation and treatment should be a thorough history including questions about the nature of the constipation.
- It is important to ascertain whether the patient perceives the problem as infrequent bowel movements, stools of insufficient size, a feeling of fullness, or difficulty and pain on passing stool.
- The patient should be asked about the frequency of bowel movements and the chronicity of constipation. The patient also should be carefully questioned about usual diet and laxative regimens. Does the patient have a diet consistently deficient in high-fiber items and containing

mainly highly refined foods? What laxatives or cathartics has the patient used to attempt relief of constipation?

- It should be noted that laxative abusers frequently deny laxative use.
- The patient should be questioned about other concurrent medications, with interest toward agents that might cause constipation.
- Chronic constipation can result in a more complex picture. Patients may have long-standing complaints of GI irregularities with a variety of symptoms.
- The laxative abuser may present with contradictory findings, sometimes diarrhea or weight loss. Laxative abusers may also have vomiting, abdominal pain, lassitude, thirst, edema, and bone pain (due to osteomalacia). With prolonged abuse, patients may have fluid and electrolyte imbalances (most commonly hypokalemia), protein losing gastroenteropathy with hypoalbuminemia, and syndromes resembling colitis.

▶ DESIRED OUTCOME

A major goal for treatment of constipation is initiation of measures (such as proper diet) to prevent constipation. For acute constipation the goal is to relieve symptoms and restore normal bowel function.

▶ TREATMENT

GENERAL PRINCIPLES

- General measures believed to be beneficial in managing constipation include dietary modification to increase the amount of fiber consumed daily, exercise, adjustment of bowel habits so that a regular and adequate time is made to respond to the urge to defecate, and increasing fluid intake.
- If an underlying disease is recognized as the cause of constipation, attempts should be made to correct it. GI malignancies may be removed through a surgical resection. Endocrine and metabolic derangements are corrected by the appropriate methods.
- Potential drug causes of constipation should be identified. For some medications (e.g., antacids), nonconstipating alternatives exist. If no reasonable alternatives exist to the medication thought to be responsible for constipation, consideration should be given to lowering the dose. If a patient must remain on constipating medications, then more attention must be paid to general measures for prevention of constipation, as discussed next.

DIETARY MODIFICATION AND BULK-FORMING AGENTS

- The most important aspect of the therapy for constipation for the majority of patients is dietary modification to increase the amount of fiber consumed.

- Patients should be advised to include at least 14 g of crude fiber in their daily diets.
- Fruits, vegetables, and cereals have the highest fiber content.
- A trial of dietary modification with high-fiber content should be continued for at least 1 month before effects on bowel function are determined.
- The patient should be cautioned that abdominal distention and flatus may be particularly troublesome in the first few weeks, particularly with high bran consumption.

SURGERY

- In a small percentage of patients presenting with complaints of constipation, surgical procedures (such as intestinal resection) are necessary. Surgery is usually necessary with most colonic malignancies and with GI obstruction from a number of causes.

PHARMACOLOGIC THERAPY

- The various types of laxatives are discussed in this section. The agents are divided into three general classifications: (1) those causing softening of feces in 1 to 3 days (bulk-forming laxatives, docusates, and lactulose); (2) those that result in soft or semifluid stool in 6 to 12 hours (diphenylmethane derivatives and anthraquinone derivatives); and (3) those causing water evacuation in 1 to 6 hours (saline cathartics, castor oil, and polyethylene glycol–electrolyte lavage solution).
- Dosage recommendations for laxatives and cathartics are provided in Table 20.1.

EMOLLIENT LAXATIVES

- These surfactant agents, docusate in its various salts, work by facilitating the mixing of aqueous and fatty materials within the intestinal tract. They may increase water and electrolyte secretion in the small and large bowel.
- These products result in a softening of stools within 1 to 3 days.
- Emollient laxatives are not effective in treating constipation but are used mainly to prevent constipation. They may be helpful in situations where straining at stool should be avoided, such as after recovery from myocardial infarction, with acute perianal disease, or after rectal surgery.
- It is unlikely that these agents are very effective in preventing constipation if major causative factors (e.g., heavy opiate use, uncorrected pathology, inadequate dietary fiber) are not concurrently addressed.

Lubricants

- Mineral oil is the only lubricant laxative in routine use and acts by coating stool and allowing easier passage. It inhibits colonic absorption of water, thereby increasing stool weight and decreasing stool transit time.
- Generally, the effect on bowel function is noted after 2 or 3 days of use.

TABLE 20.1. Dosage Recommendations for Laxatives and Cathartics

Agent	Recommended Dose
Agents That Cause Softening of Feces in 1–3 d	
Bulk-forming agents	
Methylcellulose	4–6 g/d
Polycarbophil	4–6 g/d
Psyllium	Varies with product
Emollients	
Docusate sodium	50–360 mg/d
Docusate calcium	50–360 mg/d
Docusate potassium	100–300 mg/d
Lactulose	15–30 mL orally
Sorbitol	30–50 g/d orally
Mineral oil	15–30 mL orally
Agents That Result in Soft or Semifluid Stool in 6–12 h	
Bisacodyl (oral)	5–15 mg orally
Phenolphthalein	30–270 mg orally
Cascara sagrada	Dose varies with formulation
Senna	Dose varies with formulation
Magnesium sulfate (low dose)	<10 g orally
Agents That Cause Watery Evacuation in 1–6 h	
Magnesium citrate	18 g in 300 mL water
Magnesium hydroxide	2.4–4.8 g orally
Magnesium sulfate (high dose)	10–30 g orally
Sodium phosphates	Varies with salt used
Bisacodyl	10 mg rectally
Polyethylene glycol–electrolyte preparations	4 L

V

- Mineral oil is helpful in situations similar to those suggested for docusates: to maintain a soft stool and avoid straining for relatively short periods of time (a few days to 2 weeks).
- Mineral oil may be absorbed systemically and cause a foreign-body reaction in lymphoid tissue. Also, in debilitated or recumbent patients, mineral oil may be aspirated causing lipoid pneumonia.

Lactulose and Sorbitol

- Lactulose is a disaccharide that causes an osmotic effect retained in the colon.
- Lactulose is generally not recommended as a first-line agent for the treatment of constipation because it is costly and not necessarily more effective than agents such as milk of magnesia. It may be justified as an alternative for acute constipation and been found to be particularly useful in elderly patients.
- Occasionally, the use of lactulose may result in flatulence, cramps, diarrhea, and electrolyte imbalances.
- Sorbitol, a monosaccharide, is occasionally used as a laxative, exerting its effect by osmotic action. It is as effective as lactulose and much less expensive.

Diphenylmethane Derivatives

- The two commonly used agents in this class are bisacodyl and phenolphthalein.
- Bisacodyl stimulates the mucosal nerve plexus of the colon; the mechanism of action of phenolphthalein is poorly understood.
- The dose of these agents for effective use in various individuals appears to vary greatly. A dose that causes no effects in one patient may result in excessive cramping and fluid evacuation in another.
- Their use is acceptable intermittently (every few weeks) to treat constipation or as a bowel preparation before diagnostic procedures in which cleansing of the colon is necessary.
- The patient taking phenolphthalein-containing laxatives should be cautioned that it may turn urine pink.

Anthraquinone Derivatives

- The agents in this class are cascara sagrada, sennosides, and casanthrol.
- Effects are limited to the colon, and stimulation of Auerbach's plexus may be involved.
- Recommendations for the use of these agents are similar to those for the diphenylmethane derivatives. In most cases, intermittent use is acceptable; daily use should be strongly discouraged.

Saline Cathartics

- Saline cathartics are composed of relatively poorly absorbed ions such as magnesium, sulfate, phosphate, and citrate, which produce their effects primarily by osmotic action to retain fluid in the GI tract.
- These agents may be given orally or rectally.
- A bowel movement may result within a few hours after oral doses and in 1 hour or less after rectal administration.
- These agents should be used primarily for acute evacuation of the bowel, which may be necessary before diagnostic examinations, after poisonings, and in conjunction with some anthelmintics to eliminate parasites.
- Agents such as milk of magnesia (an 8% suspension of magnesium hydroxide) may be used occasionally (every few weeks) to treat constipation in otherwise healthy adults.

- Saline cathartics should not be used on a routine basis to treat constipation. With fecal impactions, the enema formulations of these agents may be helpful.

Castor Oil

- Castor oil is metabolized in the GI tract to an active compound, ricinoleic acid, which stimulates secretory processes, decreases glucose absorption, and promotes intestinal motility, primarily in the small intestine.
- Castor oil usually results in a bowel movement within 1 to 3 hours of administration.
- Because the agent has such a strong purgative action it should not be used for the routine treatment of constipation.

Glycerin

- This agent is usually administered as a 3-g suppository and exerts its effect by osmotic action in the rectum.
- As with most agents given as suppositories, the onset of action is usually less than 30 minutes.
- Glycerin is considered a very safe laxative, although it may occasionally cause rectal irritation. Its use is acceptable on an intermittent basis for constipation, particularly in children.

Polyethylene Glycol–Electrolyte Lavage Solution

- Whole-bowel irrigation with polyethylene glycol–electrolyte lavage solution (PEG-ELS) has become popular for colon cleansing before diagnostic procedures or colorectal operations.
- Four liters of this solution is administered over 3 hours to obtain complete evacuation of the GI tract.
- The solution is not recommended for the routine treatment of constipation and its use should be avoided in patients with intestinal obstruction.

Other Agents

- Tap-water enemas may be used to treat simple constipation. The administration of 200 mL of water by enema to an adult often results in a bowel movement within one-half hour. Soapsuds are no longer recommended for use in enemas because their use may result in proctitis or colitis.
- Cisapride is a GI prokinetic agent that is used in GI motility disorders. It has been demonstrated to be effective in relieving acute constipation in both adults and children. The agent is considerably more expensive than most alternatives.

RECOMMENDATIONS

- Treatment and prevention of constipation should consist of bulk-forming agents in addition to dietary modifications that increase dietary fiber.

- For most nonhospitalized persons with acute constipation, the infrequent use (less than every few weeks) of most laxative products is acceptable; however, before more potent laxative/cathartics are used, relatively simple measures may be tried. For example, acute constipation may be relieved by the use of a tap-water enema or a glycerin suppository; if neither is effective, the use of low doses of diphenylmethane or anthraquinone derivatives or saline laxatives (e.g., milk of magnesia) may provide relief.
- If laxative treatment is required for longer than 1 week, the person should be advised to consult a physician to determine if there is an underlying cause of constipation that requires treatment with agents other than laxatives.
- For some bedridden or geriatric patients, or others with chronic constipation, bulk-forming laxatives remain the first line of treatment, but the use of more potent laxatives may be required relatively frequently. When other than bulk-forming laxatives are used, they should be administered in the lowest effective dose and as infrequently as possible to maintain regular bowel function (more than three stools per week). Agents that may be used in these situations include diphenylmethane and anthraquinone derivatives, milk of magnesia, and lactulose.
- In the hospitalized patient without GI disease, constipation may be related to the use of general anesthesia and/or opiate substances. Most orally or rectally administered laxatives may be used. For prompt initiation of a bowel movement, a tap-water enema or glycerin suppository is recommended, or milk of magnesia. With infants and children, constipation may occur commonly.
- The approach to the treatment of constipation in young persons should consider neurologic, metabolic, or anatomic abnormalities when constipation is a persistent problem. When not related to an underlying disease, the approach to constipation is similar to that in an adult.
- Patients with chronic, intractable constipation are commonly found to have slow GI transit, pelvic floor dysfunction, both of the above, or irritable bowel syndrome. With failure of medical management, surgery may be indicated in patients with slow transit. Behavioral treatments such as biofeedback are successful in about 70% of patients with pelvic floor dysfunction.

See Chapter 36, Diarrhea and Constipation, authored by R. Leon Longe, PharmD and Joseph T. DiPiro, PharmD, FCCP, for a more detailed discussion of this topic.

Chapter 21

► DIARRHEA

► DEFINITION

Diarrhea is the abnormal frequency and liquidity of fecal discharge compared with the normal stools. Frequency and consistency are variable within and between individuals. For example, some individuals defecate as many as three times per day, while others defecate only two or three times per week.

► EPIDEMIOLOGY

- Diarrhea is most often the result of infection.
- In the United States viral and bacterial organisms account for most of the infectious diarrhea. Common bacterial organisms are *Shigella, Salmonella, Campylobacter, Staphylococcus,* and *Escherichia coli.*
- Acute viral infections are attributed mostly to Norwalk and rotavirus groups.
- In underdeveloped countries, acute diarrhea kills 5 million children annually.
- Diarrheal illness is associated with poor sanitation, poor nutrition, and age <5 years, especially infancy.

► PATHOPHYSIOLOGY

- Diarrhea is an imbalance in absorption and secretion of water and electrolytes. In normal volunteers, small intestine water has a maximum rate of absorption. If absorption decreases or secretion increases beyond normal, diarrhea results. Normally, the absorption of water and electrolytes exceeds secretory fluxes.
- Four general pathophysiologic mechanisms disrupt water and electrolyte balance, leading to diarrhea. These four mechanisms are the basis of diagnosis and therapy:

  1. A change in active ion transport by either decreased sodium absorption or increased chloride secretion
  2. Change in intestinal motility
  3. Increase in luminal osmolarity
  4. Increase in tissue hydrostatic pressure

- These mechanisms have been related to four broad clinical diarrheal groups: secretory, osmotic, exudative, and altered intestinal transit.

▶ CLINICAL PRESENTATION

- Diarrhea is divided into acute and chronic diarrheal disorders. Usually, acute diarrheal episodes subside within 72 hours of onset. Chronic diarrhea involves frequent attacks during two to three extended periods.
- With acute diarrhea, the patient complains of abrupt onset of frequent watery, loose stools, flatulence, malaise, and abdominal pain. Intermittent periumbilical or lower right quadrant pain with cramps and audible bowel sounds is characteristic of small intestinal disease. When pain is present in large intestinal diarrhea, it is a gripping, aching sensation with tenesmus (straining ineffective and painful stooling). In chronic diarrhea, previous bouts, weight loss, anorexia, and chronic weakness are important findings.
- Americans traveling abroad may experience traveler's or parasitic diarrhea. Environmental conditions such as the recent ingestion of bacteria contaminated foods identifies "food poisoning" as a possible etiology. An attentive dietary history identifies offending foods (e.g., dairy products with lactose intolerance). With AIDS patients, opportunistic pathogens may cause diarrheal illness. Recent gastrointestinal (GI) surgery may cause a dumping syndrome.
- Many agents, including antibiotics and other drugs, cause diarrhea (Table 21.1). Laxative abuse for weight loss may also result in diarrhea.

TABLE 21.1. Drug-Induced Diarrhea

Laxatives
Antacids (magnesium-containing)
Antibiotics
Clindamycin
Tetracyclines
Sulfonamides
Any broad-spectrum antibiotic
Antihypertensives
Reserpine
Guanethidine
Methyldopa
Guanabenz
Guanadrel
Cholinergics
Bethanechol
Metoclopramide
Neostigmine
Cardiac agents
Quinidine
Digitalis
Digoxin

- With diarrhea, physical examination of the abdomen may detect hyper-peristalsis with borborygmi (growling stomach sounds) and generalized or local tenderness. A rectal examination detects masses or possibly fecal impaction, a common cause of diarrhea in the elderly.
- For unexplained diarrhea, especially in chronic situations, special tests are used, including stool examination for parasites and ova, blood, mucus, or fat. Stool osmolality, pH, and electrolytes may also be assessed. Direct endoscopic visualization and biopsy can be used to diagnose conditions such as colitis. Radiographic studies are helpful in diagnosing neoplastic and inflammatory conditions.

▶ DESIRED OUTCOME

The therapeutic goals of diarrhea treatment are to prevent excessive water, electrolyte, and acid–base disturbances, provide symptomatic relief, treat curable causes of diarrhea, and manage secondary disorders causing diarrhea. Clinicians must clearly understand that diarrhea, like a cough, may be a body defense mechanism for ridding itself of harmful substances or pathogens. The correct therapeutic response is not neces-sarily to stop diarrhea at all costs!

▶ TREATMENT

GENERAL PRINCIPLES

- Management of the diet is a first priority for treatment of diarrhea (Fig-ures 21.1 and 21.2). Most clinicians recommend stopping solid foods for 24 hours and avoiding dairy products.
- When nausea or vomiting is mild, digestible low-residue diet is admin-istered for 24 hours.
- If vomiting is present and uncontrollable with antiemetics, nothing is taken by mouth. As bowel movements decrease, a bland diet is begun. Feeding should continue in children with acute bacterial diarrhea.
- Overzealous laxative use in the elderly, whether self- or physician-pre-scribed, is a common cause of diarrhea and must be identified and stopped. Other drugs that may cause or worsen diarrhea should be stopped or the dosage reduced.
- Repletion and maintenance of water and electrolytes are the primary treatment measures until the diarrheal episode ends. If vomiting and dehydration are not severe, enteral feeding is the less costly and pre-ferred method. In the United States many commercial oral rehydration preparations are available (Table 21.2).

PHARMACOLOGIC THERAPY

- Various drugs have been used to treat diarrhea (Table 21.3). These drugs are grouped into several categories: antimotility, adsorbents, anti-

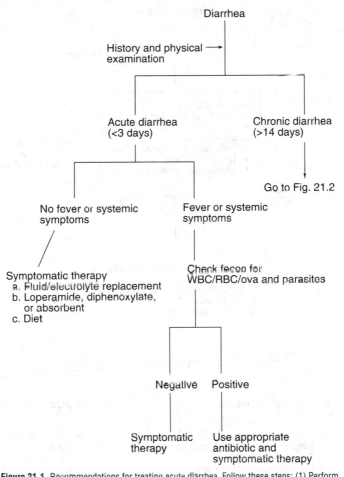

Figure 21.1. Recommendations for treating acute diarrhea. Follow these steps: (1) Perform a complete history and physical examination. (2) Is the diarrhea acute or chronic? If acute diarrhea, check for fever and/or systemic signs and symptoms (i.e., toxic patient). If systemic illness (fever, anorexia, volume depletion), check for infectious source. If positive for infectious diarrhea, use appropriate antibiotic/anthelminthic drug, and symptomatic therapy. If negative for infectious cause, use only symptomatic treatment. (3) If no systemic findings, then use symptomatic therapy, based on severity of volume depletion, oral or parenteral fluid/electrolytes, antidiarrheal agents (see Table 21.3), and diet.

V

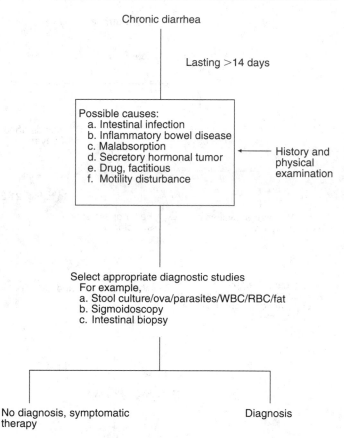

Figure 21.2. Recommendations for treating chronic diarrhea. Follow these steps: (1) Perform a careful history and physical examination. (2) The possible causes of chronic diarrhea are many. These can be classified into intestinal infections (bacterial, protozoal), inflammatory (Crohn's disease, ulcerative colitis), malabsorption (lactose intolerance), secretory hormonal tumor (intestinal carcinoid tumor, VIPoma), drug (antacid), factitious (laxative abuse), or motility disturbance (diabetes mellitus, irritable bowel syndrome, hyperthyroidism). (3) If the diagnosis is uncertain, selected appropriate diagnostic studies should be ordered. (4) Once diagnosed, treatment is planned for the underlying cause with symptomatic antidiarrheal therapy. (5) If no specific cause can be identified, symptomatic therapy is prescribed.

TABLE 21.2. Oral Rehydration Solutions

	WHO–ORS[a]	Lytren (Mead Johnson)	Pedialyte (Ross)	Rehydralyte (Ross)	Ricelyte (Mead Johnson)	Resol (Wyeth)
Osmolality (mOsm/L)	333	220	249	304	200	269
Carbohydrates[b] (g/L)	20	20	25	25	30[c]	20
Calories (cal/L)	77	85	100	100	126	80
Electrolytes (mEq/L)						
Sodium	90	50	45	75	50	50
Potassium	20	25	20	20	25	20
Chloride	80	45	35	65	45	50
Citrate	—	30	30	30	34	34
Bicarbonate	30	—	—	—	—	—
Calcium	—	—	—	—	—	4
Magnesium	—	—	—	—	—	4
Sulfate	—	—	—	—	—	—
Phosphate	—	—	—	—	—	5

[a] World Health Organization Oral Rehydration Solution.
[b] Carbohydrate is glucose.
[c] Rice syrup solids is carbohydrate source.

V ◄

257

secretory compounds, antibiotics, enzymes, and intestinal microflora. Usually, these drugs are not curative but palliative.

- Opiates and opioid derivatives delay the transit of intraluminal content or increase gut capacity, prolonging contact and absorption. The limitations of the opiates are addiction potential (a real concern with long-term use) and worsening of diarrhea in selected infectious diarrheas.
- Adsorbents are used for symptomatic relief (Table 21.3). Adsorbents are nonspecific in their action; they adsorb nutrients, toxins, drugs, and digestive juices. Coadministration with other drugs reduces their bioavailability.
- *Lactobacillus* preparation is a controversial treatment that is intended to replace colonic microflora. This supposedly restores intestinal functions and suppresses the growth of pathogenic microorganisms. However, a dairy-product diet containing 200–400 g of lactose or dextrin is equally effective in recolonization.

TABLE 21.3. Selected Antidiarrheal Preparations

	Dose Form	Adult Dose
Antimotility		
Diphenoxylate	2.5 mg/tablet 2.5 mg/5 mL	5 mg QID; do not exceed 20 mg/d
Loperamide	2 mg/capsule	Initially 4 mg, then 2 mg after each loose stool; do not exceed 16 mg/d
Paregoric	1 mg/5 mL	5–10 mL 1–4 times daily
Opium tincture	2 mg/5 mL (morphine)	0.6 mL QID
Atropine	5 mg/mL (morphine) 0.3, 0.4, 0.6 mg/tablet	0.4–0.6 mg every 4–6 h
Adsorbents		
Kaolin–pectin mixture	0.98 g kaolin + 21.7 mg pectin per 5 mL	30–120 mL after each loose stool
Polycarbophil	500 mg/tablet	Chew 2 tablets QID or after each loose stool; do not exceed 12 tablets a day
Antisecretory (bismuth subsalicylate)	300/mg tablet 525 mg/30 mL	Two tablets or 30 mL every 30 min as needed up to 8 doses per day
Enzymes (lactase)	1250 neutral lactase units per 4 drops	3–4 drops taken with milk or dairy product
	3300 FCC lactase units per tablet	1 or 2 tablets as above
Bacterial replacement (*Lactobacillus acidophilus*, *L. bulgaricus*)		2 tablets or 1 granule packet 3 to 4 times daily; give with milk, juice, or water

- Anticholinergic drugs, such as atropine, block vagal tone and prolong gut transit time. Their value in controlling diarrhea is questionable and limited by side effects.
- Bismuth subsalicylate blocks copious fluid flow in secretory diarrheas. It is effective and safe in treatment and prevention of traveler's diarrhea.
- The role of antibiotics for treatment of diarrhea is controversial. Antibiotics are curative if the causative organism is susceptible, but most infectious diarrheas are self-limiting and treated with supportive therapy.
- Octreotide, a synthetic octapeptide analogue of endogenous somatostatin, is prescribed for the symptomatic treatment of carcinoid tumors and vasoactive intestinal peptide-secreting tumors (VIPomas). Octreotide is used in selected patients with carcinoid syndrome. Octreotide blocks the release of serotonin and other active peptides and is effective in controlling diarrhea and flushing. Dosage range is 100–600 μg/d in two to four divided doses subcutaneously.

▶ EVALUATION OF THERAPEUTIC OUTCOMES

- With the urgency/emergency situation, evaluation of the volume status of the patient is the most important outcome.
- Toxic patients (those with fever, dehydration, hematochezia, hypotensive) require hospitalization; they need intravenous electrolyte solutions and empiric antibiotics while awaiting cultures. With quick management, they usually recover within a few days.
- Therapeutic outcomes are directed to key symptoms, signs, and laboratory studies. The constitutional symptoms usually improve within 24 to 72 hours.
- One should check the frequency and character of bowel movements each day along with the vital signs and improving appetite.
- The clinician also needs to monitor body weight, serum osmolality, serum electrolytes, complete blood cell count, urinalysis, and cultures (if appropriate).

See Chapter 36, Diarrhea and Constipation, authored by R. Leon Longe, PharmD and Joseph T. DiPiro, PharmD, FCCP, for a more detailed discussion of this topic.

Chapter 22

► GASTROESOPHAGEAL REFLUX DISEASE

► DEFINITION

Gastroesophageal reflux refers to the retrograde movement of gastric contents from the stomach into the esophagus. Gastroesophageal reflux disease (GERD) refers to any symptomatic clinical condition or histologic alteration that results from episodes of gastroesophageal reflux. When the esophagus is repeatedly exposed to refluxed material for prolonged periods of time, inflammation of the esophagus (i.e., reflux esophagitis) can occur. Gastroesophageal reflux must precede the development of GERD or reflux esophagitis.

► EPIDEMIOLOGY

- Gastroesophageal reflux disease occurs in both adults and children.
- The true prevalence and incidence of GERD is difficult to assess because of several factors: (1) many patients do not seek medical treatment, (2) symptoms do not always correlate well with severity of disease, and (3) there is no standardized definition or universal gold standard method for diagnosing the disease.
- In general, the prevalence increases in adults >40 years of age.
- Except for pregnant women, there does not appear to be a major difference in incidence between men and women.
- A national survey estimated that approximately 44% of adult Americans experience heartburn at least once every month and that 13% of the adult population take medications for indigestion at least a few times per week.
- The overall prevalence of esophagitis in the general population is approximately 2–4%. However, of the 20–40% of patients who experience heartburn, approximately 30–79% of these patients will have evidence of esophagitis.

► PATHOPHYSIOLOGY

- The body of the esophagus lies within the negative-pressure thoracic cavity, while the abdominal cavity has a positive pressure gradient. Without normal defense mechanisms, the pressure gradients would favor continual reflux of gastric material into the esophagus.
- In many patients with GERD, the problem is not that they produce too much acid, but that the acid produced spends too much time in contact with the esophageal mucosa.

ANATOMIC FACTORS

- Patients with hypotensive lower esophageal sphincter pressures and large hiatal hernias are more likely to experience gastroesophageal reflux following abrupt increases in intra-abdominal pressure as compared to patients with hypotensive lower esophageal sphincter and no hiatal hernia.
- The presence of a hiatal hernia may impair esophageal clearance and predispose a patient to GERD.

LOWER ESOPHAGEAL SPHINCTER PRESSURE

- A primary factor influencing the occurrence of esophageal reflux is the lower esophageal sphincter pressure (Table 22.1). Patients with gastroesophageal reflux usually have decreased basal lower esophageal sphincter pressures, frequently <10 mm Hg and often <6 mm Hg. There is significant overlap between pressure values of normal healthy individuals and those of patients with gastroesophageal reflux.
- Mechanisms by which gastroesophageal reflux may occur are three-fold. Reflux may occur following spontaneous transient lower esophageal sphincter relaxations that are not associated with swallowing. It may also occur following transient increases in intra-abdominal pressure (stress reflux), or third, the lower esophageal sphincter may be atonic thus permitting free reflux.

ESOPHAGEAL CLEARANCE

- The symptoms and/or severity of damage produced by gastroesophageal reflux are partially dependent on the duration of contact between the gastric contents and the esophageal mucosa which is, in turn, dependent on the rate at which the esophagus clears the noxious material and the frequency of reflux.
- Decreased esophageal clearance of gastric acid has been observed in some patients who have symptomatic gastroesophageal reflux.

COMPOSITION OF REFLUXATE

- The composition and volume of the refluxate are the most important aggressive factors in determining the consequences of gastroesophageal reflux. The combination of acid, pepsin, and bile has been shown to be a potent refluxate in producing esophageal damage.

GASTRIC EMPTYING

- Delayed gastric emptying can also contribute to gastroesophageal reflux. An increase in gastric volume may increase both the frequency of reflux and the amount of gastric fluid available to be refluxed. It is theorized that patients with gastroesophageal reflux have a defect in antral motility.

Gastrointestinal Disorders

TABLE 22.1. Factors that Affect Lower Esophageal Sphincter Pressures

Decrease Lower Esophageal Sphincter	Increase Lower Esophageal Sphincter
Foods	
Carminatives (peppermint, spearmint)	Protein meal
Chocolate	
Fatty meal	
Drugs	
Atropine	Bethanechol
Barbiturates	Cisapride
Calcium channel blockers	Edrophonium
Diazepam	Methacholine
Dopamine	Metoclopramide
Estrogen	Norepinephrine
Ethanol	Pentagastrin
Isoproterenol	Phenylephrine
Meperidine	
Morphine	
Nicotine (smoking)	
Phentolamine	
Progesterone	
Theophylline	
Hormones/Physiologic Factors	
Cholecytokinin	Gastric alkalinization
Estrogen	Gastrin
Gastric acidification	Prostaglandin F_2
Glucagon	
Progesterone	
Prostaglandins (E_1, E_2, A_2)	
Secretin	
Vasoactive intestinal peptide (VIP)	

Adapted from Castell DO. Ann Intern Med 1975;83:396, with permission.

▶ CLINICAL PRESENATION

- The hallmark symptom of gastroesophageal reflux and esophagitis is heartburn or pyrosis. It is classically described as a substernal sensation of warmth or burning that may radiate to the neck. It is waxing and waning in character, and is often aggravated by activities that potentiate gastroesophageal reflux (i.e., supine position, bending over).
- Other symptoms that may occur in patients with GERD include regurgitation, water brash (hypersalivation), dysphagia (difficulty swallowing), odynophagia (pain on swallowing), and hemorrhage.

- Symptoms that are more atypical of GERD include pulmonary symptoms, cough, hoarseness, and hiccups.
- The severity of the symptoms of gastroesophageal reflux does not usually correlate with the degree of esophagitis, but it does correlate with the duration of reflux.
- Gastroesophageal reflux may lead to many severe complications, including esophageal ulceration, stricture formation, esophageal perforation, pharyngeal/oral disturbances, hemorrhage, and Barrett's esophagus.

▶ DIAGNOSIS

- The most useful tool in the diagnosis of gastroesophageal reflux is the clinical history, including both presenting symptomology and associated risk factors.
- Figure 22.1 depicts an algorithm that can be used to direct the selection of diagnostic tests based on the patient's clinical presentation.
- A commonly used grading scale for esophagitis is depicted in Table 22.2.
- Twenty-four hour ambulatory pH monitoring, considered the gold standard by many, documents the percentage of time the intraesophageal pH is low. It is very effective at determining the frequency and severity of reflux. Continuous pH monitoring is performed by passing a small electrode pH probe intranasally and placing it approximately 5 cm above the lower esophageal sphincter.
- Patients who present with atypical chest pain often require both cardiac and esophageal evaluations. The diagnosis is complicated because esophageal pain may cause electrocardiographic disorders, and both esophageal and cardiac disorders may occur simultaneously.

▶ DESIRED OUTCOME

The multifold goals of treatments are to alleviate/eliminate the patient's symptoms, decrease the frequency and duration of gastroesophageal reflux, promote healing of the injured mucosa, and prevent the development of complications.

▶ TREATMENT

GENERAL PRINCIPLES

- Therapeutic modalities utilized in the treatment of gastroesophageal reflux are targeted at reversing the various pathophysiologic abnormalities.
- Therapy is directed at augmenting defense mechanisms that may prevent reflux and/or decreasing the aggressive factors that potentiate reflux or mucosal damage (Figure 22.2).
- Specifically, therapy is directed at increasing lower esophageal sphincter pressure, enhancing esophageal acid clearance, improving gastric

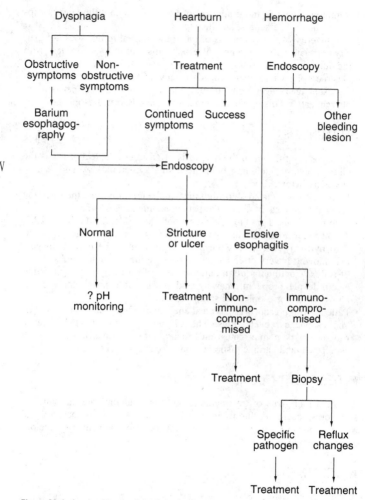

Figure 22.1. An algorithm to direct the selection of diagnostic tests based on the patient's clinical presentation. *(From Pope CE. New Engl J Med 1994;331[10]: 656–660, with permission)*

TABLE 22.2. Endoscopic Classification of Esophagitis

Grade 0	Normal esophageal mucosa
Grade 1	Erythema or diffusely red mucosa, edema causing accentuated folds
Grade 2	Isolated round or linear erosions extending from the gastroesophageal junction upwards, not involving entire circumference
Grade 3	Confluent erosions extending around entire circumference or superficial ulceration without stenosis
Grade 4	Complicated cases; erosions as above plus deep ulcerations, stricture, or columnar epithelium-lined esophagus

Adapted from Savary M, Miller G. Handbook and Atlas of Endoscopy. Solothurn, Gassman, 1978, with permission.

V

emptying, protecting the esophageal mucosa, decreasing the acidity of the refluxate and the gastric volume available to be refluxed.

- Treatment is categorized into the following modalities: lifestyle changes, pharmacologic interventions, and surgical interventions.
- The initial therapeutic modality used is, in part, dependent on the condition of the patient (degree of esophagitis, presence of complications, etc.). However, historically, a stepwise approach has been used, starting with noninvasive lifestyle modifications (Table 22.3 and 22.4).

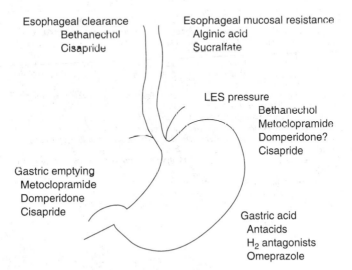

Figure 22.2. Therapeutic interventions in the management of gastroesophageal reflux disease. Pharmacologic interventions are targeted at improving defense mechanisms or decreasing aggressive factors. LES, lower esophageal sphincter.

TABLE 22.3. Therapeutic Approach to Gastroesophageal Reflux Disease

Phase I	Lifestyle changes/antacids/OTC H_2 antagonists[a]
Phase IIa	A. Standard doses of H_2 antagonists for 8–12 weeks (usually first-line therapy after phase I).

- Cimetidine 400 mg four times daily or 800 mg twice daily[b]
- Ranitidine 150 mg twice daily[c]
- Famotidine 20 mg twice daily[d]
- Nizatidine 150 mg twice daily[e]

OR

B. Mucosal protective agents (alternative to H_2 antagonist)
Sucralfate 1 g after meals and at bedtime

OR

C. Prokinetic agents[f,g]

- Metoclopramide 10 mg before meals and at bedtime (up to 15 mg four times daily)
- Cisapride 10 mg four times daily (up to 20 mg four times daily)
- Bethanechol 25 mg four times daily

Phase IIb[h]   A. Titration of H_2 antagonists to 1.5–2× standard dose

OR

B. Proton pump inhibitors

- Omeprazole 20 mg daily for 8 weeks[i]
- Lansoprazole 30 mg daily for 8 weeks[i]

Phase III   Surgery

[a]Low-dose H_2 antagonists: famotidine 10 mg taken up to twice daily; cimetidine 200 mg taken up to twice daily.
[b]FDA labeled dosage regimens and indications: erosive esophagitis, cimetidine 800 mg twice daily or 400 mg four times daily for up to 12 weeks. Cimetidine 400 mg twice daily may also be effective in patients with mild disease, however, this dose is lower than the FDA approved dose.
[c]FDA labeled dosage regimens and indications: GERD symptoms, ranitidine 150 mg twice daily for up to 6 weeks; erosive esophagitis, ranitidine 150 mg four times daily for up to 12 weeks; maintenance of healing erosive esophagitis, ranitidine 150 mg twice daily.
[d]FDA labeled dosage regimens and indications: GERD symptoms, famotidine 20 mg twice daily for up to 6 weeks; esophagitis, famotidine 20–40 mg twice daily for up to 12 weeks.
[e]FDA labeled dosage regimen and indication: esophagitis, nizatidine 150 mg twice daily for up to 12 weeks.
[f]Concurrent use of an H_2 antagonist + prokinetic agent may be considered in those patients refractory to single-agent therapy or in those patients who have multifactoral problems contributing to their disease state. (e.g., esophagitis + motor dysfunction).
[g]Use in the presence of motor dysfunction, such as decreased lower esophageal sphincter pressure or decreased gastric emptying.
[h]Phase IIb therapy is often reserved for those patients who fail on phase I or IIa therapy or in those patients who present with even more severe disease (grade 3 or 4 esophagitis).
[i]Higher dosage regimens or longer durations of therapy may be used in refractory patients.

TABLE 22.4. Phase I Treatment Modalities

- Elevate the head of the bed (increases esophageal clearance)
  - Use 6–8 1-inch blocks or 1 6- to 8-inch block under the head of the bed
  - Sleep on a foam wedge
- Dietary changes
  - Avoid foods that may decrease lower esophageal sphincter pressure (fats, chocolate, alcohol, peppermint, and spearmint)
  - Avoid foods that have a direct irritant effect on the esophageal mucosa (spicy foods, orange juice, tomato juice, and coffee)
  - Include protein-rich meals in diet (augments lower esophageal sphincter pressure)
  - Eat small meals and avoid eating immediately prior to sleeping (decreases gastric volume)
  - Weight reduction (reduces symptoms)
- Stop smoking (decreases spontaneous esophageal sphincter relaxation)
- Avoid alcohol (increases amplitude of the lower esophageal sphincter, peristaltic waves, and frequency of contraction)
- Avoid tight-fitting clothes
- Discontinue drugs that may promote reflux, if possible
- Take drugs that have a direct irritant effect on the esophageal mucosa with plenty of liquid if they cannot be avoided (tetracyclines, quinidine, KCL, iron salts, aspirin, NSAIDs)
- Take antacids or over-the-counter H_2 antagonists as directed to relieve symptoms

V

ANTACIDS AND ANTACID–ALGINIC ACID PRODUCTS

- Antacids are commonly used in the treatment of gastroesophageal reflux because of their acid-neutralizing ability. While antacids are commonly used to treat gastroesophageal reflux and esophagitis, documentation of their efficacy in placebo-controlled clinical trials is lacking.
- Antacids and/or antacid combination products are frequently used in the treatment of gastroesophageal reflux without complications.
- Antacids are generally used to provide symptomatic relief in patients who have mild to moderate intermittent symptoms.
- Patients with significant symptoms and/or severe disease often require more aggressive pharmacologic intervention with H_2 antagonists, prokinetic agents, mucosal protectants, or proton pump inhibitors. However, antacids are sometimes employed as adjunctive therapy to provide symptomatic relief.

H_2 ANTAGONISTS: CIMETIDINE, RANITIDINE, FAMOTIDINE, AND NIZATIDINE

- The H_2 antagonists have historically been the mainstay in the treatment of GERD. These agents decrease gastric acid secretion which results in a less irritating refluxant. In addition, inhibition of gastric acid secretion results in a lower volume of gastric fluid available to be refluxed.
- The clinical trials clearly indicate that the efficacy of H_2 antagonists in the management of GERD is extremely variable and is frequently lower than desired.

- Response to the H_2 antagonists appears to be dependent on the severity of disease, duration of therapy, and dosage regimen used. The more severe the esophageal damage, the poorer the response to H_2 antagonists.
- Based on the contribution of duration of therapy to the efficacy of H_2 antagonists, prolonged therapy (8 weeks or more) is frequently used when treating patients with GERD.
- In general, standard-dose H_2 antagonists provide improvement in the degree of esophagitis in 45–80% of patients. Because of the somewhat disappointing healing rates observed with standard dosages of H_2 antagonists, many recent studies have evaluated the efficacy of higher doses.
- It is prudent to recommend starting a patient on standard doses (cimetidine 400 mg four times a day or 800 mg twice daily, ranitidine 150 mg twice daily, famotidine 20 mg twice daily, or nizatidine 150 mg twice daily). If the patient fails to respond to standard regimens or if the patient has severe disease, higher dose regimens may be recommended.
- Since all of the H_2 antagonists are efficacious, selection of the specific agent to be used in the management of GERD should be based on other factors such as differences in pharmacokinetics and safety profiles, as well as cost. In general, these agents are extremely safe.

PROKINETIC AGENTS: BETHANECHOL, METOCLOPRAMIDE, AND CISAPRIDE

- Bethanechol, metoclopramide, and cisapride have been shown to increase lower esophageal sphincter pressure and thereby may minimize the number of reflux episodes.
- Bethanechol and cisapride have also been shown to improve esophageal clearance.
- Metoclopramide and cisapride promote gastric emptying and thus may be of benefit in patients with GERD, many of whom have delayed gastric emptying. Bethanechol does not improve gastric emptying.
- Although bethanechol has been shown to increase lower esophageal sphincter pressure and improve esophageal clearance, its side-effect profile severely limits its use.
- Oral bethanechol may cause abdominal cramps, urinary frequency, malaise, blurred vision, and diarrhea.
- Cisapride is thought to increase lower esophageal sphincter pressure and accelerate gastric emptying through the facilitation of acetylcholine release at the myenteric plexus. Unlike metoclopramide, this newer prokinetic agent is devoid of antidopaminergic effects and, therefore, does not cause extrapyramidal side effects or prolactin secretion.

METOCLOPRAMIDE

- Metoclopramide, a dopamine antagonist, increases lower esophageal sphincter pressure in a dose-related manner and has also been shown to accelerate gastric emptying in gastroesophageal reflux.

- Based on metoclopramide's ability to increase lower esophageal sphincter pressure and improve gastric emptying, it may be useful in the treatment of gastroesophageal reflux.
- A limiting factor with metoclopramide therapy is the high incidence of adverse effects. Most commonly reported adverse reactions were somnolence (9%), nervousness (9%), fatigue (8%), dizziness (5%), weakness (3%), depression (2%), diarrhea (2%), and rash (2%). Other possible adverse reactions include anxiety, insomnia, and extrapyramidal reactions.

MUCOSAL PROTECTANTS: SUCRALFATE

- Sucralfate is a nonabsorbable aluminum salt of sucrose octasulfate that is effective in the treatment of duodenal ulcer disease.
- In general, sucralfate appears effective in some patients and may therefore be a suitable alternative to standard-dose H_2 antagonists or antacid–alginic acid therapy for treating mild esophagitis.

PROTON PUMP INHIBITORS: OMEPRAZOLE AND LANSOPRAZOLE

- Omeprazole and lansoprazole inhibit gastric acid secretion by inhibiting gastric H^+/K^+-adenosine triphosphatase.
- Omeprazole and lansoprazole have been shown to be efficacious in patients who are refractory to standard doses of H_2 antagonists and in those with gastroesophageal reflux complications, such as Barrett's esophagitis.
- Clinical trials clearly indicate that omeprazole and lansoprazole are effective in providing symptomatic relief and esophageal healing in a significant percentage of patients with severe GERD.

COMBINATION THERAPY

- Combination therapy should be reserved for those patients failing to respond to traditional single-agent therapy or for those patients who obviously have multifactorial problems contributing to their disease (e.g., esophagitis + motor dysfunction). The most frequently used combinations include H_2 antagonists with prokinetic agents.

MAINTENANCE THERAPY

- Although healing and/or symptomatic improvement may be achieved via many different therapeutic modalities, 70–90% of patients will relapse within 1 year of discontinuation of therapy.
- Because of the high rate of relapse, several maintenance regimens have been used.
- The primary goal of maintenance therapy is to keep the patient in remission using lower dosages than those routinely used therapeutically.
- Maintenance therapy with the H_2 antagonists is extremely effective in preventing duodenal ulcer recurrence; however, their efficacy in maintaining GERD patients in remission is somewhat disappointing.

- Neither cimetidine 300 mg twice daily nor cimetidine 400 mg at bedtime was significantly superior to placebo in preventing recurrence over the 12-month study period.
- Emerging data suggest that cisapride may be effective in preventing relapse in certain patients.
- Proton pump inhibitors appear to be more effective than H_2 antagonists in preventing recurrence of GERD.

SURGERY

- Surgical intervention (Nissen, Belsey Mark IV, or Hill operations) is indicated when the patient fails to respond to conservative and pharmacologic treatment modalities, strictures are present, major bleeding occurs, and pulmonary complications exist.

▶ EVALUATION OF THERAPEUTIC OUTCOMES

- Pharmacists should take an active role in educating patients about potential adverse effects and drug interactions that may occur with drug therapy.
- The frequency and severity of symptoms should be monitored; and patients should be counseled on symptoms that may suggest the presence of complications requiring immediate medical attention, such as dysphagia or odynophagia.
- Patient compliance is another factor that will affect the outcome of drug therapy. Drug regimens that are easily managed will improve compliance and therefore outcome for the patient.

See Chapter 31, Gastroesophageal Reflux Disease, authored by Dianne B. Williams, PharmD and Lynda S. Welage, PharmD, for a more detailed discussion of this topic.

Chapter 23

► HEPATITIS, VIRAL

► DEFINITION

Viral hepatitis refers to the clinically important hepatotrophic viruses responsible for hepatitis A (HAV), hepatitis B (HBV), delta hepatitis (HDV), hepatitis C (HCV), and hepatitis E (HEV). Those viruses that cause hepatitis as part of a generalized illness, such as Epstein–Barr virus, herpes simplex virus, measles virus, and cytomegalovirus, are not discussed in this chapter. Viral hepatitis has several clinical forms (acute, fulminant, chronic), defined by duration or severity of infection.

Acute viral hepatitis is a systemic viral infection of up to but not exceeding 6 months in duration that produces inflammatory necrosis of the liver. Chronic viral hepatitis describes prolongation or continuation of the hepatic necroinflammatory process 6 months or more beyond the onset of the acute illness.

► EPIDEMIOLOGY

- Viral hepatitis is a major cause of morbidity and mortality in the United States. Several distinct viruses are responsible for the 56,000 cases of hepatitis reported yearly. The actual number of patients infected is closer to 600,000.
- Hepatitis A causes an estimated 300,000 infections, while hepatitis B is responsible for 120,000 to 200,000 cases.
- Six to ten percent of all patients infected with hepatitis B develop chronic hepatitis, while chronic disease develops in >50% of patients infected with hepatitis C. Many of these patients ultimately die of complications of chronic hepatitis such as cirrhosis or hepatocellular carcinoma (HCC).
- More than 300 million people are infected with hepatitis B worldwide. The World Health Organization (WHO) lists hepatitis B as the ninth leading cause of death in the world.
- Hepatitis A is the primary etiologic agent of worldwide hepatitis epidemics throughout recorded history. HAV, an RNA virus, remains a significant cause of clinical hepatitis worldwide, although HEV plays a role in many epidemics.
- There are more than 1 million chronic carriers of Hepatitis B virus in the United States alone. In highly endemic areas (China, Southeast Asia, the Middle East, and parts of Africa and South America), HBV spread is predominantly by mother-to-infant perinatal transmission and child-to-child transmission. In parts of the world where the endemicity of HBV is relatively low (North America, Australia, Western Europe, and temperate South America), HBV transmission occurs either through intimate contact or by the parenteral route. High-risk groups in these

areas include intravenous drug abusers, multitransfused patients, health care providers, male homosexuals, heterosexual partners of HBV-infected people, and heterosexual partners of human immunodeficiency virus (HIV)-infected individuals.

- Patients at risk for Hepatitis C virus infection in the United States include those who receive blood products, intravenous drug users, and health care workers. Up to 40% of all cases of hepatitis C report no known risk factors, and the mechanism(s) of transmission for these sporadically occurring cases is poorly understood.

- Hepatitis delta virus (HDV) parallels the transmission patterns and areas of endemicity of HBV, with only a few differences. Three forms of HDV infection have been identified and are designated acute HDV–HBV coinfection, acute HDV superinfection, and HDV chronic infection. Coinfection describes simultaneous infection with both HBV and HDV, while superinfection occurs when HDV is transmitted after the patient has been exposed to HBV. HDV infection in the United States is strongly associated with intravenous drug abuse, exposure to infected blood, and/or fulminant hepatitis.

- HEV is endemic in Africa, Southeast and Central Asia, Mexico, and Central and South America. Many sporadic cases of acute hepatitis in areas endemic for HEV are also attributed to HEV. To date, Western travelers to endemic areas provide the reported cases of HEV in developed countries.

▶ PATHOPHYSIOLOGY

ACUTE VIRAL HEPATITIS

- Once virions gain access to the circulation, they accumulate in hepatic sinusoids and are internalized by the hepatocytes.

- The internalized viral particles replicate within the hepatocyte. Infective viral particles are then shed into blood, bile, and other body secretions.

- The duration of the incubation stage is virus specific and varies (Table 23.1). The host is essentially asymptomatic during the incubation stage of the infection.

- The hepatotrophic viruses cause hepatic injury either because of the host immune response or from direct viral damage to hepatocytes. Cellular and humoral immune response is directed against viral antigens found on the host hepatocyte membranes and/or circulating within the vascular compartment.

- This acute hepatitis stage begins with a preicteric phase (before the onset of jaundice), which parallels initiation of the host immune response and occurs before significant liver cell injury.

- The preicteric phase is frequently associated with nonspecific influenza-like symptoms consisting of anorexia, nausea, fatigue, and malaise.

- Clinical symptoms are accompanied by moderate to marked elevations of the serum bilirubin, gamma globulin, and hepatic transaminases (4–10 times normal).

TABLE 23.1. Important Features of HAV, HBV, HCV, HDV and HEV

	Hepatitis A	Hepatitis B	Hepatitis C	Hepatitis D	Hepatitis E
Virus	HAV	HBV	HCV	HDV	HEV
Family	Picornavirus	Hepadnavirus	Flavivirus	Satellite	Calicivirus
Size (nm)	27	42	30–60	40	32
Genome	ssRNA	dsDNA	ssRNA	ssRNA	ssRNA
Incubation (days)	14–45	40–180	35–84	40–180 coinf 14–45 superinf	14–42
Transmission	Fecal-oral	Parenteral Sexual Perinatal	Parenteral Sexual (?)	Parenteral Sexual (?)	Fecal-oral
Serologic markers					
Antigens	HAVAg	HBsAg HBcAg HBeAg	HCVAg	HDVAg	HEVAg
Antibodies	Anti-HAV	Anti-HBs Anti-HBc Anti-HBe	Anti-HCV	Anti-HDV	Anti-HEV
Viral markers	HAV RNA	HBV DNA DNA polymerase	HCV RNA	HDV RNA	Viruslike particles
Clinical illness					
Children	Anicteric	Anicteric 70%	Anicteric 75%	Not known	High % anicteric
Adults	Icteric	Icteric 30%	Most icteric	Icteric 25%	Not known
Acute mortality (%)	0.2	0.2–1	0.2	2–20	0.2 (pregnancy)
Chronicity	No	2–7% Neonates 90%	50–70%	2–70%	No
HCC	No	Yes	Yes	Yes	No

coinf, coinfection; superinf, superinfection; HAVAg, hepatitis A antigen; HCC, hepatocellular carcinoma.
Adapted from Sem Liver Dis, 1991;11:74, with permission.

V

- Viral serologic markers and host antibodies are detectable during this stage of the illness.
- HBV is not cytopathic.
- The liver injury (like HAV infection) is immune related and T lymphocytes are important for both the host cellular and humoral responses.

CHRONIC VIRAL HEPATITIS

- A weak cell-mediated immune response has been demonstrated in patients with persistent HBV infection. In healthy carriers, an absent or poor cell-mediated response results in persistent viral replication but only minimal liver damage. Patients with chronic HBV infection are deficient in producing, or responding to, interferon (IFN), which results in incomplete direction of the lymphocyte to the target infected cell.
- If persistent viral replication and subsequent hepatocyte inflammatory destruction continue unabated, the number of functioning hepatocytes gradually decreases over time, and fibrosis resulting from cellular repair mechanisms distorts the basic cellular architecture. Hepatic nodules are thus formed.
- When widespread, the hepatic fibrosis with nodule formation is termed cirrhosis.
- The consequences of cirrhosis do not differ with regard to initial etiologies and can produce portal hypertension and ascites.

▶ CLINICAL PRESENTATION

- The natural history of the infection is divided into three stages based on viral serologic markers: incubation, acute hepatitis, and convalescence.
- Clinical severity of illness varies widely from asymptomatic, anicteric hepatitis to fulminant hepatitis, a rapidly fatal disease.
- Most patients with acute viral hepatitis develop only a few, mild symptoms and minimal hepatocyte damage. This mild disease is called *acute anicteric hepatitis.*
- The minimal degree of liver cell damage is reflected by mild elevations of serum bilirubin, gamma globulin, and hepatic transaminases (ALT, AST) values to about twice normal.
- A subset of patients experiences enough hepatocyte destruction to produce significant liver function derangement characterized by interruption of bilirubin metabolism and flow, resulting in jaundice.
- The icteric phase is generally accompanied by fever, right upper quadrant abdominal pain, nausea, vomiting, dark urine, acholic stools, and worsening of systemic symptoms.
- Clinical symptoms are accompanied by moderate to marked elevations of serum bilirubin, gamma globulin, and hepatic transaminase (4–10 times normal).
- Viral serologic markers and host antibodies are detectable during this stage of the illness.

- Most patients with either acute anicteric or icteric hepatitis go through the convalescence stage to complete recovery without developing complications or chronic sequelae.
- The duration of disease stages and the risk for developing chronic sequelae are virus-specific phenomena (Table 23.1).

HEPATITIS A

- HAV infection usually produces a mild, self-limited illness, and rarely re-sults in fulminant hepatitis or death.
- Clinical symptoms are age dependent, with children <6 years old generally displaying a mild, influenza-like illness without clinical jaundice.
- In contrast, infected adults display the characteristic clinical syndrome of acute hepatitis with elevated hepatic transaminase levels and jaundice. Pruritus may be the primary complaint of this latter patient group.
- No cases of a chronic carrier state or chronic hepatitis have been reported. However, up to 20% of patients relapse with acute hepatitis 2–8 weeks after the initial illness.
- The diagnosis of acute HAV infection depends on clinical suspicion, characteristic symptoms (if present), elevated aminotransferases and bilirubin, and a positive anti-HAV IgM (Table 23.1).

HEPATITIS B

- In the typical case of acute HBV infection, the incubation period is followed by a symptomatic prodromal phase consisting of malaise, fatigue, weakness, anorexia, myalgias, and arthralgias.
- Jaundice develops in about one-third of patients as liver cell destruction increases. Jaundice may persist for several weeks.
- Clinical manifestations of HBV infection are age dependent. Newborns infected with HBV are generally asymptomatic, while about one-third of adult patients with acute HBV infection have symptoms.
- Of the approximately 65% of adults with subclinical infection, most recover completely.
- Twenty-five percent have symptomatic illness with jaundice and 1% develop fulminant hepatic failure during the acute illness.
- Approximately 10% of adult patients develop chronic or persistent infection. Chronicity is more likely to occur in patients with mild, anicteric forms of acute hepatitis, and is much more likely to occur when the infection is acquired as a newborn or infant.
- Over a period of years, about 25% of adults with chronic HBV infection develop chronic active hepatitis (CAH), and a smaller percentage progress to cirrhosis.
- Extrahepatic manifestations such as neuropathies, glomerulonephritis, pancreatitis, and hematopoietic stem cell suppression (aplastic anemia, thrombocytopenia) are occasionally seen.
- HBV has four potential gene regions: the nucleocapsid region (HBcAg and HBeAg), the envelope region (HBsAg), the P region (DNA poly-

merase), and the poorly understood X region. In typical acute HBV infection, serologic markers proceed in sequence from the development of HBsAg followed by HBeAg (30–60 days prior to onset of clinical symptoms) through to the appearance of anti-HBs in late convalescence.

HEPATITIS C

- Acute hepatitis C is clinically indistinguishable from other types of viral hepatitis.
- The clinical course is generally mild with <25% of patients developing jaundice. Major complaints are frequently limited to fatigue and malaise.
- Similar to other types of viral hepatitis, the hepatic transaminase values in HCV hepatitis vary from mildly to markedly elevated.
- Unlike the other types, HCV infections characteristically demonstrate a pattern of widely fluctuating enzyme values over the course of the infection.
- An important feature of this form of hepatitis is that 60–70% of cases progress to chronic infection.
- Within 5 years, 30–35% develop CAH and 20–33% progress to cirrhosis. Others who eventually develop cirrhosis and hepatic failure do so after up to 20 years of indolent, asymptomatic infection. Chronic HCV infection-related cirrhosis is an etiologic factor in the development of HCC.
- Seroconversion to anti-HCV appears from 3–6 months following initial exposure and, in rare instances, can take up to 12 months. This lag time is a major limitation in testing for hepatitis C. HCV RNA is detectable by PCR as early as 1 week after infection.
- Viral RNA remains positive and histologic progression continues in those who develop chronic infection with HCV. However, serum aminotransferase levels can fluctuate, or even normalize, confounding the diagnosis of chronic HCV infection.
- To assess chronic HCV, liver biopsy is the only reliable indicator of disease progression. It is not uncommon for a patient to present to the physician with cirrhosis or portal hypertension secondary to HCV infection years to decades prior, yet to have had few or no clinical signs or symptoms during the intervening years.

DELTA HEPATITIS VIRUS

- Because of the dependence of HDV on HBV for its infectivity, the natural course of HDV coinfection and superinfection differ significantly.
- In coinfection, the acute delta hepatitis is almost always self-limited and follows the usual course of HBV infection. A biphasic rise in liver transaminase levels may be seen, the first peak attributable to HBV and the second to HDV.
- In HDV superinfection, delta viral replication occurs rapidly due to the persistent HBV infection, providing a ready supply of HBsAg. Liver

injury and clinical symptoms appear quickly and may be severe, leading to a fulminant course. Many of these patients develop chronic liver disease and some develop HCC.

- In acute superinfection of a chronic HBV carrier, markers for acute HBV are negative. HBsAg, HDVAg, and anti-HDV IgM are usually present. In acute coinfection, HDVAg, anti-HDV IgM, and markers for acute HBV are usually present. Anti-HDV IgG follows. Currently, only a test for total anti-HDV is commercially available.

HEPATITIS E VIRUS

- Infection with HEV follows a benign course, except in pregnant women; women who contract HEV during the third trimester are at considerable risk for developing fulminant hepatitis. The diagnosis is made on clinical grounds in conjunction with exclusion of other viruses.

FULMINANT HEPATITIS

- Liver injury that results in fulminant hepatic necrosis and hepatic failure is relatively rare. When it occurs, death results in a few days or weeks in nearly 80% of cases.
- In the United States, fulminant hepatitis is mainly due to HBV, and occasionally, HCV.
- Acute hepatitis B leads to acute liver failure in 1% of patients.
- Patients with fulminant hepatic necrosis typically develop signs and symptoms of viral hepatitis, then rapidly develop evidence of hepatic failure. The clinical syndrome is usually a 1- to 3-week course of hepatic failure and encephalopathy with coma developing within a few weeks of the onset of acute hepatitis.
- Manifestations of hepatic failure include metabolic encephalopathy, coma, coagulation defects, ascites, and edema. In fulminant liver failure, complications include gastrointestinal hemorrhage, sepsis, cerebral edema, renal failure, lactic acidosis, and disseminated coagulopathy, with death resulting from bleeding, cerebral edema, hypoglycemia, infection, and/or multisystem organ failure.

CHRONIC HEPATITIS

- The clinical findings, course, and histologic features are similar in all patients with chronic hepatitis regardless of the etiologic agent. Sixty to eighty percent of all cases are related to HBV or HCV infection.
- Complications of chronic hepatitis include cirrhosis, hepatic failure, and HCC.
- HBV carriers have a relative risk of acquiring HCC that is more than 100-fold that of noncarriers.
- Chronic HBsAg carriers with markers of ongoing viral replication (HBcAb–IgM, HBeAg, and HBV DNA) display persistent hepatic injury.
- Unlike acute hepatitis, physical symptoms do not correlate well with the severity of liver injury. Many patients are asymptomatic and there-

fore are diagnosed only after elevated serum liver transaminases and/or HBsAg are found in patients' serum upon routine testing.

- In either chronic HBV or chronic HCV, if the patient is symptomatic, fatigue, malaise, anorexia, and weight loss are common. Many patients have a history of jaundice.
- On physical examination, hepatomegaly is usually present, but the stigmata of chronic liver disease (spider nevi, splenomegaly, palmar erythema, testicular atrophy, caput medusa, female escutcheon) are generally absent until late in the disease course.
- Mild but persistent elevations of the serum aminotransferases, bilirubin, and gamma globulin levels are most commonly seen.
- In chronic hepatitis C, the patient is often asymptomatic, yet liver biopsy demonstrates ongoing liver injury and progressive histologic changes. Serum enzymes can be normal or only mildly elevated; unfortunately, the patient is on an insidious course that progresses to complications after a period of 15–20 years.

V

▶ TREATMENT

GENERAL PRINCIPLES

- Management of acute viral hepatitis is primarily supportive. General measures include a healthy diet, rest, maintaining fluid balance, and avoidance of hepatotoxic drugs and alcohol.
- The patient should avoid becoming fatigued; bed rest may be required during the acute phase of the illness.
- Management includes monitoring for development of chronic liver disease and preventing disease spread.
- Treatments that offer no benefit include special diets, corticosteroids, and antiemetics. Vitamin K is recommended only if the patient has a prolonged prothrombin time. Hospitalization is necessary only for those who have prolonged vomiting, coagulation defects, or fulminant hepatitis.
- Preliminary trials and case reports of the use of IFN-α and IFN-β as therapy in acute HBV and HCV infections are promising. Because not all studies have demonstrated IFN to be useful, further studies are ongoing to define the role of IFN in acute hepatitis treatment.
- The role of antiviral agents is undefined.

FULMINANT HEPATITIS

- There is no specific treatment for fulminant hepatic failure. Management of fulminant hepatitis focuses on recognition, prevention of complications, and aggressive treatment of complications.
- Measures that improve survival of patients include intensive supportive care plus early referral for liver transplantation. Specific measures include:
  - Fresh frozen plasma administered for bleeding
  - H_2 blocker therapy given to prevent gastrointestinal (GI) bleeding
  - Aggressive antibiotic therapy used for infections

- Management of cerebral edema including intracranial-pressure monitoring and administration of mannitol (0.3–0.4 g/kg body weight as a 20% solution)
- Urgent liver transplantation is the therapy of choice for patients with fulminant hepatic failure.
- Patients do not benefit from administration of corticosteroids, heparin, insulin, or glucagon.
- The role of antiviral therapy is not clear.

CHRONIC VIRAL HEPATITIS

- General therapeutic measures in patients with compensated chronic hepatitis include exercise as tolerated, avoidance of potentially hepatotoxic drugs and chemicals (e.g., alcohol), and a healthy diet.
- Patients should not donate blood; serum monitoring for exacerbations of disease or spontaneous seroconversion should be done periodically.
- Sexual partners and children of patients with chronic HBV should be vaccinated against hepatitis B.
- Effective treatment of chronic viral hepatitis should decrease morbidity and mortality and prevent infected patients from serving as reservoirs of infection.
- The decision to treat patients with chronic hepatitis should not be made based on the presence or absence of symptoms or the degree of abnormality of biochemical tests. The activity and extent of the liver disease do not correlate with the level of serum aminotransferases or the patient's symptoms. Rather, a systematic approach to the treatment should be made, such as the management approach shown in the algorithm in Figure 23.1.

Interferons

- IFN is now the treatment of choice for patients with chronic HBV, HCV, and HDV infection. Unfortunately, only a proportion of patients respond favorably; considerably fewer have lasting response; very few are cured.
- Recombinant IFNs (alfa-2A, Roferon A, Hoffmann-LaRoche; α-2B, Intron A, Schering) and lymphoblastoid IFN (α-n1, Wellferon, Burroughs Wellcome) are effective in relieving symptoms and halting progression of chronic hepatitis B in one-third to one-half of immunocompetent patients from Western countries. Remissions are marked by loss of HBV DNA, HBeAg, normalization of serum aminotransferases, and improvement in liver histology.
- Effective dosing regimens of IFN in clinically stable patients with chronic HBV are 5 million units (MU) daily or 10 MU subcutaneously three times weekly for 4–6 months. One specific regimen (FDA-approved) for IFN-α 2b is 5 MU 5 days per week or 10 MU every other day for 16 weeks. Therapy should be started as early as possible after diagnosis. Mildly or moderately decompensated patients should receive only 2 MU daily or 2–5 MU three times weekly, if IFN is used at all.

V

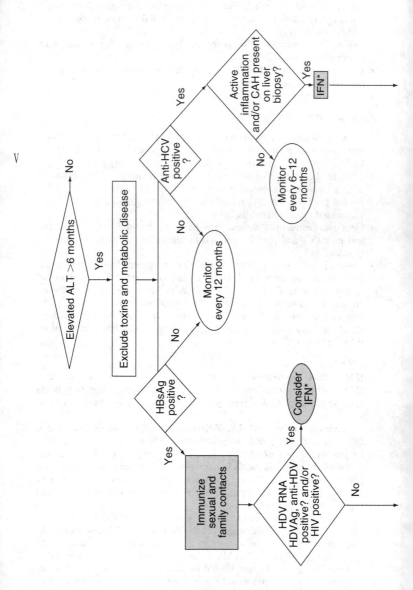

Elevated ALT >6 months → No

Yes

Exclude toxins and metabolic disease

HBsAg positive?

Yes → Immunize sexual and family contacts → HDV RNA HDVAg, anti-HDV positive? and/or HIV positive? → Yes → Consider IFN*

No

No → Monitor every 12 months

Anti-HCV positive? → Yes → Active inflammation and/or CAH present on liver biopsy? → Yes → IFN*

No → Monitor every 12 months

No → Monitor every 6–12 months

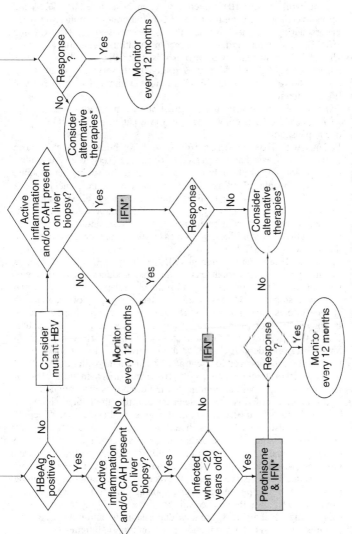

Figure 23.1. Algorithm for the management of chronic viral hepatitis. *See text for IFN dosing and alternative therapies.

V

- It is important to measure the markers of chronic HBV infection (HBeAg and HBV DNA) immediately prior to initiating treatment because a few patients with chronic HBV infection spontaneously lose HBV DNA and seroconvert each year without treatment. Laboratory monitoring parameters during treatment include the aminotransferases, HBeAg, and HBV DNA. Clinical vigilance for decompensation is essential.
- Use of IFN in patients with cirrhosis is controversial. These patients appear to respond to IFN at rates similar to those with less advanced disease; however, IFN side effects are more common and severe—even life-threatening.
- Extreme caution must be used in treating patients with cirrhosis with IFN and should be attempted only in those patients with mild or early decompensation.
- Patients with HBV in whom IFN should not be used include those whose liver disease has progressed to end stage (very low serum albumin, prolonged prothrombin time, elevated bilirubin, leukopenia, thrombocytopenia, bleeding esophageal varices, ascites, encephalopathy, and/or progressive jaundice), those with liver disease of other causes, patients on immunosuppressive therapy, patients actively abusing drugs, those with significant psychiatric illness, and those with significant other medical illnesses such as cardiac, renal, or thyroid disease that are not successfully treated.
- In chronic delta hepatitis, high-dose IFN-α treatment (5 MU daily or 9 MU three times weekly for at least 12 months) produces disease improvement in about 50% of patients. Unfortunately, relapse is common when therapy is stopped, and these patients have a high rate of drug-related adverse effects necessitating dosage reduction or termination of therapy. Prolonged IFN therapy may be necessary to achieve a sustained response.
- IFN-α therapy may lead to complete eradication of HCV infection in long-term responders. IFN-α-2b at a dose of 3 MU three times weekly for 24 weeks is approved for treatment of chronic hepatitis C. One-third to one-half of treated patients improve, but approximately 50% of responders relapse within 6 months when therapy is discontinued.
- The side effects of IFN are frequent enough that the patient should be informed about them before treatment begins. Early side effects include fatigue, malaise, muscle aches, headaches, changes in appetite, fever, chills, nausea, and sleep disturbance. Late adverse reactions include those previously mentioned plus mild myelosuppression, bacterial infection, weight loss, loss of libido, thyroiditis, alopecia, IFN-induced autoimmune hepatitis (very rarely), exacerbation of other autoimmune phenomena, development of a variety of autoantibodies (e.g., antinuclear antibody, smooth muscle antibody, or antibody to thyroid microsomal antigen), irritability, anxiety, depression, attention span deficits, seizures, psychosis, delirium, and, most commonly, fatigue.
- Ongoing monitoring of IFN toxicity includes complete blood counts weekly during the first 2 weeks of therapy and monthly thereafter.

- Patients should be asked about level of performance, mood changes, and symptoms.
- The dose of IFN should be decreased by 50% if any of the following develop: fatigue that interferes with the daily routine, daily nausea with occasional vomiting, granulocytopenia (less than $750/mm^3$), and/or thrombocytopenia (less than $50,000/mm^3$).
- IFN should be immediately discontinued if any of the following develop: fatigue that requires bed rest, vomiting more than twice daily, profound granulocytopenia (less than $500/mm^3$), or thrombocytopenia (less than $30,000/mm^3$).

Corticosteroids, Antiviral Agents, and Immunostimulants

- Corticosteroids lead to reduced hepatic inflammation, but also result in dramatic increases in viral replication. In addition, withdrawal of the steroids causes a flare in hepatitis disease activity. Thus, corticosteroids can cause further decompensation and death in patients with clinically unstable disease.
- Chinese patients and those patients with mild disease and low levels of HBV DNA can be tried on a 4- to 8-week tapering course of prednisone (e.g., decreasing daily doses of 60, 40, and 20 mg, each for 2 weeks) followed by IFN-α 3 to 5 MU daily for 16 weeks.

Liver Transplantation

- Liver transplantation is an option for patients with end-stage chronic liver disease secondary to viral infection. Recurrent viral hepatitis B infection in the transplanted liver almost always occurs.
- The primary strategy to protect the graft from reinfection is to transplant HBV DNA negative patients and then treat them for life with HBIG.

PREVENTION OF VIRAL HEPATITIS

- The mainstays of hepatitis prevention are risk reduction, education, passive immunization with immune globulins, and, for hepatitis B, active immunization through vaccination programs.
- The spread of HAV can be controlled by cautious handling of fomites contaminated with feces coupled with good handwashing techniques. Universal precautions are used to prevent hepatitis spread within the hospital setting.
- HBV and HCV spread are reduced, but not eliminated, through screening of blood donors and testing for HBsAg and anti-HCV.

HEPATITIS A PREVENTION

- Prevention of HAV has traditionally focused on avoiding exposure as well as preexposure and postexposure prophylaxis with immune globulin (IG).
- A single dose of IG of 0.02 mL/kg intramuscularly (IM) is recommended for travelers to high-risk areas if travel is for <3 months. For lengthy stays, 0.06 mL/kg IM should be given every 3 to 5 months. Dosing is the same for adults and children.

TABLE 23.2. Groups Recommended for Postexposure Prophylaxis of Hepatitis A

Household or sexual contacts

Staff and children in day care centers where cases of hepatitis A are diagnosed (or identified in households of children attending the center)

Members of households that have children in diapers attending a day care center where cases of hepatitis A are identified

Residents and staff of prisons and facilities for developmentally disabled

Hospital personnel exposed to feces of infected patients

Food handlers and patrons of restaurants if the (1) infected food handler is directly involved in handling foods, without gloves, that will not be cooked; (2) source has deficient hygienic practices; and (3) exposed patrons can be identified and treated within 2 weeks of exposure

- The postexposure prophylactic benefit from IG is greatest early in the incubation period and is of no benefit more than 2 weeks after exposure. A single IG dose of 0.02 mL/kg IM is used for postexposure prophylaxis of hepatitis A.
- Some groups recommended to receive postexposure prophylaxis are listed in Table 23.2.
- An inactivated HAV vaccine, Havrix (SmithKline Beecham) demonstrates protective efficacy in at least 94% of vaccinees within 1 month after vaccination. It is indicated for immunization of individuals 2 years of age or greater who are at increased risk of hepatitis A infection.
- Groups considered at increased risk of infection with hepatitis A are listed in Table 23.3.

TABLE 23.3. People at Increased Risk of Hepatitis A Infection

Persons traveling to areas of high endemicity for hepatitis A[a]

Residents of a community experiencing an outbreak of hepatitis A

Military personnel

Persons engaging in high-risk sexual activity (including bisexual and homosexual males)

Native peoples of Alaska and the Americas

Users of illicit injectable drugs

Institutional workers, such as caretakers for the developmentally disabled

Employees of child day care centers

Laboratory workers who handle live hepatitis A virus

Handlers of primate animals that may be harboring HAV

People living in, or relocating to, areas of high endemicity

[a]Africa, Asia (except Japan), the Mediterranean basin, Eastern Europe, the Middle East, Central and South America, Mexico, and parts of the Caribbean.

HEPATITIS B PREVENTION

- Two products are available for prevention of hepatitis B infection: hepatitis B vaccine, which provides active immunity, and HBIG, which provides temporary passive immunity.
- The goals of immunization against viral hepatitis include prevention of the short-term viremia that can lead to transmission of infection, clinical disease, and chronic HBV infection.

Hepatitis B Immune Globulin (HBIG)

- Postexposure prophylaxis for HBV is recommended for perinatal exposure of infants of HBV-carrier mothers, sexual exposure to HBsAg-positive persons, accidental percutaneous or permucosal exposure to HBsAg-positive blood, and exposure of an infant to a care giver who has acute hepatitis B.
- HBIG is used only in postexposure prophylaxis. The recommended dose is 0.06 mL/kg administered intramuscularly. Guidelines for use are listed in Tables 23.4 and 23.5.

Hepatitis B Vaccine

- Hepatitis B vaccines contain 5–40 g HBsAg protein per mL adsorbed onto aluminum per mL of vaccine, with thimerosal added as preserva-

TABLE 23.4. Recommended Schedule of Immunoprophylaxis to Prevent Perinatal or Sexual Transmission of HBV Infection

Vaccine Recipient	Immunoprophylaxis	Timing
Infant born to HBsAg positive mother	Vaccine dose 1	Within 12 hours of birth
	HBIG[a]	Within 12 hours of birth
	Vaccine doses 2 and 3[b]	Usual schedule
Infant born to mother not screened for HBsAg	Vaccine dose 1[c]	Within 12 hours of birth
	HBIG	If mother is found to be HBsAg-positive, administer dose to infant as soon as possible, but no later than 1 week after birth
	Vaccine doses 2 and 3[h]	Usual schedule
Sexual exposure	HBIG[d]	Single dose within 14 days of sexual contact
	Vaccine dose 1	At time of HBIG treatment[e]

[a]0.5 mL, intramuscularly, at a site different from that used for the vaccine.
[b]The four-dose schedule for Engerix-B can also be used.
[c]The first dose of vaccine is the same as that for the infant of an HBsAg-positive mother. If the mother is found to be HBsAg-positive, that dose is continued. If the mother is found to be HBsAg-negative, the remaining vaccine doses are those appropriate for other infants and children.
[d]0.06 mL/kg intramuscularly.
[e]The first dose can be given at the same time as the HBIG dose but in a different site; subsequent doses should be given as recommended in Table 23.6.

TABLE 23.5. Recommendations for Hepatitis B Prophylaxis Following Percutaneous or Permucosal Exposure

Exposed Person	Treatment When Source Is Found to Be:		Source Not Tested or Unknown
	HBsAg-Positive	HBsAg-Negative	
Unvaccinated	HBIG × 1[a] and initiate HB vaccine[b]	Initiate HB vaccine[b]	Initiate HB vaccine[b]
Previously vaccinated			
Known responder	Test exposed for anti-HBs 1. If adequate,[c] no treatment 2. If inadequate, HB vaccine booster dose	No treatment	No treatment
Known nonresponder	HBIG × 2 or HBIG × 1 plus 1 dose HB vaccine	No treatment	If known high-risk source, may treat as if source were HBsAg-positive
Response unknown	Test exposed for anti-HBs 1. If inadequate,[c] HBIG × 1 plus HB vaccine booster dose 2. If adequate, no treatment	No treatment	Test exposed for anti-HBs 1. If inadequate,[c] HB vaccine booster dose 2. If adequate, no treatment

[a]HBIG dose 0.06 mL/kg IM.
[b]HB vaccine dose; see Table 23.6.
[c]Adequate anti-HBs is ≥10 sample ratio units by radioimmunoassay or enzyme immunoassay.

tive. Side effects of the vaccine are soreness at the injection site, headache, fatigue, and fever.

- The dose of HBsAg to induce the desired antibody response/protective effect varies between the two available vaccines (Table 23.6).
- HBV vaccine is given as a series of three IM doses into the deltoid (anterolateral thigh in infants), given over a period of months.
- A pediatric formulation is available that contains 5 μg/mL.
- Specific dosing guidelines for all age groups are listed in Tables 23.6 and 23.7.
- Hepatitis B vaccines are inactivated and can be simultaneously administered with other vaccines.
- Postvaccination testing for immunity is not routinely done. It is recommended for those whose management depends on their immune status and those in whom a suboptimal response is expected (hemodialysis patients, HIV-infected patients, certain public safety personnel, smokers, the extremely obese, and those who receive intradermal vaccine administration).
- Nonresponders and inadequate responders should be immediately revaccinated with one or two injections of vaccine (Table 23.8).
- Hemodialysis patients have decreased seroconversion rates, decreased antibody titers to surface antigens, and a faster rate of loss of antibody after HBV vaccination. These patients require higher vaccine doses or an increased number of doses. A special formulation of Recombivax

TABLE 23.6. Recommended Doses and Schedules of Currently Licensed HB Vaccines

Group	Recombivax HB[a] dose, μg (mL)	Engerix-B[a,b] dose, μg (mL)
Infants of HBsAg-positive mothers	Adult formulation: 5 (0.5) Pediatric formulation: 5 (1)[c]	10 (0.5)
Other infants and children <11 years	Adult formulation: 2.5 (0.25) Pediatric formulation: 2.5 (0.5)[c]	10 (0.5)
Children and adolescents 11–19 years	5 (0.5)	20 (1.0)
Adults >19 years	10 (1.0)	20 (1.0)
Dialysis patients and other immunocompromised persons	40 (1.0)[d]	40 (2.0)[e,f]

V

[a]Usual schedules: three doses given at 0, 1, and 6 months or, for infants, with other routine immunizations at 2, 4, and 6 months.
[b]Alternative schedule: four doses at 0, 1, 2, and 12 months.
[c]A special pediatric formulation of Recombivax HB is available that contains 5 μg/mL.
[d]Special formulation for dialysis patients.
[e]Two 1.0-mL doses given at different sites.
[f]Four-dose schedule recommended at 0, 1, 2, and 6 months.

TABLE 23.7. Recommended Schedule for Routine Hepatitis B Vaccination of Infants and Children

Hepatitis B Vaccination[a]	At Birth (Before Hospital Discharge)	1–2 Months	4 Months	6–18 Months
Option 1[b]	X	X		X
Option 2[b]		X	X	X

[a]For use among infants born to HBsAg-negative mothers. The first dose should be administered during the newborn period, no later than age 2 months. Premature infants of HBsAg-negative mothers should receive the first dose of the hepatitis B vaccine series at the time of hospital discharge or when the other routine childhood vaccines are initiated. (All infants born to HBsAg-positive mothers should receive immunoprophylaxis for hepatitis B as soon as possible after birth.)
[b]Hepatitis B vaccine can be administered simultaneously at the same visit with DTP (or DTaP), OPV, Hib, and/or MMR.

TABLE 23.8. Guidelines for Booster Dose Inoculations Following Hepatitis B Immunization

Type of Response	Anti-HBs Level (IU/L)	Booster Dose Recommendations
Nonresponse	Negative	Immediate
Inadequate response	<10	Immediate
Low response	10–100	1–2 years
Good or adequate response	>100	5–10 years or none

From Hollinger FB. Am J Med 1989;87 (suppl 3A):38S, with permission.

TABLE 23.9. High-Risk Groups Recommended for Preexposure Hepatitis B Vaccination[a]

Health care and public safety workers who have occupational exposure to blood

Parenteral drug abusers

Individuals with multiple sexual partners (homosexual, bisexual, or heterosexual)

Hemodialysis patients

Recipients of certain blood products, i.e., uninfected patients with hemophilia and other clotting disorders

Clients and staff of institutions for the developmentally disabled

Household and sexual contacts of HBV carriers

Adoptees from countries where HBV is highly endemic

Populations where HBV is highly endemic (e.g., Alaskan Eskimos)

Inmates of long-term correctional facilities

International travelers to highly endemic HBV regions for >6 months

Unvaccinated infants under 12 months of age exposed to acute HBV infection through primary caregiver

Household contacts with blood exposure to a patient with acute HBV infection

[a]CDC recommendations are that all newborns be vaccinated against hepatitis B.

HB (40 μg/mL) is available for these patients. A more rapid rise in antibody concentration is observed with a 0-, 1-, 2-, and 6-month vaccination schedule in these patients, although overall conversion rate is similar whether the final (fourth) dose is given 6 or 12 months after the series begins.

Groups Recommended for Preexposure Vaccination

- The primary eradication strategy for hepatitis B is routine infant vaccination, which, over several decades, could eliminate transmission of the virus.
- The groups currently recommended for preexposure vaccination are listed in Table 23.9.

Postexposure Prophylaxis for Hepatitis B

- HBIG and HBV are recommended in combination for postexposure prophylaxis. The antibody response to the vaccine is not attenuated by administration of HBIG.
- Hepatitis B vaccination is recommended for any person not previously vaccinated who is exposed to blood potentially containing HBsAg. The source should be tested for HBsAg. If positive, the exposed person should receive HBIG.
- Current recommendations also include administration of both HBIG and HBV vaccine to neonates with HBV exposure, although vaccination without HBIG may be effective.

See Chapter 40, Viral Hepatitis, authored by Marsha A. Raebel, PharmD, FCCP, BCPS, for a more detailed discussion of this topic.

Chapter 24

▶ INFLAMMATORY BOWEL DISEASE

▶ DEFINITION

There are two forms of idiopathic inflammatory bowel disease (IBD): ulcerative colitis, a mucosal inflammatory condition confined to the rectum and colon, and Crohn's disease, a transmural inflammation of gastrointestinal (GI) mucosa that may occur in any part of the GI tract. The etiologies of both conditions are unknown, but they may have a common pathogenetic mechanism.

▶ EPIDEMIOLOGY

- At least 1 million Americans are believed to have IBD, with 15,000 to 30,000 new cases diagnosed annually.
- The incidence of new cases per year for ulcerative colitis is 3 to 6 per 100,000 and with a prevalence (number of cases at any point in time) of 35 to 70 cases per 100,000 Americans.
- Crohn's disease has a reported incidence of 4.3 to 6.8 and a prevalence of 20 to 40 per 100,000 people.
- The peak incidence occurs in the second or third decade of life, but infants and the elderly may present with either disorder.

▶ PATHOPHYSIOLOGY

- The major theories of the cause of IBD involve infectious or immunologic causes. The infectious theory assumes that the body is reacting normally to an unrecognized pathogen, whereas the immunologic theory assumes that the immune system is acting inappropriately to antigens to which most people are exposed (Table 24.1).
- Ulcerative colitis and Crohn's disease differ in two general respects: anatomic sites and depth of involvement within the bowel wall. There is, however, overlap between the two conditions, with a small fraction of patients showing features of both diseases (Table 24.2). Confusion can occur, particularly when the inflammatory process is limited to the colon.

ULCERATIVE COLITIS

- Ulcerative colitis is confined to the colon and rectum, and affects primarily the mucosa and the submucosa. The primary lesion occurs in the crypts of the mucosa (crypts of Lieberkuhn) in the form of a crypt abscess.

TABLE 24.1. Proposed Etiologies for Inflammatory Bowel Disease

> **Infectious Agents**
> Viruses
> L-forms of bacteria
> *Mycobacteria*
> *Chlamydia*
>
> **Genetics**
> Metabolic defects
> Connective tissue disorders
>
> **Environmental Factors**
> Diet
>
> **Immune Defects**
> Altered host susceptibility
> Immune-mediated mucosal damage
>
> **Psychologic Factors**
> Stress
> Emotional or physical trauma
> Occupation

Complications

- Ulcerative colitis can be accompanied by complications that may be local (involving the colon) or systemic (not directly associated with the colon). With either type the complications may be mild, serious, or even life-threatening.

- Local complications occur in the majority of ulcerative colitis patients. Relatively minor complications include hemorrhoids, anal fissures, or perirectal abscesses.

- A major complication is toxic megacolon, a severe condition that occurs in 1–3% of patients with ulcerative colitis or Crohn's disease. The risk of colonic carcinoma is much greater in patients with ulcerative colitis as compared with the general population.

- Approximately 11% of patients with ulcerative colitis have been reported to have hepatobiliary complications including fatty liver, pericholangitis, chronic active hepatitis, cirrhosis, sclerosing cholangitis, cholangiocarcinoma, and gallstones.

- Arthritis is found to be present in about 5% of patients. Arthritis is typically migratory and involves one or a few joints. The joints most often affected, in decreasing frequency, are the knees, hips, ankles, wrists, and elbows.

- Ocular complications, including iritis, uveitis, episcleritis, or conjunctivitis, occur in about 10% of patients with IBDs. The most commonly reported symptoms include blurred vision, headaches, eye pain, and photophobia.

TABLE 24.2. Comparison of the Clinical and Pathologic Features of Crohn's Disease and Ulcerative Colitis

Feature	Crohn's Disease	Ulcerative Colitis
Intestinal		
Malaise, fever	Common	Uncommon
Rectal bleeding	Intermittent about 50%	Common
Abdominal tenderness	Common	May be present
Abdominal mass	Very common (especially with ileocolitis)	Not present
Abdominal pain	Very common	Unusual
Abdominal wall and internal fistulas	Very common	Rare
Endoscopic		
Rectal disease	About 20%	Almost 100%
Diffuse, continuous symmetric involvement	Uncommon	Very common
Aphthous or linear ulcers	Common	Rare
Radiologic		
Continuous disease	Rare	Very common
Ileal involvement	Very common	Rare
Asymmetry	Very common	Rare
Strictures	Common	Rare
Fistulas	Very common	Rare
Pathologic		
Discontinuity	Common	Rare
Rectal involvement	Rare	Common
Intense vascularity	Rare	Common
Ileal involvement	Common	Nonexistent
Transmural involvement	Common	Rare
Crypt abscesses	Rare	Very common
Granulomas	Common	Rare

Adapted from Rumming KF. In Sabiston DC (ed): Essentials of Surgery. Philadelphia, WB Saunders, 1987:483, with permission.

V

- A number of different skin and mucosal lesions are associated with IBDs, including erythema nodosum, pyoderma gangrenosum, and aphthalous ulceration. Overall, most studies report 5–10% of IBD patients experience dermatologic or mucosal complications.

CROHN'S DISEASE

- Crohn's disease is best characterized as a transmural inflammatory process. The terminal ileum is the most common site of the disorder (14–30%), but it may occur in any part of the GI tract.
- About two-thirds of patients have some colonic involvement, and 15–25% of patients have only colonic disease.

- Patients often have normal bowel separating segments of diseased bowel; that is, the disease is often discontinuous.
- Complications of Crohn's disease may involve the intestinal tract or organs unrelated to it. Small-bowel stricture and subsequent obstruction is a complication that may require surgery. Fistula formation is common and occurs much more frequently than with ulcerative colitis.
- Systemic complications of Crohn's disease are common, and similar to those found with ulcerative colitis. Arthritis, iritis, skin lesions, and liver disease often accompany Crohn's disease.

▶ CLINICAL PRESENTATION

V
ULCERATIVE COLITIS

- Although a typical clinical picture of ulcerative colitis can be described, there is a very wide range of presentation. Symptoms may range from mild abdominal cramping with frequent small-volume bowel movements to profuse diarrhea.
- Most patients with ulcerative colitis experience intermittent bouts of illness after varying intervals with no symptoms.
- Mild disease has been defined as less than four stools daily without anemia, tachycardia, weight loss, or hypoalbuminemia, and severe disease as greater than six stools daily with the signs just listed.
- Patients with moderate disease have more prominent abdominal discomfort and usually present with diarrhea as the major complaint. They may be noted to have a low-grade fever.
- With severe disease the patient is usually found to be in acute distress, has profuse bloody diarrhea, and often has a high fever with leukocytosis and hypoalbuminemia. Often the patient is dehydrated and therefore may be tachycardic and hypotensive.

CROHN'S DISEASE

- As with ulcerative colitis, the presentation of Crohn's disease is highly variable. A single episode may not be followed by further episodes, or the patient may experience continuous, unremitting disease. Commonly, a patient may first present with a perirectal or perianal lesion.
- The course of Crohn's disease is characterized by periods of remission and exacerbation. Some patients may be free of symptoms for years, while others experience chronic problems in spite of medical therapy.

▶ DESIRED OUTCOME

Goals of treatment may vary considerably among patients and include resolution of acute inflammatory processes and attendant complications (e.g., fistulas, abscesses), alleviation of systemic manifestations (e.g., arthritis), maintenance of remission from acute inflammation, or surgical palliation or cure. The approach to the therapeutic regimen differs considerably with varying goals as well as with the two diseases, ulcerative colitis and Crohn's disease.

▶ TREATMENT

- Treatment of IBD centers on agents used to lessen the inflammatory process. Salicylates, corticosteroids, antimicrobials, and immunosuppressive agents such as azathioprine and 6-mercaptopurine are commonly used to treat active disease and, for some agents, to lengthen remission from disease.
- In addition to the use of drugs, surgical procedures are sometimes performed when active disease is not adequately controlled or when the required drug dosages pose an unacceptable risk of adverse effects.

NONPHARMACOLOGIC TREATMENT
Nutritional Support
- Proper nutritional support is an important aspect of the treatment of patients with IBD, not because specific types of diets are useful in alleviating the inflammatory conditions but because patients with moderate to severe disease are often malnourished.
- Many patients with IBD, although not the majority, have lactase deficiency and therefore, diarrhea may be associated with milk intake. In these patients, avoidance of milk or supplementation with lactase generally improves their symptoms.
- The nutritional needs of the majority of patients can be adequately addressed with enteral supplementation. Patients who have severe disease may require a course of parenteral nutrition to attain a reasonable nutritional status or in preparation for surgery.
- Parenteral nutrition is an important component of the treatment of severe Crohn's disease or ulcerative colitis. The use of parenteral nutrition allows complete bowel rest in patients with severe ulcerative colitis, which may alter the need for proctocolectomy. Parenteral nutrition has also been valuable in Crohn's disease because remission may be achieved with parenteral nutrition in about one-half of patients.

Surgery
- For ulcerative colitis, colectomy may be performed when the patient has disease uncontrolled by maximum medical therapy or when there are complications of the disease such as colonic perforation, toxic dilatation (megacolon), uncontrolled colonic hemorrhage, or colonic strictures.
- Although surgery (proctocolectomy) is curative for ulcerative colitis, this is not the case for Crohn's disease.
- The indications for surgery with Crohn's disease are not as well established as they are for ulcerative colitis, and surgery is usually reserved for the complications of the disease. Surgery may be appropriate in

well-selected patients who are documented to continue to have severe or incapacitating disease in spite of aggressive medical management.

PHARMACOLOGIC THERAPY

- Drug therapy plays an integral part in the overall treatment of IBD. None of the drugs used for IBD is curative; at best they serve to control the disease process. Therefore, a reasonable goal of drug therapy is resolution of disease symptoms such that the patient can carry on normal daily functions.
- The major types of drug therapy used in IBD include aminosalicylates, corticosteroids, immunosuppressives (azathioprine, mercaptopurine, cyclosporin A), antimicrobials (metronidazole), and other agents used investigationally, such as immune enhancers (e.g., levamisole or bacillus Calmette-Guérin, BCG) and mast cell stabilizers (cromolyn sodium).
- Sulfasalazine, an agent that combines a sulfonamide (sulfapyridine) antibiotic and 5-aminosalicylic acid (5-ASA, mesalamine) in the same molecule, has been used for many years to treat IBD. The active component of sulfasalazine is 5-ASA (mesalamine), which has a local anti-inflammatory effect on the lumen of the intestine; however, other mechanisms are still considered (Table 24.3).
- Corticosteroids and adrenocorticotropic hormone (ACTH) have been widely used for the treatment of ulcerative colitis and Crohn's disease and are used in moderate to severe disease.
- Immunosuppressive agents such as azathioprine and 6-mercaptopurine (a metabolite of azathioprine) are sometimes used for the treatment of IBDs. These agents are generally reserved for cases that are refractory to steroids and may be associated with serious adverse effects such as lymphomas, pancreatitis, or nephrotoxicity.

TABLE 24.3. Mesalamine Derivatives for Treatment of Inflammatory Bowel Disease

Product	Trade Name(s)	Formulation	Dose/Day	Site of Action
Sulfasalazine	Azulfidine	Tablet	1–4 g	Colon
Mesalamine	Rowasa, Salofalk, Claversal, Pentasa	Enema	1–4 g	Rectum, terminal, colon
	Rowasa	Suppository	1 g	Rectum
	Asacol	5-ASA coated with Eudragit-S (delayed release acrylic resin)	2.4 g	Distal ileum and colon
	Claversal (Salofalk)	5-ASA coated with Eudragit-L (delayed release acrylic resin)	1–4 g	Ileum and colon
	Pentasa	5-ASA encapsulated in ethylcellulose microgranules (oral tablet)	1–4 g	Small bowel and colon
Olsalazine	Dipentum	Dimer of 5-ASA oral capsule	1–3 g	Colon
Balsalazide	Colazide	Capsule	2.16 g	Colon

- Antimicrobial agents, particularly metronidazole, are frequently used in attempts to control Crohn's disease. Metronidazole has been demonstrated to be of value in some patients with active Crohn's disease, particularly when it involves the perineal area or fistulas.

Ulcerative Colitis

Mild to Moderate Disease
- The first line of drug therapy for the patient with mild to moderate colitis is oral sulfasalazine or an oral mesalamine derivative.
- For proctitis the preferred therapy is rectally administered steroids or mesalamine.
- Sulfasalazine therapy should be instituted at 500 mg/d and increased every few days up to 4 g or the maximum tolerated (up to 8 g/d).
- Oral mesalamine derivatives (such as those listed in Table 24.3) are reasonable alternatives to sulfasalazine for treatment of ulcerative colitis.
- Steroids have a place in the treatment of moderate to severe ulcerative colitis. Oral steroids (usually up to 1 mg/kg/d of prednisone equivalent) may be used for patients who do not have an adequate response to sulfasalazine. Prednisone dosages in the range of 40–60 mg/d have been superior to regimens of 20 mg/d in producing remission.
- Overall, steroids and sulfasalazine appear to be equally efficacious; however, the response to steroids may be evident sooner.
- Rectally administered steroids or mesalamine can be used as initial therapy for ulcerative proctitis or distal colitis.
- Transdermal nicotine has been shown to improve symptoms of patients with active ulcerative colitis (when given along with mesalamine).

Severe or Intractable Disease
- Patients with uncontrolled severe colitis or incapacitating symptoms require hospitalization for effective management. Under these conditions, patients generally receive nothing by mouth to put the bowel at rest; however, the benefit of enteral nutrition in these patients has been demonstrated. Most medication is given by the parenteral route.
- With severe colitis, there is a much greater reliance on parenteral steroids and surgical procedures. Sulfasalazine or mesalamine derivatives have not been proven beneficial for treatment of severe colitis.
- Steroids have been valuable in the treatment of severe disease because the use of these agents may allow some patients to avoid colectomy. A trial of steroids is warranted in most patients before proceeding to colectomy, unless the condition is grave or rapidly deteriorating.
- A major development in the treatment of severe ulcerative colitis refractory to steroids has been intravenous cyclosporine. Continuous intravenous infusion of cyclosporine (4 mg/kg/d) has been recommended for all patients with active ulcerative colitis refractory to steroids.

Maintenance of Remission
- Once remission from active disease has been achieved, the goal of therapy is to maintain remission.
- The major agents used for maintenance of remission are sulfasalazine and the mesalamine derivatives; steroids usually do not have a role. The value of sulfasalazine in preventing recurrences has been documented in placebo-controlled trials.
- Steroids do not have a role in the maintenance of remission with ulcerative colitis because they have been demonstrated to be ineffective. Steroids should be gradually withdrawn after remission is induced (over 3 to 4 weeks). If they are continued, the patient will be exposed to steroid side effects without likelihood of benefits.
- Azathioprine has been demonstrated effective in preventing relapse of ulcerative colitis for periods of up to 2 years. However, 3 to 6 months may be required for beneficial effect.

Crohn's Disease
- Management of Crohn's disease often proves more difficult than that of ulcerative colitis, partly because of the greater complexity of presentation with Crohn's disease.
- There is a greater reliance on drug therapy with Crohn's disease, because resection of all involved intestine may not be possible and recurrence after surgery is possible.

Active Crohn's Disease
- The goal of treatment for active Crohn's disease is to achieve remission; however, in many patients, reduction of symptoms so that the patient may carry out normal activities or reduction of the steroid dose required for control is a significant accomplishment.
- In the majority of patients, active Crohn's disease is treated with sulfasalazine, mesalamine derivatives, or steroids, although azathioprine, 6-mercaptopurine, or metronidazole are frequently used.
- Sulfasalazine is more effective when Crohn's disease involves the colon and in patients who have not undergone surgery for their disease.
- Other mesalamine derivatives (such as Pentasa or Asacol) that release mesalamine in the small bowel may be more effective than sulfasalazine for ileal involvement.
- Steroids are frequently used for the treatment of active Crohn's disease, particularly with more severe presentations. Steroids are preferred for treatment of severe Crohn's disease, mainly because these agents can be given parenterally and response to therapy may occur sooner.
- Once remission is achieved, however, it may prove difficult to reduce steroid dosage without reintroduction of active disease.
- Metronidazole may be useful in some patients with Crohn's disease, particularly in patients with colonic involvement or those with perineal disease.
- The immunosuppressive agents (azathioprine and 6-mercaptopurine) are generally limited to use in patients not achieving adequate response

to standard medical therapy, or to reduce steroid doses when toxic doses are required.

- Azathioprine has been determined effective for active disease when added to a steroid regimen.
- Cyclosporine has also demonstrated benefit in active Crohn's disease. It appears that the dose of cyclosporine is important in determining efficacy. An oral dose of 5 mg/kg/d was not effective, whereas 7.9 mg/kg/d was effective. However, toxic effects limit application of the higher dosage.

Maintenance of Remission

- Prevention of recurrence of disease is clearly more difficult with Crohn's disease than with ulcerative colitis. In the past few years there has been increasing evidence that some agents, particularly sulfasalazine and oral mesalamine derivatives, are effective in preventing acute recurrences in quiescent Crohn's disease.
- Steroids also have no place in the prevention of recurrence of Crohn's disease; these agents do not appear to alter the long-term course of the disease.
- Although the published data are not consistent, there is evidence to suggest that azathioprine and 6-mercaptopurine are effective in maintaining remission in Crohn's disease.

SELECTED COMPLICATIONS

Toxic Megacolon

- The treatment required for toxic megacolon includes general supportive measures to maintain vital functions, consideration for early surgical intervention, and drugs (steroids and antimicrobials).
- Aggressive fluid and electrolyte management is required for dehydration.
- When the patient has lost significant amounts of blood (through the rectum), blood replacement is also necessary.
- Opiates and anticholinergics should be discontinued because these agents enhance colonic dilatation, thereby increasing the risk of bowel perforation.
- Steroids in high dosages should be administered intravenously to reduce acute inflammation. Doses as high as 2 mg/kg/d of prednisone equivalent have been recommended (generally administered as hydrocortisone).
- Antimicrobial regimens that are effective against enteric aerobes and anaerobes (e.g., aminoglycoside with clindamycin or metronidazole, imipenem, or extended-spectrum penicillin with a β-lactamase inhibitor) should be administered from the time of diagnosis and continued until patient improvement is assured.
- Surgical intervention, mainly an abdominal colectomy with formation of an ileostomy, is an important consideration in patients with toxic megacolon and prevents death in some patients.

Systemic Manifestations

- The common systemic manifestations of IBD include arthritis, anemia, skin manifestations such as erythema nodosum and pyoderma gangrenosum, uveitis, and liver disease.
- Anemia may be a common problem where there is significant blood loss from the GI tract. When the patient can consume oral medication, ferrous sulfate should be administered.
- For arthritis associated with IBD, aspirin or other NSAIDs may be beneficial, as well as steroids.

▶ SPECIAL CONSIDERATIONS

PREGNANCY

- Drug therapy for IBD is not a contraindication for pregnancy, and most pregnancies are well managed in patients with these diseases. The indications for medical and surgical treatment are similar to those in the nonpregnant patient. If a patient has an initial bout of IBD during pregnancy, a standard approach to treatment should be initiated.

ADVERSE DRUG REACTIONS TO AGENTS USED FOR TREATMENT OF IBD

- Sulfasalazine is often associated with adverse drug effects and these effects may be classified as either dose related or idiosyncratic. Dose-related side effects usually include GI disturbances such as nausea, vomiting, diarrhea, or anorexia, but may also include headache and arthralgia.
- Non–dose-related adverse effects of sulfasalazine include rash, fever, or hepatotoxicity most commonly (20–50% of patients), as well as relatively uncommon but serious reactions such as agranulocytosis, pancreatitis, thrombocytopenia, and toxic epidermal necrolysis.
- Oral mesalamine derivatives may impose a lower frequency of adverse effects compared with sulfasalazine. Many patients who are intolerant to sulfasalazine will tolerate oral mesalamine derivatives.
- The well-appreciated adverse effects of corticosteroids include hyperglycemia, hypertension, osteoporosis, fluid retention and electrolyte disturbances, myopathies, psychosis, and reduced resistance to infection. In addition, corticosteroid use may cause adrenocortical suppression. Specific regimens for withdrawal of corticosteroid therapy have been suggested.
- Immunosuppressants such as azathioprine and 6-mercaptopurine have a significant potential for adverse reactions including bone marrow suppression and have been associated with lymphomas (in renal transplant patients) and pancreatitis.

▶ ASSESSMENT OF THERAPEUTIC OUTCOMES

- The success of therapeutic regimens to treat IBDs can be measured by patient-reported complaints, signs, and symptoms, direct physician examination (including endoscopy), history and physical examination, selected laboratory tests, and quality of life measures.

- Evaluation of IBD severity is difficult since much of the assessment is subjective.

- To create more objective measures, disease-rating scales or indices have been created. The Crohn's Disease Activity Index (CDAI) is a commonly used scale, particularly for evaluation of patients during clinical trials. The scale incorporates eight elements: (1) number of stools in the past 7 days, (2) sum of abdominal pain ratings from the past 7 days, (3) rating of general well-being in the past 7 days, (4) use of antidiarrheals, (5) body weight, (6) hematocrit, (7) finding of abdominal mass, and (8) a sum of symptoms present in the past week. Elements of this index provide a guide for those measures that may be useful in assessing the effectiveness of treatment regimens.

- Standardized assessment tools have also been constructed for ulcerative colitis. Elements in these scales include (1) stool frequency, (2) presence of blood in the stool, (3) mucosal appearance (from endoscopy), and (4) physician's global assessment based on physical examination, endoscopy, and laboratory data.

See Chapter 34, Inflammatory Bowel Disease, authored by Joseph T. DiPiro, PharmD, FCCP and Talmadge A. Bowden, Jr., MD, for a more detailed discussion of this topic.

Chapter 25

▶ NAUSEA AND VOMITING

▶ DEFINITION

Nausea is usually defined as the inclination to vomit or as a feeling in the throat or epigastric region alerting an individual that vomiting is imminent. Vomiting is defined as the ejection or expulsion of gastric contents through the mouth, often requiring a forceful event.

▶ ETIOLOGY

- Nausea and vomiting may be associated with a variety of clinical presentations. Specific etiologies associated with nausea and vomiting are presented in Table 25.1.
- Nausea and/or vomiting may occur in as many as 70% of patients with inferior myocardial infarction or diabetic ketoacidosis. As many as 80–90% of patients with an Addisonian crisis, acute pancreatitis, or acute appendicitis may present with nausea and vomiting.
- Drug-induced nausea and vomiting have been of particular interest, especially when caused by cytotoxic agents. Table 25.2 presents specific cytotoxic agents categorized by their emetogenic potential. Although some agents may have greater emetogenic potential than others, combinations of agents, high doses, clinical settings, psychologic conditions, prior treatment experiences, and unusual stimuli to sight, smell, or taste may alter a patient's response to a drug treatment.
- A variety of other common etiologies have been proposed for the development of nausea and vomiting in cancer patients. These are presented in Table 25.3.

▶ PATHOPHYSIOLOGY

- The three consecutive phases of emesis include nausea, retching, and vomiting. Nausea, the imminent need to vomit, is associated with gastric stasis and may be considered a separate and singular symptom. Retching is the labored movement of abdominal and thoracic muscles before vomiting. The final phase of emesis is vomiting, the forceful expulsion of gastric contents due to gastrointestinal (GI) retroperistalsis.
- Vomiting is triggered by afferent impulses to the vomiting center, a nucleus of cells in the medulla. Impulses are received from sensory centers, such as the chemoreceptor trigger zone (CTZ), cerebral cortex, and visceral afferents from the pharynx and GI tract. When excited, afferent impulses are integrated by the vomiting center, resulting in efferent impulses to the salivation center, respiratory center, and the pharyngeal, GI, and abdominal muscles, leading to vomiting.

TABLE 25.1. Specific Etiologies of Nausea and Vomiting

Gastrointestinal Mechanisms
  Mechanical gastric outlet obstruction
    Peptic ulcer disease
    Gastric carcinoma
    Pancreatic disease
  Motility disorders
    Gastroparesis
    Drug-induced gastric stasis
    Chronic intestinal pseudo-obstruction
    Postviral gastroenteritis
    Irritable bowel syndrome
    Postgastric surgery
    Idiopathic gastric stasis
    Anorexia nervosa
  Intra-abdominal emergencies
    Intestinal obstruction
    Acute pancreatitis
    Acute pyelonephritis
    Acute cholecystitis
    Acute cholangitis
    Acute viral hepatitis
  Acute gastroenteritis
    Viral gastroenteritis
    Salmonellosis
    Shigellosis
    Staphylococcal gastroenteritis (enterotoxins)

Cardiovascular Diseases
  Acute myocardial infarction
  Congestive heart failure
  Shock and circulatory collapse

Neurologic Processes
  Midline cerebellar hemorrhage
  Increased intracranial pressure
  Migraine headache
  Vestibular disorders
  Head trauma

Metabolic Disorders
  Diabetes mellitus (diabetic ketoacidosis)
  Addison's disease
  Renal disease (uremia)

Psychogenic Causes
  Self-induced
  Anticipatory

Therapy-Induced Causes
  Cytotoxic chemotherapy
  Radiation therapy
  Theophylline preparations (intolerance, toxic)
  Anticonvulsant preparations (toxic)
  Digitalis preparations (toxic)
  Opiates
  Amphotericin
  Antibiotics

Drug Withdrawal
  Opiates
  Benzodiazepines

Miscellaneous Causes
  Pregnancy
  Any swallowed irritant (foods, drugs)
  Noxious odors
  Operative procedures

TABLE 25.2. Emetogenic Potential of Cytotoxic Chemotherapy

Most Emetogenic	Moderate	Least Emetogenic
Amsacrine	Azacytidine	Asparaginase
Cisplatin	Etoposide	Bleomycin
Cyclophosphamide	Mitomycin O	Busulfan
Dacarbazine	Procarbazine	Chlorambucil
Dactinomycin	Thiotepa	Cytarabine
Daunorubicin		Diaziquone
Doxorubicin		Estramustine
Hexamethylmethamine		Floxuridine
Mechlorethamine		Fluorouracil
Mitoxantrone		Hydroxyurea
Nitrosoureas		Melphalan
Streptozocin		Mercaptopurine
		Methotrexate
		Teniposide
		Thioguanine
		Vinca alkaloids

TABLE 25.3. Nonchemotherapy Etiologies of Nausea and Vomiting in Cancer Patients

Fluid and electrolyte abnormalities
   Hypercalcemia
   Volume depletion
   Water intoxication
   Adrenocortical insufficiency
Drug induced
   Opiates
   Antibiotics
Gastrointestinal obstruction
Increased intracranial pressure
Peritonitis
Metastases
   Brain
   Meninges
   Hepatic
Uremia
Infections (septicemia, local)
Radiation therapy

Adapted from Frytak S, Moertel CG. JAMA 1981;245:393–396, with permission.

V

- The CTZ, located in the area postrema of the fourth ventricle of the brain, is a major chemosensory organ for emesis and is usually associated with chemically induced vomiting.
- Numerous neurotransmitter receptors are located in the vomiting center, CTZ, and GI tract. Examples of such receptors include cholinergic and histaminic, dopaminergic, opiate, serotonin, and benzodiazepine receptors.
- It is theorized that chemotherapeutic agents, their metabolites, or other emetic compounds trigger the process of emesis through stimulation of one or more of these receptors.
- Anticipatory nausea and vomiting may be elicited either by specific stimuli associated with the administration of noxious, often cytotoxic, agents or by the anxiety associated with such treatments.

▶ CLINICAL PRESENTATION

- Nausea and vomiting may be classified as either simple or complex. The term *simple* applies to those episodes of nausea and/or vomiting described by one of the following criteria: (1) occur occasionally and are self-limiting or relieved by the minimal use of antiemetic methods or medications; (2) account for little patient deterioration such as fluid–electrolyte imbalances, pain, or noncompliance with prescribed therapies; or (3) are not related to the administration of or exposure to noxious agents.
- The term *complex* is used when describing a patient's clinical course as including symptoms that are not adequately or readily relieved by the administration of a single antiemetic method or medication, lead to pro-

gressive patient deterioration secondary to fluid–electrolyte imbalances, pain, or noncompliance with prescribed therapies, or are caused by noxious agents or psychogenic events.

- Anticipatory nausea and vomiting is a somewhat unique problem sometimes associated with cytotoxic chemotherapy. As many as one in four cancer patients may experience this condition during repeated courses of therapy.

- Nausea and vomiting occur frequently after operative procedures; those of the abdomen, eye, ear, nose, and throat are generally associated with higher incidences of nausea and vomiting than other procedures. Women experience a three-fold higher incidence of nausea and vomiting as compared to men, independent of the type of operation or anesthetic. Children are about twice as susceptible as adults.

- Other risk factors that may be associated with an increase in postoperative symptoms include patient variables such as obesity, increased age, a history of motion sickness or prior postoperative emesis, as well as drug therapy variables such as the choice of premedication or general anesthetic agent.

- A variety of clinical conditions may be associated with vertigo and dizziness. The etiology of these complaints may include diseases that are infectious, postinfectious, demyelinative, vascular, neoplastic, degenerative, traumatic, toxic, psychogenic, or idiopathic. Whether associated with a minor or complex disorder, motion sickness may be associated with nausea and vomiting.

- Many women experience nausea and vomiting during pregnancy; however, the etiology of hyperemesis gravidarum is not well understood.

▶ TREATMENT

GENERAL PRINCIPLES

- Most cases of nausea and vomiting are self-limiting, resolve spontaneously, and require only symptomatic therapy.

- Antiemetic therapy is indicated in patients with electrolyte disturbances secondary to vomiting, severe anorexia or weight loss, or progression of disease either owing to refusal of continued therapy or poor nutritional status.

- Although many approaches to the treatment of nausea and vomiting have been suggested, antiemetic drugs [over-the-counter (OTC) and prescription] are most often recommended. Provided a patient can and will adhere to oral dosing, a suitable and effective agent can often be selected; however, for certain other patients, oral medications may be inappropriate because of their inability to retain any appreciable oral ingestion. In these patients, rectal or injectable route of administration might be preferred.

- Information concerning commonly available antiemetic preparations is compiled in Table 25.4.

TABLE 25.4. Common Antiemetic Preparations and Adult Dosage Regimens

Drug (Brand Name)	Adult Dosage Regimen	Dosage Form/Route	Availability
Antacids			
Antacids (various)	15–30 mL every 2–4 h prn	Liquid	OTC
Antihistaminic–Anticholinergic Agents			
Benzquinamide (Emete-Con)	25–50 mg every 3–4 h prn	IM, IV	Rx
Buclizine (Bucladin-S)	50 mg twice daily	Tab	Rx
Cyclizine (Marezine)	50 mg every 4–6 h prn	Tab, IM	Rx/OTC
Dimenhydrinate (Dramamine)	50–100 mg every 4–6 prn	Tab, chew tab, cap, liquid, IM, IV	Rx/OTC
Diphenhydramine (Benadryl)	10–50 mg every 4–6 prn	Tab, cap, liquid, IM, IV	Rx/OTC
Hydroxyzine (Vistaril, Atarax)	25–100 mg every 6 h prn	Tab, cap, liquid, IM	Rx
Meclizine (Bonine, Antivert)	25–50 mg every 24 h prn	Tab, chew tab, cap	Rx/OTC
Promethazine (Phenergan)	12.5–25 mg every 4–6 h prn	Tab, liquid, IM, IV, supp	Rx
Pyrilamine (Nisaval)	25–50 mg three to four times daily	Tab	Rx/OTC
Trimethobenzamide (Tigan)	200–250 mg three to four times daily prn	Cap, IM, supp	Rx
Phenothiazines			
Chlorpromazine (Thorazine)	10–25 mg every 4–6 prn	SR cap, tab, liquid, IM, IV	Rx
	50–100 mg every 6–8 h prn	Supp	Rx
Fluphenazine (Prolixin)	1.25–2.5 mg every 6–8 h prn	Tab, liquid, IM	Rx
Perphenazine (Trilafon)	8–30 mg/d divided prn	Tab, liquid, IM, IV	Rx
Prochlorperazine (Compazine)	5–10 mg three to four times daily prn	SR cap, tab, liquid, IM, IV	Rx
	25 mg twice daily prn	Supp	Rx
Promazine (Sparine)	25–50 mg every 4–6 h prn	Tab, IM	Rx
Thiethylperazine (Torecan)	10 mg three times daily	Tab, IM, supp	Rx
Cannabinoids			
Dronabinol (Marinol)	5–7.5 mg/m^2 every 2–4 h prn	Cap	Rx (C–II)

V

Drug	Form	Dose	Status
Nabilone (Cesamet)	Cap	1–2 mg two to three times daily prn	Rx (C-II)
Butyrophenones			
Droperidol (Inapsine)	IM, IV	2.5–5.0 mg every 4–6 h prn	Rx
Haloperidol (Haldol)	Tab, liquid, IM, IV	1–5 mg every 12 h prn	Rx
Corticosteroids			
Dexamethasone (Decadron)	IV	10 mg prior to chemotherapy, repeat with 4–8 mg every 6 h for total of four doses	Rx
Methylprednisolone (SoluMedrol)	IV	125–500 mg every 6 h for total of four doses	Rx
Benzodiazepines			
Diazepam (Valium)	Tab	2–5 mg every 6 h	Rx (C-IV)
Lorazepam (Ativan)	IV	0.5–4.0 mg prior to chemotherapy	Rx (C-IV)
Selective Serotonin Antagonists			
Granisetron (Kytril), for CINV diluted, give over 5 min	IV	10 µg/kg prior to chemotherapy	Rx
Ondansetron (Zofran), for CINV, IV diluted, give over 15 min	IV	32 mg prior to chemotherapy as a single dose, or 0.15 mg/kg prior to chemotherapy, repeat at 4 and 8 h	Rx
Ondansetron (Zofran), for CINV, oral	Tab	8 mg 30 min prior to chemotherapy, repeat at 4 and 8 h and every 8 h for 1–2 days after chemotherapy completion	Rx
Ondansetron (Zofran), for PONV, IV undiluted, give over 2–5 min	IV	4 mg prior to induction of anesthesia or postoperative	Rx
Miscellaneous Agents			
Dextrose, fructose, phosphoric acid (Emetrol)	Liquid	15–30 mL every 1–3 h prn	OTC
Diphenidol (Vontrol)	Tab	25–50 mg every 4 h prn	Rx
Metoclopramide (Reglan)	IV	1–2 mg/kg every 2 h × 2, then every 3 h × 3	Rx

V

Key: Rx, prescription; OTC, over the counter; cap, capsule; chew tab, chewable tablet; IM, intramuscular; IV, intravenous; liquid, oral syrup, concentrate, suspension; SR cap, sustained-release capsule; supp, rectal suppository; tab, tablet; CINV, chemotherapy-induced nausea and vomiting; PONV, postoperative nausea and vomiting.

- For most conditions, a single-agent antiemetic is preferred; however, for those patients not responding to such therapy and those receiving highly emetogenic chemotherapy, multiple-agent regimens are usually recommended.
- The treatment of simple nausea and vomiting usually requires minimal therapy. Both OTC and prescription drugs useful in the treatment of simple nausea and vomiting are usually effective in small, infrequently administered doses.
- The management of complex nausea and vomiting may require aggressive drug therapy, possibly with more than one antiemetic agent.
- For patients receiving highly emetogenic chemotherapy, antiemetic regimens may include one or more of the following agents: prochlorperazine, metoclopramide, ondansetron, granisetron, dexamethasone, or lorazepam (see section on Chemotherapy-Induced Nausea and Vomiting [CINV]).

ANTACIDS

- Single or combination OTC antacid products, especially those containing magnesium hydroxide, aluminum hydroxide, and/or calcium carbonate, may provide sufficient relief of simple nausea/vomiting, primarily through gastric acid neutralization.
- Common antacid dosage regimens for the relief of nausea and vomiting include one or more small doses of single- or multiple-agent products.

ANTIHISTAMINES, ANTICHOLINERGICS

- Antiemetic drugs from the antihistaminic–anticholinergic category may be appropriate in the treatment of simple symptomology. However, when used alone, each provides little efficacy in patients with more complex complaints such as those caused by cytotoxic chemotherapy.
- Adverse reactions that may be apparent with the use of the antihistaminic–anticholinergic agents primarily include drowsiness or confusion, blurred vision, dry mouth, urinary retention, and possibly tachycardia, particularly in elderly patients.

PHENOTHIAZINES

- Phenothiazines appear to block dopamine receptors, most likely in the CTZ.
- Rectal administration is most preferred in patients in whom parenteral administration is impractical or oral medications cannot be retained and are therefore ineffective.
- In many patients, low doses of phenothiazine drugs may not be effective, while larger doses may produce unacceptable risks.
- Phenothiazines are most useful in patients with simple nausea and vomiting or in those receiving mildly emetogenic doses of chemotherapy.
- Problems associated with these drugs include troublesome and potentially dangerous side effects, including extrapyramidal reactions, hypersensitivity reactions with possible liver dysfunction, marrow aplasia, and excessive sedation.

BUTYROPHENONE

- Two butyrophenone compounds have antiemetic activity, haloperidol and its congener droperidol.
- Preoperative doses may range from 2.5–10 mg, while dosage regimens during cytotoxic chemotherapy have been documented as low as 0.5–2.5 mg by intermittent injection to as great as 1.0–1.5 mg/h by IV infusion.
- Adverse reactions resulting from the use of the butyrophenone compounds include primarily sedation and the possibility of dystonic reactions.

CORTICOSTEROIDS

- Corticosteroids have been used successfully in the management of CINV with few problems.
- Reported adverse effects have included mood changes ranging from anxiety to euphoria as well as headache, a metallic taste in the mouth, abdominal discomfort, hyperglycemia, and itchy throat.

METOCLOPRAMIDE

- Metoclopramide, procainamide's congener, has been studied for its antiemetic effects.
- Metoclopramide increases lower esophageal sphincter tone, aids gastric emptying, and accelerates transit through the small bowel, possibly through the release of acetylcholine.
- Because the adverse reactions to metoclopramide include extrapyramidal effects, IV diphenhydramine 25–50 mg should be prophylactically administered or provided on-call for its anticipated need.

SEROTONIN ANTAGONISTS

- 5-HT_3 selective serotonin antagonists act by blocking serotonin receptors located in the area postrema and possibly vagal afferent fibers in the upper GI tract.
- Although potentially important agents for cancer patients, 5-HT_3 serotonin receptor antagonists have provided no beneficial effects in reducing motion sickness when compared with placebo.

OTHER AGENTS

- Phosphorated carbohydrate solutions (mixtures of fructose, dextrose, and phosphoric acid) are available OTC and may be administered in 15- to 30-mL doses as often as every 3 hours or as needed. This combination is safe and effective in patients with morning sickness.

CHEMOTHERAPY-INDUCED NAUSEA AND VOMITING

Droperidol

- Droperidol, usually given intravenously, has been documented as safe and effective, even in ambulatory cancer patients.

- Although the optimal antiemetic dose of droperidol for patients receiving chemotherapy is not well established, many patients benefit from small doses, particularly when combined with other antiemetic drugs.

Corticosteroids

- During therapy with mildly to moderately emetogenic agents, dexamethasone appears to be comparable to metoclopramide and superior to prochlorperazine when each is used alone; however, metoclopramide has shown greater efficacy with highly emetogenic regimens, especially those including cisplatin.
- Dexamethasone has often been administered parenterally as a single dose of 8–20 mg prior to chemotherapy, followed by oral doses of 4–12 mg up to 24 hours after completion of chemotherapy. Usually, methylprednisolone has been administered prior to chemotherapy in a dose of 250 mg. After chemotherapy, up to four subsequent doses have been given.

Metoclopramide

- Metoclopramide is commonly prescribed in multiagent combination protocols for the prevention and treatment of complex nausea and vomiting in response to chemotherapy administration, particularly cisplatin.
- Metoclopramide is given in high doses (1–2 mg/kg intravenously), with one dose administered approximately 30 minutes prior to chemotherapy. Up to four subsequent doses are given at 2-hour intervals after chemotherapy.

5-HT$_3$ Serotonin Antagonists

- Several selective 5-HT$_3$ serotonin antagonists, including ondansetron, granisetron, and tropisetron are safe and effective in the treatment of nausea and vomiting associated with cytotoxic chemotherapy and radiation therapy.
- Ondansetron is usually administered intravenously 30 minutes prior to chemotherapy at a dose of 0.15 mg/kg over 15 minutes. Similar subsequent doses are given 4 and 8 hours after the first dose.
- In adults and children at least 2 years of age, granisetron should be intravenously infused in a dose of 10 µg/kg over 5 minutes, beginning within 30 minutes before the initiation of chemotherapy, only on the day(s) chemotherapy is given.
- Some patients have experienced a reduction of efficacy with multiple-day chemotherapy or after several cycles of chemotherapy. In this situation, some clinicians recommend the addition of a corticosteroid to the regimen to increase the response rate.

Cannabinoids

- The cannabinoids are effective antiemetic agents, even in patients in whom other regimens have failed. Dronabinol, Δ-9-tetrahydrocannabinol (THC), is the major psychoactive substance present in marijuana.
- Cannabinoids are only indicated for nausea and vomiting associated with cancer chemotherapy.

- There is a strong correlation between a subjective "high" and antiemetic efficacy. Nabilone has been associated with less euphoric effects than dronabinol.
- Administration of the cannabinoids should be initiated the night before chemotherapy because failure to achieve adequate blood concentrations will likely result in vomiting.

Benzodiazepines

- Benzodiazepines (particularly lorazepam) represent the best of the therapeutic alternatives in the treatment of anticipatory nausea and vomiting. Dosage regimens include one dose before and multiple doses after each treatment with cytotoxic chemotherapy.

POSTOPERATIVE NAUSEA AND VOMITING

- A variety of pharmacologic approaches are available and may be prescribed as single or combination therapy for nausea/vomiting following an operative procedure.
- Antiemetic medications with value in the management of postoperative nausea and vomiting include promethazine, prochlorperazine, scopolamine, diphenhydramine, lorazepam, and ephedrine.
- With or without antiemetic therapy, nonpharmacologic methods (including assisting patients with movement and providing particularly close attention to adequate hydration and pain management) may be effective in reducing the potential for emesis and should be universally applied.
- Metoclopramide has been of inconsistent value for postoperative nausea and vomiting. The selective serotonin antagonists ondansetron has generally provided favorable outcomes when compared to placebo, metoclopramide, and droperidol. The true role of serotonin antagonists is presently unknown, with many clinicians preferring the use of older, more traditional and less expensive antiemetic therapy.

DISORDERS OF BALANCE

- Beneficial therapy for patients with nausea and vomiting associated with disorders of balance can reliably be found among the antihistaminic–anticholinergic agents.
- Neither the antihistaminic nor the anticholinergic potency appears to correlate well with the ability of these agents to prevent or treat the nausea and vomiting associated with motion sickness.

COMBINATION ANTIEMETIC PROTOCOLS

- The management of complex nausea and vomiting may require various combinations of from two to five antiemetic drugs.
- The primary goal of combination antiemetic regimens is to select beneficial agents that have different pharmacologic mechanisms as well as toxic effects that are not considered additive or synergistic. Combinations often include metoclopramide, diphenhydramine, and dexamethasone.

- Other agents that may be added to the regimen include droperidol, diazepam, thiethylperazine, secobarbital, pentobarbital, chlorpromazine, or prochlorperazine.
- Dexamethasone may be combined with ondansetron or granisetron.
- The ideal multiagent antiemetic protocol has not been well defined. Protocols utilizing injectable metoclopramide or a serotonin antagonist appear to have a high degree of efficacy in preventing nausea and vomiting, even in patients receiving cisplatin.

ANTIEMETIC USE DURING PREGNANCY

- Agents that have commonly been prescribed during pregnancy include phenothiazines (prochlorperazine and promethazine), the antihistaminic–anticholinergic agents (dimenhydrinate, diphenhydramine, meclizine, and scopolamine), metoclopramide, and pyridoxine.
- The efficacy of antiemetics has been questioned while the importance of other management plans (including emphasis on fluid and electrolyte management, vitamin supplements, and efforts aimed at reducing psychosomatic complaints) has been addressed.
- Presently, cyclizine and meclizine are considered the drugs of choice for the treatment of nausea and vomiting during pregnancy.
- Teratogenicity is a major consideration for the use of antiemetic drugs during pregnancy and is the primary factor that dictates the drug of choice. Of the agents commonly used, those that have demonstrated teratogenicity in animals include diphenhydramine, meclizine, prochlorperazine, and thiethylperazine; however, in humans meclizine has not been shown to have these same effects.
- Most authors currently do not recommend metoclopramide because its use during pregnancy requires further study. In addition, serotonin antagonists cannot be recommended in this setting, even though animal studies to date have revealed no harm.

NON-PHARMACOLOGIC MANAGEMENT

- Non-pharmacologic management of nausea and vomiting may include a variety of dietary, physical, or psychologic changes consistent with the etiology of symptoms.
- For patients with simple complaints, perhaps resulting from excessive or disagreeable food or beverage consumption, avoidance or moderation in dietary intake may be preferable.
- Patients suffering symptoms of systemic illness may improve dramatically as their underlying condition resolves. Finally, patients in whom these symptoms result from labyrinthine changes produced by motion may benefit quickly by assuming a stable physical position.
- Various techniques involving relaxation have been studied for anticipatory vomiting. These techniques include hypnosis, behavior modification, and guided mental imagery.

EVALUATION OF THERAPEUTIC OUTCOMES

- The etiology of a patient's nausea and vomiting determines the expected outcome of antiemetic therapy. Depending on their ability to tolerate antiemetics, symptomatic relief is often unattainable until definitive therapy can be instituted (i.e., delivery of fetus, GI surgery, correction of metabolic disorders, or removal of emetogenic agents).
- If nausea and vomiting persist despite maximal and frequent dosing of an antiemetic agent, an agent with a different mechanism of action is administered. In addition, the patient should be examined closely to elicit any signs of volume contraction and assess the need for aggressive fluid replacement.
- In accordance with the above information concerning age and clinical condition, individualized therapy is possible through drug selection and dosage adjustment.
- Monitoring criteria for drug therapy includes the subjective assessment of the severity of nausea as well as objective parameters such as the number of vomiting episodes each day, the volume of vomitus lost, and evaluation of fluid, acid–base balance, and electrolyte status, with particular attention to serum sodium, potassium, and chloride concentrations. In addition, evaluation of renal function may become important, particularly in patients with volume contraction and progressive electrolyte disturbances. Specific parameters include daily urine volume, urine specific gravity, and urine electrolyte concentrations.
- Physical assessment of patients should include evaluation of mucous membranes and skin turgor, since dryness of these tissues may be indicative of significant volume loss.

See Chapter 35, Nausea and Vomiting, authored by A. Thomas Taylor, PharmD and Eileen G. Holland, PharmD, for a more detailed discussion of this topic.

Chapter 26

▶ PANCREATITIS

▶ DEFINITION

Acute pancreatitis (AP) is an inflammatory disorder of the pancreas resulting from premature activation of proteolytic enzymes within the pancreas. It is characterized by a discrete episode of symptoms, with restoration of normal exocrine and endocrine function when the cause is removed.

Chronic pancreatitis (CP) results in functional and structural damage to the pancreas that persists after the causative factor is eliminated. The disease is often progressive and loss of pancreatic function is irreversible.

▶ EPIDEMIOLOGY

- The prevalence of pancreatitis varies in different geographic areas and depends primarily on etiologic factors. The incidence of AP in the United States is <1%, while the number of patients with CP is largely undefined.
- The overall male-to-female ratio appears to be nearly equal; however, there is an increased incidence of alcoholic pancreatitis in younger men and of gallstone-related disease in older women.

▶ PATHOPHYSIOLOGY

- The etiologic factors associated with AP are presented in Table 26.1. Ethanol abuse and gallstone-associated biliary tract disease (choledocholithiasis) together account for 60–80% of all cases; however, the frequency varies depending on the patient population and geographic location.
- A number of medications have been implicated in AP, but a causal association is difficult to confirm because ethical and practical considerations prevent rechallenge with the suspected agent.
- Table 26.2 lists drugs according to their certainty to cause AP. A definite association is based on the temporal relationship of drug administration to abdominal pain and hyperamylasemia or on a positive response to rechallenge with the offending agent. Suggestive evidence exists for drugs with a probable association, whereas evidence is inadequate or contradictory for drugs having a questionable association.

ACUTE PANCREATITIS

- The pathophysiology of AP is related to autodigestion of the pancreas as a result of premature intrapancreatic activation of proteases. Pancreatic juice contains less than 10% protein; more than 90% of the protein consists of enzymes or proenzymes secreted by the pancreatic acinar cells.

TABLE 26.1. Etiologic Factors in Acute Pancreatitis

Obstruction	Trauma
Choledocholithiasis	Accidental abdominal trauma
Pancreatic tumors	Abdominal surgery
Infection	ERCP[a]
Mumps/rubella	**Metabolic Abnormalities**
Hepatitis	Hypertriglyceridemia
Human immunodeficiency virus	Hypercalcemia
Mycoplasma	**Vascular Abnormalities**
Mycobacterium tuberculosis	Vasculitis
Toxins	Ischemia postcardiac surgery
Ethanol	
Scorpion venom	**Miscellaneous**
Organophosphorous insecticides	Crohn's disease
Medications	Cystic fibrosis
	Idiopathic Causes

[a]ERCP, endoscopic retrograde cholangiopancreatography.
Modified from Steinberg WS, Tenner S. N Engl J Med 1994;330:1198–1210.

- The four major enzyme groups are identified in Table 26.3.
- Several mechanisms may initiate enzymatic activation within the pancreas, including reflux of duodenal contents containing enterokinase, activated pancreatic enzymes, and bile salts into the pancreatic duct; disruption of the pancreatic ducts and extravasation of juice as a result of gallstone-induced ductal hypertension; and intracellular activation of proteases by lysosomal enzymes such as cathepsin B.
- The manifestations of enzymatic activation on the pancreas include inflammation, edema, and ischemia, which combine to produce a local and regional necrosis.
- When digestive enzymes enter the systemic circulation, widespread necrosis of extra-abdominal organs occurs. Vasoactive substances (histamine, prostaglandins, kinins) are released from the inflamed pancreas into the circulation causing increased vascular permeability, vasodilation, and edema.

CHRONIC PANCREATITIS

- Chronic pancreatitis results in functional and structural damage to the pancreas that persists after the causative factor is eliminated. In contrast to ethanol-induced CP, structural and functional changes may improve in obstructive CP when the obstruction is removed.
- In most individuals, CP is progressive and loss of pancreatic function is irreversible. Permanent destruction of pancreatic tissue usually leads to exocrine and endocrine insufficiency.
- Cystic fibrosis is a cause of pancreatic exocrine insufficiency in children.

TABLE 26.2. Drugs Associated with Acute Pancreatitis

Definite Association

5-Aminosalicylic acid	Metronidazole
Azathioprine	Pentamidine
Didanosine	Sulfonamides
Estrogens	Sulindac
Furosemide	Tetracycline
6-Mercaptopurine	Thiazide diuretics
Methyldopa	Valproic acid

Probable Association

Ampicillin	Corticosteroids
Asparaginase	Cytarbine
Bumetamide	Ethacrynic acid
Calcium	Phenformin
Cimetidine	Piroxicam
Chlorthalidone	Procainamide
Cisplatin	Salicylates
Clozapine	Zalcitabine
Colaspase	

Questionable Association

Acetaminophen	Isotretinoin
β-Adrenergic blockers	Ketoprofen
Amiodarone	Lipid emulsions
Amoxapine	Lisinopril
Carbamazepine	Mefenamic acid
Cholestyramine	Metolazone
Clonidine	Nitrofurantoin
Cyclosporine	Octreotide
Cyproheptadine	Opiates
Danazol	Oxyphenbutazone
Diazoxide	Phenolphthalein
Diphenoxylate	Potassium permanganate
Enalapril	Propoxyphene
Ergotamine	Rifampicin
Erythromycin	Ranitidine
Gold therapy	Roxithromycin
Ibuprofen	Sodium stibogluconate
Indomethacin	Ticarcillin/clavulanic acid
Interleukin-2	L-Tryptophan
Isoniazid	Warfarin

V

TABLE 26.3. Digestive Enzymes in the Pancreatic Acinar Cell

Proteolytic Enzymes
Trypsinogen
Chymotrypsinogen
Proelastase
Procarboxypeptidase A
Procarboxypeptidase B

Amylolytic Enzymes
Amylase

Lipolytic Enzymes
Lipase
Prophospholipase A_2
Caroboxylesterase lipase

Nucleases
Deoxyribonuclease (DNAse)
Ribonuclease (RNAse)

Others
Procolipase
Trypsin inhibitor

From Pandol SJ. In Sleisenger MH, Fordtran JS (eds): Gastrointestinal Disease: Pathophysiology/Diagnosis/Management, 5th ed. Philadelphia, WB Saunders, 1993:1587, with permission.

- Prolonged ethanol consumption is the main cause of CP in the United States, accounting for approximately 70% of all cases, while half of the remaining 30% of nonethanol cases are idiopathic.
- Infrequent causes of CP include hyperparathyroidism (and other chronic hypercalcemic states), protein-calorie malnutrition, heredity, trauma, pancreatic divisum, and obstruction of the main pancreatic duct by tumors, scars, stenosis, and pseudocysts. Although cholelithiasis may coexist with CP, gallstones rarely lead to chronic disease.

▶ CLINICAL PRESENTATION

ACUTE PANCREATITIS

- The spectrum of acute pancreatitis varies from mild, which is usually self-limiting, to severe, in which the severity of the attack correlates with the degree of the pancreatic involvement and complications.
- Typical signs and symptoms are listed in Table 26.4.
- The initial presentation ranges from mild abdominal discomfort to excruciating pain, shock, and respiratory distress. Abdominal pain, the major symptom of nearly all patients, is usually epigastric, often radiating to either of the upper quadrants or the back. The onset is usually sudden and the intensity is often described as "knifelike" or "boring."

TABLE 26.4. Clinical Findings in Acute Pancreatitis

Observation	Incidence (%)
Abdominal pain	95
Radiation of pain to back	50
Abdominal distention	75
Nausea and vomiting	80
Low-grade fever	75
Hypotension	30
Mental aberrations	25
Jaundice	20

V

Generally, the pain of AP tends to be steady and usually persists for several days.
- The gold standard for diagnosis of AP is surgical examination of the pancreas or pancreatic histology. In the absence of these procedures, the diagnosis depends on the recognition of an etiologic factor, the clinical signs and symptoms, abnormal laboratory tests, and imaging techniques that predict the severity and course of the disease.
- Laboratory Tests
  - Acute pancreatitis and its complications may be associated with leukocytosis, hyperglycemia, hypoalbuminemia, and mild hyperbilirubinemia.
  - Elevations in serum alkaline phosphatase and liver transaminases are common.
  - Dehydration may lead to hemoconcentration with elevated hemoglobin, hematocrit, blood urea nitrogen (BUN), and serum creatinine concentration.
  - Marked hypocalcemia is an indication of severe necrosis.
  - Some patients with severe pancreatitis develop thrombocytopenia and a prolongation in the prothrombin time.
  - The serum amylase concentration usually rises within 24 hours of the onset of symptoms and returns to normal over the next 3–5 days. Serum amylase elevations do not correlate with either the etiology or severity of the disease.
  - Serum lipase is specific to the pancreas and concentrations are usually elevated in AP. Serum lipase persists longer than serum amylase elevations and can be detected in the serum after the amylase has returned to normal.
  - Urine amylase is increased in AP and may be elevated for 7–10 days after serum values have returned to normal.
- The majority of patients with AP recover uneventfully. Mortality rates appear to be influenced by the etiology of the disease and whether the acute attack is an initial or recurrent episode. Patients with ethanol-

related AP appear to have a decreased mortality rate when compared to patients with pancreatitis from other causes.

- Local complications, including phlegmon (mass of inflamed pancreas containing patchy areas of necrosis), pseudocyst (fluid collections of necrotic debris, blood, and pancreatic enzymes without an epithelial lining), hemorrhage, abscess, and ascites, usually occur within 2–4 weeks after the initial attack.
- Systemic complications include shock, which is the main cause of death, hypoxia which occurs in >50% of patients, and acute respiratory distress syndrome, which usually occurs within a week after the onset of AP.

CHRONIC PANCREATITIS

- The main features of CP are abdominal pain, malabsorption, weight loss, and diabetes. Prolonged jaundice occurs in about 10% of patients. Other findings are as follows:
  - Abdominal pain is the most prominent clinical feature of CP and is classically described by many patients as dull, constant, epigastric, and radiating to the back.
  - Permanent destruction of the pancreas and obstruction of the pancreatic ducts leads to a decrease in the amount of pancreatic enzymes that reach the proximal duodenum.
  - Steatorrhea (excessive loss of fat in the feces) and azotorrhea (excessive loss of protein in the feces) are seen in the majority of patients once significant pancreatic destruction occurs.
  - Diarrhea may occur secondary to fat malabsorption.
  - Nausea, vomiting, anorexia, and weight loss are often seen in CP patients.
  - Pancreatic diabetes is usually a late manifestation commonly associated with pancreatic calcification.
- The classic triad of calcification, steatorrhea, and diabetes usually confirms the diagnosis of CP.
- Total serum amylase and the amylase-to-creatinine clearance ratio are not useful in diagnosing and monitoring the course of CP.
- The quantitative fecal fat test is of value in assessing the efficacy of pancreatic enzyme treatment.
- Imaging techniques are helpful in detecting calcification of the pancreas, other causes of pain (ductal obstruction secondary to stones, strictures, or pancreatic pseudocysts), and in differentiating CP from pancreatic cancer.
- ERCP may assist in the diagnosis and permits the identification of surgically correctable lesions.
- Patients with alcoholic CP usually present with an initial acute attack followed by successive attacks that are slower to resolve. Continued ethanol use leads to chronic abdominal pain and progressive exocrine and endocrine insufficiency.

- In 50% of patients, the pain diminishes in about 5–10 years after the onset of symptoms.
- Steatorrhea, calcification, and diabetes usually develop after 10–20 years of heavy ethanol ingestion.
- A minority of patients with CP will develop a pancreatic pseudocyst, ascites, or abscess; common bile duct obstruction leading to cholangitis or secondary biliary cirrhosis; or gastrointestinal (GI) bleeding resulting from multiple sources, including gastritis, peptic ulcer, and splenic/portal vein thrombosis.

▶ DESIRED OUTCOME

V
- The primary goal of treatment of acute pancreatitis is resolution of the inflammatory process such that patient symptoms are relieved and irreversible pancreatic damage does not occur.
- An immediate goal of therapy is to replace fluid and electrolyte losses that result from a "chemical burn" induced by the pancreatic exudate.
- The goal of treatment of uncomplicated CP is directed at the control of chronic pain and the correction of malabsorption.

▶ TREATMENT

ACUTE PANCREATITIS
General Principles
- Initial treatment should be aimed at relieving pain, minimizing complications, and preventing subsequent episodes.
- In the early phase of the attack, most patients are treated by withholding food or liquids in order to minimize exocrine stimulation of the pancreas.
- Nasogastric (NG) aspiration is beneficial in patients with profound pain, severe disease, paralytic ileus, and intractable vomiting.
- IV fluids may be required to maintain intravascular volume and blood pressure in severe pancreatitis.
- Intravenous potassium, calcium, and magnesium should be used to correct deficiency states.
- Insulin may be needed to treat hyperglycemia.
- Parenteral nutrition is indicated in patients with severe, protracted pancreatitis who are unable to tolerate enteral feedings.
- Secondary infections require the use of antibiotics and surgical intervention.
- Analgesics should be administered to reduce the severity of abdominal pain. Begin therapy with parenteral meperidine (50–100 mg) at regular intervals. Theoretically it causes less spasm of the sphincter of Oddi than other narcotic medications.

Other Treatment Principles
- In patients with mild to moderate AP, the inhibition of gastric acid secretion by antisecretory drugs does not appear to be more effective

than NG suction or withholding food when these modalities are used to diminish the pain associated with pancreatic exocrine secretion.

- The use of prophylactic antibiotics does not offer any therapeutic advantage in patients with mild to moderate ethanol-induced AP.
- There is no conclusive support for or against the use of somatostatin and its analogue octreotide in the treatment of AP.

Recommendations for Treatment of Acute Pancreatitis

- Discontinue medications listed in Table 26.2, whenever possible.
- Administer IV fluids to maintain intravascular volume and analgesics to control pain.
- Measures to reduce pancreatic secretions should be initiated.
- Nasogastric aspiration is indicated if pain is severe and if ileus or intractable vomiting are present.
- Patients with a prolonged course or severe AP should be treated with NG suction and parenteral nutrition.
- Antisecretory agents do not appear to be of benefit, but may be used to prevent stress-bleeding.
- Antibiotics should not be used in the absence of signs of infection except in patients with choledocholithiasis or when pancreatic necrosis or abscess is likely.
- Octreotide or glucagon may be tried, but their efficacy remains unproven.

CHRONIC PANCREATITIS

- In patients with ethanol-induced CP, abstinence is the most important factor in the prevention of chronic pain in the early stages of the disease.
- Small and frequent meals (six meals per day) and a diet restricted in fat (50–75 g/d) is recommended to minimize postprandial pancreatic secretion and resulting pain.
- Non-narcotic analgesics such as aspirin or acetaminophen should be tried initially, preferably before meals, to prevent postprandial exacerbation of pain.
- Frequently, severe pain relief necessitates the use of opiate analgesics. Narcotics should not be withheld because of the risk of inducing addiction. Oral agents (e.g., codeine derivatives) should be added to the non-narcotic drug regimen before parenteral narcotics are administered.
- Exogenous pancreatic enzymes may be attempted prior to narcotics.
- If all nonsurgical measures fail and severe pain continues, surgery is indicated.
- The administration of large doses of pancreatic enzymes early in the course of the disease may afford pain relief by suppressing pancreatic enzyme secretion through a negative feedback mechanism involving proteases present in the duodenum.
- If enzymes are ineffective in reducing pain after 1–2 months, the addition of an H_2 receptor antagonist (H_2RA) may enhance their efficacy.

- The standard therapy for malabsorption resulting from exocrine pancreatic insufficiency is the use of pancreatic enzyme supplements that contain lipase. The combination of enzyme supplementation and a reduction in dietary fat (to <25 g per meal) enhances the patient's nutritional status, reduces (but does not totally correct) steatorrhea, and may alleviate other symptoms. Approximately 30,000 IU of lipase and 10,000 IU of trypsin should be administered during a 4-hour postprandial period.
- Oral pancreatic enzyme supplements are available as powders, uncoated or coated tablets, capsules, enteric-coated spheres (ECS) and microspheres (ECMS), or enteric-coated microtablets (ECMT) encased in a cellulose capsule (Table 26.5). Controversy exists over the optimal dosage schedule, although the consensus is that tablets/capsules should be taken with meals.

Recommendations for Treatment of Chronic Pancreatitis

- Pain management should begin with simple analgesics such as aspirin or acetaminophen (Figure 26.1). If pain persists, the response to exoge-

TABLE 26.5. Enzyme Content of Selected Pancreatic Enzyme Preparations

Product	Dosage Form[b]	Enzyme Content (Units)[a]		
		Lipase	Amylase	Protease
Cotazym	C	8000	30,000	30,000
Cotazym-S	ECS	5000	20,000	20,000
Creon-5	ECMS	5000	16,600	18,750
Creon-10	ECMS	10,000	33,200	37,500
Creon-20	ECMS	20,000	66,400	75,000
Ku-Zyme HP	C	8000	30,000	30,000
Pancrease	ECMS	4000	20,000	25,000
Pancrease MT-4	ECMT	4000	12,000	12,000
Pancrease MT-10	ECMT	10,000	30,000	30,000
Pancrease MT-16	ECMT	16,000	48,000	48,000
Pancrease MT-20	ECMT	20,000	56,000	44,000
Ultrase MT-6	ECMT	6000	19,500	19,500
Ultrase MT-12	ECMT	12,000	39,000	39,000
Ultrase MT-18	ECMT	18,000	58,500	58,500
Ultrase MT-20	ECMT	20,000	65,000	65,000
Viokase	UCT	8000	30,000	30,000
Viokase[c]	P	16,800	70,000	70,000
Zymase	ECS	12,000	24,000	24,000

[a]All listed products contain pancrealipase. Pancrealipase contains not less than 24 USP units of lipase activity, not less than 100 USP units of amylase activity, and not less than 100 USP units of protease activity per mg.
[b]C, powder encased in a cellulose capsule; ECS, enteric-coated sphere encased in a cellulose capsule; ECMS, enteric-coated microspheres encased in a cellulose capsule; ECMT, enteric-coated microtablets encased in a cellulose capsule; UCT, uncoated tablet; P, powder.
[c]Units of 0.7 g of powder.

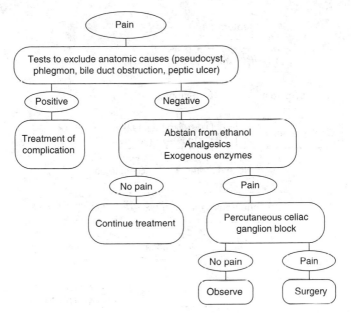

Figure 26.1. Algorithm for treatment of pain. *(Modified from DiMagno EP, Layer P, Clain JF: In Go VLW, Gardner JD, Brooks FP, et al (eds): The Pancreas: Biology, Pathobiology, and Diseases, 2nd ed. New York, Raven Press, 1993:676, with permission.)*

nous pancreatic enzymes is evaluated in patients with mild to moderate nonalcoholic pancreatitis.

- Parenteral narcotics are reserved for those patients with severe pain unresponsive to oral analgesics.
- An initial prandial dose of 30,000 IU of lipase is given with each meal; however, the lipase dose should be titrated to a reduction in steatorrhea.
- Addition of an H_2RA is reserved for those occasional patients resistant to enzyme therapy (Figure 26.2).

SURGERY

- Surgery may be necessary in AP to treat a pseudocyst or abscess or to drain the pancreatic bed if hemorrhagic or necrotic pancreatitis is present. Surgical correction of biliary tract disease may reduce the risk of recurrent episodes of AP.
- The most common indication for surgery in CP is abdominal pain refractory to medical therapy. Although the pain may diminish as the gland deteriorates, it is unreasonable that a patient wait years for spontaneous relief.

V

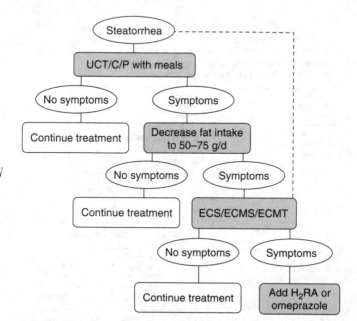

Figure 26.2. Algorithm for treatment of malabsorption. UCT, uncoated tablet; C, capsule; P, powder; ECS, enteric-coated sphere; ECMS, enteric-coated microsphere; ECMT, enteric-coated microtablet; H_2RA, H_2-receptor antagonist *(Modified from DiMagno EP, Layer P, Clain JE. In Go VLW, Gardner JD, Brooks FP, et al (eds): The Pancreas: Biology, Pathobiology, and Diseases, 2nd ed. New York, Raven Press, 1993:684, with permission.)*

- Surgical procedures that alleviate pain include a subtotal or total pancreatectomy, drainage of the pancreatic duct, or interruption of the splanchnic nerves.

See Chapter 39, Pancreatitis, authored by Rosemary R. Berardi, PharmD, FASHP and Lisa M. Henderson, PharmD, for a more detailed discussion of this topic.

Chapter 27

▶ PEPTIC ULCER DISEASE

▶ DEFINITION

Peptic ulcer disease (PUD) refers to a group of ulcerative disorders of the upper gastrointestinal (GI) tract that require acid and pepsin for their formation. Ulcers differ from superficial mucosal erosions in that they extend deeper into the muscularis mucosa.

▶ EPIDEMIOLOGY

- Approximately 10% of Americans will develop PUD during their lifetimes.
- The occurrence of PUD has been declining in young men while increasing in women.
- Since 1960, ulcer-related hospitalizations, operations, and deaths in the United States have declined.
- PUD remains one of the most common GI diseases.

▶ PATHOPHYSIOLOGY

- The pathogenesis of duodenal (DU) and gastric ulcer (GU) is multifactorial and most likely reflects a combination of pathophysiologic abnormalities, environmental, and genetic factors.
- Most peptic ulcers occur in the presence of acid and pepsin when *Helicobacter pylori* (HP), NSAIDs, or other possible factors disrupt normal mucosal defense and healing mechanisms. Factors responsible for acid hypersecretion include increased parietal cell mass, increased basal secretory drive [high basal acid output/maximal acid output (BAO/MAO) ratio], and increased postprandial secretory drive.
- A strong association exists between HP (formerly *Campylobacter pylori*) and PUD. Virtually all patients with DU and GU who are not taking NSAIDs have evidence of HP infection and antral gastritis.
- HP may cause ulcer by impairing mucosal defense by elaboration of toxins and enzymes, or increasing antral gastrin release which leads to increased acidity.
- There is overwhelming evidence linking chronic NSAID (including aspirin) use and gastroduodenal ulcers. Chronic NSAID therapy produces gastroduodenal injury by two mechanisms: a direct action on the mucosa and a systemic effect whereby endogenous prostaglandin synthesis is inhibited.
- The association between adrenocorticoids and PUD remains controversial.

- Cigarette smoking increases the risk for the development and recurrence of DU and GU, and the risk appears to be proportional to the amount smoked.
- Although clinical observation supports the belief that ulcer patients are adversely affected by stressful life events, controlled studies have failed to document a cause-and-effect relationship.
- The causal association between specific dietary substances and PUD has not been substantiated. Ethanol may cause acute gastric mucosal damage, but is not clearly the cause of ulcers.

▶ CLINICAL PRESENTATION

V
- Patients with a PUD usually present with dyspeptic symptoms such as nausea, vomiting, belching, and bloating in addition to heartburn or epigastric pain.
- Epigastric pain is the classic and most frequent symptoms of peptic ulcer disease. The pain is often described as burning but can present as a vague discomfort, abdominal fullness, or cramping (Table 27.1). Many patients with DU describe a typical nocturnal pain that awakens them at night.

TABLE 27.1. Clinical Features of Gastric and Duodenal Ulcer[a]

Feature	Gastric Ulcer	Duodenal Ulcer
Pain	+ + + +	+ + + +
Epigastric	+ + +	+ + + +
Frequently severe	+ + +	+ + +
Radiation to back	+ +	+ +
Episodic (clusters)	+	+ + +
Nocturnal	+ + +	+ + + +
Within 30 minutes of food	+ +	+
Food relief	+ +	+ + +
Relieved by antacids	+ + + +	+ + + +
Anorexia	+ + +	+ +
Weight loss	+ + +	+ +
Nausea	+ + + +	+ + +
Vomiting	+ + + +	+ + +
Heartburn	+	+ + +
Bloating	+ + +	+ + +
Belching	+ + +	+ + +
Ulcer recurrence	+ + +	+ + + +

[a]Frequencies represent estimates and are categorized as being consistent (+ + + +), frequent (+ + +), infrequent (+ +), or rare (+). None of the features is always present or always absent.

- The severity of symptoms varies from patient to patient and, in some patients, symptoms may be seasonal, occurring more frequently in the spring or fall.
- Patients consuming NSAIDs and the elderly are often symptom free prior to bleeding or perforation.
- Nausea, vomiting, anorexia, and weight loss are more common in patients with GU.
- The physical examination usually reveals epigastric tenderness which occurs between the umbilicus and the xiphoid process and less commonly radiates to the back.
- The natural history of PUD is characterized by periods of exacerbations and remissions. Most ulcers will eventually heal on their own, but the healing process is accelerated with treatment.

V

▶ DIAGNOSIS

- Routine laboratory tests are not helpful in establishing a diagnosis of uncomplicated PUD.
- The hematocrit, hemoglobin, and stool hemoccult tests are used to detect bleeding.
- The diagnosis of HP can be made using invasive or noninvasive tests. The invasive methods require upper GI endoscopy with a mucosal biopsy taken for histology, culture, gram stain, or detection of urease activity. The ^{13}C and ^{14}C urea breath tests are noninvasive methods that require that patients ingest radiolabeled urea, which, in the presence of urease, forms ammonia and radiolabeled bicarbonate.
- The diagnosis of PUD depends on visualizing the ulcer crater. DU should be distinguished from other acid-peptic diseases, and benign GU must be distinguished from those that are malignant. Therefore, the diagnosis depends on radiologic or endoscopic findings. Fiber optic endoscopy detects more than 90% of peptic ulcers.

▶ DESIRED OUTCOME

The ultimate goals of PUD treatment are relief of ulcer pain, acceleration of ulcer healing, reduction of ulcer recurrence, and ulcer-related complications.

▶ TREATMENT

GENERAL PRINCIPLES

- The patient should stop or reduce smoking.
- Treatment can be initiated with either an H_2 receptor antagonist (H_2RA), sucralfate, or a proton pump inhibitor (PPI). Therapy with an H_2RA or sucralfate usually is continued for 6–8 weeks, while therapy with a PPI usually is continued for 4 weeks (Figure 27.1).

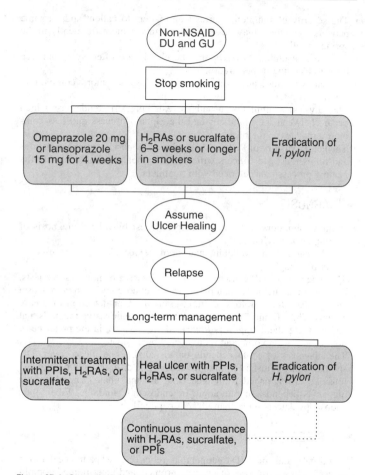

Figure 27.1. Strategies for managing non-NSAID duodenal and gastric ulcers. *(Modified from Freston JW. Scand J Gastroenterol 1994;29:(suppl 201):51.)*

- In patients with GU, treatment with and H_2RA (8 weeks) or PPI (4 weeks), should be initiated.
- The H_2RAs (cimetidine, famotidine, nizatidine, and ranitidine), PPIs (omeprazole and lansoprazole), sucralfate, and antacids are all effective in healing peptic ulcers but do not alter the underlying ulcer diathesis.
- H_2RAs can be used in single daily dose (bedtime) regimens (Table 27.2).

TABLE 27.2. Oral Antiulcer Drug Treatment Regimens[a]

Drug	DU Healing (mg/dose)	GU Healing (mg/dose)	DU Maintenance (mg/dose)	GU Maintenance (mg/dose)
H₂ Receptor Antagonists				
Cimetidine	300 qid	300 qid	400 hs	400 hs
	400 bid	800 hs		
	800 hs			
Famotidine	20 bid	20 bid[a]	20 hs	20 hs[a]
	40 hs	40 hs		
Nizatidine	150 bid	150 bid	150 hs	150 hs[a]
	300 hs	300 hs		
Ranitidine	150 bid	150 bid	150 hs	150 hs[a]
	300 hs	300 hs[a]		
Proton Pump Inhibitors				
Omeprazole	20 qd	20 qd[a]		
Lansoprazole	15 qd	15 qd		
Enhances Mucosal Defense				
Sucralfate[b]	1 qid	1 qid[a]	1 bid	1 bid[a]
	2 bid[a]	2 bid[a]		

[a]Not a Food and Drug Administration (FDA)-approved indication/dose regimen.
[b]Dose = (g/dose).

- Famotidine and nizatidine will pose fewer drug interactions with drugs metabolized by the hepatic P-450 enzymes compared with cimetidine.
- PPIs heal DU and GU more rapidly than conventional doses of H₂RAs.
- Anti-HP treatment should be instituted in HP positive patients. There is a strong belief among most gastroenterologists that all patients with non-NSAID-induced DU or GU should be initially treated with one of the more effective anti-HP regimens, although the optimal regimen has not been identified (Tables 27.3 and 27.4). A 2-week course of clarithromycin and either a PPI or ranitidine bismuth citrate permits almost all DU to heal and affords a cure of about 80%. A one-week course of metronidazole, clarithromycin or amoxicillin and a PPI also provides excellent eradication rates and ulcer healing.
- Patients who do not warrant anti-HP therapy include those with mild disease, the elderly or those who may not tolerate the antimicrobials, patients with a history of bleeding or perforation, those with NSAID-induced ulcers, and patients with Zollinger-Ellison syndrome.

▶ LONG-TERM STRATEGIES

- If symptoms persist or recur after initial treatment (regardless of the initial ulcer-healing regimen), a second course of antiulcer therapy should be instituted.

TABLE 27.3. *Helicobacter Pylori* Eradication Rates with Single Agents and Combination Therapy

Regimen	Eradication Rate (%)[a]
Monotherapy	
Bismuth subsalicylate, antibiotics (most), ciprofloxacin, or H$_2$-receptor antagonists (H$_2$RA), proton pump inhibitors alone	0–10
Colloidal bismuth subcitrate, amoxicillin, erythromycin base, or furazolidone alone	10–40
Clarithromycin	40–60
One Antimicrobial Plus an Antisecretory Agent	
Amoxicillin + PPI	30–90
Clarithromycin + PPI	70–90
Two Antimicrobials Plus an Antisecretory Agent	
Bismuth + amoxicillin + H$_2$RA	30–60
Bismuth + metronidazole + H$_2$RA	30–75
Metronidazole + amoxicillin + H$_2$RA	55–90
Metronidazole + clarithromycin + PPI	90–95
Metronidazole + amoxicillin + PPI	90–95
Three Antimicrobials Plus an Antisecretory Agent	
Bismuth + metronidazole + tetracycline + H$_2$RA	90–95
Bismuth + metronidazole + amoxicillin + H$_2$RA	80–90
Bismuth + metronidazole + tetracycline + PPI	>95

[a]Eradication rates are dependent on individual drug doses and duration of therapy.

- High-risk patients who relapse early (within 3–6 months of ulcer healing) or frequently (two or more relapses per year) after ulcer healing and those with a history of ulcer complications or multiple risk factors may be placed on continuous maintenance therapy.
- Low-dose therapy with an H$_2$RA, sucralfate, or possibly a PPI keeps a majority of ulcers healed and patients symptom free.

▶ EVALUATION OF THERAPEUTIC OUTCOMES

- Patients should be monitored for symptomatic relief of ulcer pain as well as potential adverse effects and drug interactions related to drug therapy.
- Most patients with uncomplicated PUD will be rendered symptom-free after appropriate treatment with any one of the recommended antiulcer regimens. Symptoms, however, cannot be used to guide therapeutic decisions in patients taking NSAIDs.
- Follow-up endoscopy to determine if ulcers or HP are present can be justified in patients with frequent symptomatic recurrence, refractory dis-

TABLE 27.4. Drug Regimens Frequently Used in the Treatment of *Helicobacter Pylori*-Associated Peptic Ulcer Disease[a]

Regimen	Drug
1.	Bismuth subsalicylate 525 mg qid × 2 weeks Metronidazole 250 mg tid/qid × 2 weeks Tetracycline/Amoxicillin 500 mg qid × 2 weeks H₂RA (e.g., ranitidine 300 mg/d) × 4–6 weeks
2.	Bismuth subsalicylate 525 mg qid × 2 weeks Metronidazole 500 mg qid × 1 week Tetracycline/Amoxicillin 500 mg qid × 1 week PPI (e.g., omeprazole 20 mg bid) × 1 week
3.	Metronidazole 500 mg bid × 1 week Omeprazole 20 mg bid × 1 week Clarithromycin 250–500 mg bid × 1 week Metronidazole 500 mg tid × 12–14 days H₂RA (e.g., ranitidine 300 mg/d) × 6–10 weeks
4.	Omeprazole 20 mg bid × 2 weeks then 20 mg/day × 2 weeks Amoxicillin 1 g bid or 500 mg qid × 2 weeks
5.	Omeprazole 20 mg bid × 2 weeks; then 20 mg/day × 2 weeks Clarithromycin 1000–1500 mg/d × 2 weeks
6.	Metronidazole 500 mg bid × 1 week Omeprazole 20 mg bid × 1 week Amoxicillin 250–500 mg bid × 1 week

[a]Selection of a specific treatment regimen should take into account drug efficacy/resistance, compliance, adverse effects, and cost.

case, complications, or suspected hypersecretory states. Alternatively, the urea breath test can be performed to confirm eradication of HP.
• A second course of therapy should be considered in patients with recurrent disease.

See Chapter 32, Peptic Ulcer Disease and Zollinger–Ellison Syndrome, authored by Rosemary R. Berardi, PharmD, FASHP, for a more detailed discussion of this topic.

Gynecologic and Obstetric Disorders
Edited by Barbara G. Wells, PharmD, FASHP, FCCP

Chapter 28

► CONTRACEPTION

► EFFECTIVENESS

- Failure inherent in the proper use of the contraceptive alone is called a "method failure" or "perfect use failure." "User failure" or "typical use failure" takes into account inaccuracies in the user's abilities to follow directions, such as skipping an oral contraceptive pill (Table 28.1).

► HORMONAL METHODS OF CONTRACEPTION

COMPOSITION AND FORMULATIONS

- Estrogens and/or progestins inhibit ovulation and alter cervical mucous and the endometrium by suppressing the production of follicle-stimulating hormone (FSH) and the lutenizing hormone (LH) surge.
- The progestin-only "minipill" is generally used for women who have contraindications or intolerance to estrogens, smokers older than 35 years of age, and women who are breast feeding, as it is less effective than the combination pill and is associated with irregular bleeding and increased frequency of functional ovarian cysts.
- Mestranol is considered to be 50% less potent than ethinyl estradiol (EE). Mestranol is converted to EE, which is pharmacologically active, in the liver.
- Progestins vary in progestational, estrogenic, antiestrogenic, and androgenic activity.
- The composition and activity of oral contraceptives (OCs) are shown in Table 28.2.

CONSIDERATIONS WITH ORAL CONTRACEPTIVE USE

- Absolute and relative contraindications to the use of OCs are shown in Tables 28.3 and 28.4. Guidelines for use of OCs in patients with selected medical problems are shown in Table 28.5.
- Generally, OCs are an acceptable form of birth control for women younger than 50 years of age who do not smoke.
- Patients who may benefit from OC use include those at risk for pelvic inflammatory disease and those with ovarian cysts, benign breast disease, or severe dysmenorrhea.
- When an OC is prescribed for a patient with a history of glucose intolerance, a product containing one of the new progestins (i.e., desogestrel or norgestimate) or a low dose of a norethindrone-type progestin is recommended.

TABLE 28.1. Comparison of Reversible Methods of Contraceptives

| | | | | Failure Rates (%)[a] | |
				Perfect Use	Typical Use
Method	Contraindications	Advantages	Disadvantages		
Episodic Contraceptive Methods					
Spermicides alone	Allergy to spermicide Abnormal vaginal anatomy	Inexpensive No office visit required Some protection against STDs	May enhance HIV transmission High user failure rate Must be reapplied before each act of intercourse May cause local irritation in either partner	6	21
Condoms, male	Allergy to latex	Inexpensive Readily available STD protection, including HIV (latex only) No office visit required	Poor acceptance Possibility of breakage Efficacy decreased by oil-based lubricants Latex can cause allergic reactions in either partner	3	12
Condoms, female (Reality)	Allergy to polyurethane Hx of toxic shock syndrome (?)	Stronger than latex STD protection, including HIV Protects outside the vagina and base of penis Not affected by oil-based lubricants No office visit required Can be inserted up to 8 hours before intercourse	Dislike ring hanging outside vagina Cumbersome	5	21

VI

331

TABLE 28.1. continued

Method	Contraindications	Advantages	Disadvantages	Failure Rates (%)[a]	
				Perfect Use	Typical Use
Sponge	Allergy to spermicide Hx of toxic shock syndrome	Moderate cost No office visit required Can be inserted just before intercourse or ahead of time; provides protection for 24 hours	Decreased efficacy with parity Difficulty in removal Causes vaginal dryness Increased incidence of vaginal yeast and UTI infections Increased incidence of toxic shock syndrome USA manufacturer stopped production in early 1995	20 (parous) 9 (nulliparous)	36 (parous) 18 (nulliparous)
Diaphragm with spermicide	Allergy to rubber or spermicide Recurrent UTIs Hx of toxic shock syndrome Abnormal gynecologic anatomy	Low cost Decreased incidence of cervical neoplasia STD protection, including HIV Can be inserted up to 6 hours before intercourse	Office visit required Decreased efficacy with increased frequency of intercourse Increased incidence of vaginal yeast and UTI infections Increased incidence of toxic shock syndrome Efficacy affected by oil-based lubricants Cervical irritation	6	18
Cervical cap (Prentif)	Allergy to rubber or spermicide Hx of toxic shock syndrome Abnormal gynecologic anatomy Abnormal Pap smear	Low cost STD protection, including HIV Can be inserted just before intercourse or ahead of time; provides protection for 48 hours	Office visit required May be difficult for patient to use correctly Decreased efficacy with parity Not possible to fit all patients	26 (parous) 9 (nulliparous)	36 (parous) 18 (nulliparous)

Hormonal Methods

Method	Contraindications	Advantages	Disadvantages		
OCPs	Hepatic adenomas Thromboembolic disorders or history thereof Cerebrovascular or coronary artery disease Known or suspected breast cancer Undiagnosed abnormal gynecologic bleeding Cardiovascular risk factors (relative contraindication) Jaundice with pregnancy or previous pill use	Decreased menstrual flow Decreased menstrual cramping Decreased rate of ectopic pregnancy Decreased rate of PID (except chlamydia) Protection against ovarian and endometrial cancer Protection against iron deficiency anemia, fibrocystic breast disease, and ovarian cysts	Increased risk of benign hepatocellular adenomas Mild increased risk of thromboembolism and stroke Increased elevation of blood pressure No protection against most STDs Estrogenic side effects (nausea, breast tenderness, fluid retention) Progestogen side effects (acne, increased appetite, depression) Increased risk of myocardial infarction in older smokers, nausea, headache, depression	0.1	3
Progestin-only OCPs	Undiagnosed abnormal gynecologic bleeding	May be used by lactating women and women with cardiovascular risk Allows avoidance of estrogen-related side effects Protection against PID, iron deficiency anemia, and dysmenorrhea	Frequent spotting/amenorrhea Increased risk of ectopic pregnancy Must take every day at the same time	0.5	3
Norplant (Levonorgestrel)	Undiagnosed abnormal gynecologic bleeding Acute liver disease Hx of MI, cerebrovascular accident or breast cancer Active thrombophlebitis or pulmonary emboli Relative contraindications: diabetes mellitus, migraine, epilepsy, depression, gallbladder or kidney disease, predisposition to SBE	Passive contraception Effective for 5 years Effects are quickly reversible Less menstrual cramping/mittelschmerz pain No suppression of lactation No metabolic disturbances	Requires outpatient surgical procedure Irregular menstrual bleeding, headaches, weight gain, acne Progestin side effects Local infection or bruising on insertion; removal may be difficult Expensive initially High discontinuation rate Unacceptable in patients using some anticonvulsants	0.09	0.09

VI

TABLE 28.1. continued

				Failure Rates (%)[a]	
Method	Contraindications	Advantages	Disadvantages	Perfect Use	Typical Use

Hormonal Methods (cont.)

Depo-Provera

Contraindications:
Breast cancer
Liver disease
Thrombophlebitis
Undiagnosed abnormal gynecologic bleeding

Advantages:
No suppression of lactation
No increased risk of thromboembolism
Passive contraception
No drug interactions
May decrease seizures
Effective for 3 months

Disadvantages:
Irregular menstrual bleeding, headache, weight gain, acne
Possible increased risk of breast cancer in younger users
Decreased HDL
Progestin side effects
Decreased bone density in long term users
Office visit required

Perfect Use: 0.3
Typical Use: 0.3

**Intrauterine Devices
(Hormonal and Nonhormonal)**

Copper-T 380
(Paragard)

Contraindications:
Multiple sexual partners/ partner with multiple partners (high risk for STDs)
Hx of PID or ectopic pregnancy, acute pelvic infection
Abnormal uterine cavity/pelvic surgery/undiagnosed vaginal bleeding
Uterine or cervical cancer
Postpartum endometritis or infected abortion in previous 3 months

Advantages:
Passive contraception
Long-term contraception (can remain in place up to 10 years)
Less expensive per year and easier for some patients

Disadvantages:
Increased fertility rate after removal
Increased heavy bleeding
Spotting between periods
Increased cramping and dysmenorrhea
Increased risk of ectopic pregnancy
Office visit required
Rarely uterine perforation

			%[a]
Progesterone T (Progestasert)	Acute cervicitis or vaginitis, (including BV) until infection controlled Conditions associated with increased susceptibility to infections, including leukemia, AIDS, IV drug abuse, and corticosteroid use	Remains in place for 1 year Decreased cramping and dysmenorrhea Decrease in menstrual blood loss	Office visit required Must be changed each year Increased risks of ectopic pregnancy Rarely uterine perforation	<2
Levonorgestrel IUD	Valvular heart disease (+/-) Nulliparity (+/-) Genital actinomyces Wilson's disease Allergy to copper	Constant rate of hormone release for 5 years Possibly, the single most effective reversible contraceptive method over 5-year period Decreased cramping and dysmenorrhea Reduces incidence of PID and menorrhagia Combines benefits of Norplant and Copper-T	Office visit required Irregular menstrual bleeding (?) Rarely uterine perforation	<2

[a]% failure during first year of use.
[b]Contraindicated with Copper-T IUD.

VI

TABLE 28.2. Composition and Activity of Commonly Prescribed Oral Contraceptives[a]

Product	Composition				Relative Activities			
	Estrogen	µg	Progestin	mg	Estrogenic	Progestational	Androgenic	Spotting & BTB[b] (%)
50 µg Estrogen								
Ovral	E. estradiol	50	Norgestrel	0.5	+++	+++	++	4.5
Norlestrin 2.5/50	E. estradiol	50	Nor. acetate	2.5	+	++++	++++	5.1
Genora/Norethin/Norinyl/ Ortho-Novum 1/50	Mestranol	50	Norethindrone	1.0	++	++	++	10.6
Ovcon 50	E. estradiol	50	Norethindrone	1.0	+++	+++	++	11.9
Demulen 50	E. estradiol	50	Ethy. diacetate	1.0	++	+++	++	13.9
Norlestrin 1/50	E. estradiol	50	Nor. acetate	1.0	+++	+++	+++	13.6
Sub 50 µg Estrogen Monophasic								
Lo-Ovral	E. estradiol	30	Norgestrel	0.3	++	++	++	9.6
Desogen/Ortho-Cept	E. estradiol	30	Desogestrel	0.15	++	+++	+	9.9
Ovcon 35	E. estradiol	35	Norethindrone	0.4	+++	+	+	11.0
Levlen/Nordette/Min-Ovral[c]	E. estradiol	30	Levonorgestrel	0.15	++	++	++	14.0
Ortho-Cyclen	E. estradiol	35	Norgestimate	0.25	+++	+	+	14.3
Brevicon/Modicon/Nelova 0.5/35 Brevicon/Ortho 0.5/35[c]	E. estradiol	35	Norethindrone	0.5	+++	+	+	14.6
Genora/Nelova/Norethin/Norinyl/ Ortho-Novum 1/35 Ortho 1/35[c]	E. estradiol	35	Norethindrone	1.0	+++	+++	++	14.7
Loestrin 1.5/30	E. estradiol	30	Nor. acetate	1.5	+	++++	++	25.2
Loestrin/Minestrin[c] 1/20	E. estradiol	20	Nor. acetate	1.0	+	+++	+++	29.7
Demulen 1/35	E. estradiol	35	Ethy. diacetate	1.0	+	+++	++	37.4

VI

Sub 50 µg Estrogen Multiphasic[d]

Ortho Novum 7/7/7	E. estradiol	35(7)	Norethindrone	0.5(7)	+++	++	12.2
	E. estradiol	35(7)	Norethindrone	0.75(7)			
	E. estradiol	35(7)	Norethindrone	1.0(7)			
Jenest	E. estradiol	35(7)	Norethindrone	0.5(7)	++	++	14.1
	E. estradiol	35(14)	Norethindrone	1.0(14)			
Tri-Levlen/TriPhasil	E. estradiol	30(6)	Levonorgestrel	.05(6)	++	+	15.1
Triquilar[c]	E. estradiol	40(5)	Levonorgestrel	.075(5)			
	E. estradiol	30(10)	Levonorgestrel	.125(10)			
Tri-Norinyl	E. estradiol	35(7)	Norethindrone	.5(7)	+++	++	14.7
Synphasic[c]	E. estradiol	35(9)	Norethindrone	1.0(9)			
	E. estradiol	35(7)	Norethindrone	.5(5)			
Tri-Cyclen	E. estradiol	35(7)	Norgestimate	0.180(7)	++	+	17.5
	E. estradiol	35(7)	Norgestimate	0.215(7)			
	E. estradiol	35(7)	Norgestimate	0.250(7)			
Ortho Novum 10-11	E. estradiol	35(10)	Norethindrone	0.5(10)	+++	++	19.6
	E. estradiol	35(11)	Norethindrone	1.0(11)			
Progestin Only							
Ovrette	none		Norgestrel	0.075	—	+	34.9
Micronor/Nor Q.D.	none		Norethindrone	0.35	—	+	42.3

Key: E. estradiol, ethinyl estradiol; Ethy. diacetate, ethynodiol diacetate; Nor. acetate, norethindrone acetate; BTB, breakthrough bleeding; +, very low; ++, low; +++, moderate; ++++, high; +++++, very high.

[a] Oral contraceptives containing greater than 50 µg of estrogen are not included in this chart. These products are generally not necessary to prevent conception and are associated with an increase in serious complications. Women who may need to use the higher strength estrogen include women who have had a contraceptive failure while *properly* taking a product containing 50 µg of estrogen, women who are concomitantly taking a medication which decreases the efficacy of the estrogen or in women who have severe acne. The higher dose estrogen products are also used to treat other conditions such as ovarian cysts, endometriosis, and dysfunctional uterine bleeding.

[b] Reported prevalence of breakthrough bleeding (BTB) and spotting in the third cycle of use. Information should not be precisely compared.

[c] Canadian trade name.

[d] Number in parentheses indicates number of tablets (days) in each phase.

VI

337

TABLE 28.3. Absolute Contraindications to the Use of Oral Contraception

1. Thrombophlebitis, thromboembolic disorders, cerebral vascular disease, coronary occlusion, or a past history of these conditions, or conditions predisposing to these problems.

2. Markedly impaired liver function. Steroid hormones are contraindicated in patients with hepatitis until liver function tests return to normal.

3. Known or suspected breast cancer.

4. Undiagnosed abnormal vaginal bleeding.

5. Known or suspected pregnancy.

6. Smokers over the age of 35.

From Speroff L, Darney P. A Clinical Guide for Contraception. Baltimore, Williams & Wilkins, 1992:70–71, with permission.

VI

- Generally, synthetic progestins decrease high-density lipoprotein (HDL) and increase low-density lipoprotein (LDL). Estrogens have the opposite effect. Studies of low-dose estrogen-progestin formulations found no adverse alterations in levels of HDL, LDL, or total cholesterol. Triphasic products with norgestrel may lower HDL.
- The increased incidence of venous and arterial cardiovascular disease, including myocardial infarction, is believed to be the result of thrombosis, not atherosclerosis. Venous thrombosis and pulmonary embolism appear to be directly related to the dose of estrogen. Both thrombotic and hemorrhagic stroke are associated with OC use. Myocardial infarction primarily occurs in OC users who have additional risk factors for cardiovascular disease (e.g., cigarette smoking, advancing age).

SELECTING AN ORAL CONTRACEPTIVE

- Most clinicians routinely prescribe a combination OC that possesses hormonal activity equivalent to 50 μg or less of EE.
- Women with a history of migraine, heavy menstrual cramps, or severe nausea during pregnancy may be estrogen-sensitive and may benefit from an OC containing a very low dose of estrogen. However, she should be cautioned that spotting may occur and that missed pills could result in breakthrough ovulation.
- Women with a history of weight gain, tiredness, varicose veins, or toxemia during pregnancy may be progestin-sensitive and may benefit from an OC with low progestational activity.
- Women with a history of irregular heavy menses, oily skin, hirsutism, and acne may be androgen-sensitive and may benefit from a pill with high progestational and low androgenic activity.
- Women taking anticonvulsants may have more effective contraception with an OC containing greater estrogenic activity; however, other forms of contraception are strongly recommended.
- OCs should be stopped immediately if serious symptoms occur (e.g., loss of vision; diplopia; papilledema; unilateral numbness, weakness, or

TABLE 28.4. Relative Contraindications to the Use of OCs Requiring Clinical Judgment and Informed Consent

1. Migraine headaches. In retrospective studies of high-dose pills, migraine headaches have been associated with an increased risk of stroke, however some women report an improvement in their headaches.

2. Hypertension. A woman under 35 who is otherwise healthy and whose blood pressure is controlled by medication can elect to use oral contraception.

3. Uterine leiomyoma. This is no longer a contraindication with the low-dose formulations. There is evidence that the risk of leiomyomas is decreased by 31% in women who used higher dose oral contraception for 10 years.

4. Gestational diabetes. Low-dose formulations do not produce a diabetic glucose tolerance response in women with previous gestational diabetes, and there is no evidence that oral contraception increases the incidence of overt diabetes mellitus. We believe that women with previous gestational diabetes can use oral contraception with annual assessment of the fasting glucose level.

5. Elective surgery. The recommendation that oral contraception should be discontinued 4 weeks before elective surgery to avoid an increased risk of postoperative thrombosis is based on data derived from high-dose pills. If possible, it is safer to follow this recommendation, but it is probably less critical with low-dose oral contraceptives. It is more prudent to maintain contraception right up to the performance of a sterilization procedure, and this short, outpatient operation probably carries very minimal risk.

6. Epilepsy. Oral contraceptives do not exacerbate epilepsy, and in some women, improvement in seizure control has occurred. Antiepileptic drugs, however, may decrease the effectiveness of oral contraception.

7. Obstructive jaundice in pregnancy. Not all patients with this history will develop jaundice on oral contraception, especially with the low-dose formulations.

8. Sickle cell disease or sickle C disease. Patients with sickle cell trait can use oral contraception. The risk of thrombosis in women with sickle cell disease or sickle C diseases is theoretical (and medical-legal). We believe effective protection against pregnancy in these patients warrants the use of low-dose oral contraception.

0. Diabetes mellitus. Effective prevention of pregnancy outweighs the small risk in diabetic women who are under age 35 and otherwise healthy.

10. Gallbladder disease.

From Speroff L, Darney P. A Clinical Guide for Contraception. Baltimore, Williams & Wilkins, 1992:70–71, with permission.

tingling; severe pains in chest, left arm, or neck; hemoptysis; severe pains, tenderness or swelling, warmth, or palpable cord in legs; slurring of speech; hepatic mass or tenderness).

DRUG INTERACTIONS

- Table 28.6 shows a summary of clinically significant drug interactions.

PATIENT INSTRUCTIONS

- If the patient forgets to take one pill, instruct her to take it as soon as she remembers. If she does not remember to take the pill until the next

TABLE 28.5. OC Use and Medical Problems

Gestational Diabetes. There is no contraindication to oral contraceptive use following gestational diabetes.

Diabetes Mellitus. Oral contraception can be used by diabetic women less than 35 years old, who do not smoke and are otherwise healthy (especially an absence of diabetic vascular complications).

Hypertension. Low-dose oral contraception can be used in women less than 35 years old with hypertension controlled by medication, and who are otherwise healthy and do not smoke.

Pregnancy-Induced Hypertension. Women with pregnancy-induced hypertension can use oral contraception as soon as the blood pressure is normal in the postpartum period.

Gallbladder Disease. Oral contraception use may precipitate a symptomatic attack in women known to have stones or a positive history for gallbladder disease, and therefore, should either be used very cautiously or not at all.

Obesity. An obese woman who is otherwise healthy can use low-dose oral contraception.

Hepatic Disease. Oral contraception can be utilized when liver function tests return to normal. Follow-up liver function tests should be obtained after 2–3 months of use.

Seizure Disorders. There is no impact of oral contraceptives on pattern or frequency of seizures. The concern is that anticonvulsant-induced hepatic enzyme activity can increase the risk of contraceptive failure. Some clinicians advocate the use of higher dose (50 μg estrogen) products.

Mitral Valve Prolapse. Oral contraception use is limited to patients who have only the echocardiographic diagnosis and are free of the clinical findings of mitral regurgitation.

Systemic Lupus Erythematosus. Oral contraceptive use can exacerbate systemic lupus erythematosus, and the vascular disease associated with lupus represents a contraindication to estrogen-containing oral contraceptives. The progestin-only methods can be considered.

Migraine Headaches. Low-dose oral contraception can be tried with careful surveillance. Daily administration can prevent menstrual migraine headaches.

Sickle Cell Disease. Patients with sickle cell trait can use oral contraception. The risk of thrombosis in women with sickle cell disease or sickle C diseases is theoretical (and medical-legal). We believe effective protection against pregnancy in these patients warrants the use of low-dose oral contraception.

Benign Breast Disease. Benign breast disease is not a contraindication for oral contraception; with 2 years of use, the condition can improve.

Congenital Heart Disease or Valvular Heart Disease. Oral contraception is contraindicated only if there is marginal cardiac reserve or a condition that predisposes to thrombosis.

Hyperlipidemia. Because low-dose oral contraceptives have negligible impact on the lipoprotein profile, hyperlipidemia is not a contraindication, with the exception of very high levels of triglycerides (which can be made worse by oral contraception). Of course, if vascular disease is already present, oral contraception should be avoided.

Depression. Low-dose oral contraceptives have minimal, if any, impact on mood.

Smoking. Oral contraception is absolutely contraindicated in smokers over the age of 35. In patients 35 years old and less, heavy smoking (15 or more cigarettes per day) is a relative contraindication. The data indicate no increased risk of dying of a cardiovascular event in smokers under the age of 30. An ex-smoker should be regarded as a nonsmoker. Risk is only linked to active smoking.

Pituitary Prolactin-Secreting Adenomas. Low-dose oral contraception can be used in the presence of microadenomas.

Infectious Mononucleosis. Oral contraception can be used as long as liver function tests are normal.

Ulcerative Colitis. There is no association between oral contraception and ulcerative colitis; women with this problem can use oral contraceptives. Oral contraceptives are absorbed mainly in the small bowel.

From Speroff L, Darney P. A Clinical Guide for Contraception. Baltimore, Williams & Wilkins, 1992:80–82, with permission.

VI

TABLE 28.6. Pill Interactions with Other Drugs

Interacting Drugs	Adverse Effects (Probable Mechanism)	Comments and Recommendations
Acetaminophen (Tylenol and others)	Possible decreased pain-relieving effect (increased metabolism)	Monitor pain-relieving response
Alcohol	Possible increased effect of alcohol	Use with caution
Anticoagulants (oral)	Decreased anticoagulant effect	Use alternative contraceptive
Antidepressants (Elavil, Norpramin, Tofranil, and others)	Possible increased antidepressant effect	Monitor antidepressant concentration
Barbiturates (phenobarbital and others)	Decreased contraceptive effect	Avoid simultaneous use; use alternative contraceptive for epileptics
Benzodiazepine tranquilizers (Ativan, Librium, Serax, Tranxene, Valium, Xanax, and others)	Possible increased or decreased tranquilizer effects including psychomotor impairment	Use with caution Greatest impairment during menstrual pause in oral contraceptive dosage
Beta blockers (Corgard, Inderal, Lopressor, Tenormin)	Possible increased blocker effect	Monitor cardiovascular status
Carbamazepine (Tegretol)	Possible decreased contraceptive effect	Use alternative contraceptive
Corticosteroids (cortisone)	Possible increased corticosteroid toxicity	Clinical significance not established
Griseofulvin (Fulvicin, Grifulvin V, and others)	Decreased contraceptive effect	Use alternative contraceptive
Guanethidine (Esimil, Ismelin)	Decreased guanethidine effect (mechanism not established)	Avoid simultaneous use
Hypoglycemics (Tolbutamide, Diabinese, Orinase, Tolinase)	Possible decreased hypoglycemic effect	Monitor blood glucose
Methyldopa (Aldoclor, Aldomet, and others)	Decreased antihypertensive effect	Avoid simultaneous use
Penicillin	Decreased contraceptive effect with ampicillin	Low but unpredictable incidence; use alternative contraceptive
Phenytoin (Dilantin)	Decreased contraceptive effect Possible increased phenytoin effect	Use alternative contraceptive Monitor phenytoin concentration
Primidone (Mysoline)	Decreased contraceptive effect	Use alternative contraceptive
Rifampin	Decreased contraceptive effect	Use alternative contraceptive
Tetracycline	Decreased contraceptive effect	Use alternative contraceptive
Theophylline (Bronkotabs, Marax, Primatene, Quibron Tedral, Theor-Dur, and others)	Increased theophylline effect	Monitor theophylline concentration
Troleandomycin (TAO)	Jaundice (additive)	Avoid simultaneous use
Vitamin C	Increased serum concentration and possible increased adverse effects of estrogens with 1 g or more per day of vitamin C	Decrease vitamin C to 100 mg/d

From Hatcher RA, Trussell J, Stewart F, et al. Contraceptive Technology, 16th ed. New York, Irvington, 1994, with permission.

scheduled pill, she may take two pills at once. If she misses two pills in a row, she may take two pills for the next 2 days. If she misses more than two pills, she should call her physician. If she misses one or more pills in any given cycle, an additional (barrier) method should be used for the rest of that cycle. An additional method of contraception should be recommended during use of the initial pack of pills and during any time that she experiences severe diarrhea or vomiting for several days. If she received antibiotics, she may need to use an additional method of contraception for the course of antibiotics and the rest of that cycle.

▶ POSTCOITAL "MORNING-AFTER" PILLS

- Although not approved by the Food and Drug Administration (FDA) for this use, Ovral is recommended by some practitioners as a "morning-after" pill. It has a low failure rate when two tablets are taken within 72 hours (preferably within 12–24 hours) after unprotected intercourse and two more tablets are taken 12 hours later or two pills daily for 2 days.

▶ LONG-ACTING INJECTABLE OR IMPLANTABLE PROGESTINS

- Sustained progestogen exposure blocks the LH surge, thus preventing ovulation. Should ovulation occur, progestogens reduce ovum motility in the fallopian tubes, thin the endometrium, and thicken cervical mucous.

MEDROXYPROGESTERONE ACETATE

- Depomedroxyprogesterone acetate (DMPA), 150 mg administered by deep intramuscular (IM) injection in the gluteal or deltoid muscle within 5 days after the onset of menstrual bleeding, inhibits ovulation for more than 3 months.
- Compared to the 100 mg/mL strength, the 400 mg/mL concentrated form has inconsistent bioavailability, may be less effective, is more painful, and is not approved for contraception.
- DMPA can be used in lactating women and in women with sickle-cell disease. It does not alter blood pressure nor increase the risk of thromboembolic disorders. It may be used in women with seizure disorders and may even decrease the frequency of seizures.
- The median time to conception from the first omitted dose is 6 months.
- The most frequent adverse effects are menstrual irregularities. The incidence of irregular bleeding decreases from 30% in the first year to 10% thereafter. After 12 months of therapy, 57% of women report amenorrhea. Because estrogen concentrations may be lower than normal, women can lose some bone density. Other side effects are breast tenderness, weight gain, and depression. Minor elevations in serum total triglycerides and decreases in serum HDL have need noted.

- If any relationship exists between breast cancer and DMPA use, DMPA may enhance the growth of already existing tumors.

NORPLANT

- Norplant contraceptive system is a set of six implantable, non-biodegradable, soft, silicone rubber capsules, each filled with 35 mg of crystalline levonorgestrel. These capsules are inserted just under the skin to provide continuous long-term contraception.
- Norplant is not recommended for use by women heavier than 154 pounds. The system may be less effective in heavy women in the fourth and fifth years of use. The system should be replaced after 5 years.
- Like other progestin-only methods of contraception, the most common side effect is irregular menstrual bleeding, which occurs in 60–70% of women during the first year.
- Most women return to baseline ovulatory patterns within one month of removal of the system.
- Drugs that increase hepatic enzymes, including most antiseizure medications and rifampin, lower the efficacy of Norplant.

▶ BARRIER TECHNIQUES AND SPERMICIDES

- These methods include the diaphragm, cervical cap, sponge, condom, and spermicide.
- They can reduce the rate of transmission of sexually transmitted diseases.
- The diaphragm may be inserted as long as 6 hours before intercourse and must be left in place for at least 6 hours after intercourse. If intercourse occurs more than once within 6 hours, more spermicide must be inserted.
- Diaphragm users appear to have a lower incidence of cervical neoplasia, but an increased incidence of urinary tract infections.
- The Prentif cervical cap is a soft rubber cup that fits over the cervix like a thimble. It is used with a spermicide. It is less messy to use than a diaphragm and remains effective for more than one episode of intercourse (up to 48 hours) without adding more spermicide. Women should not wear the cap for more than 48 hours.
- Most condoms made in the United States are made of latex rubber and are impermeable to viruses; however, condoms made of lamb intestine are not.
- When used with any other barrier method, the effectiveness of condoms theoretically approaches 95%. Water-soluble lubricants are preferable, as mineral oil-based lubricants can decrease the barrier strength of latex.
- The condom for women (Reality) appears to be as effective as the diaphragm in preventing pregnancy. It may be more effective than the male condom in preventing transmission of diseases such as herpes because it protects the labia from contact with the base of the penis.

- Most spermicides contain nonoxynol-9, a surfactant that destroys sperm cell walls and offers some protection against sexually transmitted diseases and cervical cancer.
- Additional spermicides must be used each time intercourse is repeated.

▶ EVALUATION OF THERAPEUTIC OUTCOMES

- It is critical that patients be provided adequate information to participate in the selection and proper use of contraceptive methods.
- Initial OC use should be reevaluated during the first 3–6 months of therapy to determine if the patient is experiencing any adverse effects and if they wish to continue.
- All users of OCs should have blood pressure monitored regularly.
- Glucose tolerance should be periodically monitored when an OC is prescribed for a patient with a history of glucose intolerance.
- OC users should receive at least annual cytology screening for cervical cancer.

VI

See Chapter 77, Contraception, authored by Kathryn K. Bucci, PharmD, BCPS, and Deborah Stier Carson, PharmD, BCPS, for a more detailed discussion of this topic.

Chapter 29

▶ HORMONE REPLACEMENT THERAPY

▶ DEFINITIONS

Menopause is usually defined as the loss of ovarian function leading to a state of permanent amenorrhea. The climacteric spans several years and includes a series of physiologic and psychologic changes. A period of amenorrhea lasting at least 1 year is used clinically to define the onset of menopause.

▶ PHYSIOLOGY

ESTROGENS

- The major circulating estrogen during the reproductive years is 17β-estradiol (E_2) produced primarily by the ovaries. Estrone has approximately one-third the estrogenic potency of estradiol. In the postmenopausal period, virtually all circulating estradiol is derived from conversion of estrone. Estrone concentrations exceed estradiol by about four-fold after menopause.

GONADOTROPINS

- Postmenopausal decline in estradiol production causes diminished negative-feedback on the anterior pituitary, and there is a compensatory increase in secretion of the gonadotropins, follicle-stimulating hormone (FSH), and luteinizing hormone (LH). This results in the level of FSH exceeding LH which is the inverse of the ratio found in the premenopausal period.
- The remaining follicles generally do not respond to gonadotropin stimulation because of their relative gonadotropin insensitivity.

▶ CLINICAL PRESENTATION

GENITOURINARY ATROPHY

- Atrophy of the vagina, vulva, urethra, and trigone of the bladder begins with diminished estrogen concentrations and continues over many years. There is also thinning of hair of the mons, and shrinkage of the labia minora.
- Vaginal epithelium becomes pale and thin, and there is reduced secretion. The vaginal pH becomes alkaline. Atrophic vaginitis characterized by itching, bleeding, or dyspareunia may occur.
- Postmenopausal women are more prone to the urethral syndrome (e.g., a recurrent, nonbacterial urethritis) and to bacteriuria.

- Estrogen therapy often relieves symptoms of vaginitis and improves urinary frequency, dysuria, nocturia, urgency, dribbling, and stress urinary incontinence.

VASOMOTOR INSTABILITY

- Hot flushes (or flashes) are experienced by 75–85% of women following natural menopause and by 37–50% of premenopausal women who undergo bilateral oophorectomy. They are most common 12–24 months after the last menstrual period and gradually subside thereafter.
- Symptoms of the hot flash may include increased skin temperature, increased heart rate, nausea, dizziness, headache, palpitations, and diaphoresis.
- Estrogen is the traditional treatment for relieving hot flashes, but medroxyprogesterone in relatively high doses and some ergot alkaloids are also effective.

VI OSTEOPOROSIS

- Osteoporosis is a gradual loss of bone mass that eventually compromises the skeleton and results in fractures after minimal trauma. Bone loss is associated with declining estrogen levels in the perimenopausal and menopausal periods.
- Vertebral crush fractures are most common, but hip fractures have the most serious sequelae. Ten percent of patients who suffer a hip fracture die from surgical complications within 6 months.
- The greatest risk of postmenopausal osteoporosis occurs in slender, sedentary females of Caucasian or Asian descent. Other risk factors include smoking, alcohol use, positive family/medical history, and chronic use of certain drugs (e.g., corticosteroids).

CARDIOVASCULAR DISEASE

- After natural or surgical menopause, the incidence of coronary artery disease increases.

OTHER SYMPTOMS

- Other symptoms include insomnia, fatigue, irritability, depression, crying spells, anxiety, and impaired memory.
- Most women experience some change in sexual function in the years immediately before and after menopause.

▶ DIAGNOSIS

- The diagnosis of menopause should involve a comprehensive medical history and thorough physical examination with complete blood count and measurement of serum FSH. In the absence of other disease processes, a serum FSH of 30 pg/mL or greater indicates that the woman is menopausal.
- Altered thyroid function and pregnancy must be excluded.

▶ DESIRED OUTCOME

The goal of hormone replacement therapy (HRT) is relief of vasomotor, genitourinary, and associated symptoms, and prevention of osteoporosis and cardiovascular disease. Patients should understand the nature of menopause and HRT and participate in their treatment decisions and the monitoring process.

▶ TREATMENT

NONHORMONAL TREATMENT

- Nonpharmacologic measures are generally not very helpful, but aerobic exercise and resistance training may help with cardiovascular disease, obesity, muscle weakness, and osteoporosis. Behavioral symptoms may respond to psychiatric counseling.
- Refer to the chapter on Osteoporosis for treatment and prevention.
- For the treatment of vaginal dryness and dyspareunia, a mucoadherent lubricant, polycarbophil, is available without a prescription. It is long-acting and lowers pH.
- Exercise and diet, along with smoking cessation and no more than moderate alcohol consumption are the foundation of prevention of cardiovascular disease.

VI

ESTROGEN REPLACEMENT

- In symptomatic patients with either elevated (>30 pg/mL) or borderline (15–30 pg/mL) FSH serum concentrations, HRT may be considered. A growing body of clinical data now supports the use of HRT for prevention or treatment of osteoporosis and for its cardioprotective benefits.

Pharmacology

- Estrogens attach to receptor proteins in the cytoplasm of target organs including the ovaries, uterus, fallopian tubes, vagina, bladder, urethra, and breast. Other target organs are the skin, adrenals, cardiovascular system, gastrointestinal tract, and the central nervous system (CNS). The estrogen-protein complex diffuses through the nuclear membrane and ultimately binds to materials in the cell nucleus. Synthesis of DNA, RNA, and other proteins increases, resulting in characteristic changes in response tissue.
- Exogenous estrogen products are shown in Table 29.1. Injectable estrogens are not generally used for menopausal symptoms because of poor patient acceptance and fluctuating plasma concentrations.
- Conjugated equine estrogens are a mixture of estrogen compounds, mostly sulfates and glucuronides, some of which are not found in humans.
- Absorption of oral estradiol tablets has become more reliable with micronized formulations, but estradiol is metabolized significantly on first pass through the liver to other less active metabolites.

TABLE 29.1. Estrogen Products

VI

Agent	Dosage Form	Dose	Indications
Estrone aqueous suspension	Injection	0.1–5 mg IM 2–3 times/week	A,B
Estrogenic substance or estrogen aqueous suspension (primarily estrone) injection	Injection	0.1–1.0 mg IM 2–3 times/week	A,B
Estradiol cypionate (in oil)	Injection	1–5 mg/d IM every 3–4 weeks	C
Estradiol valerate (in oil)	Injection	10–20 mg every 4 weeks	A,B,C
Conjugated estrogens	Oral	0.03–1.25 mg/d[a]	A,B,C,D
Conjugated estrogens/medroxyprogesterone acetate	Oral	0.625 mg/2.5 mg per day[b]	C,D
Conjugated estrogens/medroxyprogesterone acetate	Oral	0.625 mg per day for 14 days,[b] then 0.625 mg/5 mg per day for 14 days[b]	C,D
Micronized estradiol	Oral	0.5–2 mg/d[a]	A,B,C,D
Esterified estrogens (75–85% estrone sulfate and 6–15% sodium equilin)	Oral	0.3–1.25 mg/d[a]	A,B,C,D
Estropipate (piperazine estrone sulfate)	Oral	0.75–6 mg/d[a]	A,B,C
Ethinyl estradiol	Oral	0.02–1.5 mg/d[a]	A,C
Quinestrol	Oral	0.1 mg/d for 7 days, then 0.1 mg once weekly	A,B,C
Chlorotrianisene	Oral	12–25 mg/d for 21 days	A,B,C
Estropipate vaginal cream	Topical	3–6 mg daily for 3 weeks	B
Micronized estradiol vaginal cream	Topical	Daily[c]	B
Conjugated estrogens vaginal cream	Topical	1.25–2.5 mg daily for 3 weeks	B
Dienestrol vaginal cream	Topical	Once or twice daily[c]	B
Estrone vaginal cream	Topical	2–4 mg daily	B
Estradiol transdermal	Transdermal	0.05–0.1 mg system twice weekly	A,B,C,D

Key: A, replacement therapy of estrogen deficiency-associated conditions (i.e., female hypogonadism); B, senile vaginitis and Kraurosis vulvae; C, moderate to severe vasomotor symptoms associated with menopause; D, osteoporosis.

[a]May administer continuously or cyclically with 3 weeks of daily estrogen followed by 1 week off.

[b]Blister pack dosage cards used for single prescription convenience in continuous or cyclic combination regimens.

[c]Typical regimen: Initial therapy one dose daily for 2 weeks, followed by daily therapy at one-half dose, followed by maintenance therapy of one dose 1–3 times/week for three weeks. Check drug information references for specific regimens.

- Estrogen in vaginal creams is a feasible treatment for urogenital symptoms and for other menopausal symptoms. Estradiol is metabolized very little as it is absorbed from the vagina, resulting primarily in increased estradiol concentrations. Unfortunately, these concentrations return to baseline in approximately 6 hours; they are not widely used.
- The transdermal patch is applied to the skin, usually on the lower trunk. This dosage form offers parenteral therapy with little metabolism of estradiol, convenient administration, and precise dosing.
- Transdermal administration of estrogens, such as 17β-estradiol, results in estradiol levels equivalent to those in the early to mid-follicular phase and an estrone-to-estradiol ratio of approximately 1:1, which closely resembles the premenopausal state. Unlike oral estrogen replacement, transdermal estrogen delivery has no significant effect on production of certain hepatic proteins, renin substrate, sex-hormone–binding globulin, thyroxine-binding globulin, and cortisol-binding globulin. Although controversial, the effects of transdermal estrogen administration on the lipid profile appear to be less favorable than with orally administered estrogens.
- Administration of transdermal estrogen may be either continuous, or in 3-week cycles with 1 week estrogen free. The addition of a progestin is recommended for the last 10–13 days of the cycle in women receiving cyclic therapy who have an intact uterus.

Clinical Use
- The presence of any estrogen-dependent cancer should be ruled out before the initiation of ERT. If not recently done, mammography should be performed.

Vasomotor Instability
- The symptoms of vasomotor instability respond to exogenous estrogen therapy. These symptoms typically last 3–5 years.
- The addition of a progestin (e.g., medroxyprogesterone acetate, norethindrone, norgestrel, or micronized oral progesterone) is standard therapy in women with an intact uterus to counter the increased risk of endometrial cancer.
- For women in whom cyclical bleeding is unacceptable, an alternative involves the continuous administration of estrogens with the addition of a progestin for 10–12 days during the calendar month. Some clinicians advocate the continuous administration of estrogens and lower dose progestins (2.5–5 mg daily medroxyprogesterone acetate) as an effective alternative to cyclic therapy which also avoids withdrawal bleeding.

Urogenital Atrophy
- Therapy is generally initiated with the smallest dose to restore the vaginal epithelium, usually 2–4 g of estradiol cream given once daily for 1–2 weeks initially. Therapy is tapered to half-doses for an additional 2 weeks. Maintenance therapy can be continued with 1 g given one to three times weekly in the usual cyclic manner.

VI

- Alternatives to estradiol cream include dienestrol, conjugated estrogens, or estropipate cream given in the same cyclic manner as estradiol.
- Oral or transdermal administration of estrogens may also be used to treat the symptoms in the same doses discussed for vasomotor instability.

Osteoporosis

- The response of bone to estrogen therapy is reduced rate of resorption with normal mineralization of the remodeling unit.
- HRT should be begun soon after menopause (preferably within 3 years) to prevent loss of bone density. If HRT is discontinued, bone loss begins immediately. Estrogen therapy should continue for at least the next 10–15 years.
- The dose of estrogen required to prevent bone loss is 0.625 mg daily. Lower doses of conjugated estrogen, e.g., 0.312 mg/d, may prevent bone loss if used in conjunction with high daily doses of elemental calcium (1500 mg/d). Alternative regimens are esterified estrogens (0.625 mg/d), oral ethinyl estradiol (0.02 mg/d), micronized 17β-estradiol (1 mg/d), and transdermal estrogen patches (delivering estradiol 0.05–0.10 mg administered as one patch twice weekly).
- Adequate intake of calcium and regular weight-bearing exercise are also important adjunctive treatments.

Cardiovascular Disease

- Estrogens lower low-density lipoprotein (LDL) cholesterol and increase high-density lipoprotein (HDL) cholesterol. Other mechanisms such as platelet effects and direct effects on vessel wall physiology may also be cardioprotective. While triglycerides may be higher in estrogen users, blood pressure and fasting blood glucose levels are unchanged or lower.
- Estrogen therapy has shown a 50% or greater reduction in cardiovascular disease and related mortality.
- Progestins may attenuate the benefits on HDL. However, cardiovascular benefits of combined treatment on HDL cholesterol have been confirmed in a well-controlled trial.
- The most effective regimen has not been established.

PROGESTIN THERAPY

- Progestins alone are as effective as estrogens for relief of vasomotor symptoms. These agents are also useful in the treatment and prevention of osteoporosis, by increasing the formation of new bone.
- Administration of a progestin for 10 days each month with ERT serves three purposes: (1) decreases the risk of estrogen-induced irregular bleeding, endometrial hyperplasia, and carcinoma; (2) protects against breast carcinoma; and (3) enhances estrogen prophylaxis of osteoporosis.
- Synthetic forms of 17α-hydroxyprogesterone and 19-nortestosterone are used clinically. The 19-nortestosterone derivatives possess androgenic activity and are used primarily in oral contraceptives. The 17α-hydroxyprogesterone derivatives are associated with depression and anxiety. Medroxyprogesterone acetate is the progestin generally used.

Clinical Use

- Usual dose of medroxyprogesterone acetate is 2.5–5 mg/daily with ERT to prevent endometrial hyperplasia.
- Medroxyprogesterone acetate (20 mg/d) orally has been used alone to treat vasomotor instability. Alternatively, depot medroxyprogesterone acetate 50–100 mg intramuscularly given every 2–3 months is as effective as conjugated estrogens.

Adverse Effects

- When used alone or with ERT, a premenstrual tension-like syndrome may occur. Breast tenderness, bloating, edema, cramping, anxiety, depression, and irritability are frequent complaints. Weight gain, headache, and drowsiness may occur. Dosage reduction or change to another progestin may help.
- Progestins cause a dose-related decrease in HDL cholesterol and an increase in LDL cholesterol. They should be used in the minimum dosage required for endometrial protection when prescribed with estrogen.

▶ EVALUATION OF THERAPEUTIC OUTCOMES

- Routine follow-up visits with regular breast examinations and PAP smear are indicated in women taking HRT.
- All women receiving ERT should practice regular breast self-examination along with annual physician breast examinations and routine mammography.
- Blood pressure should be checked regularly, especially in women receiving progestins.

▶ RISKS AND BENEFITS

- Estrogen users have a four-fold to eight-fold increase in risk of developing endometrial cancer relative to the risk in the normal population.
- The addition of progestin to estrogen therapy confers protection against endometrial hyperplasia and is generally recommended for at least 10 days per month or continuously in patients with an intact uterus.
- A history of thromboembolism is a relative contraindication to estrogen therapy.
- Progestins produce a dose-related elevation in blood pressure by causing sodium and water retention.

See Chapter 79, Hormone Replacement Therapy, authored by Patricia Moynahan Mullins, PharmD, Mark C. Pugh, PharmD, and Andrea O. Moore, PharmD, for a more detailed discussion of this topic.

Chapter 30

▶ PREGNANCY AND LACTATION: THERAPEUTIC CONSIDERATIONS

▶ DIAGNOSIS OF PREGNANCY

- Pregnancy may be confirmed by the presence of human chorionic gonadotropic (HCG). Serum tests such as radioimmunoassay (RIA) and enzyme-linked immunosorbent assay (ELISA) can detect concentrations as low as 5 mIU/mL (present about 6–10 days after implantation). Urine tests using monoclonal antibodies can usually detect concentrations of HCG in the 20–40 mIU/mL range (1–2 weeks after conception). Ectopic pregnancies may not produce enough HCG to be detected by urine tests.
- Quantitative serum assays for HCG should be used in the diagnosis of ectopic pregnancies or suspected pregnancy loss.
- Home pregnancy tests using monoclonal antibodies are very sensitive and specific and are useful for detecting normal pregnancies when used correctly. Home tests fail to detect 50% of ectopic pregnancies. A negative test should be repeated in 7 days if menses has not begun.

▶ PHYSIOLOGIC CHANGES IN PREGNANCY

- Total blood volume in pregnancy increases 30–40%. The cellular components increase about 20%, and the fluid portion about 40–50%. During the second and third trimester, the extravascular volume also increases. These changes could cause a decrease in plasma concentrations of some drugs.
- Serum proteins are often 1–1.5 grams lower in pregnancy, and the albumin-to-globulin ratio falls by about 50%.
- Renal blood flow increases about 30%, and the glomerular filtration rate is increased about 50%.
- Serum urea, creatine, and uric acid are decreased.
- Cardiac output increases about 32% due to an increased heart rate and stroke volume.
- Motility and acidity of the gastrointestinal tract (GI) are decreased. Constipation is common.
- Vomiting early in pregnancy may contribute to the decreased absorption of medications, and the decreased motility of the GI tract may delay the fecal excretion of some drugs.

▶ NORMAL COURSE OF PREGNANCY

- The normal gestation period is 267 days from conception or 280 days from the first day of the last menstrual period. The average weight gain during pregnancy is 24 pounds, 3 pounds during the first trimester and 1 pound per week during the last 16 weeks.

- During pregnancy it is common to give a multivitamin, and 200 mg of elemental iron is included in most prenatal vitamins. Pregnant women should also ingest at least 1.2 grams of elemental calcium daily either in their diet or with calcium supplementation.

- All women of childbearing age who are capable of becoming pregnant should take at least 0.4 mg of folic acid daily to reduce the incidence of neural tube defects. Patients should never take more than 0.8 mg of folic acid daily without physician supervision.

▶ PREGNANCY-INDUCED ILLNESSES

NAUSEA AND VOMITING

- Half of all pregnant patients experience some degree of nausea and vomiting during the first trimester, especially upon arising. For some women nausea lasts throughout the day and throughout pregnancy. Hyperemesis gravidarum (i.e., severe nausea and vomiting) that cannot be controlled and results in dehydration and malnutrition can be life-threatening and requires immediate therapy, usually with intravenous fluids, electrolytes, and antiemetics. Total parenteral nutrition has been effective.

- Medication must be considered for patients whose nausea persists despite dietary alterations. Medications used most often include phenothiazines, meclizine, cyclizine, dimenhydrinate, doxylamine, and pyridoxine.

HEARTBURN

- Heartburn during the latter half of pregnancy is common and results from relaxation of the cardiac sphincter and increased pressure in the stomach caused by the enlarging uterus. Smaller, more frequent meals, avoiding food and liquids other than water for at least 3 hours before bedtime, and elevating the head of the bed with blocks often helps.

- Magnesium and/or aluminum hydroxides are usually effective for relieving the pain, and their duration of activity is several hours. Sucralfate is poorly absorbed by the GI tract and has been suggested as a reasonable treatment for heartburn in pregnancy.

CONSTIPATION

- Constipation is common, and pregnant women should be encouraged to add high-fiber foods to their diet, increase their fluid intake, and exercise moderately (e.g., walking).

- Surfactants and bulk laxatives are the agents of choice. Adequate fluid intake is critical with fiber laxatives. Mineral oil should be avoided.

HEMORRHOIDS

- Hemorrhoids often develop or worsen during pregnancy as a result of constipation and increased venous pressure below the uterus.

- Correction of constipation and use of stool softeners and sitz baths are usually helpful.
- External medications are preferred over those inserted into the rectum because many drugs are absorbed rectally. Topical anesthetics and steroids should be avoided except under supervision of a physician, as they may be absorbed and affect the fetus.

COAGULATION DISORDERS

- Thromboembolic phenomena are uncommon during pregnancy.
- About 30% of pregnancies exposed to oral anticoagulants result in fetal malformations, developmental deficiencies, stillbirths, or hemorrhage. Teratogenic risk is greatest during the first trimester, but ophthalmic abnormalities and mental retardation are associated with the use of coumarin anticoagulants in the second and third trimesters. Fetal hemorrhage is a concern if delivery occurs while the mother is taking oral anticoagulants.
- The anticoagulant of choice during pregnancy is subcutaneous (SQ) heparin. No congenital defects have been reported, and the effect of heparin can be antagonized by administering protamine sulfate. This is advantageous, as the onset of labor and necessity of an operative delivery are not always predictable.
- Conversion from oral anticoagulants to SQ heparin should be considered for those desiring to become pregnant.

PREGNANCY-INDUCED HYPERTENSION

- Pregnancy-induced hypertension can be a serious and life-threatening complication.
- Gestational hypertension is diagnosed when the blood pressure exceeds 140/90 mm Hg in the absence of proteinuria or pathologic edema.
- Mild preeclampsia is hypertension accompanied by proteinuria (≥300 mg/24 h or 100 mg/dL in two random samples 6 hours apart) and/or pathologic edema.
- Preeclampsia is severe when proteinuria exceeds 4 g/24 h or persistent dipstick values of 2+ are present, blood pressure is 160/110 mm Hg, and/or severe headache, visual disturbances, or epigastric pain is noted.
- Eclampsia is the development of generalized tonic-clonic seizures in a patient with pregnancy-induced hypertension.
- Pregnancy-aggravated hypertension is diagnosed in a patient with preexisting essential hypertension who experiences a 15 mm Hg increase in diastolic or 30 mm Hg increase in systolic blood pressure after the 24th week of gestation.
- Eighty-five percent of patients diagnosed with preeclampsia are primiparas, particularly those who are very young or at the upper end of the reproductive age range. Other risk factors include essential hypertension, diabetes, and multiple fetuses.
- The only cure for preeclampsia/eclampsia is termination of the pregnancy.

- Prevention of preeclampsia with low-dose aspirin has been suggested for patients at high risk for developing the disorder. The recommended dose is 60 mg/d and is usually initiated at the 24th to 28th week of gestation and continued until the onset of labor. Low-dose aspirin has not been shown to be useful in the treatment of existing preeclampsia/ eclampsia.
- Patients exhibiting mild preeclampsia should be placed on bedrest. Diuresis usually begins within 36–48 hours with regression of symptoms in 4–5 days. Patients who remain at home should be instructed to measure urine protein daily and check blood pressure twice daily. Patients unable to comply with instructions should be hospitalized.
- Severely preeclamptic women must be hospitalized and begun on a regimen of parenteral magnesium sulfate intramuscularly or intravenously to prevent seizures, and plans for delivery should be discussed. If IV administration is chosen, a loading dose of 4 g is followed by an infusion of 1–3 g/h and a controlled infusion pump used. Another regimen begins with a 4 g IV loading dose with simultaneous IM injection of 10 g (5 g in each buttock) followed by 5 g IM every 4 hours. The large volume IM injections are painful, and lidocaine may be used to minimize discomfort.
- Patients receiving magnesium must be closely monitored for signs of toxicity. The optimum serum concentration for prevention of convulsions is 4–7 mEq/L. Reflexes should be checked every 30 minutes. Urine output should be >25 mL/h, and respirations should be >10/min. IV administration of 1 gm of calcium gluconate (10 mL of 10% solution) usually reverses mild magnesium toxicity. Magnesium levels should be determined in "floppy" neonates exposed to magnesium prior to delivery.
- Convulsions not controlled by adequate serum concentrations of magnesium may respond to IV diazepam or phenytoin.
- A systolic reading of 160–180 mm Hg or greater or a diastolic reading of 110 mm Hg or greater should be treated with an IV antihypertensive to prevent cerebral hemorrhage. Parenteral hydralazine often produces tachycardia, palpitations, flushing, and headache; propranolol may be useful in opposing the cardiac side effects of hydralazine but should not be used alone for treatment of hypertension. Labetalol, an α- and β- adrenergic blocking agent, may be an alternative to hydralazine, as it has a faster onset of effectiveness with less reflex tachycardia. Hydralazine, however, tends to be somewhat more effective.
- Neither diazoxide, nitroprusside, nor diuretics are recommended in these patients. Calcium channel blockers may be useful for acute hypertensive episodes in pregnancy, but further investigation is required.
- Generally, the response to any treatment is temporary.

ANEMIAS

- Iron deficiency anemia is the most common anemia that occurs during pregnancy.
- Hemoglobin values normally drop during pregnancy because of increased blood volume.

- Iron deficiency anemia should be ruled out when the hemoglobin falls below 10 g/dL or the hematocrit below 30%. Decreased blood levels of serum iron and total iron binding capacity are diagnostic.
- All pregnant patients should receive approximately 30–60 mg of elemental iron daily.

▶ CHRONIC MEDICAL DISORDERS IN PREGNANCY

DIABETES

- The incidence of congenital abnormalities in diabetics is 3–22% (depending on the degree of glycemic control) compared with 2% in the normal population.
- It is important that patients be normoglycemic before conception and during the first trimester, as congenital malformations associated with diabetes seem to be related to poor control during the first 8 weeks. Patients with highest risk of complications include those with vasculopathy, poor glucose control, a previous stillbirth, and noncompliance.
- Complications of diabetic pregnancies include fetal macrosomia, polyhydramnios, malformations, and respiratory distress syndrome.
- During pregnancy, diabetic patients have an increased risk of hypoglycemia and ketoacidosis.
- Glucose tests using whole blood are preferred over urine tests. Glucose should be monitored fasting, before meals, and at bedtime daily. Some physicians ask for monitoring 1 hour after a meal once weekly, as well. Evaluation of glycosylated hemoglobin once each trimester also helps assess control.
- Rigid glucose control is the goal, and most women should be able to maintain glucose levels between 60–120 mg/dL.
- Pregnant patients usually require a diabetic diet of 35 kcal/kg ideal body weight daily, or about 2200–2400 calories. Only intermediate-acting and fast-acting insulins should be used. NPH or Lente insulin, combined with regular insulin, should be given SQ in two divided doses daily. Optimal control is usually achieved by administering two-thirds the total dose of each insulin before breakfast and the remaining one-third before the evening meal. Split dosing includes using a 2:1 ratio of NPH to regular insulin in the morning injection and a 1:1 mixture in the evening.
- About 70% of pregnant patients have increased insulin requirements after the 24th week, and requirements usually double by the end of pregnancy.
- Oral hypoglycemic agents are contraindicated during pregnancy, as they can cause fetal and neonatal hypoglycemia and have teratogenic effects. They should be discontinued before conception if possible.
- Glucose intolerance of pregnancy (gestational diabetes) develops during the second half of pregnancy in about 2–3% of patients. If a diabetic diet does not control glucose, insulin therapy should be started.

VI

- Tight glucose control should be maintained during labor and delivery. An IV infusion of 1 L of 5% dextrose injection with 10 units of regular insulin given at a rate of 100 mL/h may be given. Additional glucose or insulin may be given to maintain glucose at approximately 100 mg/dL. An alternative regimen is IV administration of 50 g of glucose every 6 hours, with regular insulin given SQ as needed. Blood glucose should be checked every 1–2 hours.
- Immediately after delivery of the placenta, insulin requirements drop and remain lower for 24–72 hours, and hypoglycemic shock is common during this period.
- Breastfeeding is encouraged; lower insulin requirements during lactation are expected.

THYROID DISEASE

- Preeclampsia, maternal heart failure, and stillbirths are more common in hyperthyroid pregnancies than normal pregnancies or those adequately treated.
- Methimazole and propylthiouracil (PTU) are equally effective. PTU is generally preferred, as it may cross the placenta to a lesser degree. The dose should be adequate to maintain the total serum T_4 level in the upper range of normal and the patient clinically minimally thyrotoxic.
- Hypothyroidism in pregnancy should be treated with thyroxine replacement.

CHRONIC HYPERTENSION

- Chronic hypertension in pregnancy is described as hypertension present at conception or developing before the 20th week of gestation. These patients are considered high risk.
- About one-third of hypertensive patients have superimposed preeclampsia, which occurs earlier and progresses more rapidly than in normal pregnancies.
- Cerebral hemorrhage is a more common cause of maternal mortality than preeclampsia in these patients.
- It is common for blood pressure to decrease in the second trimester.
- Most chronic hypertension is mild and with minimal sequelae. Mild hypertension should be treated with bedrest for at least 1 hour at lunch time and 1 hour in the afternoon in addition to 10 hours of bedrest each night.
- Patients not responding satisfactorily may be treated with methyldopa which is effective without significant fetal or neonatal problems. Either propranolol or hydralazine is the second-line drug. There are reports of intrauterine growth retardation, bradycardia, neonatal respiratory distress syndrome, and hypoglycemia with propranolol use.
- If propranolol becomes necessary, it should be discontinued 1–2 weeks before delivery when possible and the neonate observed closely for adverse effects.
- Oral hydralazine may be less effective than propranolol.

VI

- Diuretics are avoided during pregnancy as they cause a 5–10% decrease in plasma volume, electrolyte imbalance, and decreased carbohydrate tolerance in the mother.
- Until more data are available, calcium channel blockers should be avoided during pregnancy. Angiotensin-converting enzyme (ACE) inhibitors are contraindicated.

EPILEPSY

- About 40–50% of epileptic patients experience an exacerbation of the disease, and 5–10% improve during pregnancy.
- Patients with epilepsy, whether medicated or not, are more likely to deliver an infant with congenital abnormalities and mental retardation. Most evidence supports a role of anticonvulsants in causing congenital problems including orofacial clefts, skeletal anomalies, central nervous system (CNS) malformations, cardiac abnormalities, and mental retardation. Although teratogenicity occurs with anticonvulsants, the risk of maternal seizures is considered more harmful to the fetus.
- Patients who have been seizure-free for several years should undergo a trial of medication withdrawal before becoming pregnant. Patients with recurrent epilepsy who are on medication should be advised that they have a 90% chance of having a normal child, but that the risk of congenital abnormalities and mental retardation is twice that of the normal population.
- Treatment with one antiepileptic drug (AED) is preferred, but if monotherapy fails, a second drug should be initiated and the first drug gradually withdrawn during the course of 7 days. A trial using a third drug may be tried, but if monotherapy with the third drug does not succeed, then a trial with two medications concurrently is indicated.
- Serum concentrations of most AEDs are lower during pregnancy, but seizure frequency may not increase because free concentrations of the drug do not decline proportionally with total concentrations. Serum concentrations should be evaluated at least bimonthly and the dose adjusted according to concentration, seizures frequency, and side effects.
- With use of phenytoin, teratogenicity, coagulopathy, and vitamin deficiencies occur, but neonatal CNS depression and withdrawal do not occur. About 10% of infants exposed in utero to phenytoin will manifest the full syndrome of fetal hydantoin syndrome, and about 30% will have some features. Fetal hydantoin syndrome includes craniofacial abnormalities, growth retardation, limb defects, cardiac lesions, hernias, and distal digital and nail hypoplasias. Phenytoin is probably more teratogenic than phenobarbital.
- A large percentage of neonates exposed to AEDs have a severe coagulopathy during the first 24 hours after delivery. This is caused by a deficiency of the vitamin K-dependent clotting factors, and all exposed infants should be treated with 2 mg vitamin K_1 at birth. Some physicians give pregnant patients receiving AEDs prophylactic oral vitamin

VI

K during the last 3 weeks before delivery. Folate deficiency also occurs in patients on AEDs, and prophylaxis is recommended to prevent megaloblastic anemia.

- Phenobarbital is the anticonvulsant of choice in women of childbearing age as it appears to have less teratogenic potential than phenytoin. Higher doses are usually required during pregnancy to maintain serum levels. Coagulopathy and folate deficiency can occur as discussed above. Neonates may experience CNS depression and withdrawal at delivery, and withdrawal symptoms do not usually begin for 4–7 days after delivery and may last 2–6 months. Withdrawal may be characterized by neuromuscular excitability, hyperactivity, sleep disturbances, excessive crying, tremulousness, vomiting, or diarrhea.
- Primidone is associated with the same problems as phenobarbital; phenobarbital is a metabolite of primidone.
- Carbamazepine is teratogenic, and defects include spina bifida, craniofacial defects, nail hypoplasia, and developmental delays.
- Valproic acid is associated with cleft palate, renal defects, and neural tube defects, and it should be avoided in women of childbearing age.
- Trimethadione is the most potent teratogen of the AEDs, and it is contraindicated in pregnancy.

ASTHMA

- During pregnancy, one-third of asthmatics experience improvement of their disease and one-third worsen. Severe asthma with medical complications may have an adverse effect on pregnancy outcome.
- Of drugs used to treat asthma, only the iodides are contraindicated in pregnancy. Cromolyn sodium is not recommended by the manufacturer for use in pregnancy.
- For patients with mild and/or infrequent attacks, aerosol albuterol, metaproterenol, or isoetharine should be chosen.
- Patients with more severe or more frequent asthma attacks may receive oral theophylline, although fetal serum concentrations approximate maternal levels. Oral terbutaline may be added to theophylline if symptoms persist.
- Aerosolized steroids are added if necessary. When steroids are required, prednisone and prednisolone are suggested.
- Severe attacks and status asthmaticus are managed as in the nonpregnant population.

▶ TREATMENT OF PRETERM LABOR

- Uterine contractions with cervical changes beginning before the 37th week of gestation are considered premature labor.
- Labor occurring before the 20th week of amenorrhea usually results in expulsion of an imperfect fetus; inhibition of labor should not be attempted before the 20th week.

- Drug therapy is most successful when the cervix is dilated <4 cm and membranes are intact. Premature rupture of membranes is usually considered a contraindication to inhibition of labor, but it may be advantageous to administer pharmacologic agents to delay delivery 24–48 hours to allow glucocorticoids to enhance fetal lung maturity.
- Although some investigators have questioned the efficacy of tocolytic agents (β agonists, specifically) to prolong gestation and decrease perinatal mortality, most clinicians choose to treat preterm labor.

BETA AGONISTS

- Ritodrine is the only β-adrenergic drug approved in the United States for the treatment of premature labor, but terbutaline is also used. There are no clear advantages of either drug, but terbutaline is as effective as ritodrine and much less expensive.
- Side effects of both drugs include hypotension, tachycardia, hypokalemia (occurs with parenteral therapy and is due to an intracellular shift), palpitations, tremor, nervousness, angina, hyperglycemia, pulmonary edema, and headache. Hyperglycemia is usually not clinically important unless the patient is a diabetic. The incidence of pulmonary edema is greater when the infusion solution is isotonic saline. The fluid of choice is 5% dextrose in water. Limiting the fluid intake to 2500 mL/24 hours may also decrease the likelihood of pulmonary edema.
- The IV infusion of ritodrine or terbutaline is usually continued for 12 hours after contractions cease. Oral medication is initiated 30 minutes before the infusion is stopped. Terbutaline has also been given by SQ pump for maintenance.

MAGNESIUM SULFATE

- Magnesium sulfate is also effective in suppressing uterine contractions at serum levels of 6–8 mEq/L. In addition to monitoring the patellar reflex, urine output, and respirations, some protocols require serial magnesium levels every 6 hours. It may be the agent of choice for the diabetic patient.
- Serious neonatal effects are uncommon unless the treatment fails and the delivery occurs during the infusion. Respiratory depression in the mother can be reversed by administration of 10 mL of 10% calcium gluconate.

PROSTAGLANDIN SYNTHETASE INHIBITORS

- Oral and rectal indomethacin are effective in the treatment of preterm labor, but it can potentially cause serious fetal side effects including premature closure of the ductus arteriosus, poor cardiopulmonary adaptation after delivery, necrotizing enterocolitis, intracranial hemorrhage, and renal dysfunction.

VI

▶ INDUCTION OF LABOR

- Indications for induction of labor include severe maternal infection, uterine bleeding, preeclampsia/eclampsia or chronic hypertension, diabetes mellitus, maternal renal insufficiency, premature rupture of membranes after the 36th week, polyhydramnios, evidence of placental insufficiency, isoimmunization, and postdate pregnancy.
- The ergot alkaloids are used to terminate pregnancy, not to induce labor.
- The prostaglandin suppositories and solution that are currently available are used only for the termination of pregnancy, because their effects on the fetus are unknown.
- Oxytocin is the drug used most often to induce labor, augment inadequate labor, and decrease postpartum bleeding. The initial dose is 2 mU/minute by IV infusion. A controlled pump must be used. The dose may be increased by 2 mU/min every 15–20 minutes if needed. The dose should not exceed 20 mU/min. The goal of treatment is contractions lasting 45–60 seconds at intervals of 2–3 minutes.
- Close monitoring of uterine contractions and fetal heart rate is essential. Resting uterine contractions must be monitored, as a resting pressure >15–20 mm H_2O increases the incidence of complications such as uterine rupture and fetal distress from hypoxia. If resting pressure exceeds this level, oxytocin should be discontinued. Maternal blood pressure and pulse should also be monitored.
- Side effects of oxytocin include uterine rupture (infrequent), fetal hypoxia (reduced uteroplacental blood flow), maternal hypotension, hypoglycemia, and fluid retention.
- Contraindications to oxytocin include abnormal fetal positions or presentations, cephalopelvic disproportion, repeat cesarean section or other previous uterine surgery, or a firm, closed, uneffaced, posterior cervix. Patients with functional class III or IV heart disease are not good candidates for oxytocin use.

▶ LACTATION SUPPRESSION

- Breast engorgement is usually self-limiting, begins about the third to fourth day postpartum, and resolves within 48–72 hours. Nondrug treatment includes application of ice packs and binding of the breasts.
- Most obstetric centers have discontinued the pharmacologic suppression of lactation.
- Although many estrogenic and androgenic substances were once used, chlorotrianisene, a synthetic proestrogen and a testosterone enanthate/estradiol valerate combination injection were the most frequently used. Concern for side effects have limited their use.
- Bromocriptine mesylate is also effective, but several side effects are associated with its use, and the incidence of rebound lactation after discontinuation is as high as 40%.

▶ DRUG EFFECTS ON THE FETUS

- The incidence of major structural abnormalities in the fetus in the United States is 2–4%. If minor malformations, such as ear tags or extra digits are included, this could increase to as much as 10%. About 25% of abnormalities are probably due to genetic predisposition, while 2–3% are drug-induced.
- The Food and Drug Administration (FDA) requires that all drugs marketed after 1983 be assigned a pregnancy risk category (Table 30.1). Therefore, most drugs currently available are not required to have risk categories assigned.
- Drug exposure around the time of conception and implantation may kill the fetus, and the patient may never know that she was pregnant. If exposure occurs in the first 12–15 days after conception, when the cells are still totipotential (i.e., if one cell is damaged or killed, another can assume its function), the fetus may not be damaged. The first 3 months are the most critical in terms of malformations. Functional and behavioral defects have been associated with drug exposure later in gestation.
- If drugs are to be given, the lowest effective dose should be prescribed for the shortest possible duration.
- Many drugs reach fetal blood levels that are 50–100% of maternal levels. The proportion of free drug is often higher in the fetus. Fetal clearance may be slower than in adults.
- Factors that influence teratogenicity include genotypes of mother and fetus, embryonic stage at exposure, dose, specificity of the agent, and simultaneous exposure to other drugs or environmental agents.
- Teratogens may cause spontaneous abortion, congenital abnormalities, intrauterine growth retardation, mental retardation, carcinogenesis, and mutagenesis.

VI

TABLE 30.1. FDA Categories for Drug Use in Pregnancy

Category A: Controlled studies in women fail to demonstrate a risk to the fetus in the first trimester, and the possibility of fetal harm appears remote.

Category B: Either animal studies do not indicate a risk to the fetus and there are no controlled studies in pregnant women or animal studies have indicated fetal risk, but controlled studies in pregnant women failed to demonstrate a risk.

Category C: Either animal studies indicate a fetal risk and there are no controlled studies in women or there are no available studies in women or animals.

Category D: There is positive evidence of fetal risk but there may be certain situations where the benefit might outweigh the risk (life-threatening or serious diseases where other drugs are ineffective or carry a greater risk).

Category X: There is definite fetal risk based on studies in animals or humans or based on human experience and the risk clearly outweighs any benefit in pregnant women.

From Federal Register 1980;44:37434–37467.

- Effects of medication on labor and delivery should be considered. Salicylate use late in gestation can cause increased bleeding at delivery or even delay the onset of labor.

PLACENTAL TRANSPORT

- Drugs with molecular weights of <400, highly unionized, and lipophilic drugs cross the placenta more readily. Most drugs have molecular weights between 250 and 400 and thus have considerable potential to enter the fetal circulation. Other factors influencing placental transfer are degree of protein binding, maternal and fetal blood flow, the area available for exchange, and the amount of placental metabolism.
- Most drugs cross the placenta by simple diffusion (driven by concentration gradient), and fetal serum concentrations usually equal maternal levels. However, fetal levels may be lower or higher than maternal levels.

SPECIFIC AGENTS

VI

The following is not a complete list of drugs affecting the fetus, and the reader is referred to the primary literature. Drugs with known, suspected, and no known teratogenic effects are listed in Tables 30.2, 30.3, 30.4, and 30.5.

Benzodiazepines

- These drugs are associated with congenital malformations (particularly facial clefts), especially when administered during the first trimester.
- Floppy infant syndrome, neonatal CNS depression, and withdrawal may occur following chronic benzodiazepine use during the last trimester and when large doses are given shortly before delivery.

TABLE 30.2. Medications Known to be Teratogens

ACE inhibitors
Alcohol
Androgens
Anticonvulsants
Antineoplastics
Cocaine
Diethylstilbestrol
Iodides
Isotretinoin
Lithium
Live vaccines
Tetracycline
Warfarin

TABLE 30.3. Medications Suspected to be Teratogens

Benzodiazepines
Estrogens
Methimazole
Quinolones
Oral hypoglycemic agents
Progestogens
Tricyclic antidepressants

Lithium

- Infants exposed to lithium during the first trimester of pregnancy have an increased risk of developing abnormalities, 75% of which are cardiovascular (e.g., Epstein's anomaly).
- When administered late in pregnancy, manifestations of neonatal toxicity include cyanosis, hypotonia, bradycardia, and electrocardiographic abnormalities.

Sex Hormones

- Progestins and androgens are associated with masculinization of the female fetus.
- Progestins, primarily those in oral contraceptives, may produce the VACTERL syndrome, characterized by vertebral, anal, cardiovascular, esophageal, renal, and limb defects. This is a rare event, and the more likely problem resulting from progestin exposure is abnormal sex organ development.

TABLE 30.4. Medications with No Known Adverse Effects in Pregnancy[a]

Acetaminophen
Cephalosporins
Corticosteroids
Docusate sodium
Erythromycin
Multiple vitamins
Narcotic analgesics
Penicillin
Phenothiazines
Thyroid hormones

[a]No drug is absolutely without risk during pregnancy. These drugs appear to have a minimal risk when used judiciously in usual doses under the supervision of a medical professional.

TABLE 30.5. Medications with Nonteratogenic Adverse Effects in Pregnancy

Antithyroid drugs
Aminoglycosides
Aspirin
Barbiturates (chronic use)
Beta blockers
Benzodiazepines (chronic use)
Caffeine
Chloramphenicol
Cocaine
Diuretics
Isoniazid
Narcotic analgesics (chronic use)
Nicotine
Nonsteroidal anti-inflammatory agents
Oral hypoglycemic agents
Propylthiouracil
Sulfonamides

VI

- Diethylstilbestrol (DES) causes a number of reproductive tract abnormalities in both female and male offspring exposed in utero, the most common being vaginal clear cell adenocarcinoma in daughters of mothers taking DES.
- Estrogens and progestogens are contraindicated during pregnancy.

Isotretinoin
- Isotretinoin, a vitamin A isomer, is a potent teratogen. Women of childbearing age should have a negative pregnancy test before initiating treatment and must use at least two reliable methods of contraception during therapy and for 1 month after the last dose. Major malformations reported include craniofacial, CNS, and cardiac defects.

Antineoplastic Agents
- All antineoplastic agents except cyclosporin A have teratogenic potential in animals. The highest rate of malformations occurs with first trimester exposure.

▶ MEDICATION USE DURING LACTATION

- Drugs that decrease milk production include sympathomimetics, nicotine, levodopa, bromocriptine, ergot alkaloids, pyridoxine, monoamine oxidase inhibitors, and androgens.

365

- Drugs that increase milk production and may cause galactorrhea include antipsychotics, cimetidine, metoclopramide, reserpine, amoxapine, and methyldopa.
- To minimize the effects of drugs during breastfeeding, sustained-release products or drugs with long half-lives should be avoided. Scheduling a dose immediately after a feeding or before a long sleep would help decrease the dose reaching the infant depending on the half-life of the drug.
- The infant should be monitored closely if a nursing mother is taking medication.
- Drugs contraindicated by nursing mothers include amphetamines, bromocriptine, cocaine, ergotamine, lithium, nicotine, most antineoplastic drugs, and drugs of abuse.

SELECTED DRUGS

- Ingestion of large quantities or chronic use of alcohol may cause sedation, CNS depression, weakness, and abnormal growth.
- Caffeine can cause irritability and sleeplessness in breast-fed infants. Moderate use (1–2 cups/day) of coffee is considered acceptable if tolerated by the infant.
- Nicotine should be avoided by lactating women, as it is excreted in breast milk and can cause decreased milk production. Nausea, vomiting, diarrhea, tachycardia, and restlessness may occur in nursing infants exposed to nicotine.
- Most analgesics are excreted in breast milk in low concentrations that should not be harmful to the baby; large doses or chronic use should be considered with caution.
- All antibiotics cross into breast milk, but at less than pharmacologic doses. There is potential to cause candidiasis, diarrhea, and thrush in the nursing infant. Penicillins, cephalosporins, and erythromycin are usually considered to be permissible for nursing mothers. Sulfonamides are permitted if the nursing infant is healthy and full-term. Chloramphenicol, tetracycline, and isoniazid should be avoided. If metronidazole is required, a single 2-gm dose should be used, and the breasts should be pumped for 24–48 hours to allow for excretion of the drug before nursing is resumed.

Anticonvulsants

- Anticonvulsants are generally considered permissible during breastfeeding, but the infant should be observed for sedation and poor feeding.

Hypoglycemic Agents/Insulin

- Diabetic mothers using insulin may breast-feed because the large molecular weight of insulin prevents its excretion into breast milk.

See Chapter 75, Therapeutic Considerations in Pregnancy and Lactation, authored by Janet McCombs, PharmD, for a more detailed discussion of this topic.

Hematologic Disorders

Edited by Cindy W. Hamilton, PharmD

Chapter 31

▶ ANEMIAS

▶ DEFINITION

Anemias are a group of diseases characterized by a decrease in either hemoglobin or red blood cells (RBCs), resulting in a decrease in the oxygen-carrying capacity of blood.

▶ PATHOPHYSIOLOGY

- Anemias can be classified on the basis of RBC morphology, etiology, or pathophysiology (Table 31.1). The most common anemias are included in this chapter.
- Morphologic classifications are based on cell size. Megaloblasts are large nucleated precursors that typically are associated with deficiencies of folate or vitamin B_{12}. Microcytes are small cells that typically are associated with iron deficiency; corresponding iron concentrations may be normal (normochromic) or decreased (hypochromic).
- Iron-deficiency anemia accounts for 25% of anemias and is usually caused by inadequate dietary intake, inadequate gastrointestinal absorption, increased iron demands (e.g., pregnancy), blood loss, and chronic diseases.
- Vitamin B_{12}- and folate-deficiency anemias are caused by inadequate intake, decreased absorption, and inadequate utilization. Deficiency of intrinsic factor may cause decreased absorption of vitamin B_{12} (i.e., pernicious anemia). Celiac disease is the most common cause of folate malabsorption. Folate-deficiency anemia also may be caused by hyper-utilization (e.g., pregnancy or hemolytic anemia), myelofibrosis, malignancy, chronic inflammatory disorder, dialysis-dependent renal failure, or growth spurt. Drugs may cause megaloblastosis by reducing absorption of vitamin B_{12} or folate, or by interfering with corresponding metabolic pathways (Table 31.2).
- Anemia of chronic disease is a hypoproliferative anemia associated with infectious, inflammatory, or neoplastic diseases that last >1–2 months. Anemia of renal failure is addressed separately. Although the cause of anemia of chronic disease is uncertain, the etiology may involve blocked iron release from marrow reticuloendothelial cells, which may be mediated by cytokines that inhibit the production or action of erythropoietin or that inhibit RBC production.
- The etiology of anemia of chronic renal failure is multifactorial. Decreased renal production of erythropoietin is the primary mechanism.

TABLE 31.1. Classification Systems for Anemias

I. Morphology. Classifies anemias based on the red blood cell's size (microcytic, normocytic, macrocytic) and hemoglobin content (hypochromic, normochromic, hyperchromic)

Macrocytic
  Megaloblastic anemias
    Vitamin B_{12} deficiency
    Folic acid deficiency anemia
Hypochromic, microcytic
  Iron deficiency anemia
  Genetic anomaly
    Sickle cell anemia
    Thalassemia
    Other hemoglobinopathies (abnormal hemoglobins)
Normocytic anemias
  Recent blood loss
  Hemolysis
  Bone marrow failure
  Anemias of chronic disease
  Renal failure
  Endocrine disorders
  Myeloplastic anemias

II. Etiology. Classifies anemias on the basis of three fundamental mechanisms

Deficiency
  Iron
    Vitamin B_{12}
    Folic acid
    Pyridoxine
Central—caused by impaired bone marrow function
  Anemia of chronic disease
  Anemia of the elderly
  Malignant bone marrow disorders
Peripheral
  Bleeding (hemorrhage)
  Hemolysis (hemolytic anemias)

III. Pathophysiology. Classifies anemias based on an evaluation of the pathophysiologic etiology

Excessive blood loss
  Recent hemorrhage
    Trauma

Excessive blood loss (cont.)
  Recent hemorrhage (cont.)
    Peptic ulcer
    Gastritis
    Hemorrhoids
  Chronic hemorrhage
    Vaginal bleeding
    Peptic ulcer
    Intestinal parasites
    Aspirin and other nonsteroidal anti-inflammatory agents
Excessive red cell destruction
  Extracorpuscular (i.e., outside the cell) factors
    RBC antibodies
    Drugs
    Physical trauma to RBC (artificial valves)
    Excessive sequestration in the spleen
Intracorpuscular factors
  Heredity
  Disorders of hemoglobin synthesis
Inadequate production of mature RBCs
  Deficiency of nutrients (B_{12}, folic acid, iron, protein)
  Deficiency of erythroblasts
    Aplastic anemia
    Isolated (often transient) erythroblastopenia
    Folic acid antagonists
    Antibodies
  Conditions with infiltration of bone marrow
    Lymphoma
    Leukemia
  Myelofibrosis
    Carcinoma
  Endocrine abnormalities
    Hypothyroid
    Adrenal insufficiency
    Pituitary insufficiency
  Chronic renal disease
  Chronic inflammatory disease
    Granulomatous diseases
    Collagen-vascular diseases
  Hepatic disease

TABLE 31.2. Drug-Induced Megaloblastosis[a]

Impaired absorption or folate inactivation
 Phenytoin
 Phenobarbital
 Primadone
 Alcohol
 Oral contraceptives
 Sulfasalazine
Inhibition of dihydrofolate reductase necessary for conversion of DHF to THF, the metabolically active folate cofactor for nucleic acid synthesis
 Methotrexate
 Trimethoprim
 Triamterene
Inadequate or inactive vitamin B_{12}
 Neomycin
 Colchicine

[a]Only phenytoin, phenobarbital, primidone, and methotrexate have a frequent incidence of reported megaloblastosis.

VII

Other factors include decreased RBC life span caused by uremia, increased folate demand plus depleted body stores, and dialysis-induced blood and iron loss.

- Anemia is one of the most common clinical problems in the elderly. Age-related reductions in bone marrow reserve may render the elderly patient more susceptible to anemia that is caused by multiple minor and often unrecognized diseases (e.g., nutritional deficiencies) that negatively affect erythropoiesis. The most common type of anemia in the elderly is iron-deficiency anemia followed by macrocytic anemia, which is more likely to be caused by vitamin B_{12} than folate deficiency.
- Hemolytic anemia, one of the least common anemias, occurs when the RBC life span is shorter than its normal length of 120 days. Of the many potential etiologies, the most common are RBC membrane defects (e.g., hereditary spherocytosis), altered hemoglobin solubility or stability (e.g., sickle cell anemia and thallasemias), and changes in intracellular metabolism (e.g., glucose-6-phosphate dehydrogenase [G6PD] deficiency). Hemolysis results from the action of the spleen and reticuloendothelial system on damaged RBCs. Depending on the mechanism, hemolytic anemia can be mild, chronic, compensated, and lifelong, or it may be acute, severe, and life threatening. Sickle cell anemia is discussed in Chapter 33.
- Sideroblastic anemia is caused by defective hemoglobin synthesis or acquired defects in precursor cell metabolism that produce a (usually) macrocytic cell with excess nonheme iron in its cytoplasm. Another defect in heme synthesis, porphyria, can lead to overproduction of heme precursors. No further consideration is given to these anemias in this chapter.

▶ CLINICAL PRESENTATION

- Signs and symptoms of anemia depend on the onset and cause of the anemia. Anemia of recent onset usually is manifested by cardiorespiratory symptoms such as tachycardia, light-headedness, and breathlessness. Chronic anemia is manifested by fatigue, headache, vertigo, faintness, sensitivity to cold, pallor, and loss of skin tone.
- Iron-deficiency anemia is manifested by spooning of the nails (koilonychia), angular stomatitis and glossitis, and craving for substances low in iron (pica); however, symptoms do not appear until hemoglobin concentrations fall below 8 or 9 g/dL.
- Vitamin B_{12}- and folate-deficiency anemias are manifested by cardiorespiratory symptoms. Vitamin B_{12} anemia is distinguished by neuropsychiatric abnormalities, especially paresthesias and ataxia, which are absent in patients with folate-deficiency anemia.
- Pernicious anemia in the elderly is manifested by weakness, fatigue, anorexia, reduced drive, sore tongue and mouth, and lemon-yellow discoloration of the skin. Neurologic manifestations include ataxia, loss of position sense, peripheral neuropathy, urinary incontinence, impotence, paresthesias, and visual disturbances. Neuropsychiatric symptoms do not correlate well with vitamin B_{12}-deficiency anemia in the elderly.
- Patients who have hereditary spherocytosis are at risk of developing cholelithiasis or cholecystitis, pigment bile stones, mild jaundice, and splenomegaly.

▶ DIAGNOSIS

- Evaluation of anemia involves a complete blood count including RBC indices, reticulocyte index, examination of the peripheral blood smear, and stool for occult blood (Table 31.3).
- The earliest laboratory change associated with iron-deficiency anemia is decreased serum ferritin (<15 ng/mL), which is followed by further decreases in serum ferritin (<12 ng/mL), decreased serum iron concentrations, increased total iron-binding concentration (TIBC >400 μg/dL), and only slightly decreased hemoglobin. Hemoglobin, hematocrit, and RBC indices usually remain normal until later stages of iron-deficiency anemia.
- Vitamin B_{12}- and folate-deficiency anemias are associated with decreased RBC counts, hemoglobin values, and hematocrit values. Macrocytic anemias are characterized by mean corpuscular volume (MCV) of >100 μm³. One of the earliest and most specific indications of macrocytic anemia is hypersegmented polymorphonuclear leukocytes on the peripheral blood smear.
- Vitamin B_{12} and folate concentrations can be measured to differentiate between the corresponding deficiency anemias. A vitamin B_{12} value of <150 pg/mL, together with appropriate peripheral smear and clinical symptoms, is diagnostic of vitamin B_{12}-deficiency anemia. The Schilling

TABLE 31.3. Normal Hematologic Values

Test	Reference Range (yr)			
	2–6	*6–12*	*12–18*	*18–49*
Hemoglobin (g/dL)	11.5–13.0	11.5–15.5	M 13.0–16.0	M 13.5–17.5
			F 12.0–16.0	F 12.0–16.0
Hematocrit (%)	34.0–40.0	35.0–45.0	M 37.0–49.0	M 41.0–53.0
			F 36.0–46.0	F 36.0–46.0
MCV (μm^3)	75–87	77–95	M 78–98	80–100
			F 78–102	
MCHC (%)	—	31–37	31–37	31–37
MCH (pg)	24–30	25–33	25–35	26–34
RBC (million/mm^3)	3.9–5.3	4.0–5.2	M 4.5–5.3	M 4.5–5.9
Reticulocyte count, absolute (%)				0.5–1.5
Serum iron ($\mu g/dL$)		50–120	50–120	M 50–160
				F 40–150
TIBC ($\mu g/dL$)	250–400	250–400	250–400	250–400
Ferritin (ng/mL)	7–140	7–140	7–140	M 15–200
				F 12–150
Folate (ng/mL)				1.8–16[a]
Vitamin B$_{12}$ (pg/ml)				100–900[a]
Erythropoietin (U/mL)				0.01–0.03

[a]Varies by assay method.

MCV, mean corpuscular volume; MCHC, mean corpuscular hemoglobin concentration; MCH, mean corpuscular hemoglobin; RBC, red blood cell; TIBC, total iron-binding capacity.

test, which is usually abnormal in patients with pernicious anemia, should be performed if the vitamin B$_{12}$ value is <200 pg/mL. The vitamin B$_{12}$ determination should be repeated in 1–3 months, if the value is 200–300 pg/mL. With folate-deficiency anemia, RBC folate concentrations are more predictive of tissue concentrations than serum folate concentrations because the latter are sensitive to acute changes in folate balance.

- Diagnosis of anemia of chronic disease is usually one of exclusion, with consideration of iron-deficiency anemia as the primary or coexisting anemia. Serum iron is usually decreased, but, unlike iron-deficiency anemia, serum ferritin is normal or increased and TIBC is increased. The bone marrow reveals an abundance of iron; the peripheral smear reveals normocytic anemia. The hematocrit may be as low as 25% in 20% of patients.
- Diagnosis of anemia in the elderly is analogous to that in younger adults except as indicated below. A serum ferritin value of <18 ng/mL is highly suggestive of iron-deficiency anemia. If the peripheral smear is consistent with macrocytic anemia, a vitamin B$_{12}$ concentration of <100 pg/mL indicates vitamin B$_{12}$ deficiency, while a serum folate con-

centration of <2 ng/mL or RBC folate concentration of <100 ng/mL indicates folate-deficiency anemia.

▶ DESIRED OUTCOME

The ultimate goals of treatment in the anemic patient are to (1) alleviate signs and symptoms, (2) correct the underlying etiology (e.g., restore depleted stores of iron or other elements required for RBC production), and (3) prevent recurrence of anemia.

▶ TREATMENT

IRON-DEFICIENCY ANEMIA

- Treatment of iron-deficiency anemia consists of dietary supplementation and administration of therapeutic iron preparations. Oral iron therapy with soluble ferrous iron salts that are not enteric coated and not slow- or sustained-release is recommended at a daily dosage of 200 mg elemental iron in two or three divided doses (Table 31.4). Food also plays a significant role because iron is poorly absorbed from vegetables, grain products, dairy products, and eggs; iron is best absorbed from meat, fish, and poultry.
- Patients with iron-deficiency anemia may require parenteral iron therapy if there is iron malabsorption, intolerance of oral iron therapy, or noncompliance. Iron dextran may be given intramuscularly by Z-tract administration or intravenously by multiple slow injections of the undiluted solution, or by infusion of the diluted solution. Dosage is determined by the etiology of the anemia (Table 31.5). After an initial test dose of 25 mg intramuscularly or intravenously (or 5 to 10 minutes of the diluted intravenous infusion solution), patients should be monitored for 1 hour for adverse reactions such as allergic reactions, including anaphylaxis.

VITAMIN B_{12}-DEFICIENCY ANEMIA

- Vitamin B_{12}-deficiency anemia is treated with replacement therapy. Cyanocobalamin or hydroxycobalamin 800–1000 µg is injected daily

VII

TABLE 31.4. Iron Products

Salt	Elemental Iron (%)
Ferrous sulfate	20
Ferrous sulfate, exsiccated	30
Ferrous gluconate	12
Ferrous fumarate	33
Ferric pyrophosphate	12
Ferrous carbonate	48

TABLE 31.5. Equations for Calculating Doses of Iron Dextran

In patients with iron deficiency anemia:

$$\text{mg of iron} = W \times (100 - \%Hb) \times 0.3$$

where W is the patient's weight in pounds and $\%Hb$ is the patient's observed hemoglobin expressed as a percentage of the normal hemoglobin concentration (assuming 14.8 g of hemoglobin per 100 mL is equivalent to 100% concentration).

If the patient weighs 13.6 kg (30 lb) or less, the dose is 80% of the calculated amount.

In patients with anemia secondary to blood loss (hemorrhagic diathesis or long-term dialysis):

$$\text{mg of iron} = \text{blood loss} \times \text{hematocrit}$$

where blood loss is in milliliters and hematocrit is expressed as a decimal fraction.

---

for 1–2 weeks until symptoms subside, followed by 100–1000 µg once weekly until hemoglobin and hematocrit values return to normal. Thereafter, 100–1000 µg is injected monthly for life. Oral vitamin B_{12} is rarely indicated unless the individual has a nutritional deficiency; very large doses are required to provide adequate absorption by the intrinsic-factor–independent method for the patient with pernicious anemia.

FOLATE-DEFICIENCY ANEMIA

- Treatment of folate-deficiency anemia is initiated with oral folate 0.5 mg daily for 2 days, followed by 2 mg orally twice weekly, or 0.5–1 mg daily for approximately 4 months. Long-term therapy may be required if the etiology is a chronic condition that can not be corrected.

ANEMIA OF CHRONIC DISEASE, RENAL FAILURE, AND OLD AGE

- Treatment of anemia of chronic disease is less specific than that of other anemias. This type of anemia usually subsides when the inflammation subsides. Iron therapy is not effective when the inflammation is present. RBC transfusions are effective but should be limited to episodes of inadequate oxygen transport. Erythropoietin may be indicated because erythropoietin concentrations are low relative to the severity of anemia; however, studies of patients with rheumatoid arthritis yielded mixed results.

- Recombinant human erythropoietin or *epoetin alfa* reverses the anemia of chronic renal failure in essentially all patients, circumvents the inherent risks of RBC transfusions, and therefore has become the mainstay of treatment. *Epoetin alfa* should be initiated at a dosage of 50–100 U/kg three times weekly until the hematocrit approaches 36%; the dosage should be titrated to maintain a hematocrit of 30–36%. Although *epoetin alfa* may be administered intravenously or subcutaneously, the latter method may be preferred because it provides more sustained concentrations. The agent of choice for preventing concomitant iron deficiency is oral ferrous sulfate, 325 mg once daily at bedtime.

373

- Treatment of anemia in the elderly is analogous to that in younger adults except as indicated below. Elderly adults who have iron-deficiency anemia and difficulty swallowing tablets may require a pediatric elixir, or even parenteral iron therapy. The initial dosage of cyanocobalamin for vitamin B_{12}-deficiency anemia is 200 μg by weekly injection until stores are replenished, followed by 1000 μg every 1 or 3 months.

HEMOLYTIC ANEMIA

- Treatment of hemolytic anemias is determined by etiology. The treatment of choice for hereditary spherocytosis is splenectomy. Because there is no specific therapy to compensate for G6PD deficiency, treatment consists of avoiding oxidant medications and chemicals.

▶ EVALUATION OF THERAPEUTIC OUTCOMES

- In patients with iron-deficiency anemia, therapeutic doses of iron should raise hemoglobin by 1–2 g/dL per week. The patient should be reevaluated if hemoglobin does not increase by 2 g/dL in the course of 3 weeks or if reticulocytosis does not occur within 7–10 days. Iron therapy is continued until iron stores are restored to normal, which usually requires at least 3–6 months.
- Signs and symptoms of megaloblastic anemia usually subside soon after starting vitamin B_{12} or folate therapy. The patient should be reevaluated if the bone marrow does not become normoblastic after 24 hours, reticulocytosis does not occur after 2–3 days, hemoglobin does not rise after 1 or 2 weeks, or leukocyte and platelet counts do not normalize after 1 week.
- In patients with anemia of chronic failure, the goal of *epoetin alfa* therapy is to maintain a hematocrit of 30–36%. Iron depletion is a major reason for failure to respond to epoetin therapy; iron therapy is considered if the transferrin saturation is at least 20% and the serum ferritin is <100 ng/mL. Blood pressure is monitored because approximately 30–47% of patients receiving *epoetin alfa* experience elevated diastolic blood pressure; antihypertensive therapy may need to be adjusted.

See Chapter 93, Anemias, authored by William J. Spruill, PharmD, and William E. Wade, PharmD, FASHP, for a more detailed discussion of this topic.

VII

Chapter 32

► COAGULATION DISORDERS

► DEFINITION

Coagulation disorders are a group of diseases characterized by altered regulation of hemostasis (i.e., spontaneous arrest of bleeding from damaged vessels), resulting in an increased risk of bleeding. This chapter focuses on hemophilia, von Willebrand's disease, disseminated intravascular coagulation, and other coagulopathies; thrombotic disorders are not included.

► PATHOPHYSIOLOGY

- The exact mechanisms that regulate the balance between clot formation and lysis are not completely understood. The major components of normal hemostasis are blood vessel walls, platelets, the coagulation system, and the fibrinolytic system (Figure 32.1). Disturbances in these components can cause a wide variety of congenital and acquired coagulopathies.

- Vessel walls contribute to primary hemostasis by vasoconstriction, formation of platelet plugs, and regulation of coagulation and fibrinolysis. Platelets respond to vascular injury in four phases: adhesion, aggregation, secretion, and elaboration of procoagulant activity.

- Coagulation and fibrinolytic systems provide interrelated and opposing functions. Clotting is initiated by an intrinsic or extrinsic pathway, with subsequent factor interactions that converge at the common pathway in which thrombin promotes fibrin activation (Figure 32.2). The 12 coagulation factors can be divided into groups based on their biochemical properties: vitamin K-dependent factors (II or prothrombin, VII, IX, and X), contact activation factors (XI, XII, prekallikrein, and high molecular weight kininogen), and thrombin-sensitive factors (I or fibrinogen, V, VIII, and XIII). During fibrinolysis, plasmin enzymatically digests fibrin, dissolves the clot, and releases fibrin degradation or split products.

- The entire factor VIII molecule consists of factor VIII coagulant material and a larger molecule, von Willebrand's factor, which mediates platelet adhesion to injured vessel walls and also serves as a carrier for factor VIII.

- The most common congenital coagulopathy is von Willebrand's disease, followed by hemophilia. Von Willebrand's disease is usually an autosomal dominant disorder caused by a deficiency of the larger part of the factor VIII molecule. Hemophilia is a recessive sex-linked disease that is caused by a deficiency of factor VIII coagulant material (hemophilia A or classic hemophilia) in 85% of affected patients or by a deficiency of factor IX (hemophilia B) in nearly all of the remaining patients.

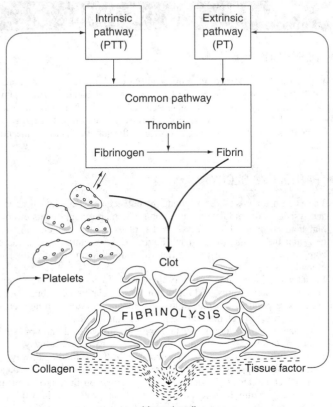

Figure 32.1. Simplified scheme of the hemostatic system, showing interaction of vessel wall, platelets, coagulation pathways, and fibrinolytic system. Not shown are regulatory and inhibitory mechanisms. *(From Stead RB. In Goldhaber SZ (ed): Pulmonary Embolism and Deep Vein Thrombosis. Philadelphia, WB Saunders, 1985:28, with permission.)*

- The degree of the genetic defect determines the severity of the congenital coagulopathy. Variants are possible depending on whether the affected molecule is completely absent, deficient, or defective.
- Pseudo von Willebrand's disease results from a platelet abnormality instead of from a deficiency of von Willebrand's factor.
- Acquired von Willebrand's disease may occur in patients with connective tissue diseases, monoclonal gammopathies, lymphoproliferative disease, or Wilms' tumor.

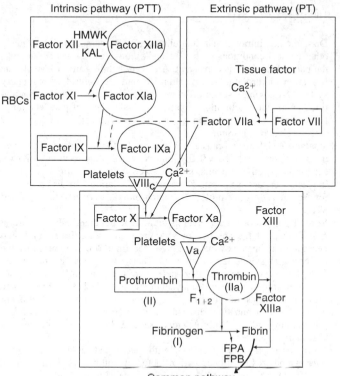

Intrinsic pathway (PTT) Extrinsic pathway (PT)

Figure 32.2. The coagulation pathways. Important features include the contact activation phase, vitamin K-dependent factors (affected by warfarin), the activated serine proteases that are inhibited by heparin: antithrombin III, and the role of platelets and calcium. Factors VIIIc and Va are nonenzymatic cofactors that are inactivated by protein C. The protime (PT) measures the function of the extrinsic and common pathways; the partial thromboplastin time (PTT or APTT) measures the function of the intrinsic and common pathways. HMWK, high molecular weight kininogen; KAL, kallikrein *(From Stead RB. In SZ Goldhaber (ed): Pulmonary Embolism and Deep Vein Thrombosis. Philadelphia, WB Saunders, 1985:32, with permission.)*

- Disseminated intravascular coagulation (DIC) is associated with many other clinical conditions (Table 32.1). Although the causes are diverse, the pathophysiology is consistent. An overwhelming insult leads to the formation of thrombin and plasmin beyond the control of regulatory systems. A complex series of events triggers consumption of coagulation factors during clotting, depletion or dysfunction of platelets, interference with fibrin formation by fibrinogen degradation products, and lysis of clots by plasmin.
- Vitamin K deficiency causes a bleeding diathesis because of marked deficiency of factors II, VII, IX, and X, which require vitamin K_1 for activation. Inactive precursors of these coagulation factors accumulate in plasma and act as vitamin K antagonists. Vitamin K is also necessary for the active form of protein C, which inhibits activated factor V and VIII.
- Several populations may develop vitamin K deficiency. Infants are at risk because of the absence of vitamin K in human breast milk and because their intestines may not have had time to be colonized by the bacteria that synthesize vitamin K. Their livers may not be mature enough to synthesize vitamin K-dependent coagulation factors. Broad-spectrum antibiotic therapy may also sterilize the large intestine and prevent synthesis of vitamin K. Finally, malabsorption may occur because of poor nutrition; diseases of the small intestine such as celiac disease, amyloidosis, Whipple's disease, and short-bowel syndrome; or obstructive jaundice.
- Liver disease may be associated with bleeding disorders because the liver synthesizes most coagulation factors including I or fibrinogen, II, V, VII, IX, X, XII, and XIII. Hepatic cells also regulate clotting inhibitors of the fibrinolytic system such as plasminogen, α_2-antiplasmin, and α_2-macroglobulin. Furthermore, a fibrinolytic state may occur if clearance of activated clotting or fibrinolytic factors is impaired. Finally, thrombocytopenia and platelet dysfunction are common in patients with liver disease.

► CLINICAL PRESENTATION

- Hemophilia is usually manifested by joint and muscle hemorrhage and prolonged bleeding after trauma or surgery. Joint hemorrhages frequently involve large, especially weight-bearing, joints; they are often spontaneous, begin in childhood, and can lead to disabling arthropathies. Minor trauma and abrasions, which are controlled with platelet plugs, do not pose clinical problems.
- Von Willebrand's disease is manifested by mucosal bleeding such as epistaxis, gingival bleeding, easy bruising, menorrhagia, and postoperative bleeding especially after operations on mucosal surfaces (e.g., tonsillectomy, vaginal surgery, and dental surgery). Von Willebrand's disease is rarely manifested by the joint and muscle bleeding characteristic of hemophilia.

TABLE 32.1. Conditions Associated with Disseminated Intravascular Coagulation

Infectious
  Bacterial
    Gram-negative
    Gram-positive
  Mycoplasmal
  Rickettsial
    Rocky Mountain Spotted Fever
  Viral
    Cytomegalovirus
    Hepatitis
    Varicella
  Chlamydial
    Psittacosis
  Fungal
    Aspergillosis
    Candidiasis
    Histoplasmosis
  Mycobacterial
  Protozoal
    Malaria (falciparum)

Tissue Injury
  Burns
  Extensive surgery
  Crush injuries
  Multiple trauma
  Head trauma

Obstetrics
  Amniotic fluid embolism
  Placental abruption
  Missed abortion
  Eclampsia

Malignancy
  Leukemia
  Most carcinomas
  Other
    Pheochromocytoma
    Myeloma
    Sarcomas
    Neuroblastoma
    Histiocytosis X
    Polycythemia vera

Intravascular Hemolysis
  Hemolytic transfusion reaction
  Minor hemolysis
  Massive transfusion

Cardiovascular
  Postcardiac arrest
  Aortic aneurysm
  Prosthetic device (aortic balloon)
  Giant hemangiomas
  Acute myocardial infarction
  Peripheral vascular disease

Pulmonary
  Adult respiratory distress syndrome
  Pulmonary embolism
  Pulmonary infarction
  Hyaline membrane disease

Miscellaneous
  Snake bite
  Heat stroke
  Hypothermia/hyperthermia
  Organic solvent poisoning
  Aspirin poisoning
  Fat embolism
  Severe anoxia
  Liver disease
  Hematologic
    Sickle cell crisis
    Paroxysmal nocturnal hemoglobinuria
  Collagen vascular disease
  Immune complex
    Anaphylaxis
    Systemic lupus

VII

From Gilbert JA, Scalzi RP. Emerg Med Clin North Am 1993; 11:475, with permission.

- DIC is manifested by bleeding from many sites, including oozing from intravenous lines or from invasive procedures. Massive bleeding from the gastrointestinal tract or genitourinary system, peripheral cyanosis of the extremities, renal or cardiopulmonary failure or both, or purpura fulminans may dominate the clinical picture.
- Clinical manifestations of vitamin K deficiency depend on the etiology. Infants may bleed from the umbilical cord, from the gastrointestinal tract, or occasionally into the brain after birth. Malabsorption syndromes typically exhibit manifestations of the underlying disease such as abnormal development in children, weight loss, muscle wasting, and steatorrhea.
- Patients with coagulation disorders caused by liver disease usually have clinical manifestations of their underlying disease. In fact, such patients may have profoundly abnormal coagulation parameters without bleeding. Conversely, major bleeding may occur despite normal coagulation parameters in patients with esophageal varices or peptic ulcer disease.

▶ DIAGNOSIS

VII
- The initial diagnosis of coagulation disorders is established from a detailed clinical history, physical examination, and laboratory tests (Table 32.2).
- Activated partial thromboplastin time (aPTT) is an excellent test for screening deficiencies in the coagulation pathways because it is very sensitive. For example, aPTT detects hemophilia A in 99–100% of patients. Additional laboratory tests are needed to distinguish between hemophilia A, hemophilia B, and variants of von Willebrand's disease (Table 32.3).
- Von Willebrand's factor activity is measured as the bleeding time and by the ristocetin cofactor test (Table 32.3). Von Willebrand's antigen can be quantified by electrophoresis with precipitating antibody to von Willebrand's factor or by radioimmunoassay. Genetic variants are defined by the relative proportions of large and small multimers demonstrated by electrophoresis.
- DIC should be considered when clinical manifestations occur in a patient whose underlying condition is a risk factor (Table 32.1). A complete battery of laboratory tests is required to confirm the diagnosis. Routine testing of blood coagulation usually reveals prolonged prothrombin time (PT), variable or even normal aPTT, and prolonged thrombin time [TT]. Although not specific for DIC, fibrinogen is <150 mg/dL and platelet counts are <150,000 mm^3 in 95% of patients; 75% of patients have red blood cell fragments or schistocytes. The most specific findings are low platelet counts associated with elevated fibrin split products and depressed antithrombin III and fibrinogen levels.
- In patients with liver disease, PT, aPTT, and TT are useful screening tests for deficiency of liver-dependent factors. Platelet count should also be determined. Clotting time can be measured using snake venom to

TABLE 32.2. Laboratory Procedures

Procedure	Reagent Content	Normal Range	System Tested	Disease Detected and Therapy Monitored
Template bleeding time	None	1–8 min	Platelets and capillaries	Thrombocytopathy, von Willebrand's disease, and thrombocytopenia
Activated partial thromboplastin time (APTT)	Phospholipid contact activator	<42 s	Intrinsic	Mild (40–50%) deficiencies of factors VIII, IX, and XI (hemophilias); deficiency of factor XII; von Willebrand's disease; disseminated intravascular coagulation; inhibitors; heparin therapy
Prothrombin time (PT)	Tissue thromboplastin	10–12 s	Extrinsic	Factor VII deficiency (acquired or hereditary); vitamin K deficiency; DIC; inhibitors; warfarin therapy
Thrombin time (TT)	Thrombin	20–24 s	Conversion of fibrinogen to fibrin	Hypofibrinogenemia and dysfibrinogenemia; fibrin split products; presence of heparin

Modified from Triplett DA. *Hemostasis: A Case Oriented Approach.* New York, Igaku-Shoin, 1985:E6, with permission

VII

TABLE 32.3. Tests in Patients with Hemophilia A, Hemophilia B, and von Willebrand's Disease

	Hemophilia[a]		von Willebrand's Disease			
	A	B	I	II-A	II-B	III
APTT	A	A	A	A/N	A/N	A
PT	N	N/A[b]	N	N	N	N
Factor VIII	A	N	A	A/N	A/N	A
vWF:Ag	N	N	A	A/N	A/N	A
vWF:R	N	N	A/N	A	A	A
RIPA	N	N	A/N	A	A[c]	A
vWF multimers						
In plasma	N	N	Reduced, absent	Largest absent	Largest absent	None
In platelets	N	N	N	Largest absent	All present	None
Factor IX	N	A	N	N	N	N
TT	N	N	N	N	N	N
Bleeding time	N	N	A	A	A	A
Platelet adhesion	N	N	A	A	A	A
Other factors	N	N	N	N	N	N

[a]A, abnormal; N, normal.
[b]Prothrombin time is abnormal in hemophilia B_m.
[c]Platelet aggregation with ristocetin is increased.

VII

test the degree of dysfibrinogenemia and obtain an indication of the degree of liver dysfunction. Factor V can be measured; this factor is independent of the vitamin and is synthesized by liver cells.

▶ DESIRED OUTCOME

- In patients with coagulopathies, bleeding episodes should be prevented through education.
- The main goal of treating hemophilia is to control and prevent bleeding episodes and their long-term sequelae, such as arthropathies.
- The main goal of treating von Willebrand's disease is to improve factor VIII concentrations and bleeding time.
- The main goal of treating DIC is to minimize morbidity and prevent mortality.

▶ TREATMENT

GENERAL PRINCIPLES

- Total care of hemophilia requires a multitude of medical and paramedical personnel, including pharmacists. Federal funding enables regional comprehensive treatment programs, which also cover the high cost of treatment.

- Patients should be educated from birth about physical protection during usual play and other preventive measures.
- Genetic counseling should be offered to patients and potential carriers.
- To achieve independence, patients should learn to self-administer medications. Patients should be educated about proper storage, handling, and administration techniques (e.g., initiation of therapy at onset of bleeding symptoms). Patients should be educated about side effects, including unlikely complications, because unwarranted fear of acquiring viral infections, particularly HIV, can lead to poor compliance.
- Nonsteroidal anti-inflammatory drugs (NSAIDs) should be avoided in patients with coagulopathies.

HEMOPHILIA A

- Treatment is determined by the severity of hemophilia A. Severe or moderate disease can be treated with factor VIII concentrate or cryoprecipitate. Mild factor VIII deficiency may be treated with 1-desamino-8-D-arginine vasopressin (desmopressin acetate, DDAVP), a synthetic analogue of antidiuretic hormone or vasopressin that transiently increases factor VIII (and von Willebrand factor) and shortens prolonged bleeding time. VII
- All factor VIII preparations (Table 32.4) are equally effective and have similar rates of antibody development. Cost and personal preference influence choice. Plasma-derived products carry a small potential for transmission of blood-borne viruses other than HIV and hepatitis, and may or may not have immunosuppressant effects.
- The approach to replacement therapy is empiric and should be individualized. The general goal is to achieve a factor VIII concentration of 30–50% to maintain hemostasis. Each unit of factor VIII infused per kilogram of body weight increases plasma levels by 2%. Therefore, the initial dose can be calculated as follows: Factor VIII (units) = (desired level – actual level) × 0.5 (patient's weight in kilograms). Alternatively, dose can be based on body weight and on the site and severity of bleeding (Table 32.5).
- Because the half-life of factor VIII is 8–12 hours, it must be administered at least twice daily or as a continuous infusion. Continuous infusion may be more convenient than bolus therapy.
- Cryoprecipitate contains factor VIII, fibrinogen, and von Willebrand factor; however, it has generally been replaced with factor VIII concentrate. Although the potency varies, each 10- to 20-mL bag of cryoprecipitate contains approximately 70-100 units of factor VIII activity. Dose determination is analogous to that for factor VIII concentrate.
- DDAVP may be administered by several routes. Intravenous injection over 15–30 minutes increases factor VIII levels four-fold to six-fold, with peak levels at 90–120 minutes and persistent activity for >6 hours. DDAVP can be repeated within 12–24 hours, but the response is attenuated with frequent dosing. Subcutaneous administration is as effective as the intravenous route and more practical for self-administration.

TABLE 32.4 Factor VIII Preparations

Manufacturer	Brand Name	Viral Inactivation or Exclusion Method	Annual Cost[a] ($)
Alpha	Profilate-OSD[b]	Solvent-detergent	72,000
American Red Cross	AHF-M[b]	Solvent-detergent	28,000
Armour	Humate-P[b]	Pasteurized	104,000
	Monoclate-P[b]	Pasteurized/ monoclonal antibody	
Baxter	Hemophil M[b]	Solvent-detergent/ monoclonal antibody	72,000
	Recombinate[c]	Affinity chromatography	94,000
Miles/Bayer	Koate HP[b]	Solvent-detergent	72,000
	Kogenate[d]	Affinity chromatography	94,000

[a]Based on 1994 average wholesale price *(Red Book)*, and consumption of 80,000 units/yr.
[b]Plasma derived.
[c]Hamster ovary cell derived.
[d]Hamster kidney cell derived.
Adapted from Anonymous. Med Lett Drugs Ther 1993;35(898):51.

Intranasal DDAVP is a convenient alternative, but it increases factor VIII levels to a lesser extent than does parenteral administration.

HEMOPHILIA B

- High purity factor IX plasma concentrate is the treatment of choice for hemophilia B. The half-life is 24 hours. Each unit infused per kg of body weight raises the plasma level by 1%. A plasma concentration of 10–25% is recommended to achieve normal hemostasis. Levels of 40% are recommended for severe muscle and joint bleeding. Levels of 60% are recommended for major surgery, and infusion should be continued for at least a week.
- Alphanine and Alphanine-SD (Alpha Therapeutic) contain 50 U/mg protein; Mononine (Armour) contains 150 U/mg protein. These products provide excellent hemostasis and are not associated with thromboembolic complications.

SPECIAL CONSIDERATIONS FOR HEMOPHILIA

- Up to one-half of hemophiliacs develop inhibitors or IgG antibodies to factor VIII or IX, which prevent the calculated dose from producing the expected plasma level. Product selection (plasma-derived versus recombinant factor VIII) does not affect the development of inhibitors.

VII

TABLE 32.5. Factor VIII Replacement Therapy For Severely Affected Hemophiliacs[a]

Site of Hemorrhage	Desired Factor VIII Level (% of normal)	Factor VIII Dose (units/kg body weight[b])	Frequency of Dose[c] (interval in hours)	Duration (days)
Hemarthroses	30–50	≈25	24	1–2
Superficial intramuscular hematoma	30–50	≈25	24	1–2
Gastrointestinal tract	50–100	≈25–50	12	7–10
Epistaxis	30–50	≈25	12	Until resolved
Oral mucosa	30–50	≈25	12	Until resolved
Hematuria	30–100	≈25–50	12	Until resolved
Central nervous system	75–100	50	8–12	7–10 days or until healing occurs
Retropharyngeal	75–100	50	8–12	7–10 days or until healing occurs
Retroperitoneal	75–100	50	8–12	7–10 days or until healing occurs

[a] Mild or moderately affected patients may respond to DDAVP which should be used in lieu of blood or blood products whenever possible.

[b] The factor VIII may be administered in a continuous infusion if the patient is hospitalized. After initial bolus, about 150 units factor VIII per h is usually sufficient in an average-sized adult.

[c] Both the frequency of dosing and duration of therapy may be adjusted in keeping with the severity and duration of each patient's bleeding episode.

From Roberts HR, Jones MR., in Williams WJ, Beutler E, Erslev AJ, Lichtman MA (eds): Hematology. New York, McGraw-Hill, 1990:1450, with permission.

VII

385

- There are several approaches to inhibitors to factor VIII (Figure 32.3) and IX. Inhibitor concentrations may be reduced by prophylactic administration of immunosuppressive agents, gamma globulin infusions, or plasmapheresis; or immune tolerance may be induced by repeated or high-dose infusions of the factor. An alternative method is designed to induce hemostasis during acute bleeding or surgery. If the patient has low inhibitor titers (<5 BU/mL), high-dose factor therapy (e.g., twice the calculated dose) may induce hemostasis. If the patient has high inhibitor titers (>10 BU/mL), prothrombin complex concentrate (PCC), activated prothrombin complex concentrate (APCC), or porcine factor VIII may be required. PCC and APCC should be administered at twice the calculated dose. Porcine factor VIII is only indicated for hemophilia A and is administered at the calculated dose.
- Surgical candidates, regardless of whether the procedure is minor or major, require a factor VIII level of 100% 1 hour before the procedure. Guidelines should be followed to avoid potentially life-threatening hemorrhage (Table 32.6). Antifibrinolytic agents such as ε-aminocaproic acid (EACA) and tranexamic acid are effective adjuncts for controlling bleeding after some surgical procedures.
- Pain is a common complication of hemophilia. Chronic pain may require acetaminophen, narcotic analgesics, and even nonpharmacologic intervention such as surgery.

VON WILLEBRAND'S DISEASE

- Cryoprecipitate, which contains von Willebrand factor along with factor VIII and fibrinogen, is the usual treatment for severe bleeding. Unfortunately, cryoprecipitate may be contaminated with blood-borne viruses.
- Selection of cryoprecipitate dose is generally empiric because of both disease and potency variability, and also because of the lack of reliable laboratory tests for monitoring replacement therapy. In general, one bag of cryoprecipitate/10 kg body weight is sufficient.
- Although most factor VIII concentrates are not suitable, Humate-P contains sufficient von Willebrand's factor to provide adequate hemostasis. Koate-HS and Koate-HP have also been reported to achieve clinical hemostasis before surgery.
- DDAVP may be used in place of cryoprecipitate in mild von Willebrand's disease or as adjunct therapy. However, DDAVP should not be used in patients with an unknown variant because DDAVP may cause platelet aggregation and worsen thrombocytopenia in patients with type II-B or pseudo von Willebrand's disease. DDAVP is not beneficial in patients with type II-C or II-D disease.
- Intravenous DDAVP, 0.3–0.4 μg/kg over the course of 15–30 minutes, usually increases von Willebrand's factor and factor VIII four-fold to six-fold. The dose may be repeated in 8–12 hours, but the response

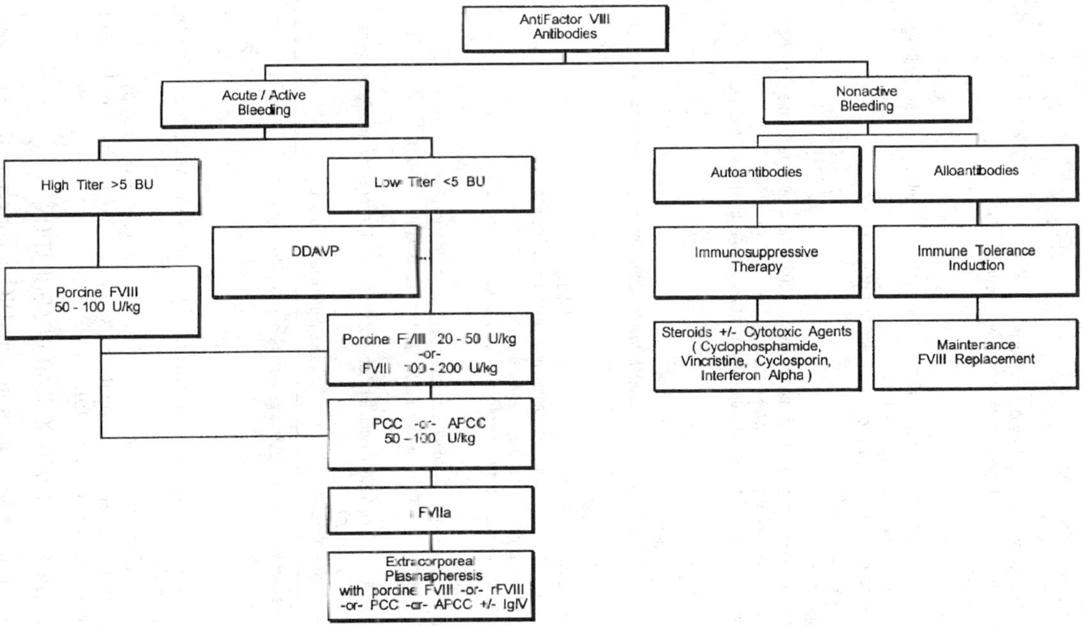

Figure 32.3. Treatment algorithm for the management of patients with hemophilia and factor VIII antibodies. (Adapted from: Kessler CM. Semin Hematol 1994;31:33–36, with permission.)

TABLE 32.6. Guidelines for Managing Hemophilic Patients Who Require Surgery

Before surgical procedure
1. Complete coagulation workup
2. Incubate test for inhibitors
3. Calculate needs and stockpile therapeutic material in hospital
4. Survival study for recovery and half-life of therapeutic material
5. Red cell type, crossmatch

Minor surgical procedures
1. Give dose calculated to bring patient's plasma level to 100% 1 hour before procedure (50 IU/kg)
2. Maintain plasma level about 60% for 4 days
3. Maintain plasma level above 20% for the subsequent 4 days
4. Assay daily prior to dose

Major surgical procedures
1. Give dose calculated to bring patient's plasma level to 100% 1 hour before procedure (50 IU/kg)
2. Maintain plasma level above 60% for 4 days
3. Maintain plasma level above 20% for the subsequent 4 days or until all drains and sutures are removed
4. Assay daily prior to dose

Orthopedic surgical procedures
1. Give dose calculated to bring patient's plasma level to 100% 1 hour before procedure (50 IU/kg)
2. Maintain plasma level above 80% for 4 days
3. Assay daily prior to dose
4. Maintain plasma level above 40% for the subsequent 4 days
5. If patient is casted, discontinue replacement until rehabilitation program is begun
6. If not casted, maintain above 20% for ambulation
7. For rehabilitation program, maintain above 10% for 3 weeks

Dental procedures
1. Give EACA 100 mg/kg IV 4 hours before surgery or tranexamic acid 10mg/kg
2. Give factor replacement dose calculated to bring patient's plasma level to 100% 1 hour before procedure
3. Continue EACA 100 mg/kg orally q6h for 7 days or tranexamic acid for 7 days (adults, 2 g three times a day for 7 days)
4. Repeat one dose of replacement therapy in 3 days if procedure is extensive

From Hilgartner MW. In Hilgartner MW, Pochedly C (eds): Hemophilia in the Child and Adult. New York, Raven Press, 1989:14, with permission.

VII

diminishes with repeated treatment. The intranasal route may also be considered.
- Menorrhagia may be controlled with oral contraceptive therapy.
- If inhibitors develop in patients with severe type III disease, PCC or plasmapheresis may be useful.

DISSEMINATED INTRAVASCULAR COAGULATION

- The most important step in treating DIC is correcting the underlying disease. If this is not possible or effective, then deficient factors may be replaced or anticoagulant therapy may be attempted (Table 32.7).

TABLE 32.7. Sequential Therapy for Disseminated Intravascular Coagulation

Individualize therapy
Site(s) and severity of hemorrhage
Site(s) and severity of thrombosis
Hemodynamic status
Age
Treat or remove triggering process
Component therapy as indicated
Fresh-frozen plasma
Antithrombin concentrate
Platelet concentrates
Packed red cells
Cryoprecipitate
Stop intravascular clotting problem
Subcutaneous or intravenous heparin
Antithrombin concentrate
Antiplatelet agents?
Inhibit residual fibrino(geno)lysis
EACA
Tranexamic acid

Adapted from Bick RL. Med Clin North Am 1994;78:531, with permission.

VII

- Fresh-frozen plasma provides volume to expand intravascular space and replaces clotting factors including fibronogen. If hypofibrinogenemia is severe, cryoprecipitate may be useful.
- Anticoagulation is controversial in patients with DIC. Heparin is thought to prevent further consumption of hemostatic factors by interfering with thrombin activity, but anticoagulation may not be prudent therapy for a bleeding disorder. No controlled trials are available to settle this controversy. Conditions in which heparin may be useful include progressive organ dysfunction, evidence of dermal necrosis or ischemia, retained-dead-fetus syndrome, aortic aneurysm, and hemangioma. Heparin may also be added to replacement therapy, especially in patients with acute progranulocytic leukemia. Heparin is contraindicated if there is bleeding into a closed space.
- Heparin may be given intravenously by bolus every 4 hours or by continuous infusion. The dose is controversial, ranging from full-dose regimens (e.g., 5000 U by bolus followed by continuous infusion of 1000 U/hour) to low-dose regimens (e.g., 500 U/h).
- Antifibrinolytic therapy is controversial and is probably contraindicated more often than not. EACA is usually reserved for use in conjunction with heparin, except in the two clinical conditions in which isolated fibrinolysis may occur without thrombin generation, namely cardiopulmonary bypass surgery and carcinoma of the prostate.

VITAMIN K DEFICIENCY

- Vitamin K_1 is the treatment of choice for vitamin K deficiency. The dose, frequency, and duration depend on the severity of the deficiency and the patient's response. The dose ranges from 2–25 mg and may be administered orally, intramuscularly, subcutaneously, or intravenously. An oral dose increases blood coagulation factors 6–12 hours later. Even when administered parenterally, vitamin K_1 takes 24–48 hours to normalize PT.
- Infants with vitamin K deficiency usually respond to a parenteral dose of 1 mg on the first day, which can be repeated every 8 days until clotting-test results normalize.
- Disease severity and etiology may influence the selection of route. Intramuscular administration should be avoided in severe hypothrombinemia because of the risk of hematoma. Because of the rare anaphylactic reaction associated with intravenous administration, this method is restricted to patients who cannot absorb the drug from the gastrointestinal tract and who are thrombocytopenic.
- Fresh-frozen plasma may be used to immediately correct vitamin K-dependent factors in the event of severe hemorrhage.

LIVER DISEASE

- Liver disease-induced coagulopathy should only be treated if overt bleeding is present or if the patient requires an invasive procedure.
- Aggressive management with blood products is required to stop overt bleeding. In a seriously ill patient 1–2 units (250–500 mL) of fresh-frozen plasma may be necessary every 6 hours.
- Vitamin K_1, 10–25 mg, may be administered for 1 or 2 days to rule out vitamin K deficiency.
- Prothrombin complex concentrates may be administered, but this approach may increase the risk of DIC.
- The use of heparin and antifibrinolytic agents is controversial.
- Platelet transfusions may be necessary if thrombocytopenia occurs.

▶ LONG-TERM STRATEGIES

- Life-long patient education and multidisciplinary intervention are required to achieve desired outcomes.
- Bleeding episodes can be nearly eliminated in patients with hemophilia A if they receive prophylactic factor VIII 24–40 IU/kg three times weekly to maintain a level of >1% beginning at 1 year of age. Pharmacokinetic dosing models have been proposed as a cost-saving approach to prophylaxis.
- Patients who are at risk for vitamin K deficiency should be identified and treated accordingly. For example, newborns should receive prophylactic vitamin K_1. Patients receiving long-term total parenteral nutrition should receive vitamin K_1 weekly.

▶ EVALUATION OF THERAPEUTIC OUTCOMES

- Successful replacement treatment of hemophilia requires achieving appropriate factor VIII or IX levels, which in turn requires monitoring with corresponding assays.
- Surveillance for the development of inhibitors to factors VIII and IX should be performed, especially in hemophiliacs with severe disease who require high usage of factor concentrates. Patients who require PCC or APCC should be monitored clinically and closely because of the lack of corresponding assays.
- Patients with von Willebrand's disease must be monitored clinically because there is no standard method for determining whether ristocetin cofactor concentrations are adequate to achieve hemostasis. There is often a discrepancy between von Willebrand's factor activity and factor VIII levels 24 hours after the infusion, if additional cryoprecipitate is not given. Bleeding time can be unreliable because it may only be transiently shortened.
- In patients with DIC, monitoring heparin therapy is confounded because the aPTT value may be elevated before initiation of anticoagulant therapy. Consequently, it is best to follow fibrin degradation products and fibrinogen levels.
- Before initiating antifibrinolytic therapy for DIC, defibrination should be distinguished from fibrinolysis.
- Patients with vitamin K deficiency should be monitored closely. If the PT value does not become normal 48 hours after treatment, another etiology should be considered (e.g., liver disease).
- In patients with liver disease and bleeding, PT or aPTT should be repeated after infusing fresh-frozen plasma. If the values are >1.5 times the upper limits of control values, extra units may be needed. The patient should also be monitored for signs and symptoms of fluid overload, especially if multiple units of fresh-frozen plasma are required.

See Chapter 94, Coagulation Disorders, authored by Mariela Diaz-Linares, PharmD, Keith A. Rodvold, PharmD, FCCP, BCPS, and William R. Friendenberg, MD, for a more detailed discussion of this topic.

VII

Chapter 33

▶ SICKLE CELL ANEMIA

▶ DEFINITION

Sickle cell disease is a group of hemolytic anemias caused by genetic defects in hemoglobin, which result in sickle-shaped red blood cells (RBCs).

▶ PATHOPHYSIOLOGY

- The biochemical defect causing development of sickle cell disease involves an amino acid in the β polypeptide chain of the hemoglobin molecule; the α chain is normal.
- The most common abnormal hemoglobin in the United States is hemoglobin S, where sickle cell trait occurs in 8% of the black population and sickle cell anemia occurs in 0.3%. Hemoglobin C can be detected in 3% of the corresponding population. Other abnormal hemoglobins are E, which is found in the Far East, and D, which is found in India, Pakistan, Afghanistan, and Iran.
- Two genes for hemoglobin S result in a homozygote with sickle cell anemia, while only one results in a heterozygote with sickle cell trait. It should be noted, however, that the heterozygotes may experience pathology, especially if they are double heterozygotes with hemoglobin S and either hemoglobin C or thalassemia.
- Clinical manifestations of sickle cell disease are attributable to impaired circulation, RBC destruction, and stasis of blood flow.
- When RBCs contain hemoglobin S, their membranes become damaged, which cause cells to lose potassium and water. This dehydrated state enhances the formation of sickle-shaped RBCs. With repeated episodes, these RBCs retain calcium, become more rigid, and eventually assume irreversible sickle shapes.
- The presence of sickle-shaped RBCs increases blood viscosity and encourages sludging in the capillaries and small vessels. Such obstructive events lead to local tissue hypoxia, which accentuates the pathologic process.
- Not all clinical manifestations are readily attributable to sickling of RBCs. For example, reticuloendothelial function may be impaired because of functional asplenia, which in turn increases the risk of bacterial infection and of disseminated intravascular coagulation (DIC).

▶ CLINICAL PRESENTATION

- Sickle cell disease is associated with many clinical manifestations (Table 33.1). Symptoms do not appear until after 4–6 months of age

TABLE 33.1. Manifestations of Sickle Cell Disease: Crises and Complications

Crisis	Characteristic
Vaso-occlusive	Infarction/pain
Hemolytic	Massive hemolysis
Splenic sequestration	Sequestration of red blood cells
Aplastic	Bone marrow failure
Organ system	Complication
Pulmonary	Acute chest syndrome
Neurologic	Various, including cerebrovascular accident
Dermatologic	Chronic ulcers
Cardiovascular	Hypertrophy
Genitourinary	Priapism, hematuria, hyposthenuria
Skeletal	Aseptic necrosis, osteomyelitis
Ocular	Retinal problems
Hepatic	Cholelithiasis

VII ◀

because of the oxygen-carrying capability of fetal hemoglobin and because hemoglobin F is less likely to sickle.

- Common initial findings are pneumonia or pain and swelling of the hands and feet (e.g., hand-and-foot syndrome or dactylitis). Splenomegaly is also common in children.
- Usual clinical signs and symptoms of sickle cell disease are chronic anemia, fever and pallor, arthralgia, scleral icterus, abdominal pain, weakness, anorexia, fatigue, and hematuria.
- Children experience delayed growth and sexual maturation. Additional physical findings are protuberant abdomen and exaggerated lumbar lordosis, asthenic appearance with long extremities and tapered fingers, and barrel-shaped chest.
- Sickle cell crisis may be precipitated by fever, infection, dehydration, hypoxia, acidosis, sudden temperature change, or a combination of factors. The most common type of crisis is vasoocclusive or infarctive, which is manifested by pain over the involved areas without changes in hemoglobin or other laboratory values. This type of crisis may affect hands and feet, joints and extremities, abdomen, liver, and lungs. Less common types of crises are aplastic, hemolytic, and splenic sequestration (see Table 33.1).
- Complications of sickle cell disease include acute chest syndrome, neurologic abnormalities due to cerebrovascular occlusion, chronic ulcers of the inner aspect of the lower leg, cholelithiasis, cardiovascular abnormalities, priapism, destructive bone and joint problems, ocular

complications, and renal complications. Acute chest syndrome is characterized by cough, dyspnea, chest pain, fever, pulmonary infiltration, and equivocal response to antibiotic therapy; the etiology may or may not be pulmonary infarction.

- Patients with sickle cell trait are usually asymptomatic, except for impaired renal function and dilute urine, increased risk of dehydration, and hematuria.

▶ DIAGNOSIS

- The diagnosis should be considered in any black patient with hemolytic anemia, especially if there is a history of painful crises, arthropathies, ankle ulcers, or other clinical manifestations.
- Evaluation of a blood sample from a patient with sickle cell anemia will reveal reduced hemoglobin, increased reticulocyte count, usually increased platelet and leukocyte counts, and sickle forms on the peripheral smear.
- The screening test for hemoglobin disorders is electrophoresis on cellulose acetate, followed by solubility testing for sickling.
- The presence of abnormal hemoglobin is confirmed by citrate agar electrophoresis, quantifying of hemoglobin fractions, alkali denaturation, and family studies.

▶ DESIRED OUTCOME

The goal of treatment is to decrease the number of sickle cell crises, prevent complications, and improve the quality of life.

▶ TREATMENT

GENERAL PRINCIPLES

- Treatment is primarily supportive.
- Patients with sickle cell disease should receive pneumococcal and hemophilus b conjugate vaccines at appropriate ages.

SICKLE CELL CRISIS

- Hydration and analgesics are the core interventions for sickle cell crisis, but there is no consensus on specific guidelines.
- Daily hydration may consist of ≥ 4 L in hospitalized adults, 2.5 L/m^2 in hospitalized children, and 2–3 L in outpatients.
- Morphine is replacing meperidine as the narcotic analgesic of choice because morphine has a longer duration of action and avoids problems resulting from accumulation of metabolites that may be toxic, especially in patients with sickle cell disease.
- There is no consensus regarding the selection between scheduled versus as-needed dosing of analgesic therapy. Patient-controlled analgesia

TABLE 33.2. Representative Protocol for PCA

	Morphine	Meperidine
Suggested concentration	1–5 mg/mL	10 mg/mL
PCA bolus dose	0.5–1 mg	5–10 mg
Lock-out interval	10–20 min	10–20 min
Loading dose	1–2 mg	5–10 mg
Continuous rate/hour	1–2 mg/h	10–20 mg/h
Titration	10–20% increase or decrease/h	

From Barbaccia JB. Pharmacy and Therapeutics Committee monograph: Patient controlled analgesia. Washington, DC, Washington Hospital Center, 1989, with permission.

(PCA) combines the advantages of providing steady analgesic blood concentrations with the ability to administer additional bolus doses (Table 33.2).

- Although oxygen is widely utilized, there are no controlled clinical studies. Occlusion prevents oxygen from reaching the areas where it is most needed. If oxygen is indicated for hypoxemia, it should be used intermittently rather than continuously.
- Because crises may be precipitated by infection, an infectious etiology should be considered. *Streptococcus pneumoniae, Haemophilus influenzae,* and *Salmonella* are the most likely pathogens.
- Dextran has been advocated because it may improve microcirculation by decreasing erythrocyte aggregation and blood viscosity; however, its benefit has not been established in controlled trials.
- Mild cases may be treated on an outpatient basis with rest, hydration, warmth, and oral analgesics. Oral analgesic options include nonsteroidal anti-inflammatory drugs (NSAIDs) or acetaminophen, generally in combination with codeine or a codeine derivative.
- Splenic sequestration crisis is a major cause of mortality in young patients. Treatment includes whole-blood transfusion to correct hypovolemia, and broad-spectrum antibiotic therapy including coverage for *S. pneumoniae* and *H. influenzae*. Although controversial, splenectomy is probably merited after a life-threatening crisis or after repetitive episodes.
- Treatment of aplastic crisis is primarily supportive. Blood transfusion may be indicated for severe anemia. Antibiotic therapy is generally not warranted because an infectious etiology is probably viral rather than bacterial.
- There is no specific treatment for hemolytic crises. Treatment is primarily supportive and may include blood transfusions.

395

ADDITIONAL INTERVENTIONS

- Transfusion therapy has been used to treat life-threatening complications of sickle cell disease, such as central nervous system infarction or multiorgan failure associated with sickle cell crisis. Transfusion has also been used before childbirth and before surgery. After a stroke, chronic transfusion may reduce the risk of subsequent stroke and halt clinical progression.

- The risks of transfusion therapy include iron overload, acquired viral infection, and sensitization to transfusion products. The conventional dosage of the iron chelator, deferoxamine, is 1–2 g by subcutaneous infusion over 10–12 hours. A higher dosage, such as 6 g/day intravenously at a rate of 15 mg/kg/hour, may be required for large iron stores or noncompliance.

- Conventional therapeutic approaches to priapism are often ineffective in patients with sickle cell disease. Options that have occasionally been successful include stilbestrol, pentoxifylline, terbutaline, and gonadotropin-releasing hormone analogue. More invasive approaches, such as aspiration of the corpora cavernosa or surgery, may be required.

VII

- In patients with idiopathic unilateral renal hematuria, high fluid intake is indicated to prevent clotting and urethral colic. Iron therapy and possibly transfusions should be used as needed for blood loss. Nephrectomy may be required for massive hemorrhaging.

▶ LONG-TERM AND NEW STRATEGIES

- Current therapeutic interventions do not necessarily prevent complications. Folic acid, 1 mg daily, is given empirically because of increased demand caused by accelerated erythropoiesis; however, there are no controlled clinical trials indicating that supplementation is essential.

- Prophylactic penicillin prevents pneumococcal septicemia and meningitis, but this approach has been criticized because of the risk of promoting development of drug-resistant strains, compliance problems, and uncertainty about the duration of therapy.

- New strategies that are being considered to decrease gelation of sickle cells include hydroxyurea, azacytadine, cytarabine, and butyrate. Oral hydroxyurea rapidly increases fetal hemoglobin-containing reticulocytes; recently evaluated regimens using conservative doses of approximately 10–20 mg/kg/day have avoided the problem of bone marrow suppression observed in earlier studies.

- Studies of pentoxifylline yielded mixed results regarding the ability of this agent to decrease the number and severity of sickle cell crises.

- Bone marrow transplantation produces dramatic results in patients with sickle cell disease. The procedure involves marrow ablation followed by transplantation of marrow harvested from a matched sibling donor. This procedure is limited by the shortage of suitable donors and by substantial toxicity.

▶ EVALUATION OF THERAPEUTIC OUTCOMES

- Patients receiving hydration for sickle cell crisis should be monitored to prevent overhydration and subsequent pulmonary edema.
- Folate levels and mean corpuscular volume (MCV) should be monitored to detect possible folate deficiency and megaloblastic anemia.
- The number, severity, and duration of sickle cell crises should be monitored to evaluate the effectiveness of long-term interventions such as gelation inhibitor therapy or pentoxifylline.
- The effectiveness of analgesic therapy is evaluated by subjective assessments by patients and health care practitioners.
- Patients should be monitored for bacterial infections, especially infections caused by *S. pneumoniae, H. influenzae,* and *Salmonella.* When infections occur, appropriate antibiotic therapy should be initiated.

See Chapter 95, Sickle Cell Anemia, authored by Clarence E. Curry, Jr., PharmD, and Eula D. Beasley, PharmD, for a more detailed discussion of this topic.

VII ◀

Chapter 34

► ANTIMICROBIAL REGIMEN SELECTION

A generally accepted systematic approach to the selection and evaluation of an antimicrobial regimen is shown in (Table 34.1).

► CONFIRMING THE PRESENCE OF INFECTION

FEVER

- Fever is defined as a controlled elevation of body temperature above the normal range of 36–37.8°C. Fever is a manifestation of many disease states other than infection. In particular, many collagen vascular (autoimmune) disorders and several malignancies may have fever as a manifestation.
- Many drugs have been identified as causes of fever. Drug-induced fever is defined as persistent fever in the absence of infection or other underlying condition. The fever must coincide temporally with the administration of the offending agent and disappear promptly upon its withdrawal, after which it remains normal.
- Fever patterns are believed by some to be helpful in establishing the etiology of the increased temperature. For example, high-spiking fevers are believed to be more consistent with an infectious process, whereas sustained fevers are associated with collagen vascular disease or malignancy. Although these guidelines may be generally true, there are reports of high-spiking fever due to drugs. Overall, characterization of the fever pattern probably offers little in the general assessment of the patient.

SIGNS AND SYMPTOMS

White Blood Cell Count

- Most infections result in elevated white blood cell (WBC) counts (leukocytosis) because of the mobilization of granulocytes and/or lymphocytes to ingest and destroy invading microbes. The generally accepted range of normal values for WBC counts is between 4000 and 10,000/mm³.
- Classically, bacterial infections are associated with elevated granulocyte counts (neutrophils, basophils), often with immature forms (band neutrophils) seen in peripheral blood smears (left-shift). With infection, peripheral leukocyte counts may be very high, but are rarely higher than 30,000 to 40,000/mm³. Low leukocyte counts after the onset of infec-

TABLE 34.1. Systematic Approach for Selection of Antimicrobials

A. Confirm the presence of infection
  1. Fever
  2. Signs and symptoms
  3. Predisposing factors

B. Identification of the pathogen
  1. Collection of infected material
  2. Stains
  3. Serologies
  4. Culture

C. Selection of presumptive therapy
  1. Host factors
  2. Drug factors

D. Monitor therapeutic response
  1. Clinical assessment
  2. Laboratory tests
  3. Assessment of therapeutic failure

tion indicate an abnormal response and are generally associated with a poor prognosis of bacterial infection.

- Relative lymphocytosis, even with normal or slightly elevated total WBC counts, is generally associated with viral or fungal infections.
- Many types of infections, however, may be accompanied by a completely normal WBC count and differential.

Pain and Inflammation

- The classic signs of pain and inflammation may accompany infection and are manifested by swelling, erythema, tenderness, and purulent drainage. Unfortunately, these are visibly apparent only if the infection is superficial or in a bone or joint.
- The manifestations of inflammation in deep-seated infections such as meningitis, pneumonia, endocarditis, and urinary tract infection must be ascertained by examining tissues or fluids. For example, the presence of polymorphonuclear leukocytes (neutrophils) in spinal fluid, lung secretions (sputum), and urine is highly suggestive of bacterial infection.

Other Factors

- Table 34.2 lists factors that predispose patients to infection. Generally, immunosuppressive disease states lead to a wide variety of infections (e.g., AIDS), while other diseases may predispose the patient to a certain type of infectious disease (e.g., recurrent meningococcal infection with complement deficiency). Information from the patient's history regarding underlying disease is vitally important, since the presence of an underlying condition may not only predispose patients to infection, but also may modify the likely offending pathogen.

VIII

TABLE 34.2. Factors Predisposing to Infection

Alterations in normal flora of the host
Disruption of natural barriers
    Skin/mucous membranes
    Cilia of respiratory tract
    pH and motility of bowel
Age
Immunosuppression secondary to:
    Malnutrition
    Underlying disease (hereditary or acquired)
    Hormones (e.g., pregnancy, corticosteroids)
    Drugs (e.g., cytotoxic agents)

- Many factors predisposing to infection are related to disruption of the host's integumentary barriers. For example, trauma, burns, and iatrogenic wounds induced in surgery may lead to a substantial risk of infection depending on the severity and location of the injury or disruption.

VIII ▶ IDENTIFICATION OF THE PATHOGEN

- Infected body materials must be sampled, if at all possible or practical, before institution of any antimicrobial therapy, for two reasons. First, Gram stain of the material may rapidly reveal bacteria, or acid-fast stain may detect mycobacteria or actinomycetes. Second, delay in obtaining infected fluids or tissues until after therapy is started may result in false-negative culture results or alterations in the cellular and chemical composition of infected fluids.
- Less accessible fluids or tissues must be obtained based on localized signs or symptoms (e.g., spinal fluid in meningitis, joint fluid in arthritis). Abscesses and cellulitic areas should also be aspirated. Finally, blood cultures should nearly always be performed in the acutely ill, febrile patient.
- Once positive Gram stain and/or culture results are obtained, the clinician must be cautious in determining whether the organism recovered is a true pathogen, a contaminant, or is part of the normally expected flora from the site of specimen collection.
- Cultures of specimens from purportedly infected sites that are obtained by sampling from or through one of these contaminated areas, may contain significant numbers of the normal flora.
- Caution must also be taken in the evaluation of positive culture results from normally sterile sites (e.g., blood, cerebrospinal fluid, joint fluid). The recovery of bacteria normally found on the skin in large quantities (e.g., coagulase-negative staphylococci, diphtheroids) from one of these

sites may be a result of contamination of the specimen rather than a true infection.

▶ SELECTION OF PRESUMPTIVE THERAPY

- To select rational antimicrobial therapy for a given clinical situation, a variety of factors must be considered. These include the severity and acuity of the disease, host factors, factors related to the drugs used, and the necessity for use of multiple agents.
- There are generally accepted drugs of choice for the treatment of most pathogens (see Table 34.3). The drugs of choice are compiled from a variety of sources and are intended as guidelines rather than specific rules for antimicrobial use.
- Local susceptibility data should be considered whenever possible rather than information published by other institutions or national compilations.
- Therapy is often begun empirically or without knowledge of the exact infecting organism(s). Empiric therapies are directed at organisms that are frequently known to cause the infection in question. The severity and/or acuity of the infectious process dictates the necessity for use of empiric antimicrobial therapy.

HOST FACTORS

- In evaluating a patient for initial or empiric therapy, the factors listed in Table 34.4 should be considered.
- Patients with diminished renal and/or hepatic function will accumulate certain drugs unless dosage is adjusted. Table 34.5 lists drugs by antimicrobial class, identifies their route of elimination, and the dose-related toxicity to be avoided.
- Any concomitant therapy the patient is receiving may influence both the selection of drug therapy, the dosage, and monitoring.
- A list of selected drug interactions involving antimicrobials and antimicrobial interference with laboratory tests is provided in Table 34.6.

DRUG FACTORS

- In selecting an antimicrobial agent for empiric therapy, the kinetic disposition of the agent is an important consideration. This is partly because of cost considerations (less frequent dosing is less costly) and also because drugs should be selected that are best suited for the elimination capacity of the patient.
- The relevance of tissue concentrations of antimicrobials has long been disputed. The central nervous system (CNS) is one body site where antimicrobial penetration is relatively well defined and correlations with clinical outcomes are established. Cerebrospinal fluid (CSF) concentrations of antimicrobial agents necessary to eradicate bacterial meningitis have been defined, and drugs that do not reach significant concentrations in CSF should be avoided in treating meningitis.

TABLE 34.3. Drugs of Choice

Key
First choice
Alternative(s)

Gram-Positive Cocci

Streptococcus (groups A, B, C, G, and *S. bovis*)
Penicillin G[a] or V[b] or ampicillin
Erythromycin, FGC,[c,d] vancomycin

Streptococcus pneumoniae
Penicillin G or V or ampicillin
Erythromycin, FGC,[c,d] cefotaxime or ceftriaxone,[d,e] chloramphenicol[e]

Streptococcus, viridans group
Penicillin G ± gentamicin[f]
Vancomycin ± gentamicin

Enterococcus
Ampicillin (or penicillin G) + gentamicin[g] (in serious infection)
Vancomycin and gentamicin (UTI: nitrofurantoin, tetracycline, or fluoroquinolone) ampicillin–sulbactam (for β-lactamase-producing strains)

Staphylococcus aureus
Penicillinase-negative
  Penicillin G or V
  FGC,[c,d] clindamycin, vancomycin
Penicillinase-positive
  PRP[h]
  FGC,[c,d] vancomycin, clindamycin,[i] BLIC[j]
Methicillin-resistant
  Vancomycin ± rifampin or gentamicin
  Trimethoprim–sulfamethoxazole or fluoroquinolone,[k] both ± rifampin

Gram-Negative Cocci

Moraxella catarrhalis
Trimethoprim–sulfamethoxazole
Amoxicillin/clavulanate, erythromycin, tetracycline, TGC

Neisseria gonorrhoeae
Uncomplicated infection
  Ceftriaxone or fluoroquinolone[k]
  APPG,[l] cephamycin,[m] tetracycline, amoxicillin/probenecid
DGI[n]
  Ceftriaxone + doxycycline
  TGC,[o] cephamycin

Neisseria meningitidis
Penicillin G
TGC,[o] chloramphenicol

Gram-Positive Bacilli

Clostridium perfringens
Penicillin G

Clindamycin, metronidazole

Clostridium tetani
TIG[p]
Penicillin, tetracycline

Clostridium difficile
Metronidazole or vancomycin[q]
Bacitracin

Corynebacterium diphtheriae
Antitoxin + erythromycin
Penicillin G

Listeria monocytogenes
Ampicillin ± gentamicin
Trimethoprim–sulfamethoxazole

Gram-Negative Bacilli

Acinetobacter spp.
Imipenem
Aminoglycoside, ESP,[r] fluoroquinolone, trimethoprim– sulfamethoxazole, ampicillin/sulbactam

Aeromonas hydrophila
Trimethoprim–sulfamethoxazole
Gentamicin, fluoroquinolone, imipenem

Bacteroides fragilis (and others)
Metronidazole
BLIC,[s] clindamycin, cephamycin,[m] imipenem, ESP[r]

Bordetella pertussis
Erythromycin
Trimethoprim–sulfamethoxazole

Campylobacter sp.
Fluoroquinolone or erythromycin
Tetracycline, gentamicin

Enterobacter sp.
Fluoroquinolone, imipenem, or cefepime
Gentamicin + ESP,[r] trimethoprim–sulfamethoxazole, TGC[o]

Escherichia coli
FGC[c]
Gentamicin, TGC,[o] ampicillin, fluoroquinolone

Gardnerella vaginalis
Metronidazole
Ampicillin

Haemophilus influenzae
TGC,[o,t] trimethoprim–sulfamethoxazole
BLIC,[j] cefuroxime, chloramphenicol, ampicillin/amoxicillin, sulfa/erythromycin

VIII

TABLE 34.3. continued

Klebsiella pneumoniae
FGC,^{c,d} aminoglycoside
TGC,^{o,t} trimethoprim–sulfamethoxazole,
fluoroquinolone^k

Legionella sp.
Erythromycin ± rifampin
Trimethoprim–sulfamethoxazole, ciprofloxacin,
clarithromycin

Pasteurella multocida
Penicillin G
Tetracycline, BLIC^j

Proteus mirabilis
Ampicillin
FGC,^{c,d} gentamicin, trimethoprim–sulfamethoxazole,
fluoroquinolone

Proteus (indole-positive) (including
Providencia rettgeri, Morganella
morganii, Proteus vulgaris)
TGC^o
Aminoglycoside, trimethoprim–sulfamethoxazole,
fluoroquinolone,^{k} imipenem, ESP

Providencia stuartii
TGC^o
Aminoglycoside, trimethoprim–sulfamethoxazole,
fluoroquinolone,^{k} imipenem, ESP

Pseudomonas aeruginosa
Aminoglycoside + ESP^f or ceftazidime
Ciprofloxacin, aztreonam + aminoglycoside,
imipenem

Pseudomonas cepacia
Trimethoprim–sulfamethoxazole
Ceftazidime, chloramphenicol

Salmonella typhi
Fluoroquinolone^k or TGC^o
Trimethoprim–sulfamethoxazole, ampicillin,
chloramphenicol

Salmonella (non-typhi)
TGC^{o,u}
Trimethoprim–sulfamethoxazole, fluoroquinolone^k

Serratia marcescens
TGC^o
Aminoglycoside, trimethoprim–sulfamethoxazole,
fluoroquinolone,^{k} imipenem, ESP

Shigella
Fluoroquinolone^k
Trimethoprim–sulfamethoxazole, ampicillin,
ceftriaxone

Xanthomonas maltophilia
Trimethoprim–sulfamethoxazole
Minocycline, ceftazidime, fluoroquinolone

Miscellaneous Organisms
Actinomyces israelii
Penicillin G
Tetracycline

Afipia felis (cat scratch fever)
Ciprofloxacin
Trimethoprim–sulfamethoxazole

Nocardia
Trimethoprim–sulfamethoxazole
Sulfonamide,^{v} amikacin, minocycline,
imipenem

Chlamydiae
Tetracycline or erythromycin
Sulfonamide, ofloxacin, clarithromycin

Mycoplasma pneumoniae
Erythromycin
Tetracycline, clarithromycin

Rickettsia
Tetracycline
Chloramphenicol, fluoroquinolone

Rochalimaea henselae bacillary
angiomatosis
Erythromycin
Tetracycline

Treponema pallidum
Penicillin G
Tetracycline, ceftriaxone

Borrelia burgdorferii
Doxycycline
Ceftriaxone, azithromycin, clarithromycin

Fungi
Aspergillus sp.
Amphotericin B
Itraconazole

Blastomycosis
Itraconazole or amphotericin B
Ketoconazole

Candida sp.
Amphotericin B or fluconazole
Ketoconazole,^{w} flucytosine^x

Coccidioides immitis
Amphotericin B
Fluconazole, ketoconazole, itraconazole

Cryptococcus neoformans
Amphotericin B ± flucytosine
Fluconazole, itraconazole

Histoplasma capsulatum
Amphotericin B or itraconazole
Ketoconazole

VIII

TABLE 34.3. continued

Mucormycosis	***Human immunodeficiency virus*** (HIV)
Amphotericin B	Zidovudine
None	*Didanosine, zalcitabine, stavudine,*
Sporothrix schenkii	*saguinavir, ritonavir, indinavir*
Itraconazole, Iodides[y]	***Influenza A***
Amphotericin B	Amantadine
Viruses	*Rimantadine, ribavirin*
Cytomegalovirus	***Respiratory syncitial virus***
Ganciclovir	Ribavirin
Foscarnet	*None*
Herpes simplex	***Varicella-zoster***
Tri-fluridine,[z] acyclovir,[aa] or famciclovir	Acyclovir
Vidarabine, idoxuridine,[z] foscarnet	*Vidarabine*

[a] Either aqueous penicillin G or benzathine penicillin G (pharyngitis only).

[b] Only for soft tissue infections or upper respiratory infections (pharyngitis, otitis media).

[c] First-generation cephalosporins—cefazolin, cephalexin, cephradine, or cefadroxil.

[d] Some penicillin-allergic patients may react to cephalosporins.

[e] For the treatment of meningitis.

[f] Gentamicin should be added if tolerance or "moderately susceptible" (MIC ≥ 0.1 g/mL) organisms are encountered; streptomycin is used but may be more toxic.

[g] Must be added for synergy in cases of endocarditis, meningitis, and perhaps bacteremic pyelonephritis.

[h] Penicillinase-resistant penicillin: nafcillin or oxacillin; methicillin is probably more nephrotoxic.

[i] Not reliably bactericidal, so should not be used for endocarditis.

[j] β-Lactamase inhibitor combination: ampicillin/sulbactam, amoxicillin/clavulanate.

[k] Ciprofloxacin, ofloxacin, fleroxacin.

[l] Aqueous procaine penicillin G.

[m] Cefoxitin, cefotetan, cefmetazole.

[n] Disseminated gonococcal infection.

[o] Third-generation cephalosporins—cefotaxime, ceftizoxime, ceftriaxone.

[p] Tetanus immune globulin.

[q] Oral administration only.

[r] Extended-spectrum penicillin—ticarcillin, mezlocillin, or piperacillin.

[s] β-lactamase inhibitor combination: ampicillin/sulbactam, ticarcillin/clavulanate, piperacillin/tazobactam

[t] Should only be used in serious infections.

[u] Antibiotics should not be given for gastroenteritis, because the carrier state may be prolonged without significant clinical benefit.

[v] Sulfisoxazole, sulfadiazine (preferred for CNS disease), trisulfapyrimidines.

[w] Mucocutaneous disease only.

[x] May be added to amphotericin for potential synergy, but only if *in vitro* susceptibility is documented. Resistance develops frequently if used alone.

[y] Lymphocutaneous disease only.

[z] Keratitis only.

[aa] Topical form for primary genital disease only; oral form to treat severe genital disease and to prevent recurrence of genital infections; IV form for severe mucocutaneous, disseminated, or meningoencephalitic disease.

TABLE 34.4. Host Factors in Selection of Antimicrobial Therapy

Allergy or history of adverse drug reactions

Age of patient

Pregnancy

Genetic or metabolic abnormalities

Renal and hepatic function

Site of the infection

Concomitant drug therapy

Underlying disease state(s)

- Apart from the bloodstream, other body fluids where drug concentration data are clinically relevant include urine, synovial fluid, and peritoneal fluid.
- Caution must be taken in selecting an antimicrobial agent for clinical use on the basis of tissue/fluid penetration. With the exception of CNS penetration data, more attention should be paid to clinical efficacy, antimicrobial spectrum, toxicity, and cost than to comparative data on penetration into a given body site.
- Certain basic pharmacokinetic parameters such as area under the concentration-vs-time curve (AUC) and maximal plasma concentration (C_{max}) can be predictive of treatment outcome when specific ratios of AUC or C_{max} to the minimum inhibitory concentration (MIC) are achieved. This is relevant for those antimicrobials that produce concentration-dependent bactericidal effects, for example, aminoglycosides and fluoroquinolones.
- When such concentration-dependent killing is coupled with a prolonged postantibiotic effect (PAE) (a prolonged lag period of growth following a brief exposure to an antimicrobial), it is possible to modify dosage regimens to take advantage of these effects.
- Antimicrobials that affect cell wall synthesis (e.g., β-lactams) do not produce concentration-dependent killing nor do they produce prolonged PAE, but rather time-dependent bactericidal effects. Therefore, the most important pharmacodynamic relationship for these antimicrobials is the duration that drug concentrations exceed the MIC.
- If one has the choice of two drugs that are equally efficacious yet one is less toxic, the less toxic drug, even if more costly, should be selected.
- The costs of drug therapy are increasing dramatically, especially as new products derived from biotechnology are introduced. The total cost of antimicrobial therapy includes much more than just the acquisition cost of the drugs. The total economic impact of antimicrobial therapy is detailed in Table 34.7.
- Many ancillary costs affect the true cost of therapy. These include factors such as storage, preparation, and administration, as well as all of

405

TABLE 34.5. Routes of Antimicrobial Elimination and Dose-Related Toxicities

Drugs	Primary Route of Elimination	Degree of Accumulation[a]	Dose-Related Toxic Effect(s)
Penicillins			
Ampicillin	Renal	Significant	CNS (seizures, etc.)
Carbenicillin	Renal	Significant	Platelet dysfunction, CNS toxicity, sodium overload
Methicillin	Renal	Moderate	?Nephritis
Mezlocillin	Renal/hepatic[b]	Moderate	?Platelet dysfunction
Nafcillin	Renal/hepatic[b]	Insignificant	?Neutropenia
Oxacillin	Renal/hepatic[b]	Insignificant	?Neutropenia
Penicillin G	Renal	Significant	CNS toxicity; hyperkalemia (with K+ salt)
Piperacillin	Renal/hepatic[b]	Moderate	?Platelet dysfunction
Ticarcillin	Renal	Significant	CNS toxicity, platelet dysfunction
Cephalosporins			
Cefamandole	Renal	Significant	Hypoprothrombinemia
Cefepime	Renal	Significant	None
Cefazolin	Renal	Significant	CNS toxicity
Cefmetazole	Renal	Significant	Hypoprothrombinemia
Cefonicid	Renal	Significant	None
Cefoperazone	Hepatic/renal[b]	Moderate	Hypoprothrombinemia
Cefotaxime	Renal/hepatic[b]	Moderate	None
Cefotetan	Renal	Significant	Hypoprothrombinemia
Cefoxitin	Renal	Significant	None
Ceftazidime	Renal	Significant	None
Cefizoxime	Renal	Significant	None
Ceftriaxone	Renal/hepatic[b]	Insignificant	None
Cefuroxime	Renal	Significant	None
Aminoglycosides	Renal	Significant	Nephrotoxicity, ototoxicity
Tetracyclines	Renal (except	Significant	Exacerbation of azotemia, doxycycline) possible hepatotoxicity
Miscellaneous			
Aztreonam	Renal	Moderate	None
Chloramphenicol	Hepatic	Moderate	Gray baby syndrome, marrow suppression
Ciprofloxacin	Renal/hepatic	Moderate	CNS toxicity

Miscellaneous *(cont.)*

Clindamycin	Hepatic	Moderate	None
Erythromycin	Hepatic	Insignificant	Ototoxicity
Fleroxacin	Renal	Moderate	CNS toxicity
Imipenem	Renal	Significant	CNS toxicity
Lomefloxacin	Renal	Moderate	CNS toxicity
Metronidazole	Hepatic/renal	Moderate	Encephalopathy, neuropathy
Ofloxacin	Renal	Significant	CNS toxicity
Polymyxins	Renal	Significant	Nephrotoxicity, neuropathy, neuro-muscular blockade
Sulfonamides	Renal/hepatic[b]	Moderate	Kernicterus
Trimethoprim	Renal	Moderate	Megaloblastic anemia

Antifungal Agents

Amphotericin B	Unknown	Insignificant	Most adverse effects increase in frequency with cumulative dose, not individual dosage size
Fluconazole	Renal	Significant	?Hepatotoxicity
Flucytosine	Renal	Significant	Marrow suppression, ?hepatoxicity
Itraconazole	Hepatic	Insignificant	?None
Miconazole	Hepatic	Insignificant	?Hepatoxicity
Ketoconazole	Hepatic	Insignificant	None

Antiviral Agents

Acyclovir	Renal	Significant	CNS toxicity, nephrotoxicity
Foscarnot	Renal	Significant	Nephrotoxicity, CNS toxicity
Ganciclovir	Renal	Significant	Marrow suppression
Vidarabine	Hepatic/renal[b]	Insignificant	?CNS toxicity
Ribavirin	Hepatic	Insignificant	?

Antitubercular Agents

Isoniazid	Hepatic	Insignificant	Neuropathy
Ethambutol	Renal	Moderate	Optic neuritis
Pyrazinamide	Hepatic	Moderate	?None
Rifampin	Hepatic	Insignificant	?None

VIII

[a]Accumulation of parent compound and/or active/toxic metabolites in patients with decreased capacity of primary route of elimination.

[b]Accumulation is probably significant in combined hepatic and renal failure, but data are sparse.

TABLE 34.6. Antimicrobial Interactions

Antimicrobial	Other Agent(s)	Results of Interaction
Aminoglycosides	Neuromuscular blocking drugs	Increased neuromuscular blockade
	Other nephrotoxins or ototoxins (e.g., cisplatin amphotericin B, ethacrynic acid, vancomycin, cyclosporine)	Increased nephrotoxicity or ototoxicity
	Penicillins	Inactivation of both drugs (a particular problem in renal failure and when obtaining drug levels)
Sulfonamides	Sufonylureas	Hypoglycemia
	Phenytoin	Increased serum concentration of phenytoin leading to toxicity
	Oral anticoagulants (warfarin derivatives)	Enhanced hypoprothrombinemia
Chloramphenicol	Phenytoin, tolbutamide, ethanol	Increased serum concentration of other agents and enhanced pharmacologic effect or increased toxicity
Metronidazole (also cefamandole, moxalactam, cefoperazone)	Ethanol (including ethanol-containing medications)	Disulfiram-like reaction
Macrolides, azalides	Theophylline	Increased serum theophylline concentration
	Terfenadine, astemizole	Cardiac arrhythmias
Fluconazole	Phenytoin, warfarin	Inhibits metabolism of these drugs
	Rifampin	Enhances metabolism of fluconazole
Itraconazole	Astemizole, terfenadine	Cardiac arrhythmias
	Phenytoin, warfarin	Inhibits metabolism of these drugs
	Rifampin	Enhances metabolism of itraconazole
Quinolones (norfloxacin, ciprofloxacin, ofloxacin, lomefloxacin, enoxacin)	Multivalent cations (antacids, iron, sucralfate, zinc)	Decreased absorption of quinolone
	Theophylline	Inhibits metabolism of theophylline (ciprofloxacin and enoxacin)
Rifampin	Coumarin anticoagulants	Decreased anticoagulant effect (increased metabolism of drug)
	Quinidine	Decreased effect of quinidine
	Digoxin	Decreased effect of digoxin
	Methadone	Narcotic withdrawal
	Propranolol	Decreased effect of propranolol
	Oral contraceptives	Decreased effect (pregnancy)
	Fluconazole; ketoconazole	Decreased antifungal effect
Tetracyclines	Antacids, iron, calcium	Inhibit intestinal absorption of tetracycline
Penicillins and cephalosporins	Uricosuric agents (probenecid, high-dose aspirin, etc.)	Block excretion of β-lactams, causing higher serum levels
	Copper reduction test for glycosuria (Clinitest tablets)	False-positive test for glycosuria (not seen with glucose oxidase method)
Isoniazid	Phenytoin	Increased serum concentrations of both

VIII

TABLE 34.7. Total Economic Impact of Antimicrobial Therapy

Drug acquisition cost
Storage/inventory cost
Preparation
Distribution
Administration
Monitoring
Adverse effects
Impact on length of stay
Cost of control systems

the costs incurred from adverse effects, and also factors such as length of hospitalization, readmissions, and all directly provided health care goods and services.

▶ COMBINATION ANTIMICROBIAL THERAPY

- Combinations of antimicrobials are generally used to broaden the spectrum of coverage for empiric therapy, achieve synergistic activity against the infecting organism, and prevent the emergence of resistance.

VIII

BROADENING THE SPECTRUM OF COVERAGE

- Increasing the coverage of antimicrobial therapy is generally necessary in mixed infections where multiple organisms are likely to be present. This is the case in intra-abdominal and female pelvic infections in which a variety of aerobic and anaerobic bacteria may produce disease.
- The other clinical situation in which increased spectrum of activity is desirable is in nosocomial infection. Hospital-acquired infections, except as previously noted, are generally caused by only one organism, but many different organisms may be possible.

SYNERGISM

- The achievement of synergistic antimicrobial activity is advantageous for infections caused by enteric gram-negative bacilli in immunosuppressed patients.
- Traditionally, combinations of aminoglycosides and β-lactams have been used since these drugs together generally act synergistically against a wide variety of bacteria. However, the data supporting superior efficacy of synergistic over nonsynergistic combinations is weak.
- Synergistic combinations may produce better results in infections caused by *Pseudomonas aeruginosa,* in certain infections caused by

409

Enterococcus sp. and, perhaps, in patients with profound, persistent neutropenia.

PREVENTING RESISTANCE

- The use of combinations to prevent the emergence of resistance is widely applied but not often realized. The only circumstance where this has been clearly effective is in the treatment of tuberculosis.

DISADVANTAGES OF COMBINATION THERAPY

- Although there are potentially beneficial effects from combining drugs, there also are potentially serious liabilities. Examples include additive nephrotoxicity from drugs such as aminoglycosides, amphotericin, and possibly vancomycin. Inactivation of aminoglycosides by penicillins may be clinically significant when excessive doses of penicillin are given to a patient in renal failure.
- Some combinations of antimicrobials are potentially antagonistic. Such combinations should probably be avoided whenever possible, unless the clinical situation warrants the use of both drugs for different pathogens.
- Of more current relevance is the increasing use of β-lactam antimicrobials in combination. Agents that are capable of inducing β-lactamase production in bacteria such as *Enterobacter cloacae* and *P. aeruginosa* (e.g., imipenem, cephamycins) may antagonize the effects of enzyme-labile drugs such as penicillins.

VIII

FAILURE OF ANTIMICROBIAL THERAPY

- A variety of factors may be responsible for apparent lack of response to therapy. Factors include those directly related to the host, those related to the pathogen, and, although unlikely, laboratory error in identification and/or susceptibility testing. Factors directly related to the antimicrobial agents being utilized are only a small proportion of the possibilities.

Failures Caused by Drug Selection

- Factors directly related to the drug selection include an inappropriate selection of drug, dosage, or route of administration. Malabsorption of a drug product because of gastrointestinal disease (e.g., short-bowel syndrome) or a drug interaction (e.g., complexation of fluoroquinolones with multivalent cations resulting in reduced absorption) may lead to potentially subtherapeutic serum concentrations.
- Accelerated drug elimination is also a possible reason for failure. This may occur in patients with cystic fibrosis or during pregnancy, when more rapid clearance or larger volumes of distribution may result in low serum concentrations, particularly for aminoglycosides.
- Inactivation of antimicrobial agents by other drugs may occur, as in the case of aminoglycoside inactivation by penicillins.

- Finally, a common cause of failure of therapy is poor penetration into the site of infection. This is especially true for the so-called "privileged" sites such as the CNS, the eye, and the prostate gland.

Failures Caused by Host Factors

- Patients who are immunosuppressed (e.g., granulocytopenia from chemotherapy, AIDS) may respond poorly to therapy because their own defenses are inadequate to eradicate the infection despite seemingly adequate drug regimens. A good example is the poor response in granulocytopenic patients that occurs when WBC counts remain low during therapy.
- Other host factors are related to the necessity for surgical drainage of abscesses or removal of foreign bodies and/or necrotic tissue. If these situations are not corrected, they result in persistent infection and, occasionally, bacteremia, despite adequate antimicrobial therapy.

Failures Caused by Microorganisms

- Factors related to the pathogen include the development of drug resistance during therapy. Primary resistance refers to the intrinsic resistance of the pathogens producing the infection. However, acquisition of resistance during treatment has become a major problem as well (discussed later in this chapter).
- The increase in resistance among pathogenic organisms is believed to be due, in large part, to continued overuse of antimicrobials in the community, as well as in hospitals, and the increasing prevalence of immunosuppressed patients receiving long-term suppressive antimicrobials for the prevention of infections. VIII

Host Abnormalities

- Host abnormalities may be responsible for predisposition to or persistence of infection, including cardiac or pulmonary disease, immunosuppressive disorders, and structural abnormalities of various organ systems.
- Administration of various adjunctive measures such as colony-stimulating factors, immunoglobulins, antibodies, antitoxins, and immunostimulatory agents may be beneficial depending on the circumstances. Obviously, prevention of infection is more desirable than treating an established disease. Therefore, active or passive immunization is often used to either prevent or abort many infectious diseases.

See Chapter 98, Selection of Antimicrobial Regimens, authored by Steven L. Barriere, PharmD, FCCP, for a more detailed discussion of this topic.

Chapter 35

▶ BONE AND JOINT INFECTIONS

There are three general types of osteomyelitis: (1) *hematogenous osteomyelitis,* which refers to infection that results from spread through the bloodstream; (2) *contiguous osteomyelitis,* which refers to infection resulting from organisms reaching the bone from an adjoining soft tissue infection or osteomyelitis that results from direct inoculation such as from trauma, puncture wounds, or surgery; and (3) osteomyelitis resulting from peripheral vascular disease. Osteomyelitis may also be classified based on the duration of the disease. Acute osteomyelitis constitutes an infection of recent onset, usually several days to 1 week, and chronic osteomyelitis is an infection with symptoms for more than 1 month before therapy or relapse of an initial infection.

▶ EPIDEMIOLOGY

- Acute hematogenous osteomyelitis has an estimated annual incidence of 4.5 per 100,000 population.
- Osteomyelitis caused by contiguous spread, including postoperative, direct puncture, and that associated with adjacent soft tissue infections, comprises about one-half of infections.
- Hematogenous osteomyelitis comprises about 20% of infections.
- Acute osteomyelitis constitutes 56% of patients, and chronic disease constitutes 44% of patients.
- Infectious arthritis most commonly occurs in patients >30 years of age; 20% of cases occur in children.

▶ PATHOPHYSIOLOGY

HEMATOGENOUS OSTEOMYELITIS

- Table 35.1 summarizes the primary characteristics of osteomyelitis.
- Once infection is initiated, exudate begins to form within the bone, which produces increased pressure.
- If there is significant periosteal damage, a soft tissue abscess may develop.
- Impairment of blood flow to the outer portion of the cortical bone may occur, producing dead bone that separates from healthy bone, termed *sequestra.*
- Children most commonly develop infections within the femur, tibia, humerus, and fibula. Vertebral infections are more common in patients >50 years of age. Neonatal infections commonly involve multiple bones.
- *Staphylococcus aureus* is isolated from 60–90% of the hematogenous infections in children. In one report of children with acute osteomyelitis

TABLE 35.1. Types of Osteomyelitis, Age Distribution, Common Sites, and Risk Factors

Type of Osteomyelitis	Typical Age (yr)	Site(s) Involved	Risk Factors
Hematogenous	Less than 1	Long bones and joints	Prematurity, umbilical catheter or venous cutdown, respiratory distress syndrome, perinatal asphyxia
	1–20	Long bones (femur, tibia, humerus)	Infection (pharyngitis, cellulitis, respiratory infections), sickle cell disease, puncture wounds to feet
	Older than 50	Vertebrae	Diabetes mellitus, blunt trauma to spine, urinary tract infection
Contiguous	Older than 50	Femur, tibia, mandible	Hip fractures, open fractures
Vascular insufficiency	Older than 50	Feet, toes	Diabetes mellitus, peripheral vascular disease, pressure sores

during a 7-year period, *S. aureus, Haemophilus influenzae* type b, and *Pseudomonas aeruginosa* were responsible for 45%, 21%, and 10%, respectively.

- The three most common etiologic agents of neonatal osteomyelitis are *S. aureus*, group B *streptococcus*, and *Escherichia coli*.
- Vertebral osteomyelitis most commonly occurs in adults, and staphylococci cause approximately 60% of these infections.
- More than 50% of the osteomyelitis infections in intravenous drug abusers are found in the vertebral column.
- *Pseudomonas aeruginosa*, either singly or in combination with other organisms, is cultured in 78% of all infections in intravenous drug abusers.
- Patients with sickle cell anemia and related hemoglobinopathies have a much higher rate of infection with *Salmonella* compared with other populations.

VIII

▶ CONTIGUOUS-SPREAD OSTEOMYELITIS

- Penetrating wounds (e.g., trauma), open fractures, or various invasive orthopedic procedures may result in direct inoculation of organisms into the bone. More than 80% of cases of postoperative osteomyelitis are known to occur following open reductions of fractures.
- Contiguous-spread osteomyelitis most commonly occurs in patients >50 years of age.
- Although *S. aureus* is still the most common organism isolated from contiguous-spread disease, infections with multiple organisms, including gram-negative bacilli, frequently occur. *Pseudomonas aeruginosa, Proteus, Streptococcus, E. coli, Staphylococcus epidermidis,* and anaerobes all may be isolated.

- Patients with osteomyelitis in association with severe vascular insufficiency are generally between the ages of 50 and 70 years. Frequently, there is an adjacent area of infection such as cellulitis or dermal ulcers.
- Infections in patients with osteomyelitis and severe vascular insufficiency almost always include multiple organisms (*Staphylococcus* and *Streptococcus,* or the combination of *Staphylococcus, Streptococcus,* and Enterobacteriaceae).

▶ INFECTIOUS ARTHRITIS

- Infectious arthritis is usually acquired by hematogenous spread.
- In addition, organisms also may gain access to the joint from a deep penetrating wound, an intra-articular steroid injection, arthroscopy, prosthetic-joint surgery, and contiguous osteomyelitis expansion into the joint.
- Table 35.2 summarizes the risk factors associated with adult infectious arthritis.
- *S. aureus* is found in 40% of cases of nongonococcal bacterial arthritis. Streptococcal infections account for 33% of cases and gram-negative organisms comprise 23% of infections.

▶ CLINICAL PRESENTATION

VIII

SIGNS AND SYMPTOMS

- Most patients with hematogenous osteomyelitis complain of significant tenderness of the infected area, pain, swelling, fever, chills, decreased motion, and malaise.
- The most frequent symptom of osteomyelitis caused by spread of infection from a contiguous focus is simply pain in the area of infection. Less commonly, patients also may develop a fever and elevated white blood cell (WBC) count.

TABLE 35.2. Risk Factors for Adult Infectious Arthritis (More than One Factor May Be Present)

Systemic corticosteroid use
Preexisting arthritis
Arthrocentesis
Distant infection
Diabetes mellitus
Trauma
Other diseases

Adapted from Esterhai JL, Gelb I. Orthop Clin North Am 1991;22:504, with permission.

- A patient with contiguous-spread osteomyelitis may have an area of localized tenderness, warmth, edema, and erythema over the infected site.
- Patients with significant vascular insufficiency usually have local symptoms such as pain, swelling, and redness.
- Non-gonococcal bacterial arthritis almost always involves only a single joint, most commonly the knee.
- The most frequent initial sign of disseminated gonococcal infections is a migratory polyarthralgia. Small papules on the trunk or extremities are the most frequent skin lesions seen in gonococcal infection, but only 30–40% of patients present with the classic hot, swollen, purulent joint.
- Infections that result from intraoperative contamination usually become apparent within 1 year of surgery.
- *S. epidermidis* is responsible for 40% of prosthetic-joint infections, and *S. aureus* is responsible for 20% of infections.

► DIAGNOSIS

- Bone changes characteristic of osteomyelitis are not seen by radiography for at least 10–14 days after the onset of the infection.
- Often, the erythrocyte sedimentation rate and the WBC count are the only laboratory abnormalities.
- Bone aspiration is valuable in determining an accurate bacteriologic diagnosis.
- Approximately 50% of patients with hematogenous osteomyelitis will have positive blood cultures.
- Joint aspiration with subsequent analysis of the synovial fluid is extremely important. The synovial fluid WBC count is usually 50,000 to 200,000/mm^3 and a glucose level usually <40 mg/dL when an infection is present.
- Gram stains of joint fluid demonstrate bacteria in 50% of patients with septic arthritis; however, such stains may be positive in only 25% of patients with gonococcal arthritis infections.

► TREATMENT

GENERAL PRINCIPLES

- The most important treatment modality of acute osteomyelitis is the early administration of appropriate antibiotics in adequate doses for a sufficient length of time.
- Following the initiation of adequate antibiotic therapy, if the patient does not respond by having a decrease in fever, local swelling, redness, and pain, the patient should undergo surgical debridement of the infected area.

VIII

PHARMACOLOGIC TREATMENT

- Antibiotics used in the management of acute osteomyelitis are generally given in high doses (adjusted for weight and renal and/or hepatic function) so that adequate antimicrobial concentrations are reached within the infected bone.
- The standard treatment for osteomyelitis has been parenteral antibiotics for 4–6 weeks. If signs or symptoms are still present at 6 weeks, therapy should be extended.
- Oral antibiotics may be used to complete parenteral therapy. Table 35.3 identifies requirements for the use of oral outpatient antibiotic therapy for osteomyelitis.
- Children responding to initial parenteral therapy may be excellent candidates to receive follow-up oral therapy with an agent such as dicloxacillin, cephalexin, or ampicillin. Adults with an infecting organism sensitive to a fluoroquinolone may also benefit from oral therapy.
- Oral antibiotics are equally effective as parenteral antibiotics, except in patients with diabetes mellitus or severe peripheral vascular disease.
- Ciprofloxacin is effective in the treatment of osteomyelitis caused by gram-negative strains such as *Enterobacter cloacae, Serratia marcescens,* and *P. aeruginosa.* However, an important limitation of the drug is that it should not be used in children younger than 16–18 years of age or in pregnant women because of its potential to cause cartilage damage.

VIII

SELECTION OF ANTIBIOTICS

- Empiric therapy must be selected on the basis of the most likely infecting organism while the results of culture and sensitivity data are pending. Empiric therapy recommendations are summarized in Table 35.4.
- Because *S. aureus,* streptococci, and *E. coli* are the most common infecting organisms in newborns, cefazolin in an IV dosage of 100 mg/kg/d (given in four divided doses) is appropriate.
- If patients are allergic to penicillins or cephalosporins, vancomycin or clindamycin may be used for *S. aureus* coverage. Children with

TABLE 35.3. Requirements for Oral Outpatient Therapy for Osteomyelitis

Confirmed osteomyelitis

Organism identified

Antibiotic sensitivity determined

Suitable oral agent available

Compliance assured

Suitable candidates:
    Children with good clinical response to IV therapy
    Adults without diabetes mellitus or peripheral vascular disease

TABLE 35.4. Empiric Treatment of Osteomyelitis

Patient Subtype	Likely Infecting Organism	Antibiotic[a]
Newborn	S. aureus, streptococci, E. coli	Cefazolin 100 mg/kg/d IV
Children 5 years of age or younger	S. aureus, H. influenzae type b, streptococci	Cefuroxime 100 mg/kg/d IV
Children older than 5 years of age	S. aureus	Nafcillin 40 mg/kg/d IV or cefazolin 100 mg/kg/d IV
Adults	S. aureus	Nafcillin 2 g IV every 4 hours or cefazolin 2 g IV every 8 hours
Intravenous drug abusers	Pseudomonas	Ciprofloxacin 750 mg PO twice daily or ceftazidime 2 g IV every 8 hours plus tobramycin 5 mg/kg/d IV
Postoperative or post-trauma patients	Gram-positive and gram-negative organisms	Nafcillin 2 g IV every 4 hours plus ceftazidime 2 g IV every 8 hours or ticarcillin–clavulanate 3.1 g IV every 4 hours
Patients with vascular insufficiency	Gram-positive and gram-negative organisms	Nafcillin 2 g IV every 4 hours or cefazolin 2 g IV every 8 hours plus ceftazidime 2 g IV every 8 hours
	If anaerobes suspected	Cefotetan 2 g IV every 12 hours or clindamycin 900 mg IV every 8 hours plus ceftazidime 2 g IV every 8 hours

[a]Dosage should be adjusted for some agents in patients with renal and/or hepatic dysfunction.

VIII ◄

osteomyelitis usually can be successfully treated with 4 weeks of parenteral therapy.

- Parenteral antibiotic therapy should be initiated and continued until there has been a resolution in the erythema, swelling, tenderness, and until the patient is afebrile.
- An oral regimen may be a reasonable alternative in many cases of osteomyelitis in children.
- Dicloxacillin, cloxacillin, and cephalexin (100 mg/kg/d) are effective oral agents.
- If peak serum bactericidal titers are used in monitoring oral therapy, the antibiotic dose may be increased, or probenecid may be added if the titer is not at least 1:8.
- Patients should be monitored with periodic WBC counts, erythrocyte sedimentation rates, and radiographic findings.
- Empiric antibiotics of first choice in a patient with a hemoglobinopathy, such as sickle cell anemia are a penicillinase-resistant penicillin plus ampicillin. Alternatives to ampicillin are a third-generation cephalosporin, chloramphenicol, or ciprofloxacin (in adults).

At-Home Therapy

- Acute osteomyelitis is one of the more common infectious diseases that may be treated with home intravenous (IV) antibiotics.

- Patients considered for home IV therapy must be screened to include those patients who are receiving a stable treatment program, who are interested in participating and are motivated, with good venous access, who have support from family members or neighbors, and who have home facilities for storage and refrigeration.
- Long-acting cephalosporins such as cefonicid or ceftriaxone, although more expensive, may allow patients to receive a regimen that is easier to administer at home.

INFECTIOUS ARTHRITIS

- The specific antibiotic selected for infectious arthritis depends on the most likely infecting organism.
- In infants <1 month old, empiric therapy must provide broad-spectrum coverage. A penicillinase-resistant penicillin, such as nafcillin or oxacillin (150 mg/kg/d), plus an aminoglycoside is appropriate.
- Children <5 years of age may be infected with *H. influenzae,* for which ampicillin therapy is indicated.
- The substitution of cefuroxime or addition of chloramphenicol may be required if the patient is located in a geographic area with a high level of ampicillin resistance.
- In children >5 years of age, and in adults, initial therapy with a penicillinase-resistant penicillin is appropriate to provide the necessary coverage against *S. aureus.*
- Therapy should be changed to vancomycin if the *S. aureus* is resistant to methicillin.

VIII

TABLE 35.5. Monitoring Protocol

Parameter	Frequency	Notes
Culture and sensitivity	At initiation of treatment	
White blood cell count	1–2 times/week until within normal range	
Erythrocyte sedimentation rate	Weekly	May not decrease to normal range until several weeks of therapy
Clinical signs of inflammation (redness, pain, swelling, tenderness, fever)	Daily during initiation of therapy	
Compliance of outpatient therapy	Reinforce before starting oral therapy and with each health care visit	Compliance is critical if treatment sois to be successful

- Two to three weeks of antibiotic therapy is generally adequate in non-gonococcal infections.
- Ceftriaxone 1 g/d for 7–10 days is the treatment of choice for disseminated gonococcal infections. If the organism is sensitive, therapy can be switched on the fourth day to either oral amoxicillin, doxycycline, or tetracycline to complete the 7- to 10-day course of antibiotic therapy.

▶ EVALUATION OF THERAPEUTIC OUTCOMES

- Patients with bone and joint infections must be monitored closely (Table 35.5).
- The clinical signs of inflammation such as swelling, tenderness, pain, redness, and fever should resolve with appropriate therapy.
- The WBC count is usually obtained once or twice per week until it returns to the normal range.
- Elevations in the erythrocyte sedimentation rate may not return to normal for several weeks of therapy.

See Chapter 111, Bone and Joint Infections, authored by Edward P. Armstrong, PharmD, BCPS and Victor A. Elsberry, PharmD, BCNSP, for a more detailed discussion of this topic.

VIII

Chapter 36

► CENTRAL NERVOUS SYSTEM INFECTIONS

► DEFINITION

Central nervous system (CNS) infections include a wide variety of clinical conditions and etiologies: meningitis, meningoencephalitis, encephalitis, brain and meningeal abscesses, and shunt infections. The focus of this chapter is meningitis.

► EPIDEMIOLOGY AND ETIOLOGY

- CNS infections may be caused by a variety of bacteria, fungi, viruses, and parasites. The most common causes of bacterial meningitis include *Streptococcus pneumoniae, Haemophilus influenzae,* and *Neisseria meningitidis.*
- CNS infections are divided into two categories: septic and aseptic. Septic or bacterial infections are the result of hematogenous spread from a primary site of infection, parameningeal seeding from a localized infection, or trauma or congenital defects in the CNS. Aseptic infection is a term broadly used to describe chemical irritants, viral, fungal, parasitic, tuberculous, sarcoid, neoplastic, and syphilitic processes of the CNS.

► PATHOPHYSIOLOGY

- The critical first step in the acquisition of acute bacterial meningitis is nasopharyngeal colonization of the host by the bacterial pathogen. The bacteria must first attach themselves to nasopharyngeal epithelial cells with bacterial surface structures called lectins. The bacteria are then phagocytized across nonciliated columnar nasopharyngeal cells into the host's bloodstream.
- A common characteristic of most CNS bacterial pathogens (e.g. *H. influenzae, Escherichia coli,* and *N. meningitidis*) is the presence of an extensive polysaccharide capsule that is resistant to neutrophil phagocytosis and complement opsonization.
- The mechanism and exact site of bacterial invasion into the CNS are currently unknown, but recent studies suggest that invasion into the subarachnoid space is accomplished by continuously exposing the CNS to large bacterial inocula.
- Bacteria replicate freely within the CSF until either bacterial overgrowth occurs or an effective antibiotic regimen is administered that terminates the process.
- Bacterial cell death then causes the release of cell wall components such as lipopolysaccharide (LPS), lipid A (endotoxin), lipoteichoic acid,

teichoic acid, and peptidoglycan depending on whether the pathogen is gram positive or gram negative. These cell wall components cause capillary endothelial cells and CNS macrophages to release cytokines (interleukin-1 [IL-1] and tumor necrosis factor [TNF]).

- Inflammatory cytokines interact with capillary endothelial cells and CNS leukocytes to release products of the cyclooxygenase–arachidonic acid pathway (prostaglandins and thromboxanes) and platelet activating factor (PAF). PAF activates the coagulation cascade, and arachidonic acid metabolites stimulate vasodilatation. These events propagate other sequential events and cytokines that lead to cerebral edema, elevated intracranial pressure, CSF pleocytosis, disseminated intravascular coagulation (DIC), inappropriate antidiuretic hormone secretion (SIADH), decreased cerebral blood flow, cerebral ischemia, and death.

▶ CLINICAL PRESENTATION

- Signs and symptoms of CNS infection have clinical features similar to those of a variety of infectious diseases. Fever, peripheral leukocytosis with a left shift, and malaise are common observations.
- Usually the cerebrospinal fluid (CSF) pattern of pleocytosis (an increasing number of leukocytes, especially lymphocytes, in the CSF), increased protein concentration, and decreased glucose concentration with respect to time can be used to help differentiate viral, fungal, and bacterial etiologies (Table 36.1).
- On initial presentation, differentiation of patients with bacterial, viral, or fungal meningitis is virtually impossible.
- The clinical signs and symptoms of meningitis are variable and dependent on the age of the patient. Adult patients will present with variable complaints of fever, stiffness of the neck and/or back, nuchal rigidity, positive Brudzinski's sign and/or positive Kernig's sign. Later in the

VIII

TABLE 36.1. Typical Components of Normal and Abnormal Cerebrospinal Fluid

Type	Normal	Bacterial	Viral	Fungal	Tuberculosis
WBC (mm³)	<10[a]	400–100,000	5–500	40–400	100–1000
Differential	>90%[a]	>90 PMN[b]	50[c,d]	>50[c]	>80[c,d]
Protein (mg/dL)	<50	80–500	30–150	40–150	≥40–150
Glucose (mg/dL)	½–⅔ serum	<½ serum	<30–70	<30–70	<30–70

[a]Monocytes.
[b]PMN = polymorphonuclear cells.
[c]Lymphocytes.
[d]Initial CSF WBC may reveal a predominance of PMNs.
Adapted from Maxson S, Jacobs RF. Postgrad Med 1993;93(8): 153–166, with permission.

course of the disease, the patient may experience seizures, focal neurologic deficits, and hydrocephalus.

- Young infants infected with bacterial meningitis may reveal only nonspecific symptoms such as irritability, altered sleep patterns, vomiting, high-pitched crying, decreased oral intake, or seizures. Symptoms in the elderly may resemble stroke or endocarditis.
- The diagnosis of bacterial meningitis is usually made on the basis of examination of CSF collected soon after the diagnosis is suspected. In addition to CSF examination, blood cultures should be performed because meningitis can frequently arise via hematogenous dissemination. Elevated CSF protein ≥50 mg/dL and a CSF glucose concentration <50% of the simultaneously obtained peripheral value suggest bacterial meningitis (Table 36.1).
- Gram stain and aerobic culture of the CSF are the most important laboratory tests performed when attempting to diagnose bacterial meningitis. When performed before antibiotic therapy is initiated, Gram stain is both rapid and sensitive and can confirm the diagnosis of bacterial meningitis in 60–90% of cases. The sensitivity of Gram stain decreases to 40–60% in patients receiving prior antibiotic therapy.
- Several rapid diagnostic methods are available for identifying potential bacterial pathogens from CSF. Latex fixation, latex coagglutination, and enzyme immunoassay (EIA) tests provide for the rapid identification of *S. pneumoniae,* Group B *Streptococci, N. meningitidis,* type B *H. influenzae,* and *E. coli* (K1).

VIII

▶ TREATMENT

GENERAL PRINCIPLES

- The administration of fluids, electrolytes, antipyretics, analgesia, and other supportive measures are indicated as needed for patients presenting with acute bacterial meningitis.

PHARMACOLOGIC TREATMENT

- Appropriate antibiotic therapy (empiric or definitive) should be started as soon as possible. Isolation and identification of the causative agent can direct the selection of the most appropriate antimicrobial therapy for the patient (Tables 36.2, 36.3 and 36.4).
- Peak CSF antibiotic concentrations should be approximately 10 times the minimum bactericidal concentration (MBC) of the microorganism causing bacterial meningitis.

Penetration of Antimicrobials into the Central Nervous System

- Several factors influence the transfer of antibiotic from capillary blood into the CNS. With increased meningeal inflammation, there will be greater antibiotic penetration (see Table 36.2). Problems of CSF penetration may be overcome by direct instillation of antibiotics by intrathecal, intracisternal, or intraventricular routes of administration (see Table

TABLE 36.2. Penetration of Antimicrobial Agents into the Cerebrospinal Fluid

Therapeutic Levels in CSF with or without Inflammation

Sulfonamides	Trimethoprim
Chloramphenicol	Isoniazid
Rifampin	Pyrazinamide
Ethionamide	Cycloserine
Metronidazole	

Therapeutic Levels in CSF with Inflammation of Meninges

Penicillin G	Ampicillin ± sulbactam
Carbenicillin	Ticarcillin ± clavulanic acid
Nafcillin	Mezlocillin
Piperacillin	Cefuroxime
Cefotaxime	Ceftizoxime
Ceftriaxone	Ceftazidime
Imipenem	Aztreonam
Vancomycin	Ciprofloxacin
Ofloxacin	Ethambutol
Flucytosine	Fluconazole
Pyrimethamine	Ganciclovir
Acyclovir	Foscarnet
Vidarabine	

Nontherapeutic Levels in CSF with or without Inflammation

Aminoglycosides	First-generation cephalosporins [VIII]
Cefoperozone	Second-generation cephalosporins[a]
Clindamycin[b]	Ketoconazole
Amphotericin B[c]	Itraconazole[c]

[a]Cefuroxime is an exception.
[b]Achieves therapeutic brain tissue concentrations.
[c]Achieves therapeutic concentrations for *C. neoformans* therapy.

36.3). The advantages of direct instillation, however, must be weighed against the risks of invasive CNS procedures.

Dexamethasone as an Adjunctive Treatment for Meningitis

- In addition to antibiotics, dexamethasone has now become a commonly used therapy for the treatment of pediatric meningitis. In general, clinical trials have shown a significant improvement in markers of active infection such as CSF glucose concentrations, as well as CSF protein and lactate concentrations, when corticosteroids are administered as adjunctive treatment. Consistently, the trials have detected a significantly lower incidence of neurologic sequella commonly associated with bacterial meningitis. Some authors have advocated that all infants (>2 months) and children with suspected bacterial meningitis receive dexamethasone.
- Currently, the American Academy of Pediatrics suggests that the use of dexamethasone be considered for infants and children 2 months of age or older with proven or strongly suspected bacterial meningitis. If dexamethasone is used, the commonly utilized intravenous (IV) dose is 0.15

TABLE 36.3. Intraventricular and Intrathecal Antibiotic Dosage Recommendations

Antibiotic	Adult Dose (mg)	Expected CSF Concentration[a] (mg/L)
Ampicillin	10–50	60–300
Methicillin	25–100	160–600
Nafcillin	75	500
Cefazolin	1–2 mg/kg, 50 mg maximum	300
Cephalothin	25–100	160–600
Chloramphenicol	25–100	160–600
Gentamicin	1–10	6–60
Tobramycin	1–10	6–60
Amikacin	5–10	60
Vancomycin	5	30
Amphotericin B	0.05–0.25 mg/d to 0.05–1 mg 1–3 times weekly	—

[a]Assumes adult CSF volume = 150 mL.

mg/kg every 6 hours for 4 days. Alternatively, prospective randomized, double-blind studies have found dexamethasone 0.15 mg/kg every 6 hours for 2 days or dexamethasone 0.4 mg/kg every 12 hours for 2 days to be equally effective and potentially less toxic regimens. Dexamethasone should be administered prior to the first antibiotic dose, and serum hemoglobin and stool guaiac should be monitored for evidence of gastrointestinal (GI) bleeding.

Neisseria Meningitidis (Meningococcus)

- *N. meningitidis* meningitis is most commonly found in children and young adults. The source of the infection is usually an asymptomatic carrier. Most cases usually occur in the winter or spring, at a time when viral meningitis is relatively uncommon.

Clinical Presentation

- Approximately 10–14 days after the onset of the disease and despite successful treatment, the patient develops a characteristic immunologic reaction of fever, arthritis (usually involving large joints), and pericarditis. At this time, examination of synovial fluid will reveal a large number of polymorphonuclear cells, elevated protein concentrations, and normal glucose concentration. Cultures of synovial fluid at this time will be sterile.
- Approximately 50% of patients die within the first 24 hours as a result of an acute fulminant course associated with meningococcemia. Other patients develop a picture of chronic meningococcemia that is characterized by episodes of fever, arthritis, and a morbilliform rash that recurs every 48–72 hours.

TABLE 36.4. Bacterial Meningitis: Most Likely Bacteria and Empiric Therapy by Age Group

Age Commonly Affected	Most Likely Organisms	Empiric Therapy	Risk Factors for All Age Groups
Newborn–1 month	Gram negative enterics[a] Group B streptococcus Listeria monocytogenes	Ampicillin + CTX or CRT or CZ[b] or AG[c]	Respiratory tract infection Otitis media Mastoiditis Head trauma Alcoholism
1 month–4 years	Haemophilus influenzae Neisseria meningitidis Streptococcus pneumoniae	CTX or CRT or CZ or ampicillin + chloramphenicol	High-dose steroids Splenectomy Sickle cell disease immunoglobulin deficiency
5–29 years	N. meningitidis S. pneumoniae H. influenzae	CTX or CRT or CZ or ampicillin + chloramphenicol	Immunosuppression
30–60 years	S. pneumoniae N. meningitidis	CTX or CRT or CZ	
>60 years	S. pneumoniae Gram-negative enterics Listeria monocytogenes	Ampicillin + CTX or CRT or CZ or AG[c]	

[a] E. coli, Klebsiella spp., Enterobacter spp. common.
[b] CTX, cefotaxime; CRT, ceftriaxone; CZ, ceftizoxime.
[c] Aminoglycoside—gentamicin used most frequently.

VIII

425

- Deafness unilaterally, or more commonly bilaterally, may develop early or late in the disease course.
- Approximately 50% of patients with meningococcal meningitis have purpuric lesions, petechiae, or both. Patients may have an obvious or subclinical picture of DIC, which may progress to infarction of the adrenal glands and renal cortex and cause widespread thrombosis.

Treatment and Prevention
- Aggressive, early intervention with high-dose intravenous crystalline penicillin G, 50,000 units/kg every 4 hours intravenously, is usually recommended for treatment of *N. meningitidis* meningitis.
- Chloramphenicol is bactericidal for *N. meningitidis* and may be used in place of penicillin G. Several third-generation cephalosporins (e.g., cefotaxime) approved for the treatment of meningitis are acceptable alternatives to penicillin G (Table 36.4).
- Close contacts of patients contracting *N. meningitidis* meningitis are at an increased risk of developing meningitis (200 to 1000 times that of the general population). Prophylaxis of contacts should be started without delay and, therefore, without the aid of culture and sensitivity studies.
- Adult patients should receive 600 mg of rifampin orally every 12 hours for four doses. Children 1 month to 12 years of age should receive 10 mg/kg of rifampin orally every 12 hours for four doses, and children younger than 1 month should receive 5 mg/kg orally every 12 hours for four doses. Alternatives to rifampin include ciprofloxacin (single dose) in adults and ceftriaxone 125–250 mg (single dose, intramuscularly).
- Patients receiving rifampin should be counseled as to the expected red-to-orange color change in urine and other body secretions.

Streptococcus Pneumoniae (Pneumococcus or Diplococcus)
- Pneumococcal meningitis occurs in the very young (1–4 months) and the very old. It is the most common cause of meningitis in adults and accounts for 12% of meningitis episodes in children 2 months to 10 years.

Treatment (Table 36.5)
- The treatment of choice until susceptibility of the organism is known is vancomycin (15 mg/kg every 6 hours up to 2 g per day) plus a broad-spectrum cephalosporin (cefotaxime 50 mg/kg every 6 hours intravenously in neonates and ceftriaxone 50–100 mg/kg every 12 hours intravenously in children (2 g every 12 hours in adults). If adjunctive dexamethasone is given in adults the preferred regimen is ceftriaxone plus rifampin (600 mg per day).
- If the pathogen is found to be susceptible to penicillin and ceftriaxone, either agent may be used alone (penicillin given at 200,000–300,000 units/kg/day given every 4 hours intravenously). If the pathogen is resistant to penicillin (≥0.1 µg/mL) but susceptible to ceftriaxone or cefotaxime, either alone may be continued. If it is resistant to penicillin and ceftriaxone, combination therapy as above should be continued.

VIII

TABLE 36.5. Antimicrobial Agents of First Choice and Alternative Choice in Treatment of Meningitis Caused by Gram-Positive Microorganisms

Organism	Antibiotic of First Choice[a]	Alternative Antibiotics[a]
Streptococcus pneumoniae		
Penicillin susceptible	Penicillin G 200,000–300,000 units/kg/d, every 6 h IV max: 4 million units every 4 h IV	Chloramphenicol 100 mg/kg/d, every 6 h max: 1.5 g IV every 6 h Cefotaxime 200 mg/kg/d every 4 h max: 2 g IV every 4 h Ceftriaxone 100 mg/kg/d every 24 h[b] max: adults 2 g IV every 12 Ceftizoxime 200 mg/kg/d every 6–8 h max: 3–4 g IV every 8 h
Low-level penicillin resistance[c]	Cefotaxime or ceftriaxone	Vancomycin 30–40 mg/kg/d IV
High-level penicillin resistance[d]	Vancomycin ± ceftriaxone	Imipenem 80 mg/kg/d max: 1 g IV every 6 h
Group B *Streptococcus*	Penicillin	Cefotaxime Ceftriaxone Ceftizoxime Chloramphenicol
Staphylococcus aureus		
Penicillin resistant	Nafcillin 200 mg/kg/d every 4 h max: 2 g every 4 h IV	Vancomycin
Methicillin resistant	Vancomycin	—
Staphylococcus epidermidis		
Penicillin resistant	Nafcillin	Vancomycin
Methicillin resistant	Vancomycin	
Listeria monocytogenes	Ampicillin 200–400 mg/kg/d, every 6 h IV or Pen G max: 2 g every 4 h IV plus aminoglycoside IV—usually gentamicin	Trimethoprim 10 mg/kg/d and sulfamethoxazole 50 mg/kg/day, every 6 h

[a]Recommended doses for adults and pediatric patients with normal renal and/or hepatic function.
[b]Pediatrics.
[c]Incidence of low-level resistance is 10–20%.
[d]Incidence of high-level resistance is 1–2%; therapeutic recommendations for this infection have not been clearly defined.

VIII

427

- Virtually all serotypes of *S. pneumoniae* exhibiting intermediate or complete resistance to penicillin are found in the current 23 serotype pneumococcal vaccine, and clinicians need to universally immunize appropriate patients. Unfortunately, the efficacy of this product in children <2 years and compromised adults limits this strategy as a solution to the problem of penicillin-resistant pneumococci.
- Chemoprophylaxis and vaccination for close contacts of an index case with *S. pneumoniae* meningitis are generally not recommended because the risk of acquiring secondary pneumococcal disease is similar to the infection rate in the general population. However, vaccination and chemoprophylaxis with oral penicillin reduce the incidence of pneumococcal septicemia and meningitis in young patients with sickle cell disease.

Gram-Negative Bacillary Meningitis

- During the last 20 years, the incidence of gram-negative bacillary meningitis, excluding *H. influenzae* has been increasing in both children and adults. Gram-negative organisms are the fourth leading cause of meningitis, with only *S. pneumoniae, H. influenzae,* and *N. meningitidis* having a higher incidence.
- In the postneonatal period, the two most common organisms causing gram-negative meningitis are *E. coli* and *K. pneumoniae* together, which are responsible for 60–70% of cases.

Treatment (Table 36.6)

- Meningitis caused by *P. aeruginosa* is treated with ceftazidime plus an aminoglycoside, usually tobramycin.
- If the pseudomonad is initially suspected to be antibiotic resistant or becomes resistant during therapy, an intraventricular aminoglycoside (preservative-free) should be considered along with IV aminoglycoside. Intraventricular aminoglycoside dosages are adjusted to the estimated CSF volume (0.03 mg of tobramycin or gentamicin/mL of CSF and 0.1 mg of amikacin/mL of CSF every 24 hours). Ventricular levels of aminoglycoside are monitored every 2 or 3 days, just prior to the next intraventricular dose, and "trough levels" should approximate 2–10 mg/L.
- Gram-negative organisms, other than *P. aeruginosa,* that cause meningitis can also be treated with a third-generation cephalosporin such as cefotaxime, ceftizoxime, ceftriaxone, or ceftazidime in combination with an IV aminoglycoside. In adults, daily doses of 8–12 g/d of these third-generation cephalosporins or 2 g of ceftriaxone should produce CSF concentrations of 5–20 mg/L.
- Therapy for gram-negative meningitis is continued for 21 days. CSF cultures may remain positive for 10 days or more on a regimen that will eventually be curative. Therapeutic efficacy is monitored through bacterial colony counts every 2 or 3 days, and colony counts should progressively decrease over the period of therapy.

TABLE 36.6. Antimicrobial Agents of First Choice and Alternative Choice in Treatment of Meningitis Caused by Gram-Negative Organisms

Organism	Antibiotic of First Choice[a]	Alternative Antibiotics[a]
Neisseria meningitidis (meningococcal)	Penicillin G 200,000–300,000 u/kg/d IV	Cefotaxime 200 mg/kg/d every 4 h max: 2 g IV every 4 h Ceftriaxone 100 mg/kg/d every 24 h[b] max: adults 2 g IV every 12 h Ceftizoxime 200 mg/kg/d every 6–8 h max: 3–4 g IV every 8 h Chloramphenicol 100 mg/kg/d max: 1.5 g IV every 6 h
Escherichia coli	Cefotaxime	Ceftriaxone Ceftizoxime Chloramphenicol
Haemophilus influenzae		
β-Lactamase positive	Cefotaxime	Ceftriaxone Ceftizoxime
β-Lactamase negative	Ampicillin	Cefotaxime Ceftriaxone Ceftizoxime
Pseudomonas aeruginosa	Ceftazidime 85 mg/kg/d max: 2 g IV every 8 h plus tobramycin 5–7.5 mg/kg/d IV[c]	Imipenem 80 mg/kg/d max: 1 g IV every 6 h Piperacillin 200–300 mg/kg/d max: 3 g every 4 h IV plus Tobramycin
Enterobacteriaceae	Cefotaxime	Ceftriaxone Ceftizoxime Piperacillin plus aminoglycoside Imipenem

[a]Recommended doses for adults and pediatric patients with normal renal and/or hepatic function.   [c]Direct CNS administration may be added; see Table 36.3 for dosage
[b]Pediatrics.

VIII

429

Haemophilus Influenzae

- In the past, *H. influenzae* was the most common cause of meningitis in children 6 months to 3 years. The disease is often a complication of primary infectious involvement of the middle ear, paranasal sinuses, or lungs.
- Coma and seizures commonly occur early in the course of the disease. Morbiliform and petechial rashes are very uncommon, but may resemble the rash seen with meningococcal infection.

Treatment

- Approximately 30–40% of *H. influenzae* are ampicillin resistant. For this reason, many clinicians use a third-generation cephalosporin (cefotaxime or ceftriaxone) for initial antimicrobial therapy. Once bacterial susceptibilities are available, ampicillin may be used if the isolate proves ampicillin sensitive.

Prevention

- Because cases of *H. influenzae* meningitis occur in clusters, treatment of close contacts (household members, individuals sharing sleeping quarters, crowded confined populations, day care attendees, and nursing home residents) of patients is usually recommended. The goal of prophylaxis is to eliminate nasopharyngeal and oropharyngeal carriage of *H. influenzae*.
- VIII • Prophylaxis for *H. influenzae* is not recommended when at least one member of the same household as the patient is <4 years of age, if all contacts <4 years old are fully immunized. Households with children <12 months (regardless of vaccination status) or with children ages 1–3 years who are not adequately vaccinated should all receive rifampin prophylaxis in order to eliminate nasopharyngeal carriage and the subsequent spread of disease to others. Chemoprophylaxis should be initiated as soon as possible after exposure. The patient should also receive chemoprophylaxis prior to discharge from the hospital because there have been reports of recolonization after successful antibiotic therapy.
- Adults receive 600 mg of rifampin daily for 4 days. Children 1 month to 12 years receive 20 mg/kg (maximum 600 mg) per day for 4 days, and children <1 month receive 10 mg/kg/d for 4 days.
- Guidelines regarding the use of HIB conjugate vaccines are as follows:

  1. Any of the conjugate vaccines, with the exception of ProHIBIT, are indicated for the primary vaccination series in infants older than 2 months of age.
  2. Three doses of HbOC or PRP-T and two doses of PRP-OMP should be administered to infants younger than 6 months; ideally at 2, 4, and 6 months.
  3. Two doses of the previously mentioned vaccines should be given to infants first seen between 7 and 11 months of age.
  4. One dose of these vaccines should be administered to infants first seen between 12 and 14 months of age.

5. All infants should receive a booster dose at 15 months of age or 2 months after their last vaccination. Any of the currently licensed conjugate vaccines (HbOC, PRP-T, PRP-OMP, PRP-D) can be used for the dose at 15 months, because they all appear to be effective at that age.

- The Centers for Disease Control (CDC) recommends completion of the primary series with the same Hib conjugate vaccine, if possible. If different vaccines are administered, a total of three doses is necessary to assure adequate response.

Listeria monocytogenes

- *Listeria monocytogenes* is a gram-positive diphtheroid-like organism and is responsible for 3% of all reported cases of meningitis. The disease affects primarily neonates, immunocompromised adults, and the elderly. In the immunocompromised patient, the CSF resembles that found in bacterial meningitis.

Treatment

- The combination of penicillin G or ampicillin with gentamicin results in a bactericidal effect. Patients should be treated for 2–3 weeks after defervescence to prevent the possibility of relapse.
- Trimethoprim–sulfamethoxazole may be an effective alternative, because adequate CSF penetration is achieved with these agents. VIII ◄

Mycobacterium tuberculosis

- *Mycobacterium tuberculosis* var. *hominis* is the primary cause of tuberculous meningitis. Tuberculous meningitis may exist in the absence of disease in the lung or extrapulmonary sites. The tuberculin skin test (purified protein derivative [PPD]) is negative in 5–50% of cases.
- Upon initial examination, CSF usually contains from 100–1000 WBC/mm^3, which may be 75–80% polymorphonuclear cells. Over time, the pattern of WBC in the CSF will shift to lymphocytes and monocytes.
- One potentially useful diagnostic sign unique to tuberculous meningitis is paralysis of the VIth cranial nerve, which initially may be unilateral and then progress to become bilateral.
- Cultures of CSF may be positive in 45–90% of cases depending on the quantity of CSF used in the culture, pathogen density, and the experience in the laboratory culturing *M. tuberculosis*. Positive culture results may take up to 8 weeks, providing little help with initial diagnosis.
- Isoniazid is the mainstay in virtually any regimen to treat *M. tuberculosis*. In children, the usual dose of isoniazid is 10–20 mg/kg/d (maximum 300 mg/d). Adults usually receive 5–10 mg/kg/d or a daily dose of 300 mg.
- Supplemental doses of pyridoxine hydrochloride (vitamin B$_6$) 50 mg/d are recommended to prevent the peripheral neuropathy associated with isoniazid administration.

- Concurrent administration of rifampin is recommended at doses of 10–20 mg/kg/d (maximum 600 mg/d) for children and 600 mg/d for adults. The addition of pyrazinamide (children and adults 15–30 mg/kg/d; maximum in both 2 g/d) to the regimen of isoniazid and rifampin is now recommended. The duration of concomitant pyrazinamide therapy should be limited to 2 months in order to avoid hepatotoxicity.
- As of 1993, the CDC recommends a regimen of four drugs for empiric treatment of *M. tuberculosis,* unless resistance to isoniazid in the area is <4%. This regimen should consist of isoniazid, rifampin, pyrazinamide, and ethambutol 15–25 mg/kg/d (maximum 2.5 g/d) or streptomycin 15–30 mg/kg/d (maximum 1 g/d) for the first 2 months, generally followed by isoniazid plus rifampin for the duration of therapy. Therapy after the first 2 months should be individualized based on susceptibility patterns.
- Patients with *M. tuberculosis* meningitis should be treated for a duration of 9 months or longer with multiple drug therapy.
- The use of steroids for tuberculous meningitis remains controversial. In some cases administration of steroids as oral prednisone 40–60 mg/d or 0.2 mg/kg/d of IV dexamethasone has resulted in a dramatic clearing of sensorium, remission of CSF abnormalities, reduction in fever, and elimination of headaches.

VIII *Cryptococcus neoformans*

- In the United States, cryptococcal meningitis is the most common form of fungal meningitis and is a major cause of morbidity and mortality in immunosuppressed patients. Patients with HIV are at a 5–10% risk of developing cryptococcus during their lifetime. *Cryptococcus neoformans* is a soil fungus acquired by inhalation of spores from the environment.
- Fever and a history of headaches are the most common symptoms of cryptococcal meningitis, although altered mentation and evidence of focal neurologic deficits may be present. Examination of CSF usually reveals small numbers of WBCs (<150/mm^3), which are primarily lymphocytes. Diagnosis is based on the presence of a positive CSF, blood, sputum, or urine culture for *C. neoformans.*
- CSF cultures are positive in more than 90% of cases. The organism can be seen microscopically when stained with India ink. An additional rapid test helpful in diagnosis is latex agglutination, which detects the presence of cryptococcal antigens.

Treatment

- Amphotericin B has long been the drug of choice for treatment of acute *C. neoformans* meningitis. Amphotericin B 0.5–1 mg/kg/d combined with flucytosine 100 mg/kg/d is more effective than amphotericin alone, with successful outcomes in 75% of non-AIDS patients and in 50% of AIDS patients. In the AIDS population, flucytosine is often poorly tolerated, causing bone marrow suppression and GI distress.

- Intraventricular amphotericin B in addition to IV amphotericin B plus flucytosine has been suggested as initial therapy, but intraventricular amphotericin is generally reserved for patients who fail to respond to systemic therapy.
- Due to the high relapse rate following acute therapy for *C. neoformans*, AIDS patients require lifelong maintenance or suppressive therapy. The standard of care for AIDS-associated cryptococcal meningitis is primary therapy, generally using amphotericin B with or without flucytosine or fluconazole alone, followed by maintenance therapy with fluconazole for the life of the patient.

Viral Meningitis

- Meningitis typically is characterized as being either purulent or aseptic. While purulent meningitis refers to a bacterial etiology, aseptic meningitis historically was defined by diagnosis of exclusion.
- At least 70% of aseptic meningitis cases are caused by viruses; however, unusual bacterial organisms such as *M. tuberculosis, Brucella* spp., and *Borrelia burgdorferi* can cause aseptic meningitis.
- The clinical syndrome seen with viral meningitis is generally independent of the particular viral etiology and may vary depending on the patient's age.
- Common signs in adults include headache, mild fever (<40°C), nuchal rigidity, malaise, drowsiness, nausea, vomiting, and photophobia. Only fever and irritability may be evident in the infant, and meningitis must be ruled out as a cause of fever when no other localized findings are observed in a child.
- The duration of symptoms is generally 1 to 2 weeks, and specific manifestations outside of the meninges can also occur depending on the particular viral etiology.
- Laboratory examination of CSF usually reveals a pleocytosis with 10–1000 WBCs/mm^3, which are primarily lymphocytic; however, 20–75% of patients with viral meningitis may have a predominance of polymorphonuclear cells on initial examination of the CSF, especially in enteroviral meningitis. Upon repeat lumbar puncture, 90% of patients initially presenting with a predominance of neutrophils experience a shift to a predominance of mononuclear cells.
- Other laboratory findings include normal to mildly elevated protein concentrations and normal or mildly reduced glucose concentrations (Table 36.1).
- Although there are numerous pathogenic causes of viral meningitis, much of the clinical presentation, diagnosis, and treatment is similar for different viral pathogens.
- Acyclovir is the drug of choice for herpes simplex encephalitis. In patients with normal renal function, acyclovir is usually administered as 10 mg/kg every 8 hours. Herpes virus resistance to acyclovir has been reported with increasing incidence, particularly from immunocompromised patients with prior or chronic exposures to acyclovir.

VIII

- The alternative treatment for acyclovir-resistant herpes simplex virus is vidarabine. Vidarabine is used intravenously in a dose of 15 mg/kg/d. Because of its poor solubility in water, the drug must be mixed in large volumes of parenteral fluid and infused over a 12-hour period. In addition, patients receiving vidarabine should be monitored for leukopenia, megaloblastic anemia, thrombocytopenia, and a parkinsonin-like neurologic syndrome.

See Chapter 99, Central Nervous System Infections, authored by Karl J. Madaras-Kelly, PharmD, Beth E. Ostergaard, PharmD, and John C. Rotschafer, PharmD, FCCP, for a more detailed discussion of this topic.

VIII

Chapter 37

▶ ENDOCARDITIS

▶ DEFINITION

Endocarditis is an inflammation of the endocardium, the membrane lining the chambers of the heart and covering the cusps of the heart valves. *Infective endocarditis* (IE) refers to infection of the heart valves by various microorganisms.

Endocarditis is often referred to as either acute or subacute depending on the clinical presentation. Acute bacterial endocarditis is a fulminating infection associated with high fevers, systemic toxicity, and death within a few days to weeks if untreated. Subacute bacterial endocarditis (SBE) is a more indolent infection caused by less invasive organisms such as *viridans streptococci,* usually occurring in a setting of prior valvular heart disease.

▶ EPIDEMIOLOGY

- Infective endocarditis accounts for approximately 1 of every 1000 hospital admissions. Most persons with IE have evidence of preexisting cardiac valvular abnormalities or other risk factors, although a predisposing factor may be absent in up to 25% of cases.
- Most types of structural heart disease resulting in turbulence of blood flow will increase the risk for IE. Some of the most important include:
  - Congenital heart disease accompanied by cyanosis (such as patent ductus arteriosus and ventricular septal defects)
  - Rheumatic heart disease following rheumatic fever
  - Mitral valve prolapse with regurgitation
  - Degenerative valvular lesions in the elderly, such as valvular stenosis and regurgitation
  - Presence of a prosthetic valve
  - IV drug abuse
- Three groups of organisms cause most cases of IE: streptococci (50–60%), staphylococci (25%), and enterococci (10%) (Table 37.1).

▶ PATHOPHYSIOLOGY

- The development of IE via hematogenous spread, the most common route, requires the sequential occurrence of several factors

    1. The endothelial surface of the heart must be damaged. This occurs with turbulent blood flow associated with the valvular lesions previously described.
    2. Platelet and fibrin deposition occurs on the abnormal epithelial surface. These deposits are referred to as nonbacterial thrombotic endocarditis (NBTE).

Infectious Diseases

TABLE 37.1. Etiologic Agents in Infective Endocarditis

Agent	Percentage of Cases
Streptococci	60–80
Viridans streptococci	30–40
Other	15–25
Enterococci	5–18
Staphylococci	20–35
Coagulase-positive	10–27
Coagulase-negative	1–3
Gram-negative aerobic bacilli	1.5–13
Fungi	2–4
Miscellaneous	<5
Culture-negative	<5–24

From Scheld WM, Sande MA. In Mandell GL, Douglas RG, Bennett JE (eds): Principles and Practice of Infectious Diseases, 4th ed. New York, Churchill Livingstone, 1995:681, with permission.

VIII

3. Bacteremia results in colonization of the endocardial surface. Most often, bacteremia is the result of trauma to a mucosal surface having a high concentration of resident bacteria, such as the oral cavity and gastrointestinal tract. Transient bacteremia commonly follows certain dental and gastrointestinal procedures.
4. Staphylococci, *viridans streptococci,* and enterococci are most likely to adhere to NBTE, probably because of production of specific adherence factors, such as dextran production by some oral streptococci.
5. After colonization of the endothelial surface, fibrin, platelets, and bacteria continue to aggregate and a "vegetation" forms. The protective cover of fibrin and platelets allows unimpeded bacterial growth to concentrations as high as 10^9–10^{10} per gram of tissue. Bacteria within the vegetation grow slowly and are protected from antibiotics and host defenses.

▶ CLINICAL PRESENTATION

- The clinical presentation of patients with IE is highly variable (Table 37.2).
- Important clinical signs, especially prevalent in subacute illness, may include the following peripheral manifestations ("stigmata") of endocarditis:
  - Osler nodes
  - Janeway lesions
  - Splinter hemorrhages
  - Petechiae

TABLE 37.2. Clinical Manifestations of Infective Endocarditis

Symptoms	Percentage of Patients	Physical Findings	Percentage of Patients
Fever	80	Fever	90
Chills	40	Heart murmur	85
Weakness	40	Changing murmur	5–10
Dyspnea	40	New murmur	3–5
Sweats	25	Embolic phenomenon	>50
Anorexia	25	Skin manifestations	18–50
Weight loss	25	Osler nodes	10–23
Malaise	25	Splinter hemorrhages	15
Cough	25	Petechiae	20–40
Skin lesions	20	Janeway lesion	<10
Stroke	20	Splenomegaly	20–57
Nausea/vomiting	20	Septic complications (pneumonia, meningitis, etc.)	20
Headache	15		
Myalgia/arthralgia	15		
Edema	15	Mycotic aneurysms	20
Chest pain	15	Clubbing	12–52
Abdominal pain	15	Retinal lesion	2–10
Delirium/coma	10	Signs of renal failure	10–15
Hemoptysis	10		
Back pain	10		

VIII

From Scheld WM, Sande MA. In Mandell GL, Bennett JE, Dolin R (eds): Principles and Practices of Infectious Diseases, 4th ed. New York. Churchill Livingstone, 1995:748, with permission.

- Clubbing of the fingers
- Roth spot
- Emboli
- Patients with IE virtually always have some laboratory abnormalities; however, there are none specific for endocarditis.
- Without appropriate antimicrobial therapy and surgery if required, IE is usually fatal. With proper management, recovery can be expected in most patients.
- Factors associated with increased mortality include:

  1. Congestive heart failure
  2. Culture-negative endocarditis
  3. Endocarditis caused by resistant organisms such as fungi and gram-negative bacteria
  4. Left-sided endocarditis caused by *S. aureus*
  5. Prosthetic valve endocarditis.

LABORATORY AND DIAGNOSTIC FINDINGS

- The hallmark of IE is a continuous bacteremia caused by shedding of bacteria from the vegetation into the bloodstream. More than 95% of patients with IE have a positive blood culture when three samples are obtained during a 24 hour period.
- Two-dimensional echocardiography, using either the transthoracic (TTE) or transesophageal (TEE) technique, is increasingly important in identifying and localizing valvular lesions in patients suspected of having IE. TEE is more sensitive for detecting vegetations ($\geq$90%), compared to TTE (~50%).

▶ TREATMENT

GENERAL PRINCIPLES

- The most important approach to treatment of IE includes isolation of the pathogen followed by high-dose, bactericidal antibiotics for an extended period.
- For some pathogens, such as enterococci, the use of synergistic antimicrobial combinations is essential to obtain a bactericidal effect.
- For most patients, 4–6 weeks of therapy are required.
- Specific recommendations for treating IE caused by the most common organisms are discussed here and are summarized in Tables 37.3 through 37.8.

SURGERY

- Surgery is an important adjunct to management of endocarditis in certain patients. The major causes of death in patients with IE are heart failure and infection of vital organs from septic embolization. In most cases, valvectomy and valve replacement are performed to remove infected tissues and restore hemodynamic function.

VIII

- The most important indications for surgery include the following:
  - Moderate to severe congestive heart failure
  - Valvular obstruction
  - Local suppurative complications such as a myocardial abscess
  - Endocarditis caused by resistant organisms (e.g., most cases of endocarditis caused by Enterobacteriaceae, *Pseudomonas,* or fungi)
  - Almost all cases of early prosthetic valve endocarditis (PVE)
  - Persistent bacteremia or other evidence of failure of appropriate medical therapy.

VIRIDANS STREPTOCOCCAL ENDOCARDITIS

- The term *viridans streptococcus* refers to a large number of different species, such as *S. mutans, S. sanguis,* and *S. mitior* and are the most common cause of IE, especially in cases involving native valves. *Streptococcus bovis* is not a *viridans streptococcus,* but is included here because it is penicillin sensitive and treatment regimens are the same as for *viridans streptococci.*
- Approximately 10–20% of *viridans streptococci* are "moderately" susceptible to penicillin, MIC = 0.1–0.5 µg/mL. This difference in in vitro susceptibility has led to recommendations that the minimum inhibitory concentration (MIC) should be determined for all viridans streptococci, and the results be used to guide therapy. Although some streptococci are "tolerant" to the killing effects of penicillin, this has not been demonstrated to be clinically important, and treatment is the same as for nontolerant organisms. VIII
- Recommended therapy in the uncomplicated case caused by fully susceptible strains is 2 weeks of combined therapy with penicillin G and gentamicin (Table 37.3 and 37.4).
- Therapy for the patient with penicillin allergy is relatively straightforward. Vancomycin is effective and is the drug of choice (Table 37.5).

STAPHYLOCOCCAL ENDOCARDITIS

- *Staphylococcus aureus* is the most common organism causing IE both among IV drug abusers and in persons with venous catheters. Coagulase-negative staphylococci (CNST, usually *S. epidermidis*) are prominent causes of PVE.
- Management requires consideration of several factors:

  1. Is the organism methicillin resistant?
  2. Should combination therapy be used?
  3. Is the infection on a native valve or a prosthetic valve?
  4. Is the patient an intravenous drug abuser?
  5. Is the infection on the left or right side of the heart?

- The recommended therapy for patients with left-sided IE caused by methicillin-sensitive *S. aureus* (MSSA) is 4–6 weeks of oxacillin or nafcillin, often combined with a short course of an aminoglycoside (Table 37.6).

TABLE 37.3. Suggested Regimens for Therapy for Endocarditis Due to Penicillin-Susceptible Viridans Streptococci and *Streptococcus bovis* (MIC ≤ 0.1 μg/mL)

Antibiotic	Adult Dose and Route	Pediatric Dose and Route	Duration (wk)
1. Aqueous crystalline penicillin G[a]	12–18 million U/24 h IV either continuously or in 6 equally divided doses	150,000–200,000 U/kg per 24 h IV (not to exceed 20 million U/24 h) either continuously or in 6 equally divided doses	4
or			
Ceftriaxone	2 g once daily IV or IM		4
2. Aqueous crystalline penicillin G	12–18 million U/24 h IV either continuously or in 6 equally divided doses	150,000–200,000 U/kg per 24 h IV (not to exceed 20 million U/24 h) either continuously or in 6 equally divided doses	2
With gentamicin[b]	1 mg/kg IM or IV (not to exeed 80 mg) every 8 h	2–2.5 mg/kg IV (not to exceed 80 mg) every 8 h	2
3. Vancomycin[c]	30 mg/kg per 24h IV in two equally divided doses, not to exceed 2 g/24 h unless serum levels are monitored.		4

[a]Preferred in most patients older than 65 years of age and in those with impairment of the eighth nerve or of renal function.

[b]When obtained 1 h after a 20–30 minute IV infusion or IM injection, serum concentration of gentamicin of approximately 3 μg/mL is desirable; trough concentration should be <1 μg/mL. Dosing of aminoglycosides on a milligram per kilogram basis will produce higher serum concentrations in obese than in lean patients. Therefore, in obese patients, dosing should be based on ideal body weight. Relative contraindications to use of aminoglycosides are age greater than 65 years or renal or eighth nerve impairment.

[c]Vancomycin dosage should be reduced in patients with impaired renal function. In obese patients dosing should be based on ideal body weight.

From Wilson WR, Karchmer AW, Dajani AS, et al. *Antibiotic treatment of adults with infective endocarditis due to streptococci, enterococci, and staphylococci, and HACEK organisms. JAMA 1995; 274:1706–1713, with permission. Copyright 1989, American Medical Association.*

TABLE 37.4. Therapy for Endocarditis Due to Strains of Viridans Streptococci and *Streptococcus bovis* Relatively Resistant to Penicillin G (MIC > 0.1 μg/mL and < 0.5 μg/mL)[a]

Antibiotic	Adult Dose and Route	Pediatric Dose and Route	Duration (wk)
1. Aqueous crystalline penicillin G[a]	18 million U/24 h IV either continuously or in 6 equally divided doses	200,000–300,000 U/kg per 24 h IV (not to exceed 20 million U/24 h) given continuously or in 6 equally divided doses	4
or			
With gentamicin[b]	1 mg/kg IM or IV (not to exceed 80 mg) every 8 h	2–2.5 mg/kg IM or IV (not to exceed 80 mg) every 8 h	2
2. Vancomycin[c]	30 mg/kg per 24 h IV in two equally divided doses, not to exceed 2 g/24 h unless serum levels are monitored		4

[a]Cephalothin or cefazolin (with an aminoglycoside for the first 2 weeks) can be used in patients whose penicillin hypersensitivity is not of the immediate type. Antibiotic doses should be modified appropriately for patients with impaired renal function.

[b]Gentamicin should be given in addition to penicillin for the first 2 weeks. Aminoglycosides given on a milligram per kilogram basis will produce higher serum concentrations in obese than in lean patients. Therefore, in obese patients, dosing should be based on ideal body weight.

[c]Vancomycin dosage should be reduced in patients with impaired renal function. In obese patients dosing should be based on ideal body weight.

From Wilson WR, Karchmer AW, Dajani AS, et al. Antibiotic treatment of adults with infective endocarditis due to streptococci, enterococci, and staphylococci, and HACEK organisms. JAMA 1995; 274:1706–1713, with permission. Copyright 1989, American Medical Association.

VIII

441

TABLE 37.5. Therapy for Endocarditis due to Penicillin-Susceptible Viridans Streptococci and *Streptococcus bovis* (MIC ≤ 0.1 μg/mL) in Patients Allergic to Penicillin[a]

Antibiotic	Adult Dose and Route	Pediatric Dose and Route	Duration (wk)
Cephalothin[b,c]	2 g IV every 4 h	100–150 mg/kg per 24 h IV (not to exceed 12 g/24 h) in equally divided doses every 4 to 6 h	4
or			
Cefazolin[b,c]	1 g IM or IV every 8h	80–100 mg/kg per 24 h IM or IV (not to exceed 3.0 g/24 h) in equally divided doses every 8 h	4
Vancomycin[d]	30 mg/kg per 24 h IV in 2 or 4 equally divided doses, not to exceed 2 g/24 h unless serum levels are monitored	40 mg/kg per 24 h IV in 2 or 4 equally divided doses, not to exceed 2 g/24 h unless serum levels are monitored	4

[a]Vancomycin dose should be reduced in patients with renal dysfunction; cephalosporin dose may need to be reduced in patients with moderate to severe renal dysfunction.

[b]Streptomycin or gentamicin may be added to cephalothin or cefazolin for first 2 weeks in doses recommended in Table 37.3.

[c]There is potential cross-allergenicity between penicillins and cephalosporins. Cephalosporins should be avoided in patients with immediate-type hypersensitivity to penicillin.

[d]Peak serum concentrations of vancomycin should be obtained 1 h after infusion and should be in the range of 30–45 μg/mL for twice daily dosing and 20–35 μg/mL for four times daily dosing. Vancomycin or aminoglycosides given on a milligram per kilogram basis will produce higher serum concentrations in obese than in lean patients. Each dose of vancomycin should be infused over 1 h.

From Wilson WR, Karchmer AW, Dajani AS, et al. Antibiotic treatment of adults with infective endocarditis due to streptococci, enterococci, and staphylococci, and HACEK organisms. JAMA 1995; 274:1706–1713, with permission.

TABLE 37.6. Therapy for Endocarditis due to *Staphylococci* in the Absence of Prosthetic Material[a]

Antibiotic	Adult Dose and Route	Pediatric Dose and Route	Duration
Methicillin-Susceptible Staphylococci			
Regimen for non–penicillin-allergic patients			
Nafcillin	2 g IV every 4 h	150–200 mg/kg per 24 h IV (not to exceed 12 g/24 h) in 4 to 6 equally divided doses	4–6 wk
or			
Oxacillin	2 g IV every 4 h	150–200 mg/kg per 24 h IV (not to exceed 12 g/24 h) in 4 to 6 equally divided doses	4–6 wk
With optional addition of gentamicin[b,c]	1 mg/kg IM or IV (not to exceed 80 mg) every 8 h	2–2.5 mg/kg IV (not to exceed 80 mg) every 8 h	3–5 d
Regimen for penicillin-allergic patients			
Cefazolin[d] (or other first generation cephalosporin in equivalent dosages)	2 g IV every 8 h	80–100 mg/kg per 24 h IV (not to exceed 6 g/24 h) in equally divided doses every 8 h	4–6 wk
With optional or addition of gentamicin[b]	Same as for non–penicillin-allergic patient	Same as for non–penicillin-allergic patient	3–5 d
or			
Vancomycin[b,e]	30 mg/kg per 24 h IV in 2 equally divided doses not to exceed 2 g/24 h unless serum levels are monitored	40 mg/kg per 24 h IV in 2 or 4 equally divided doses, not to exceed 2 g/24 h unless serum levels are monitored	4–6 wk
Methicillin-Resistant Staphylococci			
Vancomycin[b,e]	30 mg/kg per 24 h IV in 2 equally divided doses, not to exceed 2 g/24 h unless serum levels are monitored	40 mg/kg per 24 h IV in 2 or 4 equally divided doses, not to exceed 2 g/24 h unless serum levels are monitored	4–6 wk

[a]Antibiotic doses should be modified appropriately for patients with impaired renal function. For treatment of endocarditis due to penicillin-susceptible staphylococci (MIC <0.1 mg/mL), aqueous crystalline penicillin G (Tab 37.3, first regimen) should be used for 4–6 weeks instead of nafcillin or oxacillin. Shorter antibiotic courses have been effective in some drug addicts with right-sided endocarditis due to *Staphylococcus aureus*.

[b]Dosing of aminoglycosides and vancomycin on a milligram per kilogram basis will give higher serum concentrations in obese than in lean patients.

[c]Benefit of additional aminoglycoside has not been established. Risk of toxic reactions due to these agents is increased in patients who are older than age 65 years or who have renal or eighth nerve impairment.

[d]There is potential cross-allergenicity between penicillins and cephalosporins. Cephalosporins should be avoided in patients with immediate-type hypersensitivity to penicillin.

[e]Peak serum concentration of vancomycin should be obtained 1 h after infusion and should be in the range of 30–45 mg/mL for twice daily dosing. Each dose of vancomycin should be infused over 1 h. See text for consideration of optional addition of gentamicin.

From Wilson WR, Karchmer AW, Dajani AS, et al. Antibiotic treatment of adults with infective endocarditis due to streptococci, enterococci, and staphylococci, and HACEK organisms. *JAMA* 1995; 274:1706–1713, with permission.

VIII

443

- If a patient has a mild allergy to penicillin, first-generation cephalosporins have also been effective.
- The use of cephalosporins, particularly cefazolin, has been somewhat controversial for MSSA endocarditis. In the majority of studies, these agents appear effective; however, there are reports of failures with cephalosporins despite in vitro susceptibility.
- If there is a history of immediate hypersensitivity to penicillin, vancomycin is the agent of choice. Vancomycin, however, only slowly kills *S. aureus* and is generally regarded as inferior therapy to penicillinase-resistant penicillins for MSSA.
- Rifampin may be added to vancomycin in refractory or complicated infections in patients with left-sided IE and, in some cases, addition of rifampin appeared to result in dramatic patient improvement. Generally, antibiotic therapy should be continued for 4–6 weeks.

Treatment of Methicillin-Resistant Staphylococcal Endocarditis
- Vancomycin is the drug of choice for methicillin-resistant staphylococci since all methicillin-resistant *S. aureus* (MRSA) and most CNST are susceptible (Table 37.7).

Treatment of Staphylococcus Endocarditis in the Intravenous Drug Abuser

- IE in the IV drug abuser is most frequently (60–80%) caused by *S. aureus,* although other organisms may be more common in certain geographic locations.
- Standard treatment for MSSA consists of 4 weeks of therapy with a penicillinase-resistant penicillin (Table 37.6).
- In contrast to treatment of left-sided IE, addition of an aminoglycoside to penicillin does not improve outcome in *S. aureus* IE in addicts with right-sided disease.

PROSTHETIC VALVE ENDOCARDITIS
- PVE that occurs within 1 year of surgery is usually caused by staphylococci implanted at the time of surgery. Since this is a nosocomial infection, methicillin-resistant organisms are common, and vancomycin is the cornerstone of therapy.
- Surgery is often a more essential component of management than are antibiotics.
- Because of the high morbidity and mortality associated with PVE and refractoriness to therapy, combinations of antimicrobials are usually recommended.
- For methicillin-resistant staphylococci (both MRSA and CNST), vancomycin is used with rifampin for 6–8 weeks (Table 37.7). An aminoglycoside is added for the first 2 weeks if the organism is susceptible.
- For methicillin-susceptible staphylococci, a penicillinase-stable penicillin is used in place of vancomycin.

TABLE 37.7. Treatment of Staphylococcal Endocarditis in the Presence of a Prosthetic Valve or Other Prosthetic Material[a]

Antibiotic	Adult Dose and Route	Pediatric Dose and Route	Duration (wk)
Regimen for Methicillin-Resistant Staphylococci			
Vancomycin[b,c]	30 mg/kg per 24 h IV in 2 equally divided doses, not to exceed 2 g/24 h unless serum levels are monitored	40 mg/kg per 24 h IV in 2 or 4 equally divided doses, not to exceed 2 g/24 h unless serum levels are monitored	≥6
With rifampin[d]	300 mg PO every 8 h	20 mg/kg per 24 h PO (not to exceed 900 mg/24 h) in 2 equally divided doses	≥6
and			
With gentamicin[c,e,f]	1.0 mg/kg IM or IV (not to exceed 80 mg) every 8 h	2–2.5 mg/kg per 24 h IV (not to exceed 80 mg) every 8 h	2
Regimen for Methicillin-Susceptible Staphylococci			
Nafcillin or oxacillin[g]	2 g IV every 4 h	150–200 mg/kg per 24 h IV (not to exceed 12 g/24 h) in 4 to 6 equally divided doses	≥6
With rifampin[d]	300 mg PO every 8 h	20 mg/kg per 24 h PO (not to exceed 900 mg/24 h) in 2 equally divided doses	≥6
and			
With gentamicin[c,e,f]	1.0 mg/kg IM or IV (not to exceed 80 mg) every 8 h	2–2.5 mg/kg IV (not to exceed 80 mg) every 8 h	2

[a]Vancomycin and gentamicin doses must be modified appropriately in patients with renal failure

[b]Peak serum concentrations of vancomycin should be obtained 1 h after infusion and should be in the range of 30–45 mg/mL for twice daily dosing. Each dose should be infused over 1 h.

[c]Aminoglycosides or vancomycin given on a milligram per kilogram basis will produce higher serum concentrations in obese than in lean patients.

[d]Rifampin is recommended for therapy of infections due to coagulase-negative staphylococci. Its use in coagulase-positive staphylococcal infections is controversial. Rifampin increases the amount of warfarin sodium required for antithrombotic therapy.

[e]Serum concentration of gentamicin should be monitored and dose should be adjusted to obtain a peak level of approximately 3 mg/mL.

[f]Use during initial 2 weeks. See text on alternative aminoglycoside therapy for organisms resistant to gentamicin

[g]First-generation cephalosporins should be used in penicillin-allergic patients. Cephalosporins should be avoided in patients with immediate-type hypersensitivity to penicillin and in patients infected with methicillin-resistant staphylococci.

From Wilson WR, Karchmer AW, Dajani AS, et al. Antibiotic treatment of adults with infective endocarditis due to streptococci, enterococci, and staphylococci, and HACEK organisms. JAMA 1995; 274:1706–1713, with permission.

VIII

445

ENTEROCOCCAL ENDOCARDITIS

- Enterococci cause 5–18% of endocarditis cases and are noteworthy for the following reasons:

    1. No single antibiotic is bactericidal.
    2. MICs to penicillin are relatively high (1–25 µg/mL).
    3. They are intrinsically resistant to all cephalosporins and relatively resistant to aminoglycosides (i.e., "low-level" aminoglycoside resistance).
    4. They are killed only by a combination of a cell wall active agent, such as a penicillin or vancomycin, plus an aminoglycoside.
    5. Resistance to all available drugs is increasing.

- Enterococcal endocarditis ordinarily requires 4–6 weeks of high-dose penicillin G or ampicillin, plus an aminoglycoside for cure (Table 37.8). A 6-week course is recommended for patients with symptoms lasting longer than 3 months, recurrent cases, and patients with mitral valve involvement.
- Resistance among enterococci to the preceding drugs is increasing. Enterococci that exhibit high-level resistance to streptomycin (MIC > 2000 µg/mL) are not synergistically killed by penicillin and streptomycin because the aminoglycoside either no longer binds to the ribosome or is inactivated by an aminoglycoside-modifying enzyme, streptomycin adenylase.
- In addition to isolates with high-level aminoglycoside resistance, β-lactamase-producing enterococci (especially *E. faecium*) are increasingly reported. Therapy with vancomycin is usually recommended, although penicillin-β-lactamase inhibitor combinations appear effective.

GRAM-NEGATIVE BACILLI

- Endocarditis caused by gram-negative bacilli is relatively uncommon, although the incidence may be increasing. Patients at higher risk include IV drug abusers and those with prosthetic valves.
- The organism most commonly associated with gram-negative rod endocarditis in IV drug abusers is *Pseudomonas aeruginosa.* Other gram-negative bacilli causing IE include other pseudomonads, *Serratia marcescens, Escherichia coli, Enterobacter, Salmonella,* and *Haemophilus.* Generally, these infections have a poor prognosis with mortality rates as high as 60–80%.
- Overall, there is very little clinical information on which to base solid recommendations for treatment. For most cases of IE due to *P. aeruginosa* and Enterobacteriaceae, antibiotics and valve replacement are necessary.
- Antimicrobial therapy includes the combination of an aminoglycoside and an extended-spectrum β-lactam.

VIII

TABLE 37.8. Therapy for Endocarditis Due to Enterococci (or to Viridans Streptococci with a MIC ≥0.5 mg/mL)[a]

Antibiotic	Adult Dose and Route	Pediatric Dose and Route	Duration (wk)
Regimen for Non-Penicillin-Allergic Patients			
1. Aqueous crystalline penicillin G	18–30 million U/24 h IV given continuously or in 6 equally divided doses	200,000–300,000 U/kg per 24 h IV (not to exceed 30 million U/24 h) given continuously or in 6 equally divided doses	4–6
With gentamicin[b,c,d]	1 mg/kg IM or IV (not to exceed 80 mg) every 8 h	2–2.5 mg/kg IM or IV (not to exceed 80 mg) every 8 h	4–6
2. Ampicillin	12 g/24 h IV given continuously or in 6 equally divided doses	300 mg/kg per 24 h IV (not to exceed 12 g/24 h) in 4 to 6 equally divided doses	4–6
With gentamicin[b,c,d]	1 mg/kg IM or IV (not to exceed 80 mg) every 8 h	2–2.5 mg/kg IM or IV (not to exceed 80 mg) every 8 h	4–6
Regimen for Penicillin-Allergic Patients (desensitization should be considered; cephalosporins are not satisfactory alternatives)			
Vancomycin[e]	30 mg/kg per 24 h IV in 2 equally divided doses, not to exceed 2 g/24 h unless serum levels are monitored	40 mg/kg per 24 h IV in 2 equally divided doses, not to exceed 2 g/24 h unless serum levels are monitored	4–6
With gentamicin[b,c,d]	1 mg/kg IM or IV (not to exceed 80 mg) every 8 h	2–2.5 mg/kg IM or IV (not to exceed 80 mg) every 8 h	4–6

[a]Antibiotic doses should be modified appropriately in patients with impaired renal function.

[b]Choice of aminoglycoside depends on resistance level of infecting strain (see text). Enterococci should be tested for high-level resistance (MIC ≥2000 mg/mL).

[c]Serum concentration of gentamicin should be monitored and dose adjusted to obtain a peak level of approximately 3 mg/mL.

[d]Dosing of aminoglycosides and vancomycin on a milligram per kilogram basis will give higher serum concentrations in obese than in lean patients.

[e]Peak serum concentrations of vancomycin should be obtained 1 h after infusion and should be in the range of 30–45 mg/mL for twice daily dosing and 20–35 mg/mL for four times daily dosing. Each dose should be infused over 1 h.

From Wilson WR, Karchmer AW, Dajani AS, et al. Antibiotic treatment of adults with infective endocarditis due to streptococci, enterococci, and staphylococci, and HACEK organisms. *JAMA* 1995; 274:1706–1713, with permission.

VIII

- The appropriate regimen for the treatment of gram-negative bacillary endocarditis caused by Enterobacteriaceae depends on the results of in vitro susceptibility testing. For *Klebsiella pneumoniae, E. coli,* and *Proteus mirabilis,* a third-generation cephalosporin is frequently combined with an aminoglycoside. Treatment should generally be continued for 6 weeks.

▶ EVALUATION OF THERAPEUTIC OUTCOMES

- The evaluation of patients treated for IE includes assessment of signs and symptoms, reculture of blood, in vitro microbiologic tests (e.g., MIC, minimum bactericidal concentration (MBC), or serum bactericidal titers), antimicrobial serum-concentration determinations, and other tests that may be necessary in the evaluation of organ function.

SIGNS AND SYMPTOMS

- Persistence of fever may indicate ineffective antimicrobial therapy, emboli, infections of intravascular catheters that have been in place for long periods of time, or a drug reaction. In some patients, low-grade fever may persist even with appropriate antimicrobial therapy. With defervescence the patient should begin to feel better and other symptoms, such as lethargy or weakness, should subside.

VIII
BLOOD CULTURES AND BACTERIAL SUSCEPTIBILITY

- With effective therapy, blood cultures should be negative within a few days, although microbiological response to vancomycin may be unusually slow.
- After the initiation of therapy, blood cultures should be rechecked, possibly daily, until they are found negative. During the remainder of therapy, frequent blood culturing is not necessary.

SERUM BACTERICIDAL TITER (SBT)

- At present, SBTs have little value in the treatment of common types of IE. This test may be useful when the causative organisms are only moderately susceptible to antimicrobials, when less well-established regimens are used, or when response to therapy is suboptimal and dosage escalation is considered. In addition, an extremely high SBT may suggest that a decrease in antimicrobial dose is acceptable when the patient is at high risk of drug toxicity.

SERUM DRUG CONCENTRATION

- Serum concentrations of the antimicrobial should generally exceed the MBC of the organism, however, in practice this principle is usually not helpful in monitoring patients with endocarditis.
- In IE caused by *P. aeruginosa,* clinical trials previously discussed suggest that higher aminoglycoside concentrations (e.g., 15–20 μg/mL) improve the outcome to therapy.

▶ PREVENTION OF ENDOCARDITIS

- Antimicrobial prophylaxis is used to prevent IE in patients believed to be at high risk.
- The use of antimicrobials for this purpose requires consideration of the types of patients who are at risk, the procedures causing bacteremia, the organisms that are likely to cause endocarditis, and the pharmacokinetics, spectrum, cost, and ease of administration of available agents. The objective of prophylaxis is to diminish the likelihood of IE in high-risk individuals who are undergoing procedures that cause transient bacteremia (Table 37.9).

PATIENTS AT RISK

- Patients with certain cardiac lesions, particularly those with a history of rheumatic heart disease and prosthetic heart valves, are at risk for developing endocarditis (Table 37.10). However, only 15–25% of patients who develop IE are in a definable high-risk category, and only a small proportion of high-risk patients (estimated to be 1 of 53–115,500 persons) will develop IE if prophylaxis is not given.

PROCEDURES CAUSING BACTEREMIA

- For dental procedures of the gums and oral structures which cause bleeding, *viridans streptococci* frequently (~40%) cause bacteremia, VIII

TABLE 37.9. Dental or Surgical Procedures for Which Endocarditis Prophylaxis Is Recommended[a]

Dental procedures known to induce gingival or mucosal bleeding, including professional cleaning
Tonsillectomy and/or adenoidectomy
Surgical operations that involve intestinal or respiratory mucosa
Bronchoscopy with a rigid bronchoscope
Sclerotherapy for esophageal varices
Esophageal dilatation
Gallbladder surgery
Cystoscopy
Urethral dilatation
Urethral catheterization if urinary tract infection is present
Urinary tract surgery if urinary tract infection is present
Prostatic surgery
Incision and drainage of infected tissue
Vaginal hysterectomy
Vaginal delivery in the presence of infection

[a]This table lists selected procedures but is not meant to be all inclusive.
From Dajani AS, Bisno AL, Chung KJ. JAMA 1990;264:2919–2922, with permission.

TABLE 37.10. Cardiac Conditions[a]

Endocarditis Prophylaxis Recommended

Prosthetic cardiac valves, including bioprosthetic and homograft valves

Previous bacterial endocarditis, even in the absence of heart disease

Most congenital cardiac malformations

Rheumatic and other acquired valvular dysfunction, even after valvular surgery

Hypertrophic cardiomyopathy

Mitral valve prolapse with valvular regurgitation

Endocarditis Prophylaxis Not Recommended

Isolated secundum atrial septal defect

Surgical repair without residua beyond 6 mo of secundum atrial septal defect, ventricular septal defect, or patent ductus arteriosus

Previous coronary artery bypass graft surgery

Mitral valve prolapse without valvular regurgitation[b]

Physiologic, functional, or innocent heart murmurs

Previous Kawasaki disease without valvular dysfunction

Previous rheumatic fever without valvular dysfunction

Cardiac pacemakers and implanted defibrillators

[a]This table lists selected conditions but is not meant to be all inclusive.
[b]Individuals who have a mitral valve prolapse associated with thickening and/or redundancy of the valve leaflets may be at increased risk for bacterial endocarditis, particularly men who are 45 years of age or older.
From Dajani AS, Bisno AL, Chung KJ. *JAMA* 1990;264:2919–2922, with permission.

TABLE 37.11. Recommended Standard Prophylactic Regimen for Dental, Oral, or Upper Respiratory Tract Procedures in Patients Who Are at Risk[a]

Drug	Dosing Regimen[b]
Standard regimen	
Amoxicillin	3 g orally 1 h before procedure; then 1.5 g 6 h after initial dose
Amoxicillin/penicillin-allergic patients	
Erythromycin	Erythromycin ethylsuccinate, 800 mg, or erythromycin stearate, 1 g, orally 2 h before procedure; then half the dose 6 h after initial dose
or	
Clindamycin	300 mg orally 1 h before procedure and 150 mg 6 h after initial dose

[a]Includes those with prosthetic heart valves and other high-risk patients.
[b]Initial pediatric doses are as follows: amoxicillin, 50 mg/kg; erythromycin ethylsuccinate or erythromycin stearate, 20 mg/kg; and clindamycin, 10 mg/kg. Follow-up doses should be one half the initial dose. Total pediatric dose should not exceed total adult dose. The following weight ranges may also be used for the initial pediatric dose of amoxicillin: <15 kg, 750 mg; 15 to 30 kg, 1500 mg; and >30 kg, 3000 mg (full adult dose).
From Dajani AS, Bisno AL, Chung KJ. *JAMA* 1990;264:2919–2922, with permission.

VIII

TABLE 37.12. Alternate Prophylactic Regimens for Dental, Oral, or Upper Respiratory Tract Procedures in Patients Who Are at Risk

Drug	Dosing Regimen[a]
Patients unable to take oral medication	
Ampicillin	Intravenous or intramuscular administration of ampicillin, 2 g, 30 min before procedure; then intravenous or intramuscular administration of ampicillin, 1 g, or oral administration of amoxicillin, 1.5 g, 6 h after initial dose
Ampicillin/amoxicillin/penicillin-allergic patients unable to take oral medications	
Clindamycin	Intravenous administration of 300 mg 30 min before procedure and an intravenous or oral administration of 150 mg 6 h after initial dose
Patients considered high risk and not candidates for standard regimen	
Ampicillin, gentamicin, and amoxicillin	Intravenous or intramuscular administration of ampicillin, 2 g, plus gentamicin, 1.5 mg/kg (not to exceed 80 mg), 30 min before procedure; followed by amoxicillin, 1.5 g, orally 6 h after initial dose; alternatively, the parenteral regimen may be repeated 8 h after initial dose
Ampicillin/amoxicillin/penicillin-allergic patients considered high risk	
Vancomycin	Intravenous administration of 1 g over 1 h, starting 1 h before procedure; no repeated dose necessary

[a]Initial pediatric doses are as follows: ampicillin, 50 mg/kg; clindamycin, 10 mg/kg; gentamicin, 2.0 mg/kg; and vancomycin, 20 mg/kg. Follow-up doses should be one half the initial dose. Total pediatric dose should not exceed total adult dose. No initial dose is recommended in this table for amoxicillin (25 mg/kg is the follow-up dose).
From Dajani AS, Bisno AL, Chung KJ. JAMA 1990;264:2919–2922, with permission.

whereas instrumentation and surgery of the gastrointestinal and genitourinary tracts more often result in enterococcal bacteremia.

ANTIBIOTIC REGIMENS

- A 3-g dose of amoxicillin is recommended for adult patients at risk, given 60 minutes prior to undergoing procedures associated with bacteremia. This is to be followed by 1.5 g 6 hours later (Table 37.11). For penicillin-allergic patients or those undergoing gastrointestinal surgery, alternative prophylaxis is recommended (Tables 37.12 and 37.13).

See Chapter 104, Infective Endocarditis, authored by Ron E. Polk, PharmD, for a more detailed discussion of this topic.

TABLE 37.13. Regimens for Genitourinary/Gastrointestinal Procedures

Drug	Dosage Regimen[a]
Standard regimen	
Ampicillin, gentamicin, and amoxicillin	Intravenous or intramuscular administration of ampicillin, 2 g, plus gentamicin, 1.5 mg/kg (not to exceed 80 mg), 30 min before procedure; followed by amoxicillin, 1.5 g, orally 6 h after initial dose; alternatively, the parenteral regimen may be repeated once 8 h after initial dose
Ampicillin/amoxicillin/penicillin-allergic patient regimen	
Vancomycin and gentamicin	Intravenous administration of vancomycin, 1 g, over 1 h plus intravenous or intramuscular administration of gentamicin, 1.5 mg/kg (not to exceed 80 mg), 1 h before procedure; may be repeated once 8 h after initial dose
Alternate low-risk patient regimen	
Amoxicillin	3 g orally 1 h before procedure; then 1.5 g 6 h after initial dose

[a]Initial pediatric doses are as follows: ampicillin, 50 mg/kg; amoxicillin, 50 mg/kg; gentamicin 2 mg/kg; and vancomycin, 20 mg/kg. Follow-up doses should be half the initial dose. Total pediatric dose should not exceed total adult dose.

From Dajani AS, Bisno AL, Chung KJ. JAMA 1990;264:2919–2922, with permission.

Chapter 38

► FUNGAL INFECTIONS

Systemic mycoses caused by primary or "pathogenic" fungi, such as histoplasmosis, coccidioidomycosis, cryptococcosis, blastomycosis, paracoccidioidomycosis, and sporotrichosis, can cause disease in both healthy and immunocompromised individuals. In contrast, mycoses caused by opportunistic fungi such as *C. albicans*, *Aspergillus* species, *Trichosporon*, *Torulopsis (Candida) glabrata*, *Fusarium*, *Alternaria*, and *Mucor* are generally found only in the immunocompromised host.

► EPIDEMIOLOGY

- Systemic fungal infections are a major cause of morbidity and mortality in the immunocompromised patient.
- Fungal infections account for 20–30% of fatal infections in patients with acute leukemia, 10–15% of fatal infections in patients with lymphoma, and 5% of fatal infections in patients with solid tumors.
- The frequency of fungal infections among transplant recipients ranges from 0–20% for kidney and bone marrow to 10–35% for heart and 30–40% for liver transplant recipients.

► SPECIFIC FUNGAL INFECTIONS

HISTOPLASMOSIS

- Histoplasmosis is caused by inhalation of dust-borne microconidia of the dimorphic fungus *Histoplasma capsulatum*.
- In the United States, most disease is localized along the Ohio and Mississippi river valleys.

Clinical Presentation

- In the vast majority of patients, low-inoculum exposure to *H. capsulatum* results in *asymptomatic infection* or an acute, self-limited illness with flu-like pulmonary symptoms, including fever, chills, headache, myalgia, and a nonproductive cough.
- *Chronic pulmonary histoplasmosis* generally presents as an opportunistic infection imposed on a preexisting structural abnormality such as lesions resulting from emphysema. Patients demonstrate chronic pulmonary symptoms and apical lung lesions that progress with inflammation, calcified granulomas, and fibrosis. Progression of disease over a period of years, seen in 25–30% of patients, is associated with cavitation, bronchopleural fistulas, extension to the other lung, pulmonary insufficiency, and often death.

- In patients exposed to a large inoculum and in immunocompromised hosts, progressive illness, *disseminated histoplasmosis,* occurs. The clinical severity of the four diverse forms of disseminated histoplasmosis (Table 38.1) generally parallels the degree of macrophage parasitization observed.
- *Acute (infantile) disseminated histoplasmosis* is seen in infants and young children and (rarely) in adults with Hodgkin's disease or other lymphoproliferative disorders. It is characterized by unrelenting fever, anemia, leukopenia or thrombocytopenia, enlargement of the liver, spleen, and visceral lymph nodes, and gastrointestinal symptoms, particularly nausea, vomiting, and diarrhea. Untreated disease is uniformly fatal in 1–2 months.
- Most adults with disseminated histoplasmosis demonstrate a mild, chronic form of the disease. Untreated patients are often ill for 10–20 years, demonstrating long asymptomatic periods interrupted by relapses of clinical illness, characterized primarily by weight loss, weakness, and fatigue.
- Adult patients with AIDS demonstrate an acute form of disseminated disease that resembles the syndrome seen in infants and children.

Diagnosis

- Detection of single, yeast-like cells 2–5 μm in diameter with narrow-based budding in direct examination or histologic study of blood smears or tissues should raise strong suspicion of infection with *H. capsulatum.*
- Identification of mycelial isolates from clinical cultures can be made by conversion of the mycelium to the yeast form (requires 3–6 weeks), via commercially available exoantigen test kits, or by the more rapid (2 hours) and 100% sensitive DNA probe.
- In most patients, serologic evidence remains the primary method in the diagnosis of histoplasmosis. A four-fold rise in the CF titer is usually indicative of recent infection, although some patients with severe disease or profound immunosuppression may demonstrate a weaker antibody response.
- In the AIDS patient with progressive disseminated histoplasmosis, the diagnosis is best established by bone marrow biopsy and culture, which yield positive cultures in >90% of patients.

Treatment

- Recommended therapy for the treatment of histoplasmosis is summarized in Table 38.1.
- In AIDS patients, intensive primary (induction) antifungal therapy is followed by lifelong suppressive (maintenance) therapy.
- In patients with underlying immunosuppression, including AIDS patients with progressive disseminated histoplasmosis, amphotericin B remains the drug of choice for induction therapy.
- Amphotericin B dosages of 50 mg/d (up to 1 mg/kg/d) should be administered to a cumulative dose of 15–35 mg/kg (1–2 grams) and until negative fungal cultures are achieved.

TABLE 38.1. Clinical Manifestations and Therapy of Histoplasmosis

Type of Disease and Common Clinical Manifestations	Approximate Frequency (%)[a]	Therapy/Comments
Acute Pulmonary Histoplasmosis		
Asymptomatic histoplasmosis	50–99	Asymptomatic disease: No therapy generally required.
Self-limited disease	1–50	Self-limited disease: High-dose corticosteroids plus AmB[b] 0.3–0.5 mg/kg/d × 2–4 weeks or ketoconazole 400 mg orally daily × 3–6 months may be beneficial in patients with severe hypoxia following inhalation of large inocula. Antifungal therapy generally not useful for arthritis, or pericarditis. NSAIDs[c] or corticosteroids may be useful in some cases. Mediastinal granulomas: Most lesions resolve spontaneously. Surgery or antifungal therapy with AmB 40–50 mg/d × 2–3 weeks or ketoconazole 400 mg orally × >30 months may be beneficial in some cases.
Inflammatory/fibrotic histoplasmosis	0.02	Fibrosing mediastinitis: Antifungal therapy generally not helpful; surgery may be of benefit if disease is detected early; late disease may not respond to therapy. Sarcoid-like: NSAIDs or corticosteroids may be of benefit for some patients.
Chronic Pulmonary Histoplasmosis	0.05	Chronic pulmonary histoplasmosis: Antifungal therapy generally recommended for immunosuppressed patients with either persistent cavitation, cavitary wall thickness >2 mm, or progressive symptoms (including weight loss, cough, sputum production, low-grade fever. Ketoconazole 400 mg/d orally for 1 year; increase to 600–800 mg/d if no favorable response or AmB >35 mg/kg over 10 weeks.
Disseminated Histoplasmosis		Disseminated histoplasmosis: Untreated mortality 33–93%; relapse 5–23% in non-AIDS patients.
Acute	0.02–0.05	Nonimmunosuppressed patients: Ketoconazole 400 mg orally × 6–12 months or AmB 35 mg/kg.
Subacute		Immunosuppressed patients (non-AIDS) or + endocarditis or CNS disease: AmB ≥35 mg/kg.
Chronic (adult-type)		
Progressive disease of AIDS	25–50[d]	AIDS patients: AmB 15–30 mg/kg (1–2 g over 4–10 weeks); followed by chronic itraconazole for initial therapy. Treat relapses with AmB.

[a]As a percentage of all patients presenting with histoplasmosis.
[b]AmB, amphotericin B.
[c]NSAIDs, nonsteroidal anti-inflammatory drugs.
[d]As a percentage of AIDS patients presenting with histoplasmosis as the initial manifestation of their disease.

VIII

455

- Response to therapy should be measured by resolution of radiologic, serologic, and microbiologic parameters, and improvement in signs and symptoms of infection.
- Once the initial course of therapy for histoplasmosis is completed, life-long suppressive therapy with oral azoles or amphotericin B (1–1.5 mg/kg weekly or biweekly) is recommended, because of the frequent recurrence of infection.

BLASTOMYCOSIS

- North American blastomycosis is a systemic fungal infection caused by *Blastomyces dermatitidis.*
- Pulmonary disease probably occurs by inhalation. It may be acute or chronic and can mimic infection with tuberculosis, pyogenic bacteria, other fungi, or malignancy.
- Blastomycosis can disseminate to virtually every other body organ, and approximately 40% of patients with blastomycosis present with skin, bone and joint, or genitourinary tract involvement without any evidence of pulmonary disease.

Clinical Presentation
- Acute pulmonary blastomycosis is generally an asymptomatic or self-limited disease characterized by fever, shaking chills, and a productive cough.
- Pulmonary blastomycosis may present as a more chronic or subacute disease, with low-grade fever, night sweats, weight loss, and a productive cough that resembles tuberculosis rather than bacterial pneumonia.
- Chronic pulmonary blastomycosis is characterized by fever, malaise, weight loss, night sweats, and cough.
- The most common sites for disseminated disease include the skin and bony skeleton, although less commonly the prostate, oropharyngeal mucosa, and abdominal viscera are involved.

Diagnosis
- The simplest and most successful method of diagnosing blastomycosis is by direct microscopic visualization of the large, multinucleated yeast with single, broad-based buds in sputum or other respiratory specimens, following digestion of cells and debris with 10% potassium hydroxide.
- Early and rapid definitive diagnosis of blastomycosis can be achieved by demonstration of *B. dermatitidis* in tissue or specimen culture or histopathology, or by a positive exoantigen or fluorescent antibody (FA) assay.
- An ELISA titer of 1:8 to 1:16 plus a positive immunodiffusion test or an ELISA of ≥32 plus a positive or negative immunodiffusion test is considered diagnostic for blastomycosis.

VIII

Treatment

- Acute pulmonary blastomycosis may not require therapy in patients with mild illness, but patients must be followed carefully for many years for evidence of reactivation or progressive disease.
- Some authors recommend ketoconazole therapy for the treatment of self-limited pulmonary disease, with the hope of preventing late extra-pulmonary disease.
- Ketoconazole (400 mg/day) appears to be as effective as amphotericin B for non–life-threatening, nonmeningeal, mild to moderate blastomy-cosis in immunocompetent hosts.
- The dosage of ketoconazole should be increased to 600–800 mg orally per day in the absence of a favorable clinical response.
- Patients with CNS disease, progressive or life-threatening disease, or those experiencing toxicity while on ketoconazole should receive amphotericin B (40–50 mg/d) until clinical improvement is observed, followed by administration three times weekly until a total dose of 1.5–2 grams is achieved.
- All patients with chronic pulmonary blastomycosis and those with extrapulmonary disease require therapy (ketoconazole 400 mg orally per day for 6 months).
- Patients with genitourinary tract disease should be treated initially with 600–800 mg/d of ketoconazole because low concentrations of drug are achieved in the urine and prostate tissue.
- CNS disease should be treated with amphotericin B for a total dose of 30–35 mg/kg.

COCCIDIOIDOMYCOSIS

- Coccidioidomycosis is caused by infection with *Coccidioides immitis*.
- The endemic regions encompass the semi-arid regions of the south-western United States from California to Texas known as the Lower Sonoran Zone.

Clinical Presentation

- Sixty percent of subjects are asymptomatic or have nonspecific symp-toms that are often indistinguishable from ordinary upper respiratory infections, including fever, cough, headache, sore throat, myalgias, and fatigue.
- "Valley fever" is a syndrome characterized by erythema nodosum and erythema multiforme of the upper trunk and extremities in association with diffuse joint aches or fever. Valley fever occurs in approximately 25% of patients although, more commonly, a diffuse mild erythroderma or maculopapular rash is observed.
- Some patients present with an acute pneumonia as the primary mani-festation of disease. They have a productive cough that may be blood-streaked.

- Pulmonary coccidioidomycosis can also develop into a chronic, persistent pneumonia complicated by hemoptysis, pulmonary scarring, and the formation of cavities or bronchopleural fistulas.
- Disseminated infection occurs in <1% of infected patients. Dissemination may occur to the skin, lymph nodes, bone, meninges, spleen, liver, kidney, and adrenal gland.
- CNS infection with *C. immitis* is a particularly devastating complication that develops in approximately 16% of patients with disseminated coccidioidomycosis.

Diagnosis

- Most patients develop a positive skin test within 3 weeks of the onset of symptoms.
- Early infection is characterized by the development of IgM antibody (detected by tube precipitin or immunodiffusion techniques), which peaks within 2–3 weeks of infection then declines rapidly.
- Recovery of *C. immitis* from infected tissues or secretions for direct examination and culture provides an accurate and rapid method of diagnosis.

Treatment

- Candidates for therapy include those with severe primary pulmonary infection or increasing CF antibody titers (particularly ≥1:16 to 1:32), immunocompromised patients, and those with persistent (>6 weeks) fever, prostration, or worsening pulmonary disease. Any patient with evidence of disseminated disease should receive therapy.
- Almost all patients with disease located outside the lungs should receive amphotericin B in dosages of 1–1.5 mg/kg/d, tapering to 1–1.5 mg/kg three times a week to a total dose of 0.5–1.5 grams over 2–4 weeks, based on clinical response.
- A minimum of 2–3 grams of amphotericin B is probably necessary for the treatment of persistent pulmonary infection or miliary coccidioidomycosis.
- Ketoconazole at a dosage of 400 mg orally per day is efficacious in patients with infiltrative pulmonary disease, soft tissue infection, or skeletal involvement.
- Limited data also suggest that fluconazole may prove beneficial in the treatment of coccidiomycosis.
- Initial studies suggest that itraconazole is effective in the treatment of nonmeningeal coccidioidomycosis.
- Optimal therapy for the treatment of coccidioidal meningitis has not been established. The best dose of intrathecal amphotericin B is unclear, although therapy is generally initiated with very low dosages (0.025–1.5 mg) and increased cautiously to a maximum of 0.5–0.7 mg three to four times weekly.
- Ketoconazole cannot be routinely recommended for the treatment of coccidioidal meningitis due to its poor CNS penetration following oral administration.

VIII

CRYPTOCOCCOSIS

- Cryptococcosis is a noncontagious, systemic mycotic infection caused by the ubiquitous encapsulated soil yeast *Cryptococcus neoformans*.
- Cryptococcosis is the fourth most common infectious complication of AIDS and the second most common fungal pathogen.

Clinical Presentation

- Primary cryptococcosis in humans almost always occurs in the lungs.
- Symptomatic infections are usually manifested by cough, rales, and shortness of breath that generally resolve spontaneously.
- Disease may remain localized in the lungs or disseminate to other tissues, particularly the CNS, although the skin can also be affected.
- In the non-AIDS patient, the symptoms of cryptococcal meningitis are nonspecific. Headache, fever, nausea, vomiting, mental status changes, and neck stiffness are generally observed.
- In AIDS patients, fever and headache are common, but meningismus and photophobia are much less common than in non-AIDS patients. Approximately 10–12% of AIDS patients have asymptomatic disease, similar to the rate observed in non-AIDS patients. Cryptococcal disease is present in 7.5–10% of AIDS patients.

Diagnosis

- Examination of CSF in patients with cryptococcal meningitis generally reveals an elevated opening pressure, CSF pleocytosis (usually lymphocytes), leukocytosis, a decreased CSF glucose, an elevated CSF protein, and a positive cryptococcal antigen.
- Antigens to *C. neoformans* can be detected by latex agglutination.
- *C. neoformans* can be detected in approximately 60% of patients by India ink smear of CSF, and cultured in more than 96% of patients.

Treatment

- The use of large (1–1.5 mg/kg) daily doses of amphotericin B results in cure rates of approximately two-thirds of patients.
- When amphotericin B is combined with fluorocytosine (150 mg/kg/day) for 6 weeks, a smaller dose of amphotericin B (0.3 mg/kg/day) can be used due to the in vitro and in vivo synergy between the two antifungal agents.
- The use of intrathecal amphotericin B is not recommended for the treatment of cryptococcal meningitis except in patients who fail to respond to amphotericin B alone. The dosage of amphotericin B employed is usually 0.5 mg administered via the lumbar, cisternal, or intraventricular (via an Ommaya reservoir) route two or three times weekly.
- Treatment of cryptococcal meningitis in patients with AIDS has been discouraging.
- Amphotericin B with or without fluorocytosine remains the treatment of choice for acute therapy of cryptococcal meningitis in AIDS patients. Many clinicians will initiate therapy with amphotericin B 0.4–0.7 mg/kg/d IV (with or without oral fluorocytosine 75–100 mg/kg/d). After

VIII

1 week, therapy may be changed to oral fluconazole 400 mg daily for the remaining 9 weeks of therapy.

- Relapse of *C. neoformans* meningitis occurs in approximately 50% of AIDS patients after completion of primary therapy. Fluconazole (200 mg daily) is currently recommended for chronic suppressive therapy of cryptococcal meningitis in AIDS patients.

▶ CANDIDA INFECTIONS

- Eight species of candida are regarded as clinically important pathogens in human disease, including *C. albicans, C. tropicalis, C. parapsilosis, C. krusei, C. stellatoidea, C. guilliermondi, C. lusitaniae,* and *C. rugosa.*

MUCOCUTANEOUS CANDIDIASIS

- Mucocutaneous candidiasis can generally be divided into several categories: oropharyngeal candidiasis (thrush), esophageal candidiasis, gastrointestinal candidiasis, and vaginal candidiasis.
- Oral candidiasis is often the first sign of infection in patients with AIDS.

Chronic Mucocutaneous Candidiasis

- Chronic mucocutaneous candidiasis refers to a collection of syndromes characterized by chronic or recurrent infections of the skin, nails, and mucous membranes by *C. albicans.*

Oral Candidiasis (Thrush)

- Oral candidiasis occurs in as many as 5% of all newborn infants, >35% of patients with acute leukemia or those receiving chemotherapy for solid tumors, patients undergoing organ transplantation, and approximately 10% of all hospitalized, debilitated, elderly patients.
- Oral candidiasis is characterized by the presence of creamy, white plaques on the tongue and buccal mucosa that generally leave a painful, raw, ulcerated surface when scraped.
- The diagnosis of oral candidiasis is based on the clinical appearance of the lesions and by scraping of lesions, using either 10% potassium hydroxide digestion of this material to reveal the presence of pseudohyphae and yeast forms or the presence of gram-positive staining yeast forms.
- Topical (local) therapy with a variety of antifungal agents, including nystatin suspension and clotrimazole troches are generally efficacious in the prophylaxis and therapy of oral candidiasis.
- Nystatin has been utilized as a "swish and swallow" regimen in dosages ranging from 0.5 million units (MU) four times daily to 1.5 MU six times daily.
- In oncology patients, ketoconazole in dosages of 200–400 mg daily is as efficacious as nystatin in dosages of 0.5–3 MU four times daily for the treatment of oral candidiasis.

VIII

- Fluconazole 100 mg orally appears to be as efficacious as ketoconazole 400 mg daily, clotrimazole troches 10 mg five times daily, or amphotericin B 400 mg (as 200-mg tablets plus 200-mg suspension) administered four times daily in the prophylaxis or therapy of oropharyngeal candidiasis.

Esophageal Candidiasis
- *Candida* esophagitis is most commonly associated with the treatment of malignancies and in AIDS patients.
- Although a definitive diagnosis is made by endoscopy with brush biopsy, a barium swallow can often reveal a characteristic "shaggy mucosa" appearance.
- Generally, systemic antifungal agents, such as ketoconazole 200–400 mg daily or fluconazole 100–200 mg daily are required.
- A lack of response to antifungal therapy can be due to altered absorption of drugs such as ketoconazole. In patients who do not respond to oral therapy with ketoconazole or fluconazole, a low dose (10–15 mg) of IV amphotericin B is often successful.

Vaginal Candidiasis
- Vulvovaginal candidiasis is characterized by the presence of a thick, curdlike vaginal discharge, intense pruritus, and the presence of masses of epithelial cell, hyphae, and pseudohyphae on KOH smear of the vaginal discharge.
- Vulvovaginal candidiasis is a common infection in women; approximately one-fourth of women in their childbearing years develop an infection.
- Although treatment with 7-day topical regimens have been traditionally employed, recent studies have demonstrated success utilizing 1- and 3-day topical regimens.
- A single oral dose of fluconazole (150 mg) is generally effective.

Hematogenous Candidiasis
- "Hematogenous candidiasis" describes the clinical circumstances in which hematogenous seeding to deep organs such as the eye, brain, heart, and kidney occurs.
- Risk factors for hematogenous disease include prior therapy with antibiotics, the presence of indwelling urinary or IV catheters, recent surgery, concomitant bacterial infections, extensive burns, and administration of total parenteral nutrition.
- No test has demonstrated reliable accuracy in the clinical setting for the diagnosis of disseminated infection with Candida.
- Only 25–45% of neutropenic patients with disseminated candidiasis at autopsy have a positive blood culture with *C. albicans* prior to death.
- Three distinct presentations of disseminated *C. albicans* have been recognized: (1) patients present with the acute onset of fever, tachycardia, tachypnea, and occasionally chills or hypotension, (2) intermittent fevers, and (3) progressive deterioration with or without fever.

VIII

- Administration of fluconazole 400 mg daily is as efficacious as intravenous amphotericin B 0.5 mg/kg/d in non-neutropenic patients with blood cultures with *C. albicans.* Since fluconazole has poor activity against *Aspergillus* spp. and some non-*albicans* strains of *Candida,* amphotericin B remains the therapy of choice in patients with suspected fungemia.
- In some patients, particularly those patients with a relatively intact immune system and in whom candidemia is clearly associated with the presence of an indwelling venous catheter, removal of the catheter will result in spontaneous resolution.
- Currently, most clinicians recommend amphotericin B in total dosages of 0.5–1 gram administered over approximately 1–2 weeks in patients with *Candida* endophthalmitis and in all neutropenic patients with candidemia.
- Many clinicians advocate early institution of empiric intravenous amphotericin B in patients with neutropenia and persistent (>5–7 days) fever.

CANDIDURIA

- Within the urinary tract, most common lesions are either *Candida* cystitis or hematogenously disseminated renal abscesses.
- In most patients, the infection is asymptomatic and clears spontaneously without specific antifungal therapy.
- Initial therapy of candidal cystitis should focus on removal of urinary catheters whenever possible. If this is not feasible, local irrigation may be used.
- Amphotericin B (50 mg in 500 mL of sterile water) can be instilled twice daily into the bladder via a three-way catheter.
- Oral therapy with fluorocytosine or fluconazole can be considered for short courses of therapy since high urinary concentrations are achieved.

▶ ASPERGILLUS

- Of over 300 species of *Aspergillus,* 3 are most commonly pathogenic: *A. fumigatus, A. flavus,* and *A. niger.*
- The term "aspergillosis" may be broadly defined as a spectrum of diseases attributed to allergy, colonization, or tissue invasion caused by members of the fungal genus *Aspergillus.*
- Aspergillosis is generally acquired by inhalation of airborne conidia that are small enough (2.5–3 μm) to reach alveoli or the paranasal sinuses.

SUPERFICIAL INFECTION

- Superficial or locally invasive infections of the ear, skin, or appendages can often be managed with topical antifungal therapy.

ALLERGIC BRONCHOPULMONARY ASPERGILLOSIS

- Allergic manifestations of *Aspergillus* range in severity from mild asthma to allergic bronchopulmonary aspergillosis (BPA) characterized by severe asthma with wheezing, fever, malaise, weight loss, chest pain, and a cough productive of blood-streaked sputum.
- Therapy is aimed at minimizing the quantity of antigenic material released in the tracheobronchial tree.
- Antifungal therapy is generally not indicated in the management of allergic manifestations of aspergillosis, although some patients have demonstrated a decrease in their corticosteroid dose following therapy with itraconazole.

ASPERGILLOMA

- In the nonimmunocompromised host, *Aspergillus* infections of the sinuses most commonly occur as saprophytic colonization (aspergillomas or "fungus balls") of previously abnormal sinus tissue. Treatment consists of removal of the aspergilloma. Therapy with corticosteroids and surgery is generally successful.
- Pulmonary aspergillomas are fungus balls arising in preexisting cavities due to tuberculosis, histoplasmosis, lung tumors, or radiation fibrosis, although occasionally no previous pulmonary disease is present.
- Although intravenous amphotericin B is generally not useful in eradicating aspergillomas, intracavitary instillation of amphotericin B has been employed successfully in a limited number of patients. Hemoptysis generally ceases when the aspergilloma is eradicated.
- Prolonged neutropenia appears to be the most important predisposing factor to the development of invasive aspergillosis, accounting for the high frequency of disease in patients with acute leukemia.

VIII

CLINICAL PRESENTATION

- Patients often present with classic signs and symptoms of acute pulmonary embolus: pleuritic chest pain, fever, hemoptysis, a friction rub, and a wedge-shaped infiltrate on chest radiographs.

DIAGNOSIS

- Demonstration of *Aspergillus* by repeated culture and microscopic examination of tissue provides the most firm diagnosis.
- In the immunocompromised host, aspergillosis is characterized by vascular invasion leading to thrombosis, infarction, and necrosis of tissue.
- Serologic tests (immunoprecipitation, immunodiffusion, and counterimmunoelectrophoresis) to detect antibody production to *Aspergillus* are generally helpful only in the diagnosis of allergic BPA and aspergilloma.

TREATMENT OF INVASIVE ASPERGILLOSIS

- Administration of amphotericin B appears to decrease mortality from >90% to approximately 45%.
- Antifungal therapy should be instituted in any of the following conditions: (1) persistent fever or progressive sinusitis unresponsive to antimicrobial therapy; (2) an eschar over the nose, sinuses, or palate; (3) the presence of characteristic radiographic findings, including wedge-shaped infarcts, nodular densities, new cavitary lesions; or (4) any clinical manifestation suggestive of orbital or cavernous sinus disease or an acute vascular event associated with fever. Isolation of *Aspergillus* sp. from nasal or respiratory tract secretions should be considered confirmatory evidence in any of the previously mentioned clinical settings.
- Since *Aspergillus* is only moderately susceptible to amphotericin B, full doses (1–1.5 mg/kg/d) are generally recommended, with response measured by defervescence and radiographic clearing.
- Although the addition of fluorocytosine and/or rifampin is advocated by some authors, controlled clinical studies verifying the efficacy of these combination therapies are lacking.
- Itraconazole should be reserved as a second-line agent for patients intolerant or not responding to high-dose amphotericin B. If itraconazole is used, a loading dose of 200 mg three times daily with food for 2–3 days should be employed, followed by itraconazole 200 mg twice daily with food for a minimum of 6 months.
- The use of prophylactic antifungal therapy to prevent primary infection or reactivation of aspergillosis during subsequent courses of chemotherapy is controversial.

See Chapter 113, Invasive Fungal Infections, authored by Peggy L. Carver, PharmD, for a more detailed discussion of this topic.

Chapter 39

▶ GASTROINTESTINAL INFECTIONS

Gastrointestinal infections are among the more common causes of morbidity and mortality around the world. In underdeveloped and developing countries, acute gastroenteritis involving diarrhea is the leading cause of mortality in infants and young children under 4 years of age. In the United States, more than 210,000 children per year are hospitalized for gastroenteritis.

▶ REHYDRATION THERAPY

- The mainstay of therapy for gastrointestinal infections is rehydration, most often, oral rehydration therapy (ORT).
- Initial assessment of fluid loss is essential for rehydration. Weight loss is the most reliable means of determining the extent of water loss. Clinical signs such as changes in skin turgor, sunken eyes, dry mucous membranes, decreased tearing, decreased urine output, altered mentation, and changes in vital signs can be helpful in determining approximate deficits (Table 39.1).
- Although ORT may be successful in reversing severe dehydration, parenteral replacement is indicated as initial treatment for the patient in shock or a comatose state, the patient unable to tolerate oral fluids, the patient with ileus, and the patient with persistent vomiting or stool output >100 mL/kg/h
- The necessary components of ORT solutions include glucose, sodium, potassium, chloride, and water (Table 39.2).
- The rehydration phase should provide replacement of estimated fluid deficits in 4–6 hours.
- The maintenance phase should not exceed 150 mL/kg/d and is generally adjusted to equal stool output and insensible water loss.
- Guidelines for parenteral fluid replacement of severe fluid loss are shown in Table 39.3.
- Early initiation of feeding has shortened the course of diarrhea. Initially, easily digested foods, such as bananas, applesauce, and cereal may be added as tolerated. Foods high in fiber, sodium, and sugar should be avoided.

▶ BACTERIAL INFECTIONS

- The bacterial species most commonly associated with gastrointestinal infection and infectious diarrhea in the United States are *Shigella* sp., *Salmonella* sp., *Campylobacter* sp., *Yersinia* sp., *Escherichia* sp., *Clostridium* sp., and *Staphylococcus* sp.

TABLE 39.1. Signs of Dehydration

% body weight loss as water	Clinical signs
Adults and Older Children	
<4 (mild)	Decreased tearing, thirsty, alert, restless
4–8 (moderate)	Decreased skin turgor, sunken eyes, tachycardia, reduced urine flow, postural hypotension, dry mucous membranes, thirsty
>8 (severe)	Hypotension, muscle cramps, variable alertness, cold, sweaty, cyanotic, wrinkled skin, usually conscious
Infants and Young Children	
<5 (mild)	Thirsty, alert, restless, moist mucous membranes, normal urine flow, tearing
5–10 (moderate)	Thirsty, restless, lethargic, irritable, tachycardia, hypotension, deep respirations, sunken fontanelle, sunken eyes, absent tearing, dry mucous membranes, reduced and dark urine
>10 (severe)	Drowsy, limp, cold, sweaty, cyanotic, comatose, tachycardia, tachypnea, very sunken fontanelles, hypotension, sunken eyes, absent tears, dry mucous membranes, no urine production

VIII

- The two most commonly recognized mechanisms of bacterial-induced infectious diarrhea involve enterotoxin-stimulated hypersecretion (secretory diarrhea) and mucosal invasion (invasive diarrhea). Antibiotic choices for bacterial infections are given in Table 39.4.

▶ ENTEROTOXIGENIC (CHOLERA-LIKE) DIARRHEA

CHOLERA *(VIBRIO CHOLERAE)*

- The two species most often causing human illness are *Vibrio cholerae* and *Vibrio parahemolyticus*. Four mechanisms for transmission have been proposed, including animal reservoirs, chronic carriers, asymptomatic or mild disease victims, or water reservoirs.
- Most pathology of cholera is thought to result from an enterotoxin that increases cyclic AMP-mediated secretion of chloride ion into the intestinal lumen that results in isotonic secretion (primarily in the small intestine) exceeding the absorptive capacity of the intestinal tract (primarily the colon).
- The incubation period of *V. cholerae* is 6–48 hours.
- Cholera is characterized by a spectrum from the asymptomatic state to the most severe typical cholera syndrome. In the most severe state, this disease can progress to death in a matter of 2–4 hours if not treated.
- Most signs and symptoms are a direct result of fluid and electrolyte loss. These frequently include poor skin turgor, sunken eyes, cyanosis, shallow or absent pulses, tachycardia, hypotension, and tachypnea.

TABLE 39.2. Comparison of Solutions Used in Oral Rehydration and Maintenance

Product	Electrolytes (mEq/L)					Carbohydrate (g/L)	Osmolarity (mOsm/L)
	Na	K	Cl	Base	Other Cations		
Infalyte (Penwalt)	50	20	40	30	—	20	251
Lytren (Mead Johnson)	50	25	45	30		20	583
Pedialyte (Ross)	45	20	35	30	—	25	388
Pedialyte RS (Ross)	75	20	65	30	—	25	314
Ricelyte (Mead Johnson)	50	25	45	34	—	30	200
WHO (Unicef)	90	20	80	30	—	20	333
Resol (Wyeth)	50	20	50	34	4 Ca, 4 Mg, 5 PO4	20	
Rehydralyte (Ross)	75	20	65	30		25	
EquaLYTE (Ross)	78.2	22.3	67.6	30.1		25	305
Less Desirable Alternatives							
Cola	0–6.5	0–4	—	13	—	100–120	390–750
Gatorade	20–24	3	17	30	—	46–58	305
Grape juice	3	31–34	—	32	—	156	1180
Jell-O (½ strength)	6–17	0.2	0–5			70 80	600
Kool-Aid	1	1	—		—	102	250–590
7-Up	5–7	2	—		—	74–102	535

VIII

TREATMENT

- The mainstay of treatment for cholera consists of fluid and electrolyte replacement. Rice-based rehydration formulations are the preferred ORT for cholera patients. Intravenous (IV) therapy is usually required only in severe cases.

TABLE 39.3. Parenteral Replacement of Fluid Deficit for Severely Dehydrated (>10% of Body Weight) Children

Type of Dehydration	Replacement Solution	% Replaced During Noted Period		
		0–12 h	12–24 h	24–48 h
Isonatremic (130–150 mEq/L)	D_5 ⅓ NS	50	50	—
Hyponatremic (<130 mEq/L)	D_5 ½ NS	75	25	—
Hypernatremic (>150 mEq/L)	D_5 ¼ NS	25	25	50

Key: D_5, dextrose 5%; NS, normal saline (0.9% sodium chloride).

TABLE 39.4. Antibiotic Selection

Organism	First Choice	Alternatives
Clostridium difficile	Metronidazole	Vancomycin, bacitracin, cholestyramine
Campylobacter	Fluoroquinolone[a]	Erythromycin, clindamycin, aminoglycoside, doxycycline
Escherichia coli	Fluoroquinolone	TMP–SMX,[b] aminoglycoside chloramphenicol, ampicillin
Salmonella	Ciprofloxacin, ceftriaxone, cefoperazone, TMP–SMX	
Shigella	Fluoroquinolone, norfloxacin	TMP–SMX, ampicillin
Vibrio cholerae	Fluoroquinolone, doxycycline	TMP–SMX
Yersinia enterocolitica	Ciprofloxacin, norfloxacin, ofloxacin	TMP–SMX, antipseudomonal aminoglycoside

Dosing Guidelines		
Drug	Children	Adults
Amikacin (IV)	15–22.5 mg/kg/d every 8 h	15 mg/kg/d divided every 8–12 h
Ampicillin (IV)	100–200 mg/kg/d divided every 6 h	150–200 mg/kg/d divided every 6 h
(PO)	50 mg/kg/d divided every 6 h	250–500 mg every 6 h
Bacitracin (PO)	800–1200 units/kg/d every 8 h	25,000 units every 6 h
Cefoperazone (IV)	100–150 mg/kg/d divided every 8–12 h	4–16 g/d divided every 6–12 h
Ceftriaxone (IV)	50–100 mg/kg/d divided every 12–24 h	1–2 g/d divided every 12–24 h
Chloramphenicol (PO)	50–75 mg/kg/d divided every 6 h	50 mg/kg/dose every 6 h
Ciprofloxacin (IV)	NR	200–400 mg every 12 h
(PO)		500–750 mg every 12 h
Clindamycin (PO)	20–30 mg/kg/d divided every 6 h	150–450 mg every 6 h
(IV)	25–40 mg/kg/d divided every 6–8 h	150–900 mg every 8 h
Doxycycline (PO)	NR	100 mg every 12–24 h
Enoxacin (PO)	NR	600–800 mg/d divided every 12–24 h
Erythromycin (PO)	30–40 mg/kg/d divided every 6–8 h	250–500 mg every 6 h
Gentamicin (IV)	3–7.5 mg/kg/d divided every 8 h	3–5 mg/kg/d divided every 8 h
Lomefloxacin (PO)	NR	400 mg every 24 h
Metronidazole (PO)	15–35 mg/kg/d divided every 8 h	500 mg every 6 h
Netilmicin (IV)	3–7.5 mg/kg/d divided every 8 h	4–6.5 mg/kg/d divided every 8 h
Norfloxacin (PO)	NR	400 mg every 12 h
Ofloxacin (PO)	NR	200–400 mg every 12 h
TMP–SMX (PO)	8–12 mg/kg/d TMP divided every 12 h	160 mg TMP every 12 h
Tobramycin (IV)	3–6 mg/kg/d divided every 8 h	3–5 mg/kg/d divided every 8 h
Vancomycin (PO)	10–50 mg/kg/d divided every 6 h, max 125 mg per dose	125 mg every 6 h

Key: NR, not recommended.

[a]Fluoroquinolone: ciprofloxacin, ofloxacin, lomefloxacin, enoxacin (fluoroquinolones are not approved for children).

[b]TMP–SMX, trimethoprim–sulfamethoxazole.

VIII

- Antibiotics shorten the duration of diarrhea, decrease the volume of fluid lost, and shorten the duration of the carrier state (Table 39.4). The tetracyclines or fluoroquinolones should be avoided during pregnancy or in young children, and cotrimoxazole is an appropriate alternative. Antibiotics need only be given for 3–5 days in most cases.

ESCHERICHIA COLI

- *Escherichia coli* gastrointestinal disease may be caused by enterotoxigenic *E. coli* (ETEC), enteroinvasive *E. coli* (EIEC), enteropathogenic *E. coli* (EPEC), enteroadhesive *E. coli* (EAEC), and enterohemorrhagic *E. coli* (EHEC). ETEC is now incriminated as being the most common cause of traveler's diarrhea.
- ETEC are capable of producing two plasmid-mediated enterotoxins: heat-labile toxin (HLT) and heat-stable toxin (HST). The net effect of this toxin on the mucosa is production of a cholera-like secretory diarrhea.
- Diarrhea caused by ETEC is often characterized by abrupt onset of watery diarrhea, with or without abdominal cramping. Usually, there is no blood or pus in the stool. Most ETEC diarrhea resolves within 24–48 hours without complication.
- Most cases respond readily to ORT and although antibiotic therapy is seldom necessary, prophylaxis has been shown to effectively prevent the development of ETEC diarrhea.
- Effective prophylactic agents include tetracycline, cotrimoxazole, neomycin, furazolidone, norfloxacin, and ciprofloxacin. Nonantibiotic regimens, including bismuth subsalicylate and cholestyramine, have also been recommended as effective prevention or treatment regimens.

VIII

PSEUDOMEMBRANOUS COLITIS *(CLOSTRIDIUM DIFFICILE)*

- Pseudomembranous colitis (PMC) has increasingly been associated with antibiotic administration. PMC results from toxins produced by *Clostridium difficile*. It occurs most often in epidemic fashion and affects high-risk groups such as the elderly, debilitated patients, cancer patients, surgical patients, or any patient receiving antibiotics.
- PMC has been associated most often with broad-spectrum antimicrobials, including clindamycin, ampicillin, or cephalosporins.
- Symptoms can occur from several days after the start of antibiotic therapy to several weeks after antibiotics are discontinued.
- PMC is characterized by vomiting, fever, cramping, abdominal pain and tenderness, and profuse greenish diarrhea (watery or mucoid). Fevers of 103–105°F, marked leukocytosis, and hypoalbuminemia are also common. Pseudomembranous lesions, which look like whitish-yellow raised plaques, can be found anywhere in the colon.
- Diagnosis is made by colonoscopic visualization of pseudomembranes. Cytotoxins can be demonstrated in stools.

- The patient should be supported with fluid and electrolyte replacement. If the patient has not improved within 72 hours, has severe disease, requires continuation of the inducing antibiotic, or is a high-risk patient (pediatric, elderly, debilitated), antibiotic therapy should be promptly initiated. *Clostridium difficile* is usually susceptible in vitro to vancomycin, metronidazole, bacitracin, and cephalosporins.
- Metronidazole (1 g/day orally) is the agent of choice for treatment of PMC. Because of its mutagenic and tumorigenic potential in laboratory animal experiments, metronidazole should not be used indiscriminately in pregnant women. Vancomycin, 125 mg every 6 hours orally, is as effective but should be avoided to reduce emergence of vancomycin-resistant enterococci.
- Clinical response is generally observed within the first 4 days of therapy.
- Drugs that inhibit peristalsis, such as diphenoxylate, are contraindicated. Some patients have become worse after use of these drugs.

▶ INVASIVE (DYSENTERY-LIKE) DIARRHEA

BACILLARY DYSENTERY (SHIGELLOSIS)

- Four species of *Shigella* are most often associated with disease, *S. dysenteriae* type I, *S. flexneri, S. bovdii,* and *S. sonnei.*
- Poor sanitation, poor personal hygiene, inadequate water supply, malnutrition, and increased population density are associated with increased risk of shigella gastroenteritis epidemics, even in developed countries. The majority of cases are thought to result from fecal–oral transmission.
- Shigellosis is primarily a disease of children, with the highest incidence between ages 6 months and 5 years. The reported incidence in the United States ranges from 15,000–20,000 cases per year.
- *Shigella* sp. causes dysentery upon penetrating the epithelial cells lining the colon. Microabscesses may eventually coalesce, forming larger abscesses. Some *Shigella* species produce a cytotoxin, or shigatoxin, the pathogenic role of which is unclear although it is thought to damage endothelial cells of the lamina propria, resulting in microangiopathic changes that can progress to hemolytic uremic syndrome. Watery diarrhea commonly precedes the dysentery and may be a result of these toxins.
- Shigellosis is generally a self-limiting disease. Patients most often become afebrile and completely recover within 4–7 days. Approximately 10% experience a recurrence.
- Signs and symptoms are initially nonspecific: nausea, fever, malaise, abdominal tenderness of the lower quadrants, and hyperactive bowel sounds. Frequent watery stools, 10–25 per day, appear within 48 hours, and are followed by bloody diarrhea and dysentery within a few days.

VIII

Stools are greenish in color and often contain mucus and/or blood, as well as many leukocytes. If untreated, bacillary dysentery usually lasts about 1 week (range 1–30 days).

- White blood cell counts are inconsistent and range from a leukopenia to a pronounced leukocytosis with a left shift. Fluid and electrolyte loss may be significant, particularly in infants and elderly patients. Stool culture will establish *Shigella* species as the causative agent.

- Treatment of bacillary dysentery generally includes correction of fluid and electrolyte disturbances and occasionally, antimicrobials in the very young and elderly.

- Fluid and electrolyte losses can generally be replaced with oral therapy, as dysentery is generally not associated with significant fluid loss. Intravenous replacement is necessary only for those patients with severe illness.

- Because shigellosis is usually a self-limiting disease and antibiotic resistance is an increasing concern, some clinicians feel antibiotics should be reserved for the severely ill. However, because antibiotic therapy has been shown to shorten the period of fecal shedding (usually 1–4 weeks in patients not receiving antimicrobials) and attenuate the clinical illness, many clinicians prefer to treat with antibiotics (Table 34.4).

- Antispasmodics and agents that inhibit intestinal peristalsis are not used because they may prolong fever and diarrhea, worsen the dysentery, and possibly contribute to development of toxic megacolon. VIII

SALMONELLOSIS

- Human disease caused by salmonella generally falls into four categories: acute gastroenteritis (enterocolitis), bacteremia, extraintestinal localized infection, and enteric fever (typhoid and paratyphoid fever). *S. typhimurium* is the most common cause of salmonellosis. Salmonellosis is a disease primarily of infants, children, and adolescents. Contaminated food (particularly poultry, poultry products, beef, pork, and dairy products) or water has been implicated in the majority of cases.

- Salmonellae enterocolitis appears to occur secondary to mucosal invasion of microorganisms, but it may involve enterotoxin production, or local inflammatory exudates as possible mechanisms of pathology. Organisms may invade beyond the mucosa and enter the mesenteric lymphatics which then carry bacteria to the general circulation via the thoracic duct. Bacteria not cleared by the reticuloendothelial system may cause metastatic infection in various organs.

- With enterocolitis, patients often complain of nausea and vomiting within 24 hours of ingestion followed by crampy abdominal pain, fever, and diarrhea, although the actual presentation is quite variable.

- Stool cultures inevitably yield the causative organism, if obtained early. However, recovery of organisms continues to decrease with time so that by 3–4 weeks, only 5–15% of adult patients are passing salmonella.

- Some patients may continue to shed salmonella for a year or longer. These "chronic carrier" states are rare for serotypes other than *S. typhi.*

- Salmonellae can produce bacteremia without classic enterocolitis or enteric fever. The clinical syndrome is characterized by persistent bacteremia and prolonged intermittent fever with chills. Stool cultures are frequently negative.

- Extraluminal infection and/or abscess formation can occur at any site. They may follow any of the other syndromes or may be the primary presentation. Metastatic infections have been reported to involve bone, cysts, heart, kidney, liver, lungs, pericardium, spleen, and tumors.

- Enteric fever caused by *S. typhi* is called typhoid fever. If caused by any other serotype, it is referred to as paratyphoid fever. The onset of symptoms is gradual. Nonspecific symptoms of fever, dull headache, malaise, anorexia, and myalgias are most common. Initially, fever tends to be remittent, but gradually progresses over the first week to temperatures that are often sustained over 104°F. Other frequently encountered symptoms include chills, nausea, vomiting, cough, weakness, and sore throat.

VIII
- About 80% of patients have positive blood cultures. Bacteremia persists in about one-third of patients for several weeks if not treated. Diagnostic tests other than culture are unreliable.

Treatment

- Most patients with enterocolitis require no therapeutic intervention. When required, the most important part of therapy for salmonella enterocolitis is fluid and electrolyte replacement.

- Antimicrobials have not been shown to shorten the course of this self-limiting disorder. Antibiotic therapy should be considered if there is suspected transition to one of the other salmonella syndromes (bacteremia, localized infection, or enteric fever) or if underlying conditions predispose to systemic spread. Both cotrimoxazole and ciprofloxacin have been used to treat salmonella enterocolitis.

- Chloramphenicol or ampicillin is most frequently used for the treatment of bacteremia and localized infections. Cotrimoxazole is considered when the organism is resistant to both chloramphenicol and ampicillin. The duration of antibiotic therapy is dictated by the site; for example, osteomyelitis is treated for 4–6 weeks or longer.

- Chloramphenicol has been the mainstay of therapy for enteric fever in most areas of the world. Ampicillin, amoxicillin, and cotrimoxazole are also effective, although response is not as predictable as with chloramphenicol. Therapy should be continued for at least 2 weeks.

- Clinical response to antibiotics is often seen within 2 days; however, temperatures slowly normalize within 3–5 days.

- Antidiarrheal agents or laxatives are not used because they may prolong illness or precipitate perforation.
- Live oral attenuated vaccine Ty21a and parenteral v: polysaccharide vaccine have been shown to confer 60–90% efficacy for a duration of 2 and 3 years, respectively.

CAMPYLOBACTERIOSIS

- *Campylobacter* species are now thought to be a major cause of diarrhea, comparable to *Salmonella* and *Shigella.*
- Approximately 80% of cases reported to the CDC surveillance program were in persons less than 35 years old.
- Transmission of infection appears to be by the fecal–oral route or by ingestion of contaminated food or water.
- Incubation usually ranges from 1–12 days with an average of 2–4 days.
- The most common symptoms include diarrhea of varying consistency and severity, abdominal pain, and fever. Nausea, vomiting, headache, myalgias, and malaise may also occur. Bowel movements may be numerous, bloody (dysentery-like), foul smelling, melenic, and range from loose to watery (cholera-like).
- The disease is self-limiting and signs and symptoms usually resolve in about a week, but may persist longer in 10–20% of patients.
- As with other acute diarrheal illnesses, fluid and electrolyte support is a mainstay of therapy mainly with ORT.
- Antibiotic therapy is not necessary in the majority of cases. Antibiotics should be considered in the very young and the very old and when the patient has severe bloody diarrhea, continued fever (>102°F), persistence of symptoms beyond 7 days, worsening symptoms, or a compromised immune system.
- Currently, erythromycin is the agent of choice.

VIII

YERSINIOSIS

- *Yersinia enterocolitica* and *Yersinia pseudotuberculosis* are associated with intestinal infection. The organisms have been isolated from a variety of food sources, including raw goat and cow milk.
- These bacteria cause a wide spectrum of clinical syndromes.
- The majority of cases present with enterocolitis that is mild and self-limiting. Symptoms, generally lasting 1–3 weeks, include vomiting, abdominal pain, diarrhea, and fever.
- A clinical syndrome seen in older children and adolescents presenting with mesenteric adenitis, fever, right lower quadrant pain, and leukocytosis may be clinically indistinguishable from appendicitis.
- Development of chronic abdominal pain following *Yersinia* enteritis has been reported.
- As many as one-third of adults with *Y. enterocolitica* may have an immunologically mediated polyarthritis within 1 month of the onset of diarrhea.

- These diseases are generally self-limiting and are easily managed with oral rehydration solutions.
- In severe disease, bacteremia, or localizing forms of the disease, antibiotic treatment is indicated.
- *Y. enterocolitica* is generally susceptible to third-generation cephalosporins, aminoglycosides, chloramphenicol, tetracycline, and cotrimoxazole.
- Suggested antibiotics of choice are shown in Table 39.4.

▶ ACUTE VIRAL GASTROENTERITIS

- Rotavirus accounts for the majority of morbidity and even mortality among children with gastroenteritis, while Norwalk and Norwalk-like viruses account for the majority of adult cases.

ROTAVIRUSES

- Although rotaviruses have been isolated from a variety of mammals and birds, the exact mechanism of transfer or principal vectors of infection are poorly understood. Water, food, or inspired droplets have been suspected; however, it is generally thought that the primary route is fecal–oral.
- Rotaviruses have been associated with up to 50% of enteritis in hospitalized children. The highest frequency of rotavirus-associated diarrhea appears between ages of 6 and 24 months. The exact mechanism by which the rotaviruses cause diarrhea is not known.
- Clinical manifestations of rotavirus infections vary from asymptomatic (which is common in adults) to severe nausea, vomiting, and diarrhea with dehydration. Symptoms are characterized initially by nausea and vomiting. Diarrhea occurs in most patients and lasts from 1–9 days, but some patients experience only loose stool with no increase in frequency. Other signs and symptoms include fever, respiratory symptoms, irritability, lethargy, pharyngeal erythema, rhinitis, red tympanic membranes, and palpable cervical lymph nodes. Dehydration and electrolyte disturbances occur more frequently in children.
- Treatment of rotavirus-associated vomiting and/or diarrhea is directed at prevention or correction of dehydration.

NORWALK AND NORWALK-LIKE AGENTS

- The epidemiology of the Norwalk-like agents is poorly understood. The disease can affect all age groups and is nonseasonal. The exact mechanisms of virus-induced vomiting or diarrhea are unknown.
- Norwalk-like viral gastroenteritis is characterized by sudden onset of abdominal cramps with nausea and/or vomiting. Although adults frequently experience nonbloody diarrhea, children experience vomiting more often. Other frequent complaints are myalgias, headache, and

VIII

malaise, which are accompanied by fever in about 50% of cases. Signs and symptoms generally last only 12–60 hours.

• The disease is generally self-limiting and does not require therapy. On occasion, oral rehydration may be required. Rarely is parenteral hydration necessary.

See Chapter 106, Gastrointestinal Infections and Enterotoxigenic Poisonings, authored by Tom A. Larson, PharmD, and Russel E. Seay, PharmD, for a more detailed discussion of this topic.

VIII

Chapter 40

▶ HIV/AIDS

▶ DEFINITION

The acquired immunodeficiency syndrome (AIDS) refers to the group of conditions caused by infection with human immunodeficiency virus type 1 (HIV-1). The exact case definition, along with the therapeutic approach, is being updated continuously as more information becomes available. Because of the dynamic nature of this research, the reader should supplement this chapter with the most current information.

▶ EPIDEMIOLOGY AND ETIOLOGY

- Approximately 18.5 million people worldwide are believed to have been infected with HIV, and 4.5 million have developed AIDS.
- 50,000–60,000 new persons are infected with HIV in the United States each year.
- By the year 2000, an estimated 30–40 million persons worldwide will be infected with HIV.
- HIV-1 is the primary cause of AIDS. A second retrovirus is a far less common cause of AIDS, and it may have different clinical manifestations and antiretroviral susceptibilities.
- There are three major modes for HIV transmission: sexual, parenteral (injection drug use; receipt of infected blood, blood products, or organs), and perinatal transmission from an HIV-infected mother. Of these, sexual contact is the most common and is estimated to account for almost 90% of cases.
- There is a small but definite occupational risk of parenteral HIV transmission among health care workers through accidental injury. The risk of HIV infection after percutaneous exposure is approximately 0.4%.

▶ PATHOPHYSIOLOGY

- HIV attacks immunologic cells resulting in many abnormalities (eg, both immune activation and immunosuppression). Progressive loss of immunologic function leads to opportunistic infections and malignancies. Although the course of HIV infection varies among individuals, a general pattern has emerged.
  - Primary infection is associated with a high viral burden and development of an immune response that suppresses, but may not eliminate, viral replication for a period of time. HIV becomes widely disseminated during primary infection.
  - Clinical latency (median duration: 10 years) follows primary infection. This period, however, is not virologically latent, because viral replication and gradual immune system deterioration are ongoing

(eg, increase in viral load and persistent decrease in CD4 lymphocytes).

- Late symptomatic phase includes many conditions, such as severe persistent constitutional signs and symptoms, opportunistic infections, and neoplasms.
- Opportunistic infections, which are responsible for almost 90% of deaths, usually represent reactivation of quiescent infections. Major opportunistic infections include *Pneumocystis carinii* pneumonia (PCP), candidal esophagitis, central nervous system (CNS) toxoplasmosis, cryptococcosis, mycobacterial disease, and herpes virus infections.

▶ CLINICAL MANIFESTATIONS

HIV INFECTION

- Signs and symptoms may be due to infectious or neoplastic complications in addition to HIV itself.
- Initial clinical presentation of HIV infection varies. The 1993 classification scheme of the Centers for Disease Control and Prevention (CDC) divides HIV infection into a matrix of nine categories based on the CD4 cell count (see section on Diagnosis) and clinical conditions (Table 40.1 and Table 40.2).

  VIII

  - Category A consists of asymptomatic infection, persistent generalized lymphadenopathy, and acute retroviral syndrome.
  - Category B consists of mild to moderate symptomatic conditions that are not AIDS-defining conditions. This category includes AIDS-related complex (ARC) and conditions such as bacillary angiomatosis; oropharyngeal candidiasis; vulvovaginal candidiasis that is persistent, frequent, or poorly responsive to therapy; cervical dysplasia; unexplained constitutional symptoms (fever >38.5°C, diarrhea lasting >1 month); oral hairy leukoplakia; recurrent or multidermatomal varicella-zoster infection; idiopathic thrombocytopenia purpura; listeriosis; pelvic inflammatory disease; and peripheral neuropathy.
  - Category C includes clinical conditions from the AIDS surveillance case definition (Table 40.2), which are generally severe, life-threatening opportunistic diseases.
- Clinical manifestations of AIDS are different in children (including CD4+ cell counts), but they are not covered separately, because medical management involves principles analogous to those for adults.

OPPORTUNISTIC INFECTIONS

- Clinical presentation of PCP differs in patients with versus without AIDS in that it is often more subacute in patients with AIDS. Characteristic symptoms include fever and dyspnea; clinical signs are tachypnea with or without rales or rhonchi and nonproductive or mildly productive cough. Chest radiographs may show florid or subtle infiltrates

TABLE 40.1. Conditions Included in the Centers for Disease Control and Prevention 1993 AIDS Surveillance Case Definition

Candidiasis of bronchi, trachea, or lungs

Candidiasis, esophageal

Cervical cancer, invasive[a]

Coccidioidomycosis, disseminated or extrapulmonary

Cryptococcosis, extrapulmonary

Cryptosporidiosis, chronic intestinal (>1 month duration)

Cytomegalovirus disease (other than liver, spleen, or nodes)

Cytomegalovirus retinitis (with loss of vision)

Encephalopathy, HIV-related

Herpes simplex: chronic ulcer(s) (>1 month duration); or bronchitis, pneumonitis, or esophagitis

Histoplasmosis, disseminated or extrapulmonary

Isosporiasis, chronic intestinal (>1 month duration)

Kaposi's sarcoma

Lymphoma, Burkitt's

Lymphoma, immunoblastic

Lymphoma, primary, of brain

Mycobacterium avium complex or *M. kansasii*, disseminated or extrapulmonary

Mycobacterium tuberculosis, any site (pulmonary or extrapulmonary)

Mycobacterium, other species or unidentified species, disseminated or extrapulmonary

Pneumocystis carinii pneumonia

Pneumonia, recurrent[a]

Progressive multifocal leukoencephalopathy

Salmonella septicemia, recurrent

Toxoplasmosis of brain

Wasting syndrome due to HIV

[a]Added in the 1993 expansion of the AIDS surveillance case definition.

or occasionally may be normal, although infiltrates are usually interstitial and bilateral.
- Clinical signs and symptoms of toxoplasmosis are most frequently associated with involvement of the CNS. Clinical presentation often includes fever, headache, seizures (in 10–25% of patients), focal neurologic abnormalities (in 60–90%), and mental status changes.
- Usual clinical presentation of cryptococcal infection is meningitis; clinical features may be subtle, nonspecific, and not localized to the CNS. Fever, headache, and malaise are the most frequent symptoms.

TABLE 40.2. Centers for Disease Control and Prevention 1993 Revised Classification System for HIV Infection in Adults

CD4+ T-cell Categories (absolute number and percentage)	Clinical Categories		
	(A) Asymptomatic, Acute (Primary) HIV or PGL[a]	*(B) Symptomatic, Not (A) or (C) Conditions*	*(C) AIDS-Indicator Conditions*
1. ≥500/μL or ≥29%	A1	B1	C1
2. 200–499/μL or 14–28%	A2	B2	C2
3. <200/μL or <14% (AIDS-indicator T-cell count)	A3	B3	C3

[a]PGL, persistent generalized lymphadenopathy.

- In patients with advanced HIV disease, *Mycobacterium avium* complex (MAC) causes a widely disseminated infection. The associated clinical syndrome includes high spiking fevers, diarrhea, night sweats, malaise, weight loss, anemia, and neutropenia. Persistent diarrhea and abdominal pain, a malabsorption syndrome, and extrahepatic biliary obstruction are manifestations of MAC gastrointestinal infection.
- Cytomegalovirus (CMV) infection is associated with numerous manifestations, including retinitis, esophagitis, hepatitis, gastrointestinal involvement, and, less commonly, radiculopathy, encephalitis, and pneumonitis. CMV retinitis, the most common disease, is usually associated with a painless progressive loss of vision. Patients may initially complain of blurry vision, loss of visual acuity, or "floaters." Gastrointestinal CMV can involve sites from the esophagus and stomach to the colon and rectum. CMV colitis may be characterized by abdominal pain, fever, weight loss, and diarrhea—common symptoms even in the absence of CMV infection. Characteristic symptoms of CMV esophagitis are dysphagia and substernal chest pain.
- Manifestations of herpes simplex virus (HSV) disease include orolabial, genital, anorectal mucocutaneous disease, esophagitis, and, less commonly, encephalitis. Symptoms of anorectal disease, the most common HSV disease in homosexual men with AIDS, include pain, itching, and painful defecation.
- Varicella-zoster virus (VZV) infection usually begins as radicular pain followed by localized erythematous rash and characteristic vesicles. VZV usually remains confined to a limited number of dermatomes, but complications such as widespread cutaneous involvement and disseminated visceral zoster may occur.

VIII

▶ DIAGNOSIS

HIV INFECTION

- AIDS is defined by a combination of laboratory and clinical findings (see Table 40.2). The 1993 case definition expanded the definition to include not only persons with serious symptomatic disease but also all HIV-infected people who have <200 CD4 lymphocytes/µL or a CD4 T-lymphocyte percentage of total lymphocytes <14. The 1993 definition retained 23 clinical conditions (eg, *P. carinii* pneumonia, CMV retinitis) from previous definitions and added pulmonary tuberculosis, recurrent pneumonia, and invasive cervical cancer (see Table 40.1).
- Patients with HIV infection show decreased numbers and percentages of CD4 cells, often increased CD8 cells, and decreased CD4:CD8 ratios. Normal number of CD4 cells is approximately 800; normal percentages are 31–61% for CD4 lymphocytes and 18–39% for CD8 lymphocytes. The absolute number is more variable than the percentage of CD4 cells, because the number is derived from the white blood cell (WBC) differential.
- Progression to AIDS and death in patients with HIV infection is related to viral load, which is a quantification of HIV ribonucleic acid (RNA) in plasma. Viral load determinations can be used to make decisions regarding initiation of therapy and to determine whether current antiretroviral therapy is effective.

OPPORTUNISTIC INFECTIONS

- Diagnosis of PCP is usually made by identification of *P. carinii* in induced sputum or in specimens obtained from bronchoalveolar lavage. Less commonly, transbronchial biopsy is used for diagnosis.
- Brain biopsy is required for definitive diagnosis of toxoplasmic encephalitis, but presumptive diagnosis is commonly made in *Toxoplasma gondii*–seropositive patients with typical CNS lesions. Radiographic abnormalities on computed tomography (CT) or magnetic resonance imaging (MRI) have also contributed to the diagnosis of CNS toxoplasmosis.
- Diagnosis of cryptococcal meningitis should be considered when HIV-infected individuals with advanced disease or low CD4+ lymphocyte count present with nonspecific symptoms or pulmonary or CNS findings. Diagnostic methods include serum and cerebrospinal fluid (CSF) fungal cultures and testing for cryptococcal antigen.
- Diagnosis of MAC infection is usually based on culture or organisms from blood; biopsies of liver, bone marrow, and lymph nodes are also highly sensitive and specific.
- Diagnosis of CMV retinitis is made by funduscopic examination and identification of characteristic findings (eg, fluffy white perivascular exudates frequently associated with hemorrhage). Definitive diagnosis of CMV gastrointestinal infection requires endoscopy and biopsy with

histologic identification of CMV inclusions or in situ antigen detection.

▶ DESIRED OUTCOME

The goals of therapy are to prevent and treat opportunistic infections and neoplastic complications, delay the progression of immunodeficiency, prolong survival, and maintain a high quality of life. Although eradication of HIV is the ultimate goal, this is not currently possible.

▶ TREATMENT

GENERAL PRINCIPLES

- Medical management of HIV-infected patients involves combinations of antiretroviral drugs, prophylaxis and treatment of opportunistic infections, and supportive care. Specific principles are discussed separately after these general principles.
- The complex life cycle of HIV provides many potential targets for antiretroviral therapy, including binding and entry, reverse transcriptase (RT), transcription and translation, protease inhibition, and viral maturation and budding (Figure 40.1).
- Widespread chronic use of antiretroviral agents raises concern about the potential for development of HIV resistance and treatment failure. Contributing factors include increased viral burden, length of therapy, low CD4+ lymphocyte counts, increased virulence as a result of RT mutations, and noncompliance. VIII
- Combination antiretroviral therapy is the accepted standard, because this approach enables use of agents that exploit various targets of HIV replication, minimize drug induced toxicities, and decrease emergence of antiretroviral resistance. Combinations include two nucleoside RT inhibitors (NRTIs) with a protease inhibitor or two NRTIs with a non-nucleoside RT inhibitor (NNRTI).
- Management of HIV infection is determined by the presence of symptoms, viral load, and CD4 cell counts. Viral load may be measured by target amplification assays (eg, RT polymerase chain reaction [RT-PCR] or signal amplification assays [branched deoxyribonucleic acid (bDNA]). The former may give HIV RNA levels twice the latter.
- The decision to initiate antiretroviral therapy will continue to be revised. At present, there are two guideline statements that may be used. There are some differences in guidelines and each is presented below:

  1. Guidelines for consideration of initiating antiretroviral therapy from the International AIDS Society–USA Panel (see Carpenter CCJ, Fischl MA, Hammer SM, et al. Antiretroviral therapy for HIV infection in 1997. *JAMA* 1997;277:1962–1969).
     - All patients with HIV RNA levels above 5000–10,000 copies/mL plasma regardless of the CD4+ cell count. Therapy

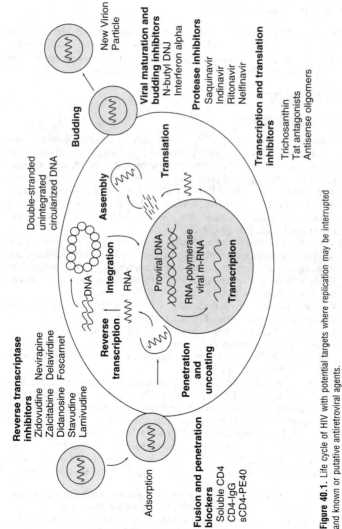

Figure 40.1. Life cycle of HIV with potential targets where replication may be interrupted and known or putative antiretroviral agents.

should be considered for all HIV-infected patients with detectable HIV RNA in plasma who request it and are committed to lifelong adherence to necessary treatment.

- Therapy might be safely deferred in patients at low risk of progression (low plasma HIV RNA level and high CD4+ count), particularly those who are not committed to complex antiretroviral regimens. These patients should be reevaluated every 3–6 months.
- Patients with symptomatic HIV disease or with CD4+ cell counts below $0.5 \times 10^9/L$, particularly below $0.35 \times 10^9/L$.

2. Guidelines for consideration of initiating antiretroviral therapy from the Department of Health and Human Services Panel on Clinical Practices and Treatment of HIV Infection (*Federal Register* draft document obtained on internet at http://www.hivatis.org/guidelin.html).

- Some experts would delay therapy and observe, whereas others would treat patients with CD4+ T cells >500/mm^3 and HIV RNA <10,000 copies/mL (bDNA) or <20,000 copies/mL (RT-PCR).
- Treatment should be offered to asymptomatic patients with CD4+ T cells >500/mm^3 or HIV RNA >10,000 copies/mL plasma (bDNA) or >20,000 copies/mL plasma (RT-PCR).
- Symptomatic patients should be treated regardless of the CD4+ VIII T-cell count or HIV RNA value.

- Guidelines for initial antiretroviral regimens are as follows:
  - Patients should be begun on two NRTIs (eg, zidovudine with lamivudine, didanosine, or zalcitabine, or stavudine combined with lamivudine or didanosine) with a protease inhibitor (indinavir, ritonavir, or nelfinavir).
  - When the primary regimen is not practical, the alternative is two NRTIs with a NNRTI (eg., nevirapine).
  - It is essential that the patient be fully committed to a complex, costly, and potentially toxic regimen, as less than excellent adherence may result in virus breakthrough and emergence of drug-resistant strains.
- Changes in antiretroviral therapy may be required for the reasons listed below:
  - Treatment failure, as suggested by a confirmed rising plasma HIV RNA level or failure to achieve the desired reduction in plasma viral load; declining CD4+ cell count; or clinical disease progression.
  - Unacceptable toxicity of, intolerance of, or nonadherence to the regimen.
  - Current use of suboptimal treatment regimens; that is, antiretroviral monotherapy.
- The following are guidelines for changes in initial antiretroviral regimens:

- When treatment failure occurs, it is recommended to change all drugs in the regimen or at least to include a minimum of two new drugs in the revised regimen.
- Recommendations for alternative antiretroviral regimens for treatment failure are found in Table 40.3.
- Measures should be instituted for prevention and treatment of opportunistic infections as shown below (see Centers for Disease Control and Prevention. 1997 USPHS/IDSA guidelines for the prevention of opportunistic infections in persons infected with human immunodeficiency virus. *MMWR* 1997;46(No. RR-12):1–46).

TABLE 40.3. Examples of Alternative Antiretroviral Regimens for Treatment Failure

Initial Regimen	Alternative
Zidovudine-lamivudine-protease inhibitor-1	Stavudine-didanosine-protease inhibitor-2 Stavudine-didanosine-NNRTI Ritonavir-saquinavir-NRTI
Stavudine-lamivudine-protease inhibitor-1	Zidovudine-didanosine-protease inhibitor-2 Zidovudine-didanosine-NNRTI Ritonavir-saquinavir-NRTI
Zidovudine-didanosine-protease inhibitor-1	Stavudine-lamivudine-protease inhibitor-2 Stavudine-lamivudine-NNRTI Ritonavir-saquinavir-NRTI
Stavudine-didanosine-protease inhibitor-1	Zidovudine-lamivudine-protease inhibitor-2 Zidovudine-lamivudine-NNRTI Ritonavir-saquinavir-NRTI
Zidovudine-didanosine-NNRTI	Stavudine-lamivudine-protease inhibitor-1 Zidovudine-lamivudine-protease inhibitor-1
Zidovudine-didanosine	Zidovudine-lamivudine-protease inhibitor Stavudine-lamivudine-protease inhibitor Ritonavir-saquinavir-NRTI
Zidovudine-zalcitabine	Zidovudine-lamivudine-protease inhibitor Stavudine-lamivudine-protease inhibitor Stavudine-didanosine-protease inhibitor Ritonavir-saquinavir-NRTI
Zidovudine-lamivudine	Stavudine-didanosine-protease inhibitor Ritonavir-saquinavir-NRTI
Stavudine-didanosine	Zidovudine-lamivudine-protease inhibitor Ritonavir-saquinavir-NRTI
Stavudine-lamivudine	Zidovudine-didanosine-protease inhibitor Ritonavir-saquinavir-NRTI

NNRTI, nonnucleoside reverse transcriptase inhibitor; NRTI, nucleoside reverse transcriptase inhibitor.
Data from Carpenter CCJ, Fischl MA, Hammer SM, et al. Antiretroviral therapy for HIV infection in 1997. *JAMA* 1997;277:1962–1969.

VIII

- *Pneumocystis carinii*
  - Prophylaxis is strongly recommended when the CD4+ count <200/µL or oropharyngeal candidiasis of unexplained fever ≥2 weeks. The preferred agent is trimethoprim-sulfamethoxazole (TMP-SMX) 1 DS once daily or 1 SS once daily. Alternatives include dapsone, dapsone plus pyrimethamine and leucovorin, or aerosolized pentamidine.
  - TMP-SMX may also be used in children who are HIV infected or HIV indeterminant. Total daily dose should not exceed 320 mg of TMP with 1600 mg of SMX in children.
  - The preferred treatment of PCP pneumonia is TMP-SMX (20 mg/kg/day of trimethoprim with sulfamethoxazole 100 mg/kg/day in three to four divided doses) given PO or IV. Adverse effects, including rash, fever, hepatotoxicity, and bone marrow suppression, occur commonly (50–80% of patients).
  - Alternative treatment is pentamidine 4 mg/kg/day IV over 1 h once daily every 21 days.
  - Dosage modification or pharmacokinetic monitoring can somewhat reduce the toxicity of both pentamidine and TMP-SMX. For example, pentamidine-associated hypotension and tachycardia appear to be infusion-rate related and can be minimized by infusion durations of 1 h.
  - Adjunctive corticosteroid therapy has been shown to decrease the risk of respiratory failure and improve survival in patients with AIDS and moderate to severe PCP (PaO$_2$ ≤75 mm Hg or A-a gradient ≥35 mm Hg). Oral prednisone should be initiated within 24–72 h of antipneumocystis therapy at a dosage of 40 mg twice daily on days 1–5; 40 mg once daily on days 6–10; and 20 mg once daily on days 11–21, or for the duration of therapy.
  - Clinical improvement is often slower in patients with AIDS than in non-AIDS patients. Nonetheless, continued worsening after 4 days or lack of improvement after 7–10 days is an indication for a change in therapy.
- *Mycobacterium tuberculosis*
  - Prophylaxis is strongly recommended in patients with purified protein derivative (PPD) >5 mm induration to, other evidence of latent infection, or contact with infected patients.
  - The preferred prophylactic regimen is isoniazid 300 mg once daily with pyridoxine 25–50 mg/day for 12 months with isoniazid-sensitive organisms. Alternatives include rifampin 600 mg/day.
  - For isoniazid-resistant organisms, rifampin 600 mg PO daily for 12 months should be used.
  - Standard, multidrug treatment regimens for drug-susceptible or drug-resistant tuberculosis should be used for treatment of active disease in HIV-infected patients.
- *Toxoplasma gondii*
  - Prophylaxis is strongly recommended in HIV-infected patients with immunoglobulin G (IgG) antibody titer to *Toxoplasma* and CD4+ count <100/µL.

VIII

- The preferred prophylactic regimen is TMP-SMX, 1 DS PO daily. Alternatives are TMP-SMX 1 SS PO daily and dapsone plus pyrimethamine plus leucovorin.
- Combination of oral pyrimethamine (loading doses of 50–200 mg and maintenance doses of 25–50 mg/day) and sulfadiazine (6–8 g/day) is considered the most effective regimen for acute therapy of AIDS-related CNS toxoplasmosis. Although agreement on optimal doses is lacking, acute therapy should be continued for at least 3 weeks and for up to 6 weeks in severely ill patients.
- Pyrimethamine plus clindamycin (300–1200 mg PO or IV every 6 h) appears to be less effective compared with pyrimethamine and sulfadiazine but is slightly less toxic.
- Because of the high relapse rate after stopping therapy, lifelong maintenance therapy is recommended. Although there is no general agreement, lower doses may be satisfactory if patients respond favorably to primary therapy. Pyrimethamine (25–50 mg/day with folinic acid 5–10 mg/day) plus 2 g/day (1 g every 12 h) of sulfadiazine has been recommended.

- *Mycobacterium avium* complex
  - Prophylaxis with clarithromycin (500 mg PO twice daily) or azithromycin (1200 mg PO once weekly) is strongly recommended in patients with a CD4+ count <50/μL.
  - Alternative prophylactic agents include rifabutin or azithromycin with rifabutin.
  - Treatment regimens should contain at least two antimycobacterial agents, including clarithromycin or azithromycin. Of these, clarithromycin is preferred because of greater clinical experience. Of the many choices for the second agent, ethambutol is preferred by many experts. Many clinicians would add a third and even a fourth drug (ie, rifabutin or rifampin, ciprofloxacin, or amikacin).
  - Clinical responses usually occur within 2–8 weeks of the start of therapy. If clinical and microbiologic responses are observed, lifelong therapy should be continued.

- *Streptococcus pneumoniae*
  - All HIV-infected patients should receive pneumococcal vaccine (0.5 mL).

- Varicella-zoster virus
  - Prophylaxis is strongly recommended for patients exposed to chickenpox or shingles who have no history of either condition or, if available, negative antibody to VZV.
  - Varicella-zoster immune globulin (five vials, 1.25 mL each given intramuscularly) should be administered less than 96 h after exposure, ideally within 48 h.
  - An alternative regimen for prophylaxis is acyclovir 800 mg PO five times daily for 3 weeks.
  - AIDS patients with disseminated cutaneous or visceral zoster should receive intravenous acyclovir 30 mg/kg/day for at least 7 days or until

all lesions are crusted. Milder disease can be treated with oral acyclovir or valacyclovir.

- Hepatitis B
  - Prophylaxis is generally recommended in all susceptible (anti-HBc–negative) patients. Engerix or Recombivax vaccine should be used.
- Influenza virus
  - It is generally recommended that all HIV-infected patients receive whole or split virus vaccine annually before the influenza season.
  - An alternative is rimantadine 100 mg PO twice daily or amantadine 100 mg PO three times daily.
- Cryptococcal meningitis
  - Standard therapeutic approach to cryptococcal meningitis has been amphotericin B for both acute and maintenance therapy, although introduction of azole compounds is changing the therapeutic approach for clinically stable patients.
  - Most patients with cryptococcal meningitis should probably receive amphotericin B in an intravenous dose of at least 0.5 mg/kg/day for a minimum of 2 weeks as acute therapy. Flucytosine in doses of 100–150 mg/kg/day can be considered for combination with amphotericin B; serum concentrations should be monitored and peak levels kept below 100 µg/mL to minimize hematologic adverse reactions.
  - Other triazole compounds (eg, itraconazole) are undergoing evaluation for treatment of cryptococcal disease.
  - Maintenance therapy is necessary to prevent relapse. Fluconazole is superior to amphotericin for maintenance therapy and can be considered the drug of choice. Although there are no known advantages for combining fluconazole and amphotericin B therapy, there are theoretical reasons to avoid this combination.
- A summary of therapies recommended for treatment of opportunistic infections is provided in Table 40.4.
- Treatment of cytomegalovirus infections
  - CMV therapy is traditionally divided into two phases, induction and long-term maintenance.
  - The choice between ganciclovir and foscarnet for initial therapy of CMV retinitis is largely dictated by adverse reaction profiles, concomitant medications, and underlying disease.
  - Ganciclovir-associated neutropenia and thrombocytopenia necessitate dose reduction or interruption of therapy in up to 50% of patients. Ganciclovir is poorly tolerated by individuals receiving zidovudine owing to additive hematologic toxicity; erythropoietin and granulocyte-macrophage colony-stimulating factor (GM-CSF) may ameliorate adverse hematologic effects.
  - Foscarnet is a pyrophosphate analog with both anti-HIV and anti-CMV activity. Although foscarnet appears less likely to cause neutropenia than ganciclovir, it is associated with many other adverse

VIII

TABLE 40.4. Therapies for Common Opportunistic Pathogens in HIV-Infected Individuals

Clinical Disease	Selected Therapies for Acute Infection in Adults	Common Drug or Dose Limiting Adverse Reactions
Fungi		
Candidiasis, oral	Nystatin 500,000 units PO swish 4–6 times daily for 7–10 days *or* Clotrimazole 10 mg (1 troche) PO 5 times daily for 7–10 days	Taste, patient acceptance
Candidiasis, esophageal	Ketoconazole 400 mg/d PO for 10–14 days *or*	Elevated liver function tests, hepatotoxicity, nausea and vomiting
	Fluconazole 200 mg PO or IV on the first day then 100 mg/d for 10–14 days	Elevated liver function tests, hepatotoxicity, rash, nausea and vomiting
Pneumocystis carinii pneumonia	Trimethoprim–sulfamethoxazole IV or PO 12–20 mg/kg/d as TMP component in 3–4 divided doses for 21 days[a] *or*	Skin rash, fever, leukopenia, thrombocytopenia
	Pentamidine IV 3–4 mg/kg/d for 21 days[a]	Azotemia, hypoglycemia, hyperglycemia
	Mild episodes: Atovaquone 750 mg PO thrice daily for 21 days[a]	Rash, elevated liver enzymes, diarrhea
Cryptococcal meningitis	Amphotericin B IV 0.5–0.7 mg/kg/d for minimum of 2 weeks *with* or *without*	Nephrotoxicity, hypokalemia, anemia, fever, chills
	Flucytosine 100–150 mg/kg/d PO in 4 divided doses *followed by*	Bone marrow suppression, elevated liver enzymes
	Fluconazole 100–200 mg/d, PO[a]	Same as above
Histoplasmosis	Amphotericin B 0.5–1 mg/kg/d IV for 6–8 weeks[a] *or*	Same as above
	Itraconazole 200–400 mg/d for 3 months[a]	Elevated liver function tests, hepatotoxicity, nausea and vomiting, hypertension
Coccidiodomycosis	Amphotericin B 0.5–1 mg/kg/d IV for 6–8 weeks[a]	Same as above
Protozoa		
Toxoplasmic encephalitis	Pyrimethamine 200 mg PO once then 50–100 mg/d *plus*	Bone marrow suppression
	Sulfadiazine 1–1.5 g PO four times daily *and*	Allergy, rash, drug fever
	Folinic acid 10–20 mg PO daily for a minimum of 28 days[a]	

[a]Maintenance therapy is recommended.

TABLE 40.4. continued

Clinical Disease	Selected Therapies for Acute Infection in Adults	Common Drug or Dose Limiting Adverse Reactions
Isosporiasis	Trimethoprim and sulfamethoxazole: 640 mg TMP and 3200 mg SMX per day PO in 2–4 divided doses per day for 2–4 weeks	Same as above

Bacteria
Organisms associated with T-cell defects

Mycobacterium avium complex	Clarithromycin 0.5–1 g PO twice daily *plus*	Gastrointestinal intolerance
	Ethambutol 15 mg/kg/d PO to a maximum of 1000 mg/d *may also add*	Optic neuritis, peripheral neuritis
	Rifampin 10 mg/kg/d PO to a maximum of 600 mg/d for 12 weeks *or*	Hepatitis, discoloration of secretions
	Clofazimine 100–200 mg PO daily *or*	Discoloration of skin and eyes, gastrointestinal intolerance
	Ciprofloxacin 500–750 mg PO twice daily	Gastrointestinal Intolerance
Salmonella enterocolitis or bacteremia	Ciprofloxacin 500–750 mg PO twice daily for 14 days *or*	Same as above
	Trimethoprim (320 mg)–sulfamethoxazole (1600 mg) PO in 2 divided doses/d for 14 days	Same as on previous page

Organisms associated with B cell defects

Campylobacter enterocolitis	Ciprofloxacin 500 mg PO twice daily for 7 days *or*	Same as above
	Erythromycin 250–500 mg PO four times daily for 7 days	Gastrointestinal intolerance, colitis, ototoxicity
Shigella enterocolitis	Ciprofloxacin 500 mg PO twice daily for 5 days	Same as above

Viruses

Mucocutaneous herpes simplex	Acyclovir 1–2 g/d PO in 3–5 divided doses, for 7–10 days	Gastrointestinal intolerance
Varicella-zoster	Acyclovir 30 mg/kg/d IV in 3 divided doses or 4 g/d PO for 7–10 days	Obstructive nephropathy, CNS symptomatology
Cytomegalovirus	Ganciclovir 7.5–10 mg/kg/d in 2–3 divided doses for 14 days[a] *or*	Neutropenia, thrombocytopenia
	Foscarnet 180 mg/kg/d in 2–3 divided doses for 14 days[a]	Nephrotoxicity, hypo–hypercalcemia, hypo–hyperphosphatemia, anemia

VIII

[a]Maintenance therapy is recommended.

effects, especially renal insufficiency and metabolic disturbances. Hydration may prevent serum creatinine elevations. Foscarnet doses must be adjusted in individuals with renal insufficiency.

- After induction, ganciclovir maintenance therapy is usually 5–6 mg/kg once daily, 5–7 days/week for an indefinite period of time. Maintenance foscarnet doses are 90–120 mg/kg intravenously once daily.
- Alternative administration routes for ganciclovir include oral (as maintenance therapy despite poor oral bioavailability) and intravitreal routes (as salvage therapy).
- Newer drugs are being considered for treatment of CMV infection, including cidofovir.
- Treatment of herpes simplex virus infections
  - Acyclovir is the initial drug of choice for HSV disease. Daily oral doses range from 1000 to 1200 mg for mild to moderate mucocutaneous disease to 2000 mg for more severe disease. Treatment should be continued until all lesions have crusted.
  - Daily intravenous doses of acyclovir range from 15 mg/kg for severe mucocutaneous disease or intolerance of oral medication (HSV esophagitis) to 30 mg/kg for viscerally disseminated disease and HSV encephalitis.
  - Individuals with recurrent HSV disease can often be managed with low-dose suppressive oral acyclovir therapy, such as 200 mg four times daily or 400 mg twice daily.

ANTIRETROVIRAL AGENTS

- Antiretroviral agents, doses, and primary adverse effects are listed in Table 40.5.
- Zidovudine has been available since 1987, and consequently, the greatest experience has been with this drug. Other available NRTIs are didanosine, zalcitabine, stavudine, and lamivudine.
- The NNRTI nevirapine is less hematologically toxic than NRTIs; however, resistance may develop rapidly, and this agent should not be used alone. Another NNRTI is delavirdine.
- Saquinavir has very low bioavailability when taken alone, but this is improved significantly when taken with food. The alternate protease inhibitors ritonavir and nelfinavir have excellent bioavailability.
- Ritonavir has significant inhibitory effects on cytochrome P450 (3A4) and can increase concentrations of drugs metabolized by this system (saquinavir, benzodiazepines). Ritonavir and other protease inhibitors should not be used with terfenadine, astemizole, and cisapride because of the increased risk of fatal arrhythmias that may occur from decreased metabolism of these agents.
- Indinavir should be taken on an empty stomach, as its absorption is inhibited by protein or fat in foods.
- Nelfinavir should be taken with food to obtain optimum bioavailability.

VIII

TABLE 40.5. Antiretroviral Agents

Drug	Adult Dose	Primary Side Effects
Nucleoside reverse transcriptase inhibitors		
Zidovudine	200 mg orally every 8 h	Anemia, neutropenia, headache, insomnia, nausea
Didanosine	<60 kg: powder 167 mg PO q12h tablets 125 mg PO q12h ≥60 kg: powder 250 mg PO q12h tablets 200 mg PO q12h	Peripheral neuropathy, pancreatitis, diarrhea
Zalcitabine	0.75 mg PO q8h	Peripheral neuropathy, fever, rash, oral ulcers
Stavudine	<60 kg: 30 mg PO q12h ≥60 kg: 40 mg PO q12h	Peripheral neuropathy, increased hepatic enzymes
Lamivudine	150 mg PO q12h	Headache, GI irritation, cough, malaise
Nonnucleoside reverse transcriptase inhibitors		
Nevirapine	200 mg PO qd × 14 days, if no rash develops, increase to 200 mg PO q12h	Rash, increased hepatic enzymes
Delavirdine	400 mg PO tid	Rash, increased hepatic enzymes
Protease inhibitors		
Saquinavir	600 mg PO q8h	Nausea, diarrhea, headache, increased hepatic enzymes, elevated CPK
Ritonavir	600 mg PO q12h	Paresthesias, GI irritation, altered taste, elevated liver enzymes, cholesterol, and triglycerides
Indinavir	800 mg PO q8h	Hyperbilirubinemia, nephrolithiasis
Nelfinavir	750 mg PO q8h	Diarrhea, asthenia, GI irritation, increased hepatic enzymes

CPK, creatine phosphokinase; GI, gastrointestinal.

VIII

▶ EVALUATION OF THERAPEUTIC OUTCOMES

- Viral load and immunologic monitoring (eg, CD4 lymphocyte counts) should be performed prospectively to evaluate the therapeutic outcome of antiretroviral therapy and to determine if changes in therapy are needed.
- Patient education contributes to successful management of HIV.
  - Compliance with drug therapy, especially complex antiviral regimens, is mandatory. Noncompliance may contribute to the development of drug resistance to HIV.

- Patients should be taught to recognize opportunistic infections and adverse drug reactions.
- Patients should also be taught methods to prevent spreading HIV to other individuals.
- Patient interviews and appropriate laboratory tests should be performed to monitor for drug-induced toxicity (eg, hematologic parameters, renal function).
- To minimize the potential for acquiring HIV, health care workers and patients should follow "universal blood and body substance isolation techniques."

Refer to Chapter 117, Principles and Management of Human Immunodeficiency Virus Infection, authored by Courtney V. Fletcher, PharmD, and Ann C. Collier, MD, for a more detailed discussion.

VIII

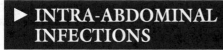

Chapter 41

▶ INTRA-ABDOMINAL INFECTIONS

▶ DEFINITION

Intra-abdominal infections are those contained within the peritoneum or retroperitoneal space. Two general types of intra-abdominal infection are discussed throughout this chapter: peritonitis and abscess.

- Peritonitis is defined as the acute, inflammatory response of peritoneal lining to microorganisms, chemicals, irradiation, or foreign body injury. Peritonitis may be classified as either primary or secondary. With primary peritonitis an intra-abdominal focus of disease may not be evident. In secondary peritonitis a focal disease process is evident within the abdomen.
- An abscess is a purulent collection of fluid separated by a more or less well-defined wall from surrounding tissue. It usually contains necrotic debris, bacteria, and inflammatory cells.

▶ EPIDEMIOLOGY AND ETIOLOGY

- Primary peritonitis occurs in 10–20% of patients with cirrhotic ascites, in other immunocompromised patients, and in patients undergoing peritoneal dialysis.
- Sixty percent of all patients on chronic ambulatory peritoneal dialysis (CAPD) will have at least one episode of peritonitis during the first year.
- Table 41.1 summarizes many of the potential causes of bacterial peritonitis. The causes of intra-abdominal abscess somewhat overlap those of peritonitis and, in fact, both may occur sequentially or simultaneously.
- Appendicitis is the most frequent cause of abscess.

▶ PATHOPHYSIOLOGY

- Intra-abdominal infection results from entry of bacteria into the peritoneal or retroperitoneal spaces or from bacterial collections within intra-abdominal organs. In primary peritonitis the route of bacterial spread is often not apparent. When peritonitis results from peritoneal dialysis, skin surface flora are introduced via the peritoneal catheter.
- In secondary peritonitis, bacteria most often enter the peritoneum or retroperitoneum as a result of disruption of the integrity of the gastrointestinal tract caused by diseases or traumatic injuries.
- When bacteria become dispersed throughout the peritoneum, the inflammatory process involves the majority of the peritoneal lining.

TABLE 41.1. Causes of Bacterial Peritonitis

Primary Bacterial Peritonitis
Peritoneal dialysis
Cirrhosis with ascites

Secondary Bacterial Peritonitis
Miscellaneous causes
Diverticulitis with perforation
Appendicitis
Inflammatory bowel diseases
Salpingitis
Biliary tract infections
Necrotizing pancreatitis

Neoplasms
Intestinal obstruction
Perforation

Mechanical gastrointestinal problems
Any cause of small bowel obstruction

Vascular causes
Mesenteric arterial or venous occlusion
Mesenteric ischemia without occlusion

Trauma
Blunt abdominal trauma with rupture of intestine
Penetrating abdominal trauma
Iatrogenic intestinal perforation

Intraoperative events
Peritoneal contamination during abdominal operation
Leakage from gastrointestinal anastomosis

VIII

- Peritonitis often results in mortality because of the effects on multiple organ systems. Fluid shifts and endotoxins may cause hypotension and shock. Fluid loss from the vasculature with generalized peritonitis is similar to that which occurs after a 50% second-degree burn.
- An abscess begins by the combined action of inflammatory cells (such as neutrophils), bacteria, fibrin, and other inflammatory components. A mature abscess may have a fibrinous capsule that isolates bacteria and the liquid core from antimicrobials and immunologic defenses.

MICROBIOLOGY

- Primary bacterial peritonitis is often caused by a single organism. In children, the pathogen is usually *Streptococcus pneumoniae* or a group A *streptococcus.* When peritonitis occurs in association with cirrhotic ascites, enteric organisms (such as *Escherichia coli*) are usually responsible.

- Peritonitis in patients undergoing peritoneal dialysis is most often caused by common skin organisms: *S. epidermidis, S. aureus,* streptococci, and diphtheroids.
- Secondary intra-abdominal infections are often polymicrobial. The mean number of isolates of microorganisms from infected intra-abdominal sites has ranged from 2.5 to 5.0, including an average of 1.4 to 2.0 aerobes and 2.4 to 3.0 anaerobes. The frequencies with which specific bacteria were isolated in intra-abdominal infections are given in Table 41.2.
- The combination of aerobic and anaerobic organisms appears to greatly increase pathogenicity. In intra-abdominal infections, facultative bacteria may provide an environment conducive to the growth of anaerobic bacteria. Although many bacteria isolated in mixed infections are nonpathogenic by themselves, their presence may be essential for the pathogenicity of the bacterial mixture.
- Aerobic enteric bacteria and anaerobic bacteria are both pathogens in intra-abdominal infection. Aerobic bacteria, particularly *E. coli,* appear responsible for the early mortality from peritonitis, whereas anaerobic bacteria are major pathogens in abscesses, with *B. fragilis* predominating.
- The role of enterococcus as a pathogen was not clear, because it fails to produce peritonitis or abscesses when given alone.

▶ CLINICAL PRESENTATION

PERITONITIS

- With generalized bacterial peritonitis the patient most often presents in acute distress. The patient lies still, usually on his or her back, possibly

TABLE 41.2. Pathogens Isolated from 900 Patients with Intra-abdominal Infections from Six Independent Studies

Aerobic Bacteria	Percent of Patients	Anaerobic Bacteria	Percent of Patients
E. coli	51	*Bacteroides* sp.	72
Klebsiella sp.	14	Fusobacteria	7
Enterobacter sp.	6	Veillonela	2
Proteus sp.	16	Propionbacteria	5
Pseudomonas sp.	7	Clostridiae	23
Streptococci	12	Peptostreptococci	13
Enterococci	17	Peptococci	8
Staphylococci	5	Others	21
Others	8		

From Wittmar DH. Intra-Abdominal Infections: Pathophysiology and Treatment. New York, Marcel Dekker, 1991:69, with permission.

with hips slightly flexed. The patient exhibits voluntary guarding of the abdomen, and respirations are shallow and frequent. There is generalized abdominal tenderness on examination, and after a short period of time the abdominal muscles become rigid ("board-like abdomen"). Because of the fluid loss into the peritoneum and vomiting, the patient may appear dehydrated, and a decreased urine output is noted. Temperature may progress from normal up to 103°F.

- If peritonitis continues untreated the patient may go into hypovolemic shock from fluid loss into the peritoneum. This may be accompanied by generalized sepsis.
- Laboratory evaluations with peritonitis usually demonstrate leukocytosis (15,000–20,000 WBC/mm^3). The hematocrit and the blood urea nitrogen may be elevated because of dehydration. Serum lactic acid will probably be elevated.
- Abdominal radiographs may be useful, as free air in the abdomen (indicating intestinal perforation) or distention of the small or large bowel is often evident.
- Primary peritonitis can develop over a period of days to weeks, evident as an acute febrile illness. Usually the patient has nausea, vomiting (sometimes with diarrhea), abdominal tenderness, and hypoactive bowel sounds, although the abdominal signs are variable. The patient's temperature or WBC count may be only mildly elevated. The cirrhotic patient may have worsening encephalopathy.
- Patients with peritonitis related to chronic peritoneal dialysis usually have abdominal pain and tenderness, possibly with nausea and vomiting, but fever is not a consistent finding. In these patients a cloudy dialysate drainage is often noted as a first sign of peritonitis indicating the presence of bacteria and inflammatory cells.

Abscess

- Intra-abdominal abscesses pose a more difficult diagnostic challenge because the symptoms are often neither specific nor dramatic. The patient may complain of abdominal pain or discomfort, but these symptoms are not reliable.
- A number of radiographic methods are used to make the diagnosis of an intra-abdominal abscess. Plain radiographs may show air–fluid levels or may demonstrate the shift of normal intra-abdominal contents by the abscess mass. Computed tomography (CT) and magnetic resonance imaging may be used to locate some intra-abdominal abscesses.

▶ DESIRED OUTCOME

The goals of treatment are the correction of intra-abdominal disease processes or injuries that have caused infection and the drainage of collections of purulent material (e.g., abscess). Secondary goals are the prevention of dissemination of infection to sites outside the abdomen or reinfection in the abdomen. Ideally, treatment would be effected without significant complications such as organ dysfunction or adverse drug reactions.

VIII

▶ TREATMENT

GENERAL PRINCIPLES

- The three major modalities for the treatment of intra-abdominal infection are prompt drainage, support of vital functions, and appropriate antimicrobial therapy.
- Antimicrobials are an important adjunct to surgical procedures in the treatment of intra-abdominal infections; however, the use of antimicrobial agents without surgical intervention is usually inadequate. For some specific situations (e.g., most cases of primary peritonitis), drainage procedures may not be required, and antimicrobial agents become the mainstay of therapy.
- With generalized peritonitis, large volumes of intravenous fluids are required to restore vascular volume and improve cardiovascular function.
- Respiratory function can be assisted by a variety of methods including ventilatory support in severely ill patients. Often, the critically ill patient with intra-abdominal infection will require intensive-care monitoring, particularly if there is cardiovascular or respiratory instability.
- Isolation procedures may be required if the infectious process poses a threat to other hospitalized patients.

NON-PHARMACOLOGIC TREATMENT

- Secondary peritonitis requires surgical correction of the underlying pathology.
- Drainage of the purulent material, either by open surgical procedure or drained percutaneously, is the critical element in the management of an intra-abdominal abscess. Without adequate drainage of the abscess, antimicrobial therapy and fluid resuscitation can be expected to fail.
- Aggressive fluid repletion and management are required for the purposes of achieving or maintaining proper intravascular volumes and adequate urine output and correcting acidosis.
- Urine output should be continuously monitored in severely ill patients by use of a transurethral bladder catheter, quantitated hourly, and it should equal or exceed 1 mL/kg body weight per hour.
- In patients with peritonitis, hypovolemia is often accompanied by acidosis, so a reasonable intravenous fluid would be lactated Ringer's, which contains the bicarbonate precursor, lactate.
- In the initial hour of treatment a large volume of solution may need to be administered to restore intravascular volume. Although this volume may frequently approach 4 L, much more fluid may be required to restore vital functions.
- In patients with significant blood loss, blood should be given. This is generally in the form of packed red blood cells. The criteria for blood transfusion are controversial, but a hematocrit of 25% is generally accepted.

VIII

PHARMACOLOGIC THERAPY

- The goals of antimicrobial therapy are to control bacteremia and the establishment of metastatic foci of infection, to reduce suppurative complications after bacterial contamination, and to prevent local spread of existing infection.
- An empiric antimicrobial regimen should be started as soon as the presence of intra-abdominal infection is suspected based on the likely pathogens.
- Likely pathogens, those against which antimicrobial agents should be directed, are listed in Table 41.3.
- Table 41.4 presents recommended and alternative regimens for selected situations. These are general guidelines, not rules, because there are many factors that cannot be incorporated into such a table.

Recommendations

- Most patients with severe intra-abdominal infections (where there is generalized peritonitis or septic shock or where the patient has a high fever and shaking chills) should be placed on an aminoglycoside in combination with an antianaerobic agent or an agent demonstrated to be effective in this category of patients (e.g., imipenem/cilistatin). Gentamicin is the aminoglycoside of choice, based on its lower cost. The dosage for aminoglycosides should be adjusted on the basis of age, weight, and renal function.
- Ampicillin may be added to assure antimicrobial coverage for enterococci, although this is controversial.

VIII

TABLE 41.3. Likely Intra-abdominal Pathogens

Type of Infection	Aerobes	Anaerobes
Primary Bacterial Peritonitis		
Children (spontaneous)	Pneumococci, group A *Streptococcus*	—
Cirrhosis	*E. coli, Klebsiella*, pneumococci (many others)	—
Peritoneal dialysis	*Staphylococcus, Streptococcus*	—
Secondary Bacterial Peritonitis		
Gastroduodenal	*Streptococcus, E. coli*	
Biliary tract	*E. coli, Klebsiella*, enterococci	*Clostridium* or *Bacteroides* (infrequent)
Small or large bowel	*E. coli, Klebsiella*, spp., *Proteus* spp.	*Bacteroides fragilis* and other *Bacteroides, Clostridium*
Appendicitis	*E. coli, Pseudomonas*	*Bacteroides* spp.
Abscesses	*E. coli, Klebsiella*, enterococci	*B. fragilis* and other *Bacteroides, Clostridium*, anaerobic cocci
Liver	*E. coli, Klebsiella*, enterococci, staphylococci, amoeba	*Bacteroides* (infrequent)
Spleen	*Staphylococcus, Streptococcus*	

- The selection of a specific agent or combination should be based on culture and susceptibility data for peritonitis that occurs from chronic peritoneal dialysis. If microbiologic data are unavailable, empiric therapy as listed in Table 41.4 should be initiated.
- Patients with peritonitis who are undergoing chronic peritoneal dialysis (CPD) may receive parenteral as well as intraperitoneal antimicrobial agents. Intraperitoneal antimicrobial agents alone are often sufficient, unless severe infection is present. A number of agents may be instilled through peritoneal catheters. Recommended concentrations of antimicrobial agents for intraperitoneal irrigation solutions are 8 mg/L for gentamicin and tobramycin, 1–3 mg/L for clindamycin, 50,000 U/L for penicillin G, 125 mg/L for cephalosporins, 100–150 mg/L for ticarcillin or carbenicillin, 50 mg/L for ampicillin, 100 mg/L for methicillin, 30 mg/L for vancomycin, and 3 mg/L for amphotericin B.
- The usual duration of therapy for peritonitis associated with CPD is 10–14 days but may extend to 3 weeks. Antimicrobial therapy should be continued until dialysate fluid is clear, cultures are negative for 2–3 days, and the patient is asymptomatic.
- After acute bacterial contamination, such as with abdominal trauma where gastrointestinal contents enter the peritoneum, combination antimicrobial regimens are not required. If the patient is seen soon after injury (within 2 hours) and surgical measures are instituted promptly, single-agent regimens such as antianaerobic cephalosporins or extended-spectrum penicillins are effective in preventing most infectious complications.
- The necessary duration of treatment for secondary intra-abdominal infections is not clearly defined. Acute intra-abdominal contamination, such as after a traumatic injury, may be treated with a very short course (24 hours). For established infections (peritonitis or intra-abdominal abscess) an antimicrobial course of at least 7 days is justified.

Regarding selection of antimicrobial agents for secondary intra-abdominal infections:

- Single-agent regimens with β-lactams that have antianaerobic activity perform as well as combination regimens with aminoglycosides plus clindamycin or metronidazole.
- Clindamycin and metronidazole are equally effective anti-anaerobic agents when used with aminoglycosides for treatment of intra-abdominal infections.

▶ EVALUATION OF THERAPEUTIC OUTCOMES

- Whichever antimicrobial regimen is chosen, the patient should be continually reassessed to determine the success or failure of therapies. The clinician should recognize that there are many reasons for poor outcome of patients with intra-abdominal infection; improper antimicrobial administration is only one.

TABLE 41.4. Recommendations for Initial Antimicrobial Agents for Intra-abdominal Infections

Primary Bacterial Peritonitis		
Cirrhosis	Aminoglycoside plus penicillin or antistaphylococcal cephalosporin	1. Add clindamycin or metronidazole if anaerobes are suspected
		2. Third-generation cephalosporins, extended-spectrum penicillins, aztreonam, and imipenem as alternatives
Peritoneal dialysis	Regimen based on organism isolated	
	1. *Staphylococcus:* penicillinase-resistant penicillin or first-generation cephalosporin	1. Alternative for resistant staphylococci is vancomycin
	2. *Streptococcus:* penicillin G	2. Alternative for *Streptococcus* is a first-generation cephalosporin
	3. Aerobic gram-negative bacilli: aminoglycoside plus an antipseudomonal penicillin or ceftazidime	3. Alternatives for gram-negative bacilli are third-generation cephalosporins, aztreonam, and extended-spectrum penicillins with β-lactamase inhibitors
	4. *Pseudomonas aeruginosa:* aminoglycoside plus antipseudomonal penicillin or ceftazidime	
Secondary Bacterial Peritonitis		
Perforated peptic ulcer	First-generation cephalosporins	1. Antianaerobic cephalosporins[a]
		2. Possibly add aminoglycoside if patient condition is poor
Other	Aminoglycoside with clindamycin or metronidazole	1. Add ampicillin if patient is immunocompromised or if biliary tract origin of infection
		2. Aztreonam with clindamycin or imipenem/cilistatin alone
		3. Antianaerobic cephalosporins,[a] extended-spectrum penicillins with β-lactamase inhibitor

[a]Cefoxitin, cefotetan, ceftizoxime, and cefmetazole.

- Unsatisfactory outcomes in patients with intra-abdominal infections may result from complications that arise in other organ systems. A complication commonly associated with mortality after intra-abdominal infection is pneumonia.
- Once antimicrobials are initiated and other important therapies described before are used, most patients should show improvement within 2–3 days. Usually, temperature will return to near normal, vital signs should stabilize, and the patient should not appear in distress, with the exception of recognized discomfort and pain from incisions, drains, and nasogastric tube.

VIII

TABLE 41.4. continued

Abscess

General	Aminoglycoside with clindamycin or metronidazole	1. Aztreonam with clindamycin, imipenem alone, or extended-spectrum penicillins with β-lactamase inhibitor, as alternatives
Liver	As above but add a first-generation cephalosporin	2. Use metronidazole if amoebic liver abscess is suspected
Spleen	Aminoglycoside plus penicillinase-resistant penicillin	3. Alternatives for penicillinase-resistant penicillin are first-generation cephalosporins or vancomycin

Appendicitis

Normal or inflamed	Antianaerobic cephalosporins[a] (discontinued immediately post-operation)	1. Aminoglycoside with clindamycin or metronidazole
Gangrenous or perforated	Aminoglycoside with clindamycin or metronidazole	1. Aztreonam with clindamycin, or imipenem alone 2. Antianaerobic cephalosporins[a] or extended-spectrum penicillins with β-lactamase inhibitor
Acute Cholecystitis	First-generation cephalosporin	Aminoglycoside plus ampicillin if severe infection
Cholangitis	Aminoglycoside with ampicillin with or without clindamycin or metronidazole	Use vancomycin for ampicillin if patient is allergic to penicillin
Acute Contamination from Abdominal Trauma	Antianaerobic cephalosporins[a] or extended spectrum penicillins	Aminoglycoside with one of the following: clindamycin, metronidazole, or antianaerobic cephalosporins[a]

VIII

[a]Cefoxitin, cefotetan, ceftizoxime, and cefmetazole.

- At 24–48 hours, aerobic bacterial culture results should return. If a suspected pathogen is not sensitive to the antimicrobial agents being given, the regimen should be changed if the patient has not shown sufficient progress.
- If the isolated pathogen is extremely sensitive to one antimicrobial, and the patient is progressing well, concurrent antimicrobial therapy may often be discontinued.
- With present anaerobic culturing techniques and the slow growth of these organisms, anaerobes are often not identified until 4–7 days after culture, and sensitivity information is difficult to obtain. For this reason there are usually few data with which to alter the antianaerobic component of the antimicrobial regimen.
- Superinfection in patients being treated for intra-abdominal infection is often due to *Candida*, but enterococci or opportunistic gram-negative bacilli such as *Pseudomonas* or *Serratia* may be involved.

• Treatment regimens for intra-abdominal infection can be judged successful if the patient recovers from the infection without recurrent peritonitis or intra-abdominal abscess and without the need for additional antimicrobials. A regimen can be considered unsuccessful if a significant adverse drug reaction occurs, if reoperation is necessary, or if patient improvement is delayed beyond 1 or 2 weeks.

See Chapter 107, Intra-Abdominal Infections, authored by Joseph T. DiPiro, PharmD, FCCP, and David A. Rogers, MD, for a more detailed discussion of this topic.

VIII

Chapter 42

▶ RESPIRATORY TRACT INFECTIONS, LOWER

▶ DEFINITION

Lower respiratory tract infections include infectious processes of the lungs and bronchi, pneumonia, bronchitis, and lung abscess.

▶ BRONCHITIS

ACUTE BRONCHITIS

- The bronchiolitides (i.e., bronchitis and bronchiolitis) refer to an inflammatory condition of the tracheobronchial tree that is usually associated with a generalized respiratory infection. The inflammatory process does not extend to include the alveoli. The disease entity is frequently classified as either acute or chronic.

Epidemiology and Etiology

- Acute bronchitis most commonly occurs during the winter months, following a pattern very similar to those of other acute respiratory tract infections. Cold, damp climates and/or the presence of high concentrations of irritating substances such as air pollution or cigarette smoke may precipitate attacks.
- Respiratory viruses are by far the most common infectious agents associated with acute bronchitis. The common cold viruses, rhinovirus and coronavirus, and lower respiratory tract pathogens, including influenza virus, adenovirus, and respiratory syncytial virus, account for the majority of cases. *Mycoplasma pneumonia* also appears to be a frequent cause of acute bronchitis. More recently, a new *Chlamydia psittaci* strain, often denoted as TWAR or *Chlamydia pneumoniae,* has been associated with acute respiratory tract infections.

Pathophysiology

- Infection of the trachea and bronchi yields hyperemic and edematous mucous membranes with an increase in bronchial secretions. Destruction of respiratory epithelium can range from mild to extensive and may affect bronchial mucociliary function. In addition, the increase in bronchial secretions, which can become thick and tenacious, further impairs mucociliary activity. Recurrent acute respiratory infections may be associated with increased airway hyperreactivity and possibly the pathogenesis of chronic obstructive lung disease.

Clinical Presentation

- Cough is the hallmark of acute bronchitis and occurs early. The onset of cough may be insidious or abrupt and will persist despite the resolution of nasal or nasopharyngeal complaints. Frequently, the cough is initially nonproductive but progresses, yielding mucopurulent sputum. Fever, when present, rarely exceeds 39°C and appears most commonly with adenovirus, influenza virus, and *M. pneumonia* infections.

- Initial physical examination is generally unimpressive, usually revealing a variable degree of rhinitis. Chest examination may reveal rhonchi and coarse, moist rales bilaterally. Chest radiographs, when performed, are usually normal.

- Bacterial cultures of expectorated sputum are generally of limited utility due to the inability to avoid normal nasopharyngeal flora by the sampling technique. In routine cases, viral cultures are unnecessary and frequently unavailable. Cultures or serologic diagnosis of *M. pneumonia* and culture or direct fluorescent antibody detection for *Bordetella pertussis* should be obtained in prolonged or severe cases when epidemiologic considerations would suggest their involvement. The white blood cell (WBC) count is usually normal or slightly elevated ($>10,000/mm^3$) with a predominance of neutrophils in approximately one-third of the cases.

Treatment

- The treatment of acute bronchitis is symptomatic and supportive in nature. Bed rest and mild analgesic–antipyretic therapy are often helpful in relieving the associated lethargy, malaise, and fever. Aspirin or acetaminophen (650 mg in adults or 10–15 mg/kg per dose in children) or ibuprofen (200–400 mg in adults or 10 mg/kg per dose in children) is administered every 4–6 hours.

- In children, aspirin should be avoided and acetaminophen used as the preferred agent because of the possible association between aspirin use and the development of Reye's syndrome.

- Patients should be encouraged to drink fluids to prevent dehydration and possibly decrease the viscosity of respiratory secretions.

- Mist therapy and/or the use of a vaporizer may further promote the thinning and loosening of respiratory secretions.

- Persistent, mild cough, which may be bothersome, may be treated with dextromethorphan; more severe coughs may require intermittent codeine or other similar agents.

- Routine use of antibiotics in the treatment of acute bronchitis is discouraged; however, in patients who exhibit persistent fever or respiratory symptomatology for more than 4–6 days, the possibility of a concurrent bacterial infection should be suspected.

- When possible, antibiotic therapy is directed toward anticipated respiratory pathogen(s) (i.e., *Streptococcus pneumonia, Haemophilus influenzae*) and/or those demonstrating a predominant growth upon throat culture.

- *Mycoplasma pneumonia,* if suspected by history or positive cold agglutinins (titers $\geq$ 1:32), or if confirmed by culture or serology, may be treated with erythromycin or its analogues.

- During known epidemics involving the influenza A virus, amantadine or rimantadine may be effective in minimizing associated symptomatology if administered early in the course of the disease.

CHRONIC BRONCHITIS

Epidemiology and Etiology

- Chronic bronchitis is a nonspecific disease that affects primarily adults. Current estimates suggest that between 10% and 25% of the adult population 40 or older suffer from chronic bronchitis.
- The exact cause of chronic bronchitis remains unidentified. Current data and experience suggest that chronic bronchitis is a result of several contributing factors; the most prominent of these include cigarette smoking, exposure to occupational dusts, fumes, and environmental pollution, and bacterial (and possibly viral) infection.

Pathogenesis

- In chronic bronchitis, the bronchial wall is thickened and the number of mucus-secreting goblet cells in the surface epithelium of both larger and smaller bronchi is markedly increased. Hypertrophy of the mucus glands and dilatation of the mucus gland ducts are also observed.
- As a result of these changes, chronic bronchitics have substantially more mucus in their peripheral airways, further impairing normal lung defenses. This increased quantity of tenacious secretions within the bronchial tree frequently causes mucus plugging of the smaller airways.
- Accompanying these changes are squamous cell metaplasia of the surface epithelium, edema and increased vascularity of the basement membrane of larger airways, and variable chronic inflammatory cell infiltration.
- Continued progression of this pathology can result in residual scarring of small bronchi, augmenting airway obstruction and the weakening of bronchial walls.

VIII

Clinical Presentation

- The hallmark of chronic bronchitis is cough that, depending on the severity of the disease, may range from a mild "smoker's" cough to severe incessant coughing productive of purulent sputum. Coughing may be precipitated by multiple stimuli including simple, normal conversation.
- Expectoration of the largest quantity of sputum usually occurs upon arising in the morning, although many patients expectorate sputum throughout the day. The expectorated sputum is usually tenacious and can vary in color from white to yellow-green.
- The diagnosis of chronic bronchitis is based primarily on clinical assessment and history. By definition, any patient who reports the coughing up of sputum on most days for at least 3 consecutive months each year for 2 consecutive years suffers from chronic bronchitis.
- With the exception of pulmonary findings, the physical examination of patients with mild to moderate chronic bronchitis is usually unremarkable. Chest auscultation usually reveals inspiratory and expiratory rales,

rhonchi, and mild wheezing with an expiratory phase that is frequently prolonged. Normal vesicular breathing sounds are diminished. Depending on the severity of the disease, an increase in the anteroposterior diameter of the thoracic cage (observed as a "barrel chest"), hyperresonance on percussion with obliteration of the area of cardiac dullness, and depressed diaphragms with limited mobility are often observed.

- The microscopic and laboratory assessment of sputum is considered an important component in the overall evaluation of patients with chronic bronchitis. An increased number of polymorphonuclear granulocytes often suggests continual bronchial irritation, whereas an increased number of eosinophils may suggest an allergic component that should be investigated further. The most common bacterial isolates identified from sputum culture in patients experiencing an acute exacerbation of chronic bronchitis are outlined in Table 42.1.

Desired Outcome

The primary goal of the treatment of acute exacerbations of chronic bronchitis is to foster prompt resolution of symptoms and positively influence the duration of the symptom-free post-treatment time period of the patient.

Treatment

General Principles

- A complete occupational/environmental history for the determination of exposure to noxious, irritating gases, as well as cigarette smoking must be assessed.
- Humidification of inspired air may promote the hydration (liquefaction) of tenacious secretions allowing for more effective sputum production. The use of mucolytic aerosols (e.g., *N*-acetylcysteine; DNAse) is of questionable therapeutic value.

TABLE 42.1. Common Bacterial Pathogens Isolated from the Sputum of Patients with an Acute Exacerbation of Chronic Bronchitis

Pathogen	Estimated Incidence[a]
Haemophilus influenzae[b]	24–26
Haemophilus parainfluenzae	20
Streptococcus pneumoniae	15
Moraxella catarrhalis[b]	15
Klebsiella pneumoniae	4
Serratia marcescens	2
Neisseria meningitidis[b]	2
Pseudomonas aeruginosa	2

[a]Expressed as percent of cultures.
[b]Often β-lactamase positive.

VIII

- Oral or aerosolized bronchodilators (e.g., albuterol aerosol) may be of benefit to some patients during acute pulmonary exacerbations.

Pharmacologic Therapy
- The use of antimicrobials has been controversial although antibiotics are an important component of treatment. Agents should be selected that are effective against likely pathogens, have the lowest risk of drug interactions, and can be administered in a manner that promotes compliance.
- Antibiotics commonly used in the treatment of these patients and their respective adult starting doses are outlined in Table 42.2.
- Ampicillin is often considered the drug of choice for the treatment of acute exacerbations of chronic bronchitis. Unfortunately, the need for multiple repeat daily doses (four times daily) and the increasing incidence of penicillin-resistant β-lactamase–producing strains of bacteria have limited the usefulness of this safe and cost-effective antibiotic. The value of the erythromycins when mycoplasma is involved is unquestioned.
- Azithromycin and clarithromycin should be considered as second-line therapy.
- The fluoroquinolones are effective alternative agents for adults, particularly when gram-negative pathogens are involved.

VIII

TABLE 42.2. Oral Antibiotics Commonly Used for the Treatment of Acute Respiratory Exacerbations In Chronic Bronchitis

Antibiotic	Usual Adult Dose (g)	Dose Schedule (doses/d)
Preferred Drugs		
Ampicillin	0.5–1	4
Amoxicillin	0.5–1	2–3
Ciprofloxacin	0.5–0.75	2
Ofloxacin	0.2–0.4	2
Doxycycline	0.1	2
Minocycline	0.1	2
Tetracycline HCl	0.5	4
Amoxicillin–clavulanate	0.5	3
Trimethoprim–sulfamethoxazole	1 DS[a]	2
Lomefloxacin	0.4	1
Supplemental Drugs		
Erythromycin	0.5	4
Clarithromycin	0.25–0.5	2
Cephalexin	0.5	4
Cefaclor	0.25–0.5	3

[a]DS, double strength tablet (160 trimethoprim/800 mg sulfamethoxazole).

- The decision to use antibiotics for the prevention and/or treatment of an acute exacerbation of chronic bronchitis should be made on an individual patient-specific basis. In those patients whose history suggests recurrent exacerbations of their disease that might be attributable to certain specific events (i.e., seasonal-winter months), a trial of prophylactic antibiotics might be beneficial. If no clinical improvement is noted over an appropriate period (e.g., 2–3 months per year for 2–3 years), one might elect to discontinue further attempts at prophylactic therapy.

BRONCHIOLITIS

Epidemiology and Etiology

- Bronchiolitis is an acute viral infection of the lower respiratory tract of infants that shows a definite seasonal pattern (peaks during the winter months and persists through early spring). The disease most commonly affects infants during the first year of life.
- Respiratory syncytial virus is the most common cause of bronchiolitis, accounting for 45–60% of all cases. Parainfluenza viruses type 3 (10–15%), type 1 (5–10%), and type 2 (1–5%) are the second most common etiologic pathogens, constituting as a group nearly 25% of cases. Bacteria serve as secondary pathogens in only a small minority of cases.

Clinical Presentation

VIII

- The most common clinical signs of bronchiolitis are cough and coryza. As symptoms progress, infants may experience vomiting, diarrhea, noisy breathing, and an increase in respiratory rate.
- For those infants presenting to a hospital, examination reveals a rapid pulse and a respiratory rate between 40 and 80 breaths per minute. Breathing is labored with retractions of the chest wall, nasal flaring, and grunting. Chest auscultation reveals wheezing and inspiratory rales.
- As a result of limited oral intake due to coughing combined with vomiting and diarrhea, infants are frequently dehydrated.
- The diagnosis of bronchiolitis is based primarily on history and clinical findings. The isolation of a viral pathogen in the respiratory secretions of a wheezing child establishes a presumptive diagnosis of infectious bronchiolitis. However, the ability to identify specific viral pathogens is often hindered by the limited availability of special virology laboratories.
- The peripheral WBC count is usually normal or only slightly elevated.
- In those children requiring hospitalization, abnormalities in blood gas tensions are frequent and appear to relate to disease severity. Hypoxemia is common and acts to increase the respiratory drive, whereas hypercarbia is seen only in the most severe cases.

Treatment

- Bronchiolitis is a self-limiting illness and usually requires no therapy unless the infant is hypoxic or dehydrated.

- In severely affected children, the mainstays of therapy for bronchiolitis are oxygen therapy and intravenous fluids.
- Aerosolized β-adrenergic therapy appears to offer little benefit for the majority of patients, but may be useful in the child with a predisposition toward bronchospasm.
- There are no data to document the effectiveness of mist tents despite their widespread use.
- Because bacteria do not represent primary pathogens in the etiology of bronchiolitis, antibiotics should not be routinely administered. However, many clinicians frequently administer antibiotics initially while awaiting culture results, because the clinical and radiographic findings in bronchiolitis are often suggestive of a possible bacterial pneumonia.
- Ribavirin may offer an effective therapy for bronchiolitis although it is approved only in aerosolized form against respiratory syncytial virus. Use of the drug requires special equipment (small-particle aerosol generator) and specifically trained personnel for administration via oxygen hood or mist tent. Use of ribavirin should be reserved for more severely ill patients, including those with chronic lung disease (particularly bronchopulmonary dysplasia), congenital heart disease, prematurity, and immunodeficiency (especially severe combined immunodeficiency and HIV infection); ribavirin also should be considered in any patient requiring mechanical ventilation.

VIII ◀

▶ PNEUMONIA

EPIDEMIOLOGY

- Pneumonia occurs throughout the year, with the relative prevalence of disease resulting from different etiologic agents varying with the seasons. It occurs in persons of all ages, although the clinical manifestations are most severe in the very young, the elderly, and the chronically ill.

PATHOGENESIS

- Microorganisms gain access to the lower respiratory tract by three routes: they may be inhaled as aerosolized particles, they may enter the lung via the bloodstream from an extrapulmonary site of infection, or aspiration of oropharyngeal contents may occur.
- Factors that promote aspiration, such as altered sensorium and neuromuscular disease, may result in an increase in the size of the inoculum delivered to the lower respiratory tract, thereby overwhelming local defense mechanisms.
- Lung infections with viruses suppress the antibacterial activity of the lung by impairing alveolar macrophage function and mucociliary clearance, thus setting the stage for secondary bacterial pneumonia.
- The vast majority of pneumonia cases acquired in the community by otherwise healthy adults are due to one of two organisms: *S. pneumo-*

nia (*pneumococcus*) and *M. pneumoniae* (approximately 70% and 10–20% of all acute bacterial pneumonias in the United States, respectively). Community-acquired pneumonias caused by *Staphylococcus aureus* and gram-negative rods are observed primarily in the elderly, especially those residing in nursing homes, and in association with alcoholism and other debilitating conditions.

- Gram-negative aerobic bacilli and *S. aureus* are also the leading causative agents in hospital-acquired pneumonia.
- Anaerobic bacteria are the most common etiologic agents in pneumonia that follows the gross aspiration of gastric or oropharyngeal contents.
- Most pneumonias in the pediatric age group are due to viruses, especially respiratory syncytial virus, parainfluenza, and adenovirus.

CLINICAL PRESENTATION

Gram-Positive and Gram-Negative Bacterial Pneumonia

- Typically the onset of illness is abrupt or subacute, with fever, chills, dyspnea, and productive cough predominating. *Pneumococcus, staphylococcus,* the enteric gram-negative rods, and occasionally other organisms may produce local irritation or destruction of blood vessels leading to rust-colored sputum or hemoptysis.
- On physical examination the patient is tachypneic and tachycardiac, frequently with chest wall retractions and grunting respirations. There are diminished breath sounds on auscultation over the affected area accompanied by inspiratory crackles as pus-filled alveoli open during lung expansion.
- The chest radiograph and sputum examination and culture are the most useful diagnostic tests in gram-positive and gram-negative bacterial pneumonia. Gram stain of the expectorated sputum demonstrates many polymorphonuclear cells per high-powered field in the presence of a predominant organism, which is reflected in heavy growth of a single species on culture.
- The complete blood count usually reflects a leukocytosis with a predominance of polymorphonuclear cells. However, normal or mildly elevated WBC counts do not exclude bacterial pneumonic disease. The patient may also be hypoxic as reflected by low oxygen saturation on arterial blood gas or pulse oximetry.

Legionella pneumophilia

- Infection with *L. pneumophilia* is characterized by multisystem involvement, including rapidly progressive pneumonia. It has a gradual onset, with prominent constitutional symptoms such as malaise, lethargy, weakness, and anorexia occurring early in the course of the illness. A dry, nonproductive cough is initially present, which, during several days, becomes productive of mucoid or purulent sputum. Fevers exceeding 40°C develop in over half of patients and are typically unremitting and associated with a relative bradycardia. Pleuritic chest pain and progressive dyspnea may be seen, and fine rales are found on

VIII

lung exam, progressing to signs of frank consolidation later in the course of the illness. Extrapulmonary manifestations remain evident throughout the course of the illness and include diarrhea, nausea, vomiting, myalgias, and arthralgias.

- Substantial changes in a patient's mental status, often out of proportion to the degree of fever, are seen in approximately one-fourth of patients. Obtundation, hallucinations, grand mal seizures, and focal neurologic findings have also been associated with this illness. Laboratory findings include leukocytosis with predominance of mature and immature granulocytes in 50–75% of patients. Urinalysis may reveal proteinuria, hematuria, and casts; liver function tests (e.g., serum glutamic–oxaloacetic transaminase, serum glutamic–pyruvic transaminase, bilirubin) may be abnormal. Hyponatremia and hypophosphatemia have also been frequently reported.
- Because *L. pneumophilia* stains poorly with commonly used stains, routine microscopic examination of sputum is of little diagnostic value. In addition to diagnosis by culture, fluorescent antibody testing can be performed to diagnose Legionnaire's disease.

Anaerobic Pneumonia

- The course of anaerobic pneumonia is typically indolent with cough, low-grade fever, and weight loss, although an acute presentation may occur. Rigors are notably absent and bacteremia is rare. Putrid sputum, when present, is highly suggestive of the diagnosis. Chest radiographs reveal infiltrates typically located in dependent lung segments, and lung abscesses develop in 20% of patients 1–2 weeks into the course of the illness.

VIII

Mycoplasma pneumoniae

- *Mycoplasma pneumoniae* presents with a gradual onset of fever, headache, and malaise, with the appearance 3–5 days after the onset of illness of a persistent, hacking cough that initially is nonproductive. Sore throat, ear pain, and rhinorrhea are often present. Chills are only occasionally seen, and pleuritic pain is uncommon. Lung findings are generally limited to rales and rhonchi; findings of consolidation are rarely present.
- Nonpulmonary manifestations are extremely common and include nausea, vomiting, diarrhea, myalgias, arthralgias, polyarticular arthritis, skin rashes, myocarditis and pericarditis, hemolytic anemia, meningoencephalitis, cranial neuropathies, and Guillain–Barré syndrome. Systemic symptoms generally clear in 1–2 weeks, while respiratory symptoms may persist up to 4 weeks.
- Although the course of mycoplasmal pneumonia is usually benign and self-limited, severe respiratory disease may develop in patients with sickle cell disease, agammaglobulinemia, and chronic obstructive lung disease.
- Radiographic findings include patchy or interstitial infiltrates, which are most commonly seen in the lower lobes. Small unilateral, transient pleural effusions are common but large effusions and empyema are

TABLE 42.3. Empiric Antimicrobial Therapy for Pneumonia in Adults[a]

Clinical Setting	Usual Pathogen(s)	Presumptive Therapy
Previously healthy, ambulatory patient	Pneumococcus, *Mycoplasma pneumoniae*	Erythromycin, tetracycline
Elderly (nursing home residence)[b]	Pneumococcus, *Klebsiella pneumoniae*, *Staphylococcus aureus*, *Haemophilus influenzae*	Semisynthetic penicillin[c] plus aminoglycoside; or ticarcillin/clavulanate; cephalosporin[d]; imipenem
Chronic bronchitis	Pneumococcus, *H. influenzae*	Ampicillin, tetracycline, TMP-SMZ,[e] cefuroxime, amoxicillin/clavulanate
Alcoholism[b]	Pneumococcus, *K. pneumoniae*, *S. aureus*, *H. influenzae*	Semisynthetic penicillin[c] or ticarcillin/clavulanate plus aminoglycoside; cephalosporin[d]; imipenem
Aspiration		
Community	Mouth anaerobes	Penicillin or clindamycin
Hospital/residential care	Mouth anaerobes, *S. aureus*, gram-negative enterics	Penicillin or clindamycin plus aminoglycoside
Nosocomial pneumonia[b]	*K. pneumoniae*, *Enterobacter* spp., *Pseudomonas aeruginosa*, *S. aureus*, *Escherichia coli*	Ticarcillin, piperacillin, mezlocillin, aztreonam, or imipenem plus aminoglycoside, or ceftazidime

[a]See section on Treatment of Bacterial Pneumonia.
[b]Systemically effective quinolone may prove to be a viable alternative for initial therapy in these patients.
[c]Semisynthetic penicillin (e.g., nafcillin, oxacillin).
[d]Second- or third-generation cephalosporin (e.g., cefuroxime, ceftriaxone, cefotaxime, ceftazidime).
[e]TMP-SMZ, trimethoprim–sulfamethoxazole.
Adapted from Pennington JE. In Pennington JE (ed): Respiratory Infection: Diagnosis and Management. New York, Raven Press, 1983, with permission.

rare. Roentgenographic abnormalities resolve slowly, and 4–6 weeks may be required for complete resolution.

- Sputum Gram strain may reveal mononuclear or polymorphonuclear leukocytes, with no predominant organism. While *M. pneumoniae* can be cultured from respiratory secretions using specialized medium, 2–3 weeks may be necessary for culture identification.
- Indirect evidence of infection by *M. pneumoniae* is the presence of elevated levels of serum cold hemagglutinins. A definitive diagnosis can also be made by demonstrating a fourfold or greater rise in serum antibodies to *M. pneumoniae;* however, this test also requires 2–4 weeks for results.

Viral Pneumonia

- The clinical pictures produced by respiratory viruses are sufficiently variable and overlap to such a degree that an etiologic diagnosis cannot confidently be made on clinical grounds alone. Serologic tests for virus-specific antibodies are often used in the diagnosis of viral infections. The diagnostic four-fold rise in titer between acute and convalescent phase sera may require 2–3 weeks to develop; however, same-day diagnosis of viral infections is now possible through the use of indirect immunofluorescence tests on exfoliated cells from the respiratory tract.

- Radiographic findings are nonspecific and include bronchial wall thickening and perihilar and diffuse interstitial infiltrates.
- Pleural effusions may be seen especially in adenovirus and parainfluenza pneumonia.

TREATMENT

- The treatment of bacterial pneumonia initially involves the empiric use of a relatively broad-spectrum antibiotic (or antibiotics) that is effective against probable pathogens after appropriate cultures and specimens for laboratory evaluation have been obtained.
- Therapy should be narrowed to cover specific pathogens once the results of cultures are known.
- Appropriate empiric choices for the treatment of bacterial pneumonias relative to a patient's underlying disease are shown in Table 42.3 for adults and Table 42.4 for children.

VIII

TABLE 42.4. Empiric Antimicrobial Therapy for Pneumonia in Pediatric Patients

Age	Usual Pathogen(s)	Presumptive Therapy
1 month	Group B *streptococcus*, *Haemophilus influenzae* (nontypable), *Escherichia coli*, *Staphylococcus aureus*	Ampicillin/sulbactam, aminoglycoside, or cephalosporin[a]; imipenem
	CMV, RSV, adenovirus	Ribavirin for RSV
1–3 months	*Chlamydia, Ureaplasma*, CMV, *Pneumocystis carinii* (afebrile pneumonia syndrome)	Erythromycin, TMP–SMZ
	RSV	Ribavirin
	Pneumococcus, S. aureus	Semisynthetic penicillin[b] or cephalosporin[a]
3 months–6 years	Pneumococcus, *H. influenzae*, RSV, adenovirus, parainfluenza	Ampicillin or cephalosporin[c] Ampicillin/sulbactam Ribavirin for RSV
>6 years	Pneumococcus, *Mycoplasma pneumoniae*, adenovirus	Erythromycin

Key: CMV, cytomegalovirus; RSV, respiratory syncytial virus; TMP–SMZ, trimethoprim–sulfamethoxazole.
[a]Third-generation cephalosporin (e.g., ceftriaxone, cefotaxime).
[b]Semisynthetic penicillin (e.g., nafcillin, oxacillin).
[c]Second-generation cephalosporin (e.g., cefuroxime, cefprozil).

- The supportive care of the patient with pneumonia includes the use of humidified oxygen for hypoxemia, administration of bronchodilators when bronchospasm is present, and chest physiotherapy with postural drainage if there is evidence of retained secretions.
- Important therapeutic adjuncts include adequate hydration (by intravenous route if necessary), optimal nutritional support, and fever control.
- Antibiotic concentrations in respiratory secretions in excess of the pathogen minimum inhibitory concentration (MIC) are necessary for successful treatment of pulmonary infections.
- The benefit of antibiotic aerosols or direct endotracheal instillation has not been consistently demonstrated.
- Prevention of pneumonia is possible through the use of vaccines against *S. pneumoniae* and *H. influenzae* type B. In addition, amantadine may be administered for prevention of influenza A infection, beginning as soon as possible after exposure and continuing for at least 10 days.

See Chapter 100, Lower Respiratory Tract Infections, authored by Philip Toltzis, MD, Madolin K. Witte, MD, and Michael D. Reed, PharmD, for a more detailed discussion of this topic.

VIII

Chapter 43

▶ RESPIRATORY TRACT INFECTIONS, UPPER

▶ OTITIS MEDIA

DEFINITION

Otitis media is a nonspecific term describing an inflammation of the middle ear. Acute otitis media involves the rapid onset of signs and symptoms of inflammation in the middle ear that manifests clinically as one or more of the following: otalgia (denoted by pulling of the ear in some infants), hearing loss, fever, or irritability. Otitis media with effusion (accumulation of liquid in the middle ear cavity) differs from acute otitis media in that signs and symptoms of an acute infection are absent. Chronic purulent otitis media is characterized by a chronic inflammation of the middle ear and the mastoid, with purulent otorrhea, in the presence of a perforated tympanic membrane or of tympanostomy tubes.

EPIDEMIOLOGY AND ETIOLOGY

- Acute otitis media is the most frequent diagnosis in infants and children who visit physicians because of illness.
- Acute episodes are more frequent during the first 3 years of life, with the peak incidence occurring between 9 and 12 months. By the age of 7, it is estimated that >93% of the children will have experienced otitis media, and >40% will have had over three episodes.
- Risk factors contribute to the higher incidence and increased frequency of otitis media.
  - The earlier children experience their first episode of otitis media, the greater the risk of developing more severe, persistent, and recurrent episodes.
  - A history of recurrent acute otitis media or respiratory tract infections in a sibling, parental smoking, and attendance at a day-care center may increase the risk of otitis media.
  - The frequency of otitis media is greater in winter months and appears to parallel the outbreaks of viral infections of the respiratory tract.
  - Males are more prone to episodes of acute otitis media and are at a greater risk for recurrent disease.
  - The incidence of acute otitis media is more predominant in Caucasians than in the African-American population. Native Americans and Inuit represent a population in which this disease is severe, widespread, and recurrent.
  - Breast-feeding appears in most studies as a significant protective factor in the development of otitis media.

- Several studies have suggested that children with allergies, atopy, and immunoglobulin G (in particular IgG_2) deficiencies exhibit a higher risk of acute otitis media.
- A correlation between crowded living and poor sanitary conditions and middle ear disease has been noted.

Microbiology

- Bacterial cultures from the middle ear effusion of children over 1 month of age with acute, symptomatic otitis media have yielded strains of *Streptococcus pneumoniae* (30%), predominantly nontypable strains of *Haemophilus influenzae* (21%), *Moxarella catarrhalis* (12%).
- In infants younger than 1 month, *Staphylococcus* are found in higher frequency.
- The incidence of β-lactamase positive *H. influenzae* has been reported to range from 30–40% of all *H. influenzae*. A high rate of β-lactamase production (70–90%) by *M. catarrhalis* has also been documented.

PATHOPHYSIOLOGY

- With otitis media the patient has an antecedent event that results in congestion of the respiratory mucosa, causing secretions to accumulate in the middle ear.
- Bacteria present in the middle ear proliferate in the secretions resulting in acute otitis media.
- In recurrent episodes of acute otitis media or otitis media with effusion, anatomic or physiologic abnormalities of the eustachian tube are the most important factors.
- Abnormal function of the eustachian tube can cause reflux, aspiration, or insufflation of nasopharyngeal bacteria up to the middle ear.
- In infants, the difference in angulation of the eustachian tube may cause improper drainage of the middle ear as a result of decreased gravitational effects on the eustachian tube. It has also been noted that the eustachian tubes are shorter than those of adults. This can impair the capillary action needed to prevent nasopharyngeal reflux.

CLINICAL PRESENTATION

- Clinical presentation may include nonspecific symptoms such as lethargy, anorexia, vomiting, or diarrhea.
- The tympanic membrane is opaque, bulging, and has limited or no mobility to pneumatic otoscopy, all indicative of a middle ear effusion.
- Otorrhea (purulent discharge) through perforation of the tympanic membrane or through tympanostomy tubes, accompanied by otalgia and fever, is also indicative of acute otitis media.
- Redness of the tympanic membrane is not pathognomonic since it can result from sneezing, coughing, crying, or fever.
- The presence of otalgia, partial deafness (secondary to effusion), fever, and a sudden onset of irritability are symptoms that characterize acute otitis media.

VIII

- Inflammation or opacity of the tympanic membrane, the presence or absence of light reflection, and bulging of the tympanic membrane are all suggestive of otitis media.
- Complications and sequella of otitis media are categorized as intracranial (meningitis and brain abscess) and intratemporal (eardrum diseases). The latter are more frequent and can result in hearing loss.

TREATMENT

- There is no universally accepted method of management of otitis media.
- Oral antibiotics are still the mainstay of therapy. However, the common practice of antibiotic administration for otitis media has been questioned.
- The selection of the appropriate antibiotic is based on antimicrobial susceptibility, penetration into the middle ear, clinical efficacy, compliance factors, adverse effects profile, and cost.
- Amoxicillin and ampicillin, with excellent in vitro activity against *S. pneumoniae* and most *H. influenzae* isolates from the middle ear, are still the first choice in the treatment of acute otitis media in areas where the emergence of β-lactamase-producing *H. influenzae* and *M. catarrhalis* is limited (Table 43.1). The addition of the β-lactamase inhibitor clavulanic acid to amoxicillin increases its activity against aminopenicillin-resistant strains of *H. influenzae* and *M. catarrhalis*.

Penetration into the Middle Ear Fluid

- In addition to having adequate in vitro antimicrobial activity, bactericidal concentrations of the antimicrobial agent need to be present in the middle ear fluid. Table 43.2 presents the available data in terms of ratio between middle ear fluid concentrations (MEFC) of antimicrobials to minimal inhibitory concentrations (MIC_{90}), the lowest MIC required to inhibit 90% of the bacterial strains tested, of the three primary pathogens.
- Table 43.3 summarizes the recommended doses and dosing schedules of the primary antimicrobials utilized in the treatment of upper respiratory tract infections. Short dosing intervals and the recommended 10-day course of antimicrobial therapy for acute otitis media certainly represent contributory factors to noncompliance. A shortened therapy duration of 5 days with amoxicillin has shown comparable efficacy for children whose disease responds rapidly.
- Amoxicillin remains the antibiotic of choice for the treatment of acute otitis media despite the concerns about increasing incidence of β-lactamase production among *H. influenzae* and *M. cattarhalis*. In the setting of increased resistance to β-lactam agents, trimethoprim–sulfamethoxazole (TMP–SMX) and amoxicillin–clavulanate are appropriate choices. TMP–SMX may not be effective when *Streptococcus pyogenes* (group A hemolytic streptococcus) is the causative organism.
- Supportive therapy with analgesics, antipyretics, and local heat have been shown to be beneficial in the comfort of the child with otitis media.

VIII

TABLE 43.1. In Vitro Spectrum of Activity of Antibiotics Used in Upper Respiratory Tract Infections

	Streptococcus pneumoniae	Haemophilus influenzae		Moxarella catarrhalis		Group A β-Hemolytic Streptococci
		β-Lactamase Negative	Positive	β-Lactamase Negative	Positive	
Ampicillin or amoxicillin	+	+	–	+	–	+
Azithromycin	+	+	+	+	+	+
Clarithromycin/ 14-hydroxyclarithromycin	+	+	+	+	+	+
Erythromycin	+	–	–	+	+	+
Erythromycin–sulfisoxazole	+	+	+	+	+	+
Trimethoprim–sulfamethoxazole	+	+	+	+	+	–
Amoxicillin–clavulanate	+	+	+	+	+	+
Cefaclor	+	+	±|	+	+	+
Cefixime	+	+	+	+	+	+
Cefpodoxime proxetil	+	+	+	+	+	+
Cefprozil	+	+	+	+	+	+
Cefuroxime axetil	+	+	+	+	+	+
Loracarbef	+	+	+	+	+	+

Key: +, highly susceptible; ±, moderately susceptible; –, nonsusceptible.

TABLE 43.2. Relationship Between the Concentration of Antimicrobials Used in Otitis Media and the MIC$_{90}$ of the Three Primary Microorganisms

	Streptococcus pneumoniae	Haemophilus influenzae β-Lactamase		Moxarella catarrhalis β-Lactamase	
		Negative	Positive	Negative	Positive
Amoxicillin	>+++++[a]	++	0	>+++++	0
Ampicillin	>+++++	++	0	++	0
Cefaclor	+	+	+	-	+
Cefixime	+	>+++++	+	>+++++	+
Cefprozil	>+++++	++	++	0	0
Cefuroxime axetil	>+++++	>+++++	ND[b]	>+++++	ND
Clarithromycin/14-hydroxy-	>+++++	0	0	++	+++
clarithromycin	>+++++	0	0	>+++++	>+++++
Erythromycin					
-estolate	++	0	0	++	++
-ethylsuccinate	+	0	0	++	++
Loracarbef	++	+	+	>+++++	+
Trimethoprim	+	++	++	0	0
Sulamethoxazole	+	+++	++	ND	ND

[a]Relationship between the antimicrobial maximum concentration in middle ear fluid and the MIC$_{90}$; each + indicates that the antimicrobial concentration is onefold above the MIC$_{90}$; >+++++ indicates that the concentrations exceed the MIC$_{90}$ fivefold; 0 indicates that the antimicrobial concentration is less than onefold the MIC$_{90}$.

[b]ND, no data available.

VIII

519

TABLE 43.3. Pediatric Dosing Regimen and Cost of Antibiotics Used in Upper Respiratory Tract Infections

Antibiotic(s)	Total Daily Dose and Regimen	Cost ($)[a]	Liquid Formulation (mg/5 mL)
Penicillin V	50 mg/kg (every 6 h)	3.36[b]	125–250
Amoxicillin	30–40 mg/kg (every 8 h)	4.08[b]	125–250
Pivampicillin	40–50 mg/kg (every 12 h)	18.00[c]	175
Amoxicillin–clavulanate (4:1)	30 mg/kg of amoxicillin (every 8 h)	38.48	125/31.25–250/62.5
TMP–SMX (1:5)	8–10 mg/kg TMP (every 12 h)	6.05[b]	40/200
Cefaclor	40 mg/kg (every 8–12 h)	55.23	125–250
Cefixime	8 mg/kg (every 12–24 h)	46.06	100
Cefpodoxime proxetil	10 mg/kg (every 12 h)	54.00	50–100
Cefprozil	30 mg/kg (every 12 h)	60.36	125–250
Loracarbef	30 mg/kg (every 12 h)	70.20	100
Erythromycin–sulfisoxazole (1:3)	40 mg/kg of erythromycin (every 8 h)	16.12	200/600
Erythromycin ethylsuccinate	30 mg/kg (every 6–8 h)	7.86[b]	200–400
Erythromycin estolate	30 mg/kg (every 6–8 h)	13.99[b]	125–250

[a]Cost based on average wholesale price (Redbook, 1994).
[b]Cost based on generic price.
[c]Cost based on Canadian availability.

VIII

- Although antihistamines and decongestants have been used for the symptomatic relief of acute otitis media, studies have not shown them to be efficacious in the resolution of effusion or relief of symptoms.
- Until studies can support their efficacy, the use of oral decongestants such as pseudoephedrine or phenylpropanolamine should be limited to 1 or 2 days of treatment, if any.

Recurrent Acute Otitis Media

- If the signs and symptoms of acute otitis media occur within 1 month of the initial episode, it is assumed that the same microorganism caused the infection. This new episode should be treated with a different antibiotic, preferably one with β-lactamase activity.
- If the new episode occurs over 1 month after the initial infection in a child who was completely free of signs and symptoms between episodes, the management of the recurrent episodes is the same as the first episode.
- If children exhibit more than four episodes in a 6-month period or six episodes in a 12-month period, these patients can be managed by chemoprophylaxis with antimicrobials, and/or myringotomy and insertion of tympanostomy tubes.
- The most popular surgical approach to the treatment of recurrent episodes of otitis media is myringotomy and insertion of tympanostomy tubes.

Chronic Purulent Otitis Media

- On examination of an infant or child presenting with chronic otorrhetic discharge, the pus is suctioned and the external canal is cleansed prior to culturing the middle ear.
- After the invading pathogen(s) has been identified or speculated, therapy is initiated with an oral drug that is active against β-lactamase–producing organisms.
- Amoxicillin with clavulanic acid, cefuroxime axetil, cefaclor, cefixime, and erythromycin ethylsuccinate with sulfisoxazole are first-line agents. The use of fluoroquinolones, such as ciprofloxacin, can be considered in adults.
- Daily aural hygiene is useful in preventing reinfection and aiding in the healing process of the tympanic membrane. Cleansing agents such as carbamide peroxide (Debrox) and solutions containing propylene glycol should be used cautiously when perforation or transtympanic tubes are present. Hydrogen peroxide solution (3%) diluted as 1:1 or 1:3 with sterile water is a valuable aural cleanser for pus and debris removal.

Chemoprophylaxis

- Prophylactic therapy appears to have beneficial but limited effect on recurrent otitis media, should be initiated during the winter and early spring when recurrences are highest, and continued for 3 months or until there is a failure of therapy. VIII
- The following regimens have been advocated: (1) amoxicillin (20–30 mg/kg/d) in one dose at bedtime or in two divided doses every 12 hours; (2) sulfisoxazole (80–100 mg/kg/d) every 24 hours; and (3) TMP–SMX (equivalent of 4 mg/kg/d of TMP) every 24 hours.
- In children >2 years of age, the use of antipneumococcal vaccines can reduce occurrence of acute otitis media by approximately 10–20% (33% in day-care centers).

EVALUATION OF THERAPEUTIC OUTCOMES

- With proper treatment, symptoms of acute otitis media in most children will abate within 24–72 hours. When otalgia or fever persists or recurs during therapy, a β-lactamase–producing microorganism should be suspected and an agent with β-lactamase activity should be used (Figure 43.1).
- If treatment with the second-line agent fails, tympanocentesis to identify the pathogen may be indicated, particularly if the child is symptomatic or has an underlying disease.
- All children should be reexamined at the end of the 10-day antibiotic therapy. Even with an efficacious antibiotic treatment, effusion of the middle ear may be present in 50% of children following treatment with antibiotics and may persist for up to 3 months. If the middle ear effusion persists beyond the initial 10 days of antimicrobial therapy several options can be considered:

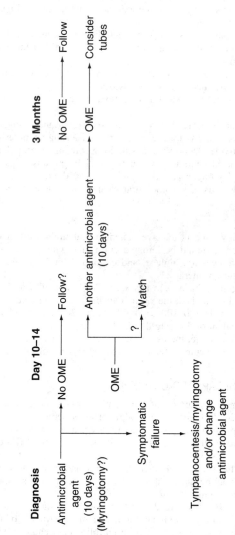

Figure 43.1. Recommended management plan for children with acute otitis media. OME, otitis media with effusion. *(From Bluestone CD. Pediatr Infect Dis J 1988;7:S129–136, with permission.)*

1. Another course of drug therapy using the same agent or an alternative antibiotic; one with β-lactamase activity is preferable if resistant strains are prevalent in the community;
2. Topical or systemic decongestants, antihistamines, or a combination of these;
3. Systemic corticosteroids or eustachian tube–middle ear inflation. If the effusion persists beyond 2–3 months, it is termed otitis media with effusion and should be treated as described in the Treatment section.

▶ PHARYNGITIS

Pharyngitis is an inflammation of the pharynx and surrounding lymphoid tissue that may be of viral or bacterial origin.

ETIOLOGY

- Viruses appear to be the cause of the majority of episodes, often as constituents of the common cold. However, a significant number are of bacterial origin, with group A β-hemolytic streptococci *(Streptococcus pyogenes)* being the most prevalent microorganism.
- In children <3 years of age, the etiology is usually viral; the peak incidence of group A β-hemolytic streptococci is between 5 and 10 years of age.
- Bacterial pathogens constitute 5–30% of all pharyngitis and the symptomatology generally overlaps that of viral pharyngitis.
- Group A β-hemolytic streptococci is the most prevalent bacterial pathogen in symptomatic pharyngitis (25–50%).

VIII

CLINICAL PRESENTATION

- In the majority of cases of acute pharyngitis, it is not possible to differentiate, on a clinical basis, between viral and bacterial etiology.
- Fever, sore throat, anterior cervical adenopathies, headache, abdominal pain, erythema of the pharynx, tonsillar exudate, lymphatic hyperplasia, and scarlatiniform rash are suggestive of group A β-hemolytic streptococci pharyngitis.
- Scarlet fever, rash, impetigo, and infected ulcers around the nostrils and the mouth are indicative of a streptococcal infection.
- The question of "to culture or not" is currently still debated. Table 43.4 lists the criteria for the identification of individuals with pharyngitis in whom a culture for identification of group A β-hemolytic streptococci is currently recommended. Rapid streptococcal tests are available for the identification of group A β-hemolytic streptococci.
- A rapid diagnosis for the prevention of acute rheumatic fever is not essential, since antibiotic therapy can be initiated as late as 9 days after the onset of streptococcal pharyngitis and still be effective.

TABLE 43.4. Conditions Where a Throat Culture is Recommended in Pharyngitis

Children aged 3–15 years, with an elevated temperature and sore throat as the primary complaint

Close contact with a person with streptococcal pharyngitis

Individuals with a history of rheumatic fever or heart disease

Epidemic of the following pathogens:
   Group A β-hemolytic streptococcus
   Corynebacterium diphtheriae

Individuals presenting with pharyngitis and one or more of the following signs and symptoms:
   Fever
   Anterior cervical adenopathy
   Tonsillar exudate
   Beefy red color of pharynx
   Lymphatic hyperplasia
   Scarlatiniform rash

TREATMENT

- The treatment of viral pharyngitis is symptomatic.
- Appropriate antibiotic therapy for group A β-hemolytic streptococci infection prevents acute rheumatic fever, reduces the period of contagion, limits the spread of infection, and reduces the incidence of suppurative complications.
- Many antimicrobial agents are appropriate choices in the treatment of group A β-hemolytic streptococci pharyngitis. These agents include penicillin, amoxicillin, ampicillin, several cephalosporins, erythromycin, and erythromycin–sulfisoxazole.
- Antibiotic selection should take into account treatment failures, the presence of copathogens, and cost.
- Penicillin remains the mainstay of therapy for patients infected with group A β-hemolytic streptococci. Children with group A β-hemolytic streptococci pharyngitis should receive penicillin V 25–50 mg/kg/d in two to four divided doses given orally for 10 days, or benzathine penicillin 25,000–50,000 U/kg intramuscularly as a single dose.
- For the penicillin-allergic patient, erythromycin estolate 20–30 mg/kg/d in two to four divided doses or erythromycin ethylsuccinate 40–50 mg/kg/d in two to four divided doses for 10 days are suitable alternatives. However, resistance of group A β-hemolytic streptococci to erythromycin has been observed in the United States in approximately 5% of the strains isolated.
- Cephalexin, taken three to four times daily, and cefadroxil, in a once-daily administration, have been demonstrated to be more effective in eradicating group A β-hemolytic streptococci than penicillin. However, penicillin V is the only agent prospectively shown to reduce the incidence of rheumatic fever due to group A β-hemolytic streptococci.

Evaluation of Therapeutic Outcomes

- Bacteriologic treatment failure rates with 10 days of oral penicillin V approximate 30–35%. A shorter course of therapy can increase the failure rate.
- For a relapse, it is appropriate to change the antimicrobial agent. Cephalosporins with β-lactamase activity are good alternatives. If a new strain is present, the initial antimicrobial can be reinstated.
- With persistent recurrent episodes, penicillin for 10 days with rifampin for the last 4 days is suggested.

▶ SINUSITIS

EPIDEMIOLOGY AND ETIOLOGY

- Sinusitis is a common condition affecting children and adults and is associated with both bacterial and viral infections of the upper respiratory tract.
- Children have between six and eight common colds per year depending on age, number of siblings, and type of day-care services. Adults experience approximately two to three common colds per year, and incidence may increase while parenting or working with young children. Of these upper respiratory infections, 1–5% will be complicated by acute sinusitis.
- The predominant organisms causing sinusitis are *S. pneumoniae* (31–36%), nontypable *H. influenzae* (21–23%), and *M. catarrhalis* (2–19%). Infrequently encountered bacteria include *S. pyogenes, S. aureus,* and anaerobic bacteria such as *Peptostreptococcus, Fusobacterium,* and *Bacteroides melaninogenicus.*

PATHOPHYSIOLOGY

- Conditions that affect patency of the sinus ostia, normal function of the mucociliary sinus epithelium, normal immune defenses of the upper respiratory tract, or events that introduce microorganisms into the sinuses predispose to sinus infections.
- Bacterial and viral infections of the respiratory tract and allergic inflammation are conditions that cause sinus ostia obstruction, and lead to retention of secretions.
- The indirect introduction of microorganisms through dental extractions and infections of the maxillary molar teeth predisposes to maxillary and chronic sinusitis.

CLINICAL PRESENTATION

- The most commonly encountered symptoms with sinusitis include mucopurulent nasal discharge, nasal congestion, tenderness over the involved sinus, and fever. An usually severe cold characterized by high fever (>39.0°C), purulent and viscous nasal discharge, hyposmia (abnormal decrease in sensitivity to odors), facial pain over the affected sinuses that worsens with movement, and periorbital swelling with or without headache may be indicative of bacterial sinusitis.

- Headaches caused by sinusitis are common. The pain corresponds to the sinuses affected and is described as a feeling of fullness or a dull ache.
- In addition to history and physical examination, the diagnosis of sinusitis may require cytologic examination of nasal aspirates, transillumination of maxillary and frontal sinuses for patients older than 10 years of age, radiography, ultrasonography, computed tomography, and magnetic resonance imaging.
- On microscopic examination of fresh nasal secretions, a high concentration of polymorphonuclear cells with intracellular bacteria is often observed.
- A differentiation between chronic sinusitis and allergic rhinitis can be made when *eosinophils* predominate. If the smear is devoid of eosinophils, chronic sinusitis can be suspected.
- Currently, the microbial etiology of patients presenting with sinusitis can only be determined by direct sinus aspiration. This procedure is recommended in the following situations:

1. Patients with sinusitis who fail conventional therapy
2. Immunosuppressed patients with sinusitis
3. Severe headache and facial pain
4. In the presence of life-threatening complications such as intraorbital or intracranial suppuration

TREATMENT

- Many symptoms of sinusitis will resolve without medical therapy within 48 hours. When they persist, pharmacotherapy should be directed toward symptomatic relief, restoring and improving sinus function, preventing intracranial complications, and eradicating the causative pathogen(s).
- Antibiotics are the mainstay of therapy of sinusitis. Amoxicillin is an appropriate agent for most uncomplicated cases of sinusitis.
- If β-lactamase–resistant strains are suspected, the patient is allergic to penicillin, the presentation is accompanied by mild periorbital edema, or if there is an apparent antibiotic failure, alternative regimens can be used, such as trimethoprim–sulfamethoxazole for group A streptococcal infections, cefaclor, erythromycin–sulfisoxazole, amoxicillin–clavulanate, loracarbef, and azithromycin.
- Acute sinusitis is treated for 10–14 days, but duration can be extended to 30 days in protracted cases.
- Vasoconstrictor sprays or drops such as xylometazoline or oxymetazoline may facilitate drainage. The use of such agents should not exceed >72 hours owing to a tolerance effect and possible rebound congestion.

VIII

► EPIGLOTTITIS AND CROUP

- Epiglottitis and croup are two distinct entities, both resulting from infections of the laryngeal area (Table 43.5). Noisy breathing is characteristic of these two clinical diseases. They both cause airway obstruction but at different anatomic sites.

EPIGLOTTITIS

- Epiglottitis is a true airway emergency in which acute airway obstruction can occur.
- It is caused primarily by *H. influenzae* type B.
- Epiglottitis is more prevalent in children ages 2–6. The onset of the disease is rapid and the evolution is often brisk. Fever, sore throat, dysphagia, dysphonia, and sialorrhea (excessive secretion of saliva) are acute signs and symptoms of the disease.
- Airway obstruction evolves rapidly and manifests by respiratory distress, irritability, fatigue, and anxiety.

Treatment

- The primary concern in the management of epiglottitis is establishing and maintaining the airway.
- Initial therapy may involve the use of a moist oxygen tent to help facilitate the breathing.

VIII

TABLE 43.5. Differentiating Clinical Features of Epiglottitis and Croup

Feature	Epiglottitis	Croup
Age	3–7 years	>3 years
Gender	Male = Female	Male > Female
Season	All seasons	Late spring and late fall
Pathogens(s)	Bacterial: *H. influenzae* B	Viral: parainfluenzae (type 1, 2 and 3)
Progression	Rapid	Slow (generally at night)
Clinical presentation	Sitting, toxic, typical posture	Supine, nontoxic, barking cough
Dysphagia	Marked, occasional drooling	None
Fever	>39.4°C (103°F)	<39.4°C (103°F)
Stridor	Rare	Frequent
WBC	>18,000 mm^3	Normal
Treatment	Parenteral antibiotics, intubation	Cool mist, racemic epinephrine
Recurrence	Rare	Common

- In severe cases, endotracheal intubation or a tracheostomy may be required.
- Antibiotic therapy should be instituted if epiglottitis is suspected and empirically directed against *H. influenzae* type B.
- The combination of ampicillin 200 mg/kg/d and chloramphenicol 100 mg/kg/d (maximum 4 g/d) both given intravenously, provides coverage of ampicillin-resistant microorganisms until sensitivities are known. The second- or third-generation cephalosporins cefuroxime (100–150 mg/kg/d given every 8 hours), cefotaxime (50–100 mg/kg/d given every 6 hours), or ceftriaxone (50–75 mg/kg/d given every 12 hours) are appropriate and often preferred.
- Recommended duration of treatment is 7–10 days.

CROUP

- In contrast to epiglottitis, croup is often preceded by a prodrome (e.g., a common cold), and its onset and progression are less rapid.
- Viral croup (acute laryngotracheobronchitis) is caused primarily by parainfluenzae (type 1 and 2).
- Typically, children <3 years of age are affected, with a majority of the cases appearing during the cold and flu season.
- Persistent spontaneous cough, stridor, hoarseness of the voice, and a barking cough are suggestive of croup.
- In the majority of episodes, the child will fully recover without any specific treatment.

Treatment

- Each episode of croup should be considered individually because some patients may benefit from simple therapy, whereas others may require a more complex approach.
- Ambient air humidification and ingestion of liquids can prevent the drying and crusting of the inflamed mucosa, and help to liquefy exudates. In minor cases, these treatments can be performed at home (the child is placed in the bathroom with a warm running shower).
- Because of its drying effect, oxygen therapy should be reserved for cyanotic children. In most serious cases, racemic epinephrine inhalation may provide relief. The recommended doses are 0.25 mL of a 2.25% solution of racemic epinephrine for children less than 6 months old and 0.5 mL for older children.
- Since croup is almost exclusively viral in nature, antibiotic therapy is not indicated. Children with persistent fever (more than 4 days) and those showing a deterioration of their condition should be empirically treated with antibiotic to prevent possible subsequent bacterial superinfection.

See Chapter 101, Upper Respiratory Tract Infections, authored by Monique Richer, PharmD, BCPS, and Marc LeBel, PharmD, FCCP, FCSHP, for a more detailed discussion of this topic.

VIII

Chapter 44

► SEPSIS AND SEPTIC SHOCK

► DEFINITION

A joint committee of the American College of Chest Physicians and the Society of Critical Care Medicine has standardized the terminology related to sepsis (Table 44.1).

► EPIDEMIOLOGY AND ETIOLOGY

- More than 200,000 episodes of gram-negative sepsis occur annually, resulting in nearly 100,000 deaths.
- The incidence of septicemia from all microorganisms (defined as systemic disease associated with the presence and persistence of pathogenic microorganisms or their toxins in the blood) increased 139% between 1979 and 1987, from 73.6 to 175.9 cases per 100,000 persons.
- The major offenders in gram-negative sepsis are the members of the families Enterobacteriaceae *(Escherichia, Klebsiella, Enterobacter, Serratia,* and *Proteus)* and Pseudomonadaceae.
- A factor important to the epidemiology of gram-negative infection is the host's loss of colonization resistance. Colonization resistance is the normal host flora that inhibits overgrowth of potentially pathogenic organisms.
- Community-acquired gram-negative infection usually arises from the endogenous flora in the biliary, urinary, or genital tracts.
- The outcome of gram-negative infection is determined by organism virulence and host susceptibility. The effect of differences in organism virulence is demonstrated in Table 44.2 for single bloodstream isolates and their corresponding frequency and mortality.

► PATHOPHYSIOLOGY

- Figure 44.1 depicts a schematic representation of the pathogenesis of gram-negative sepsis and septic shock.
- The pathophysiologic focus of gram-negative sepsis has been on the lipopolysaccharide (endotoxin) component of the gram-negative cell wall. Lipid A is a part of the endotoxin molecule that is highly immunoreactive and is responsible for most of the toxic effects. Endotoxin first associates with a protein called lipopolysaccharide binding protein in plasma. This complex then engages a specific receptor (CD14) on the surface of the macrophage which activates it and causes release of inflammatory mediators.
- Some of the mediators involved include tumor necrosis factor α (TNF-α), interleukin 1 (IL-1), interleukin 6 (IL-6) (produced by macrophages), as

TABLE 44.1. Definitions Related to Sepsis

Condition	Definition
Bacteremia	The presence of viable bacteria in the blood.
Systemic inflammatory response syndrome (SIRS)	The systemic inflammatory response to a variety of severe clinical insults. The response is manifested by two or more of the following conditions: Temperature >38°C or <36°C Heart rate >90 beats/min Respiratory rate >20 breaths/min or $Paco_2$ <32 torr (<4.3 kPa) WBC > 12,000 cells/mm^3, <4000 cells/mm^3, or >10% immature (band) forms.
Sepsis	The systemic response to infection. This systemic response is manifested by two or more of the following conditions as a result of infection: Temperature >38°C or <36°C Heart rate >90 beats/min Respiratory rate >20 breaths/min or $Paco_2$ <32 torr (<4.3 kPa) WBC >12,000 cells/mm^3, <4000 cells/mm^3, or >10% immature (band) forms.
Severe sepsis	Sepsis associated with organ dysfunction, hypoperfusion, or hypotension. Hypoperfusion and perfusion abnormalities may include, but are not limited to, lactic acidosis, oliguria, or an acute alteration in mental status.
Septic shock	Sepsis with hypotension, despite adequate fluid resuscitation, along with the presence of perfusion abnormalities that may include, but are not limited to, lactic acidosis, oliguria, or an acute alteration in mental status. Patients who are on inotropic or vasopressor agents may not be hypotensive at the time perfusion abnormalities are measured.
Hypotension	A systolic blood pressure of <90 mm Hg or a reduction of >40 mm Hg from baseline in the absence of other causes for hypotension.
Multiple organ dysfunction syndrome	Presence of altered organ function in an acutely ill patient such that homeostasis cannot be maintained without intervention.

VIII

TABLE 44.2. Gram-Negative Bacteremia

Frequency	Mortality
Escherichia coli	*Pseudomonas aeruginosa*
Klebsiella pneumoniae	*Klebsiella* sp.
Serratia[a]	*Proteus* sp.[a]
Enterobacter[a]	*E. coli*[a]
Proteus sp.[a]	*Enterobacter*[a]

[a]Rank order not significant.

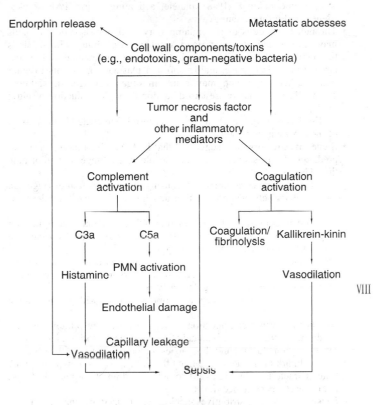

Figure 44.1. Pathogenesis of septic shock. PMN, polymorphonuclear leukocyte; ARDS, adult respiratory distress syndrome; SVR, systemic vascular resistance; CO, cardiac output.

well as interleukin 8 (IL-8), platelet activating factor (PAF), leukotrienes, and thromboxane A_2.

- Through the actions of the inflammatory mediators a variety of cells may become activated. A primary mechanism of injury with sepsis is through endothelial cells. With inflammation, endothelial cells allow circulating cells (e.g., granulocytes) and plasma constituents to enter inflamed tissues, which may result in organ damage. In addition, endothelial cells may cause vasodilatation through production of nitric oxide.
- TNF-α has received much attention because it is elevated in the plasma of most patients with sepsis.
- Some investigators have suggested that IL-6 may be a more consistent predictor of sepsis since it remains elevated for a longer period of time than TNF-α.
- Endotoxin activates complement, causing direct activation of Hageman factor, which activates coagulation and fibrinolysis and the release of vasoactive peptides.
- Disseminated intravascular coagulation (DIC), a frequent complication of gram-negative sepsis, is attributed to the activation of coagulation factor XII (Hageman factor) by endotoxin.
- Severe bleeding, thrombosis, tissue ischemia and necrosis, hemolysis, and major organ failure may result from disturbances induced by gram-negative bacteria on the coagulation systems.
- Shock is the most ominous complication associated with gram-negative sepsis.
- Another important complication of sepsis is acute respiratory distress syndrome (ARDS). Approximately 25% of patients with gram-negative sepsis develop ARDS, and this carries a mortality rate of 60–90%.
- The hallmark of the hemodynamic effect of sepsis is the hyperdynamic state characterized by high cardiac output and an abnormally low systemic vascular resistance (SVR).
- Sepsis results in distributive shock characterized by inappropriately increased blood flow to selected tissue at the expense of other tissue independent of oxygen needs.
- The pathophysiologic spectrum of sepsis is an exaggerated inflammatory response to the presence of bacteria or endotoxin in the bloodstream.

VIII

▶ DESIRED OUTCOME

The primary objective of treatment for sepsis is survival of the patient. Secondary objectives include avoidance of organ failure (renal, hepatic, cardiac, and pulmonary) and other complications. Ideally, this would be done without the occurrence of adverse drug effects. Important outcome measures include length of intensive care unit and hospital stays.

▶ TREATMENT

- The detection and elimination of septic sources, appropriate antimicrobial therapy, and comprehensive support care (including hemodynamic monitoring, adequate volume, pressor, and metabolic support) are the cornerstones in the management of sepsis and septic shock.
- An algorithmic approach to the management of sepsis is shown in Figure 44.2.

ANTIMICROBIAL THERAPY

The following principles are useful guides in initiating antimicrobial therapy.

- Empiric antimicrobial therapy must be comprehensive, it should cover all likely pathogens in the context of the clinical setting. Selection of specific agents for empiric regimens should be considered on the basis of individual institution sensitivity patterns.
- Therapy should be initiated rapidly to clear the bloodstream of bacteria before the development of the complications of sepsis.
- A seriously ill patient or one who is in shock should be treated only with intravenous antibiotics.
- Loading doses, particularly with aminoglycosides, should be given to maximize initial effect. Adjust aminoglycoside doses according to serum levels and the functional state of the kidneys.
- If the pathogen is known, targeted antimicrobial therapy should be instituted.
- Table 44.3 provides suggestions for the selection of antimicrobial regimens in the empiric treatment of sepsis.
- The average duration of therapy in the normal host with gram-negative sepsis is 10–14 days. Treatment may go considerably longer if the infection is persistent.
- In the neutropenic patient the duration of therapy is usually longer than average. These patients should be afebrile for 4–7 days, show signs of resolving infection at the source, and have rising neutrophil counts in excess of 500/μL.
- The frequent monitoring of aminoglycoside serum levels becomes imperative when this class is used. Gentamicin and also tobramycin peak levels in the range of 5.0–10.0 μg/mL are generally associated with optimal response. Amikacin peak levels of 20–40 μg/mL are likewise considered optimal. Alternatively, higher levels may be achieved with single daily dosing (15–24 μg/mL with gentamicin or tobramycin).

FLUID THERAPY AND PULMONARY SUPPORT

- Maintenance of adequate tissue oxygenation is an important consideration in the treatment of sepsis and is dependent on adequate perfusion and adequate oxygenation of the blood.

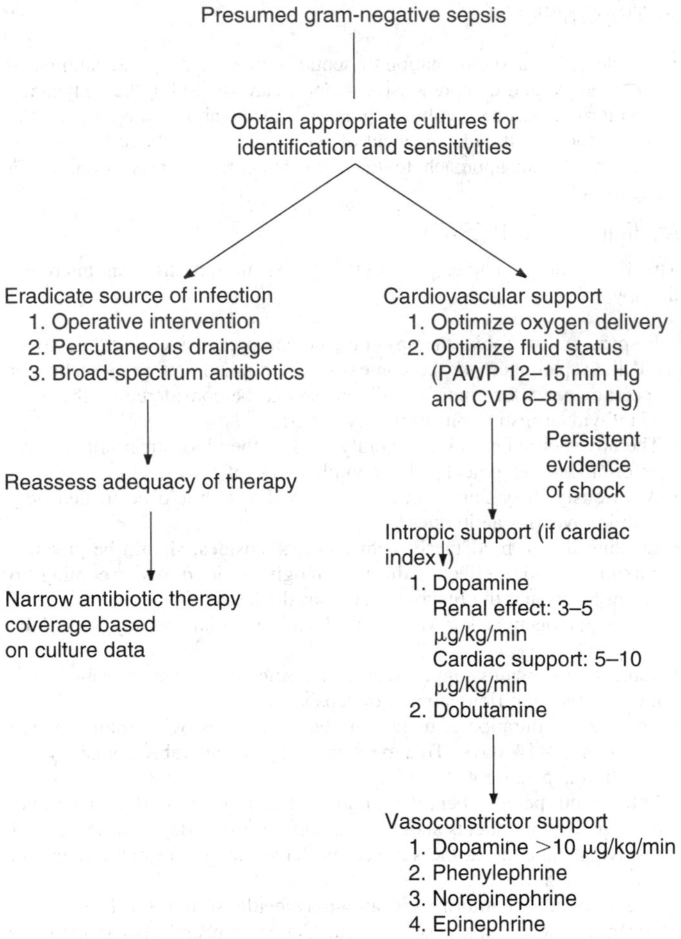

Presumed gram-negative sepsis

Obtain appropriate cultures for
identification and sensitivities

Eradicate source of infection
1. Operative intervention
2. Percutaneous drainage
3. Broad-spectrum antibiotics

Cardiovascular support
1. Optimize oxygen delivery
2. Optimize fluid status
   (PAWP 12–15 mm Hg
   and CVP 6–8 mm Hg)

Reassess adequacy of therapy

Persistent
evidence
of shock

VIII

Narrow antibiotic therapy
coverage based
on culture data

Intropic support (if cardiac
index▼)
1. Dopamine
   Renal effect: 3–5
   μg/kg/min
   Cardiac support: 5–10
   μg/kg/min
2. Dobutamine

Vasoconstrictor support
1. Dopamine >10 μg/kg/min
2. Phenylephrine
3. Norepinephrine
4. Epinephrine

Figure 44.2. Treatment algorithm for the management of gram-negative sepsis. PAWP, pulmonary artery wedge pressure.

- Rapid restoration of intravascular fluid volume and expansion of the extravascular space is an essential therapeutic intervention in the initial management of septic shock.
- The goal of fluid replacement is to maintain a systolic blood pressure >90 mm Hg and to prevent hypoperfusion to tissues and vital organs.

TABLE 44.3. Suggested Antimicrobial Regimens for the Empiric Treatment of Sepsis in Adults

Infection (Site or Type)	Antibiotic Regimen
Urinary tract or respiratory tract	Extended-spectrum penicillin + aminoglycoside or Third-generation cephalosporin ± aminoglycoside
Intra-abdominal	Metronidazole/clindamycin or } + aminoglycoside β-Lactamase inhibitor combo or Imipenem
Soft tissue	Penicillinase-resistant penicillin or Cefazolin } + aminoglycoside or Vancomycin
Central line	Vancomycin + aminoglycoside
Pseudomonas	Extended-spectrum penicillin or Ceftazidime } + aminoglycoside or Imipenem
Unknown	Extended-spectrum penicillin or Ceftazidime } + aminoglycoside or + vancomycin Imipenem

VIII

- Controversy exists regarding the optimal type of fluid (crystalloid versus colloid). An increase in pulmonary edema has been demonstrated during crystalloid volume expansion when compared with colloids, but the effects are transitory and it is not known whether there are any long-term adverse effects. Successful fluid resuscitation in sepsis usually requires a combination of crystalloid and colloid.
- Iso-oncotic colloid solutions (plasma and plasma protein fractions), such as 5% albumin and 6% hetastarch, offer the advantage of more rapid restoration of intravascular volume with less volume infused. However, they may prolong tissue edema when capillary permeability to oncotically active solutes is increased.
- Crystalloids are generally employed first with Ringer's lactate or normal saline for resuscitation purposes.
- Fluid resuscitation in sepsis usually requires hemodynamic monitoring. An acceptable PAWP is usually 12–15 mm Hg, but cardiac disease can affect this greatly.

INOTROPE AND VASOACTIVE DRUG SUPPORT

- When fluid resuscitation is insufficient to maintain tissue perfusion, the use of inotropes and vasoactive drugs is necessary. Selection and dosage are based on the pharmacologic properties of various catecholamines and how they influence hemodynamic parameters (Table 44.4).

Suggested Protocol for the Use of Inotropes and Vasoactive Agents

- Dopamine is widely used in low doses (2–3 μg/kg/min) to increase renal and mesenteric perfusion. Renal blood flow is enhanced even when used with norepinephrine.
- Dopamine in moderate doses (5–10 μg/kg/min) may be used for its selective effect on increasing cardiac output with minimal effect on the systemic vascular resistance.
- Dobutamine (5–30 μg/kg/min) has been suggested by some investigators to be superior to dopamine for maintaining tissue perfusion and oxygen consumption in critically ill, but the effect may not be significant in the septic patient.
- Amrinone administered in 1 mg/kg bolus and 10 mg/kg/min continuous infusion is an alternative to dobutamine.
- In the patient with significant hypotension (mean arterial pressure [MAP] <60 mm Hg) and a low systemic vascular resistance index (SVRI) (<500 dyne/s/cm^5/m^2) that cannot be overcome by inotropic agents, an α-adrenergic agent (norepinephrine) can be useful. It often is combined with an inotrope such as dobutamine.
- Pure α agonists such as phenylephrine can be employed either with other drugs or as single-agent therapy when SVR is markedly decreased. The goal of phenylephrine therapy is to increase SVR and MAP by increasing vasoconstriction.
- Prior to administering vasoactive agents, aggressive appropriate fluid resuscitation should occur. Vasoactive agents should not be considered an acceptable alternative to volume resuscitation.

INVESTIGATIONAL THERAPIES

- A wide variety of investigational strategies have been used to attempt to reverse or control the inflammatory process initiated with sepsis.
- One mechanism studied is direct inhibition of the effects of endotoxin from gram-negative bacteria by antibodies or with other binding substances such as bactericidal/permeability increasing protein or high density lipoprotein.
- A second general approach is inhibition of inflammatory cytokines through antibodies that bind the cytokines, through competitive inhibitors for cytokine receptor binding, or through soluble receptors that bind the cytokine but do not activate the target cells.
- Another general approach is the administration of anti-inflammatory cytokines or other substances, such as IL-10, IL-4, or IL-1 receptor antagonist.

TABLE 44.4. Cardiovascular Drugs Used in Sepsis

Agent	Dose (μg·kg/min)	Receptor	MAP	CI	SVRI	HR	PAWP
Dobutamine	2.5–40	3β₁, 1β₂	NC	I	D	NC/I	D
Dopamine	2–3	3c, 1β₁	NC	NC	NC	NC	NC
	5–10	3β₁, 2β₂	NC/I	I	NC	NC	NC
	>10	3β₁, 3α₁,₂	I	I	I	I	I
Epinephrine	0.005–0.05	3β , 1β₂	NC	NC/I	NC/D	I	NC
	>0.05	3α , 1α₂	I	I	I	I	I
Phenylephrine	0.03–2	3α₁, 5α₂	I	NC/D	I	D	I
Norepinephrine	>0.05	3α, 2β₁	I	NC/I	I	D	I
Amrinone	5–30	N/A	NC/D	I	D	NC	D

Key: HR = heart rate; I = increased; MAP = mean arterial pressure; NC = no change; NC/D = no change or slight decrease; PAWP = pulmonary artery wedge pressure.

VIII

CONTROVERSIES IN THE MANAGEMENT OF SEPTIC SHOCK

- The corticosteroids have been the subject of controversy in the management of the septic process. Multiple clinical trials have demonstrated that they are not beneficial for sepsis but may be useful for patients with ARDS (after 5–7 days).
- Heparinization for the treatment of DIC has been recommended because the paradoxical bleeding is caused by a hypercoagulable state, however there is little clinical evidence that heparin prolongs survival.
- Naloxone, through its antagonist effect on opiates and β endorphins, has been shown to raise and sustain systolic blood pressure in animals but has not been shown useful in humans with septic shock.
- It is not clear whether the aggressive use of diuretics in the early oliguric phase of acute renal failure prevents failure or makes the ensuing failure less severe. Prudent doses of diuretics are beneficial when volume expansion fails to maintain adequate urine output.

See Chapter 112, Gram-Negative Sepsis and Septic Shock, authored by Steven B. Johnson, MD, Kenneth E. Record, PharmD, and Joseph T. DiPiro, PharmD, for a more detailed discussion of this topic.

VIII

Chapter 45

► SEXUALLY TRANSMITTED DISEASES

► DEFINITION

The spectrum of sexually transmitted diseases (STDs) includes the classic venereal diseases—gonorrhea, syphilis, chancroid, lymphogranuloma venereum, and granuloma inguinale—as well as a variety of other pathogens known to be spread by sexual contact (Table 45.1). Common clinical syndromes associated with STDs are listed in Table 45.2.

► GONORRHEA

EPIDEMIOLOGY

- *Neisseria gonorrhoeae* is a gram-negative *diplococcus* responsible for an estimated 1 million infections per year in the United States.
- Gonorrheal infections occur 10 times more frequently in non-whites than whites. Other risk factors characteristic of patients with *N. gonorrhoeae* include low socioeconomic status, urban residence, unmarried marital status, and a previous history of gonorrheal infection.

CLINICAL PRESENTATION

- Infected individuals may be symptomatic or asymptomatic, have complicated or uncomplicated infections, and have infections involving several anatomic sites.
- Urethritis is the most common presenting manifestation in males, and usually develops within 2–8 days of exposure. Dysuria and urinary frequency are seen initially, followed in 1–2 days by a profuse, purulent urethral discharge.
- The majority of symptomatic patients who are not treated become asymptomatic within 6 months, with only a few becoming asymptomatic carriers of the disease.
- The majority of gonococcal urethral or cervical infections in females are either asymptomatic or produce minimal symptoms.
- In females, symptoms typically appear within 10 days following exposure. Symptoms include dysuria, urinary frequency, abnormal vaginal discharge, and abnormal uterine bleeding.
- Other sites of gonococcal infection include the rectum, oropharynx, and eye. Anorectal gonococcal infections are common in females and in homosexual males.
- Approximately 15% of women with gonorrhea develop pelvic inflammatory disease. Left untreated, PID can be an indirect cause of infertility and ectopic pregnancies.

TABLE 45.1. Sexually Transmitted Diseases

Disease	Pathogen
Bacterial	
Gonorrhea	*Neisseria gonorrhoeae*
Syphilis	*Treponema pallidum*
Chancroid	*Haemophilus ducreyi*
Granuloma inguinale (donovanosis)	*Calymmatobacterium granulomatis*
Salmonellosis	*Salmonella* sp.
Shigellosis	*Shigella* sp.
Campylobacter infection	*Campylobacter jejuni*
Nonspecific vaginitis	*Trichomonas vaginalis, Gardnerella vaginalis*
Group B streptococcal infections	Group B streptococcus
Chlamydial	
Nongonococcal urethritis	*Chlamydia trachomatis*
Lymphogranuloma venereum	*C. trachomatis*
Viral	
Herpes genitalis	Herpes simplex virus
Hepatitis B	Hepatitis B virus
Condylomata acuminata	Human papilloma virus
Molluscum contagiosum	Poxvirus
Cytomegalovirus infection	Cytomegalovirus
Mycoplasmal	
Nongonococcal urethritis	*Ureaplasma urealyticum*
Protozoal	
Trichomoniasis	*T. vaginalis*
Amebiasis	*Entamoeba histolytica*
Giardiasis	*Giardia lamblia*
Fungal	
Candidiasis	*Candida albicans*
Parasitic	
Scabies	*Sarcoptes scabiei*
Pediculosis	*Pediculus pubis*
Enterobiasis	*Enterobius vermicularis*

VIII

- In 0.5–3.0% of patients with gonorrhea, the gonococci invade the bloodstream and produce disseminated disease.
- The usual clinical manifestations of disseminated gonococcal infection are tender necrotic skin lesions, tenosynovitis, and monoarticular arthritis.

DIAGNOSIS

- Diagnosis of gonococcal infections can be made by Gram-stained smears, culture (the most reliable method), or newer methods based on the detection of cellular components of the *gonococcus* (e.g., enzymes, antigens, DNA, or lipopolysaccharide) in clinical specimens.

TABLE 45.2. Selected Syndromes Associated with Common Sexually Transmitted Pathogens

Syndrome	Commonly Implicated Pathogens	Common Clinical Manifestations[a]
Urethritis	*Chlamydia trachomatis,* herpes simplex virus, *Neisseria gonorrhoeae, Trichomonas vaginalis, Ureaplasma urealyticum*	Urethral discharge, dysuria
Epididymitis	*C. trachomatis, N. gonorrhoeae*	Scrotal pain, inguinal pain, flank pain, urethral discharge
Cervicitis/vulvovaginitis	*C. trachomatis, Gardnerella vaginalis,* herpes simplex virus, human papilloma virus, *N. gonorrhoeae, T. vaginalis*	Abnormal vaginal discharge, vulvar itching/irritation, dysuria, dyspareunia
Genital ulcers (painful)	*Haemophilus ducreyi,* herpes simplex virus	Usually multiple vesicular/pustular (herpes) or papular/pustular (*H. ducreyi*) lesions that may coalesce; painful, tender lymphadenopathy[b]
Genital ulcers (painless)	*Treponema pallidum*	Usually single papular lesion
Genital warts	Human papilloma virus	Multiple lesions ranging in size from small papular warts to large exophytic condylomas
Pharyngitis	*C. trachomatis* (?), herpes simplex virus, *N. gonorrhoeae*	Symptoms of acute pharyngitis, cervical lymphadenopathy, fever[c]
Proctitis	*C. trachomatis,* herpes simplex virus, *N. gonorrhoeae, T. pallidum*	Constipation, anorectal discomfort, tenesmus, mucopurulent rectal discharge
Salpingitis	*C. trachomatis, N. gonorrhoeae*	Lower abdominal pain, purulent cervical or vaginal discharge, adnexal swelling, fever[d]

[a]For some syndromes, clinical manifestations may be minimal or absent.
[b]Recurrent herpes infection may manifest as a single lesion.
[c]Most cases of pharyngeal gonococcal infection are asymptomatic.
[d]Salpingitis increases the risk of subsequent ectopic pregnancy and infertility.

- Rapid diagnostic tests have been developed based on detection of gonococcal antigens, enzymes, DNA, endotoxin, or lipopolysaccharide in clinical specimens and can be performed easily in an office.

TREATMENT

- Many antimicrobial regimens are effective in treating uncomplicated gonorrhea; however, no single therapeutic regimen can be recommended as optimal because of regional differences in susceptibility and the high incidence of coexistent infections (particularly *C. trachomatis*) in certain populations.
- All currently recommended regimens are single-dose treatments with various oral or parenteral cephalosporins and fluoroquinolones (Table 45.3).

VIII

VIII

TABLE 45.3. Treatment of Gonorrhea

Type of Infection	Recommended Regimen[a]	Alternative Regimen
Uncomplicated urethral, endocervical, rectal, proctitis, or epididymitis infection in adults[b,c]	Ceftriaxone 125 mg IM once; or ciprofloxacin 500 mg PO once; or cefixime 400 mg PO once; or ofloxacin 400 mg PO once plus A treatment regimen for presumptive *C. trachomatis* coinfection (see Table 45.5)	Spectinomycin 2 g IM once; or ceftizoxime 500 mg IM once; or cefotetan 1 g IM once; or cefoxitin 2 g IM once; or cefuroxime axetil 1 g PO once; or cefpodoxime proxetil 200 mg PO once; or lomefloxacin 400 mg PO once; or enoxacin 400 mg PO once; or norfloxacin 800 mg PO once plus A treatment regimen for presumptive *C. trachomatis* coinfection (see Table 45.5)
Gonococcal infections in pregnancy	Ceftriaxone 125 mg IM once[d,e] plus Erythromycin base 500 mg PO 4 times daily for 7 days	Spectinomycin 2.0 g IM once plus A treatment regimen for presumptive *C. trachomatis* coinfection (see Table 45.5)
Disseminated gonococcal infection in adults (>45 kg)[e,f,g,h]	Ceftriaxone 1 g IM or IV every 24 hours	Ceftizoxime 1 g IV every 8 hours or Cefotaxime 1 g IV every 8 hours until all symptoms resolve or Spectinomycin 2 g IM every 12 hours
Disseminated gonococcal infection in infants[i]	Ceftriaxone 25–50 mg/kg IV or IM once daily for 7 days or Cefotaxime 25 mg/kg IV or IM twice daily for 7 days	
Uncomplicated urethritis, vulvovaginitis, cervicitis, pharyngitis, or proctitis infection in children (<45 kg)	Ceftriaxone 125 mg IM once[j]	Spectinomycin 40 mg/kg IM once (not to exceed 2 g)

TABLE 45.3. continued

Gonococcal conjunctivitis	Ceftriaxone 1 g IM once[k]
Ophthalmia neonatorum	Ceftriaxone 25–50 mg/kg IV or IM once (not to exceed 125 mg)
Infants born to mothers with gonococcal infection (prophylaxis)	Ceftriaxone 25–50 mg/kg IV or IM (not to exceed 125 mg)

[a]Recommendations are those of the CDC.

[b]Treatment failures are usually due to reinfection and necessitate patient education and sex-partner referral; additional treatment regimens for gonorrhea and chlamydia infections should be administered. Epididymitis should be treated for 10 days (see Table 45.5).

[c]Patients allergic to β-lactams should receive a quinolone. Persons unable to tolerate a β-lactam (penicillin or cephalosporin) or a quinolone should receive spectinomycin.

[d]Another recommended IM or PO cephalosporin also may be used

[e]The fluoroquinolones, doxycycline, and erythromycin ethyl succinate are contraindicated during pregnancy.

[f]Patients treated with one of the recommended regimens should be treated with doxycycline or azithromycin for possible coexistent chlamydial infection.

[g]Patients with gonococcal meningitis should be treated for 10–14 days and those with endocarditis for at least 4 weeks with ceftriaxone 1–2 g IV every 12 hours.

[h]Treatment regimen should be continued for 24–48 hours after improvement begins and switched to cefixime 400 mg PO twice daily or ciprofloxacin 500 mg 2 times a day to complete a week of therapy.

[i]Treatment for 10–14 days is required if meningitis is present.

[j]Patients with bacteremia or arthritis should receive ceftriaxone 50 mg/kg (maximum 1 g) IM or IV once daily for 7 days. Patients with meningitis should be treated for 10–14 days, with a daily dose of ceftriaxone not to exceed 2 g.

[k]The eye should be lavaged one time with saline solution.

VIII

- Coexisting chlamydial infection, which is documented in ≤45% of individuals with gonorrhea, constitutes the major cause of post-gonococcal urethritis, cervicitis, and salpingitis in patients treated for gonorrhea. As a result, concomitant treatment with doxycycline or azithromycin is recommended in all patients treated for gonorrhea.
- Pregnant women infected with *N. gonorrhoeae* should be treated with either a cephalosporin or spectinomycin, since fluoroquinolones are contraindicated.
- Treatment of gonorrhea during pregnancy is essential to prevent ophthalmia neonatorum. The American Academy of Pediatrics recommends that either silver nitrate (1%), tetracycline (1%), or erythromycin (0.5%) be instilled in each conjunctival sac immediately postpartum to prevent ophthalmia neonatorum.
- Infants born to infected mothers should also receive an intramuscular or intravenous injection of ceftriaxone 50 mg/kg for 7 days.

EVALUATION OF THERAPEUTIC OUTCOMES

- Combination gonorrhea/chlamydia therapy rarely results in treatment failures, and routine follow-up of patients treated with a regimen included in the CDC guidelines is not recommended.
- Patients receiving treatment with medications other than ceftriaxone should have follow-up cultures performed 4–7 days following the completion of therapy.
- Persistence of symptoms following any treatment requires culture of the site(s) of gonorrheal infection, as well as susceptibility testing if gonococci are isolated.

VIII

▶ SYPHILIS

EPIDEMIOLOGY

- Syphilis is the fourth most frequently reported communicable disease in the United States.
- The causative organism of syphilis is *Treponema pallidum,* a spirochete.
- Syphilis is usually acquired by sexual contact with infected mucous membranes or cutaneous lesions, although on rare occasions it can be acquired by nonsexual personal contact, accidental inoculation, or blood transfusion.

CLINICAL PRESENTATION

Primary Syphilis

- After exposure and an incubation period of 10–90 days (average, 21 days), a painless lesion or chancre appears at the site of treponemal penetrance. Subsequently it develops into a papule that erodes and ulcerates.
- Chancres persist only for 1–8 weeks before spontaneously disappearing.

Secondary Syphilis

- The secondary stage of syphilis develops 2–6 weeks after the onset of the primary stage in untreated or inadequately treated patients and is characterized by a variety of mucocutaneous eruptions, resulting from widespread hematogenous and lymphatic spread of *T. pallidum.*
- Often lesions appear on the palms of the hands and the soles of the feet. In addition to the skin lesions, mild and transitory malaise, fever, pharyngitis, headache, anorexia, and arthralgia are common.
- Signs and symptoms of secondary syphilis disappear in 4–10 weeks; however, in untreated patients, lesions may recur at any time within 4 years.

Latent Syphilis

- Persons with a positive serologic test for syphilis but with no other evidence of disease have latent syphilis.
- A large percentage of untreated patients with late latent syphilis have no further sequelae; however, approximately 25–30% progress to late or tertiary syphilis.

Tertiary (Late) Syphilis

- Tertiary syphilis can affect any organ in the body and can develop 2–30 years after the onset of syphilis.
- The most common manifestations of tertiary syphilis are benign gumma, neurosyphilis, and cardiovascular syphilis.
- Neurosyphilis, found in approximately 20% of patients with tertiary disease, can produce general paresis, eighth cranial nerve deafness, optic atrophy and blindness, progressive dementia, meningovascular complications, and tabes dorsalis.
- Thirty percent of patients with tertiary disease develop cardiovascular syphilis, characterized by aortitis and aortic insufficiency.

VIII

DIAGNOSIS

- Because *T. pallidum* is difficult to culture in vitro, diagnosis is based primarily on dark-field microscopic examination of serous material from a suspected syphilitic lesion or on results from serologic testing.
- Serologic tests used in the diagnosis of syphilis are categorized as non-treponemal or treponemal. Commonly used non-treponemal tests include the Venereal Disease Research Laboratory (VDRL) slide test, rapid plasma reagin (RPR) card test, reagin screen test (RST), unheated serum reagin (USR) test, automated reagin test (ART), or the toluidine red unheated serum test (TRUST).

TREATMENT

- Treatment recommendations for syphilis from the CDC are presented in Table 45.4.
- For pregnant patients, penicillin is the treatment of choice at the dosage recommended for that particular stage of syphilis. To assure treatment success and prevent transmission to the fetus, some experts advocate an

TABLE 45.4. Drug Therapy and Follow-Up of Syphilis

Stage/Type of Syphilis	Recommended Regimen[a]	Follow-up Serology
Primary, secondary, or latent syphilis of less than 1 year's duration (early latent syphilis)	Benzathine penicillin G 2.4 million units IM in a single dose[b]	Quantitative non-treponemal tests at 3 and 6 months for primary and secondary syphilis; at 6 and 12 months for early latent syphilis[c]
Syphilis of more than 1 year's duration (includes late latent syphilis of unknown duration and late or tertiary syphilis; excludes neurosyphilis)	Benzathine penicillin G 2.4 million units IM once a week for 3 successive weeks	Quantitative non-treponemal tests at 6 and 12 months for late latent syphilis[d]
Neurosyphilis	Aqueous crystalline penicillin G 12–24 million units IV (2–4 million units every 4 hours) for 10–14 days,[f] or Aqueous procaine penicillin G 2.4 million units IM daily plus probenecid 500 mg PO four times daily, both for 10–14 days[f]	CSF[e] examination every 6 months until the cell count is normal; if it has not decreased at 6 months or is not normal by 2 years, retreatment is suggested
Congenital syphilis	Aqueous crystalline penicillin G 50,000 units/kg IV every 12 hours during the first 7 days of life and every 8 hours thereafter for 10–14 days or Procaine penicillin G 50,000 units/kg IM daily for 10–14 days	Quantitative nontreponemal tests every 2–3 months until nonreactive (6–12 months)

TABLE 45.4. continued

Penicillin-allergic patients[a]		
Primary, secondary, or latent syphilis of less than 1 year's duration	Doxycycline 100 mg PO two times daily for 2 weeks or Tetracycline 500 mg PO four times daily for 2 weeks	Same as for non-penicillin-allergic patients
Syphilis of more than 1 year's duration (except neurosyphilis)	Erythromycin 500 mg PO four times daily for 2 weeks Doxycycline 100 mg PO two times a day for 4 weeks or Tetracycline 500 mg PO four times daily for 4 weeks	Same as for non-penicillin-allergic patients

[a] Recommendations are those of the CDC.
[b] Some experts recommend multiple doses of benzathine penicillin G or other supplemental antibiotics in addition to benzathine penicillin G in HIV-infected patients with primary or secondary syphilis; HIV-infected patients with early latent syphilis should be treated with the recommended regimen for syphilis of more than 1 year's duration.
[c] More frequent follow-up (i.e. 1, 2, 3, 6, 9, and 12 months) recommended for HIV-infected patients.
[d] Minimal data exist on which to base specific follow-up recommendations for late syphilis.
[e] CSF, cerebral spinal fluid.
[f] Some experts administer benzathine penicillin G 2.4 million units IM after completion of the neurosyphilis regimens to provide a total duration of therapy comparable to that used for late syphilis in the absence of neurosyphilis.
[g] For nonpregnant patients; pregnant patients should be treated with penicillin after desensitization.

VIII

547

additional intramuscular dose of benzathine penicillin G 2.4 million units 1 week after completion of the recommended regimen.

- The majority of patients treated for primary and secondary syphilis experience the Jarisch–Herxheimer reaction beginning 2–4 hours after treatment, characterized by flu-like symptoms such as transient headache, fever, chills, malaise, arthralgia, myalgia, tachypnea, peripheral vasodilation, and aggravation of syphilitic lesions.
- The Jarisch–Herxheimer reaction should not be confused with penicillin allergy. Most reactions can be managed symptomatically with analgesics, antipyretics, and rest.

EVALUATION OF THERAPEUTIC OUTCOME

- CDC recommendations for serologic follow-up of patients treated for syphilis are given in Table 45.4. Quantitative non-treponemal tests should be performed at 3 and 6 months in all patients treated for primary and secondary syphilis and at 6 and 12 months for early and late latent disease.
- For women treated during pregnancy, monthly quantitative non-treponemal tests are recommended until the adequacy of therapy is established. Women who do not demonstrate a four-fold decrease in titer over a 3-month period or who show a four-fold increase in titer between tests should be retreated.

VIII

▶ CHLAMYDIA

EPIDEMIOLOGY

- Infections caused by *C. trachomatis* are believed to be the most common STD in the United States and the most common cause of non-gonococcal urethritis (NGU). It is estimated that more than 4 million Americans contract chlamydial infections each year.
- Coinfection with chlamydia occurs in up to 45% of individuals with gonorrhea.

CLINICAL PRESENTATION

- In males, the most common symptoms of chlamydial genital tract infections are dysuria, urinary frequency, and a mucoid urethral discharge occurring 7–21 days after exposure.
- In approximately 25% of men with chlamydial infections, no signs or symptoms are present.
- The majority of women with chlamydial infections are asymptomatic. In women with urethral infections, dysuria and frequency are uncommon.
- When symptomatic, the most common manifestation of infection is endocervicitis with a mucopurulent discharge. On examination, the cervix tends to be friable and ectopic.
- Similar to gonorrhea, chlamydia may be transmitted to an infant during contact with infected cervicovaginal secretions. Up to 70% of infants

acquire chlamydial infection after endocervical exposure, with the primary morbidity associated with seeding of the infant's eyes, nasopharynx, rectum, or vagina.

DIAGNOSIS

- Two tests that allow rapid identification of chlamydial antigens in genital secretions are the direct fluorescent antibody (DFA) test and the enzyme-linked immunoabsorbent assay (ELISA). Both tests have similar mean sensitivities and specificities in the range of 90–100% when properly performed.

TREATMENT

- Recommended regimens for treatment of chlamydial infections are given in Table 44.5.
- For prophylaxis of ophthalmia neonatorum, various groups have proposed the use of erythromycin (0.5%) or tetracycline (1%) ophthalmic ointment in lieu of silver nitrate. Although silver nitrate and antibiotic ointments are effective against gonococcal ophthalmia neonatorum, silver nitrate is not effective for chlamydial disease and may cause a chemical conjunctivitis.
- The only acceptable treatment for chlamydial ophthalmia neonatorum is systemic therapy with oral erythromycin 50 mg/kg/d in four divided doses for 10–14 days.

VIII

EVALUATION OF THERAPEUTIC OUTCOME

- Treatment of chlamydial infections with the recommended regimens is highly effective, therefore, post-treatment cultures are not routinely recommended.
- Infants with pneumonitis should receive follow-up testing, since erythromycin is only 80% effective.

▶ GENITAL HERPES

EPIDEMIOLOGY

- Genital herpes infections represent the most common cause of genital ulceration seen in the United States. It is estimated that approximately 31 million Americans have genital herpes, and this number is increasing yearly.
- The term *herpes* is used to describe two distinct but antigenically related serotypes of herpes simplex virus. Herpes simplex virus type 1 (HSV-1) is most commonly associated with oropharyngeal disease, and herpes simplex virus type 2 (HSV-2) is most closely associated with genital disease.

CLINICAL PRESENTATION

- The clinical manifestations of first episodes of genital herpes usually appear within 2–14 days after exposure.

TABLE 45.5. Treatment of Chlamydial Infections

Infection	Recommended Regimen[a]	Alternative Regimen
Uncomplicated urethral, endocervical, or rectal infection in adults	Doxycycline 100 mg PO 2 times daily for 7 days or Azithromycin 1 g once[b]	Ofloxacin 300 mg PO 2 times daily for 7 days[c] or Erythromycin base 500 mg PO 4 times daily for 7 days or Erythromycin ethyl succinate 800 mg PO 4 times daily for 7 days or Sulfasoxazole 500 mg 4 times daily for 10 days
Urogenital infections during pregnancy	Erythromycin base 500 mg 4 times PO daily for 7 days	Erythromycin base 250 mg PO 4 times daily for 14 days or Erythromycin ethyl succinate 800 mg PO 4 times daily for 7 days (or 400 mg PO 4 times daily for 14 days) or Amoxicillin 500 mg PO 3 times daily for 7 days[d]
Conjunctivitis of the newborn	Erythromycin suspension 50 mg/kg/d PO in 4 divided doses for 10–14 days	
Pneumonia in infants	Erythromycin suspension 50 mg/kg/d PO in 4 divided doses for 10–14 days	
Acute epididymo-orchitis	Ceftriaxone 250 mg IM[e] plus Doxycycline 100 mg PO 2 times daily for 10 days	

[a]Recommendations are those of the CDC.
[b]Data regarding the use of azithromycin in children ≤15 years old are not established.
[c]Ofloxacin is contraindicated during pregnancy and should not be used in patients ≤17 years old.
[d]Only if GI intolerance to erythromycin; limited data exist for efficacy.
[e]The efficacy of ceftriaxone 125 mg or azithromycin has not been studied and is unknown.

- Up to 50% of HSV-2 infections are asymptomatic, and these infections may represent the most common source of transmission of genital and neonatal herpes infections.
- More than 50% of patients with primary infections (classified as infections occurring in persons lacking antibody to either type of HSV) experience flu-like symptoms of fever, headache, malaise, and myalgias. Systemic symptoms gradually resolve over the course of a week.
- Local symptoms include development of painful pustular or ulcerative lesions on the external genitalia. Lesions usually begin as papules or

vesicles that rapidly spread over the genitalia. Clusters of the lesions coalesce into large areas of ulceration, which over 2–3 weeks, crust and/or reepithelialize.
- Other local symptoms can include itching, dysuria, vaginal or urethral discharge, and tender inguinal adenopathy.
- First-episode nonprimary genital herpes is defined as an infection in individuals who have clinical or serologic evidence of prior HSV (usually HSV-1) infection at another body site. These infections tend to be milder than true primary infections, with a lower incidence of constitutional symptoms and a shorter duration of disease reported.
- Recurrent infection is localized to the genital area and is milder and of a shorter duration (e.g., 8–12 days). Viral shedding lasts approximately 4 days.
- Symptoms of recurrent infection tend to be more severe in women, primarily as a result of the greater genital surface area involved.
- Symptoms of first-episode and recurrent infections tend to be more severe and prolonged in immunocompromised patients than in immunocompetent patients.
- A major concern is the effect of genital herpes on neonates exposed during pregnancy. Neonatal herpes is associated with a high mortality and significant morbidity.

DIAGNOSIS

VIII

- A presumptive diagnosis of genital herpes commonly is made based on the presence of dark-field–negative, vesicular, or ulcerative genital lesions. A prior history of similar lesions or recent sexual contact with an individual with similar lesions also is useful in making the diagnosis.
- Tissue culture is the most specific (100%) and sensitive method (80–90%) of confirming the diagnosis of first-episode genital herpes
- Antigen detection methods such as direct immunofluorescence, immunoperoxidase staining, and enzyme-linked immunosorbent assay have sensitivities of 70–90% compared with viral culture; however, sensitivities are significantly lower when assessing asymptomatic viral shedding.

TREATMENT

- The goals of therapy in genital herpes infection are to shorten the clinical course, prevent complications, prevent the development of latency and/or subsequent recurrences, decrease disease transmission, and eliminate established latency.
- Palliative and supportive measures are the cornerstone of therapy for patients with genital herpes.
- To prevent bacterial superinfection, lesions must be kept clean and dry.
- Specific chemotherapeutic approaches to treating genital herpes fall into six major areas: antiviral compounds, topical surfactants, photodynamic dyes, immune modulators, vaccines, and interferons (Table 45.6).
- Specific dosage recommendations for acyclovir are given in Table 45.7.

Infectious Diseases

TABLE 45.6. Agents Studied in the Treatment of Herpes Genitalis

Antiviral Compounds	Immune Modulators
Acyclovir	Inosiplex
Famciclovir	Levamisole
Valaciclovir	Transfer factor
Foscarnet	**Vaccines**
Vidarabine	BCG
Idoxuridine	Influenza
2-Deoxy-D-glucose	Polio
Lithium	Small pox
L-Lysine	**Interferons**
Phosphonoformate	Leukocyte interferon
Ribavirin	**Photodynamic Dyes**
(E)-5-(2-Bromovinyl)-2′-deoxyuridine (BVdU)	Neutral red
2′-Fluoro-5-iodoarabinosylcytosine	Acridine red
1-(2′-Fluoro-2′-deoxy-β-D-arabinofuranosyl)-thymidine	Proflavine
Topical Surfactants	**Others**
Chloroform	Butylated hydroxytoluene (BHT)
Ether	
Nonoxynol-9	
Povidone-iodine	
Intervir-A	

VIII

- Topical therapy is considered of little or no benefit in most patients. Combined use of topical acyclovir with oral therapy does not appear to offer any additional benefit over oral therapy alone.
- In humans, no acyclovir regimen is known to prevent latency or alter the subsequent frequency and severity of recurrences.
- When initiated early during the course of recurrence, oral acyclovir reduces the duration of viral shedding by approximately 1 day and diminishes the time to healing of lesions by 1–2 days. Appreciable effects on symptomology are not seen. Patients with prolonged episodes of recurrent infection are most likely to benefit from oral therapy instituted at the earliest sign of recurrence.
- Acyclovir treatment of first-episode genital herpes does not prevent later recurrences; however, chronic oral therapy reduces the frequency and the severity of recurrences in 70–90% of patients experiencing frequent recurrences.
- Patients with frequent (i.e., >6 per year) and physically or psychologically distressing recurrences are candidates for suppressive therapy with multiple daily doses of oral acyclovir.
- Both intravenous and oral acyclovir have been used to prevent reactivation of infection in patients seropositive for HSV who undergo transplantation procedures or induction chemotherapy for acute leukemia.
- The safety of acyclovir therapy during pregnancy is not established, although there is no evidence of teratogenic effects in humans.

TABLE 45.7. Treatment of Genital Herpes

Type of Infection	Recommended Regimen[a,b]	Alternative Regimen
First clinical episode of genital herpes[c]	Acyclovir 200 mg PO five times daily for 7–10 days, or until clinical resolution occurs	Acyclovir 5–10 mg/kg IV every 8 hours for 5–7 days, or until clinical resolution occurs[d]
First clinical episode of herpes proctitis	Acyclovir 400 mg PO five times daily for 10 days, or until clinical resolution occurs	Acyclovir 5–10 mg/kg IV every 8 hours for 5–7 days, or until clinical resolution occurs[d]
Recurrent infection		
Treatment	Acyclovir 200 mg PO five times daily, *or* 400 mg PO three times daily, *or* 800 mg PO twice daily for 5 days, initiated within 48 hours of onset of lesions[e]	
Suppression	Acyclovir 400 mg PO twice daily[f]	Acyclovir 200 mg PO 3–5 times daily

[a]Recommendations are those of the CDC.
[b]HIV-infected patients may require more aggressive therapy.
[c]Primary or nonprimary first episode.
[d]Only for patients with severe symptoms or complications that necessitate hospitalization.
[e]Treatment should be limited to patients with severe symptoms. Treatment is most beneficial when instituted at the earliest sign of recurrence (i.e., prodrome); therapy initiated 48 hours or more after the onset of symptoms has no effect.
[f]Indicated only for patients with frequent and/or severe recurrences; although safety and efficacy are documented in patients receiving daily therapy for as long as 5 years, it is recommended that therapy be discontinued after 1 year of continuous suppressive therapy to assess the patient's rate of recurrent episodes.

VIII

▶ TRICHOMONIASIS

EPIDEMIOLOGY

- Trichomoniasis is caused by *Trichomonas vaginalis,* a flagellated, motile protozoan.
- Trichomonal infections are much more common in women than in men.
- It is estimated that 2.5 to 3 million cases of vaginal trichomoniasis occur annually in the United States. The peak incidence in women occurs between the ages of 16 and 35, although there is a high prevalence between ages 35 and 45.

CLINICAL PRESENTATION

- The incubation period of trichomoniasis is 4–20 days, with as many as 50% of infected women remaining asymptomatic.
- When symptomatic, females can present with mild to severe vaginal discharge, vulvar pruritis, and dysuria.
- Vaginal discharge is noted in approximately 50–75% of infected women and classically has been described as malodorous, foamy, and greenish yellow in color; however, more typically the discharge is grayish and only mildly odoriferous.

- Trichomoniasis may be responsible for causing premature rupture of the membranes and preterm delivery. It can be transmitted to neonates after passage through an infected birth canal.
- In men, the majority of trichomonal infections are asymptomatic. The most common site of infection is the urethra. In symptomatic males, urethral discharge is seen most commonly, followed by pruritis and dysuria. The discharge may range from mucoid to purulent.
- For most men, trichomonal urethritis is apparently self-limited. *Trichomonas vaginalis* has been implicated in some cases of prostatitis and epididymitis.

DIAGNOSIS

- The diagnosis of *T. vaginalis* may be complicated because approximately 97% of symptomatic women are concomitantly colonized with yeast.
- The simplest and most reliable means of diagnosis is a wet-mount examination of the vaginal discharge. Trichomoniasis is confirmed if characteristic pear-shaped, flagellating organisms are observed.

TREATMENT

- Metronidazole is the only antimicrobial agent available in the United States that is consistently effective in *T. vaginalis* infections.
- Treatment recommendations for *Trichomonas* infections are given in Table 45.8.
- Gastrointestinal complaints (e.g., anorexia, nausea, vomiting, diarrhea) are the most common adverse effects with the single 2-g dose of metronidazole, occurring in 5–10% of treated patients. Some patients complain of a bitter metallic taste in the mouth.
- Patients intolerant of the single 2-g dose because of gastrointestinal adverse effects can be treated with a 7-day course of 500 mg twice daily.
- To achieve maximal cure rates and prevent relapse with the single 2-g dose of metronidazole, simultaneous treatment of infected sexual partners is necessary.
- Patients who fail to respond to an initial course usually respond to a second course of metronidazole therapy.
- Patients taking metronidazole should be instructed to avoid alcohol ingestion during therapy and for 1–2 days after completion of therapy because of a possible disulfiram-like effect.
- At present, no satisfactory treatment is available for pregnant women with *Trichomonas* infections.

EVALUATION OF THERAPEUTIC OUTCOME

- Follow-up is considered unnecessary in patients who become asymptomatic after treatment with metronidazole.
- When patients remain symptomatic, it is important to determine if reinfection has occurred. In these cases a repeat course of therapy, as well as identification and treatment or retreatment of infected sexual partners, is recommended.

VIII

TABLE 45.8. Treatment of Trichomoniasis

Type	Recommended Regimen[a]	Alternative Regimen
Symptomatic and asymptomatic infections	Metronidazole 2.0 g PO in a single dose[b]	Metronidazole 500 mg PO 2 times daily for 7 days[c]
Treatment in pregnancy	No treatment recommended unless symptoms are severe[d]	
Neonatal infections[e]	Metronidazole 10–30 mg/kg daily for 5–8 days	

[a]Recommendations are those of the CDC.

[b]Treatment failures should be treated with metronidazole 500 mg PO 2 times daily for 7 days. Persistent failures should be managed in consultation with an expert. Metronidazole 2 g PO daily for 3–5 days has been effective in patients infected with *T. vaginalis* strains mildly resistant to metronidazole, but experience is limited; higher doses also have been used.

[c]Recently the Anti-Infective Advisory Committee of the FDA recommended approval of a 375 mg twice daily for 7 days dosage regimen. This would be an alternative regimen to the 250 mg three times daily for 7 days regimen currently approved in the product labeling for metronidazole. Neither regimen is currently included in the CDC recommendations for the treatment of trichomoniasis.

[d]Metronidazole is contraindicated in the first trimester of pregnancy and generally should be avoided throughout pregnancy. A single 2-g dose may be used after the first trimester.

[e]Only infants with symptomatic trichomoniasis or with urogenital trichomonal colonization that persists beyond the fourth week of life.

VIII ◀

▶ OTHER SEXUALLY TRANSMITTED DISEASES

- Several STDs other than those previously discussed occur with varying frequency in the United States and throughout the world. While an in-depth discussion of these diseases is beyond the scope of this chapter, recommended treatment regimens are given in Table 45.9.

▶ PREVENTION

- Other than complete abstinence, the most effective way to prevent STD transmission is by using condoms with each act of sexual intercourse.
- When used correctly and consistently, latex condoms with or without spermicide are more effective in protecting against STD transmission than other condoms.
- The female condom may provide an alternative protective device for women with male sexual partners who do not desire to use a condom.
- Vaginal spermicides can reduce the risk for cervical chlamydia and gonorrhea, and some evidence exists that diaphragms may protect against cervical gonorrheal, chlamydial, and trichomonal infections.

See Chapter 110, Sexually Transmitted Diseases, authored by Leroy C. Knodel, PharmD, and Maura A. Kraynak, PharmD, for a more detailed discussion of this topic.

TABLE 45.9. Treatment Regimens for Miscellaneous Sexually Transmitted Diseases

Infection	Recommended Regimen[a]	Alternative Regimen
Chancroid *(Haemophilus ducreyi)*	Azithromycin 1 g PO in a single dose or Ceftriaxone 250 mg IM in a single dose or Erythromycin 500 mg PO four times daily for 7 days	Amoxicillin 500 mg plus clavulanic acid 125 mg three times daily for 7 days or Ciprofloxacin 500 mg PO two times daily for 3 days
Lymphogranuloma venereum	Doxycycline 100 mg PO two times daily for 21 days	Erythromycin 500 mg PO four times daily for 21 days or Sulfisoxazole 500 mg PO four times daily for 21 days or equivalent sulfonamide course
Condylomata acuminata External genital/perianal warts	Cryotherapy (e.g., liquid nitrogen or cryoprobe) or Podofilox 0.5% solution applied twice daily for 3 days, followed by 4 days of no therapy; cycle is repeated as necessary for a total of four cycles[b] or Podophyllin 10–25% in compound tincture of benzoin applied to lesions and washed off in 1–4 hours; repeat weekly for up to six applications[c] or Trichloroacetic acid 80–90% applied to warts; repeat weekly for up to six applications or Electrodesiccation[d] or electrocautery	
Vaginal warts	Cryotherapy with liquid nitrogen or Trichloroacetic acid 50–90% as for external warts or Podophyllin 10–25% in compound tincture of benzoin applied at weekly intervals[e]	

[a]Recommendations are those of the CDC.
[b]Genital warts only.
[c]Because podophyllin is systemically absorbed and toxic, use of large amounts should be avoided. Use of podophyllin is contraindicated in pregnancy.
[d]Electrodessication is contraindicated in patients with cardiac pacemakers or for lesions proximal to the anal verge.
[e]Some experts caution against vaginal use; care must be taken to ensure that the treated area is dry before removing the speculum.

VIII

Chapter 46

▶ SKIN AND SOFT TISSUE INFECTIONS

▶ DEFINITION

Bacterial infections of the skin can be classified as primary (pyodermas/cellulitis) or secondary (invasion of the wound) (Table 46.1). Primary bacterial infections are usually caused by a single bacterial species and involve areas of generally normal skin (e.g., impetigo, erysipelas). Secondary infections, however, develop in areas of previously damaged skin and are frequently polymicrobic in nature.

▶ CELLULITIS

- Cellulitis is generally an acute, spreading infectious process that initially affects the epidermis and dermis and may subsequently spread within the superficial fascia. This process is characterized by inflammation, but with little or no necrosis or suppuration of soft tissue.
- A variety of bacteria are responsible for the several types of cellulitis most commonly encountered (Table 46.1).
- Cellulitis is caused by group A β-hemolytic *streptococci* (most commonly *Streptococcus pyogenes*) or by *Staphylococcus aureus*. Occasionally, other gram-positive cocci such as *Streptococcus pneumoniae* or, in the newborn, group B streptococci can be etiologic agents.

CLINICAL PRESENTATION

- Cellulitis is characterized by erythema and edema of the skin.
- The lesion, which may be extensive, is nonelevated and has poorly defined margins. Tender lymphadenopathy associated with lymphatic involvement is common. Malaise, fever, and chills are also commonly present. There is usually a history of an antecedent wound from minor trauma, an ulcer, or surgery.
- Cellulitis of an incised wound may be caused by any microorganism, but the most aggressively spreading lesions are caused by group A *streptococci* or *Clostridium perfringens*.
- A Gram stain of a smear obtained by injection and aspiration of 0.5 mL of saline (using a small-gauge needle) into the advancing edge of the erythematous lesion may help in making the microbiologic diagnosis but often yields negative results.
- Gram-negative cellulitis can be caused by a wide variety of organisms, such as *Escherichia coli, Proteus* spp., *Klebsiella* spp., and anaerobes (especially *Bacteroides* spp.). These infections are often polymicrobic in nature (see section on Bacterial Diabetic Foot Infections) and involve *Peptostreptococcus* or other anaerobic microorganisms.

TABLE 46.1. Bacterial Classification of Important Skin and Soft Tissue Infections

Primary Infections

Cellulitis	Group A streptococcus, *S. aureus, Haemophilus influenzae* (children); occasionally other streptococci or gram-negative bacilli
Gangrenous	Group A streptococcus, anaerobic streptococci plus a second organism, cellulitis (*Staphylococcus* sp. or gram-negative bacilli, e.g., *Proteus*)
Crepitant cellulitis	*Clostridia* sp., *Bacteroides* sp., anaerobic streptococci, gram-negative bacilli *(Klebsiella, E. coli)*
Impetigo	Group A streptococcus, *S. aureus*
Erysipelas	Group A streptococcus

Secondary Infections

Bite wounds	*Pasteurella multocida, S. aureus, Eikenella corrodens,* anaerobic streptococci, *Fusobacterium* sp., *Bacteroides* sp.
Burn wounds	*Pseudomonas aeruginosa, Enterobacter* sp., other gram-negative bacilli, *S. aureus, Streptococcus* sp.
Diabetic foot infections	*Proteus* sp., *E. coli, S. aureus, Bacteroides fragilis,* anaerobic streptococci
Infections in intravenous drug abusers	*S. aureus, Streptococcus* sp., gram-negative bacilli, *Bacteroides* sp.
Decubitus ulcers	Gram-negative bacilli, *Pseudomonas aeruginosa,* various gram-positive and -negative anaerobes
Lymphangitis (acute)	Group A streptococcus, *S. aureus. Pasteurella multocida*

VIII

TREATMENT

- Antimicrobial therapy of bacterial cellulitis depends on the type of bacteria either documented to be present or suspected. In some instances the rapid identification and treatment are imperative (i.e., group A *streptococci*).
- Local care of cellulitis includes elevation and immobilization of the involved area to decrease local swelling.
- Surgical intervention (incision and drainage) as a mode of therapy is rarely indicated in the treatment of cellulitis.
- As streptococcal cellulitis is indistinguishable clinically from staphylococcal cellulitis, administration of a semisynthetic penicillin (nafcillin or oxacillin) is recommended until a definitive diagnosis, by skin or blood cultures, can be made (Table 46.2). If documented to be a mild cellulitis secondary to streptococci, oral penicillin VK 250–500 mg four times daily or intramuscular procaine penicillin for 10–14 days is adequate. For more severe streptococcal infections aqueous penicillin G should be used intravenously. Mild-to-moderate staphylococcal infections may be treated orally with dicloxacillin 250–500 mg four times daily.

TABLE 46.2. Initial Parenteral Treatment Regimens for Cellulitis Due to Various Pathogens

Staphylococcal or unknown gram-positive infection	Nafcillin or oxacillin 1–2 g every 4–6 h[a,b]
Streptococcal (documented)	Procaine penicillin G 600,000 units intramuscularly every 8–12 h[a] or Aqueous penicillin G 1–2 million units intravenously every 4–6 h[a]
Haemophilus influenzae	*Children:* Ampicillin 50–100 mg/kg/d in four divided doses[c] or Cefuroxime 75 mg/kg/d in three divided doses or a third-generation cephalosporin (i.e., ceftriaxone 75–100 mg/kg once or twice daily, or cefotaxime 200 mg/kg/d in three or four divided doses)[d] *Adults:* Ampicillin 0.5–1 g every 6 h[c] or Cefuroxime 0.75–1.5 g every 8 h or a third-generation cephalosporin (i.e., ceftriaxone 1 g once daily, or cefotaxime 1–2 g every 6–8 h)[e]
Other single gram-negative aerobes	Aminoglycoside[f] or cephalosporin (first- or second-generation depending on severity of infection or susceptibility pattern)
Polymicrobic infection without gram-positive anaerobes	Aminoglycoside[f] + penicillin G 0.6–1.0 million units every 4–6 h or a semisynthetic penicillin (i.e., nafcillin 1–2 g every 4–6 h depending on isolation of staphylococci or streptococci)
Polymicrobic infection with anaerobes	Aminoglycoside[f] + clindamycin 0.9 g every 8 h or metronidazole 0.5–0.75 g every 8 h or Single-drug therapy with second- or third-generation cephalosporin (i.e., cefoxitin 1–2 g every 6 h or ceftizoxime 1–2 every 8 h) or Single-drug therapy with imipenem/cilastatin 0.5 g every 6–8 h

[a]For penicillin-allergic patients, use erythromycin 0.5–1 g every 6 h.

[b]For methicillin-resistant staphylococci, use vancomycin 0.5–1.0 g every 6–8 h with dosage adjustments made for renal dysfunction.

[c]In areas with high incidence of β-lactamase-producing strains, a third-generation cephalosporin should be used until sensitivities are available.

[d]For penicillin-allergic children, use trimethoprim–sulfamethoxazole (4 mg/kg twice daily) or chloramphenicol 50–100 mg/kg/d in four divided doses.

[e]For penicillin-allergic adults, use trimethoprim–sulfamethoxazole (4–5 mg/kg twice daily) or a fluoroquinolone (ciprofloxacin: 200–300 mg IV or 750 mg PO twice daily; ofloxacin 400 mg IV or PO twice daily).

[f]Gentamicin or tobramycin, 2 mg/kg loading dose, then maintenance dose determined by serum concentrations.

VIII

- In penicillin-allergic patients, oral or parenteral erythromycin is used. Alternatively, a first-generation cephalosporin such as cefazolin (500 mg every 8 hours for mild infections or 1–2 g every 6–8 hours for serious infections) may be used cautiously for patients who have not experienced immediate or anaphylactic penicillin reactions and are penicillin skin test negative. In cases where an oral cephalosporin can be used, cefadroxil 500 mg twice daily or cephalexin 250–500 mg four times daily is recommended.
- When erythromycin or cephalosporins cannot be used due to methicillin-resistant staphylococci or severe allergic reactions to β-lactam antibiotics, intravenous vancomycin (for 10–14 days) should be administered. Other effective but more expensive agents include ceftriaxone, imipenem, and the β-lactamase inhibitor combination antibiotics (ampicillin/sulbactam, ticarcillin/clavulanic acid, and piperacillin/tazobactam).
- When treated promptly with appropriate antibiotics, the majority of patients with cellulitis are cured rapidly. Failure to respond to therapy may be indicative of an underlying local or systemic problem, or misdiagnosis.
- For cellulitis caused by gram-negative bacilli or a mixture of microorganisms, immediate antimicrobial chemotherapy as determined by Gram stain is essential, along with appropriate surgical excision of necrotic tissue and drainage. Usually an aminoglycoside combined with an antianaerobic cephalosporin, extended spectrum penicillin, or clindamycin will be used. Therapy should be 10–14 days in duration.

VIII

► ERYSIPELAS

- Erysipelas (Saint Anthony's fire) is a distinct type of superficial cellulitis with extensive lymphatic involvement. It is almost always due to *S. pyogenes* (group A streptococci). Other streptococci (in the newborn) and rarely *S. aureus* can cause similar skin lesions. Erysipelas most commonly occurs in infants, young children, and the elderly, and frequently in patients with nephrotic syndrome. Erysipelas manifests as a warm, painful, edematous, indurated lesion sharply circumscribed by an elevated border.
- Fever and leukocytosis are common.
- In adults it occurs most commonly on the skin of the face and involves the bridge of the nose and cheeks.
- Mild to moderate cases of erysipelas in adults are treated with procaine penicillin G 600,000 units intramuscularly twice daily or penicillin VK 250–500 mg orally four times daily for 7–10 days. Dramatic improvement is generally expected 24–48 hours after treatment has begun.
- Penicillin-allergic patients can be treated with erythromycin 250–500 mg orally every 6 hours for 7–10 days. For more serious infections, aqueous penicillin G 2–8 million units daily should be administered intravenously.

► IMPETIGO

- Impetigo is another distinctive type of superficial cellulitis caused by group A streptococci (known as streptococcal impetigo or impetigo contagiosa). *S. aureus* may be the causative agent in approximately 10% of patients.
- Impetigo manifests initially as small, fluid-filled vesicles. These lesions then rapidly develop into pus-filled blisters that readily rupture. The purulent discharges of these lesions dry to form golden-yellow crusts that are quite characteristic of impetigo. Pruritus is common, and scratching of the lesions may further spread infection through excoriation of the skin. Other systemic signs of infection are minimal.
- The drug of choice for treatment of impetigo is penicillin. It may be administered as either a single intramuscular dose of benzathine penicillin G (300,000–600,000 units in children, 1.2 million units in adults) or as oral penicillin VK (25,000–90,000 units/kg/day divided in four doses in children, 250–500 mg orally four times daily in adults) given for 7–10 days.
- Penicillin-allergic patients can be treated with oral erythromycin (30–50 mg/kg/d divided in four doses in children, 250–500 mg every 6 hours in adults) for 7–10 days.

► LYMPHANGITIS

VIII

- Acute lymphangitis refers to an inflammation involving lymphatic subcutaneous channels. This acute process is secondary to bacterial pathogens, most frequently group A streptococci, but may occasionally be caused by *S. aureus* or *Pasteurella multocida*.
- Acute lymphangitis is characterized by the rapid development of fine red linear streaks extending proximally from the extremities. These linear streaks may be a few to several centimeters wide and extend from the initial site of infection toward the regional lymph nodes, which are usually enlarged and tender. Peripheral edema of the involved extremity may often be present.
- Systemic symptoms are often prominent and include fever, chills, malaise, and headache. A peripheral leukocytosis is generally noted. Cultures of the affected lesions often yield negative results, as the infection resides within the lymphatic channels.
- Penicillin is the treatment of choice for acute lymphangitis. For mild cases 600,000 units of intramuscular procaine penicillin G once or twice daily is used initially; the patient may then (over 24–48 hours) be converted to oral penicillin VK 250–500 mg four times daily for a total of 10 days. In more severely ill patients with bacteremia, aqueous penicillin G 600,000 to 2 million units is given intravenously every 4–6 hours.
- If the suspicion is high that *S. aureus* is the causative pathogen, a semisynthetic penicillinase-resistant penicillin should be used (i.e., nafcillin

1–2 g every 4–6 hours depending on the severity of the infection). For penicillin-allergic patients, erythromycin 250–500 mg four times daily for 10–14 days may be used.

▶ INFECTED PRESSURE ULCERS

- Pressure ulcers are most frequently seen in chronically debilitated persons, in the elderly, and in persons with serious spinal cord injury. Generally, those patients who are at risk for pressure ulcers are elderly or chronically ill young patients who are immobilized either to bed or wheelchair and who may have altered mental status often associated with incontinence.

PATHOPHYSIOLOGY

- Many factors are thought to predispose patients to the formation of pressure ulcers: paralysis, paresis, immobilization, malnutrition, anemia, infection, and advanced age. Four factors thought to be most critical to their formation are pressure, shearing forces, friction, and moisture; however, there is still debate as to the exact pathophysiology of pressure sore formation.
- Without treatment an initial small localized area of ulceration can rapidly progress to 5–6 cm within days.
- Pressure sores are routinely colonized by a wide variety of microorganisms; gram-negative aerobes and anaerobes are most often associated with the infections.

CLINICAL PRESENTATION

- Pressure sores can occur anywhere on the body. More than 95% of all pressure sores are located on the lower part of the body (65% in the region of the pelvis and 3.4% on the lower extremities). The most common sites on the lower portion of the body are the sacral and coccygeal areas, ischial tuberosities, and greater trochanter.
- Pressure sores vary greatly in their severity, ranging from an abrasion to large lesions that can penetrate into the deep fascia involving both bone and muscle (Table 46.3).

PREVENTION AND TREATMENT

- Prevention is the single most important aspect in the management of pressure sores. Friction and shearing forces can be minimized by proper positioning. Skin care and prevention of soilage are important, with the intent being to keep the surface relatively free from moisture. Relief of pressure (even for 5 minutes once every 2 hours) is probably the single most important factor in preventing pressure sore formation.

Medical Management

- Medical management is generally indicated for lesions that are of moderate size and of relatively shallow depth (stage 1 or 2 lesions) and are not located over a bony prominence.

VIII

TABLE 46.3. Pressure Sore Classification

Stage 1	Pressure sore is generally reversible, is limited to the epidermis, and resembles an abrasion. It is best described as an irregularly shaped area of soft tissue swelling, with induration and heat.
Stage 2	A stage 2 sore may also be reversible; it extends through the dermis to the subcutaneous fat along with extensive undermining.
Stage 3[a]	In this instance the sore or ulcer extends further into subcutaneous fat along with extensive undermining.
Stage 4[a]	The sore or ulcer is characterized by penetration into deep fascia involving both muscle and bone.

[a]Stage 3 and 4 lesions are unlikely to resolve on their own and often require surgical intervention.

- The goal of topical therapy is to clean and decontaminate the ulcer, to promote wound healing by permitting the formation of healthy granulation tissue, or to prepare the wound for an operative procedure. The main factors to be considered for successful topical therapy (local care) are the relief of pressure, cleaning measures (debridement), disinfection, and stimulation of granulation tissue.

Debridement

- Debridement and cleansing measures are used to remove devitalized VIII tissue and reduce bacterial contamination, which can slow granulation time and therefore impede healing. Debridement can be accomplished by surgical or mechanical means (wet-to-dry dressing changes). None of the currently available debriding agents (Table 46.4) has been documented to be superior to wet-to-dry dressings.
- Collagenase is thought by many to be the most effective enzymatic debriding agent. Generally, collagenase need only be applied to a clean wound once daily, unless the wound is extremely soiled.

TABLE 46.4. Chemical Debriding Agents

Enzymes
    Sutilains (Travase)
    Collagenase (Santyl/Biozyme-C)
    Fibrinolysin and desoxyribonuclease (Elase)
    Trypsin (Granulex)
    Papin (Panafil)
    Streptokinase/streptodornase (not commercially available)
Elements
    Dextranomer (Debrisan)
    Hydrogen peroxide
    Silver nitrate

- Dextranomer appears to be effective in cleansing exudative venous stasis and decubitus ulcers. It also appears to increase tissue granulation, decrease wound inflammation, and decrease pus and debris; however, its cost and application techniques limit its usefulness.

Disinfection

- A number of agents have been used to disinfect pressure sores (Table 46.5) as well as other types of open wounds; however, objective clinical trials evaluating their efficacy are lacking.
- Most pressure sores are infected with both aerobic and anaerobic microorganisms; however, disinfectants have not been shown to penetrate tissue effectively to completely eradicate these organisms.
- Although disinfectants do not sterilize a wound and may interfere with wound healing, they may be a potential benefit by cleaning the wound (by decreasing the bacterial counts), but they should be stopped when the wound is clean and granulation appears to be occurring.

Granulation/Epithelialization

- After the pressure sore has been adequately debrided and disinfected, and pressure, friction, and moisture have been kept to a minimum, granulation and reepithelialization begin. Many agents have been suggested to aid this process, but hardly any evidence of a supportive nature exists.

VIII
- Karaya has been used successfully in the treatment of excoriated skin sites around ostomies; however, the data and number of patients evaluated are too small to draw any conclusion of possible benefit. Other agents used without documented benefit include sugar, insulin, Gelfoam, benzoyl peroxide, phenytoin, and ketaserin.

RECOMMENDATIONS

- Treatment of the wound begins with the removal of necrotic tissue via either debridement or surgery, along with elimination of any infection. The goal of therapy is to maintain a clean and moist environment. Some broad major guidelines can be recommended for the treatment of pressure sores (stages 1 and 2):

TABLE 46.5. Disinfecting Agents

Acetic acid	Topical antibiotics
Sodium hypochlorite (Dakin's)	Mupirocin ointment
Sodium oxychlorosene	Neomycin
Hydrogen peroxide	Gentamicin
Povidone-iodine	Chloramphenicol
Hexachlorophene	Bacitracin
	Polymyxin B
	Metronidazole

- Relieve pressure.
- Avoid unnecessary friction and shearing forces.
- Prevent patient from lying in a moist environment.
- Use debridement, either pharmacologic or via minor surgical approach.
- Keep the wound clean by pharmacologic means or through use of a physical barrier.
- Use occlusive dressing (may also lead to increased healing and simplify the nursing care routine) if possible.
- For stage 3 and 4 pressure sores, surgical management is most likely the major approach, with follow-up according to guidelines 1 through 6 above.

▶ INFECTED BITE WOUNDS

DOG BITES

- Dog bites account for 80–90% of all animal bite wounds requiring medical attention. Health care providers see two distinct groups of patients seeking medical attention for dog bites. The first group of patients presents 8–12 hours after the injury and require general wound care, repair of tear wounds, or rabies and/or tetanus therapy. The second group of patients presents >12 hours after the injury has occurred and usually have clinical signs of infection and seek medical attention for infection-related complaints (i.e., pain, purulent discharge, swelling).
- The infected dog bite is usually characterized by a localized cellulitis and pain at the site of injury. The cellulitis usually spreads proximally from the initial site of injury. If *Pasteurella multocida* is present, a rapidly progressing cellulitis with a gray malodorous discharge may be encountered.
- The most frequently isolated organisms from infected and noninfected wounds are *S. aureus*, α-hemolytic *streptococci*, *Streptococcus intermedius*, *P. multocida*, *Eikenella corrodens*, *Capnocytophaga canimursus*, *Bacteroides* sp., and *Fusobacterium* sp.
- Wounds should be thoroughly irrigated with a sterile saline solution or a chlorhexidine scrub solution. Proper irrigation significantly decreases the rate of subsequent infection.
- A semisynthetic penicillinase-resistant penicillin orally or amoxicillin/clavulanic acid should be used for puncture wounds, wounds to the hands, and wounds in compromised hosts.
- Tetracycline or trimethoprim–sulfamethoxazol (TMP-SMX) is recommended as an alternative form of therapy for those patients allergic to penicillins. Erythromycin may be considered an alternative for tetracycline in growing children or pregnant women.
- Prophylactic therapy should be given for 5 days. In addition to irrigation and antibiotics, when indicated, the injured area should be immobilized and elevated.

VIII

- Infections developing within the first 24 hours of a bite are most often caused by *P. multocida* and should be treated with penicillin or amoxicillin/clavulanic acid (tetracycline is an alternative for nonpregnant adult penicillin-allergic patients). Treatment should be given for 10–14 days.
- For those infections developing more than 36–48 hours after the bite, the risk of *P. multocida* being involved dramatically decreases in likelihood. Therapy in this instance includes a penicillinase-resistant penicillin (e.g., dicloxacillin) or a cephalosporin (e.g., cefuroxime axetil) and should be given for a full 10–14 days.
- If the immunization history of a patient with anything other than a clean minor wound is not known, tetanus/diphtheria toxoids (Td) and tetanus immune globulin (TIG) should be administered.
- If a patient has been exposed to rabies the treatment objectives consist of thorough irrigation of the wound, tetanus prophylaxis, antibiotic prophylaxis, if indicated, and immunization. Postexposure prophylaxis immunization consists of *both* passive antibody administration and vaccine administration.

CAT BITES

- Cats are probably the second most common cause of animal bite wounds in the United States.
- Approximately 40% of cat bites and scratches become infected. These infections are frequently caused by *P. multocida*, which has been isolated in the oropharynx of 50–70% of healthy cats.
- The management of cat bites is similar to that discussed for dog bites. Antibiotic therapy with penicillin is the mainstay and therapy is as described for dog bites.

HUMAN BITES

- Infected human bites can occur as bites from the teeth or from blows to the teeth (clenched-fist injuries). Human bites are generally more serious than animal bites and carry a higher likelihood of infection. Infections can occur in up to 50% of patients with human bites.
- Infections caused by these injuries are similar and most often caused by the normal oral flora, which include both aerobic and anaerobic microorganisms. The most frequent aerobic organisms are streptococcal species, *S. aureus, Haemophilus parainfluenzae, Klebsiella pneumoniae,* and *Eikenella corrodens.* The most common anaerobic organisms are *Bacteroides* sp., *Fusobacterium* sp., *Peptostreptococcus* sp., and *Peptococcus* sp. Anaerobic microorganisms have been isolated in the range of 40% of human bite and 55% of clenched-fist injuries.
- Management of bite wounds consists of aggressive irrigation, surgical debridement, and immobilization of the affected area. Primary closure for human bites is not generally recommended. If damage to a bone or joint is suspected, radiographic evaluation should be undertaken. Tetanus toxoid and antitoxin may be indicated.

VIII

- Patients with noninfected bite injuries should be given prophylactic antibiotic therapy. Initial therapy should consist of a penicillinase-resistant penicillin (e.g., dicloxacillin) in combination with penicillin. Prophylactic therapy should be given for 3–5 days as for dog bites. A first-generation cephalosporin is not recommended, as the sensitivity to *E. corrodens* is variable. For infected bite wounds, penicillin and a penicillinase-resistant penicillin or amoxicillin/clavulanic acid should be empirically started and changed pending the culture results. Duration of therapy for infected bite injuries should be 7–14 days.

▶ BACTERIAL DIABETIC FOOT INFECTIONS

- Infection of the lower extremities is the most common infectious problem leading to hospitalization of diabetics. Three key factors are involved in the causation of diabetic foot problems: neuropathy, ischemia, and immunologic defects. Any of these disorders can occur in isolation; however, they frequently occur together.
- Diabetic foot infections are typically polymicrobic (an average of 2.5–5.8 isolates per culture). Obligate anaerobes have a significant part in the bacterial flora of these infections. The most common aerobic isolates are *Proteus mirabilis,* group D streptococci, *E. coli,* and *S. aureus.* VIII The principal anaerobic isolate is *B. fragilis,* followed by *Peptococcus* and *Peptostreptococcus.*
- In the treatment of diabetic foot infections the use of intravenous antibiotics alone is often not adequate.
- In addition to the need for local wound care, immobilization of the extremity in question, control of hyperglycemia (maintaining serum glucose below 200 mg/dL may alleviate impairment of phagocytosis), drainage, debridement, and amputation are often necessary.
- Monotherapy with broad-spectrum parenteral antimicrobials along with appropriate medical and/or surgical management is often effective in treating moderate to severe infections (including those in which osteomyelitis is present). Initial (empiric) therapy for diabetics requiring hospitalization for lower extremity infections is similar to that for polymicrobic cellulitis with anaerobes (Table 46.2).
- The drug of choice should be cefoxitin or cefotetan, as determined by cost. Alternatives such as ticarcillin/clavulanate 3.1 g every 4–6 hours, ampicillin/sulbactam 1.5 to 3 g every 6 hours, or piperacillin/tazobactam 3.375 g every 6 hours may also be useful, although relatively little data are available and these agents may be more costly. Imipenem/cilastatin may also be an acceptable alternative, although again relatively few studies are available.
- In patients with penicillin allergies, clindamycin plus either gentamicin or a fluoroquinolone (either parenteral or oral) may be effective alternative regimens.

- Treatment of soft tissue infections in diabetic patients should generally be 10–14 days in duration. However, in cases of underlying osteomyelitis, treatment should continue for 6–12 weeks.
- Outpatient therapy with oral antimicrobials such as cefaclor, ciprofloxacin, ofloxacin, or amoxicillin/clavulanic acid may be appropriate in those diabetics with mild uncomplicated cellulitis. Oral antimicrobials should be used cautiously in serious infections, especially those complicated by osteomyelitis, extensive ulceration, and/or areas of necrosis.
- Treatment with a parenteral agent should also be considered if a mild infection being treated with an oral agent fails to show improvement within 48–72 hours of the beginning of therapy.

Recommendations for the Management of the Infected Diabetic Foot

- Initially assess the extent of the lesion.
- Obtain deep tissue cultures for both anaerobes and aerobes.
- Debride necrotic tissue and keep wound clean with dressing changes as needed (generally two to three times daily).
- Maximize diabetic control to ensure optimal healing.
- Restrict the patient initially to bedrest, leg elevation, and control of edema, if present.
- Rule out possibility of osteomyelitis via x-ray and/or bone scan.
- Mild uncomplicated infections can be treated in the outpatient setting with an oral antimicrobial regimen as previously described. Treatment should last at least 10–14 days.
- For more severe cases or those complicated by the presence of osteomyelitis, parenteral antimicrobial therapy is used. In severely infected cases, therapy is continued until healing of the wound can be documented. If improvement is seen in 7–14 days the regimen may be converted to an oral regimen. Therapy should continue for at least 6–12 weeks.
- After healing of the infected ulcer has occurred, a program for prevention should be designed.

VIII

▶ BURN WOUND INFECTIONS

- Of the approximately 1.45 million burn injuries that occur in the United States each year, a surprisingly low percentage (4%) results in a visit to the emergency department. Of these approximately half-million emergency department visits, about 100,000 are classified as severe burns, and 6000 result in death on an annual basis.
- The typical clinical features following burn injury are visible swelling with blister formation, loss of the protective epithelium resulting in wet and weeping surfaces. Due to the fluid shifts associated with these changes, major burns may result in hypovolemic shock without adequate fluid resuscitation. Overhydration of tissues may aggravate the edema formation, increasing the risk of infection and ischemia.

- Edema formation in humans is maximal around 6 hours after injury, starts to resolve by 24 hours, and is usually resolved in 6–7 days. The magnitude of the fluid shifts appears to be linearly related to the time of heat exposure and temperature of the exposure. Although a partial thickness burn and a deep full thickness burn will result in coagulation necrosis, the deep burn eliminates microcirculation and limits edema formation.
- The majority of burn wound infections are now caused primarily by gram-negative bacteria. Initially, *P. aeruginosa* was the most common bacteria identified; however, the use of potent antibiotics has reduced its overall incidence. No single microorganism is responsible for the majority of burn wound infections. Some other commonly isolated gram-negative bacteria include *Enterocbacter cloacae, Providencia stuartii, Serratia marcescens,* and *Klebsiella* sp.
- If the bacterial concentration at the burn site exceeds 10^6 microorganisms per gram of tissue, then spread to viable tissue and bacteremia usually occurs.

TREATMENT

- Following thermal injury, a variety of measures is initiated to resuscitate the patient.
    - Initially, all foreign material should be lavaged from the burn site.
    - Patients receive tetanus prophylaxis. Aseptic technique is observed by all personnel caring for the patient.
    - Aggressive nutritional replacement is instituted to meet the patient's hypermetabolic needs.
- Fluid resuscitation is the prime objective of initial burn therapy. Swift and appropriate fluid resuscitation can greatly decrease morbidity and mortality from this type of injury. The most commonly used guidelines for fluid resuscitation for burn shock consist of fluid administered through two large-bore intravenous lines at a rate adequate to produce a urine output of 30 mL/h. Ringer's lactate is administered at a dose of 4 mL per percent of total burn surface area burn per kilogram of body weight.
- Fifty percent of the fluid replacement need is administered in the first 8 hours from the time of burn. The remaining 50% is administered over the next 16 hours based on clinical evaluation. After the first 24 hours, maintenance fluid administration is then administered in amounts to account for normal basal fluid needs plus calculated evaporated water loss from the wound.
- Another major goal of burn wound therapy is to prevent the wound from becoming infected. Therapy includes prompt removal of necrotic tissue from the burn injury and immediate closure of the wound with skin grafts. One of the main methods of controlling burn wound sepsis is prevention of local burn infection via the use of topical antibiotics. Several agents are available for topical administration, including silver sulfadiazine, sodium mafenide, and silver nitrate.

VIII

Recommendations for the Management of Burn Wound Infections

- The burn wound should be kept clean and free of infection.
- Wash and debride loose eschar twice daily.
- A great deal of effort in the management of burn injuries is aimed at the prevention and treatment of infections. To control wound surface bacteria, topical antibiotics should be applied twice daily.
- Infections in the burn patient may be either at the site of the injury or at other sites. The patient should be watched closely for signs of systemic infection.
- If signs of systemic infection are present, then parenteral antibiotics should be used. Serum concentrations of drugs should be monitored closely (if possible) since the hyperdynamic state of the burn patient has been documented to alter the pharmacokinetics of drugs. Careless and indiscriminate use of antimicrobials in this setting is a problem and should be avoided to minimize the potential for the emergence of resistant strains of bacteria.

See Chapter 103, Skin and Soft Tissue Infections, authored by Larry H. Danzinger, PharmD, Douglas Fish, PharmD, and Erkan Hassan, PharmD, for a more detailed discussion of this topic.

VIII

Chapter 47

▶ SURGICAL PROPHYLAXIS

▶ DEFINITION

- *Prophylactic* antibiotics are administered prior to contamination of previously sterile tissues or fluids. The goal is to *prevent* a surgical-site infection (SSI) from developing.
- The prevention and management of postoperative complications (non-SSI) such as catheter-related urinary tract infections and atelectasis are important and occasionally require antibiotics, but that is not the goal of surgical prophylaxis.
- Antibiotics that are given when there is a strong possibility of, but as yet unproven, established infection are termed *presumptive. Therapeutic* antibiotics are required for established infection.
- SSIs are classified as either incisional or deep. Both types, by definition, occur by postoperative day 30. This period extends to 1 year in the case of deep infection associated with prosthesis implantation.

▶ RISK FACTORS FOR SURGICAL WOUND INFECTION

- The traditional classification system developed by the National Research Council (NRC) stratifying surgical procedures by infection risk is reproduced in Table 47.1. The NRC wound classification for a specific procedure is determined intraoperatively

INDIVIDUALIZING RISK FOR SURGICAL WOUND INFECTION

- The Study on the Efficacy of Nosocomial Infection Control (SENIC) analyzed >100,000 surgery cases in order to identify and validate risk factors for SSI. Abdominal operations, operations lasting >2 hours, contaminated or dirty procedures by NRC classification, and more than three underlying medical diagnoses were associated with an increased incidence of SSI. When the NRC classification was stratified by the number of SENIC risk factors present, the infection rates varied by as much as a factor of 15 within the same operative category (Table 47.2).
- The SENIC risk assessment technique has been modified to include the American Society of Anesthesiologists (ASA) preoperative assessment score (Table 47.3). An ASA score of ≥3 was associated with increased SSI risk.

▶ REDUCING SURGICAL–SITE INFECTION RISK

- Prolonged hospitalization is associated with colonization of, and occasionally, infection with, nosocomial bacteria, which increases the incidence of SSI. For this reason, elective surgery is often postponed if the patient is hospitalized for an unrelated medical problem.

TABLE 47.1. National Research Council Wound Classification, Risk of Surgical Wound Infection, and Indication for Antibiotics

Classification	SSI Rate (%)	Criteria	Antibiotics
Clean	<2	No acute inflammation or transection of gastrointestinal, oropharyngeal, genitourinary, biliary, or respiratory tracts. Elective case, no technique break	Not indicated unless high-risk procedure[a] (? high-risk patient)
Clean–contaminated	<10	Controlled opening of aforementioned tracts with minimal spillage/minor technique break. Clean procedures performed emergently or with major technique breaks	Prophylactic antibiotics indicated
Contaminated	20	Acute, nonpurulent inflammation present. Major spillage/technique break during clean–contaminated procedure	Prophylactic antibiotics indicated
Dirty	40	Obvious preexisting infection present (abscess, pus, or necrotic tissue present)	Therapeutic antibiotics required

[a]High-risk procedures include implantation of prosthetic materials and other procedures where surgical wound infection is associated with high morbidity.

VIII

- Shaving the incision site with a razor the day before surgery is associated with higher infection rates. Clipping the operative site just prior to the procedure is preferred.
- Preoperative showering with an antiseptic soap may also lower infection rates.
- Unnecessary prolongation of the surgical procedure results in a higher incidence of SSI.

TABLE 47.2. Surgical Site Infection Incidence (%) Stratified By National Research Council Wound Classification and SENIC Risk Factors[a]

No. of SENIC Risk Factors	Clean	Clean–Contaminated	Contaminated	Dirty
0	1.1	0.6	N/A	N/A
1	3.9	2.8	4.5	6.7
2	8.4	8.4	8.3	10.9
3	15.8	17.7	11.0	18.8
4	N/A	N/A	23.9	27.4

[a]SENIC risk factors include abdominal operation, operations lasting >2 hours, contaminated or dirty procedures by NRC classification, and >3 underlying medical diagnoses.

TABLE 47.3. American Society of Anesthesiologists Physical Status Classification

Class	Description
1	Normal healthy patient
2	Mild systemic disease
3	Severe systemic disease that is not Incapacitating
4	Incapacilating systemic disease that is a constant threat to life
5	Not expected to survive 24 hours with or without operation

▶ MICROBIOLOGY

- Loss of protective flora via antibiotics can upset the balance and allow pathogenic bacteria to proliferate and increase infectious risk.
- Normal flora can become pathogenic when translocated to a normally sterile tissue site or fluid during surgical procedures.
- According to the National Nosocomial Infections Surveillance System (NNIS), the five most common pathogens encountered in surgical wounds are *S. aureus, enterococci,* coagulase-negative *staphylococci, E. coli,* and *Pseudomonas aeruginosa.*

▶ ANTIBIOTIC ISSUES   VIII ◀

BASIC PRINCIPLES FOR THE USE OF ANTIMICROBIAL SURGICAL PROPHYLAXIS

- Antimicrobials are delivered to the targeted tissue site prior to the initial incision.
- Bactericidal antibiotic tissue concentrations are maintained throughout the length of the surgical procedure.
- Antimicrobials with short serum half-lives may require multiple dosing at frequent dosing intervals, especially if the surgery is prolonged or in instances of massive blood loss.
- Under ideal conditions, the antibiotic chosen for surgical prophylaxis should achieve its highest tissue concentrations at the time of initial skin incision during surgery.
- Antibiotics administered too early or after skin incision probably achieve subtherapeutic concentrations during the operation, putting the patient at high risk of infection.

ANTIMICROBIAL SELECTION

- The choice of the prophylactic antimicrobial depends on a multitude of factors, including the type of surgical procedure, the most likely pathogenic organisms, the safety and efficacy of the antimicrobial, the track record for success based on published literature, and costs.
- The antimicrobial must also take into account the susceptibility patterns of nosocomial-derived pathogens associated with the specific institution.

- Typically, gram-positive coverage is included in the choice of surgical prophylaxis since organisms such as *S. aureus* and *S. epidermidis* are commonly encountered as skin flora.
- The decision to broaden coverage to gram-negatives and anaerobic organisms is site specific (e.g., upper respiratory tract, gastrointestinal tract, genitourinary tract etc., Table 47.4) and depends on whether the operation will transect a hollow viscous or mucous membrane containing resident flora.
- Intravenous antibiotic administration is favored because of its reliability in achieving suitable tissue concentrations.
- First-generation cephalosporins (particularly cefazolin) are the preferred choice (as good as second- or third-generation cephalosporins) for most surgical procedures. Although there are some reports of failure with cefazolin in cardiac procedures associated with methicillin-sensitive *S. aureus,* the majority of concern is due to the increasing incidence of methicillin-resistant *S. aureus* (MRSA) infections.
- Vancomycin would seem to be a logical alternative to cefazolin in institutions with a high incidence of MRSA or for patients with β-lactam allergy.
- In cases where broader gram-negative and anaerobic coverage is desired, the antianaerobic cephalosporins such as cefoxitin, cefotetan, and cefmetazole are appropriate.

► VIII

► RECOMMENDATIONS FOR SPECIFIC TYPES OF SURGERY

Specific recommendations are summarized in Table 47.4.

GASTRODUODENAL SURGERY

- The risk of infection rises with conditions that increase gastric pH and subsequent bacterial overgrowth such as obstruction, hemorrhage, malignancy, or acid-suppression therapy (clean–contaminated).
- A single dose of intravenous cefazolin will provide adequate prophylaxis for most cases.
- Postoperative antibiotics may be indicated if perforation is detected during surgery, depending on whether an established infection is present.

BILIARY TRACT SURGERY

- Antibiotic prophylaxis has been proven beneficial for surgery involving the biliary tract.
- Most frequently encountered organisms include *E. coli, Klebsiella,* and *enterococci.* Single-dose prophylaxis with cefazolin is currently recommended.
- Some surgeons use *presumptive* antibiotics for cases of acute cholecystitis or cholangitis and defer surgery until the patient is afebrile, in an attempt to decrease infection rates further, but this practice is controversial.

TABLE 47.4. Most Likely Pathogens and Specific Recommendations for Surgical Prophylaxis

Type of Operation	Likely Pathogens	Recommended Prophylaxis Regimen[a]	Comments
Gastroduodenal	Enteric gram-negative bacilli, gram-positive cocci, oral anaerobes	Cefazolin 1 g × 1	High-risk patients only
Biliary tract	Enteric gram-negative bacilli, enterococci, clostridia	Cefazolin 1 g × 1	Bactobilia does not correlate well with pathogens
Colorectal	Enteric gram-negative bacilli, anaerobes	PO: neomycin 1 g + erythromycin base 1 g at 1 pm, 2 pm, + 11 pm 1 day pre-op plus mechanical bowel prep IV: cefoxitin or cefotetan 1 g × 1	Benefit of oral plus IV's controversial
Appendectomy	Enteric gram-negative bacilli, anaerobes	Cefoxitin or cefotetan 1 g × 1	3–5 days of therapeutic antibiotics post-op if established infection present
Urologic	E. coli	Cefazolin 1 g or oral antibiotic with comparable spectrum (where appropriate) × 1	Only beneficial in high-risk cases (preexisting bacteriuria, high infection rate)
Cesarean section	Enteric gram-negative bacilli, anaerobes, group B streptococci, enterococci	Cefazolin 2 g × 1	Give after cord is clamped
Hysterectomy	Same as Cesarean section	Vaginal: cefazolin 1 g × 1, may repeat q8h × 2 doses Abdominal: cefazolin 1 g × 1	Beneficial in abdominal hysterectomy regardless of risk
Head and neck	S. aureus, streptococci, oral anaerobes	Cefazolin 2 g or clindamycin 600 mg at induction and q8h × 2 more doses	Addition of gentamicin to clindamycin is controversial
Cardiac	S. aureus, S. epidermidis, corynebacterium, enteric gram-negative bacilli	Cefazolin 1 g q8h × 48 hours beginning at induction	Second-generation cephalosporins have been advocated; controversial
Vascular	S. aureus, S. epidermidis, enteric gram-negative bacilli	Cefazolin 1 g at induction and q6h × 2 more doses	Abdominal and lower extremity procedures have highest infection rate
Orthopedic	S. aureus, S. epidermidis	Joint replacement: cefazolin 1 g × 1 pre-op, then q8h × 2 more doses Hip fracture repair: same except continue for 48 hours total	Open fractures assumed contaminated with gram-negative bacilli; aminoglycosides often used
Neurosurgery	S. aureus, S. epidermidis	Cefazolin 1 g × 1	Use in CSF shunting procedures is controversial

VIII

[a]One-time doses are optimally infused at induction of anesthesia except as noted. Repeat doses may be required for long procedures.

- Detection of an active infection during surgery (gangrenous gallbladder, suppurative cholangitis) is an indication for *therapeutic* postoperative antibiotics.

COLORECTAL SURGERY

- Anaerobes and gram-negative aerobes predominate in SSIs, although gram-positive aerobes are also important (Table 47.4). Therefore, the risk of SSI in the absence of an adequate prophylactic regimen is substantial.
- Reducing bacteria load with a thorough bowel preparation regimen (4 liters of polyethylene glycol solution administered orally the day before surgery) is the single most important method to prevent SSI.
- The combination of 1 gram of neomycin plus 1 gram of erythromycin base given orally 19, 18, and 9 hours preoperatively is the most commonly used oral regimen in the United States.
- Whether perioperative parenteral antibiotics, in addition to the standard preoperative oral antibiotic regimen, will lower SSI rates further still is controversial.
- Postoperative antibiotics are unnecessary in the absence of any untoward events or findings during surgery.

APPENDECTOMY

- A cephalosporin with antianaerobic activity such as cefoxitin or cefotetan is currently recommended as a first-line agent.
- Single-dose therapy is adequate as long as the appendix is not found to be gangrenous or perforated during surgery.
- Established intra-abdominal infections require appropriate *therapeutic* postoperative antibiotics.

UROLOGIC PROCEDURES

- As long as the urine is sterile preoperatively, the risk of SSI after urologic procedures is very low and the benefit of *prophylactic* antibiotics in this setting is controversial.
- Specific recommendations are listed in Table 47.4.
- *E. coli* is the most frequently encountered organism.
- Urologic procedures requiring an abdominal approach such as a nephrectomy or cystectomy require prophylaxis appropriate for a clean–contaminated abdominal procedure.

CESAREAN SECTION

- Antibiotics are efficacious to prevent SSIs for women undergoing cesarean section regardless of underlying risk factors.
- Several types of bacteria have been implicated in SSIs (Table 47.4).
- Cefazolin remains the drug of choice.
- Providing a broader spectrum by using cefoxitin against anaerobes or piperacillin for better coverage against *Pseudomonas* or *enterococci,* for example, does not lower postoperative infection rates any further in comparative studies.

VIII

- A single 2-g dose of cefazolin has been found to be superior to a 1-g dose and thus is recommended.
- Antibiotic should be administered just after the umbilical cord is clamped, avoiding exposure of the infant to the drug.

HYSTERECTOMY

- Vaginal hysterectomies are associated with a high rate of postoperative infection when performed without the benefit of prophylactic antibiotics.
- Cefazolin is the drug of choice.
- Single-dose therapy should be adequate, but most reports used a 24-hour regimen.
- Abdominal hysterectomy SSI rates are correspondingly lower than vaginal hysterectomy rates. However, prophylactic antibiotics are still recommended regardless of underlying risk factors.
- Both cefazolin and anti-anaerobic cephalosporins (e.g., cefoxitin, cefotetan) have been studied extensively, and it is unclear which is superior.
- The antibiotic course should not exceed 24 hours in duration.

HEAD AND NECK SURGERY

- Many head and neck surgical procedures, such as parotidectomy or a simple tooth extraction, are clean procedures by NRC definition and are associated with very low rates of SSI. As expected, surgical prophylaxis has not been proven to be beneficial in these circumstances. VIII
- Head and neck procedures involving an incision through a mucosal layer (and therefore breaching primary immune system barriers) carry a high risk of SSI.
- Specific recommendations for prophylaxis are listed in Table 47.4.
- Whereas typical doses of cefazolin are ineffective for anaerobic infections, the recommended 2-g dose produces concentrations high enough to be inhibitory to these organisms. A 24-hour duration has been used in most studies, but single-dose therapy may also be effective.

CARDIAC SURGERY

- Although most cardiac surgeries are technically clean procedures, prophylactic antibiotics have been shown to lower rates of SSI.
- The usual pathogens are skin flora (see Table 47.4) and, rarely, gram-negative enteric organisms.
- Cefazolin has been extensively studied and is currently considered the drug of choice.
- The accepted duration of prophylactic antibiotics after cardiac surgery is currently 48 hours. However, there is some evidence that 24 hours is sufficient.
- It may be necessary to use vancomycin in hospitals with a high incidence of SSI with MRSA. The need for vancomycin should be evaluated carefully, as previously discussed.

NON-CARDIAC VASCULAR SURGERY

- Prophylactic antibiotics are beneficial, especially in procedures involving the abdominal aorta and the lower extremities.
- *Staphylococci* and gram-negative enterics are the most likely pathogens.
- Twenty-four hours of prophylaxis with IV cefazolin is adequate.

ORTHOPEDIC SURGERY

- Prophylactic antibiotics have been shown to be beneficial in cases involving implantation of prosthetic material (pins, plates, artificial joints).
- The most likely pathogens mirror those of other clean procedures and include *Staphylococci* and, infrequently, gram-negative aerobes.
- Cefazolin is the best studied antibiotic and is thus the drug of choice.
- Rates of SSI after total joint replacement are reduced with prophylactic antibiotics. They are also indicated for hip fracture surgery. The current accepted duration is up to 48 hours.

NEUROSURGERY

- The use of prophylactic antibiotics in neurosurgery is controversial.
- Single doses of cefazolin or, where required, vancomycin appear to lower SSI risk after craniotomy.
- Conversely, studies performed on shunting procedures do not consistently show lower infection rates with antibiotic prophylaxis.

VIII

See Chapter 115, Antimicrobial Prophylaxis in Surgery, authored by Stephen W. Janning, PharmD and Michael J. Rybak, PharmD, FCCP, BCPS, for a more detailed discussion of this topic.

Chapter 48

► TUBERCULOSIS

► EPIDEMIOLOGY

- Tuberculosis remains the leading cause of infectious deaths in the world. In the United States, approximately 13 million people are infected, with 23,000–25,000 new cases each year, resulting in an annual death rate of about 2000 patients.
- Tuberculosis is concentrated in patients who are the most difficult to treat: underprivileged patients without access to health care and who live in crowded conditions; recalcitrant patients who are noncompliant with treatment protocols; and immune-compromised patients, who are unable to ward off the disease.
- Close contacts of patients with pulmonary tuberculosis (> 40 h/week) are at particularly high risk, with an estimated infection rate of 25–30%.
- The elderly (> 65 years of age) comprise the age group with the largest number of infected persons. However, the upswing in tuberculosis case rates has occurred owing to an increased infection rate in certain younger populations, especially those in crowded living conditions with reduced access to health care.

► PATHOPHYSIOLOGY

- *Mycobacterium tuberculosis, M. bovis,* and *M. africanum* are pathogenic to normal human hosts, with *M. tuberculosis* being the most prevalent.
- Tuberculosis is invariably transmitted from person to person via micro-size droplet nuclei that are dispersed by either coughing or sneezing.
- Primary infection is initiated by the alveolar implantation of organisms in droplet nuclei that are small enough (1–5 μm) to escape the ciliary epithelial cells of the upper respiratory tract. Once implanted, the organisms multiply and are ingested by pulmonary macrophages where they continue to multiply, albeit more slowly. Tissue necrosis and calcification of the originally infected site and regional lymph nodes may occur, resulting in the formation of a radiodense area referred to as a *Ghon complex.*
- After lymph node involvement, organisms may be held in check or may spread via the bloodstream to a variety of organ systems.
- Concurrent with the proliferation of organisms is the development of delayed hypersensitivity via activation and multiplication of CD4 lymphocytes.
- The arrest of mycobacterial proliferation is characterized pathologically by formation of granulomas of two types: *proliferative* granulomas, which are stable and can effectively limit the spread of the organism, and *caseating* granulomas, so named for their cheese-like appearance.

TABLE 48.1. Likelihood of Various Clinical Presentations of Tuberculous Infection in Different Patient Groups

Status at Exposure	Asymptomatic Infection	Progressive Primary Infection	Reactivation Pulmonary	Extrapulmonary Disease	Miliary Tuberculosis
<1 yr old	++	+++	+/-	++	+
1–5 yr	++	++	+/-	++	+
6–10 yr	++	+	+	+	+
11–15 yr	+++	+/-	+	+	+/-
HIV (-) adult	+++	+/-	+	+	+/-
HIV (+) adult	+	++	+	++	+

Key: +++, predominant feature; ++, common; +, occasional; +/-, rare.

They have a necrotic center, are relatively unstable, and permit the limited growth of *M. tuberculosis* within them.

- Approximately 90% of patients who experience primary disease have no further clinical manifestations other than a positive skin test either alone or in combination with radiographic evidence of stable granulomas.

- Approximately 3–5% of patients (usually children, the elderly, or the immunocompromised) experience progressive primary disease at the site of the primary infection (usually the lower lobes) and frequently by dissemination, leading to meningitis and often to involvement of the upper lobes of the lung as well. The remaining 7–10% of patients develop reactivation disease, which arises subsequent to the hematogenous spread of the organism.

- Occasionally, a massive inoculum of organisms may be introduced into the bloodstream, causing widely disseminated disease and granuloma formation known as *miliary tuberculosis.*

- The various forms of tuberculosis infection occur at different degrees of frequency in different populations (Table 48.1).

- HIV infection increases the risk that a patient infected with *M. tuberculosis* will develop active disease. The Centers for Disease Control and Prevention (CDC) estimates an HIV-infected individual with tuberculous infection to be 113–170 times more likely to develop active diseases than an HIV seronegative patient.

VIII

▶ CLINICAL PRESENTATION

NON–HIV-INFECTED PATIENTS

- The clinical presentation of pulmonary tuberculosis is nonspecific, indicative only of a slowly evolving infectious process (Table 48.2).

TABLE 48.2. Clinical Features of Tuberculosis in HIV-Positive Versus -Negative Patients

	HIV-Negative (Immunocompetent)	HIV-Positive (AIDS)
Onset	Gradual	Abrupt
Presentation	Reactivation	Progressive primary
PPD Result	Usually positive	Usually negative
Chest radiograph	Apical infiltrate	Diffuse, lower lobes
Extrapulmonary forms	Occasional	Common
Other pathogens present	Occasional	Common
AFB-positive sputum	Usually	Usually
Response to therapy	Excellent	Fair–good

- A patient with subclinical or early disease may be completely asymptomatic. When the population of organisms increases to a certain point, however, the patient begins to complain of generalized malaise, anorexia, weight loss, and fatigue as well as intermittent fevers with alternating chills and night sweats. Subsequently, a cough with increasing sputum production develops. Hemoptysis and shortness of breath are usually indicative of advanced disease. VIII

- Physical examination is nonspecific, suggestive of progressive pulmonary disease. Dullness to chest percussion suggests consolidation in involved areas of the lung. Rales and increased vocal fremitus are frequently observed upon auscultation.

- Abnormal laboratory data are usually limited to moderate elevations in the white blood cell count with a lymphocyte predominance.

- Clinical features associated with extrapulmonary tuberculosis vary depending on the organ system(s) involved, but typically consist of slowly progressive compromise of organ function with low-grade fever and other constitutional symptoms, as mentioned previously.

HIV-INFECTED PATIENTS

- The clinical features of patients with HIV infection who develop tuberculosis may be markedly different from those classically observed in immunocompetent individuals (Table 48.2). In AIDS patients, tuberculosis is much more likely to present as the progressive primary form, to involve extrapulmonary sites, and to involve multiple lobes of the lung.

- Tuberculosis in AIDS patients is less likely to involve cavitary disease, be associated with a positive skin test, or be associated with fever. Nonspecific findings of tuberculosis such as malaise, weight loss, weakness, and fever are, in fact, the norm in AIDS patients.

▶ DIAGNOSIS

IDENTIFICATION OF INDIVIDUALS WITH ASYMPTOMATIC INFECTION

- The types of individuals who should be screened with PPD are shown in Table 48.3.
- The CDC recommends that the following individuals be screened for tuberculous infection and/or tuberculosis: HIV-infected persons; close contacts of known or suspected cases of active tuberculosis; patients with medical risk factors such as silicosis, gastrectomy, jejunoileal bypass, weight < 90% of ideal body weight, chronic renal failure, diabetes mellitus, use of high-dose corticosteroids or other immunosuppressive drugs, and hematologic or other malignancies; patients with chest radiographs showing fibrotic lesions consistent with old tuberculosis; medically underserved low-income groups, especially racial minorities; immigrants and other foreign-born individuals; alcoholics and intravenous drug users; residents and employees of long-term care facilities such as nursing homes, prisons, and mental institutions; and health care workers and trainees.

TUBERCULIN SKIN TEST

- The most widely used screening method for tuberculous infection is the tuberculin skin test, which uses purified protein derivative (PPD). Three test strengths of PPD-S are available:
  - First strength (1 TU), intermediate strength (5 TU), and second strength (250 TU). First-strength PPD-S is sometimes used for testing patients in whom a severe reaction may be expected (i.e., patients with known prior positive test), although few data exist to support this practice.

TABLE 48.3. Candidates for Screening with PPD Skin Test

Individuals	Initial Screening	Retest Periodically	Test If Local Outbreak
HIV-infected	×	If possible	N/A
Hospital employees	×	Annually–semiannually	Yes, if exposed
Nursing home staff	×	Annually	Yes, if exposed
Nursing home residents	×	Probably not	Yes, if exposed
Workers at prisons, homeless shelters, clinics, etc.	×	Annually	Yes, if exposed
Immigrants	×	If possible	N/A
Health care students	×	Annually–biannually	Yes, if exposed
General population	No	No	Yes, if exposed

VIII

- The intermediate-strength form is almost invariably used for routine screening and diagnostic purposes.
- Second-strength PPD-S may be used in testing patients with depressed cell-mediated immunity who have had a negative result with the intermediate-strength test, but appear likely to have tuberculosis on the basis of clinical criteria.
- The Mantoux method of PPD administration, which is the most reliable technique, consists of the intradermal injection of 0.1 mL of PPD containing 5 TU. The test is read 48–72 hours after injection by measuring the diameter of the zone of induration.
- A positive reaction remains for at least 5 days after the test has been administered.
- For patients with AIDS or young children with recent exposure to an index case, any extent of induration might be read as positive. For HIV-infected patients or those suspected of having HIV infection but who refuse HIV testing, as well as all others with documented recent exposure, a cutoff of 5 mm is used to initiate treatment. For individuals who were recently ($\leq$2 years ago) skin-test negative, as well as those with a reaction of unknown duration and radiographic signs of old tuberculosis, or a history of diabetes, gastrectomy, cancer, immunosuppressive therapy, or renal failure, reactions >10 mm are considered positive.
- For those with a reaction of unknown duration and with no other risk factors, a reaction size of 15 mm is considered necessary to initiate treatment. VIII
- Since HIV-infected patients are frequently anergic, a negative PPD test result cannot rule out infection. This has led the CDC to recommend that empiric preventive therapy be strongly considered for any HIV-infected patient who is anergic and in whom the incidence of new infection is 1% per year or in whom the cumulative infection prevalence is 10% or greater (see high-risk groups previously listed).

SYMPTOMATIC DISEASE

- Confirmatory diagnosis of a clinical suspicion of tuberculosis must be made via chest x-ray and microbiological examination of sputum or other infected material to rule out active disease.
- Examination of sputum is important in providing microbiologic evidence of pulmonary tuberculosis. Acid-fast bacilli (AFB) may be detected by sputum fluorochrome fluorescent stain in 50–80% of all patients with active pulmonary tuberculosis. To detect AFB by staining, 10,000 AFB/mL of specimen is necessary. Multiple sputum collections during 3 consecutive days are recommended.
- Drug susceptibility tests should routinely be performed. Agar-based susceptibility testing requires at least 4–6 weeks to complete. The BACTEC system provides information on mycobacterial identification and susceptibility in a much shorter time period.

▶ TREATMENT

GENERAL PRINCIPLES

- Selection of a treatment plan (e.g., which drugs, how many, how long) depends on a number of patient- and disease-related factors. These are listed in Table 48.4. The number of antimicrobials used in therapy depends on the estimated number of acid-fast bacilli in the body, the likelihood of resistance, and the desired duration of therapy.

PHARMACOLOGIC TREATMENT

Asymptomatic Infection

- Chemoprophylaxis should be initiated in patients who are asymptomatic and have sufficient objective evidence of infection (history of recent exposure, skin test result, underlying disease state[s]) to merit therapy, *or* are infected with HIV, are anergic, and possess other risk factors for tuberculous infection (IV drug abuser, history of recent institutionalization/incarceration, exposure to others with tuberculosis) (Table 48.5).
- A 6-month course of isoniazid (INH) administered daily is sufficient in most asymptomatic patients. Children, HIV-positive patients (or high-risk patients who refuse testing), and patients with stable abnormal chest films should still remain on therapy for 12 months. Individuals likely to be noncompliant may be treated with a regimen of 15 mg/kg (to a maximum of 900 mg) twice weekly with observation.
- If the individual has been exposed to a patient with INH-resistant *M. tuberculosis* or a patient who has failed chemotherapy, chemoprophylaxis with rifampin (RIF) alone or in combination with pyrazinamide (PZA) or ethambutol (EMB) should be initiated and continued for 12 months. If the index case has documented multiple drug resistant TB (MDR-TB), combination therapy with PZA and ofloxacin is recommended. All other patients should receive INH alone for 6 months (12

VIII

TABLE 48.4. Factors to Consider When Choosing the Number of Drugs for Therapy of Tuberculous Infection

Use Fewer Drugs	Use More Drugs
Asymptomatic disease	Symptomatic disease
Longer course of therapy	Shorter course of therapy
No cavitary disease	Cavitary disease
Pulmonary disease only	Extrapulmonary disease
HIV-negative patient	HIV-positive patient
Doubt resistance	Suspect resistance
INH- or rifampin-susceptible	INH- and rifampin-resistant

TABLE 48.5. Antimicrobial Regimens for Chemoprophylaxis of Tuberculosis in Asymptomatic Patients

Patient Type/Situation	Drug and Regimen
Child with documented recent exposure to an index case of pulmonary tuberculosis	Skin test and INH for three months; continue for 12 months if skin test positive
Adult with "positive" PPD skin test and no other confounding factors	INH for 6 months
HIV-infected patient with "positive" PPD skin test, or anergic with risk factors for tuberculosis	INH for 12 months
Positive skin test and documented exposure to INH-resistant TB	PZA/rifampin or PZA/ethambutol for 12 months
Positive skin test and documented exposure to INH- and rifampin-resistant TB	PZA/ofloxacin for 12 months

VIII

months for HIV-infected patients and children). All patients treated with INH should also receive pyridoxine, 25–50 mg daily.

Symptomatic Disease, Culture-Positive, Resistance Unlikely

- Tables 48.6 and 48.7 list drug regimen options and doses for treatment of symptomatic infection. Short-course (6 months) chemotherapy with multiple antimicrobial agents is now the standard for treating drug-susceptible tuberculosis

- Current practices of chemotherapy for tuberculosis use combinations of two classes of agents: those that rapidly eliminate extracellular organisms from the sputum and decrease infectivity (early bactericidal drugs such as INH and streptomycin [STR]), and those that slowly destroy dividing organisms within granulomas and macrophages (sterilizing drugs such as RIF and PZA).

- Two distinct phases of this short-course form of chemotherapy are employed. The 2 month initial or induction phase include INH and rifampin and constitutes the core regimen. They are used in combination with PZA with or without STR or EMB when resistance is suspected and/or more rapid killing is desired.

- The second or continuation phase is of longer duration and is designed to eliminate "persisters" from the body. Combined therapy with INH and RIF is again used here; addition of other agents appears to offer no benefit. During the continuation phase, INH and RIF may be dosed twice weekly rather than daily.

TABLE 48.6. Treatment Regimen Options for Symptomatic Tuberculosis

Option 1—Reliably Compliant Patient, Drug Resistance Unlikely	Option 2—Less Reliable Patient and/or Drug Resistance Suspected	Option 3—Unreliable Patient; Drug Resistance Likely
INH/Rif/PZA +/– EMB or STR *daily* for 2 *months*, followed by INH/RIF 2–3 times weekly for 4 months	INH/RIF/PZA/EMB or STR *daily* for 2 *weeks*, followed by same drugs 2–3 times weekly for 6 *weeks*, followed by INH/RIF 2–3 times weekly for 4 months	INH/RIF/PZA/EMB or STR 2–3 times weekly for entire 6 months

For regimens utilizing 2–3 times weekly dosing, treatment should be via directly observed therapy (DOT). While a 6-month duration of therapy is noted, therapy should continue for 3 months after culture conversion to negative. HIV-infected patients should routinely be treated for 9 months total (6 months after culture conversion) by extending the maintenance period to 7 months.

Key: INH, isoniazid; RIF, rifampin; PZA, pyrazinamide; EMB, ethambutol; STR, streptomycin.

- All patients should receive initial therapy a with daily regimen of INH/RIF/PZA. In patients who have been treated previously and/or who may have been exposed to patients with drug-resistant strains, drug resistance is suspected, and a fourth drug (either EMB or STR) is added. In patients who are documented failures to conventional (three-drug) therapy or are considered likely to be infected with MDR strains (e.g., part of a localized outbreak), both STR and EMB is added.
- When one or more of the above-mentioned first-line agents cannot be used (intolerance, drug resistance), the clinician must substitute alternative agents to achieve the same degree of efficacy. In some cases older, more toxic agents such as ethionamide, para-amino–salicylic acid, cycloserine, or capreomycin must be used.
- Patients with pulmonary tuberculosis should be placed in strict respiratory isolation. All health care workers who must come in contact with the patient while in respiratory isolation should wear a powered, half-mask respirator equipped with a high efficiency particulate air (HEPA) filter, which will filter particles of 1 μm.

Antitubercular Agents

Isoniazid

- Isoniazid (INH) remains the mainstay for treatment of patients with both asymptomatic and symptomatic infection.
- Therapy with INH results in development of adverse effects in approximately 5.5% of patients. A transient elevation in serum transaminases occurs in 12–15% of patients and usually occurs within the first 8–12 weeks of therapy. Risk factors for hepatotoxicity include patient age, pre-existing liver disease, and pregnancy/postpartum state. INH also may result in neurotoxicity, most frequently presenting as peripheral neuropathy or, in overdose, seizures and coma. Patients with pyridoxine deficiency such as alcoholics, children, and the malnourished are at

TABLE 48.7. Dosing Regimens for Common Antitubercular Agents in Adults and Children, Assuming Normal Renal and/or Hepatic Function

Drug	Doses in Adults (Maximum)	Doses in Children (Maximum)
Isoniazid	5 mg/kg (300 mg) daily, or 15 mg/kg (900 mg) 2–3 times weekly	10–20 mg/kg (300 mg) daily, or 20–40 mg/kg (900 mg) 2–3 times weekly
Rifampin	10 mg/kg (600 mg) daily or 2–3 times weekly	10–20 mg/kg (600 mg) daily or 2–3 times weekly
Pyrazinamide	15–30 mg/kg (2000 mg) daily, 50–70 mg/kg (4000 mg) 2 times weekly, or 50–70 mg/kg (3000 mg) 3 times weekly	Same as for adults
Ethambutol	15–25 mg/kg (2500 mg) daily, 50 mg/kg (2500 mg) 2 times weekly, or 25–30 mg/kg (2500 mg) 3 times weekly	Same as for adults; avoid use in children less than 6 years of age
Streptomycin	15 mg/kg (1000 mg) daily, 25–30 mg/kg (1500 mg) 2 times weekly, or 25–30 mg/kg (1000 mg) 3 times weekly	20–30 mg/kg (1000 mg) daily; same as for adults 2–3 times weekly

VIII ◄

increased risk, as are patients who are slow acetylators of INH and those predisposed to neuropathy, such as diabetics.

Rifampin
- Adverse effects associated with RIF are infrequent and rarely necessitate withdrawal of drug. Elevations in hepatic enzymes have been attributed to RIF in 10–15% of patients, with overt hepatotoxicity occurring in <1%. When INH and RIF are used together, elevations in serum transaminases occur in 20–30% of patients, usually within the first 8 weeks of therapy. More frequent adverse effects of RIF include rash, fever, and gastrointestinal distress.
- RIF's induction of hepatic enzymes may enhance the elimination of a number of drugs including theophylline, steroids, narcotics, oral hypoglycemics, zidovudine, and warfarin. Females who use oral contraceptives should be advised to use another form of contraception during therapy.
- The red colorizing effects of RIF on urine, other secretions, and contact lenses should be discussed with the patient.

Pyrazinamide
- Hepatotoxicity is the major limiting adverse effect seen with PZA therapy. PZA also frequently causes gastrointestinal irritation with nausea and vomiting.

Ethambutol

- Retrobulbar neuritis is the major adverse effect noted in patients treated with EMB. Incidence is dose related, with occurrence rates of 1–5%. Patients usually complain of a change in visual acuity and/or inability to see the color green.
- EMB should probably not be used in children who are too young to undergo testing for color blindness. Patients should have baseline tests of renal function and visual acuity, with follow-up tests of vision every 1–2 months.

Streptomycin

- Impairment of eighth cranial nerve function is the most important adverse effect of STR. Vestibular function is most frequently affected, but hearing may also be impaired.

Quinolones

- Ofloxacin has generally been favored over ciprofloxacin because of its higher serum concentrations in relationship to in vitro activity.
- Ofloxacin is usually used in combination with other agents in the treatment of documented MDR-TB. In addition, it is recommended for chemoprophylaxis (together with PZA) for patients with asymptomatic infection due to MDR-TB.
- Patients receiving full doses of PZA (15 mg/kg/d) and ofloxacin (800 mg daily) frequently experience adverse effects including headache, dizziness, confusion, joint pain, gastrointestinal distress, and/or dysuria.

Penicillin-β-Lactamase Inhibitors

- Amoxicillin–clavulanic acid may be considered a third or fourth-line agent for treating tuberculosis, in combination with other more lipophilic antitubercular drugs. It may be considered part of a therapeutic regimen for treatment of drug-resistant tuberculosis, but only in a patient with MDR-TB who is unable to take oral medications.

Rifabutin

- Rifabutin (ansamycin) is an analogue of RIF with greater activity than RIF against *M. avium* complex. It does not, however, demonstrate any advantage over RIF against *M. tuberculosis*. Because rifabutin (like RIF) will increase the metabolism of many drugs, dose modifications of these other drugs will likely be necessary.

DRUG RESISTANCE

- *M. tuberculosis* is remarkably capable of modifying its genetic make-up to develop resistance to antimicrobials. Resistance is most likely due to bacterial mutation.
- The most common mode for expression of resistance is altered bacterial target site; in this way, resistance may often arise via a single mutation.
- The resurgence of tuberculosis in the United States has been accompanied by an increase in the number of drug-resistant isolates. Since 1985,

the fraction of strains resistant to INH has more than doubled; the same may be said for strains resistant to RIF. Approximately 1 strain in 7 is resistant to at least one antitubercular agent, and 1 in 30 is resistant to both INH and RIF (i.e., multidrug-resistant *M. tuberculosis,* or MDR-TB).

- Inappropriate management (noncompliance, incorrect drug selection, reduced bioavailability) results in the emergence of MDR-TB mutants.

▶ EVALUATION OF THERAPEUTIC OUTCOMES

- Symptomatic patients should be isolated and have sputum samples sent for AFB stains every 1–2 days, until a consistent downward trend in the number of AFB observed in sputum is realized. This may typically take 10–14 days. After that time, the patient may be removed from isolation and, if symptomatically improved, discharged from the hospital.
- Once on maintenance therapy, patients should have sputum collected for AFB stain every 2 weeks until negative, and sputum cultures performed monthly until negative. It is anticipated that cultures will convert to negative within 2 months. If sputum cultures continue to be positive after 4 months, drug resistance should be suspected.

The following time line would constitute an "ideal" response to short-course chemotherapy:

- Day 0   Isolate sent for susceptibility tests; respiratory isolation VIII
                 initiated.
- Day 5   Symptomatic improvement (fever, malaise, cough)
                 noted.
- Day 14   Substantial reduction in AFB in sputum; stable chest
                 radiograph; remove from isolation, discharge.
- 2 months   Sputum is AFB negative; susceptibility results allow
                 modification of therapy.
- 4 months   Last sputum culture was negative.
- 6 months   Discontinue drug therapy.

- For patients infected with drug-susceptible strains who are treated with appropriate therapy and are compliant and/or treated with directly observed therapy (DOT), efficacy approaches 100%. Noncompliance, drug resistance, extrapulmonary disease, and concomitant disease states reduce the overall effectiveness of chemotherapy of tuberculosis to about 75%.
- Patients should have serum AST/ALT determined periodically, depending on the presence of other factors that may increase the likelihood of hepatotoxicity (advanced age, alcohol abuse, and possibly pregnancy). Hepatotoxicity should be suspected in patients whose transaminases exceed 350 U/mL or whose total bilirubin exceeds 3 mg/dL. At this point, the offending agent(s) should be discontinued, and alternatives selected.
- Audiometric testing should be performed in patients who must receive STR for more than 2 months.

- Vision testing should be performed on all patients who must receive EMB for more than 2 months. All patients diagnosed with tuberculosis should be tested for HIV infection.

PROGNOSIS

- The success of chemotherapy for tuberculosis depends on three factors, the susceptibility of the isolate, patient compliance, and patient immune status.
- For patients infected with pan-sensitive strains or strains resistant to only one drug (excluding RIF), the success rate of chemotherapy approaches 100%. In contrast, the failure rate for MDR-TB is 80 times greater than that for susceptible strains.
- To achieve at least a 75% success rate, it is important that patients receive antitubercular therapy for at least 4 months, regardless of the regimen used. Ideally, therapy should continue for 4–6 months after sputum cultures have converted to negative. In noncompliant patients, relapse and failure rates of 15–25% are not uncommon.
- HIV-infected patients with tuberculosis tend to experience worse outcomes than do seronegative individuals.

OTHER THERAPEUTIC ISSUES/SITUATIONS

Smear and/or Culture Negative

- Six months of therapy with INH and RIF appears to be adequate for smear-negative, culture-positive patients. However, some studies have demonstrated a 75% rate of progression in patients who are PPD-positive.

Drug Resistance Likely or Suspected

- Patients who require retreatment (along with those in whom therapy is failing and those with a documented exposure to drug-resistant organisms) should be considered to be infected with resistant organisms until proven otherwise.
- In patients with prior treatment, therapy should be modified to include two additional drugs that have not been used previously.
- For initial therapy in suspected drug-resistant tuberculosis, a four-drug regimen should be used (Table 48.7). These regimens may be altered when the susceptibility pattern becomes known.

Drug Resistance Proven

- Therapy needs to be modified if drug resistance is detected from the initial susceptibility report. Specific therapy depends on the susceptibility pattern observed and is outlined in Table 48.8.

Unreliable Patient

- For patients in whom compliance may be a problem (and any patient receiving STR), therapy is administered on a twice- or three-times-weekly basis, using direct observed treatment (DOT). DOT may be performed by having the patient come to a clinic or through home visits.

TABLE 48.8. Suggested Drug Regimens for Documented Drug-Resistant Tuberculosis

Documented Resistance to:	Change Therapy to (X):								Duration (months)
	Rif	PZA	EMB	Amik	Quin	Ethio	CyS	PAS	
INH,PZA,S	X	X	X	X					6-9
INH,EMB,S	X	X		X	X				6-12
INH,RIF,S		X	X	X	X				18-24
INH,RIF,EMB,S		X		X	X	X±	X±	X±	24+
INH,RIF,PZA,S			X	X	X	X±	X±	X±	24+
INH,RIF,PZA,EMB,S				X	X	X±	X±	X±	24+

Key: INH, isoniazid; RIF, rifampin; PZA, pyrazinamide; EMB, ethambutol; S, streptomycin; Amik, amikacin 15–20 mg/kg/d; Quin, quinolone such as ofloxacin 800 mg/d; Ethio, ethionamide 500–1000 mg/d; CyS, cycloserine 500–1000 mg/d; PAS, *p*-aminosalicylate 10–12 g/d. For isolates resistant to four drugs, surgical intervention (lobectomy) should be considered.

This form of therapy improves compliance and, secondarily, the frequency of favorable outcomes.

Pregnancy

- Pregnant women with active tuberculosis should probably receive INH and RIF for a period of 9 months. If a third drug is necessary, EMB may be added. Therapy with INH for asymptomatic tuberculous infection may be delayed until after pregnancy or, if recent skin test conversion has occurred, started during the second trimester of pregnancy.
- Although most antituberculous drugs are excreted in breast milk, the amount of drug received by the infant through nursing is insufficient to cause toxicity.

Children

- Tuberculosis in children may be treated with regimens similar to those used in adults. A regimen of both INH and RIF given daily for 1–2 months followed by RIF and INH daily or twice weekly for 8 months has been shown to be highly effective.

HIV Infected

- Tuberculosis in AIDS patients and other immunocompromised hosts may be managed with chemotherapeutic regimens similar to those used in immunocompetent individuals. A longer course of therapy (INH, RIF, and PZA for 2–3 months followed by INH and RIF for 6–7 months) is generally recommended.
- INH and/or RIF may interact with other medications frequently administered to AIDS patients (e.g., fluconazole, ketoconazole, zidovudine), so dose adjustments of these drugs may be necessary.

See Chapter 105, Tuberculosis, authored by Steven C. Ebert, PharmD, for a more detailed discussion of this topic.

Chapter 49

► URINARY TRACT INFECTIONS AND PROSTATITIS

► DEFINITION

- Infections of the urinary tract represent a wide variety of clinical syndromes including urethritis, cystitis, prostatitis, and pyelonephritis.
- A urinary tract infection (UTI) may be defined as the presence of microorganisms in the urine that cannot be accounted for by contamination, and have the potential to invade the tissues of the urinary tract and adjacent structures.
- Lower tract infections, such as cystitis, involve the bladder and manifest with symptoms of dysuria, frequency, urgency, and occasionally suprapubic tenderness.
- Upper tract infections involve the kidney and are referred to as pyelonephritis. Uncomplicated UTIs are not associated with structural or neurologic abnormalities that may interfere with the normal flow of urine or the voiding mechanism.
- Complicated UTIs are the result of a predisposing lesion of the urinary tract such as a congenital abnormality or distortion of the urinary tract, a stone, indwelling catheter, prostatic hypertrophy, obstruction, or neurologic deficit that interferes with the normal flow of urine and urinary tract defenses.
- Recurrent UTIs are characterized by multiple symptomatic episodes with asymptomatic periods occurring between these episodes. These infections are either due to reinfection or to relapse.
- Reinfections are caused by a new organism and account for the majority of recurrent UTIs.
- Relapse represents the development of repeated infections caused by the same initial organism.

► EPIDEMIOLOGY

- UTIs account for 7 million physician visits annually.
- They constitute the most commonly occurring nosocomial infection.
- At least 20% of all females will suffer a symptomatic urinary tract infection at some time in their lives, with many having multiple recurrences. Infections in males occur much less frequently, but a higher proportion of these infections are associated with complications, such as septicemia and pyelonephritis.
- The overall incidence of UTI increases substantially in the elderly, with the majority of these infections being asymptomatic.

▶ PATHOPHYSIOLOGY

- UTIs can be acquired via three possible routes: the ascending, hematogenous, or lymphatic pathways.
- In females, the short length of the urethra and proximity to the perirectal area make colonization of the urethra likely. Bacteria are then believed to enter the bladder from the urethra.
- Once in the bladder, the organisms multiply quickly and can ascend the ureters to the kidney.
- Infection of the kidney by hematogenous spread of organisms usually can occur as the result of dissemination of organisms from a distant primary infection in the body.
- Three factors determine the development of infection: the size of the inoculum, the virulence of the microorganism, and the competency of the natural host defense mechanisms.
- Patients who are unable to void urine completely are at greater risk of developing urinary tract infections and frequently have recurrent infections.
- An important virulence factor of bacteria is their ability to adhere to urinary epithelial cells.
- Other virulence factors include hemolysin, a cytotoxic protein produced by bacteria that lyses a wide range of cells including erythrocytes, polymorphonuclear leukocytes, and monocytes, and aerobactin which facilitates the binding and uptake of iron by *E. coli*.

VIII

MICROBIOLOGY

- The most common cause of uncomplicated urinary tract infections is *E. coli*, accounting for more than 80% of community-acquired infections followed by *Staphylococcus saprophyticus* (coagulase-negative *staphylococcus*), accounting for 5–15%.
- The urinary pathogens in complicated or nosocomial infections may include *Proteus* spp., *Klebsiella* spp., *Enterobacter* spp., *Pseudomonas* spp., *staphylococci*, and *E. faecalis* as as well as *E. coli* which accounts for <50% of these infections. *Candida* spp. have become common causes of urinary infection in the critically ill and chronically catheterized patient.
- The majority of urinary tract infections are caused by a single organism; however, in patients with stones, indwelling urinary catheters, or chronic renal abscesses, multiple organisms may be isolated.

▶ CLINICAL PRESENTATION

- The typical symptoms of lower tract infections include dysuria, urgency, frequency, nocturia, and suprapubic heaviness or pain. Fever is uncommonly associated with lower tract infections.
- The manifestations of upper tract infections classically include flank pain, costovertebral tenderness, or abdominal pain, and systemic symptoms such as fever, rigors, headache, nausea, vomiting, and malaise.

TABLE 49.1. Criteria for Defining Significant Bacteriuria

$\geq 10^2$ CFU coliforms/mL or $\geq 10^5$ noncoliforms/mL in a symptomatic female

$\geq 10^3$ CFU bacteria/mL in a symptomatic male

$\geq 10^5$ CFU bacteria/mL in asymptomatic individuals on two consecutive specimens

Any growth of bacteria on suprapubic catheterization in a symptomatic patient

$\geq 10^2$ CFU bacteria/mL in a catheterized patient

From Johnson CC. Med Clin North Am 1991;75:242 with permission.

▶ DIAGNOSIS

- The key to the diagnosis of UTI is the ability to demonstrate significant numbers of microorganisms present in an appropriate urine specimen to distinguish contamination from infection.
- A standard urinalysis should be obtained in the initial assessment of a patient. Microscopic examination of the urine should be performed by preparation of a Gram stain of unspun or centrifuged urine. The presence of at least one organism per oil-immersion field in a properly collected uncentrifuged specimen correlates with $\geq 100,000$ bacteria/mL of urine.
- ▶ VIII • Criteria for defining significant bacteriuria are listed in Table 49.1.
- The presence of >10 WBCs/mm^3 is almost always existent in symptomatic bacteriuria, but is absent in up to 30% of patients with asymptomatic bacteriuria. Patients with pyuria may or may not have infection.
- The Griess test can be used to detect the presence of nitrate reducing bacteria in the urine.
- The most reliable method of diagnosing urinary tract infections is by quantitative urine culture. Patients with infection usually have >10^5 bacteria/mL of urine, although as many as one-third of women with symptomatic infection have <10^5 bacteria/mL.
- A method to detect upper urinary tract infection is the antibody-coated bacteria (ACB) test, an immunofluorescent method that detects bacteria coated with immunoglobulin in freshly voided urine. The sensitivity and specificity of the test to detect upper tract infection has been reported to average 88% and 76%, respectively.

▶ TREATMENT

GENERAL PRINCIPLES

- The management of a patient with a UTI includes initial evaluation, selection of an antibacterial agent and duration of therapy, and follow-up evaluation.
- The initial selection of an antimicrobial agent for the treatment of UTI is primarily based on the severity of the presenting signs and symp-

toms, the site of infection, and whether the infection is determined to be complicated or uncomplicated.

PHARMACOLOGIC TREATMENT

- The ability to eradicate bacteria from the urinary tract is directly related to the sensitivity of the organism and the achievable concentration of the antimicrobial agent in the urine.
- Table 49.2 lists the most common agents used in the treatment of urinary tract infections along with comments concerning their general use.
- Table 49.3 presents an overview of various therapeutic options for outpatient therapy for UTI.
- Table 49.4 describes empiric treatment regimens for selected clinical situations.

Uncomplicated Urinary Tract Infections in Females

- These infections are predominantly caused by *E. coli,* and antimicrobial therapy should be directed against this organism initially. Other causes include *S. saprophyticus* and occasionally *Klebsiella* and *Proteus* species.
- Because the causative organisms and their susceptibilities are generally known, a cost-effective approach to management is recommended which includes a urinalysis and initiation of empiric therapy without a urine culture (Figure 49.1). VIII ◄
- Single-dose therapy provides high urinary concentrations for 12–24 hours and is highly effective in treating many women with acute cystitis. Cure rates have ranged from 82–100% using single doses of sulfisoxazole (2 g), trimethoprim–sulfamethoxazole (two double-strength [DS] tablets), and amoxicillin (3 g).
- Single dose therapy should not be considered when symptoms of upper tract infection are present or suspected, stones or other urologic abnormalities are present, there is a previous history of antibiotic resistance, or in males.
- Short-course therapy (3-day therapy with amoxicillin, trimethoprim, trimethoprim–sulfamethoxazole, fluoroquinolones, or doxycycline) may be superior to single-dose therapy for uncomplicated infection and should be the treatment of choice. Short-course therapy should be reserved for those female patients with infection limited to the bladder and with no underlying complicating factors.
- Follow-up urine cultures are not necessary in those patients who respond.

Symptomatic Abacteriuria

- In patients who present for the first time, cultures should be obtained for gonorrhea before treatment is started.
- Single-dose or short-course therapy with trimethoprim–sulfamethoxazole has been used effectively, and prolonged courses of therapy are not necessary for the majority of patients.

TABLE 49.2. Commonly Used Antimicrobial Agents in the Treatment of Urinary Tract Infections

Agents	Comments
Oral Therapy	
Sulfonamides	These agents are useful for the first episodes of infection. They have generally been replaced by more active agents due to resistance formation. Only current advantage is low cost.
Trimethoprim–sulfamethoxazole	This combination is highly effective against most aerobic enteric bacteria, except *Pseudomonas aeruginosa*. High urinary tract tissue levels and urine levels are achieved, which may be important in complicated infection treatment. Also effective as prophylaxis for recurrent infections.

Penicillins
  Ampicillin
  Amoxicillin
  Amoxicillin–clavulanic acid
  Carbenicillin indanyl
	Ampicillin is the standard penicillin that has broad-spectrum activity, including most enteric bacteria causing urinary tract infections. There have been increasing reports of areas of *E. coli* resistance. Amoxicillin is better absorbed and has fewer side effects. Amoxicillin–clavulanate therapy is preferred for resistance problems. Carbenicillin indanyl is indicated only for the treatment of urinary tract infections and is active against *Pseudomonas aeruginosa*.

Cephalosporins
  Cephalexin
  Cephradine
  Cefaclor
  Cefadroxil
  Cefuroxime
  Cefixime
	There are no major advantages of these agents over other agents in the treatment of urinary tract infections and they are more expensive. They may be useful in cases of resistance to amoxicillin and trimethoprim–sulfamethoxazole. These drugs are not as effective for single-dose therapy.

Tetracyclines
  Tetracycline
  Doxycycline
  Oxytetracycline
  Minocycline
	These agents are effective for initial episodes of urinary tract infections. Resistance, however, develops rapidly and their use should be guided by sensitivity testing. These agents also lead to candidal overgrowth. They are primarily useful for chlamydial infections.

Quinolones
  Nalidixic acid
  Oxolinic acid
  Cinoxacin
  Ciprofloxacin
  Norfloxacin
  Ofloxacin
	Nalidixic acid, oxalinic acid, and cinoxacin are effective for initial episodes of infection due to *E. coli* and other Enterobacteriaceae, but not *Pseudomonas aeruginosa*. The newer quinolones have a greater spectrum of activity, including *Pseudomonas aeruginosa*. Ciprofloxacin and ofloxacin are indicated for systemic therapy, as well.

VIII

TABLE 49.2. continued

Agents	Comments
Nitrofurantoin	This agent is effective as both a therapeutic and prophylactic agent in patients with recurrent urinary tract infections. Main advantage is the lack of resistance even after long courses of therapy. Adverse effects may limit its usefulness (e.g., GI intolerance, neuropathies, pulmonary reactions).
Azithromycin	Useful as single-dose therapy in chlamydial infections.
Methanamine hippurate Methanamine mandalate	These agents are reserved for prophylactic therapy or suppressive use between episodes of infection.
Parenteral Therapy Aminoglycosides Gentamicin Tobramycin Amikacin Netilmicin	Gentamicin and tobramycin are equally effective and gentamicin is less expensive. Tobramycin has greater pseudomonal activity which may be important in serious systemic infections. Amikacin is generally reserved for multiresistant bacteria.
Penicillins Ampicillin Carbenicillin Ticarcillin Mezlocillin Piperacillin	These agents are generally equally effective for susceptible bacteria. The extended-spectrum penicillins are more active against *Pseudomonas aeruginosa* and enterococci and are often preferred over cephalosporins. They are very useful in renally impaired patients or when an aminoglycoside is to be avoided.
Cephalosporins First, second, and third generation	Second- and third-generation cephalosporins have a broad spectrum of activity against gram-negative bacteria, but are not active against enterococci and have limited activity against *Pseudomonas aeruginosa* (ceftazidime active *P. aeruginosa*). They are useful for nosocomial infections and urosepsis due to susceptible pathogens.
Imipenem/cilastatin	Has a very broad spectrum of activity including gram-positive, gram-negative, and anaerobic bacteria. It is active against enterococci and *Pseudomonas aeruginosa* but may be associated with candidal superinfections.
Aztreonam	This monobactam is active only against gram-negative bacteria, including *Pseudomonas aeruginosa*. Generally useful for nosocomial infections when aminoglycosides are to be avoided and in penicillin-sensitive patients.

VIII

TABLE 49.3. Overview of Outpatient Antimicrobial Therapy for Lower Tract Infections in Adults

Indication	Antibiotic	Dose	Interval[a]	Duration
Lower tract infection	Trimethoprim–sulfamethoxazole double-strength tablet	2 tablets	Single dose	1 d
		1 tablet	12 h	3 d
		1 tablet	12 h	7–14 d
	Amoxicillin	6 × 500 mg	Single dose	1 d
		1 × 250 mg	8 h	7–14 d
	Amoxicillin–clavulanate	1 × 500 mg	8 h	7–14 d
	Sulfisoxazole	4 × 500 mg	Single dose	1 d
		2 × 500 mg	6 h	7–14 d
	Trimethoprim	1 × 100 mg	12 h	7–14 d
	Norfloxacin	1 × 400 mg	12 h	3 d
		1 × 400 mg	12 h	7–14 d
	Ciprofloxacin	1 × 250–500 mg	12 h	3 d
	Ofloxacin	1 × 250–500 mg	12 h	7–14 d
		1 × 200 mg	12 h	7–14 d
Acute urethral syndrome Initial therapy	Trimethoprim–sulfamethoxazole double-strength tablet	2 tablets	Single dose	1 d
		1 tablet	12 h	3 d
		100 mg	12 h	10–14 d
After failure	Doxycycline	1 g	Single dose	1 d
	Azithromycin			
Long-term prophylaxis	Trimethoprim–sulfamethoxazole single strength	½ tablet	24 h	6 mo
Recurrent infections	Nitrofurantoin	50 mg	24 h	6 mo
	Trimethoprim	100 mg	24 h	6 mo

[a]Dosing interval for normal renal function.

Asymptomatic Bacteriuria

- The management of asymptomatic bacteriuria depends on the age of the patient and whether they are pregnant.
- In children, treatment should consist of conventional courses of therapy, as described for symptomatic infections.
- In the nonpregnant female, therapy is controversial; however, it appears that treatment has little effect on the natural course of infections.
- Most clinicians feel that asymptomatic bacteriuria in the elderly is a benign disease and may not warrant treatment.

Complicated Urinary Tract Infections

Acute Pyelonephritis

- The presentation of high-grade fever and severe flank pain should be treated as acute pyelonephritis and aggressive management is warranted. Severely ill patients with pyelonephritis should be hospitalized and intravenous drugs administered initially.

TABLE 49.4. Empiric Treatment of Urinary Tract Infections/Prostatitis

Diagnosis	Pathogens	Treatment	Comments
Acute uncomplicated infection	E. coli S. saprophyticus	1. TMP–SMX × 3 days 2. Quinolone × 3 days	More effective than single-dose therapy
Pregnancy	As above	1. Amox/clav × 7 days 2. Cephalosporin × 7 days 3. TMP–SMX × 7 days	Avoid TMP–SMX during last trimester
Acute pyelonephritis			
Uncomplicated	E. coli	1. TMP–SMX × 14 days 2. Quinolone × 14 days	Can be managed as out-patient
Complicated	E. coli, P. mirabilis, K. pneumoniae, Pseudomonas aeruginosa, E. faecalis	1. Quinolone × 14 days 2. Ampicillin/sulbactam or piperacillin plus an aminoglycoside	Severity of illness will determine duration of IV therapy. Culture results should direct treatment and an oral agent may complete 14 days of therapy
Prostatitis	E. coli, Klebsiella pneumoniae, Proteus spp., Pseudomonas aeruginosa	1. TMP–SMX × 4 weeks 2. Quinolone × 4 weeks	Acute prostatitis may require IV therapy initially. Chronic prostatitis may require longer treatment periods or surgery

- At the time of presentation, a Gram stain of the urine should be performed, along with urinalysis, culture, and sensitivities.
- In the mild to moderately symptomatic patient in which oral therapy is considered, an effective agent should be administered for at least a 2-week period. Oral antibiotics that have shown efficacy in this setting include trimethoprim, trimethoprim–sulfamethoxazole, amoxicillin–clavulanic acid, norfloxacin, and ciprofloxacin. If a Gram stain reveals streptococci, *E. faecalis* should be considered and ampicillin or amoxicillin is probably the agent of choice.
- In the seriously ill patient, the traditional initial therapy has included an aminoglycoside in combination with ampicillin given intravenously. Because of the increased incidence of ampicillin resistance in the community, other agents have been proposed. These include parenteral trimethoprim–sulfamethoxazole, aztreonam, piperacillin, ampicillin–sulbactam or ticarcillin–clavulanic acid, and the third-generation cephalosporins (cefotaxime, ceftriaxone, etc.).

VIII

```
Lower tract symptoms
Urinalysis/gram-stain
Significant bacteriuria
```

├─ No ─→ Symptomatic abacteriuria

└─ Yes ─→ Upper tract symptoms acute pyelonephritis

  ├─ No ─→ Short course therapy
  │   ├─ Clinical cure
  │   └─ Clinical failure ─→ Urine culture

  └─ Yes ─→ Obtain urine culture ─→ Acutely ill high risk patient
              ├─ No ─→ Oral therapy 2 weeks
              └─ Yes ─→ Hospitalization parenteral antibiotics

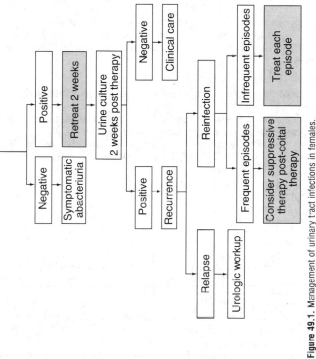

Figure 49.1. Management of urinary tract infections in females.

VIII

- If the patient has been hospitalized in the last 6 months, has a urinary catheter, or is in a nursing home, the possibility of *Pseudomonas* and *enterococcus* infection, as well as resistant organisms, should be considered. In this setting, ceftazidime, ticarcillin–clavulanic acid, aztreonam, imipenem, or piperacillin in combination with an aminoglycoside is recommended. If the patient responds to initial combination therapy, the aminoglycoside may be discontinued after 3 days.
- Follow-up urine cultures should be obtained 2 weeks after the completion of therapy to ensure a satisfactory response and to detect possible relapse.

Urinary Tract Infections in Males
- The conventional view is that therapy in males requires prolonged treatment (Figure 49.2).
- A urine culture should be obtained before treatment, since the cause of infection in men is not as predictable as in women.
- If gram-negative bacteria are presumed, trimethoprim–sulfamethoxazole or trimethoprim is a preferred agent. If a resistant organism is suspected, a fluoroquinolone such as ciprofloxacin or norfloxacin should be considered. Initial therapy is for 10–14 days. For recurrent infections in males, cure rates are much higher with a 6 week regimen of trimethoprim–sulfamethoxazole.

VIII Recurrent Infections
- Recurrent episodes of urinary tract infection (reinfections and relapses) account for a significant portion of all UTIs.
- These patients are most commonly females and can be divided into two groups: those with less than two or three episodes per year and those who develop more frequent infections.
- In those patients with infrequent infections (i.e., less than three infections per year), each episode should be treated as a separately occurring infection. Single-dose or short-course therapy should be used in symptomatic female patients with lower tract infection.
- In those patients who have frequent symptomatic infections, long-term prophylactic antimicrobial therapy may be instituted (Table 49.3). Therapy is generally given for 6–12 months with urine cultures followed periodically.
- In those women who experience symptomatic reinfections in association with sexual activity, voiding after intercourse may help prevent infection. Also, self-administered, single-dose prophylactic therapy with trimethoprim–sulfamethoxazole taken after intercourse has been found to reduce significantly the incidence of recurrent infection in these patients.
- Women who relapse after short-course therapy should receive a 2-week course of therapy. In patients who relapse after 2 weeks, therapy should be continued for another 2–4 weeks. If relapse occurs after 6 weeks of treatment, therapy for 6 months or even longer may be considered.

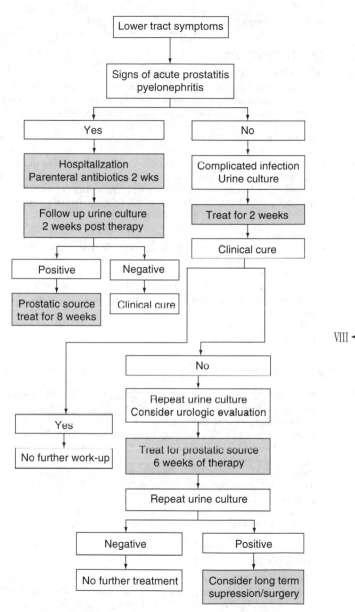

Figure 49.2. Management of urinary tract infections in males.

SPECIAL CONDITIONS

Urinary Tract Infection in Pregnancy

- In those patients with significant bacteriuria, symptomatic or asymptomatic, treatment is recommended in order to avoid possible complications during the pregnancy. Therapy should consist of an agent with a relatively low adverse effect potential (a sulfonamide, cephalexin, ampicillin, amoxicillin, nitrofurantoin) administered for 7 days.
- Tetracyclines should be avoided due to teratogenic effects and sulfonamides should not be administered during the third trimester due to the possible development of kernicterus and hyperbilirubinemia. Also, the quinolones should not be given because of their potential to inhibit cartilage and bone development in the newborn.

Catheterized Patients

- When bacteriuria occurs in the asymptomatic, short-term catheterized patient (<30 days), the use of systemic antibiotic therapy should be withheld and the catheter removed as soon as possible. If the patient becomes symptomatic, the catheter should again be removed and treatment as described for complicated infections should be started.
- There is no evidence that prophylactic antibiotic administration prevents the development of fever or acute pyelonephritis in long-term catheterized patients.

VIII

▶ PROSTATITIS

- Pathogenic bacteria and significant inflammatory cells must be present in prostatic secretions and urine to make the diagnosis of bacterial prostatitis. Typically, prostatitis is a severe illness characterized by a sudden onset of fever and urinary and constitutional symptoms. Chronic bacterial prostatitis (CBP) represents a recurring infection with the same organism (relapse).
- Nonbacterial prostatitis is typified by the presence of signs and symptoms of infection including excessive inflammatory cells, but where pathogenic bacteria cannot be isolated.
- Prostatodynia is a syndrome in which patients present with the subjective constitutional symptoms of prostatitis, but lack all objective evidence of infection.

PATHOGENESIS/ETIOLOGY

- The exact mechanism of bacterial infection of the prostate is not well understood. The possible routes of infection include ascending infection of the urethra, reflux of infected urine into prostatic ducts, invasion by rectal bacteria through direct extension or lymphatic spread, and by hematogenous spread.

- Several sexually transmitted organisms, including *Chlamydia, Ureaplasma,* and *Trichomonas* have been implicated as nonbacterial pathogens.
- Gram-negative, enteric organisms are the most frequent pathogens in bacterial prostatitis. *E. coli* is the predominate organism, occurring in 75% of cases.
- CBP is most commonly caused by *E. coli* with other gram-negative organisms isolated much less often.

CLINICAL PRESENTATION/DIAGNOSIS

- Common symptoms include high fever, chills, malaise, myalgia, localized pain (perineal, rectal, sacrococcygeal), and other urinary tract symptoms (frequency, urgency, dysuria, nocturia, retention).
- Digital palpation of the prostate via the rectum may reveal a swollen, tender, warm, tense, or indurated prostate. Massage of the prostate will express a purulent discharge, which will readily grow the pathogenic organism. However, prostatic massage is contraindicated in acute bacterial prostatis (ABP) because of a risk of inducing bacteremia and associated pain.
- CBP is characterized by recurrent urinary tract infections with the same pathogen. In fact, CBP is the most common cause of recurrent UTI in males. Presenting symptoms include the vague description of voiding difficulties such as frequency, urgency, and dysuria, along with low back pain and perineal and suprapubic discomfort.
- Urinary tract localization studies are critical to the diagnosis of CBP.
- Both ABP and CBP are characterized by the presence of numerous WBC and lipid-containing macrophages (oval fat bodies) on microscopic exam of expressed prostatic secretions.

VIII

TREATMENT

- Oral or parenteral therapy with trimethoprim–sulfamethoxazole (TMP-SMX) has been advocated as initial therapy. If patients are unable to tolerate TMP-SMX, then IV to oral sequential therapy with a fluoroquinolone, such as ciprofloxacin or ofloxacin, would be appropriate.
- If a presumptive diagnosis of ABP is made, a traditional regimen includes a combination of an aminoglycoside with a β-lactam antibiotic (e.g., gentamicin plus ampicillin).
- Parenteral therapy should be maintained until the patient is afebrile and less symptomatic. The conversion to an oral antibiotic can be considered if the patient has responded to 5–7 days of intravenous therapy. The total course of antibiotic therapy should be 4 weeks in order to reduce the risk of development of chronic prostatitis.
- The choice of antibiotics in CBP should include those agents that are capable of crossing the prostatic epithelium into the prostatic fluid in

therapeutic concentrations and which also possess the spectrum of activity to be effective.
- Trimethoprim was considered the ideal drug based on its favorable chemical characteristics and its ability to concentrate, however, the low cure rates observed call into question the current recommendation that TMP-SMX is the drug of choice.
- Fluoroquinolones may be more effective than TMP-SMX with reported cure rates ranging from 50–90%.

See Chapter 109, Urinary Tract Infections and Prostatitis, authored by Timothy A. Mullenix, PharmD, MS and Randall A. Prince, PharmD, for a more detailed discussion of this topic.

VIII

Chapter 50

► VACCINES, TOXOIDS, AND OTHER IMMUNOBIOLOGICS

► DEFINITIONS

- Vaccines are substances administered to generate a protective immune response.
- Toxoids are inactivated bacterial toxins. They retain the ability to stimulate the formation of antitoxin.
- Adjuvants are inert substances, such as aluminum salts (i.e., alum), which enhance vaccine antigenicity by prolonging antigen absorption.
- Immune sera are sterile solutions containing antibody derived from human (immune globulin) or equine (antitoxin) sources.

► VACCINE AND TOXOID RECOMMENDATIONS

- The recommended schedules for routine immunization of children and adults are shown in Tables 50.1 and 50.2, respectively. Table 50.3 lists the minimum age for initial vaccination and minimum interval between vaccine doses.
- Children should be fully immunized before 6 years of age.
- Adults should be fully immunized against diphtheria, tetanus, measles, mumps, and rubella.
- Inactivated vaccines can be simultaneously administered at separate sites. Killed and live antigens may be administered simultaneously or, if they cannot be administered simultaneously, at any interval between doses with the exception of cholera (killed) and yellow fever (live) vaccine, which should be given at least 3 weeks apart. Simultaneous administration of live attenuated vaccines should be avoided, if possible, unless specified (i.e., measles, mumps, rubella). Live vaccines should be given at least 1 month apart; however, oral polio vaccine may be given at the same time as measles, mumps, and rubella vaccine.
- Administration of live attenuated vaccines should not be done during pregnancy, and inactivated vaccines should not be given until the second trimester. However, inactivated vaccines have not been shown to be teratogenic during the first trimester.
- Those patients who are immunocompromised or with active malignant disease may receive killed vaccines or toxoids but should not be given live vaccines.
- The simultaneous administration of immune globulin (general or disease specific) and live attenuated vaccines (but not inactivated vaccines) may inhibit host antibody response owing to impairment of viral replication.

TABLE 50.1. Immunization Schedules in Children

Vaccine	At Birth (Before Hospital Discharge)	1–2 Months	2 Months[a]	4 Months	6 Months	6–18 Months	12–15 Months	15 Months	4–6 Years (Before School Entry)
Diphtheria-tetanus pertussis[b]			DTP	DTP	DTP			DTaP/DTP[c]	DTaP/DTP
Polio, live oral			OPV	OPV	OPV[d]				OPV
Measles-mumps-rubella							MMR		MMR[e]
Haemophilus influenzae type b conjugate									
HbOC/PRP-T[f,f]			Hib	Hib	Hib		Hib[g]		
PRP-OMP[f]			Hib	Hib			Hib[g]		
Hepatitis B[h]									
Option 1	HepB	HepB[i]				HepB[i]			
Option 2		HepB[i]		HepB[i]		HepB[i]			

[a]Can be administered as early as 6 weeks of age.

[b]Two DTP and Hib combination vaccines are available (DTP/HbOC [TETRAMUNE]; and PRP-T [ActHIB, OmniHIB] which can be reconstituted with DTP vaccine produced by Connaught).

[c]This dose of DTP can be administered as early as 12 months of age provided that the interval since the previous dose of DTP is at least 6 months. *Diphtheria and tetanus toxoids and acellular pertussis vaccine (DTaP) is currently recommended only for use as the fourth and/or fifth doses of the DTP series among children aged 15 months through 6 years (before the seventh birthday).* Some experts prefer to administer these vaccines at 18 months of age.

[d]The American Academy of Pediatrics (AAP) recommends this dose of vaccine at 6–18 months of age.

[e]The AAP recommends that two doses of MMR should be administered by 12 years of age with the second dose being administered preferentially at entry to middle school or junior high school.

[f]HbOC: [HibTITER] (Lederle Praxis). PRP-T: [ActHIB, OmniHIB] (Pasteur Merieux). PRP-OMP: [PedvaxHIB] (Merck, Sharp, and Dohme). A DTP/Hib combination vaccine can be used in place of HbOC/PRP-T.

[g]After the primary infant Hib conjugate vaccine series is completed, any of the licensed Hib conjugate vaccines may be used as a booster dose at age 12–15 months.

[h]The first dose should be administered during the newborn period, preferably before hospital discharge, but no later than age 2 months. Premature infants of HBsAg-negative mothers should receive the first dose of the hepatitis B vaccine series at the time of hospital discharge or when the other routine childhood vaccines are initiated. (All infants born to HBsAg-positive mothers should receive immunoprophylaxis for hepatitis B as soon as possible after birth.)

[i]For use among infants born to HBsAg-negative mothers. The first dose should be administered during the newborn period, preferably before hospital discharge, but no later than age 2 months.

[j]Hepatitis B vaccine can be administered simultaneously at the same visit with DTP (or DTaP), OPV, Hib, and/or MMR.

From Centers for Disease Control and Prevention. MMWR 1994;43 (RR-1):1–38.

▶ VIII

TABLE 50.2. Immunization Schedules in Adults

Age Group (years)		Vaccine/Toxoid[a]				
	Td[b]	Measles	Mumps	Rubella	Influenza	Pneumococcal Polysaccharide
18–24	X	X	X	X		
25–64	X	X[c]	X[c]	X		
≥65	X				X	X

[a]Refer also to sections in text on specific vaccines or toxoids for indications, contraindications, precautions, dosages, side effects, adverse reactions, and special considerations.
[b]Td = Tetanus and diphtheria toxoids, adsorbed (for adult use), which is a combined preparation containing <2 flocculation units of diphtheria toxoid.
[c]Indicated for persons born after 1956.
From Centers for Disease Control. MMWR 1991;40(RR-12):1–95.

▶ DIPHTHERIA TOXOID ADSORBED (DTA) AND DIPHTHERIA ANTITOXIN (DA)

- Primary immunization with DTA is indicated for children >6 weeks of age. Generally, DTA is given along with pertussis and tetanus vaccine (DPT) at ages 2, 4, and 6–12 months of age, then at 18 months and 4–6 years of age.
- For nonimmunized adults, a complete three-dose series of diphtheria toxoid should be administered, with the first two doses given at least 4 weeks apart and the third dose given 6–12 months after the second. The combined preparation, Td, is recommended in adults since it contains less diphtheria toxoid than DPT with fewer reactions seen to the diphtheria preparation.
- Booster doses are given every 10 years.
- Diphtheria antitoxin (DA) is a sterile antitoxin derived from hyperimmunized horses and is indicated for immediate use in patients with diphtheria. Sensitivity testing by performing an intradermal or scratch test and a conjunctival test should be performed before administration
- The usual dose of DA is 20,000–40,000 U for pharyngeal disease, 40,000–60,000 U for nasopharyngeal lesions, and 80,000–120,000 U for extensive disease of 3 or more days.

▶ TETANUS TOXOID (TT), TETANUS TOXOID ADSORBED (TTA), AND TETANUS IMMUNE GLOBULIN (TIG)

- In children, primary immunization against tetanus is usually done in conjunction with diphtheria and pertussis vaccination. The trivalent vaccine, DPT, containing TTA is given intramuscularly at 2, 4, 6, and 18 months of age.

609

TABLE 50.3. Minimum Age for Pediatric Vaccination

Vaccine	Minimum Age for First Dose[a]	Minimum Interval from Dose 1 to 2[a]	Minimum Interval from Dose 2 to 3[a]	Minimum Interval from Dose 3 to 4[a]
DTP (DT)[b]	6 weeks[c]	4 weeks	4 weeks	6 months
Combined DTP-Hib	6 weeks	1 month	1 month	6 months
DTaP[b]	15 months			6 months
Hib (primary series)				
HbOC	6 weeks	1 month	1 month	[d]
PRP-T	6 weeks	1 month	1 month	[d]
PRP-OMP	6 weeks	1 month	[d]	
OPV	6 weeks[c]	6 weeks	6 weeks[f]	
IPV[e]	6 weeks	4 weeks	6 months[f]	
MMR	12 months[g]	1 month		
Hepatitis B	Birth	1 month	2 months[h]	

DTP   Diphtheria–tetanus–pertussis
DTaP   Diphtheria–tetanus–acellular pertussis
Hib   *Haemophilus influenzae* type b conjugate
IPV   Inactivated poliovirus vaccine
MMR   Measels–mumps–rubella
OPV   Live oral polio vaccine

[a]These minimum acceptable ages and intervals may not correspond with the optimal recommended ages and intervals for vaccination.

[b]DTaP can be used in place of the fourth (and fifth) dose of DTP for children who are at least 15 months of age. Children who have received all four primary vaccination doses before their fourth birthday should receive a fifth dose of DTP (DT) or DTaP at 4–6 years of age before entering kindergarten or elementary school and at least 6 months after the fourth dose. The total number of doses of diphtheria and tetanus toxoids should not exceed six each before the seventh birthday.

[c]The American Academy of Pediatrics permits DTP and OPV to be administered as early as 4 weeks of age in areas with high endemicity and during outbreaks.

[d]The booster dose of Hib vaccine which is recommended following the primary vaccination series should be administered no earlier than 12 months of age and at least 2 months after the previous dose of Hib vaccine.

[e]See text to differentiate conventional inactivated poliovirus vaccine from enhanced-potency IPV.

[f]For unvaccinated adults at increased risk of exposure to poliovirus with <3 months but >2 months available before protection is needed, three doses of IPV should be administered at least 1 month apart.

[g]Although the age for measles vaccination may be as young as 6 months in outbreak areas where cases are occurring in children <1 year of age, children initially vaccinated before the first birthday should be revaccinated at 12–15 months of age, and an additional dose of vaccine should be administered at the time of school entry or according to local policy. Doses of MMR or other measles-containing vaccines should be separated by at least 1 month.

[h]This final dose is recommended no earlier than 4 months of age.

From Centers for Disease Control and Prevention. MMWR 1994;43(RR-1):1–38.

- Primary vaccination provides protection for at least 10 years.
- Additional doses of TTA are recommended as part of traumatic wound management if a patient has not received a dose of TTA or TT during the preceding 5 years (Table 50.4).
- In adults or children where primary immunization against tetanus alone is needed, a series of three doses of TTA is administered intra-

TABLE 50.4. Summary Guide to Tetanus Prophylaxis in Routine Wound Management[a]

	Clean, Minor Wounds		All Other Wounds[b]	
	Td[c]	TIG[d]	Td[c]	TIG[d]
Uncertain or <3	Yes	No	Yes	Yes
>3[e]	No[f]	No	No[g]	No

[a]Refer also to text on specific vaccines or toxoids for contraindications, precautions, dosages, side effects, adverse reactions, and special considerations. Important details are in the ACIP recommendations on diphtheria, tetanus, and pertussis (DTP) (MMWR 1991: 40 [RR-10]).
[b]Such as, but not limited to, wounds contaminated with dirt, feces, and saliva; puncture wounds; avulsions; and wounds resulting from missiles, crushing, burns, and frostbite.
[c]Td, tetanus and diphtheria toxoids, adsorbed (for adult use). For children <7 years old, DTP (DT, if pertussis vaccine is contraindicated) is preferred to tetanus toxoid alone. For persons ≥7 years old, Td is preferred to tetanus toxoid alone.
[d]TIG, tetanus immune globulin.
[e]If only three doses of fluid toxoid have been received, a fourth dose of toxoid, preferably an adsorbed toxoid, should be given.
[f]Yes, >10 years since last dose.
[g]Yes, >5 years since last dose. (More frequent boosters are not needed and can accentuate side effects.)
From Centers for Disease Control. MMWR 1991;40 (RR-12):1–95.

muscularly initially, followed by repeat doses at 4–8 weeks and 6–12 months.
- TT and TTA may be given to immunosuppressed patients if needed. TT or TTA may be simultaneously given with other killed and live vaccines.
- Tetanus immune globulin (TIG) is used to provide passive tetanus immunization following the occurrence of traumatic wounds in nonimmunized or suboptimally immunized persons (Table 50.4). A dose of 250–500 U is administered intramuscularly. When administered with TTA, separate sites for administration should be used.
- TIG is also used for the treatment of tetanus. In this setting a single dose of 3000–6000 U is administered intramuscularly.

▶ BACILLUS CALMETTE–GUÉRIN VACCINE (BCG)

- BCG vaccine is used for vaccination against tuberculosis.
- The vaccine is recommended for health care workers with an annual attack rate of >1% in the face of other tuberculosis control measures, groups with an excessive new infection rate in whom surveillance and treatment cannot be accomplished or have failed, and individuals in close contact with infected patients who have been ineffectively treated.
- The agent is contraindicated in immunosuppressed individuals regardless of the cause because it is a live vaccine. The vaccine should not be given to burn patients, patients on isoniazid, or pregnant women.

TABLE 50.5. *Haemophilus Influenzae* Vaccines Currently Available in the United States

Manufacturer	Abbreviated Name	Trade Name	Protein Carrier
Connaught Labs	PRP-D	ProHIBit	Diphtheria toxoid
Lederle-Praxis	HbOC[a]	HIBTITER	CRM$_{197}$ (diphtheria toxin)
Merck	PRP-OMP	PedvaxHIB	OMP (from *N. meningitidis*)
Pasteur Merieux	PRP-T	ActHIB/OmniHIB	Tetanus toxoid

Note: PRP-D is recommended by the American Academy of Pediatrics for infants age ≥12 months only. HbOC, PRP-OMP, and PRP-T are recommended for infants age ≥2 months.
[a]Available as Tetramune, a combination vaccine with DPT.

▶ HAEMOPHILUS INFLUENZAE TYPE B (Hib) VACCINES

- Hib vaccines currently in use are conjugate products, consisting of either a polysaccharide or oligosaccharide of polyribosylribitol phosphate (PRP) covalently linked to a protein carrier (Table 50.5).
- Hib conjugate vaccines are indicated for routine use in all infants and children <5 years of age.
- For infants 7–11 months who have not been vaccinated, three doses of HbOC, PRP-OMP, and PRP-T should be given: two doses, spaced 8 weeks apart, and then a booster dose at age 12–18 months (but at least 8 weeks since dose 2). For unvaccinated children ages 12–14 months, two doses should be given, with an interval of 2 months between them. In a child >15 months, a single dose of any of the four conjugate vaccines is indicated.

▶ HEPATITIS B VACCINE

- The vaccine protects against all hepatitis B serotypes (including delta viroid) but does not cross-react with other hepatitis viruses (i.e., hepatitis A, C, E).

PRIMARY VACCINATION

- The vaccine is recommended for persons with occupational risk (health care workers, public safety workers), persons in training for health care fields, clients and staff of institutions for the developmentally disabled, hemodialysis patients, recipients of clotting factor concentrate, household contacts and sex partners of hepatitis B carriers, adoptees from countries where hepatitis B is endemic, international travelers (those spending more than 6 months in areas with high rates of hepatitis B infection or high-risk, short-term travelers), injecting drug users, sexually active homosexual/bisexual men, sexually active heterosexual men and women, and inmates of long-term correctional facilities. In addi-

VIII

tion, the American Academy of Pediatrics recommends universal immunization of all newborns.

- For neonates born to mothers who are not positive for HBsAg, the primary vaccination series is 2.5 µg of RecombivaxHB or 10 µg of Engerix-B. The first dose should be given at 0–2 days of age, the second dose at 1–2 (or 2 and 4) months of age, and the third dose at 6–18 months of age.
- In infants born to HBsAg-positive mothers, vaccination with 5 µg of RecombivaxHB or 10 µg of Engerix-B is given at 12 hours after birth (but no more than 7 days after birth), 1 month, and 6 months of age. A fourth dose of vaccine is administered to infants who are anti-HB nonresponders or hyporesponders and are HBsAg negative.
- For children <11 years of age who are not born of mothers who are HBsAG positive, 2.5 µg of RecombivaxHB or 10 µg of Engerix-B is administered at 0, 1, and 6 months. Children and adolescents ages 11–19 receive 5 µg of RecombivaxHB or 20 µg of Engerix-B at 0, 1, and 6 months. An alternate four-dose schedule (0, 1, 2, and 12 months) may be used for Engerix-B.
- Adults ≥20 years of age receive 10 µg of RecombivaxHB or 20 µg of Engerix-B at 0, 1, and 6 months. An alternative schedule of 20 µg at 0, 1, 2, and 12 months may be used for Engerix-B only.
- Hemodialysis patients receive either 40 µg of RecombivaxHB or 40 µg of Engerix-B in a 0-, 1-, and 6-month schedule. Anti-HBs should be determined, and if the value is <10 mIU/mL, one to three booster doses are administered. In addition, these persons should be tested yearly and boosted with a single dose of 40 µg if anti-HBs <10 mIU/mL.
- The preferred site of administration is the deltoid muscle in adults (immunogenicity is significantly lower in adults who receive injection in the buttock) and the anterolateral thigh in infants.
- Patients who should receive postvaccination serologic testing include immunocompromised patients (owing to any cause), persons at occupational risk of exposure, and infants born of HBsAG-positive mothers.

POSTEXPOSURE PROPHYLAXIS

- Hepatitis B vaccine is also used with hepatitis B immune globulin (HBIG) in the postexposure setting. Persons for whom this regimen is recommended include susceptible individuals having percutaneous or permucosal exposure to blood containing HBsAg, sexual contacts of HBsAg carriers who will continue to be exposed, and infants born of mothers who are HBsAg carriers.
- The same dosage schedule used for primary immunization is used in the postexposure setting.
- The hepatitis B vaccine series should be initiated as soon as possible after HBIG administration. Table 50.6 illustrates the specifics of vaccine use.

TABLE 50.6. Recommendations for Hepatitis B Prophylaxis Following Percutaneous Exposure

Exposed Person	Treatment When Source Is Found to Be		
	HBsAg Positive	HBsAg Negative	Unknown or Not Tested
Unvaccinated	Administer HBIG × 1[a] and initiate hepatitis B vaccine	Initiate hepatitis B vaccine	Initiate hepatitis B vaccine
Previously Vaccinated			
Known responder	Test exposed person for anti-HBs 1. If adequate, no treatment 2. If inadequate, hepatitis B vaccine booster dose	No treatment	No treatment
Known nonresponder	HBIG × 2 or HBIG × 1, plus 1 dose of hepatitis B vaccine	No treatment	If known high-risk source, may treat as if source were HBsAg positive
Response unknown	Test exposed person for anti-HB[b] 1. If inadequate HBIG × 1, plus hepatitis B vaccine booster dose 2. If adequate, no treatment	No treatment	Test exposed person for anti-HBs[b] 1. If inadequate hepatitis B vaccine booster dose 2. If adequate, no treatment

[a]Hepatitis B immune globulin (HBIG) dose 0.06 mL/kg intramuscularly.
[b]Adequate anti-HBs is ≥10 mIU.
From Centers for Disease Control. MMWR 1991:40(RR-13):1–25.

▶ HEPATITIS B IMMUNE GLOBULIN

- HBIG is used for postexposure, and rarely pre-exposure, prophylaxis for hepatitis B infection.
- Indications for the use of HBIG include passive immunization following exposure to hepatitis B virus via percutaneous, permucosal, or oral ingestion routes (e.g., needlesticks, accidental splash, sexual contact, mouth pipetting) and for infants born to mothers who are hepatitis B carriers.
- It is currently recommended by the CDC that HBIG be given as soon as possible after acute exposures (percutaneous, permucosal, oral inges-

VIII

tion), preferably within 24 hours. It is not recommended that HBIG be given beyond 14 days after acute exposure.

▶ INFLUENZA VIRUS VACCINE

- Indications for current split-virus and whole-virus influenza vaccines are as follows: adults with chronic cardiovascular or pulmonary diseases, residents of nursing home facilities, health care personnel dealing with high-risk patients, healthy adults older than age 65, adults with chronic metabolic disease, and children with chronic metabolic or cardiopulmonary diseases. In addition, groups that can transmit influenza to high-risk people should be vaccinated (health care personnel, employees of nursing homes or chronic care facilities who have patient contact, providers of home care to high-risk patients, and household members of persons in high-risk groups).
- Individuals who should not be vaccinated are those with anaphylactic hypersensitivity to eggs or other components of the vaccine or adults with febrile illness (until the fever abates).

▶ MEASLES VACCINE

- Measles vaccine is administered for primary immunization to persons 15 months of age or older, usually as MMR (measles–mumps–rubella). A second dose is recommended prior to entry into elementary school or junior high school.
- The vaccine should not be given to immunosuppressed patients (except those infected with HIV), pregnant women, or to patients with a history of egg allergy.
- The vaccine should not be given within 6 weeks (preferably 3 months) of IM immune globulin administration, or within 8 months of IGIV given as replacement therapy for humoral immune deficiencies.
- The vaccine should not be given within 1 month of any other live vaccine except mumps, rubella, and oral polio.
- Measles vaccine is indicated in all persons born after 1956 or in those who lack documentation of wild virus infection either by history or antibody titers.
- For postexposure prophylaxis, the vaccine is effective if given within 72 hours of exposure. In addition, immune globulin may be administered intramuscularly at a dose of 0.25 mg/kg (maximum dose, 15 mL), if given within 6 days of exposure.

▶ MENINGOCOCCAL POLYSACCHARIDE VACCINE (MPV)

- MPV is indicated in high-risk populations such as those exposed to the disease, those in the midst of uncontrolled outbreaks, or travelers to an area with epidemic or hyperendemic meningococcal disease.

VIII

- In the United States, serotype B, a strain not contained in the current vaccine, causes the majority of disease, thus routine vaccination is not recommended.
- The vaccine should not be given to pregnant women unless there is a substantial risk of infection.

► MUMPS VACCINE

- The vaccine (usually given in conjunction with measles and rubella) is given beginning at age 12–15 months, with a second dose prior to entry into elementary school (or alternatively, prior to entry into junior high school). If the vaccine is given before 12 months of age, revaccination is necessary and should be given after reaching 1 year of age.
- The vaccine is also indicated in previously unvaccinated adults and in those in whom a poor history of wild virus infection or previous administration of killed mumps exists.
- Postexposure vaccination is of no benefit.
- Mumps vaccine should not be given to pregnant women or immunosuppressed patients. The vaccine should not be given within 6 weeks (preferably 3 months) of administration of immune globulin. Finally, the vaccine should not be given to neomycin-sensitive individuals.

VIII ► PERTUSSIS VACCINE

- Pertussis vaccine is usually administered in combination with diphtheria and tetanus toxoids (as DTP).
- The primary immunization series for pertussis vaccine consists of four doses given at ages 2, 4, 6, and 15–18 months. A booster dose is recommended at age 4–6 years.
- Adverse events reportedly having a temporal relationship to pertussis vaccine administration include prolonged crying (3%), unusual high-pitched cry (0.1%), convulsions (0.06%), and acute neurologic illness (0.00005%). Other authors have reported mortality in 0.05–0.1% and permanent brain damage of 0.005% of vaccine recipients. A large population-based case control study failed to find an increased risk of serious acute neurologic illness within 7 days of DTP administration.
- The American Academy of Pediatrics and the Immunization Practices Advisory Committee continue to recommend routine pertussis vaccine.
- There are only two absolute contraindications to pertussis administration: an immediate anaphylactic reaction to a previous dose, or encephalopathy within 7 days of a previous dose, with no evidence of other cause.

► PNEUMOCOCCAL VACCINE

- The pneumococcal vaccine is recommended for persons at high risk of acquiring the disease (patients who are immunosuppressed [e.g.,

Hodgkin's disease and other lymphoproliferative disorders, multiple myeloma, renal failure] and those with splenic dysfunction or anatomic asplenia). Patients with chronic illnesses of the cardiovascular and pulmonary systems, alcoholism, and the elderly, particularly those who are institutionalized, are also felt to be at increased risk.

- Recommendations for pneumococcal vaccine include adults and children >2 years of age who are at high risk for pneumococcal disease, and otherwise healthy adults >65 years of age.
- Pneumococcal vaccine is recommended for routine use in immunocompetent adults and immunocompromised adults at increased risk of pneumococcal disease (including HIV infection).
- Children 2 years of age and older with chronic disease (including HIV infection) that places them at increased risk for pneumococcal disease should be vaccinated. This does not include children with recurrent otitis media, sinusitis, or upper respiratory infection.
- When possible the vaccine should be administered at least 2 weeks before the administration of immunosuppressive therapy or splenectomy.
- Currently recommendations suggest limiting revaccination to the following individuals: (1) persons who received the 14-valent vaccine and who are at highest risk of fatal infection (e.g., asplenic patients); (2) adults at high risk who received the 23-valent vaccine 6 years or more previously and who may have significant declines in antibody levels; VIII and (3) children at high risk who would be 10 years of age or younger at revaccination (3–5 years after initial vaccination).

▶ POLIOVIRUS VACCINES

- Two types of trivalent poliovirus vaccines are currently licensed for distribution in the United States, an enhanced inactivated vaccine (eIPV) and a live attenuated, oral vaccine (OPV) which has been the primary immunizing agent for poliovirus infection.
- OPV is administered in a series of three oral doses with a second dose given 6–8 weeks after the first and the third dose 6–8 weeks after the second. In children, OPV immunization generally begins at 6–12 weeks of age, commonly with the first DTP immunization.
- OPV is not recommended for persons who are immunodeficient or for normal individuals who reside in a household where another person is immunodeficient.
- HIV-infected patients should receive eIPV in place of the live vaccine; however, in other countries of the world the live product has been used.
- OPV should not be given during pregnancy because of the small but theoretical risk to the fetus.
- Primary immunization with eIPV consists of a series of three subcutaneous injections given 4–8 weeks apart with a similar booster dose 6–12 months after the third injection.

- Primary poliomyelitis immunization is recommended for all children and young adults up to age 18. OPV is the vaccine of choice in this age group unless an immunodeficiency exists in the patient or a household contact, in which case eIPV is recommended.
- Primary immunization of adults <18 years of age is not routinely recommended because a high level of immunity already exists in this age group and the risk of exposure in developed countries is small. However, unimmunized adults who are at increased risk for exposure because of travel, residence, or occupation should receive primary immunization with eIPV.

▶ RABIES VACCINE

- Human diploid cell vaccine (HDCV) and rabies vaccine adsorbed (RVA) are killed vaccines used for preexposure and postexposure rabies virus prophylaxis.
- Preexposure indications for using HDCV or RVA include persons whose vocation or avocation place them at high risk for rabies exposure, for example, veterinarians, animal handlers, laboratory workers in rabies research labs, and field personnel (trappers, hunters, cave explorers).
- Travelers who will be in a country or area of a country where there is a constant threat of rabies, whose stay is likely to extend beyond 1 month, and who may not have readily available medical services (e.g., Peace Corps workers, missionaries) should also be considered for preexposure prophylaxis.
- HDCV for preexposure prophylaxis is administered in three doses of 1.0 mL intramuscularly or 0.1 mL intradermally on days 0 and 7 and between days 21 and 28, although intradermal HDCV may give a nonprotection rate of 7.5%.
- The vaccine is not recommended for persons who are immunocompromised.
- An intramuscular booster dose every second year is recommended for persons who will have continued exposure.
- Postexposure prophylaxis should be given after percutaneous or permucosal exposure to saliva or other infectious material from a high-risk source.
- Persons previously immunized with HDCV or RVA or those who have received postexposure prophylaxis previously should receive two 1.0-mL intramuscular doses of HDCV or RVA on postexposure days 0 and 3.
- Postexposure, individuals who have not been previously immunized should receive the recommended regimen of rabies immune globulin (see later section) and five doses of HDCV or RVA, 1.0 mL intramuscularly on days 0, 3, 7, 14, and 28 after exposure. The intradermal route should not be used for postexposure prophylaxis.

VIII

▶ RABIES IMMUNE GLOBULIN

- In persons who have not been previously immunized against rabies, rabies immune globulin is given simultaneously with rabies HDCV to provide optimal coverage in the interval before immune response to the vaccine occurs.
- Rabies immune globulin use is not recommended beyond 8 days after initiation of the vaccine series nor in persons previously immunized to rabies.
- Human rabies immune globulin is administered in a dose of 20 IU/kg (0.133 mL/kg), half to be given intramuscularly and the other half infiltrated around the wound site. This product should never be administered by the intravenous route.

▶ RUBELLA VACCINE

- The vaccine is indicated for children >1 year of age, persons 12 years or older without evidence of wild virus infection, women of childbearing potential for whom serologic testing is unavailable, and to persons at a substantial risk for exposure.
- The vaccine should not be given to immunosuppressed individuals nor used within 6 weeks (preferably 3 months) of immune globulin administration.
- While the vaccine has been shown to be safe to the fetus, its use in pregnancy is discouraged. Women should be counseled not to become pregnant for 3 weeks following vaccination.

VIII

▶ VARICELLA VACCINE

- The American Academy of Pediatrics recommends routine immunization with varicella vaccine for all children.
- The vaccine is given as two doses separated by three months.

▶ VARICELLA-ZOSTER IMMUNE GLOBULIN

- Varicella-zoster immune globulin (VZIG) is used for passive immunization of susceptible immunodeficient patients exposed to VZ infection.
- Use of VZIG should be considered in exposed children and certain adults who are immunocompromised and susceptible to VZ. Criteria for its use in children are listed in Table 50.7.
- Criteria for its use in immunocompromised adults are less clear because of difficulties in determining susceptibility status.
- For maximum effectiveness, VZIG must be given within 48 hours and not more than 96 hours following exposure.
- Administration of VZIG is by the intramuscular route (never intravenously).

TABLE 50.7. Indications for Varicella-Zoster Immune Globulin[a]

1. Susceptible to VZ infection
2. Significant exposure within 96 hours
   a. Household contact
   b. Playmate contact (more than 1 hour of play indoors)
   c. Hospital contact (in adjacent beds or same two- to four-bed room)
   d. School contact (adjacent desks in same classroom or same carpool)
   e. Transplacental contact (newborn born to mother who developed varicella less than 5 days prior to or 48 hours after delivery)
3. Age <15, with administration to immunocompromised adolescents, adults, and other older patients on an individual basis
4. One of the following underlying illnesses or conditions:
   a. Leukemia or lymphoma
   b. Congenital or acquired immunodeficiency
   c. Immunosuppressive treatment
   d. Newborn of mother with varicella (2e above)
   e. Premature infant (≥28 week gestation) whose mother lacks a prior history of chicken pox
   f. Premature infants (<28 weeks gestation or ≤1000 grams) regardless of maternal history

[a]Patients should meet all four criteria.

VIII

▶ IMMUNE GLOBULIN

- Immune globulin (IG) is available as both intramuscular (IGIM) and intravenous preparations (IGIV).
- The plasma half-life of IG averages 18–32 days. Serum IgG levels increase approximately 250 mg% for each 100 mg/kg of intravenous IG infused.
- IGIM is indicated for providing passive immunity in hepatitis A infections, as an alternative to HBIG in hepatitis B exposures (however, HBIG is significantly more effective), hepatitis C (but not hepatitis E), measles, varicella zoster, and primary immunodeficiency diseases. IGIM is not indicated for prevention of rubella, mumps, or poliomyelitis. Table 50.8 lists the suggested dosages for IGIM in various disease states.
- Currently there are many approved indications for IVIG and other non-approved disease states for which IGIV is used. Dosages vary based on the preparation used.

IVIG Uses
- Primary immunodeficiency states including both antibody deficiencies and combined deficiencies. HIV disease is not in this class.
- Idiopathic thrombocytopenia purpura (ITP).

TABLE 50.8. Indications and Dosage of Intramuscular Immune Globulin in Infectious Diseases

Primary immunodeficiency states	1.2 mL/kg IM then 0.6 mL/kg IM every 2–4 weeks
Hepatitis A exposure	0.02 mL/kg IM within 2 weeks
Hepatitis A prophylaxis	0.02 mL/kg IM if exposure <3 months
	0.06 mL/kg if exposure >3 months, every 4–6 months
Hepatitis B	0.06 mL/kg IM (HBIG is preferred in known exposures) as soon as possible
Non-A/non-B hepatitis	0.06 mL/kg IM as soon as possible (questionable effectiveness)
Measles	0.25 mL/kg IM within 6 days (maximum dose = 15 mL)
Rubella	0.55 mL/kg, single dose
Primary immunodeficiency states	1.2 mL/kg IM then 0.6 mL/kg IM every 2–4 weeks

- Chronic lymphocytic leukemia (CLL) in patients who have had a serious bacterial infection.
- A number of other proposed uses of IGIV can be identified. It is important to note that generally these are not approved indications and are not generally accepted in the medical community for routine treatment. VIII These uses include the following:
  - Kawasaki disease (mucocutaneous lymph node syndrome).
  - Neonatal sepsis.
  - Autoimmune diseases.
  - Cystic fibrosis.
  - Intractable epilepsy.
  - Thermal injury.
  - Cytomegalovirus infection.
  - HIV infection.
  - Bone marrow transplant.

▶ RH$_0$(D) IMMUNE GLOBULIN (RDIG)

- RDIG suppresses the antibody response and formation of anti-Rh$_0$(D) in Rh$_0$(D)-negative, D^u-negative women exposed to Rh$_0$(D)-positive blood and prevents the future chance of erythroblastosis fetalis in subsequent pregnancies with a Rh$_0$(D)-positive fetus.
- RDIG, when administered within 72 hours of delivery of a full-term infant, reduces active antibody formation from 12% to 1–2%.
- In addition, RDIG is also used in the case of a premenopausal woman who is Rh$_0$(D)-negative or D^u-negative and has inadvertently received Rh$_0$(D)-positive or D^u-positive blood or blood products.
- RDIG is given within 72 hours of a term delivery.

- For postpregnancy termination occurring up to 13 weeks gestation, one microdose (50-µg) vial is given within 72 hours. For pregnancy termination after 13 weeks, one standard dose (300 µg) is given within 72 hours.
- RDIG is administered intramuscularly only.

See Chapter 116, Vaccines, Toxoids, and Other Immunobiologics, authored by Joseph S. Bertino, Jr., PharmD, FCCP and Daniel T. Casto, PharmD, FCCP, for a more detailed discussion of this topic.

VIII

Neurologic Disorders

Edited by Barbara G. Wells, PharmD, FASHP, FCCP

Chapter 51

▶ EPILEPSY

▶ DEFINITIONS

The term epilepsy implies a periodic recurrence of seizures with or without convulsions. A seizure results from an excessive discharge of neurons and is characterized by changes in electrical activity as measured by the electroencephalogram (EEG). A convulsion implies a violent, involuntary contraction or series of contractions of the voluntary muscles.

▶ PATHOPHYSIOLOGY

- A seizure is traceable to an unstable cell membrane or its surrounding cells. Excess excitability spreads either locally (focal seizure) or more widely (generalized seizure).
- An abnormality of potassium conductance, a defect in the voltage-sensitive calcium channels, or a deficiency in the membrane ATP-ases linked to ion transport may result in neuronal membrane instability and a seizure.
- Normal neuronal activity depends on normal functioning of excitatory (e.g., glutamate, aspartate, acetylcholine, norepinephrine, histamine) and inhibitory (e.g., dopamine, gamma-aminobutyric acid [GABA]) neurotransmitters and an adequate supply of glucose, oxygen, sodium, potassium, calcium, and amino acids; normal pH; and normal receptor function.
- Common causes of seizures are shown in Table 51.1.
- The causes of seizures in the elderly include cerebrovascular disease, tumor, head trauma, metabolic disorders, and central nervous system (CNS) infections.
- There is no identifiable cause for seizures in most patients, and especially in children.
- Hyperventilation may precipitate absence seizures. Sleep, sleep deprivation, sensory stimuli, and emotional stress may initiate seizures. Hormonal changes occurring at the time of menses, puberty, or pregnancy have been associated with onset of or increase in seizure activity. Oral contraceptives should be given with caution to patients with epilepsy. Other precipitants include fever, lack of food, trauma, drugs (e.g., theophylline, alcohol, phenothiazines, antidepressants, cocaine, antiepileptic drugs [AEDs] in excessive concentrations), and drug withdrawal.
- The most clearly established risk factors for epilepsy are severe head trauma, CNS infections, and stroke. Children who are small for gestational age, neonates with seizures, and children with febrile seizures,

TABLE 51.1. Common Causes of Seizures

Mechanical	Sudden Withdrawal of Drugs
Trauma	Alcohol
Birth injury	Street drugs
Neoplasms	Antipsychotics
Vascular abnormalities	Antidepressants
Metabolic	Antiepileptic drugs
Electrolytes	Toxins
Water	Fever
Glucose	Infection
Amino acids	Hereditary
Lipids	Idiopathic
pH	

cerebral palsy, or mental retardation are at increased risk for developing epilepsy.

▶ CLINICAL PRESENTATION

- Partial seizures manifest as alterations in motor functions, sensory or somatosensory symptoms, or autonomic symptoms. If there is no loss of consciousness, the seizures are classified as simple partial. If there is loss of consciousness, the seizures are described as complex partial. With complex partial seizures, the patient may have automatisms, periods of memory loss, or aberrations of behavior.
- In generalized seizures, motor manifestations are bilateral, and there is a loss of consciousness.
- Absence seizures are manifested by a sudden onset, interruption of ongoing activities, a blank stare, and possibly a brief upward rotation of the eyes.
- Tonic-clonic seizures (formerly known as grand mal) may be preceded by premonitory symptoms known as an aura. A tonic-clonic seizure that is preceded by an aura is likely a partial seizure that is secondarily generalized. Tonic-clonic seizures begin with a short tonic contraction of muscles followed by a period of rigidity. The patient may lose sphincter control, bite the tongue, or become cyanotic. The episode may be followed by unconsciousness and frequently the patient goes into a deep sleep.
- Myoclonic jerks are brief shock-like muscular contractions of the face, trunk, and extremities. They may be isolated events or rapidly repetitive.
- In atonic seizures, there is a sudden loss of muscle tone that may be described as a head drop, dropping of a limb, or slumping to the ground.

IX

▶ DIAGNOSIS OF SEIZURES

- The patient and family should be interviewed to characterize the seizures for frequency, duration, precipitating factors, times of occurrence, presence of an aura, ictal activity, and postictal state.
- Physical, neurologic, and laboratory (SMA-20, complete blood cell count [CBC], urinalysis, and special blood chemistries) examination may identify an etiology. A lumbar puncture may be indicated if there is fever.
- An EEG should be done as soon after the seizure as possible. Simultaneous EEG and video monitoring may be helpful.
- Imaging studies (computed tomography [CT], positron emission tomography [PET], single photon emission CT [SPECT], and magnetic resonance imaging [MRI]) may identify structural or functional abnormalities.

▶ CLASSIFICATION OF SEIZURES

- More than 90% of seizure patients may be classified using the classification in Table 51.2.

TABLE 51.2. International Classification of Seizures

I. Partial seizures (seizures begin locally)

    A. Simple (without impairment of consciousness)

        1. With motor symptoms

        2. With special sensory or somatosensory symptoms

        3. With psychic symptoms

    B. Complex (with impairment of consciousness)

        1. Simple partial onset followed by impairment of consciousness—with or without automatisms

        2. Impaired consciousness at onset—with or without automatisms

    C. Secondarily generalized (partial onset evolving to generalized tonic–clonic seizures)

II. Generalized seizures (bilaterally symmetrical and without local onset)

    A. Absence

    B. Myoclonic

    C. Clonic

    D. Tonic

    E. Tonic–clonic

    F. Atonic

    G. Infantile spasms

III. Unclassified seizures

IV. Status epilepticus (prolonged partial or generalized seizures without recovery between attacks)

IX

- Partial seizures begin in one hemisphere of the brain and unless they become secondarily generalized, result in an asymmetric seizure.
- The EEG during an absence seizure has a characteristic 2–4 cycle/s spike and slow-wave complex.

▶ DESIRED OUTCOME

The goal of treatment is to control or reduce the frequency of seizures, allowing the patient to live as normal a life as possible. Complete suppression of seizures must be balanced against side effects, and the patient should be involved in defining this balance. An additional goal is to maximize compliance with the drug regimen and avoid side effects and drug interactions.

▶ TREATMENT

- Reasons for AED treatment failure include inappropriate drug selection, inappropriate dosing, and poor compliance. Some patients do not respond despite rational therapy.
- AED pharmacokinetic and pharmacologic summary are shown in Tables 51.3 and 51.4.

PRINCIPLES OF THERAPY

- Establish the diagnosis and exclude remedial causes.
- Select the primary drug most appropriate for the seizure type(s) (Table 51.5). Valproic acid is the only AED effective against absence and other seizure types. If valproic acid is ineffective in treating a mixed seizure disorder that includes absence, ethosuximide should be used with another AED. Serum concentrations may need to be higher to control complex partial seizures than tonic-clonic seizures.
- Initiate appropriate drug therapy early after the diagnosis. Early initiation of appropriate AED therapy enhances the likelihood of controlling seizure activity.
- Begin with monotherapy. The initial agent should be titrated to maximum benefit or intolerable side effects. A second medication may be added if seizures continue despite good plasma concentrations. The second AED may replace or be added to the initial therapy. If the initial AED is replaced, it should be gradually tapered after the second drug has been titrated to the desired dose. If two drugs are used, they generally should have differing mechanisms of action and side effect profiles.
- Titrate the AED to achieve an adequate response. Usually therapy is initiated with one-fourth to one-third the anticipated maintenance dose and gradually increased over 3 to 4 weeks to an effective dose. Serum concentrations may be useful, but the therapeutic range must be correlated with clinical outcome. Some patients need and tolerate concentrations above the range. For populations known to have altered plasma protein

IX

TABLE 51.3. Antiepileptic Drug Pharmacokinetic Data

AED	$t_{1/2}$ (h)	Time to Steady State (d)	% Unchanged	V_D (L/kg)	% Bioavailability	Clinically Important Metabolite	% Removed by Dialysis	% Protein Binding
Phenytoin	A 10–34 C 5–14	7–28	<5	0.6–8.0	90–95	No	4% (H)	90
Phenobarbital	A 46–136 C 37–73	14–21	20–40	0.6	90–100	No	30% (H)	50
Primidone	A 3.3–19 C 4.5–11	1–4	40	0.43–1.1	90–100	PB PEMA	30% (H)	80
Carbamazepine	12 h if monotherapy; 5–14 h if combination; chronic dosing undergoes autoinduction	21–28 for completion of auto-induction	<1	1–2	>75	10,11-epoxide	<20	40–90
Valproic acid	A 8–20 C 7–14	1–3	<5	0.1–0.5	100	May contribute to toxicity	—	90–95 binding saturates
Ethosuximide	A 60 C 30	6–12	10–20	0.67	Assumed 100	No	~50	0
Felbamate	22	5	50	0.73–0.82	>90[a]	No	?	~25
Gabapentin	5.3	1	0	58 L	No	No	Y	0
Lamotrigine	22	5	128	1.2	No	?	40–50	
Topiramate	20–30	5	50–80		80	?		15

A, adult; C, child; H, hemodialysis; PB, phenobarbital; PEMA, phenylethylmalonamide.

[a]The bioavailability of gabapentin is dose dependent.

IX

TABLE 51.4. Summary of Antiepileptic Drug Pharmacologic Data

AED	Initial Dose (mg/kg/d)	Therapeutic Range (μg/mL Total)	Side Effects Dose Related	Side Effects Not Dose Related	Manufacturer
Phenytoin	Loading dose; 20 in status	10–20	Nystagmus, ataxia, cognitive impairment, lethargy	Gingival hyperplasia, increase in body hair, coarsening of facial features, acne, folate deficiency, skin rash	Parke-Davis, others
Phenobarbital	Loading dose; 20 in status	15–40	Sedation, mental dullness, cognitive impairment, hyperactivity, ataxia	Hyperactivity, change in sleep problems, skin rashes	Multiple
Primidone	50–125 mg initial dose; no loading dose required	5–20			Ayerst
Carbamazepine	2–8 mg; no loading dose required	4–12	Double vision, blurred vision, lethargy	Fluid retention, leukopenia, bone marrow suppression, skin rash, GI distress	Ciba-Geigy, others
Valproic acid	7.5–15; no loading dose required	50–150(?)	GI upset, lethargy	Weight gain, nausea, alopecia, hepatitis	Abbott, others
Ethosuximide	5–7; no loading dose required	40–100	GI distress, nausea, drowsiness, hiccups	Headache	Parke-Davis
Felbamate		—	—	Anorexia, insomnia, aplastic anemia, acute liver failure	Carter Wallace
Gabapentin		—	—	CNS	Parke-Davis
Lamotrigine		—	—	CNS, rash	Glaxo Wellcome
Topiramate	50 mg/d initial dose	—	Sleepiness, fatigue, poor concentration, psychomotor slowing	—	Ortho-McNeil

TABLE 51.5. Drugs of Choice for Specific Seizure Disorders

New International	Commonly Used Major Drugs	Commonly Used Alternative Drugs
Simple partial	Carbamazepine Phenytoin	Lamotrigine Gabapentin
Complex partial	Carbamazepine Phenytoin	Lamotrigine Gabapentin
Tonic–clonic	Phenytoin Valproic acid Carbamazepine	Phenobarbital
Absence	Ethosuximide Valproic acid	Clonazepam Acetazolamide
Mixed seizures	Phenytoin Phenobarbital + ethosuximide or valproic acid	Primidone Carbamazepine + clonazepam Acetazolamide
Bilateral massive epileptic myoclonus, atonic, infantile spasms[a]	Clonazepam ACTH	Phenytoin Phenobarbital Benzodiazepines Acetazolamide

[a]Difficult group to treat; combinations are the rule.

binding (Table 51.6), free rather than total serum concentrations should be measured, if the AED is highly protein-bound.

- Provide patient education. Knowledge of epilepsy correlates with an improved quality of life. Noncompliance may be the most common reason for treatment failure.

IX

TABLE 51.6. Conditions Altering Antiepileptic Drug[a] Protein Binding

Chronic renal failure
Liver disease
Hypoalbuminemia
Burns
Pregnancy
Malnutrition
Displacing drugs
Age—neonates and elderly

[a]Phenytoin and valproic acid are highly protein bound; carbamazepine has variable binding; phenobarbital and primidone are minimally bound; and ethosuximide is not bound to plasma proteins.

- Consider discontinuing AEDs. Polypharmacy can often be reduced, and some patients can discontinue AEDs altogether. In reducing polypharmacy, the drug considered less appropriate for the seizure type should be discontinued first, and drug interactions must be considered. Withdrawal of AEDs should be gradual. Factors favoring successful withdrawal of AEDs include a seizure-free period of 2–4 years, complete seizure control within 1 year of onset, onset of seizures between age 2 and 35 years, a normal EEG, and use of AEDs for inappropriate reasons. Factors associated with poor prognosis in discontinuing AEDs are history of high frequency of seizures, repeated episodes of status epilepticus, combination of seizure types, and development of abnormal mental functioning. A 4-year seizure-free period is suggested for simple partial, complex partial, and absence associated with tonic-clonic convulsions. Follow-up monitoring for 5 years is suggested for patients withdrawn from AEDs.

SPECIFIC ANTIEPILEPTIC DRUGS

Phenytoin

- Possible mechanisms of action include blockade of post-tetanic potentiation (PTP), altering ion fluxes, altering calcium presynaptic uptake, influencing calcium-dependent protein phosphorylation and neurotransmitter release, altering sodium-potassium ATP-dependent ionic membrane pump, and preventing cyclic nucleotide buildup.
- Absorption may be saturable. Enterohepatic cycling of phenytoin occurs.

Therapeutic Range/Dosing

IX

- Several populations have altered protein binding (Table 51.6). The therapeutic range of free drug is 1–2 µg/mL.
- For many patients, metabolism changes from first order to zero order at serum concentrations within the dosing range. Empirically, doses of phenytoin may be increased by 100 mg/d if concentrations are <7 µg/mL, by 50 mg/d if concentrations are ≥7 but <12 µg/mL, and by 30 mg/d if concentrations are ≥12 µg/mL.
- Loading doses are needed only in status epilepticus. In nonacute situations, phenytoin may be initiated in doses of 3–6 mg/kg/d and titrated upward. Most (but not all) adult patients can be maintained on a single daily dose of phenytoin, but children may have more rapid elimination requiring more frequent administration.

Dosage Forms

- Phenytoin tablets and suspension contain phenytoin acid, while the capsule and parenteral solution are phenytoin sodium, which is 92% phenytoin. Clinicians should remember that there are two different strengths of phenytoin suspension.
- Some brands may be absorbed faster than others. Only preparations identified as "extended-release" should be used for single daily dosing. Switching brands requires careful monitoring.
- IM administration of phenytoin is not generally recommended.

Adverse Effects

- Initially patients may experience lethargy, lack of coordination, higher cortical dysfunction, and drowsiness. These effects may be minimized by slow dosage titration.
- Nystagmus frequently occurs at serum concentration >20 µg/mL, ataxia at concentrations >30 µg/mL, and mental status changes including coma at concentrations >40 µg/mL. Levels >30 µg/mL may induce seizures.
- Gingival hyperplasia occurs in up to 50% of patients. Other chronic side effects include suppression of cognitive abilities, vitamin D deficiency, osteomalacia, folic acid deficiency, carbohydrate intolerance, hypothyroidism, and peripheral neuropathy.
- Rarely, Steven-Johnson syndrome, pseudolymphoma, bone marrow suppression, lupus-like reactions, and hepatitis may occur.

Drug Interactions (Tables 51.7 and 51.8)

- Phenytoin may be displaced from protein binding sites by other highly bound drugs, but usually no dosage adjustment is necessary, because clearance is increased. In these situations, serum concentration of free

TABLE 51.7. Interactions Between Antiepileptic Drugs

AED	Added Drug	Effect
Phenytoin	Carbamazepine	↓ Concentration
	Methsuximide	↑ Concentration
	Valproic acid	↓ Total
	Topiramate	↑ Concentration
Phenobarbital	Phenytoin	↑ Concentration
	Valproic acid	↑ Concentration
Primidone	Carbamazepine	↑ Phenobarbital
	Phenytoin	↑ Phenobarbital
Carbamazepine	Phenobarbital	↓ Concentration
	Phenytoin	↓ Concentration
	Primidone	↓ Concentration
Valproic acid	Carbamazepine	↓ Concentration
	Phenobarbital	↓ Concentration
	Primidone	↓ Concentration
	Phenytoin	↓ Concentration
Lamotrigine	Phenytoin	↓ Concentration
	Carbamazepine	
	Valproic acid	↑ Concentration
Phenytoin	Felbamate	↑ Concentration
Carbamazepine	Felbamate	↑ Concentration of active metabolite
Phenobarbital	Felbamate	↑ Concentration

TABLE 51.8. Interactions of Antiepileptic Drugs with Other Drugs

AED	Altered by	Result	Alters	Result
Phenytoin	Antacids	↓ Absorption	Oral contraceptives	↓ Efficacy
	Disulfiram	↑ Concentration	Bishydroxycoumarin	↓ Anticoagulation
	Isoniazid	↑ Concentration	Quinidine	↓ Concentration
	Chloramphenicol	↑ Concentration	Vitamin D	↓ Concentration
	Propoxyphene	↑ Concentration	Folic acid	↓ Concentration
	Cimetidine	↑ Concentration		
	Ethanol	↓ Concentration		
Phenobarbital			Oral contraceptives	↓ Efficacy
Primidone			Quinidine	↑ Metabolism
			Tricyclics	↑ Metabolism
			Corticosteroids	↑ Metabolism
			Chlorpromazine	↑ Metabolism
			Furosemide	↓ Renal sensitivity
Carbamazepine	Propoxyphene	↑ Concentration	Warfarin	↓ Concentration
	Cimetidine	↑ Concentration	Theophylline	↓ Concentration
	Isoniazid	↑ Concentration	Doxycycline	↓ Concentration
	Erythromycin	↑ Concentration		
Valproic acid	Salicylates	↑ Free concentration		

phenytoin should be measured. Drug interactions affecting absorption, metabolism, or excretion are potentially more important.

- Presence of food in the gastrointestinal (GI) tract may slow absorption of phenytoin.
- Phenytoin decreases folic acid absorption, but folic acid replacement can reduce phenytoin serum concentrations and result in loss of seizure control.

Phenobarbital/Primidone

- Primidone is an active AED and has two active metabolites, phenobarbital and phenylethylmalonamide (PEMA). In general, phenobarbital should be tried first and primidone reserved for refractory patients.
- Phenobarbital is the drug of choice for neonatal seizures. Primidone and phenobarbital share the same indications, but primidone is less useful in partial seizures.

Pharmacokinetics

- Neonates have a longer half-life than adults, and children have a shorter half-life.
- Renal excretion of phenobarbital can be increased by giving diuretics and urinary alkalinizers.
- The half-life of primidone may become shorter after chronic therapy because the phenobarbital metabolite may induce the metabolism of primidone.

Adverse Effects
- Side effects of phenobarbital and primidone are similar. Initial complaints are fatigue, drowsiness, and depression. In children, the primary side effect is hyperactivity. Phenobarbital depresses cognitive functioning.
- Giving phenobarbital at bedtime minimizes the consequences of CNS depression.

Drug Interactions (Tables 51.7 and 51.8)
- Phenobarbital is a potent enzyme inducer and will increase the elimination of drugs metabolized by phase I oxidation.

Carbamazepine
- Carbamazepine has fewer side effects than phenytoin and phenobarbital.
- It is considered the AED of first choice for partial seizures, especially complex partial seizures. It is also useful for generalized seizures other than absence.
- Carbamazepine may depress transmission in the nucleus ventralis anterior of the thalamus, and it depresses PTP.

Pharmacokinetics
- There may be lower bioavailability at higher doses, and food may enhance bioavailability.
- There is a wide variability in time to peak (2–24 hours), with an average of 6 hours.
- The major metabolite is carbamazepine 10,11-epoxide.
- Carbamazepine induces its own metabolism, a process that begins 3–5 days after dosage initiation, is complete in 21–28 days, and rapidly reverses if therapy is discontinued.

IX

Therapeutic Range/Dosing
- Concentrations >12 µg/mL are associated with an increased incidence of CNS-related side effects.
- Carbamazepine suspension has been used to administer a loading dose of 7.4–10.4 mg/kg in critically ill patients. Oral loading has also been accomplished with a controlled-release formulation.
- CNS and GI complaints can be minimized by gradual dosage adjustment and by giving larger doses at bedtime.
- The maintenance dose range is 7–15 mg/kg/d for adults, given in two to four doses.

Dosage Forms
- If brands are switched, the patient should be carefully monitored.
- It may be necessary to administer the suspension more frequently than the tablet to prevent excessive peak-to-trough fluctuations.
- The controlled-release preparation will reduce peak-to-trough variability and may improve seizure control and patient tolerance.

Adverse Effects

- Neurosensory side effects (e.g., diplopia, blurred vision, nystagmus, ataxia, dizziness, and headache) are the most common, occurring in 35–50% of patients.
- Carbamazepine may induce hyponatremia, a condition similar to the syndrome of inappropriate antidiuretic hormone secretion. The incidence may increase with age.
- Hematologic side effects include aplastic anemia (only a few cases reported since 1964), thrombocytopenia, anemia, leukopenia (as high as 10% incidence). Leukopenia is usually transient, but may be persistent in 2% of patients. Carbamazepine may be continued unless the WBC count drops to less than 2500/mm³ and the absolute neutrophil count drops to less than 1000/mm³.

Drug Interactions (Tables 51.7 and 51.8)

- Carbamazepine may interact with other drugs by inducing their metabolism.
- Valproic acid appears to reduce the formation of the 10,11-epoxide metabolite without affecting the concentration of carbamazepine.
- The interaction of erythromycin with carbamazepine is particularly significant.

Valproic Acid

- Valproic acid is the drug of first choice for most generalized seizures and is also useful in the treatment of partial seizures. It is the only AED that is effective against absence and other types of generalized seizures, and it may also be useful in neonatal seizures.
- Valproic acid may potentiate postsynaptic GABA responses, may have a direct membrane-stabilizing effect, and may affect the potassium channel.

Pharmacokinetics

- Food delays absorption, but does not decrease the amount of valproic acid absorbed.
- The free fraction may increase as total serum concentrations increases. Protein binding is decreased in patients with head trauma.
- Some of the metabolites may be active, and may be responsible for hepatotoxicity.

Therapeutic Range/Dosing

- Although 100 μg/mL is widely used as the upper end of the therapeutic range, some patients require higher concentrations. In refractory or partially responding patients, the concentration may cautiously be titrated upward with close monitoring.
- Doses of 15–20 mg/kg daily usually produce concentrations of 75–100 μg/mL. Usually patients are started on 7.5–15 mg/kg/d in divided doses and increased in 2–3 days.
- Twice daily dosing is feasible, but children and patients taking enzyme inducers may require dosing three to four times daily.

Dosage Forms

- Valproic acid is available as a soft gelatin capsule, an enteric-coated tablet, a syrup, and a sprinkle.
- The enteric-coated tablet is sodium divalproex, which is metabolized in the intestine to valproic acid. It produces less GI distress than the capsule.
- The sprinkle has a slower rate of absorption than the capsule.

Adverse Effects

- Side effects include GI complaints (up to 20%), drowsiness (10%), ataxia (15%), tremor (10%), alopecia (usually temporary), peripheral edema, and weight gain.
- Most deaths from hepatotoxicity have occurred in patients who were <2 years old, mentally retarded, and receiving multiple therapy.
- Thrombocytopenia occurs in 6–40% of patients, but is responsive to a decrease in dose. Other hematologic toxicities include leukopenia with transient neutropenia, transient erythroblastopenia, and others.

Drug Interactions (Tables 51.7 and 51.8)

- Free fatty acids, aspirin, and phenytoin may alter valproic acid binding.

Ethosuximide

- The only indication for ethosuximide is treatment of absence seizures, and it is the drug of first choice. It may be used in combination with valproic acid in refractory patients.

Pharmacokinetics

- Ethosuximide is not bound to plasma proteins or tissues.
- Metabolites are believed to be inactive.
- There is some evidence of nonlinear metabolic processes.

IX

Therapeutic Range/Dosing

- The accepted therapeutic range is 40–100 µg/mL, but higher concentrations are sometime needed.
- Patients are started at 5–7 mg/kg/d in divided doses and increased in 1–2 week. Doses of 20 mg/kg/d usually result in concentrations of approximately 50 µg/mL. Total daily dose is usually divided into two doses.

Adverse Effects

- Common side effects are nausea, drowsiness, lethargy, dizziness, hiccups, and headaches. Rash, lupus, and blood dyscrasias are reported rarely.

NEW ANTIEPILEPTIC DRUGS

Felbamate

- Felbamate can be considered for either monotherapy or adjunctive therapy in the treatment of partial seizures, with or without generalization, in adults with epilepsy and as adjunctive therapy in the treatment of partial and generalized seizures associated with Lennox-Gastaut syndrome in children 2 years and older.

- Because of the association of aplastic anemia and acute liver failure, felbamate is recommended only for patients refractory to other AEDs.
- It displays linear pharmacokinetics and is not bound to plasma proteins.

Therapeutic Range/Dosing

- If used as monotherapy in adults, the dose is initiated at 1200 mg/day (in divided doses, three or four times daily) and increased by 600 mg every 2 weeks to a maximum of 3600 mg/d.
- When felbamate is used in combination with other AEDs, the dose of the concurrent AED should be reduced by 30–50% at the initiation of felbamate, and further reductions should occur as the dose is increased.

Adverse Effects

- Frequently reported side effects are anorexia, weight loss, insomnia, nausea, and headache. Less common side effects are diarrhea, rash, diplopia, ataxia, and rhinitis. It is also associated with aplastic anemia and acute liver failure.

Drug Interactions

- Felbamate inhibits the clearance of phenytoin, carbamazepine, and valproic acid, and doses of these drugs should be decreased by about 30% when felbamate is added.
- Interactions with phenobarbital and warfarin have also been reported.

Gabapentin

- Gabapentin is approved in adults with epilepsy for adjunctive therapy for partial seizures with or without secondary generalization.

Therapeutic Range/Dosing

- Gabapentin is initiated at 300 mg at bedtime on the first day and increased to 300 mg twice daily on the second day and 300 mg three times daily on the third day. Further titrations are then made. The manufacturer recommends doses up to 2400 or 3600 mg/d, but higher doses have been used safely.
- Gabapentin is eliminated exclusively by the kidneys. For patients with a creatinine clearance <60 mL/min, the dose is 1200 mg/d; for patients with a creatinine clearance of 30–60 mL/min, the dose is 600 mg/d; for patients with a creatinine clearance of 15–30 mL/min, the dose is 300 mg/d; and for patients with a creatinine clearance <15 mL/min, the dose is 150 mg/d (300 mg every other day).

Adverse Effects

- Most frequently reported side effects are fatigue, somnolence, dizziness, and ataxia.

Drug Interactions

- There is a 10% reduction in the clearance of gabapentin in patients taking cimetidine and a 20% reduction in the bioavailability if aluminum antacids are taken concurrently.

Lamotrigine

- Lamotrigine regulates the release of glutamate and aspartate.
- It is approved as adjunctive therapy in adults with partial epilepsy refractory to other agents.

Therapeutic Range/Dosing

- In patients who are taking enzyme-inducing drugs but not valproic acid, lamotrigine should be started at a dose of 50 mg/d for 2 weeks and then increased to 100 mg/d for 2 weeks. Then the dose can be titrated by 100 mg/d at weekly intervals up to 500 mg/d.
- In patients taking valproic acid and other enzyme inducers, the dose should be started at 25 mg every other day for 2 weeks and then increased to 25 mg/d for 2 weeks. Then the dose can be titrated if necessary to a maximum of 150 mg/d in two divided doses.

Adverse Effects

- The most frequent side effects include diplopia, drowsiness, ataxia, and headache.
- Rashes are usually mild to moderate, but Stevens-Johnson reaction has also occurred.

Topiramate

- Topiramate is recently approved for adjunctive therapy of partial onset seizures in adults.
- It blocks voltage-sensitive sodium channels, enhances GABA activity, and blocks the action of glutamate.
- Topiramate is given in a 50 mg/day dose initially, with a gradual increase during an 8-week titration period to a total of 400 mg/day in two divided doses. Usual doses are 200–600 mg/d.
- It is <20% bound to plasma proteins.
- Elimination is primarily renal; 50–80% of the drug is eliminated unchanged.
- The half-life of elimination is 20–30 hours.
- Side effects include psychomotor slowing, difficulty concentrating, sedation, and fatigue. During clinical studies, 1.5% of patients developed kidney stones.
- It occasionally causes an increase in the plasma concentration of phenytoin.

MISCELLANEOUS ANTIEPILEPTIC DRUGS

Benzodiazepines

- Clonazepam is an effective adjunctive agent in the treatment of myoclonic seizures, atonic seizures, atypical absence seizures, and infantile spasms. It may also be useful in treatment of partial seizures. Tolerance to anticonvulsant effects may occur.
- Side effects include drowsiness, ataxia, and changes in behavior.
- Dosing generally begins with 0.01–0.03 mg/kg/d given in two to three doses and is increased until the desired response or side effects occur.

IX

Acetazolamide

- Acetazolamide is effective for generalized tonic-clonic, absence, and complex partial seizures, but its use is limited by the rapid emergence of tolerance.
- Intermittent use has been more effective, and it may be particularly useful in treating the increase in seizures that sometimes occurs during menses.

Adrenocorticotropic Hormone (ACTH)

- ACTH is the standard treatment for infantile spasms.
- Dosage ranges between 5–180 U, but most clinicians recommend 20–40 U/d. Relapses are common, and duration of therapy has ranged from 2 weeks to 18 months. It can induce Cushing's syndrome.

CHRONIC SIDE EFFECTS OF AEDS

- The incidence of chronic side effects is: phenytoin (33%), phenobarbital (23%), carbamazepine (15%), and valproic acid (12%).

Cognitive and Behavioral Effects

- On balance, carbamazepine and valproate cause less impairment of cognition than phenytoin and phenobarbital.
- Phenobarbital-induced hyperactivity is nonconcentration-dependent.
- Drug-induced drowsiness and lethargy may be reduced by tolerance, gradual dosage titration, and serum-concentration monitoring.

Teratogenicity/Lactation

- The absolute risk of major malformations in infants exposed to AEDs is about 7–10%, which is 3–5% higher than in the general population.
- Barbiturates and phenytoin are associated with facial clefts, and other malformations. Valproic acid and carbamazepine are associated with spina bifida and hypospadias. Other adverse pregnancy outcomes associated with exposure to AEDs are psychomotor impairment and mental retardation.
- AEDs pass into the breast milk in low concentrations, but AED treatment is not necessarily a reason to discourage breast-feeding.

Drug-Induced Seizures

- Use of AEDs can exacerbate seizures in some situations (Table 51.9).
- Drugs most commonly reported to cause seizures are meperidine, phenothiazines, clozapine, contrast agents, flumazenil, and vaccines (febrile seizures). Seizures are also caused by anesthetics, β-lactam antibiotics, isoniazid, theophylline, and alkylating agents.

▶ SPECIAL PROBLEMS

FEBRILE CONVULSIONS

- Two to four percent of children have a febrile seizure, and they do not increase the risk of death, injury, or mental retardation.

IX

TABLE 51.9. Exacerbation of Seizures by Anticonvulsants

Acute or chronic toxicity
　High concentrations of phenytoin or carbamazepine

Use of AED in a seizure type for which it is not indicated
　Phenytoin exacerbates absence
　Phenobarbital exacerbates atonic, myoclonic, and absence
　Carbamazepine may precipitate generalized convulsive, atonic, and myoclonic seizures when used
　　in children with atypical absence seizures

Unmasking one seizure type when another is controlled
　Attributed to ethosuximide

Drug-induced somnolence
　Phenobarbital and benzodiazepines

Sudden withdrawal
　All anticonvulsants

Indirect effects
　Carbamazepine-induced water intoxication and hyponatremia secondary to inappropriate ADH
　　secretion

- Patients who have seizures only associated with fever are not epileptic. Children who have experienced a febrile seizure have a 2% chance of having epilepsy by age 7.
- Risk factors for a first febrile seizure include first- or second-degree relative with a history of febrile seizures, neonatal discharge at 28 days or later, parental report of "slow" development, and day-care attendance.
- If prophylaxis is required, intermittent prophylaxis is preferred provided it is effective. Oral or rectal diazepam, given only when fever is present is safe and reduces the risk of recurrent febrile seizures. If daily prophylaxis is used, valproic acid is the best option.

NEONATAL SEIZURES

- Phenobarbital is the most frequently used AED, but phenytoin, diazepam, paraldehyde, and primidone are also used.
- Duration of therapy is controversial, but phenobarbital is often continued for at least 1 year. Long-term treatment is often unnecessary for neonatal seizures caused by hypoglycemia, hypocalcemia, local anesthetic injections, drug withdrawal, pyridoxine deficiency, and electrolyte imbalance, but may be necessary if seizures are caused by cortical dysgenesis. In the absence of high-risk factors, phenobarbital may be discontinued after initial seizure control.

ALCOHOL WITHDRAWAL SEIZURES

- Alcohol withdrawal seizures usually occur within the first 24 hours of cessation of drinking. They are generally tonic-clonic and are frequently accompanied by signs of tremulousness, anorexia, GI disturbances, insomnia, and hallucinations.

- Liberal use of benzodiazepines in alcoholics to prevent delirium tremens may decrease the incidence of alcohol withdrawal seizures.

CEREBROVASCULAR DISEASE, CRANIOTOMY, AND STROKE

- Seizures after strokes generally occur within the first 48 hours, and tend to be single, partial, and easily controlled.
- Recent recommendations are that AED therapy be reviewed at 2–4 weeks after seizures due to stroke, and that AEDs be tapered in the absence of an underlying cortical hemorrhage, epileptiform activity on the EEG, or recurrent seizures.

SPECIAL POPULATIONS

- Neonates may metabolize drugs more slowly but eliminate unchanged drug more rapidly.
- Infants and children may metabolize drug rapidly.
- Lower doses of AEDs are required as patients age. Because of pharmacokinetic and potential pharmacodynamic changes in the elderly, seizure control rather than blood levels is the most important clinical outcome.
- Liver disease may decrease AED metabolism. If albumin levels decrease, protein binding of highly bound AEDs will decrease.
- In chronic renal failure, there may be decreased elimination of unchanged drug as well as altered protein binding.

IX

▶ ASSESSMENT OF THERAPEUTICS OUTCOMES

- Monitoring should be done in view of the therapeutic plasma concentration range of the AEDs and other monitoring parameters, including seizure control, social adjustment, drug interactions, compliance, dosage adjustments, side effects, and quality of life.
- Patients should maintain a seizure diary that documents frequency and severity.
- Patients taking felbamate should have weekly liver function tests, and a CBC should be obtained at least every other week.
- Patients taking carbamazepine should have a periodic determination of serum sodium. Autoinduction of metabolizing enzymes must be considered in adjusting the dose.

See Chapter 55, Epilepsy, authored by William R. Garnett, PharmD, for a more deatailed discussion of this topic.

Chapter 52

▶ HEADACHE: MIGRAINE AND CLUSTER

▶ MIGRAINE HEADACHES

PATHOPHYSIOLOGY

- The vascular theory is that headaches are a result of stimulation of sensory nerves in the large cerebral arteries and meningeal circulation.
- The neuronal theory focuses on the interplay between the trigeminal (fifth cranial) nerve and a variety of inflammatory neurotransmitters, resulting in plasma protein extravasation that stimulates nerve endings which results in pain. Both theories are probably applicable.
- Several factors appear to induce arterial vasoconstriction including emotions, stress, excessive afferent stimulation (lights, noise, smells), changes in the internal clock, and vasodilator therapy. This may result in ischemia sufficient to cause neurologic dysfunction including the aura. This may be followed by cerebral vasodilation and neurogenic inflammation which causes pain. The initial vasospasm may occur due to increased release and/or production of prostaglandins, epinephrine, norepinephrine, tyramine, and serotonin (5-HT).
- Platelet 5-HT concentrations decrease dramatically at the onset of a migraine, while free 5-HT concentrations in plasma may increase by as much as 100% during an attack.
- The primary 5-HT receptors in the cerebral circulation are the 5-HT$_1$ subtypes.
- The primary 5-HT receptors in the cerebral circulation are 5-HT$_{1A}$, 5-HT$_{1C}$, 5-HT$_{1D}$, and 5-HT$_{1-Like}$. The 5-HT$_{1-Like}$ receptors may mediate vasoconstriction.
- Numerous factors have been suggested to be etiologic in migraine (Table 52.1). Monosodium glutamate (MSG), a flavor enhancer, has been linked with migraines. Genetic disturbances in tyramine metabolism may also be a cause. Proposed mechanisms for drug-induced headaches include inhibition of granular reuptake and storage of 5-HT (reserpine), blocking neuronal reuptake of 5-HT (fluoxetine), altering platelet aggregation (ethinyl estradiol and mestranol), and vasodilation (nitroglycerin and nifedipine).

CLINICAL PRESENTATION

- Migraine without aura, common migraine, occurs in 85% of patients with migraines. Migraine with aura, classic migraine, occurs in approximately 10% of migraineurs. The remaining 5% are other migraine types (e.g., ophthalmologic migraine, retinal migraine, childhood periodic syndromes, complications of migraine).
- The aura or prodrome begins 15–60 minutes prior to the onset of the headache. The aura may include aphasia, visual field defects, scotomas,

TABLE 52.1. Proposed Etiologic Factors Associated with Migraine

Psychological Factors
Stress
Depression
Personality

Environmental Factors
Tobacco smoke
Sensory stimulation (e.g., light glare, odors, etc.)
Weather changes

Dietary Factors
Alcohol
Tyramine-containing foods (e.g., red wine, aged cheese)
Citrus fruit
Aspartame
Food additives
Chocolate
Caffeine

Physiologic Factors
Autonomic nervous system dysfunction
Atherosclerosis
Epilepsy
Autosomal tract defect
Immunologic response
Hypersensitivity reaction
Allergy

Medications
Cimetidine
Cocaine
Ethinyl estradiol
Fenfluramine
Fluoxetine
Histamine
Hormone replacement therapy
Indomethacin
Mestranol
Nicotine
Nifedipine
Nitroglycerin
Oral contraceptives
Reserpine

Others
Hormonal changes
Menses
Pregnancy
Hypoglycemia
Excessive or inadequate sleep
Strenuous exercise
Alterations in intracellular magnesium and calcium concentrations

hemisensory disturbances (tingling or numbness in the extremities), and alterations in mood or motor functions.

- Migraines usually occur in the early morning hours, and reach peak intensity usually within 1 hour of onset. Pain is usually unilateral (may be bilateral) and is most often in the temple. The pain may be described as pounding. Physical activity may worsen the pain, and patients may seek a dark, quiet place. There may be a sensitivity to light or sound, anorexia, nausea, vomiting, constipation or diarrhea, and changes in mood or personality. Headache duration may range from 4–72 hours.

DIAGNOSIS

- It is critical to characterize the headache with regard to time of day, presence or absence of aura, description of aura, intensity and duration of the attack, description and location of the pain, precipitating factors, factors that provide relief, and associated symptoms.
- The physical examination (including neurologic), common laboratory tests (including an erythrocyte sedimentation rate), and diagnostic pro-

cedures (computed tomography [CT scan], magnetic resonance imaging [MRI]) should be within normal limits to rule out any organic causes. Evaluation of the headache patient should also include a lumbar puncture if an infection is suspected.

TREATMENT

Abortive Therapy

- Abortive therapies must begin at the onset of the attack to achieve their full potential. Only 50–80% of patients taking abortive therapies will receive significant relief.
- Table 52.2 shows medications used for abortive therapy.

Simple Analgesics

- Initial therapy for patients with infrequent migraines should be with simple analgesics. Aspirin is considered the drug of choice, but acetaminophen can be used when aspirin is contraindicated or is not well tolerated.

Nonsteroidal Anti-inflammatory Drugs (NSAIDs)

- NSAIDs may work through inhibition of prostaglandin synthesis, inhibition of platelet aggregation, and reduction of serotonin release. They may be particularly useful to treat migraines that occur before, during, or after menstruation. They have not been associated with rebound headaches.
- Naproxen was superior to placebo and more efficacious than ergotamine in controlling acute migraine attacks. NSAIDs with rapid onset of action are preferred (e.g., naproxen, naproxen sodium, ibuprofen). Indomethacin should not be used, as it may cause headaches. Injectable ketorolac has been used in patients with drug-seeking behavior and in those with severe nausea and vomiting.

Ergotamine

- Ergotamine is a vasoconstrictor of smooth muscle in cranial blood vessels, an α-adrenergic blocker, and a nonselective 5-HT agonist.
- Ergotamine is available as an oral and sublingual tablet, suppository, dihydroergotamine injectable (DHE-45), and by inhalation. Intravenous administration is the fastest way to achieve therapeutic drug concentrations and may be preferred by some patients or in more severe attacks.
- Exceeding the maximum dosage guidelines should be avoided to prevent rebound headaches. Ergotamine addiction and dependency have been reported.
- Side effects include elevation in blood pressure, peripheral ischemia, ergotism (nausea, diarrhea, thirst, pruritis, vertigo, muscle cramps, paresthesias, and cold skin), and gastrointestinal vascular ischemia.
- Contraindications include coronary artery disease, peripheral vascular disease, hypertension, liver or kidney disease, pregnancy, and migraines with prolonged auras.

TABLE 52.2. Abortive Migraine Therapies

Medication	Dosage
Simple Analgesics	
Acetaminophen	650 mg at onset; repeat q4h as needed
Aspirin	650 mg at onset; repeat q4h as needed
Aspirin/acetaminophen with butalbital	1–2 tablets every 4–6 h, but not more than 4 tablets/day or usage more than twice per week
Aspirin/acetaminophen with narcotics	Sparingly and infrequently
NSAIDs[a]	
Diclofenac	50–100 mg at onset
Ibuprofen	400–600 mg at onset; repeat in 1–2 h
Flurbiprofen	50–100 mg at onset; repeat in 1–2 h
Ketorolac	15–60 mg IM at onset
Mefanamic acid	500 mg at onset
Meclofenamate sodium	100 mg at onset; repeat in 1 h up to 500 mg/d
Naproxen	750 mg at onset; 250 mg PRN up to 1375 mg/d
Naproxen sodium	550–750 mg at onset; repeat in 1–2 h
Ergotamine Preparations	
Ergotamine 1 mg with 100 mg caffeine	2 tablets at onset; then 1 tablet every 30 min PRN to a maximum of 6 tablets/day or 10 tablets/week
Ergotamine 2 mg SL tablets	1 tablet every 30 min as needed to a maximum of 6 tablets/day or 10 tablets/week; do not swallow, chew, or crush tablets
Ergotamine 2 mg with 100 mg caffeine suppositories	Insert 1 at onset; repeat in 1 h as needed to a maximum of 2/day or 5/week
Ergotamine MDI (0.36 mg/puff)	1 puff every 5 min as needed to a maximum of 6 puffs/day or 12–15/week
Dihydroergotamine 1 mg/mL injection	0.5–1 mg IV or IM every hour as needed to a maximum of 2 mg/day, 6 mg/week IV or 3 mg/week IM
Sumatriptan	
Sumatriptan 6 mg SQ autoinjector	6 mg SQ at onset; the maximum recommended dose in 24 hours is 2 6-mg injections separated by at least 1 hour
Sumatriptan 25 mg tablets	1 tablet at onset; the maximal single dose recommended is 100 mg. A second dose of up to 100 mg may be given after 2 hours. The maximal daily dose is 300 mg.
Miscellaneous Agents	
Butorphanol nasal spray	1 spray in 1 nostril only; repeat 1 time in 60–90 min if needed
Chlorpromazine	0.1–1 mg/kg IV at onset
Isometheptene/dichloralphenazone/acetaminophen (Midrin)	2 capsules at onset; repeat one capsule every hour to a maximum of 5/day or 12/week
Metoclopramide	10 mg IV or PO at onset
Prochlorperazine	10 mg IV at onset

[a]Usage should be limited to three times weekly.

Sumatriptan

- Sumatriptan is an agonist at the $5\text{-}HT_{1D}$ receptor (vasoconstriction) and the $5\text{-}HT_{1A}$ receptor. It also inhibits the release of tachykinins and subsequently blocks neurogenic plasma protein extravasation and inflammation.
- It is more effective than ergotamine plus caffeine and also than aspirin plus metoclopramide.
- Adverse effects associated with oral use include bad taste, nausea, vomiting, malaise, dizziness, and vertigo. Injectable sumatriptan has been associated with injection site reactions, chest tightness, and pressure.
- It is contraindicated in patients with a history of ischemic heart disease, previous myocardial infarction, uncontrolled hypertension, within 2 weeks of therapy with monoamine oxidase inhibitors, and use of ergotamine derivatives within the previous 24 hours.

Midrin

- It is a combination of a vasoconstrictor, a mild sedative, and an analgesic.
- It can be used in patients who cannot take or do not respond to ergotamine or sumatriptan.
- Side effects include dizziness, insomnia, nausea, vomiting, and transient numbness.

Metoclopramide

- It may be useful in preventing or treating nausea and vomiting associated with other abortive therapies, and may be helpful as a single agent for pain relief. It may also increase absorption of other abortive therapies.
- It should be given 15–30 minutes before the antimigraine therapy and can be repeated in 4–6 hours.

Narcotics

- Parenteral narcotics can be used for pain relief and may allow the patient to sleep through the attack. Use of narcotics should be minimized to prevent abuse. Transnasal butorphanol is an alternative to injectable narcotics.

Prophylactic Therapy

- Prophylactic therapy is used when a headache of at least moderate severity occurs more than twice monthly, when migraines are less frequent but prolonged or refractory to acute therapy, or when they are predictable in occurrence. A trial of 2–3 months is necessary before an agent can be judged ineffective. Table 52.3 summarizes medications used for prophylactic therapy.

Beta Blockers

- Those with intrinsic sympathomimetic activity are ineffective.
- Nonselective beta blockers are relatively contraindicated in patients with asthma, congestive heart failure, and diabetes.

IX

TABLE 52.3. Prophylactic Migraine Therapies

Medications	Dosage
NSAIDs/Aspirin	
Aspirin	650 mg BID
Ibuprofen	300–600 mg TID
Meclofenamate	50 mg TID
Ketoprofen	50–75 mg BID or TID
Naproxen	250–750 mg daily, or 250 mg TID
Naproxen sodium	250–750 mg daily, or 250 mg TID
Beta Blockers	
Atenolol	50–150 mg/d in divided doses
Metoprolol	50–300 mg/d in divided doses[a]
Nadolol	20–240 mg/d in divided doses
Propranolol	40–320 mg/d in divided doses[a]
Timolol	20–60 mg/d in divided doses
Calcium Channel Blockers	
Diltiazem	90–180 mg/d in divided doses[a]
Nifedipine	30–120 mg/d in divided doses[a]
Nimodipine	40 mg TID
Verapamil	120–360 mg/d in divided doses[a]
Antidepressants	
Amitriptyline	10–200 mg at bedtime
Doxepin	10–200 mg at bedtime
Fluoxetine	10–20 mg daily
Imipramine	10–200 mg at bedtime
Nortriptyline	10–150 mg at bedtime
Phenelzine	15 mg BID to QID
Miscellaneous Agents	
Clonidine	0.1 mg BID or TID
Cyproheptadine	4–8 mg daily
Ergonovine	0.2 mg BID to TID
Methysergide	4–8 mg daily
Valproic acid	250–1500 mg/d[a]

[a]Extended release preparations may be given in single daily doses.

Antidepressants
- Tertiary amine tricyclic antidepressants (e.g., amitriptyline, imipramine) are more effective than secondary amines (e.g., nortriptyline, desipramine).
- Fluoxetine is also safe and effective, but it may also trigger migraines in some patients.
- If phenelzine is used, patients must be counseled regarding dietary and drug restrictions.

Calcium Channel blockers
- Calcium channel blockers inhibit the initial vasoconstrictive phase.

NSAIDs
- Patients may benefit from daily administration or intermittent use (with predictable headaches) of aspirin or naproxen sodium.
- Long-term use should be discouraged because of gastrointestinal and renal toxicity. Monitoring of renal function and occult blood loss should be provided.

Cyproheptadine
- Cyproheptadine is an antihistamine with 5-HT$_2$ receptor antagonist activity and antiplatelet effects. Clinical response is unpredictable.

Anticonvulsants
- Phenytoin, carbamazepine, and valproic acid may be efficacious in certain migraine types, especially if there is an association with epilepsy. Rebound headaches may occur.

Calcitonin
- Salmon calcitonin and a synthetic eel-calcitonin analogue have been efficacious. Side effects include flushing and gastrointestinal disturbances.

Methysergide
- Methysergide is a potent 5-HT$_2$ receptor antagonist. It is not a first-line agent because continuous use for >7 months can cause proliferation of fibrous tissue in the retroperitoneal, pleural, pericardial, and subendocardial spaces.
- A drug holiday of 2 weeks every 3 months or 1 month every 6 months is recommended. Monitoring for flank pain, dysuria, and chest discomfort is recommended. Early recognition and discontinuation of therapy will reverse fibrotic changes. It should be tapered slowly to prevent rebound headaches.
- It is reserved for patients refractory to other therapeutic modalities.

▶ CLUSTER HEADACHES

PATHOPHYSIOLOGY

- Decreased blood flow in supraorbital and frontal arteries occurs before the headache, and vasodilation occurs during the headache phase. Extracranial vasodilation has also been observed and may distend against pain-sensitive structures.
- Stimulation of the trigeminal nerve results in release of substance P, CGRP, and other vasoactive polypeptides, resulting in vasodilation, pain, and neurogenic inflammation. Extravasation of plasma proteins may also occur.

- Triggers for cluster headaches include vasodilators and hypoxemia. High-altitude hypoxia may also induce cluster headaches.

CLINICAL PRESENTATION

- Pain is almost always unilateral and localized behind or around the eye or in the temples. Pain is described as excruciating and penetrating but not throbbing.
- Patients may appear agitated.
- Most symptoms are ipsilateral (e.g., lacrimation, nasal stuffiness, rhinorrhea, ptosis, miosis, and conjunctival injection). Scalp and facial tenderness or flushing occurs on the same side as the headache.

TREATMENT

Abortive Therapy

Ergotamine
- Ergot preparations are effective, and dosing is the same as for migraine headache.
- Oral preparations are often inadequate, but may be effective if taken an hour before the anticipated time of the attack.
- Long-term continuous therapy is not recommended.

Oxygen
- Inhalation of 100% oxygen (a cerebral vasoconstrictor) at a rate of 6–8 L/min for no longer than 15 minutes is a safe and effective alternative to ergotamine.

IX

Sumatriptan
- A reduction in the severity of headache can occur within 15 minutes of a subcutaneous injection.

Prophylactic Therapy

Lithium
- Lithium carbonate is effective in treating episodic and chronic cluster headaches. Dosage is initiated at 300–600 mg/d and increased to 600–1200 mg/d as necessary in two to four divided doses. A plasma lithium level of 0.6 to 1.2 mEq/L measured at steady state, 12 hours after the last dose, is usually sought, but optimal plasma levels for prevention of cluster headache have not been established.
- Lithium should be administered with caution to patients with renal or cardiovascular disease, dehydration, pregnancy, or concomitant diuretic use.

Ergotamine
- Ergotamine 1–2 mg in one to two daily doses has been beneficial, and ergotism is unlikely.

Methysergide
- In patients unresponsive to lithium, methysergide, 2 mg three or four times daily, is usually effective in shortening the course of headaches. Doses may be tapered after 2–3 weeks of freedom from headaches.

Corticosteroids
- Corticosteroids are effective for cluster headaches not responsive to either lithium or methysergide. High doses of injectable or oral steroids alleviate pain within 8–12 hours, with maximum effectiveness in 2–3 days. Prednisone is often given in an initial daily dose of 40–60 mg orally, administered in divided doses, and rapidly tapered over a 2-week to 1-month period. Long-term use is not recommended.

▶ EVALUATION OF THERAPEUTIC OUTCOMES

- All headache patients should be monitored for frequency, intensity, and duration of headaches, and for any change in the headache pattern.
- Therapy must be monitored to evaluate and document response and to assess for side effects. Compliance with the medication regimen must be ensured, and all drug use (prescription and over-the-counter) must be monitored. Patient counseling is essential for safe and effective drug use.

See Chapter 60, Headache Disorders, authored by Brian E Beckett, PharmD, for a more detailed discussion of this topic.

IX ◀

Chapter 53

▶ PAIN MANAGEMENT

▶ DEFINITION

Pain is defined as an unpleasant, subjective sensory and emotional experience associated with actual or potential tissue damage or described in terms of such damage.

▶ PATHOPHYSIOLOGY

AFFERENT PAIN TRANSMISSION

- H^+, K^+, prostaglandins, leukotrienes, histamine, and serotonin sensitize nociceptors. Receptor activation leads to action potentials that are transmitted along afferent nerve fibers to the spinal cord.
- Somatostatin, cholecystokinin, and substance P have been identified as possible neurotransmitters in afferent nociceptive neurons. Nociceptive transmission occurs in the A-delta (well-localized pain) or C fibers (dull, poorly localized, and persistent pain).
- *Gate Control Theory:* When large myelinated fibers are stimulated, they have an inhibitory effect on pain transmission. Therefore, perception of pain is a complex summation of non-nociceptive and nociceptive neuronal stimulation.
- Pain-initiated processes reach the brain through a complex array of ascending spinal cord pathways. The spinothalamic tract, a major ascending pathway, is divided into lateral and ventral pathways. The lateral pathway is associated with sharp localized pain, and the ventral pathway makes possible the perception of aching, dull, nonlocalized pain.

PAIN MODULATION

- Three classes of opioid peptides are known: the enkephalins, dynorphins, and β-endorphins. Each has a distinct anatomical distribution. All are generically referred to as endorphins.
- There are five opiate receptors e.g., mu (mu-1 and mu-2), delta, sigma, kappa, and epsilon (Table 53.1).
- When a given nociceptive stimulus activates both peripheral pain transmission pathways (causing pain and termed positive feedback), the brain's modulatory network (inhibiting pain and termed negative feedback) may make the sensation of pain a partial summation of these two processes.
- Other neurotransmitters that may play a role include acetylcholine, dopamine, norepinephrine, and serotonin.

EFFERENT PAIN TRANSMISSION

- This descending system for control of pain transmission influences synaptic transmission of sensory fibers at the dorsal horn.

TABLE 53.1. Opiate Receptors and Function

Opiate Receptor	Function
Mu-1	Analgesia
Mu-2	Respiratory depression
	Euphoria
	Physical dependence
	Constipation
Delta	Analgesia
Sigma	Autonomic stimulation
	Dysphoria
	Hallucinations
Kappa	Analgesia
	Sedation
	Miosis
Epsilon	Analgesia

▶ PAIN ASSESSMENT

- A comprehensive history and physical examination are imperative to thoroughly evaluate underlying diseases and possible contributing factors. A baseline description of pain can be obtained by assessing PQRST characteristics (e.g., *p*alliative and *p*rovocative factors, *q*uality, *r*adiation, *s*everity, and *t*emporal factors). Attention must also be given to mental (e.g., anxiety, depression, fatigue, anger, behavioral, cognitive, social, and cultural factors that may alter the pain threshold.
- Psychogenic pain is real, but has no known cause and is nonlocalized, ill defined, and not easily treated.

▶ DESIRED OUTCOME

The goal of therapy is to minimize pain and provide reasonable comfort for the patient at the lowest effective dose. Whenever possible, patients should participate in their own pain therapy. Close monitoring is essential to ensure effectiveness and minimize side effects. Scrupulous monitoring is also necessary to assure that the duration of therapy is no longer than that warranted by clinical needs.

▶ ACUTE PAIN

- Analgesics should be given an adequate trial and usually require individual dosage titration. In most cases, these drugs should be administered on a regular dosing schedule and not on an as-needed basis.
- Excessive sedation should be avoided.
- Placebo therapy should never be used to diagnose psychogenic pain.

- The route of administration should always be geared to the needs of the patient.

NON-NARCOTIC AGENTS

- Analgesics should be initiated with the weakest effective analgesic agent having the fewest side effects. Dosage, pharmacokinetic, pharmacodynamic, and side-effect profiles of Food and Drug Administration (FDA)-approved non-narcotic analgesics are shown in Tables 53.2, 53.3, and 53.4.
- These drugs (except acetaminophen) affect the prostaglandins produced by the arachidonic acid cascade in response to noxious stimuli, thereby decreasing the number of pain impulses.
- Caution is advised when aspirin and aspirin-like drugs are used concurrently with other peripherally acting nonsteroidal anti-inflammatory drugs (NSAIDs) because they may increase the potential for GI side effects.
- Aspirin and aspirin-like compounds should not be given to children or teenagers with influenza or chicken pox, as Reye's syndrome may result.

TABLE 53.2. Pharmacokinetic and Pharmacodynamic Profiles of FDA-Approved Non-Narcotic Analgesics

Agent	Time to Peak Concentration (h)	Elimination Half-Life (h)	Analgesic Onset (h)	Analgesic Duration (h)
Aspirin	0.25–2	0.25–0.33	0.5	3–6
Choline salicylate	1.5–2	—[a]	—[a]	4
Magnesium salicylate	1.5–2	—[a]	—[a]	4
Sodium salicylate	0.67	—[a]	—[a]	4
Diflunisal	2–3	8–12	1	8–12
Acetaminophen	0.5–2	1–4	0.5–1	3–6
Meclofenamate	0.5–2	2.3–3.3	—[a]	4–6
Mefenamic acid	2–4	2–4	—[a]	6
Etodoloc	1	7	0.5–1.0	6–8
Diclofenac potassium	0.5–1	2	0.5	6–8
Ibuprofen	1–2	1–2.5	0.5	4–6
Fenoprofen	1–2	2–3	0.25–0.5	4–6
Ketoprofen	0.5–2	2–4	1	3–4
Naproxen	2–4	12–15	1	Up to 7
Naproxen sodium	1–2	12–13	1	Up to 7
Ketorolac (parenteral)	0.5–1	4–6	0.17	6
Ketorolac (oral)	0.5–1	4–6	0.5–1	4–6

[a]Data not available.

TABLE 53.3. FDA-Approved Non-Narcotic Analgesics

Class and Generic Name	Usual Dosage Range (mg)	Maximal mg/d
Salicylates		
Acetylsalicylic acid[a] (aspirin)	325–650 every 4 h	5400
Choline[a]	870 every 3–4 h	5220
Magnesium[a]	500 every 4 h	4800
Sodium[a]	325–650 every 4 h	5400
Diflunisal	250–500 every 8–12 h	1500
***para*-Aminophenol**		
Acetaminophen[a]	325–650 every 4–6 h	4000
Fenamates		
Meclofenamate	50 every 4–6 h	400
Mefenamic acid	250 every 6 h	1000
Acetic Acid		
Etodolac	200–400 every 6–8 h	1200
Diclofenac potassium	50 three times a day	150[b]
Propionic Acids		
Ibuprofen[a]	200–400 every 4–6 h	3200
Fenoprofen	200 every 4–6 h	3200
Ketoprofen[a]	25–50 every 6–8 h	300
Naproxen	250 every 6–12 h	1250
Naproxen sodium[a]	220 every 8–12 h	660[c]
Ketorolac (parenteral)	15–30 every 6 h	120[d]
Ketorolac (oral)	10 every 4–6 h	40[d]

[a]Available both as an over-the-counter preparation and as a prescription drug.
[b]Up to 200 mg on the first day.
[c]Over the counter dose.
[d]Maximum of 5 days.

- The salicylate salts cause fewer GI side effects than aspirin and do not inhibit platelet aggregation.
- NSAIDs generally cause fewer GI problems than aspirin.
- When prostaglandin synthesis is inhibited by NSAIDs or by aspirin-like compounds in patients with poor renal function, severe renal damage may result. Patients with creatinine clearances <50 mL/min taking NSAIDs or aspirin-like compounds must be carefully monitored for further kidney damage.
- NSAIDs inhibit platelet aggregation, but only as long as plasma concentrations are sustained.
- Acetaminophen has analgesic and antipyretic activity but little anti-inflammatory action. It is highly liver toxic on overdose.

TABLE 53.4. Relative Side Effects of FDA-Approved Non-Narcotic Analgesics

Agent	GI Irritation	CNS Effects	Hepatic Toxicity	Renal Toxicity
Aspirin	++++++	+	++	++
Choline salicylate	+++	—[a]	—[a]	—[a]
Magnesium salicylate	+++	—[a]	—[a]	—[a]
Sodium salicylate	+++	—[a]	—[a]	—[a]
Diflunisal	++	++	+	+
Acetaminophen	+	+	++	+
Meclofenamate	+++	++	+	++
Mefenamic acid	++	+	+	++
Etodolac	++	++	+	++
Diclofenac potassium	++	++	+	++
Ibuprofen	++	++	+	++
Fenoprofen	++	+++	+	+++
Ketoprofen	+	+	+	++
Ketorolac[b]	++	++	+	+
Naproxen	++	++	+	++

[a]Data not available.
[b]Five-day use only.

IX

NARCOTIC AGENTS

- Usually narcotic analgesics (Tables 53.5, 53.6, 53.7, and 53.8) are considered to be the next step in the management of acute pain if non-narcotic analgesics are inadequate.
- Partial agonists and antagonists compete with agonists for opiate receptor sites and, depending on their ability to either stimulate or block these sites, exhibit mixed agonist-antagonist activity. Mixed agonist-antagonists with analgesic activity appear to exhibit selectivity for analgesic receptor sites (Table 53.1), and thus may cause analgesia with fewer side effects (Table 53.7).
- Peak analgesic effect usually occurs 1.5–2 hours after oral administration, and this must be considered when immediate relief is needed.
- The equianalgesic doses in Table 53.5 are only a guide, and doses must be individualized.
- Although caution is advised, cross sensitivity between the morphine-like agonists, meperidine-like agonists, and methadone-like agonists is

TABLE 53.5. Narcotic Analgesics

Class and Generic Name	Trade Name	Route	Equianalgesic Dose (mg)
Morphine-Like Agonists			
Morphine	Generic	IM, SQ	10
		PO	30–60
Hydromorphone	Dilaudid (generic)	IM, SQ	1.3
		PO	7.5
Oxymorphone	Numorphan	IM, SQ	1.0
		R	5
Levorphanol	Levo-Dromoran	IM, SQ	2.0
		PO	4.0
Codeine	Generic	IM	130[a]
		PO	200[a]
Hydrocodone	Generic	PO	30[a]
Oxycodone	Roxicodone (generic)	PO	30[a]
Meperidine-Like Agonists			
Meperidine	Demerol (generic)	IM, SQ	75
		PO	300[c]
Fentanyl	Sublimaze (generic)	IM	0.1–0.2
	Duragesic	Transdermal	25 μg/h[c]
Methadone-Like Agonists			
Methadone	Dolophine (generic)	IM	10
		PO	20
Propoxyphene	Darvon (generic)	PO	130[a]
Mixed Agonist–Antagonists			
Pentazocine	Talwin	IM, SQ	30–60
		PO	180[1]
Butorphanol	Stadol	IM	2.0
	Stadol NS	Intranasal	1.0[b] (one spray)
Nalbuphine	Nubain (generic)	IM	10
Buprenorphine	Buprenex	IM	0.3–0.4
Dezocine	Dalgan	IM	10
Antagonists			
Naloxone	Narcan (generic)	IV	0.4 1.2[d]
Central Analgesic (not considered a narcotic)			
Tramadol	Ultram	PO	50–100[b]

[a]Starting doses lower (codeine, 30 mg; oxycodone and hydrocodone, 5 mg; meperidine, 50 mg; propoxyphene, 65–130 mg; pentazocine, 50 mg).
[b]Starting dose only (equianalgesia not shown).
[c]Equivalent IM morphine dose = 8–22 mg day.
[d]Starting doses to be used in cases of opioid overdose.

IX ◄

TABLE 53.6. Dosing Guidelines

IX

Agent(s)	Doses (titrate up or down based on patient response)	Notes
NSAIDs/acetaminophen/aspirin	Dose to maximum before switching to another agent (see Table 53.3)	• Regular alcohol use and high doses of acetaminophen may result in liver dysfunction • Used in mild to moderate pain • May use in conjunction with narcotic agents to decrease doses of each • Care must be exercised to avoid overdose when combination products containing these agents are used
Morphine	PO 10–30 mg q 3–4 h[a] IM 5–10 mg q 3–4 h[a] IV 1–2.5 mg q 5 min PRN[a] SR 15–30 mg q 12 h (may need to be q 8 in some patients) Rectal 10–20 mg q 3–4 h[a]	• Drug of choice in severe pain • Use immediate-release product with SR product to control "breakthrough" pain
Hydromorphone	PO 2–4 mg q 3–4 h[a] IM 0.5–1 mg q 3–4 h[a] IV 0.1–0.5 mg q 5 min PRN[a] Rectal 2–4 mg q 3–4 h[a]	• Use in severe pain • More potent than morphine, otherwise no advantages
Oxymorphone	IM 1–1.5 mg q 3–4 h[a] IV 0.5 mg initially[a] Rectal 5 mg q 3–4 h[a]	• Use in severe pain • No advantages over morphine
Levorphanol	PO 2–4 mg q 6–8 h IM 2 mg q 6–8 h IV 2 mg q 6–8 h	• Use in severe pain • Extended half-life useful in cancer patients
Codeine	PO 15–60 mg q 3–4 h[a] IM 15–60 mg q 3–4 h[a] IV 15–60 mg q 3–4 h[a]	• Use in moderate pain • Weak analgesic, use with NSAIDs or aspirin or acetaminophen
Hydrocodone	PO 5–10 mg q 3–4 h[a]	• Use in moderate/severe pain • Most effective when used with NSAIDs or aspirin or acetaminophen
Oxycodone	PO 5–10 mg q 3–4 h[a]	• Use in moderate/severe pain • Most effective when used with NSAIDs or aspirin or acetaminophen

TABLE 53.6. continued

Drug	Dosing	Notes
Meperidine	PO 50–150 mg q 3–4 h[a] IM 75–100 mg q 3–4 h[a] IV 5–10 mg q 5 min PRN[a]	• Use in severe pain • Oral not recommended • Do not use in renal failure • May precipitate tremors, myoclonus, and seizures • Monoamine oxidase inhibitors can induce hyperpyrexia and/or seizures
Fentanyl	IM 0.05–0.1 mg q 1–2 h[a] Transdermal 25 μg/h	• Used preoperative, intraoperative, postoperative • Used in severe pain • Do not use transdermal in patient with acute pain
Methadone	PO 10–20 mg q 6–8 h IM 5–10 mg q 6–8 h	• Effective in severe chronic pain • Sedation can be major problem • Some patients with chronic pain can be dosed q 12 h
Propoxyphene	PO 65–100 mg q 3–4 h[a]	• Use in moderate pain • Weak analgesic, most effective when used with NSAIDs or aspirin or acetaminophen • Will cause carbamazepine levels to increase
Pentazocine	PO 50–100 mg q 3–4 h[b] IM 30 mg q 3–4 h[b]	• Third-line agent for moderate to severe pain • May precipitate withdrawal in opiate-dependent patients
Butorphanol	IM 1–4 mg q 3–4 h[a] IV 0.5–2 mg q 3–4 h[b] Intranasal 1 mg (1 spray) q 3–4 h[b]	• Second-line agent for moderate to severe pain • May precipitate withdrawal in opiate-dependent patients
Nalbuphine	IM 10 mg q 3–6 h[b] IV 10 mg q 3–6 h[b]	• Second-line agent for moderate to severe pain • May precipitate withdrawal in opiate-dependent patients
Buprenorphine	IM 0.3 mg q 6 h[b] IV 0.3 mg q 6 h[b]	• Second-line agent for moderate to severe pain • May precipitate withdrawal in opiate-dependent patients
Dezocine	IM 5–20 mg q 3–6 h[b] IV 2.5–10 mg q 2–4 h[b]	• Second-line agent for moderate to severe pain • May precipitate withdrawal in opiate-dependent patients
Naloxone	IV 0.4–1.2 mg	• When reversing opiate side effects in patients needing analgesia, dilute and titrate (0.1–0.2 mg q 2–3 minutes) so as not to reverse analgesia
Tramadol	PO 50–100 mg q 4–6 h[a]	• Maximum dose is 400 mg/24 h • Decrease dose in renal impairment and in the elderly

[a]May start with an around-the-clock regimen and switch to PRN if/when the pain/surgical signal subsides. [b]May reach a ceiling analgesic effect.

TABLE 53.7. Major Adverse Effects of the Narcotic Analgesics

Effect	Manifestation
Mood changes	Dysphoria, euphoria
Somnolence	Lethargy, drowsiness, apathy, inability to concentrate
Stimulation of chemoreceptor trigger zone	Nausea, vomiting
Respiratory depression	Decreased respiratory rate
Interference with hypothalamic function (mostly morphine)	Increase in ADH; decrease in CRF, GnRF, TSH, GH, LRF, and FSH; disordered temperature regulation
Decreased gastrointestinal motility	Constipation
Increase in sphincter tone (mostly morphine)	Biliary spasm, urinary retention
Histamine release (mostly morphine and meperidine)	Urticaria, pruritus, rarely exacerbation of asthma
Tolerance	Larger doses for same effect
Dependence	Withdrawal symptoms upon abrupt discontinuation

unlikely. With regard to cross sensitivity, the mixed agonist-antagonist class acts much like the morphine-like agonists.

IX
- In the initial stages of acute pain, analgesics should be given around the clock. As the painful state subsides, as-needed schedules can be used.
- Administration of narcotics directly into the central nervous system (CNS) (epidural and intrathecal) has shown considerable promise in controlling acute pain. Morphine given by the epidural route is dosed at 5–10 mg, the onset of pain relief is about 24 minutes, and the duration of relief is about 20 hours. One mg of hydromorphone by the same route results in pain relief in about 13 minutes and lasts for about 12 hours. Similarly, fentanyl given as a 0.1 mg epidural dose provides onset of pain relief in 4–10 minutes and lasts 2.5–6 hours.
- Patients receiving analgesics by the epidural and intrathecal route require careful monitoring, as side effects are common, and respiratory depression is a particular concern. Intrathecal doses are smaller than epidural doses, and opioids administered into the CNS should be preservative free.

Morphine and Congeners

- Many clinicians consider morphine the first-line agent for moderate to severe pain.
- These drugs may cause nausea and vomiting, especially in ambulatory patients. This may subside after the initial dose and may be

TABLE 53.8. Narcotic Analgesic Pharmacokinetics[a]

Agent	Time to Peak (h)	Half-Life (h)	Analgesic Onset (min)	Analgesic Duration (h)
Morphine	0.5–1	2–4	15–30, 60[b]	4–5
Hydromorphone	0.5–1	2–3	15–30	4–5
Oxymorphone	0.5–1	2–3	5–15	3–6
Levorphanol	0.5–1	12–16	30–90	6–8
Hydrocodone	1.3	4	—[c]	4–5
Codeine	0.5–1	2–4	15–30	4–6
Oxycodone (PO)	0.5–1	3–4	15–30	4–5
Meperidine	0.5–1	3–4	10–45	3–5
Fentanyl	—[c]	1.5–6	7–8	1–2
Methadone	0.5–1	15–40	30–60	4–5 (acute) >8 (chronic)
Propoxyphene (PO)	2.0–2.5	6–12	30–60	4–6
Pentazocine	0.25–1	4–5	15–20	3–6
Butorphanol	0.5–1	2.5–3.5	<10	4–6
Nalbuphine	1	2–3	<15	3–6
Buprenorphine	1	5	15	6
Dezocine	0.17–1.5	0.6–5	15–30	2–4
Naloxone[d]	0.5–2	0.5–1.5	2–5	0.5–1
Tramadol (PO)	2–3	6–7	<60	6

[a]Based on intramuscular data unless otherwise indicated.
[b]Data based intrathecal or epidural administration.
[c]Data not available.
[d]Narcotic antagonist.

counteracted by dopamine blocking drugs (e.g., phenothiazine deriva-tives).

- Respiratory depression is less likely in patients with severe pain, but more likely in patients with emphysema, kyphoscoliosis, and cor pulmonale. Morphine-induced respiratory depression can be reversed by pure narcotic antagonists.
- Hypovolemic patients and patients with myocardial infarction are more susceptible to morphine-induced decreases in blood pressure.
- Morphine is often considered the narcotic of choice when using opioids to treat pain associated with myocardial infarction, as it decreases myocardial oxygen demand.
- In patients with increased intracranial pressure and traumatic head injury, morphine can increase intracranial pressure, cause respiratory depression, and cloud the neurologic examination results.

IX

Meperidine and Congeners (Phenylpiperidines)

- With high doses or in patients with renal failure, the metabolite normeperidine may accumulate, causing CNS excitability (e.g., tremor, muscle twitching, seizures).
- The effects of meperidine on the cardiovascular system, GI tract, and smooth muscle are less severe than those of morphine.
- Meperidine should not be combined with monoamine oxidase inhibitors.
- In most clinical settings, meperidine offers no real advantage compared to morphine.
- Fentanyl at high doses can produce marked muscle rigidity.
- Due to its kinetic characteristics, fentanyl transdermal patch is not used for acute pain.

Methadone and Congeners

- With repeated doses, the analgesic duration of action of methadone is prolonged, but sedation may be a problem.
- It is usually used to treat chronic pain.

Mixed Narcotic Agonist-Antagonists

- This class is effective for moderate to severe pain and has a ceiling effect on respiratory depression (e.g., after a dose of 30 mg in adults, higher doses of nalbuphine do not affect respiratory rate).
- They have a low abuse potential, cause decreased constipation, and cause less biliary spasmodic effects than morphine.
- Disadvantages include psychotomimetic effects (especially with pentazocine and butorphanol), a ceiling analgesic effect, and a propensity to cause pain and initiate withdrawal in narcotic-dependent patients.
- Oral pentazocine has been melted down and used illicitly in combination with tripelennamine, but the addition of small amounts of naloxone has countered this illegitimate use by blocking the euphoric but not the analgesic effects.
- Both pentazocine and butorphanol must be used with caution in patients with myocardial ischemia.
- Nalbuphine causes a reduced myocardial oxygen demand in patients after myocardial infarction, compared to pentazocine and butorphanol. It causes little respiratory depression.
- Buprenorphine may have a longer duration of analgesic effect with less respiratory depression than previously mentioned mixed agonist-antagonists.
- Buprenorphine binds tightly to opioid receptors and large doses of narcotic antagonists may be needed to reverse its effects.
- Butorphanol, nalbuphine, and dezocine are not controlled substances.

Narcotic Antagonists

- The pure opioid antagonist naloxone binds competitively to opioid receptors, but does not produce an analgesic response.

IX

CENTRAL ANALGESIC

- Tramadol is the first centrally acting binary analgesic available in the United States. It is chemically unrelated to the opiates and NSAIDs and is indicated for moderate to moderately severe pain. It may have a role in treatment of chronic pain, but has few advantages over opiates for acute pain.
- It binds weakly to opiate receptors (predominantly to the mu-receptors) and inhibits norepinephrine and serotonin reuptake.
- It is associated with minimal dependency and tolerance, but may increase risk of seizures.

COMBINATION THERAPY

- The combination of narcotic and non-narcotic oral analgesics often results in analgesia superior to that produced by either agent alone and may allow for use of lower doses of each agent.
- Agents shown to potentiate the analgesic efficacy of parenteral narcotics include hydroxyzine and dextroamphetamine.

REGIONAL ANALGESIA

- Regional analgesia with properly administered local anesthetics can provide complete relief of pain (Table 53.9). These agents have also been applied directly onto surgical wounds and have substantially decreased postoperative narcotic requirements. They have also been used epidurally in acute and chronic pain.
- They cross the blood-brain barrier, causing CNS excitation and depression.
- Frequent administration and specialized follow-up procedures are required.

IX

TABLE 53.9. Local Anesthetics

Agent	Trade Name	Manufacturer	Onset (min)	Duration (h)
Esters				
Procaine	Novocain	SanofiWinthrop	2–5	0.25–1
	Generic	Various		
Chloroprocaine	Nesacaine	Astra	6–12	0.50
Tetracaine	Pontocaine	SanofiWinthrop	15	2–3
Amides				
Mepivacaine	Carbocaine	SanofiWinthrop	3–5	0.75–1.5
	Generic	Various		
Bupivacaine	Marcaine	SanofiWinthrop	5	2–4
	Generic	Various		
Lidocaine	Generic	Various	<2	0.5–1
Prilocaine	Citanest	Astra	<2	≥1
Etidocaine	Duranest	Astra	3–5	5–10

▶ CHRONIC PAIN

CANCER PAIN

- An algorithm for analgesic use in cancer patients is shown in Fig. 53.1.
- Non-narcotic agents are used as first-line agents, and NSAIDs are especially effective for bone pain. Strontium-89 provides partial to complete relief in 65% of patients.
- As needed schedules are to be employed in conjunction with around-the-clock regimens when patients experience breakthrough pain.
- The choice of narcotic agents remains controversial. Many clinicians prefer morphine. The fentanyl patch may provide a more convenient dosing alternative in patients on stable regimens. Meperidine is usually not recommended for long-term use because of its relatively short half-life and the CNS hyperirritability of normeperidine.

NONMALIGNANT CHRONIC PAIN

- Pharmacologic approaches to patient care do not differ from those previously described, but psychologic techniques may prove more successful.

▶ EVALUATION OF THERAPEUTIC OUTCOMES

- Hourly or daily monitoring of acute pain response and side effects may be necessary. Daily or weekly monitoring may be adequate in chronic pain patients.
- The best management of narcotic-induced constipation is prevention. Patients should be counseled on proper intake of fluids and fiber, and a laxative may be added if needed.
- If acute pain does not subside within the anticipated time frame (usually 1–2 weeks), further investigation of the cause is warranted.

See Chapter 59, Pain Management, authored by Terry J. Baumann, PharmD, for a more detailed discussion.

IX

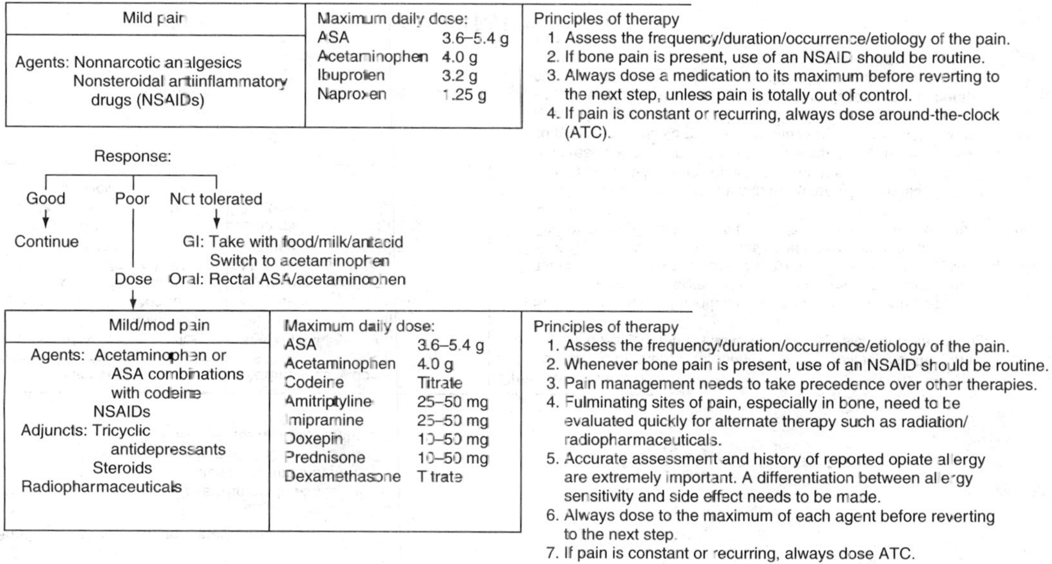

Mild pain

Agents: Nonnarcotic analgesics
Nonsteroidal antiinflammatory drugs (NSAIDs)

Maximum daily dose:
ASA 3.6–5.4 g
Acetaminophen 4.0 g
Ibuprofen 3.2 g
Naproxen 1.25 g

Principles of therapy
1. Assess the frequency/duration/occurrence/etiology of the pain.
2. If bone pain is present, use of an NSAID should be routine.
3. Always dose a medication to its maximum before reverting to the next step, unless pain is totally out of control.
4. If pain is constant or recurring, always dose around-the-clock (ATC).

Response:

Good → Continue

Poor → Not tolerated

GI: Take with food/milk/antacid
Switch to acetaminophen

Dose Oral: Rectal ASA/acetaminophen

Mild/mod pain

Agents: Acetaminophen or ASA combinations with codeine
NSAIDs
Adjuncts: Tricyclic antidepressants
Steroids
Radiopharmaceuticals

Maximum daily dose:
ASA 3.6–5.4 g
Acetaminophen 4.0 g
Codeine Titrate
Amitriptyline 25–50 mg
Imipramine 25–50 mg
Doxepin 10–50 mg
Prednisone 10–50 mg
Dexamethasone Titrate

Principles of therapy
1. Assess the frequency/duration/occurrence/etiology of the pain.
2. Whenever bone pain is present, use of an NSAID should be routine.
3. Pain management needs to take precedence over other therapies.
4. Eliminating sites of pain, especially in bone, need to be evaluated quickly for alternate therapy such as radiation/radiopharmaceuticals.
5. Accurate assessment and history of reported opiate allergy are extremely important. A differentiation between allergy sensitivity and side effect needs to be made.
6. Always dose to the maximum of each agent before reverting to the next step.
7. If pain is constant or recurring, always dose ATC.

Figure 53.1. Algorithm for pain management in oncology patients.

IX

Response:

Good → Continue

Poor → Dose

Not tolerated → GI: Take with food/antacid/milk
Switch to acetaminophen
Delete NSAID
Oral: Rectal ASA/acetaminophen

Mod/severe pain	Maximum daily dose:	
	ASA	3.6–5.4 g
Agents: ASA or acetamino-	Acetaminophen	4 g
phen combinations	Oxycodone	Titrate
with oxycodone	Morphine	Titrate
Oxycodone elixir	Hydromorphone	Titrate
Nonceiling narcotic	Methadone	Titrate
analgesics	NSAIDs	(See above)
NSAIDs	Steroids	(See above)
Adjuncts: Steroids (see note 7)	Tricyclics	(See above)
Tricyclics		

Principles of therapy
1. Assess the frequency/duration/occurrence/etiology of the pain.
2. Always dose ATC; may use narcotic analgesics for breakthrough pain.
3. Special situations of sudden onset/sudden resolution pain, especially along a nerve track, or neuralgias, may require an adjunct of an anticonvulsant (phenytoin, clonazepam, carbamazepine).
4. NSAIDs should be routine unless and until contraindicated.
5. Trial of appropriate adjuncts should be attempted before reverting to the next step.
6. Need to revert to next step when there are no intervals of adequate control or breakthrough occurs at maximum dose sooner than 3 h.
7. Pain resulting from inflammation of neural tissue in CNS (nerve-root compression or CNS metastasis) may require dexamethasone in high dose, 16 mg or more per 24 h.
8. Any time nonpharmacologic options of radiation, chemotherapy, surgical debulking, or neurological interventions are used, a total reevaluation of all drug treatment needs to be made.

Figure 53.1. continued

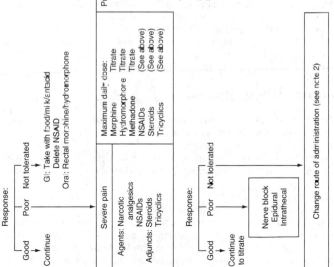

Response:

Good → Continue

Poor → Not tolerated

GI: Take with food/milk/antacid
Delete NSAID
Oral: Rectal morphine/hydromorphone

Severe pain	Maximum daily dose:	
Agents: Narcotic analgesics	Morphine	Titrate
NSAIDs	Hydromorphone	Titrate
Adjuncts: Steroids	Methadone	Titrate
Tricyclics	NSAIDs	(See above)
	Steroids	(See above)
	Tricyclics	(See above)

Response:

Good → Continue to titrate

Poor → Not tolerated

Nerve block
Epidural
Intrathecal

Change route of administration (see note 2)

Principles of therapy

1. Assess the frequency/duration/occurrence/etiology of the pain.
2. Morphine is the drug of choice in this category: (1) multiple products available; (2) multiple route of administration options, such as oral, rectal, IM, SC, IV, epidural, and intrathecal; and (3) a known equipotency between these routes that allows a much easier transition.
3. No real practical dosage limits with narcotics mentioned; can be titrated to patient response.
4. Management should be ATC dosing only, with sustained release product and as immediate release product as for breakthrough pain.
5. Utilize all possible adjuncts to minimize increases in dose.
6. Initial control may require doses higher than those needed in maintenance.
7. A fentanyl patch placed every 72 h may provide a more convenient dosing regimen when patients are on a stable oral dosing program.

IX

Figure 53.1. continued

665

Chapter 54

▶ PARKINSON'S DISEASE

▶ DEFINITION

Idiopathic Parkinson's Disease (IPD) was first described by James Parkinson in 1817. It is a disease with highly characteristic neuropathological findings and clinical presentation.

▶ PATHOPHYSIOLOGY

- Most motor deficits of IPD occur from the loss in dopaminergic nerve terminals projecting primarily to the putamen. The greatest attention for the treatment of IPD has focused on the loss of dopaminergic neurons projecting to the caudate and putamen.
- In IPD, activation of the D_2 receptor appears to be of primary importance for mediating both clinical improvements and adverse effects.
- Pathologic findings reveal a markedly decreased number of nigrostriatal dopamine neurons and a positive correlation between the degree of nigrostriatal dopamine loss and severity of disease. The threshold for onset of parkinsonism appears to be the loss of 80% of these neurons.
- Degeneration of nigrostriatal dopamine neurons results in a relative increase of striatal cholinergic interneuron activity, which contributes especially to the tremor of IPD.
- The pathogenesis of IPD is unknown, but neurotoxins highly selective to dopaminergic neurons have been considered. Cellular damage from oxyradicals is another possible mechanism.

▶ CLINICAL PRESENTATION

- IPD develops insidiously and progresses slowly. Initial complaints may include one or more sensory symptoms including aching pains, paresthesias, numbness, and coldness.
- As the disease progresses, one or more classical primary features may present (e.g., resting tremor, rigidity, bradykinesia, or change in posture).
- Bradykinesia manifested in the facial muscles results in hypomimia or a masked quality to facial expression with a staring gaze.
- Often tremor is the sole presenting feature of IPD, however, only two-thirds of IPD patients have tremor on diagnosis, and some never develop this sign. Tremor is often seen with IPD onset at a younger age, and is associated with less functional decline and decreased risk of dementia. Tremor is present most commonly in the hands, often begins unilaterally, and often has a "pill-rolling" quality. Usually, resting tremor is abolished by volitional movement, and it is absent during sleep.

- Muscular rigidity can be cog-wheel in nature. Dystonia can occur, especially in the feet.
- Other clinical characteristics of IPD are listed in Table 54.1.
- Postural instability is one of the most disabling problems in IPD, as it can lead to falls.
- Intellectual deterioration is not inevitable, but some patients deteriorate in a manner indistinguishable from Alzheimer's disease.

TABLE 54.1. Clinical Features

Primary
  Bradykinesia
  Postural instability
    Propulsion
    Retropulsion
  Resting tremor (may have postural and action components)
  Rigidity

Motor Symptoms
  Dysarthria
  Dysphagia
  Festinating gait
  Flexed posture
  "Freezing" at initiation of movement
  Hypomimia
  Hypophonia
  Micrographia
  Slow turning

Autonomic Symptoms
  Bladder and anal sphincter disturbances
  Constipation
  Diaphoresis
  Orthostatic blood pressure changes
  Paroxysmal flushing
  Sexual disturbances

Mental Status Changes
  Confusional state
  Dementia
  Psychosis (paranoia, hallucinosis)
  Sleep disturbance

Other
  Fatigue
  Oily skin
  Pedal edema
  Seborrhea
  Weight loss

IX

▶ DIAGNOSIS

- To diagnose IPD, bradykinesia should be present with at least two of the following features: limb muscle rigidity, resting tremor (at 4–6 Hz and abolished by movement), or postural instability (not caused by primary visual, vestibular, cerebellar, or proprioceptive dysfunction).
- Drug-induced parkinsonism must be ruled out (e.g., induced by antipsychotics, antiemetics, or metoclopramide). The condition most commonly mistaken for IPD is progressive supranuclear palsy.

▶ DESIRED OUTCOME

It is not possible to stop progression of the disease. The goal of treatment is to minimize disability and side effects, while ensuring the highest possible quality of life. Families and patients should be involved in treatment decisions to the greatest extent possible. Education of patients and caregivers is critical to ensure medication compliance and overall quality of care.

▶ TREATMENT

- The range of therapeutic interventions for IPD are summarized in Table 54.2.
- An algorithm for treatment of IPD is shown in Figure 54.1.
- The system developed by Hoehn and Yahr is used most frequently to stage disease severity (Table 54.3).
- Regular exercise can have a major impact on quality of life for patients with IPD. Referrals for speech, occupational, and physical therapies are sometimes quite helpful.
- In patients with mild symptoms, medications are often not needed. Some patients will never have more than mild slowness and resting tremor, and anticholinergics or amantadine may be adequate.
- The most effective drug therapies enhance dopaminergic activity (Table 54.2).
- L-dopa is the most effective medication currently available, but minimal use is widely advocated at present because of concern about possible long-term risks.
- Anticholinergics or amantadine can be used as an alternative to L-dopa for treating resting tremor. These drugs are helpful for relieving mild disabilities in the first few years after the onset of IPD. With advancing disability and ineffectiveness of these alternate medications, L-dopa therapy may be added.
- A summary of available antiparkinson medications is shown in Table 54.4.

SELEGILINE

- Selegiline, an inhibitor of monoamine oxidase B, also known as deprenyl, extends L-dopa effects. By blocking the breakdown of

TABLE 54.2. Mechanisms for Potential IPD Treatments

Increase Endogenous Dopamine
Increase tyrosine hydroxylase
  Tetrahydrobiopterin
L-dopa
  Inhibit peripheral metabolism by dopa decarboxylase
    Carbidopa
    Benserazide
  Sustained release products
  Infusions
    Intravenous
    Duodenal
  Inhibit peripheral and central metabolism by catechol-O-methyl transferase
    Entacapone (peripheral only)
    Tolcapone
  Inhibit central and peripheral metabolism by monoamine oxidase B
    Selegiline (deprenyl)

Dopamine Agonists
D_2 specific
  Bromocriptine
  Lisuride
D_1 and D_2 nonspecific
  Pergolide
  Apomorphine
    Intravenous
    Subcutaneous infusions
    Intranasal
    Sublingual
  Partial agonists
    Terguride

Anticholinergic
Benztropine
Trihexyphenidyl

Preventative
Selegiline (deprenyl)

Surgical Options
Autologous adrenal tissue transplantation
Fetal tissue transplantation
Thalamotomy
Pallidotomy
Thalamic electrical stimulation

IX

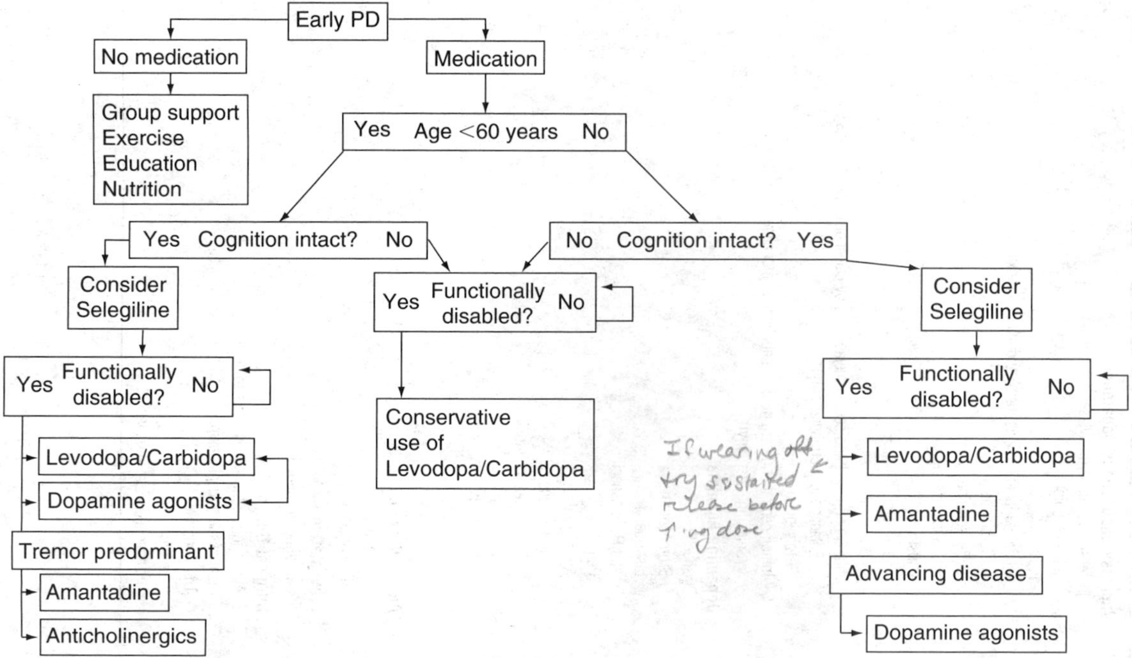

Figure 54.1. General algorithm for treating IPD.

TABLE 54.3. Hoehn and Yahr Staging of Severity of Parkinson's Disease

Stage 0:	No clinical signs evident
Stage I:	Unilateral involvement
Stage II:	Bilateral involvement but no postural abnormalities
Stage III:	Bilateral involvement with mild postural imbalance on examination or history of poor balance or falls; patient leads independent life
Stage IV:	Bilateral involvement with postural instability; patient requires substantial help
Stage V:	Severe, fully developed disease; patient restricted to bed or wheelchair

dopamine, it can extend the duration of action of L-dopa and permit reduction of L-dopa dose (by as much as one-half).

- Selegiline also increases the peak plasma concentrations of L-dopa, and so can enhance adverse reactions (e.g., worsening of preexisting dyskinesias or psychiatric symptoms such as delusions and hallucinations).
- Adverse effects of selegiline are minimal and include insomnia and jitteriness. Metabolites of selegiline are L-methamphetamine and L-amphetamine.
- When combined with fluoxetine or meperidine, selegiline may cause a reaction characterized by hypertension, diaphoresis, and shivering.
- Selegiline may have a neuroprotective effect by diverting dopamine catabolism away from generation of peroxide.

ANTICHOLINERGIC MEDICATIONS

IX

- The anticholinergic drugs can be effective for tremor and dystonia. Rarely is bradykinesia or other disabilities much improved. Tremor does not respond in all patients
- Patients with preexisting cognitive deficits and advanced age are at greater risk for central anticholinergic effects (e.g., confusion, impaired memory, sedation).
- These drugs can be used as monotherapy, or in conjunction with other antiparkinson drugs.

AMANTADINE

- Amantadine is often effective for relief of mild symptoms of IPD, especially tremor.
- A proposed mechanism of action is increased presynaptic dopamine synthesis, increased dopamine release, and inhibition of dopamine reuptake. Nondopaminergic mechanisms have also been proposed.
- Adverse effects may include sedation, vivid dreams, dry mouth, depression, hallucinations, anxiety, dizziness, psychosis, and confusion. A frequent and reversible side effect is livedo reticularis, a diffuse mottling of the skin.
- A reduced dose should be given to patients with renal dysfunction.

IX

TABLE 54.4. Drugs Used in Parkinson's Disease

Generic Name	Trade Name	Manufacturer	Dosage Range (mg/d)	Dosage Forms (mg)	Cost Index[a]
Amantadine	Symmetrel	DuPont	200–300	100, 50/5mL	8, 8
		Various generic brands			3, 7
Carbidopa/l-dopa	Sinemet	DuPont	[b]	10/100, 25/100, 25/250	6, 7, 8
	Atamet	Athena			
Controlled-release carbidopa/l-dopa	Sinemet CR	DuPont	[b]	25/100, 50/200	7, 14
L-dopa	Larodopa	Roche	[b]	100, 250, 500	2, 3, 6
	Dopar	Roberts Pharm			
Selegiline	Eldepryl	Somerset	10	5	21
Agonists					
Bromocriptine	Parlodel	Sandoz	[b]	2.5, 5	14, 22
Pergolide	Permax	Athena	[b]	0.05, 0.25, 1	2, 25, 82
Anticholinergic Drugs					
Benztropine	Cogentin	Merck and Co.	0.5–6	0.5, 1, 2	2, 2, 2
		Various generic brands			1, 1, 1
Biperiden	Akineton	Knoll	2–16	2	2
Diphenhydramine	Benadryl	Parke-Davis	25–100	25, 50	2, 3
		Various generic brands			1, 1
Procyclidine	Kemadrin	Burroughs-Wellcome	2.5–20	5	4
Trihexyphenidyl	Artane	Lederle	1–15	2.5, 2/5mL, 5 LA	1, 3, 3, 4
		Various generic brands			1, 3

[a]Cost index calculated from June 1994 Average Wholesale Price per 100. Approximate cost per 100 (or per pint for solutions) equivalent to index × $10.00.
[b]Dosage must be individualized.

L-DOPA AND CARBIDOPA/L-DOPA

- L-dopa, the most effective drug available for management of IPD, is the immediate precursor of dopamine, but unlike dopamine, it crosses the blood-brain barrier.

- L-dopa is converted to dopamine by L-amino acid decarboxylase (L-AAD). In the periphery, L-AAD can be blocked by currently administering carbidopa, which does not cross the blood-brain barrier. Carbidopa, therefore, increases the CNS penetration of exogenously administered L-dopa and decreases adverse effects (nausea, cardiac arrhythmias, postural hypotension) from peripheral L-dopa metabolism to dopamine.

- Starting L-dopa at 200–300 mg/d in combination with carbidopa often achieves adequate relief of disability. The usual maximal dose of L-dopa needed by patients even with severe parkinsonism is 800 mg/d.

- Carbidopa has a maximum effective daily dose of 100–125 mg. Carbidopa/L-dopa is most widely used in a 25 mg/100 mg tablet, but 25 mg/250 mg and 10 mg/100 mg dosage forms are also available. Controlled-release preparations of carbidopa/L-dopa are available in 50 mg/200 mg and 25 mg/100 mg strengths.

- After 3 or more years of treatment, one-third or more of L-dopa–treated patients develop involuntary movements or short-duration responses to the drug. Movement complications associated with long-term treatment with carbidopa/L-dopa treatment and their suggested treatments are listed in Table 54.5.

- End-of-dose deterioration ("wearing-off") has been related to increasing loss of neuronal storage capability for dopamine as presynaptic neurons are lost. This makes dopamine availability more dependent on dosing and pharmacokinetics of L-dopa. Instead of giving carbidopa/L-dopa more frequently, the sustained-release product can be tried. Dopamine agonists also can be added to a carbidopa/L-dopa regimen.

- "Off" periods or delayed response to carbidopa/L-dopa can be due to delayed stomach emptying or decreased absorption in the upper gastrointestinal (GI) tract. Chewing or crushing tablets and taking with a full glass of water or taking antacids may help. High protein meals may also interfere with absorption.

- Drug holiday is not currently used as a therapeutic intervention.

- Dyskinesias and dystonias are usually associated with peak anti Parkinsonian benefit.

- Dystonias are especially common in the distal lower extremities. Clenching of the toes or turning of the foot can precede the development of IPD.

- Since L-dopa and dopaminergic agonists also facilitate dopamine pathways in the mesolimbic dopaminergic projections, side effects such as delirium, agitation, paranoia, delusions, and hallucinations may occur. These reactions are more likely in older patients and those with underlying confusion or dementia. Clozapine improves psychotic symptoms without worsening Parkinsonian symptoms.

TABLE 54.5. Motor Fluctuations and Possible Interventions in IPD

Effect	Possible Treatments
End of dose deterioration ("wearing off")	Increase frequency of doses, controlled-release carbidopa/L-dopa, consider agonists, selegiline, or amantadine, duodenal or intravenous L-dopa infusions, carbidopa/L-dopa oral solution, subcutaneous apomorphine infusions, transdermal dopamine agonists
Delayed onset of response	Give on empty stomach before meals, crush or chew and take with a full glass of water, reduce dietary protein intake, antacids, morning standard-release carbidopa/L-dopa if on sustained-release carbidopa/L-dopa, infusions of L-dopa or dopamine agonists
Drug resistant "off" periods	Increase carbidopa/L-dopa dose and/or frequency, give on empty stomach before meals, crush or chew and take with a full glass of water, infusions of L-dopa or dopamine agonists, apomorphine intranasal spray
"Random" oscillations ("on-off")	Dopamine agonists, selegiline, infusions of L-dopa or dopamine agonists, consider drug holiday
Start hesitation ("freezing")	Increase carbidopa/L-dopa dose, dopamine agonists, gait modifications (tapping, rhythmic commands, stepping over objects, rocking)
Peak dose dyskinesia ("I-D-I" response[a])	Smaller more frequent doses of carbidopa/L-dopa, controlled-release carbidopa/L-dopa
Diphasic dyskinesias ("D-I-D" response[b])	Reduce anticholinergic medication
Dystonia	Baclofen, nighttime carbidopa/L-dopa, morning standard-release carbidopa/L-dopa if on sustained-release carbidopa/L-dopa, dopamine agonists, anticholinergics
Myoclonus	Decrease nighttime L-dopa doses, clonazepam
Akathisia	Benzodiazepines, propranolol

[a]I-D-I is the "improvement-dyskinesia/dystonia-improvement" pattern of response.
[b]D-I-D is the "dyskinesia-improvement-dyskinesia" pattern of response.

- Although still controversial, there is general consensus that the proper time to initiate L-dopa therapy is when the disease interferes with occupation or activities of daily living.
- There is marked intrasubject and intersubject variability in the time to peak plasma concentrations after oral L-dopa. There may be more than one peak plasma concentration after a single dose. Meals delay gastric emptying, while antacids and cisapride increase gastric emptying. L-dopa is primarily absorbed in the proximal duodenum by a saturable, large neutral amino acid (LNAA) transport system. Competition for this

site by dietary or supplemental LNAAs can reduce L-dopa plasma concentrations. LNAAs also compete with L-dopa for transport into the brain. L-dopa is not bound to plasma proteins. The elimination half-life of L-dopa is about 1 hour, and this is extended to about 1.5 hours with the addition of carbidopa.

- L-dopa should be administered cautiously with nonselective monoamine oxidase inhibitors (possible hypertensive crisis), antihypertensive agents (possible additive hypotensive effect), phenytoin (possible reversal of anti-Parkinson effect), and antipsychotic agents (possible antagonism of L-dopa effect).

DOPAMINE AGONISTS

- The dopamine agonists pergolide, bromocriptine, pramipexole, and ropinirole can prolong the effective treatment period in patients with deteriorating response to L-dopa. The dopamine agonists also decrease the frequency of "off" periods and provide an L-dopa sparing effect.
- Bromocriptine and pergolide are considered equally efficacious.
- The dopamine agonists are also effective as monotherapy in previously untreated patients, however there is a high incidence of adverse effects and treatment failure necessitating either a lower dose or the addition of L-dopa.
- A recommended initial dose of bromocriptine is 1.25 mg once or twice daily. It should be escalated slowly by 1.25 to 2.5 mg/d every week and maintained at the minimum effective dose. Average daily doses <30 mg may be effective for several years in many patients, however, some patients may require dosages of up to 120 mg/d.
- A recommended initial dose for pergolide is 0.05 mg/d for 2 days, gradually increasing by approximately 0.1–0.15 mg/d every 3 days over a 12-day period. If higher doses are needed, the dose may be increased by 0.25 mg every 3 days until symptoms are eliminated or adverse effects occur. The mean therapeutic dose in most clinical trials was approximately 3 mg/d.
- Nausea is the most frequently reported GI effect. Postural hypotension is common, but other cardiovascular effects are infrequent. Central nervous system effects are common and include confusion, hallucinations, and sedation.
- The addition of a dopamine agonist to L-dopa therapy will increase the frequency and severity of dyskinesias during periods of good functional status. Pergolide has an arrhythmogenic effect and a bradycardic effect.

IX

▶ EVALUATION OF THERAPEUTIC OUTCOMES

- Patients and caregivers should be educated regarding the disease and its treatment so that they can participate in treatment by recording medication administration times and duration of "on" and "off" periods.

- Documenting the times of day when functioning is most limited and assessing activities of daily living will help determine when L-dopa or dopamine agonists should be added.
- Side effects should be scrupulously monitored.

See Chapter 58, Parkinson's Disease, authored by Merlin V. Nelson, PharmD, MD, Richard C. Berchou, PharmD, and Peter A. LeWitt, MD, for a more detailed discussion of this topic.

IX

Chapter 55

▶ STATUS EPILEPTICUS

▶ DEFINITION

Status epilepticus (SE) is defined as >30 minutes of continuous seizure activity or two or more sequential seizures without full recovery of consciousness between seizures. SE may be convulsive or nonconvulsive, generalized or partial. The international classification of SE is provided in Table 55.1.

▶ PATHOPHYSIOLOGY AND ETIOLOGY

- The most common causes of SE in children are epilepsy, atypical febrile seizures, encephalitis, meningitis, and metabolic disease.
- The most common causes of SE in adults are withdrawal of antiepileptic drugs (AED), alcohol withdrawal, head trauma, and underlying neurologic disorder.
- The most common causes of SE in the elderly who had their first seizure after age 60 years are cerebrovascular disease, head trauma, metabolic disorders, brain tumors, and central nervous system (CNS) infection.
- Pathophysiologic underpinnings may include:
  - A diminution of γ-aminobutyric acid (GABA)-ergic inhibition after a single, short-lived seizure.
  - Excitatory neurotransmitters, free radical formation, and toxic calcium flux may also be involved in evolution of SE.

▶ DIAGNOSIS

- Diagnosis must include a clinical and electroencephalogram (EEG) exam. The diagnosis of convulsive SE should not be made until a trained clinician has witnessed at least one generalized tonic-clonic seizure occurring in a patient with a depressed state of consciousness who has a history of repeated seizures without regaining consciousness between episodes.
- The diagnosis of nonconvulsive or focal motor SE should not be made until 30 minutes of continuous seizure activity has been observed.
- The first phase of diagnostic tests includes blood sugar and serum chemistries. Hypoglycemia, hyponatremia, hypernatremia, hypomagnesemia, hypocalcemia, and renal failure can all cause seizure activity as can thyrotoxicosis. A toxicology screen and complete blood cell count (CBC) should be ordered, and women of child-bearing potential should have a pregnancy test performed.
- The second phase of diagnostic tests are done after seizures have stopped, and include EEG, lumbar puncture (especially in children with

TABLE 55.1. International Classification of Status Epilepticus

International	Traditional
Generalized SE	
Convulsive	
Tonic-clonic	Grand mal, epilepticus convulsivus
Tonic	
Clonic	
Myoclonic	
Nonconvulsive	
Absence	Spike-and-wave stupor, spike and slow-wave or 3/s spike-and-wave SE, petit mal, epileptic fugue, epilepsia minora continua, epileptic twilight state, minor SE
Partial SE	Focal motor status, focal sensory, epilepsia partialis continuans, adversive SE
Elementary	
Somatomotor	
Dysphasic	
Other types	
Complex partial	Epileptic fugue state, prolonged epileptic stupor, prolonged epileptic confusional state, temporal lobe SE, psychomotor SE, continuous epileptic twilight state
Unilateral SE	Hemicolonic SE, hemiconvulsion—hemiplegia—epilepsy, hemigrand mal SE, grand mal dimidie
Erratic SE (unclassified)	Neonatal status epilepticus

fever), brain imaging [computed tomography (CT) scan or magnetic resonance imaging (MRI)].

▶ CLINICAL PRESENTATION

- SE is a medical emergency. Table 55.2 summarizes the physiologic consequences of SE. Systemic symptoms include hyperthermia, leukocytosis, pleocytosis, hemodynamic alterations, and respiratory defects.
- Rhabdomyolysis may lead to myoglobinuria and renal failure.
- There may be increased sweating and salivation and marked elevations in plasma prolactin, glucagon, growth hormone, and adrenocorticotropic hormone.
- Some patients may recover with no discernable effects, however, others may have neurologic impairment, with decreased performance on intelligence tests, and subtle changes in neuropsychometric tests.

TABLE 55.2. Physiologic Consequences of Status Epilepticus

Phase I	Phase II
Tachycardia	Decrease in CO
Hypertension	Hypotension
Increased cardiac output	Increase in cerebral venous pressure
Pallor	Hypoglycemia
Hyperglycemia	Metabolic acidosis
Increase in central venous pressure	Hyperkalemia
Cerebral venous oxygen, raised or normal	Cerebral congestion
Lactic acidosis	Cerebral edema
Hyperkalemia or normokalemia	Increase in intracranial pressure
Hypersalivation	Increase in liver enzymes
Incontinence	Increase in plasma muscle enzymes
Vomiting (aspiration)	Water intoxication
	Hyperpyrexia
	Consumptive coagulopathy

From Brown JK, Hussain II IMI. Dev Med Child Neurol 1991;33:3–17, with permission.

▶ MORBIDITY AND MORTALITY

IX

- Estimates of mortality are 3–10% in children, 20–30% in adults, and 35% in the elderly. Predictors of mortality include seizure duration, etiology, and age.
- Of the various subtypes of SE, generalized convulsive SE clearly causes the most morbidity and mortality. Complex partial SE may continue for a prolonged period before seizures are controlled. It is imperative that focal SE and nonconvulsive SE be regarded as urgent situations requiring prompt treatment.
- Patients who have experienced SE are more likely to have continued seizures and less likely to have remission of their epilepsy.
- Patients with febrile SE may not have significant sequelea unless they have an underlying neurologic abnormality.

▶ DESIRED OUTCOMES

SE is a medical emergency, and the primary desired outcome is to stop seizure activity. However, it is similarly critical that adequate ventilation and an intact cardiovascular system be maintained and that normal blood sugar and body temperature are assured.

▶ TREATMENT

CONVULSIVE SE

- Table 52.3 summarizes the recommended management of convulsive SE.
- Table 52.4 describes some pharmacologic and pharmacokinetic parameters of AEDs used in treatment of convulsive SE. The therapeutic plasma concentrations are those specific for generalized convulsive SE, but are not based on controlled, prospective studies, and some are based only on experience. The effective half-life is an estimate of the duration of therapeutic effect after a single dose.
- AED therapy is usually initiated with a benzodiazepine (BZ), which typically has an immediate onset of activity. This is followed by another AED, usually phenytoin, which has a much longer duration of effect.

Benzodiazepines

- While BZs are used to stop SE, another AED with longer lasting effects will also be needed. Respiratory depression is more likely if the patient is also receiving phenobarbital.
- Lorazepam has a longer effective half-life than diazepam. It is effective in both generalized and partial SE, and can be rapidly administered by IV push. It is metabolized by phase II metabolic processes, and the elimination half-life of lorazepam is shorter than that of diazepam. It is frequently the initial AED that is administered because of its rapid onset and long duration of effect. Tachyphylaxis may occur with repeated doses. Adverse effects include sedation, confusion, tremor, hallucinations, and respiratory depression.
- The recommended initial dose of lorazepam in adults is 4–8 mg IV administered over 2 minutes. If the seizures do not stop within 5 minutes, the dose should be repeated. The pediatric dose of lorazepam is 0.05–0.1 mg/kg.
- Diazepam stops convulsions within 5 minutes in 80% of patients, but seizures frequently recur after 15–20 minutes. Complications associated with IV diazepam include respiratory depression, hypotension, arrhythmias, laryngospasm, and thrombophlebitis. At an infusion rate of 2 mg/min, no episodes of hypotension occurred in a series of 50 patients with SE. The maximum rate of infusion is 5 mg/min.
- The recommended initial dose of diazepam in adults is 10–20 mg IV. The expected time for seizures to stop after diazepam administration is 1–3 minutes. If seizures have not stopped after 5 minutes, another dose should be given. The maximum recommended total dose in adults is 40 mg. The pediatric dose of diazepam is 0.25–0.4 mg/kg.
- Rectal diazepam can be considered an alternative to IV diazepam for patients who cannot be given the drug intravenously. The dose rectally is 0.5 mg/kg. Rectal therapy is effective in treatment of febrile convulsions and absence SE.

TABLE 55.3. Management of Tonic–Clonic Status Epilepticus

Time[a] (min)	Action[b]
0–5	Diagnose status epilepticus by observing continued seizure activity or one additional seizure.
	Give oxygen by nasal cannula or mask; position patient's head for optimal airway patency; consider intubation if respiratory assistance is needed.
	Obtain and record vital signs at onset and periodically thereafter; control any abnormalities as necessary; initiate ECG monitoring.
	Establish an IV; draw venous blood samples for glucose level, serum chemistries, hematology studies, toxicology screens, and determinations of antiepileptic drug levels.
	Assess oxygenation with oximetry or periodic arterial blood gas determinations.
6–9	If hypoglycemia is established or a blood glucose determination is unavailable, administer glucose; in adults, give 100 mg of thiamine first, followed by 50 mL of 50% glucose by direct push into the IV; in children, the dose of glucose is 2 mL/kg of 25% glucose.
10–20	Administer either 0.1 mg/kg of lorazepam at 2 mg/min or 0.2 mg/kg of diazepam at 5 mg/min by IV; if diazepam is given, it can be repeated if seizures do not stop after 5 min; if diazepam is used to stop the status, phenytoin should be administered next to prevent recurrent status.
21–60	If status persists, administer 15–20 mg/kg of phenytoin no faster than 50 mg/min in adults and 1 mg/kg/min in children by IV; monitor ECG and blood pressure during the infusion; phenytoin is incompatible with glucose containing solutions; the IV should be purged with normal saline before the phenytoin infusion.
>60	If status does not stop after 20 mg/kg of phenytoin, give additional doses of 5 mg/kg to a maximal dose of 30 mg/kg.
	If status persists, give 20 mg/kg of phenobarbital by IV at 100 mg/min (maximum infusion rate in children is 30 mg/min), when phenobarbital is given after benzodiazepine, the risk of apnea or hypopnea is great and assisted ventilation is usually required.
	If status persists, give anesthetic doses of drugs such as phenobarbital or pentobarbital; ventilatory assistance and vasopressors are virtually always necessary.

IX ◀

[a] Time starts at seizure onset. Note that a neurologic consultation is indicated if the patient does not wake up, convulsions continue after the administration of a benzodiazepine and phenytoin, or confusion exists at any time during evaluation and treatment.
[b] ECG, electrocardiogram; IV, intravenous line.
Adapted from JAMA 1993;270(7):857 with permission.

TABLE 55.4. Pharmacokinetic and Dosing Guidelines for AEDs Commonly Used in Status Epilepticus

Drug	Usual Initial IV Dose	Administration Rate	Time to Stop SE, $t_{1/2}\alpha^a$ (min)	Mean $t_{1/2}\beta^b$ (h)	Estimated Effective Half-Life	Initial Plasma Concentration^c (µg/mL)
Diazepam	5–10 mg (0.25–0.4 mg/kg)^d	1–2 mg/min (same)	3–5	30–40	1.5 min	0.5–0.8
Phenytoin	18–20 mg/kg (same)	≤50 mg/min (0.5–1.0 mg/kg/min)	30	22^e	22 h	20–25
Phenobarbital	300–800 mg (20 mg/kg)	25–50 mg/min (same)	20	86	50–120 h	20–45
Pentobarbital	100 mg for 70 kg adult (—)	≤50 mg/min	—^{h}	15–50	—	—
Lorazepam	4–8 mg (—)	<2 mg/min (—)	3	15	2 h	0.3–1.0
Midazolam	0.15 mg/kg	Administered over 20–30 seconds	—	1.2–12.3	—	—
Lidocaine	50–100 mg (0.5–1 mg/kg)	1–2 mg/min (20–50 µg/kg/min)	1	1.5–2.5	—	—

$^a t_{1/2}\alpha$, distribution half-life.
$^b t_{1/2}\beta$, elimination half-life.
^{c}Plasma concentrations have generally not been well established for treatment of SE.
^{d}Information in parentheses for children.
^{e}Phenytoin displays nonlinear elimination; this value will change depending on the concentration.
^{f}Injectable form is no longer commercially available.
^{g}Can also be given intramuscularly at a dose of 5–10 mL for adults.
^{h}Dashes are used for data that could not be extracted from the literature.

IX

Midazolam

- Recent reports of pediatric patients have noted midazolam to be effective for seizures refractory to other AEDs. A loading dose of 0.15 mg/kg, followed by a mean dose of 2.3 µg/kg/min (range of 1–18 µg/kg/min) with a maximum total dose of 1.81 mg (range of 1.78–2.02) have been reported, with control of seizures in a mean of 0.78 hours.

Phenytoin

- Phenytoin is effective in treatment of partial and generalized convulsive SE.
- It is frequently given after a BZ because it provides a longer duration of effect. Brain phenytoin concentrations peak in 15–20 minutes, with maintenance of effective brain concentrations and subsequent seizure control for 24 hours or longer after an IV loading dose of 18–20 mg/kg.
- Hypotension and cardiac arrhythmias can be minimized by not exceeding an administration rate of 50 mg/min. Elderly patients and those with unstable cardiopulmonary function require an even slower infusion rate (e.g., ≤25 mg/min for patients with atherosclerotic cardiovascular disease). ECG monitoring and frequent blood pressure determinations should be performed during and for 1 hour after the infusion.
- Local reactions to IV phenytoin include painful sensations (burning, aching) and extravasation.
- For very obese patients, phenytoin loading doses should be calculated on the basis of ideal body weight (IBW) plus the product of 1.33 times the excess weight over IBW.
- For patients with subtherapeutic phenytoin concentrations, the following equation may be used to rapidly estimate an appropriate dose to provide therapeutic serum concentrations:

$$\text{Dose (mg)} = (Cp_d - Cp_m)(0.7)(W_{kg})$$

where Cp_d is the desired serum concentration, Cp_m is the measured subtherapeutic serum concentration, the constant 0.7 represents an approximation of the average volume of distribution, and W_{kg} is the patient's weight in kilograms.
- When interpreting phenytoin concentrations, factors altering protein binding (see Chapter 51) should be considered. Measurement of a free phenytoin concentration may be indicated in patients with decreased serum albumin or those taking other highly protein-bound drugs. A free concentration of 1–2 µg/mL is considered to be therapeutic.

Fosphenytoin

- Fosphenytoin, the water soluble disodium phosphate ester of phenytoin, is a phenytoin prodrug. Fosphenytoin, 150 mg is equivalent to phenytoin, 100 mg.
- Fosphenytoin sodium, 75 mg is equivalent to phenytoin sodium, 50 mg. The dose of fosphenytoin sodium is expressed as phenytoin sodium

IX

equivalents (PE). Fosphenytoin sodium should be infused no faster than 150 mg PE/min because of the risk of hypotension. Cardiac monitoring during IV infusion of loading doses is recommended. Maximal phenytoin concentrations occur approximately 10–20 minutes after the end of the infusion.

- The usual dose of fosphenytoin for SE is 22.5–30 mg/kg of fosphenytoin (15–20 mg PE/kg) given IV at a rate of 150–225 mg/min fosphenytoin (100–150 mg PE/min). A loading dose of 15–30 mg/kg fosphenytoin (10–20 mg PE/kg) can be given IM or IV for treatment or prophylaxis of seizures.
- Adverse reactions include nystagmus, dizziness, pruritus, paresthesias, headache, somnolence, and ataxia.

Phenobarbital

- An IV loading dose of 20 mg/kg (and possibly up to 25 mg/kg) administered at a rate not exceeding 100 mg/min is recommended. A slower rate of infusion (i.e., 30 mg/min) has been recommended for children. One author suggested a dose of 250–300 mg be given IV, and if the patient has not stopped seizing within 20–30 minutes, a second dose may be administered. Only occasionally, a third dose is given after an additional 20 minutes. Phenobarbital can be administered by IV push over several minutes.
- Therapeutic effects of phenobarbital are longer lasting than those of diazepam, but phenobarbital has a slower onset.
- For the treatment of neonatal SE, phenobarbital is the drug of choice.
- Phenobarbital may be used to induce coma for refractory generalized convulsive SE.

Lidocaine

- Lidocaine may control seizures when diazepam, phenytoin, and phenobarbital have failed. Onset of action is often noted afer 20–30 seconds.
- Most clinicians administer 50–100 mg initially, and an infusion at a rate of 1–2 mg/min is recommended, although higher rates (3–10 mg/kg/hr) may be necessary.
- Serum concentrations should be monitored and maintained between 2 and 6 μg/mL. CNS toxicity (e.g., fasciculation, visual disturbances, tinnitus) may occur at serum concentrations between 6 and 8 μg/mL.

Refractory SE

- Midazolam has recently been suggested as the third-line agent if the patient does not respond to lorazepam or phenytoin.
- If convulsive SE does not respond to recommended initial doses of a BZ, phenytoin, and phenobarbital, the condition is considered refractory, and consideration may be given to anesthetizing the patient to suppress seizures. Convulsive SE becomes harder to treat the longer it lasts.
- If the patient has not adequately responded after 24–48 hours and dosage requirements are increasing, consideration should be given to

IX

pentobarbital coma. Pentobarbital is initiated with a loading dose of 5–8 mg/kg over 40–60 minutes followed by an infusion of 3 mg/kg/h. Some pediatric centers give larger loading doses. If the patient becomes hypotensive, the rate of infusion can be slowed, or fluids or dopamine can be given. Continuous EEG monitoring is required. Intubation and respiratory support are essential. Duration of barbiturate coma in most studies has been 2–3 days.

- SE resistant to barbiturate coma has been treated with halothane and neuromuscular blockade; recently isoflurane and propofol have been used.

NONCONVULSIVE SE

- The clinical manifestations of absence SE include an altered state of consciousness and/or behavior and the classic 3 per second spike-and-wave pattern on the EEG. Correction of identifiable precipitants (e.g., structural or metabolic aberrations) may be the only therapy required. Acute absence SE, a medical emergency, can be treated by the administration of IV diazepam. Rectal valproic acid may also be useful. Acetazolamide IV (250–500 mg) has also been useful. Chronic therapy to prevent recurrent attacks should be instituted with ethosuximide or valproic acid.
- Valproic acid is probably the drug of choice for atypical absence, but combined therapy with ethosuximide or clonazepam may be useful for refractory patients. Valproic acid is probably the drug of first choice for generalized myoclonic SE.
- Complex partial SE occurs when seizure activity is focal in onset and consciousness is impaired. It is a continuous series of repeated attacks with phases of total unresponsiveness with stereotypical automatisms. Memory and behavioral alterations may occur as sequelae. Treatment is similar to that for convulsive SE, and includes removing precipitating factors and the combination of IV diazepam and phenytoin. However, phenytoin alone may be more beneficial, because it does not produce sedation. Lorazepam may be a reasonable alternative to the diazepam-phenytoin combination in treatment of nonconvulsive SE.

▶ EVALUATION OF THERAPEUTIC OUTCOMES

- Convulsive SE is a medical emergency, and therapy must be aggressive. Drug-induced side effects are less of a concern than preventing brain damage or death. Close monitoring is required to assure that interventions are effective, that seizures do not recur, and that vital functions are supported.

See Chapter 56, Status Epilepticus, authored by William R. Garnett, PharmD, for a more detailed discussion of this topic.

Chapter 56

► ASSESSMENT AND NUTRITION REQUIREMENTS

► DEFINITION

Malnutrition is a state induced by alterations in dietary intake or nutrient utilization resulting in changes in subcellular, cellular, and/or organ function that expose the individual to increased risks of morbidity and mortality. These changes can be reversed by appropriate nutrition support.

► DESIRED OUTCOME

Nutrition assessment provides a basis for determining nutrition requirements, when nutrition therapy should be initiated, and the optimal type of nutritional intervention. The principles of enteral and parenteral nutrition are covered in Chapters 57 and 58.

► CLASSIFICATION OF NUTRITIONAL DISEASES

- Deficiency states can be categorized as those involving protein and calories (protein-calorie malnutrition [PCM]) or those resulting from single nutrients (e.g., vitamins or trace minerals).
- Three types of PCM are marasmus, kwashiorkor, and mixed marasmus–kwashiorkor (Table 56.1).
- Single-nutrient deficiencies can and often do occur in combination with any PCM.

► NUTRITION SCREENING

- Checklists are often utilized to characterize a person's food and alcohol consumption habits, physical capability of buying and preparing food, and weight history. If three or more risk factors are present, a more comprehensive nutrition assessment is performed.
- The nutrition status of stable, hospitalized patients should be reevaluated every 7–14 days to avoid deterioration secondary to changes in food intake.
- By identifying individuals at risk for malnutrition, nutrition screening can be a cost-effective way to help decrease complications and length of hospital stay.

TABLE 56.1. Indicators of Protein and Energy Malnutrition (PEM)

	Marasmus	Kwashiorkor	Mixed Marasmus-Kwashiorkor
Primary deficit indicators	Energy	Protein	Protein and energy
Body weight	↓	↓	↓
Body fat	↓	WNL	↓
Somatic protein	↓	Slightly ↓	↓
Visceral protein	WNL	↓	↓
Immune function	↓	↓	↓

Key: ↓, decreased; WNL, within normal limits.
Adapted from Clinical Nutrition and Dietetics, 2E Frances J. Zeman. Macmillan College Publishing Company, 1991, with the permission of Simon & Schuster, Inc.

▶ NUTRITION ASSESSMENT

- Nutrition assessment includes medical and dietary history, physical examination, anthropometric measurements, and laboratory data. Laboratory parameters provide objective data to confirm the diagnosis, quantify degree of malnutrition, identify end organ changes that occur with malnutrition, and provide a baseline for evaluating response to nutrition therapy.
- Clinical evaluation (i.e., medical and dietary history, physical examination) remains the oldest, simplest, and probably most widely used method of identifying predisposing factors (Table 56.2).
- Physical examination should focus on assessment of lean body mass and physical findings of vitamin, trace mineral, and essential fatty acid deficiency (Table 56.3). X

ANTHROPOMETRIC MEASUREMENTS

- Anthropometric measurements (e.g., height, weight, measurements of midarm muscle or wrist circumference, and skinfold thickness) are safe, simple, and easy measures of body cell mass for both population analysis and individual long-term monitoring.
- Individual anthropometric measurements should be cautiously interpreted because (1) standards do not account for individual variations in bone size, hydration status, or skin compressibility, as well as obesity, ethnicity, and increased age; (2) technique is critical and interobserver error may be as high as 30%; (3) parameters are slow to change, often requiring weeks before significant alterations from baseline can be observed; and (4) acute changes usually reflect changes in fluid status.
- Interpretation of actual body weight (ABW) measurement should consider ideal weight for height, usual body weight, fluid status, and age. Degree of change over time can be calculated as percentage of ideal or

TABLE 56.2. Pertinent Data from Medical and Dietary History for Nutrition Assessment

Nutrition Intake and Dietary Habits
Anorexia; changes in taste
Actual intake; special diets
Supplemental vitamin or mineral intake
Food allergies or intolerance

Underlying Pathology with Nutritional Effects
Chronic infections or inflammatory states
Neoplastic diseases
Endocrine disorders
Chronic illnesses including pulmonary disease, cirrhosis, renal failure
Hypermetabolic states: trauma, burns, sepsis
Digestive or absorptive diseases
Hyperlipidemia

End-Organ Effects
Weight changes
Skin or hair changes
Exercise tolerance, fatigue
Obesity
Gastrointestinal tract symptoms: diarrhea, vomiting, constipation

Miscellaneous
Catabolic medications or therapies: steroids, immunosuppressive agents, radiation, or chemotherapy
Other medications: diuretics, laxatives
Genetic background: body habitus of parents, siblings, and family
Alcohol or drug abuse

X

usual body weight (IBW or UBW) where % change = (ABW/IBW or UBW) × 100. An absolute unintentional weight loss of >10 pounds in <6 months correlates with increased mortality in adult surgical patients.

- Body mass index (BMI) (i.e., ratio of body weight in kilograms and height in meters squared) has been used to categorize obesity and malnutrition. In patients <65 years of age, BMI values of 18.5–25 are associated with the least risk of early death, whereas values >25 are associated with obesity and values <18.5 are indicative of malnutrition.
- Skinfold-thickness measurement estimates subcutaneous fat, which is relatively insensitive to short-term changes in tissue composition. Serial measurements performed by the same trained observer on the same body site (usually triceps) with pressure-regulated calipers (Lange, Halipern) are essential for reproducibility and reliability.
- Midarm-muscle circumference (MAMC) is a noninvasive, easy, inexpensive method of assessing skeletal muscle mass. MAMC is calculated as follows: MAMC (cm) = MAC (cm) − πTSF (mm)/10. TSF is triceps skinfold thickness and MAC is midarm circumference. A decrease from the expected value (i.e., 20th percentile) suggests significant reduction in somatic protein mass.

TABLE 56.3. Physical Findings Suggestive of Malnutrition

General Appearance
　Edema
　Cachexia or obesity
　Ascites
　Signs and symptoms of dehydration: skin turgor, sunken eyes, orthostasis, dry mucous
　　membranes

Skin and Mucous Membranes
　Thin, shiny, or scaling skin
　Decubitus ulcers
　Ecchymoses, perifollicular petechiae
　Poorly healing surgical or traumatic wounds
　Pallor or redness of gums, fissures at mouth edge
　Glossitis; stomatitis; cheilosis

Musculoskeletal
　Retarded growth
　Bone pain or tenderness, epiphyseal swelling
　Muscle mass less than expected for habitus, genetic history, and level of exercise

Neurologic
　Ataxia, positive Romberg test, decreased vibratory or position sense
　Nystagmus
　Convulsions, paralysis
　Encephalopathy

Hepatic
　Jaundice
　Hepatomegaly

BIOCHEMICAL MARKERS

- Biochemical markers of lean body mass, which reflect structural and functional protein status, can be assessed by creatinine-height index (CHI) and serum visceral protein concentrations.
- CHI is obtained by calculating the ratio of the actual 24-hour urinary excretion of the patient and the ideal 24-hour excretion normalized by gender, height, and body weight (Table 56.4). CHI of ≥80% indicates no or mild somatic muscle depletion, 60–80% indicates moderate depletion, and <60% represents severe depletion.
- Visceral proteins of relevance for nutritional assessment are serum albumin, transferrin, retinol-binding protein, and thyroxine-binding pre-albumin (transthyretin) (Table 56.5). Data must be interpreted relative to individual clinical status because of the confounding effects of abnormal protein losses via renal or gastrointestinal routes, hydration status, renal and hepatic function, and metabolic stress.
  - These proteins become poor markers of nutrition status during acute stress (e.g., trauma, burn injury, sepsis).

X

TABLE 56.4. Ideal 24-Hour Urinary Creatinine Excretion by Adults of Various Heights (For Use in Calculation of the Creatinine-Height Index)

Height		Ideal Creatinine Excretion (mg)	
in.	*cm*	*Adult Women*[a]	*Adult Men*[b]
58	147.3	830	—
59	149.9	851	—
60	152.4	875	—
61	154.9	900	—
62	157.5	925	1288
63	160	949	1325
64	162.6	977	1359
65	165.1	1006	1386
66	167.6	1044	1426
67	170.2	1076	1467
68	172.7	1109	1513
69	175.3	1141	1555
70	177.8	1174	1596
71	180.3	1206	1642
72	182.9	1240	1691
73	185.4	—	1739
74	188	—	1785
75	190.5	—	1831
76	193	—	1891

[a]Creatinine coefficient (women) = 18 mg/kg of ideal body weight.
[b]Creatinine coefficient (men) = 23 mg/kg of ideal body weight.
From Blackburn GL, Bistrian RB, Maini BS, et al. Nutritional and metabolic assessment of the hospitalized patient. J Parenter Enter Nutr 1977;1:15, with permission.

- Albumin, the most commonly used, is a relatively insensitive index of early protein malnutrition because of its large body pool (4–5 g/kg), high extravascular distribution (0.6 L/kg), and long biologic half-life ($\approx$20 days).

TESTS OF IMMUNE FUNCTION

- Tests of immune function most frequently used in nutrition assessment, total lymphocyte count (TLC) and delayed cutaneous hypersensitivity (DCH) reactions, are simple to perform, readily available, and inexpensive.
- TLC of 1200–2000/mm^3 correlates with mild malnutrition, 800–1200/mm^3 with moderate malnutrition, and <800/mm^3 with severe malnutrition.

TABLE 56.5. Summary of Visceral Proteins Used for Assessment of Lean Body Mass

Serum Protein	Biosynthetic Site	Half-life (days)	Normal Value (range)[a]	Function	Factors Resulting in Increased Values[b]	Factors Resulting in Decreased Values[b]
Albumin	Hepatocyte	18–20	3.5–5.0 g/dL	Maintains plasma oncotic pressure; carrier for small molecules	Dehydration, anabolic steroids, insulin, infection	Overhydration, edema, renal insufficiency, nephrotic syndrome, poor intake, impaired digestion, burns, congestive heart failure, cirrhosis, thyroid/adrenal/pituitary hormones, trauma, sepsis
Fibronectin	Hepatocyte, fibroblasts, endothelial cells	0.5–1.0	210–300 μg/mL	A glycoprotein that in blood has opsonic activity; may exert chemotactic activity and facilitate wound healing	None currently described	Trauma, shock, burns, sepsis, disseminated intravascular coagulation; inappropriate specimen handling
Prealbumin (Transthyretin)	Hepatocyte	1–2	10–40 mg/dL	Binds T$_3$ and to a lesser extent T$_4$; carrier for REP	Renal dysfunction	Cirrhosis, hepatitis, stress, inflammation, surgery, hyperthyroidism, cystic fibrosis, renal dysfunction
Retinol-binding protein (RBP)	Hepatocyte	0.5	2.0–6.0 mg/dL	Transports vitamin A in plasma; binds noncovalently to prealbumin	Renal dysfunction, vitamin A supplementation	Same as prealbumin; also vitamin A deficiency
Somatomedin C (IGF-1)	Hepatocyte	0.1–0.3	0.5–2.0 IU/mL	An insulin-like peptide that has anabolic actions on fat, muscle cartilage and cultured cells	None currently described	Growth hormone deficiency, psychosocial growth failure, hypothyroidism, renal failure, cirrhosis, drugs (estrogens, prednisolone)
Transferrin	Hepatocyte	8	200–400 mg/dL	Binds Fe in plasma and transports to bone	Iron deficiency, pregnancy, hypoxia, chronic blood loss, estrogens	Chronic infection, cirrhosis, enteropathies, nephrotic syndrome, burns, cortisone, testosterone

[a] Normal values represent pooled subjects; ranges vary between centers; check local values.
[b] All of the listed proteins are influenced by hydration and the presence of hepatocellular dysfunction.

- DCH may be assessed as a primary response to a mitogen (e.g., phyto-hemagglutinin [PHA]) or, more commonly, as a secondary response using recall antigens (e.g., mumps, *Candida albicans,* strepto-kinase–streptodornase [SKSD], *Trichophyton,* coccidioidin, and puri-fied protein derivative [PPD]).
- Unfortunately, both TLC and DCH are affected by non-nutrition factors (e.g., infection, immunosuppressive therapy, or critical illness) and, therefore, at best are nonspecific indicators of malnutrition.

OTHER TYPES OF NUTRITION ASSESSMENT

- Bioelectric impedance analysis (BIA) is a promising, new, simple, non-invasive method of assessing body composition and fluid status. Poten-tial limitations include variability with electrolyte imbalance, interfer-ence by large fat masses, and lack of standards that reflect variations in individual body sizes.
- Hand grip strength, or forearm muscle dynamometry, and stimulation of the ulnar nerve have been used as indicators of muscle function and correlate with patient outcome. Both parameters have the advantage of indicating tissue function rather than composition. Clinical utility is hampered by lack of appropriate reference standards and limited data confirming their sensitivity and specificity as nutrition assessment tools.
- New methods to determine body composition are being utilized in clin-ical research. These clinical uses are limited by the degree of technical complexity and expensive technology.

► SPECIFIC NUTRIENT DEFICIENCIES

- Assessment of nutrition status should include evaluation of possible trace mineral, vitamin, and essential fatty acid deficiencies. Assessment includes history, physical examination, and biochemical assessment. Unfortunately, few practical methods to assess micronutrient function are currently available; most assays measure tissue or fluid concentra-tion of a nutrient, not its function.
- Essential trace minerals for which deficiency states have been described are zinc, copper, manganese, selenium, chromium, iodine, molybde-num, and iron (Table 56.6).
- Iron deficiency is usually confirmed by indirect measurements because they are noninvasive, but they may be altered by chronic illness. Direct methods (e.g., marrow staining and liver biopsy) are more accurate, but invasive and thus rarely used. More information on iron deficiency ane-mia can be found in Chapter 31.
- History and physical examination may be the most valuable means of screening patients for vitamin deficiency (Table 56.7). Laboratory assessment is primarily used to confirm clinical suspicions; the most common measurements are assays of circulating amounts in plasma or serum rather than functional measures.

X

TABLE 56.6. Assessment of Trace Mineral Status

Trace Mineral	Signs of Deficiency	Normal Serum Concentration[a]	Factors Resulting in Altered Plasma Concentrations
Chromium	Glucose intolerance, peripheral neuropathy, increased free fatty acid levels, low respiratory quotient	0.12–2.1 µg/L	Not known
Copper	Neutropenia, hypochromic anemia, osteoporosis, decreased hair and skin pigmentation, dermatitis, anorexia, diarrhea	80–155 µg/L (female) 70–140 µg/L (male)	Decreased: serum ceruloplasmin concentrations, corticosteroid therapy, Wilson's disease Increased: infection, rheumatoid arthritis, pregnancy, birth control pills
Iodine	Hypothyroid goiter, hypothyroidism	(Assessed by T_4, TSH and free T_4 index)[b]	Assays are specific to hypo- and hyperthyroid states
Manganese	Nausea, vomiting, dermatitis, color changes in hair, hypocholesterolemia, growth retardation	0.6–2.0 ng/mL (plasma)	Not known
Molybdenum	Tachycardia, tachypnea, altered mental status, visual changes, headache, nausea, vomiting	0.1–3.0 µg/L	Varies with assay method used
Selenium	Muscle weakness and pain, cardiomyopathy	46–143 µg/dL	Decreased: malignancy, liver failure, pregnancy Increased: reticuloendothelial neoplasia
Zinc	Dermatitis, hypogeusia, alopecia, diarrhea, apathy, depression	70–150 µg/dL	Decreased: infection, hypoalbuminemia, corticosteroid therapy, stress, inflammation, pregnancy Increased: tissue injury, hemolysis, contaminated collection tubes

[a]Normal values may vary between laboratories and will also depend on assay procedure.
[b]See Chapter 18, Thyroid Disorders.

TABLE 56.7. Assessment of Vitamin Status

Vitamin	Signs of Deficiency	Laboratory Assay	Normal Values	Comments
Niacin (B$_5$)	Pellagra: dermatitis, dementia, glossitis, diarrhea, loss of memory, and headaches	Urinary niacin metabolites	2.4–6.4 mg/d	Varies with age, sex, pregnancy; blood levels not done
Folate (B$_9$)	Megaloblastic anemia, diarrhea, and glossitis	Serum folate	3–16 ng/mL	Decreased in cases of increased cellular or tissue turnover (pregnancy, malignancy, hemolytic anemia)
Cyanocobalamin (B$_{12}$)	Pernicious anemia: glossitis, spinal cord degeneration, and peripheral neuropathy	Serum B$_{12}$	100–700 pg/mL	
Thiamine (B$_1$)	Paresthesias, nystagmus, impaired memory, congestive heart failure, lactic acidosis, Wernicke–Korsakoff syndrome	Red blood cell transketolase activity	850–1000 µg/mL/h	
Riboflavin (B$_2$)	Mucositis, dermatitis, cheilosis; vascularization of cornea, photophobia, lacrimation, decreased vision; impaired wound healing; normocytic anemia	Urinary riboflavin	80–120 µg/g creatinine	Varies with age, pregnancy, exercise, nitrogen balance
Pyridoxine (B$_6$)	Dermatitis, neuritis, and convulsions; microcytic anemia	Plasma B$_6$	5–30 ng/mL	Varies with age, sex

X

TABLE 56.7. continued

Pantothenic acid (B$_3$)	Fatigue, malaise, headache, insomnia, vomiting, abdominal cramps	Serum pantothenic acid	1.03–1.83 µg/mL	
Biotin	Dermatitis, depression, alopecia, lassitude, somnolence	Urinary biotin	6–50 µg/d	
Ascorbic acid (C)	Enlargement and keratosis of hair follicles; impaired wound healing; anemia, lethargy, depression, bleeding, ecchymosis	Plasma ascorbic acid	0.5–1.5 mg/dL	
A	Dermatitis, night blindness keratomalacia, xerophthalmia	Serum vitamin A	30–80 µg/dL	
D	Rickets and osteomalacia, muscle weakness	Plasma 25-hydroxy-vitamin D	13–50 ng/mL	Decreased in uremia, cirrhosis, individuals greater than 60 years old, and possibly in winter
E	Hemolysis	Serum vitamin E	5.0–13 µg/mL	Decreased with low blood lipoprotein concentrations
K	Bleeding	Serum phylloquinone	0.13–1.19 ng/mL	Decreased with hepatic disease, anticoagulants

X

- Essential fatty acid (EFA) deficiency (i.e., linoleic acid deficiency) is rare but may appear within 1 week after initiation of fat-free parenteral nutrition or with severe PCM. Symptoms include dermatitis (e.g., dry, cracked, scaly skin), alopecia, and impaired wound healing. In severe cases neurologic deficits, abnormal liver function, respiratory insufficiency, cardiac arrhythmias, and hemolysis may occur. Laboratory assessment of EFA deficiency is expensive and not readily available.
- Carnitine is a substance with vitamin-like properties for which no specific dietary requirement has been proposed. Carnitine deficiency has been associated with severe protein malnutrition, inborn errors of metabolism, insufficient dietary carnitine intake in newborn infants, and kidney and liver disease. Clinical presentation includes generalized skeletal muscle weakness, fatty liver, and reactive hypoglycemia. Carnitine status may be assessed by measuring plasma, urine, or red blood cell concentrations.

▶ ASSESSMENT OF NUTRIENT REQUIREMENTS

- Assessment of nutrient requirements must be made in the context of patient-specific factors (e.g., age, sex, size, disease state, clinical condition, nutrition status, and physical activity).

ENERGY REQUIREMENTS

- Commonly used methods for determining energy requirements (i.e., caloric needs [kcal/kg body weight]) include mathematical calculation of basal energy expenditure (BEE) and indirect calorimetry.
- Adult energy requirements are approximately 25 kcal/kg for healthy individuals with normal nutrition, 30 kcal/kg for malnourished or mildly metabolically stressed individuals, 30–35 kcal/kg for critically ill or hypermetabolic individuals, and ≥40 kcal/kg for patients with major burn injury. This approach assumes no age- or sex-related differences in energy metabolism in adults.
- The formula (below) for calculating BEE includes patient-specific factors except for stress and activity levels. BEE should be adjusted upward ranging from 20% for patients confined to bed to 80–130% for patients with severe burn injuries.

Females: BEE (kcal/d) = 655 + 9.6 (wt in kg) + 1.8 (ht in cm) − 4.7 (age in y)

Males: BEE (kcal/d) = 66 + 13.7 (wt in kg) + 5 (ht in cm) − 6.8 (age in y)

- The most accurate clinical tool for estimating energy requirements is indirect calorimetry. This noninvasive procedure determines oxygen consumption (V_{O_2}, mL/min) and carbon dioxide production (V_{CO_2}, mL/min). Resting energy expenditure (REE, kcal/d) is calculated by the abbreviated Weir equation:

$$REE = [3.9(V_{O_2}) + 1.1 (V_{CO_2})] \times 1.44.$$

X

- Data from indirect calorimetry can also be used to determine a respiratory quotient (RQ):

$$RQ = V_{CO_2}/V_{O_2}.$$

RQ values >1.0 suggest a patient is being overfed, while values <0.7 may be indicative of a ketogenic diet.

PROTEIN, FLUID, AND MICRONUTRIENT REQUIREMENTS

- The usual recommended daily protein allowance for adults is 0.8–1.3 g/kg. It increases during periods of low (1.0–1.2 g/kg for maintenance and 1.3–1.7 g/kg for anabolism) or hypermetabolic stress (1.5–2.5 g/kg). Daily protein requirements also vary in patients with renal failure (0.6–1.3 g/kg without dialysis and 1.2–2.7 g/kg with dialysis) or severe hepatic failure (0.5–1.5 g/kg).
- Daily protein requirements can be individualized by measuring urinary nitrogen excretion in a 24-hour urine collection (UUN), which measures the dietary protein required to maintain homeostasis. Nitrogen output is approximated by the following:

$$\text{Nitrogen output (g/d)} = (UUN \times 1.20) + 1.$$

- Daily adult fluid requirements are approximately 30 mL/kg or 1 mL/kcal. Fluid requirements are increased in individuals with increased insensible or gastrointestinal losses. Fluid requirements are decreased in patients with renal failure, expanded extracellular fluid volume (e.g., congestive heart failure), or hypoproteinemia with starvation.
- Requirements for micronutrients (i.e., electrolytes, trace minerals, and vitamins) vary with route of administration (Table 56.8).   X

▶ EVALUATION OF THERAPEUTIC OUTCOME

- Assessment of nutrition requirements can be an acute process; however, ongoing reassessment will be required to ascertain whether nutrition goals have been achieved.
- Initially, nutrition requirements may be based on assumptions about the patient's clinical condition and nutrition needs associated with repletion.
- The importance of history and physical examination in both nutrition screening and nutrition assessment cannot be overemphasized.
- Those markers that show the best correlation with outcome are weight and serum albumin concentration. The cost effectiveness of more extensive biochemical evaluations remains to be determined. Assessment of other anthropometric measures is probably most useful in the setting of anticipated long-term nutrition support in which these measurements will serve as a longitudinal marker of response to therapy.

Nutritional Disorders

TABLE 56.8. Recommended Adult Daily Maintenance Doses for Electrolytes, Trace Minerals, and Vitamins

Nutrient	Enteral	Parenteral
Electrolytes		
Calcium	800–1200 mg	10–15 mEq
Chloride	1700–5100 mg	—
Fluoride	1.5–4.0 mg	—
Magnesium	280–350 mg	10–20 mEq
Phosphorus	800–1200 mg	20–45 mmol
Potassium	1875–5625 mg	60–100 mEq
Sodium	1100–3300 mg	60–100 mEq
Trace Minerals		
Chromium	50–200 µg	10–15 µg[a]
Copper	1.5–3 mg	0.5–1.5 mg
Iodine	150 µg	70–140 µg
Iron	10–15 mg	0.5 mg
Manganese	2–5 mg	0.15–0.8 mg
Molybdenum	75–250 µg	100–200 µg
Selenium	55–70 µg	40–80 µg
Zinc	12–15 mg	2.5–4.0 mg[b]
Vitamins		
Biotin	30–100 µg	60 µg
Cyanocobalamin (B_{12})	2.0 µg	5.0 µg
Folic acid	200 µg	400 µg
Niacin	13–19 mg NE	40 mg NE
Pantothenic acid (B_3)	4.7 mg	15 mg
Pyridoxine (B_6)	1.6–2.0 mg	4 mg
Riboflavin (B_2)	1.2–1.7 mg	3.6 mg
Thiamin (B_1)	1.0–1.5 mg	3 mg
Vitamin A	800–100 µg RE	600 µg RE (3300 IU)
Vitamin C	60 mg	100 mg
Vitamin D	5–10 µg	5 µg (200 IU)
Vitamin E	8–10 mg TE	10 mg TE (10 IU)
Vitamin K	60–80 µg	0.7–2.5 mg

Key: NE, niacin equivalents; RE, retinol equivalents; TE, tocopherol equivalent.

[a]An additional 20 µg chromium/d is recommended in patients with intestinal losses.

[b]An additional 12.2 mg zinc/L of small-bowel fluid lost and 17.1 mg zinc/kg of stool or ileostomy output is recommended; an additional 2.0 mg zinc/d for acute catabolic stress.

Adapted from Shronts EP, Lacey JA. Metabolic support, in Gottschlich MM, Matarese LE, Shronts EP (eds): Nutrition Support Dietetics—Core Curriculum, 2nd ed. Silver Spring, MD, ASPEN, 1993, p 358, with permission.

X

See Chapter 130, Assessment of Nutrition Status and Nutrition Requirements, authored by Kathleen M. Teasley-Strausburg, MS, RPh, BCNSP, and Jan D. Anderson, PharmD, BCNSP, for a more detailed discussion of this topic.

Chapter 57

▶ ENTERAL NUTRITION

▶ DEFINITION

Enteral nutrition and tube feeding are often used interchangeably to describe an artificial feeding method that includes use of specialized feeding formulas, tubes, and pumps.

▶ PATHOPHYSIOLOGY

- Digestion and absorption are important and inseparably associated gastrointestinal (GI) processes that generate usable fuels for the body.
- Digestion is the stepwise conversion of complex chemical and physical nutrients via mechanical, enzymatic, and physicochemical processes into molecular forms, which can be absorbed from the GI tract (Figure 57.1).
- Nutrients ultimately reach the systemic circulation through portal venous or splanchnic lymphatic systems, provided they are not excreted by the GI or biliary tract.
- The GI tract (GIT) also actively defends the body from toxins and antigens by nonimmunologic and immunologic mechanisms. Nonimmunologic mechanisms include mechanical mechanisms (e.g., epithelial cell, epithelial mucus gel layer, peristalsis, gastric acid, bile salts, and salivary secretions), and indigenous microflora that limit microbial proliferation and also antagonize exogenous microbes. Immunologic mechanisms include gut-associated lymphoid tissue, secretory immunoglobulin A, and hepatic Kupffer's cells.

▶ CLINICAL PRESENTATION AND DIAGNOSIS

Clinical presentation of protein-calorie malnutrition and nutrition assessment are discussed in Chapter 56.

▶ DESIRED OUTCOME

The goals of enteral tube feeding are to reverse protein calorie malnutrition, promote growth and development of infants and children, maintain adequate nutritional state, reduce disease-related morbidity and mortality, or some combination of these goals.

▶ TREATMENT

GENERAL PRINCIPLES

- Enteral nutrition is the preferred route of nourishment if the GI tract is functioning and accessible. Advantages of enteral over parenteral nutri-

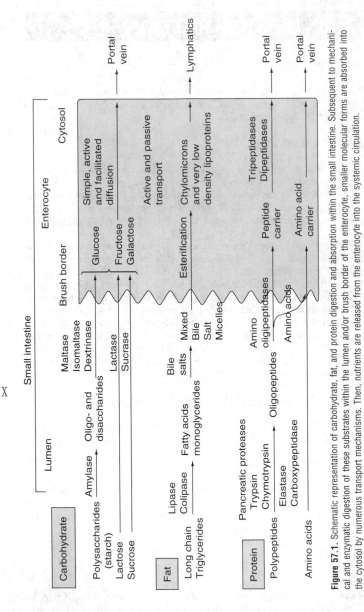

Figure 57.1. Schematic representation of carbohydrate, fat, and protein digestion and absorption within the small intestine. Subsequent to mechanical and enzymatic digestion of these substrates within the lumen and/or brush border of the enterocyte, smaller molecular forms are absorbed into the cytosol by numerous transport mechanisms. Then, nutrients are released from the enterocyte into the systemic circulation.

tion include maintaining GI tract structure and function, fewer metabolic and infectious complications, and lower costs.

- Although human data are insufficient to establish whether atrophic gut changes associated with lack of enteral nutrition lead to clinically significant translocation of gut bacteria, endotoxins, and antigenic macromolecules, these considerations currently justify the use of at least partial enteral nutrition to maintain gut mucosal function.
- Enteral nutrition is indicated for many conditions or disease states (Table 57.1). Its use is contraindicated for patients with mechanical obstruction of GI tract, diffuse peritonitis, severe diarrhea that makes metabolic management difficult, severe GI hemorrhage, intractable vomiting, chronic intestinal pseudo-obstruction, or severe malabsorption.
- Assessment of length, anatomy, and motility of GI tract is required prior to initiation of enteral therapy. Minimum length of functional small bowel required for nutrient absorption is approximately 100–150 cm of jejunum, ileum, or both.

FEEDING ROUTES

- Multiple feeding routes are available to provide enteral nutrition support, which are distinguishable by their indications, placement options, advantages, and disadvantages (Table 57.2).
- As the site of nutrient delivery is moved further away from the mouth, tube insertion becomes more difficult and invasive but, at the same time, more permanent.

TABLE 57.1. Potential Indications for Enteral Nutrition

Neoplastic Disease
  Chemotherapy
  Radiotherapy
  Upper gastrointestinal tumors
  Cancer cachexia

Organ Failure
  Hepatic
  Renal
  Cardiac cachexia
  Pulmonary
  Multiple organ system failure

Hypermetabolic States
  Closed head injury
  Burns
  Trauma
  Postoperative major surgery
  Sepsis

Gastrointestinal Disease
  Inflammatory bowel disease
  Short bowel syndrome
  Esophageal motility disorder
  Pancreatitis
  Fistulas

Neurologic Impairment
  Comatose state
  Cerebrovascular accident
  Demyelinating disease
  Severe depression
  Failure to thrive

Other Indications
  Acquired immune deficiency syndrome
  Anorexia nervosa
  Complications during pregnancy
  Geriatric patients with multiple chronic disease
  Organ transplantation

TABLE 57.2. Options and Considerations in the Selection of Tube Feeding Access

X

Access	Indications	Tube Placement Options	Advantages	Disadvantages
Nasogastric or orogastric	Short-term Intact gag reflex Normal gastric emptying	Manually at bedside	Ease of placement Allows for intermittent bolus or continuous feeding Inexpensive Multiple commercially available tubes and sizes	Potential tube displacement Increased aspiration risk Cosmetically unappealing Small bore tube
Nasoduodenal or nasojejunal	Short-term Delayed gastric emptying (early postoperative period or diabetic neuropathy) High risk gastroesophageal reflux or aspiration	Manually at bedside Fluoroscopic Endoscopic	Reduced aspiration risk Allows for early postoperative feeding Multiple commercially available tubes and sizes	Manual transpyloric passage requires greater skill Potential tube displacement Continuous (and cyclic) feeding only Cosmetically unappealing Attendant risks of complication for endoscopic placement Small bore tube
Esophagostomy or pharyngostomy	Long-term Nasopharyngeal access contraindicated Tumors or trauma of head or neck region	Bedside with local anesthesia or during surgery	Large bore tube Easy tube replacement	Dressing changes by patient more difficult due to location Cosmetically unappealing Requires stoma site care
Gastrostomy	Long-term Normal gastric emptying Swallowing dysfunction due to neuromuscular disease or central nervous system disorders Esophageal stricture or neoplasm	Surgically Endoscopically (percutaneous endoscopic gastrostomy [PEG]) Laparoscopically Fluoroscopically	Allows for intermittent, bolus, or continuous feeding Large bore tube Multiple commercially available tubes and sizes Low-profile buttons available	Cosmetically unappealing Attendant risks for complication for each method of placement Higher cost, particularly with surgical placement Aspiration risk potential Requires stoma site care
Jejunostomy	Long-term Impaired gastric emptying (diabetic neuropathy) Facilitate postoperative enteral feeding in trauma, malnourished or upper GIT surgery Inability to access upper GIT	Surgically Endoscopically (accessing jejunum via PEG) Laparoscopically Fluoroscopically	Allows for early postoperative feeding Reduced aspiration risk Multiple commercially available tubes and sizes	Cosmetically unappealing Attendant risks for complication for each method of placement Continuous (and cyclic) feeding only Requires stoma site care

- The most frequently used short-term enteral feeding routes are those accessed by inserting a tube through the nose and threading it into the stomach or upper small bowel (e.g., nasogastric, nasoduodenal, and nasojejunal routes).
- Modern feeding tubes are generally made of pliable silicone rubber or polyurethane. They are usually a small bore, which makes them lightweight and comfortable for patients. A disadvantage of small-bore tubes is that they may become clogged.
- The stomach is generally the least expensive and least labor-intensive access site for enteral feeding; however, it is not necessarily the best. Patients who have delayed gastric emptying are at higher risk for aspiration of gastric contents.
- Greater skill is required to place the feeding tube beyond the pylorus. Techniques to facilitate manual placement include use of styletted tubes, weighted tubes, placing the patient on his or her right side, and metoclopramide use.
- More permanent enteral feeding access includes esophagostomy or pharyngostomy, gastrostomy, and jejunostomy placement.

ADMINISTRATION METHODS

- Administration methods for tube feeding are continuous, continuous-cyclic, intermittent, and intermittent-bolus (Table 57.3). The choice depends on anatomic location of feeding tube, patient's clinical condition, environment in which patient resides, intestinal function, and patient's tolerance to tube feeding.
- Continuous tube feeding, which accounts for >80% of enteral feedings, provides maximal tolerance by minimizing abdominal distention or diarrhea. Continuous feeding is also beneficial for patients who have limited absorption capacity because of rapid GI transit time or severely impaired digestion.   X
- Cyclic enteral feedings allow physical and psychological breaks from being connected to the enteral infusion system, greater rehabilitation, and return to activities of daily living, especially if feeds are administered nocturnally. Cyclic feedings may require higher nutrient densities or higher infusion rates to compensate for periods when tube feedings are discontinued.
- Intermittent feeding should only be administered if the feeding tube tip is within the stomach because the stomach is capable of handling large and more rapid volumes of feeding formula. Patients who receive intermittent feeding may be at higher risk for complications such as nausea, vomiting, and aspiration.
- Bolus feedings have the advantage of requiring little administration time and minimal equipment. Unfortunately, bolus feedings may not be well tolerated and can result in cramping, nausea, vomiting, aspiration, and diarrhea.

TABLE 57.3. Administration Methods for Tube Feeding

Method	Equipment	Indication	Infusion Example
Continuous	Infusion pump generally recommended Enteral formula container Administration set	Gastric tube feeding Postpyloric tube feeding Critically ill patient Limited absorption capacity Limited feeding tolerance via intermittent and bolus methods	Full strength isotonic formula infused at 20 cc/h, advanced by 20 cc/h increments every 8 hours to desired goal rate as tolerated
Continuous-cyclic	Infusion pump generally recommended Enteral formula container Administration set	Gastric or postpyloric tube feeding Home tube feeding Rehabilitation patient Nocturnal tube feeding Potential transition to oral intake during daytime Limited feeding tolerance via bolus or intermittent method	Formula infused over 10–14 h daily at desired goal rate to achieve nutrient requirements
Intermittent	Infusion pump or gravity flow Enteral formula container Administration set	Gastric tube feeding Home tube feeding Rehabilitation patient Patient unlikely to transition to oral intake Limited feeding tolerance via bolus method	240–480 cc formula infused over 20–40 min 4–6 times daily
Intermittent-bolus	Large syringe (60 cc)	Gastric tube feeding Home tube feeding Rehabilitation patient Patient unlikely to transition to oral intake	240–280 cc formula infused over <10 min 4–6 times daily

X

EQUIPMENT AND FORMULAS

- Feeding equipment should be adaptable to multiple infusion sets and distinguishable from intravenous equipment. Feeding containers should be leakproof, unbreakable, and easy to clean; they should be equipped with reliable closures and easy-to-read volume markings. Administration sets should be long enough to easily connect the feeding container and patient, and equipped with an infusion control regulator. Enteral feeding pumps should be lightweight, easy to operate, and low maintenance; pumps should have long-lasting batteries and alarm systems.

- Modern enteral formulas are highly sophisticated and can include formula enhancements to optimize biological value and nutrient utilization. Macronutrient content (i.e., protein, carbohydrate, and fat) varies in nutrient complexity. Nutrient complexity refers to the amount of hydrolysis and digestion that a substrate source requires prior to intestinal absorption. Polymeric or intact substrates are of similar molecular form as the food we eat; other enteral formulas contain partially hydrolyzed or elemental substrates.

  - Osmolality is a function of size and quantity of ionic and molecular particles, and is primarily related to macronutrient and mineral content. Enteral formulas with partially hydrolyzed or elemental substrates have higher osmolality than formulas containing polymeric or intact substrate forms. Symptoms of gastric retention, diarrhea, abdominal distention, nausea, and vomiting have been ascribed to the relative osmolality; however, concurrent antibiotic therapy, delivery method, and other factors also affect tolerance.

  - Partially digested protein entities are the most readily absorbable form of nitrogen. Further reductions in the molecular form of protein increases osmotic load and prevalence of amino acids containing free sulfur, which in turn imparts a bitter flavor and foul odor to feeding solutions.

  - Conditionally essential amino acids (e.g., glutamine and arginine) are added to some formulas to maintain GI tract integrity and enhance nitrogen retention.

  - Partially digested carbohydrates are preferred over elemental sugars as the primary source of nonprotein calories because partially digested carbohydrates contribute less to osmolality. Glucose polymers are also useful because they have minimal osmotic loads and are easily absorbed in the intestine; however, glucose polymers are not as sweet or palatable as simple glucose. X

  - Fat provides a concentrated calorie source and serves as a carrier for fat-soluble vitamins. Most formulas contain some long-chain triglycerides (LCTs) to provide essential fatty acids. Potential advantages of medium-chain triglycerides over LCTs are greater water solubility; more rapid hydrolysis; and minimal requirement for pancreatic lipase, bile salt, or chylomicron formation for absorption.

  - Most commercially prepared formulas contain micronutrients (e.g., electrolytes, vitamins, and trace elements) to make them nutritionally complete.

  - Fiber provides several benefits including trophic effects on large bowel mucosa, promotion of sodium and water absorption in the colon, source of energy from resultant short-chain fatty acids, and possibly regulation of bowel motility.

  - Formulas with greater solute load increase the obligatory water loss via the kidney. Patients receiving high nitrogen enteral formulas may

TABLE 57.4. Enteral Formula Classification System

Category	Subcategories	Indication	Features	Product Examples
Polymeric (normal GIT digestive and absorptive capacity required)	Lactose-free	Standard oral supplement Complete tube feeding	Iso-osmolar, high nitrogen, fiber enhanced, and highly concentrated formulas available	Osmolite Resource IsoSource VHN Ultracal Deliver 2.0
	Lactose-containing	Oral supplement Lactose tolerant	Palatable, hyperosmolar	Sustogen Meritene
	Blenderized	Complete tube feeding	May contain lactose, high viscosity and may require infusion pump	Complete modified
Monomeric (less digestion and absorption required)	Chemically defined	Complete tube feeding and some use as oral supplements Disease states that alter digestive or absorptive surface capacity	Nutrients hydrolyzed to varying degrees Osmolarity varies	Peptamen Reabilan HN
	Elemental	Complete tube feeding, rarely as an oral supplement Disease states that alter digestive or absorptive surface capacity Fat malabsorption	Free amino acids, >80% of kcal as oligosaccharides, <15% fat content as long-chain fat	Vivonex Plus Tolerex

X

TABLE 57.4. continued

Specialized (monomeric or polymeric)	Organ failure	Complete ($\pm^a$) tube feeding, rarely as an oral supplement Specific products for pulmonary, renal, hepatic, and endocrine failure	Composition varies; nutrient requirements modified to a specific disorder	Pulmocare Travasorb Renal Nutrihep DiabetiSource
	Metabolic disorders	Complete ($\pm$) tube or oral feeding Management of inherited metabolic disorders such as tyrosinemia, phenylketonuria		Lofenalac Maxamaid XP
	Immune support	Complete tube feeding, rarely as an oral supplement Enhance immune competency during critical illness or sepsis	Specific nutrients modified for immunopharmacologic function	Immun-Aid Impact
Modular (majority are polymeric)	Protein Carbohydrate Fat	Generally feeding tube, can be used to compound complete ($\pm$) formulas or to supplement enteral or oral feeding	May be labor intensive Micronutrients available to make complete formulas	ProMod Polycose MCT oil
Hydration	Glucose Electrolytes	Feeding tube or oral Dehydration, severe or chronic diarrhea		Equalyte

^{a}: May or may not be complete nutrient composition.

X

707

be at risk for significant dehydration especially if they are elderly, have altered mental status, or are otherwise unable to ingest water.

- Enteral formulas categorized on the basis of composition and general indication for product prototypes can provide a template for enteral product formulary (Table 57.4).
  - Polymeric enteral feeding products contain macronutrients in the form of intact protein, triglycerides, and carbohydrate polymers. Polymeric products are used in numerous settings including patients who are critically ill, undergoing rehabilitation, and receiving home enteral nutrition support.
  - Monomeric enteral formulas have partially hydrolyzed and/or elemental macronutrients, which requires less digestive/absorptive capacity. Monomeric diets are not recommended for routine use in patients with normal GI function, those requiring early postoperative enteral feeding, or those with only mildly impaired pancreatic exocrine function, partial gastrectomy, and minor small intestinal resections. However, in pancreatectomized patients or those with markedly reduced GI surface area, the potential clinical benefit of monomeric products warrants a therapeutic trial.
  - Specialized enteral formulas containing arginine, ribonucleic acids, and omega-3 polyunsaturated fatty acids have been formulated to enhance immune competency during critical illness or sepsis. Glutamine has also been supplemented in some of these formulas to promote intestinal mucosal integrity and reduce infectious complications.
  - Modular formulas allow the clinician to enhance specific substrate content of readily available solutions by adding a single nutrient component (e.g., carbohydrate, protein, or fat).
  - Oral rehydration formulas may be used in dehydrated patients to reduce diarrheal sequelae or replenish ostomy drainage fluid and electrolyte losses.

INITIATION AND TITRATION OF ENTERAL NUTRITION REGIMEN

- Although advancement of enteral feeding should be individualized, one may start half-strength dilution at a rate of 25–50 mL/h, regardless of the actual formula employed. The rate is increased in 25 mL/h increments every 6–8 hours to a maximal rate with subsequent increase of formula strength for no more than 3 days.
  - Many patients tolerate more rapid advancement of a full-strength feeding formula from a rate of 20–25 mL/h with increments of 20–25 mL/h every 6–8 hours.
  - Hyperosmolar formulas may require slower advancement to prevent development of dumping syndrome.

DRUG COMPATIBILITY

- Mixing of commercially available liquid medications with selected enteral nutrition products has been associated with physical incompatibilities that may inhibit drug absorption and potentially clog small-bore enteral feeding tubes. Physical incompatibility is more common with formulas that contain intact protein (versus hydrolyzed protein) and with medications that are formulated as acidic syrups. Mixing of commercial liquid medications and enteral nutrition formulas should be avoided whenever possible, especially nonaqueous preparations and syrups.

- Problems may arise when medications are administered through enteral feeding tubes such as the degradation and/or inactivation of nutrient components or altered bioavailability of a drug that may compromise therapeutic efficacy (Table 57.5).
- Selecting the proper medication dosage form for administration by enteral feeding tubes is crucial to avoid drug inactivation and altered bioavailability (Table 57.6).
- The most significant drug and nutrient interactions that can occur during continuous enteral nutrition are those in which the bioavailability of the drug is reduced and the desired pharmacologic effect is not achieved (Table 57.7).

PREVENTION OF OTHER COMPLICATIONS

- Several factors responsible for metabolic complications associated with enteral nutrition are similar to those associated with parenteral nutrition. However, GI, technical, and infectious complications are unique to the enteral route of therapy (Table 57.8).

TABLE 57.5. General Considerations for Medication Administration by Enteral Feeding Tubes

1. Administer medications by mouth when feasible; consider enteral feeding tube as an alternative route.
2. Determine location of the feeding tube tip, because pre- or postpyloric drug instillation can alter effectiveness.
3. Use liquid dosage forms if available. Dosage and frequency adjustment are required if changing from a sustained-release drug to administer a non-sustained-release liquid form.
4. Dilute hyperosmolar medications.
5. Administer the contents of hard or soft gelatin capsules reconstituted with 10–15 mL of water and crushed compressed tablets reconstituted with 15–30 mL of water when a liquid form is unavailable.
6. Do not crush and administer sustained-release or enteric-coated medications.
7. Flush the feeding tube with water prior to administering a medication. Do not mix medications. Administer each medication separately, flushing with water between medications. Flush with water after medication administration completed.
8. In general, do not add medications to the enteral formula. Exceptions exist for the adding of hypertonic electrolyte injection to enteral formulas. Be aware of specific drug–enteral product incompatibilities.

TABLE 57.6. Guidelines for Medication Administration by Enteral Feeding Tubes

Dosage Form	Administered by Enteral Feeding Tube	Comment
Sublingual or buccal tablets	No	Low dosage of drug not designed for gastric or intestinal administration Altered drug bioavailability and potency due to first-pass effect
Sustained-release capsules or tablets	Not preferred Do not crush	Crushing can destroy its time-release effect Altered therapeutic drug response and gastrointestinal irritation can occur
Enteric-coated tablets	Not preferred Do not crush	Crushing can result in gastrointestinal irritation and drug inactivation
Compressed tablets (sugar or film coated)	Yes	May be crushed and administered without altering therapeutic drug response May clog small-bore feeding tubes
Hard or soft gelatin capsules	Yes	Powders from hard capsules and oils from soft capsules may be administered without altering therapeutic drug response

Liquid preparations
  Solutions
  Suspensions
  Elixirs
  Emulsions
	Yes
	Preferred
		Frequently recommended, however, drug form can be hyperosmolar requiring dilution
		Strong acid syrups may interact with enteral formulas and clog tubes

X
- Patients should be monitored for complications of enteral nutrition (Table 57.9), such as dumping syndrome, which is manifested clinically as nausea, cramping, lightheadedness, and diarrhea.
  - Pharmacologic intervention is occasionally indicated to control severe diarrhea. The primary agents employed are opiates, diphenoxylate, and loperamide.
  - Nausea and vomiting may be reduced by advancing the feeding tube beyond the pylorus.
  - Constipation may be reduced by using enteral formulas with enhanced fiber.
  - Techniques for clearing obstructed tubes include instilling water, meat tenderizer, or pancreatic enzymes, as well as passing an endoscopic cytology brush. Feeding tubes should be flushed during continuous tube feeding and medication administration to prevent occluded feeding tubes (Table 57.5).
  - Methods for preventing bronchopulmonary aspiration of gastric contents include use of small-bore feeding tubes, avoiding accumulation of large volumes in the stomach, keeping the head of the bed at

TABLE 57.7. Medications with Special Considerations for Enteral Feeding Tube Administration

Drug	Interaction	Comments
Phenytoin	Reduced bioavailability demonstrated when administered during continuous tube feeding. Results of in vitro studies suggest that protein (caseinate salts) and calcium chloride may reduce phenytoin bioavailability.	Limited data from clinical studies and case reports provide basis for suggestions to overcome incompatibility. Suggestions include holding tube feeding 2 h before and after phenytoin; administering phenytoin capsules rather than the suspension during continuous feeding; and using a meat-based enteral formula rather than a protein hydrolysate containing formula. Monitor patient's clinical response and serum drug level closely.
Antibiotics (selected)	Reduced bioavailability demonstrated between food and penicillin, tetracycline, isoniazid, rifampin, enoxacin, norfloxacin, and ofloxacin. Interaction also theoretically applied to continuous tube feeding.	Existence of clinical studies documenting enteral formula interaction with selected antibiotics is lacking. Holding tube feeding administration for specified time periods before and after drug administration has been recommended. Monitor patients clinical response closely.
Warfarin	Pharmacologic interaction demonstrated between warfarin and the vitamin K contained in enteral feeding formulas, resulting in reduced anticoagulation effect.	Vitamin K is contained in most enteral products in doses less than 200 μg per 1000 kcal. Adjust warfarin dose based on monitoring the INR and observing the vitamin K content of the enteral formula.
Antacids	Altered pharmacologic effect of antacid if administered into the small bowel. A physical incompatibility has been reported with aluminum-containing antacids causing an esophageal plug formation.	Administer antacids only into feeding tubes with the tip placed in the stomach. Administer aluminum-containing antacids after holding the tube feeding formula to prevent physical incompatibility formation.

X ◄

TABLE 57.8. Complications of Tube Feeding

Complications	Potential Causes
Metabolic	
Dehydration	Insufficient fluid intake or excessive fluid losses
Hyperglycemia	Underlying disease (diabetes mellitus)
	Drug induced (corticosteroids)
	Overfeeding
Increased serum electrolytes	Organ dysfunction (hepatic, renal, cardiac)
	Dehydration
Decreased serum electrolytes	Fluid overload due to excessive intake or organ dysfunction (hepatic, renal, cardiac)
	Extraordinary fluid losses (diarrheal, nasogastric)
	Refeeding syndrome
Decreased trace elements	Extraordinary fluid losses (diarrheal)
	Drug induced (diuretics)
Gastrointestinal	
Diarrhea	Drug related (antibiotic-induced bacterial overgrowth, antacids containing magnesium)
	Malabsorption (inadequate GIT surface area, rapid GIT transit)
	Tube feeding related (rapid formula administration, formula hyperosmolality)
Nausea and vomiting	Gastric dysmotility (surgery, anticholinergic drugs, diabetic gastroparesis)
	Rapid infusion of hyperosmolar formula
Constipation	Dehydration
	Drug induced (anticholinergics)
	Inactivity
	Low residue (fiber) content
	Obstruction/fecal impaction
Abdominal distention/cramping	Rapid formula administration
Technical	
Occluded feeding tube lumen	Insoluble complexation of enteral formula and medication(s)
	Inadequate flushing of feeding tube
	Undissolved feeding formula
Tube displacement	Self extubation
	Vomiting or coughing
	Inadequate fixation (jejunostomy)
Nasolabial, nasopharyngeal, or esophageal irritation	Prolonged local pressure of large-bore polyvinylchloride tube
Aspiration	Improper patient or feeding tube position
	Gastroparesis/atony causing regurgitation
	Compromised lower esophageal sphincter
	Diminished gag reflex
Peristomal excoriation	Improper skin and tube care
	GIT secretions leaking peristomally
Infectious	
Aspiration pneumonia	Same as technical-aspiration comments
Acute otitis media or sinusitis	Prolonged use of large-bore polyvinylchloride tube
Microbial contamination	Improper preparation, storage, or administration

X

TABLE 57.9. Suggested Monitoring of Enteral Nutrition (EN) to Prevent Complications

Parameter	During Initiation of EN or for a Critically Ill Patient	During Stable EN Therapy or for a Rehabilitating Patient	During Long-Term Home EN Therapy
Vital signs Temperature, respirations, pulse, blood pressure	Every 4–6 h	Every 12–24 h	Tailored to patient's clinical state, routinely done once or twice weekly
Physical exam[a] Abdomen, lung fields, extremities, mucous membranes, skin turgor	Every 4–6 h	Every 12–24 h	Tailored to patient's clinical state, routinely done once or twice weekly
Clinical assessment Weight Total intake/output Urine, gastrointestinal and extraordinary fluid losses Stool frequency/consistency/volume Nausea or vomiting	Daily	Daily	Tailored to patient's clinical state, routinely done once or twice weekly
Concurrent medications and administration route	Daily	Daily	Tailored to patient's clinical state, routinely done once or twice weekly
Verification of nasal or oral tube placement with x-ray	Prior to initiating EN	N/A[b]	N/A
Ongoing assessment by tube placement	Every 8 h	Every 12 h	Tailored to patient's clinical state, routinely done once or twice weekly

X

713

TABLE 57.9. continued

Parameter	During Initiation of EN or for a Critically Ill Patient	During Stable EN Therapy or for a Rehabilitating Patient	During Long-Term Home EN Therapy
Gastric residual checks	Every 8–12 h	Every 8–12 h	Daily by patient and/or caregiver
Enterostomy tube site assessment for leakage and/or skin irritation/redness	Daily	Daily	Daily by patient and/or caregiver
Patient compliance with feeding procedures and feeding tube/ostomy care	N/A	Daily	Tailored to patient's clinical state, routinely done once or twice weekly
Serum electrolytes, BUN/Cr, serum glucose[c]	Daily	2–3 times/wk	Tailored to patient's clinical state, routinely done weekly
Serum calcium, magnesium, and phosphorus	4–5 times/wk	2–3 times/wk	Tailored to patient's clinical state, routinely done weekly
Liver function tests	Weekly	Monthly	Tailored to patient's clinical state, routinely done monthly
Urine glucose/acetone[c]	Every 6 h	Daily	Tailored to patient's clinical state, routinely done 2–3 times/wk
Trace elements, vitamins	Frequency tailored to patient-specific situations	Frequency tailored to patient-specific situations	Frequency tailored to patient-specific situations

[a]Includes eyes, ear, nose, and throat exam for patients with nasoenteric feeding tubes.
[b]Not applicable.
[c]Frequency of glucose assessment for the nondiabetic patient.

X

TABLE 57.10. Suggested Monitoring of Enteral Nutrition (EN) to Promote Nutritional Efficacy

Parameter	During Initiation of EN or for a Critically Ill Patient	During Stable EN Therapy or for a Rehabilitating Patient	During Long-Term Home EN Therapy
Anthropometrics			
Weight	Daily	Weekly	Weekly
Triceps skinfold	N/A[a]	N/A	Every 1–2 months
Midarm muscle circumference	N/A	N/A	Every 1–2 months
Muscle function			
Level of physical endurance	N/A	Weekly	Weekly to monthly, then frequency tailored to the patient situation
Metabolic			
Albumin	Monthly	Monthly	Monthly, then frequency tailored to the patient response
Transferrin	Weekly	Weekly	Once to twice monthly, then frequency tailored to the patient response
24-h urine urea nitrogen	Weekly	Once or twice monthly	Frequency tailored to patient-specific situations
Indirect calorimetry	Frequency tailored to patient-specific situations	Frequency tailored to patient-specific situations	Frequency tailored to patient-specific situations
Nutritional intake			
Calories	Daily	2–3 times weekly	Weekly, then frequency tailored to the patient situation
Protein, fluid, electrolytes, trace elements, vitamins	Daily	2–3 times weekly	Weekly, then frequency tailored to the patient situation
Skin integrity Wound healing Pressure sore(s)	Daily	Daily	Weekly

[a]Not applicable.

X

715

30–45° during feeding and for 30–60 minutes after intermittent infusion, and infusing feedings into the small intestine instead of the stomach.

▶ EVALUATION OF THERAPEUTIC OUTCOMES

• Assessing outcome includes monitoring objective measures of body composition, protein and energy balance as well as subjective outcome for physiologic muscle function and wound healing (Table 57.10). Readers can find additional details on assessment in Chapter 56.

See Chapter 134, Enteral Nutrition, authored by Douglas D. Janson, PharmD, for a more detailed discussion of this topic.

▶ X

Chapter 58

▶ PARENTERAL NUTRITION

▶ DEFINITION

Parenteral nutrition (PN) provides macronutrients and micronutrients by central or peripheral venous access to meet specific nutritional requirements of the patient, promote positive clinical outcomes of an illness, or improve quality of life. Use of the intravenous route for nutrition support is also commonly referred to as total parenteral nutrition (TPN) or hyperalimentation.

▶ PATHOPHYSIOLOGY, CLINICAL PRESENTATION, AND DIAGNOSIS

- Pathophysiology of digestion and absorption is discussed in Chapter 57.
- The principles of nutrition assessment (see Chapter 56) are utilized to define nutrition goals for each patient.
- Although consensus reports do not fully agree and lack specificity in describing appropriate candidates for PN, guidelines established by the American Society for Parenteral and Enteral Nutrition (ASPEN) (Table 58.1) should facilitate development of institutional guidelines for selecting the appropriate route of delivery.
- The largest group of patients on home PN has cancer; the number with AIDS is increasing rapidly. Other candidates for home PN have Crohn's disease, ischemic bowel disease, severe gastrointestinal (GI) motility disorders, extensive intestinal obstruction, radiation enteritis, or congenital bowel dysfunction.

▶ DESIRED OUTCOME

- The overall objective of nutrition support therapy is to promote positive clinical outcomes of an illness or improve quality of life. Four fundamental steps for optimizing care are defining nutrition goals, determining nutrient requirements for achieving nutrition goals, delivering required nutrients, and assessing the nutrition regimen.
- Goals of nutrition support include correction of caloric and nitrogen imbalances, fluid or electrolyte abnormalities, and any known vitamin or trace element abnormalities, without causing or worsening other metabolic complications.
- Specific caloric goals include energy equilibrium and preservation of fat calorie stores in well-nourished individuals and positive energy balance in malnourished patients with depleted endogenous fat stores.
- Specific nitrogen goals are positive nitrogen balance or nitrogen equilibrium and improvement in serum concentration of protein markers (e.g., transferrin or prealbumin).

TABLE 58.1. Indications for TPN

1. Inability to absorb nutrients via the gastrointestinal tract because of one or more of the following:
   a. Massive small bowel resection.
   b. Intractable vomiting when adequate enteral intake is not expected for 5–7 days.
   c. Severe diarrhea not expected to resolve in 5–7 days.
   d. Inflammatory bowel disease (Crohn's disease, ulcerative colitis)
      PN may benefit patients with acute exacerbations of ulcerative colitis when surgery is being considered and when preservation of lean body mass and functional capacity with enteral nutrition is impossible.
   e. Bowel obstruction

2. Cancer—antineoplastic therapy, radiation therapy, bone marrow transplantation.
   Parenteral nutrition support may benefit some severely malnourished cancer patients or those in whom gastrointestinal or other toxicities are anticipated to preclude adequate oral nutritional intake for more than 1 week. If indicated, nutrition support should ideally be initiated in conjunction with oncologic therapy.
   Specialized nutrition support is not routinely indicated for well-nourished or mildly malnourished patients undergoing surgery, chemotherapy, or radiation treatment and in whom adequate oral intake is anticipated.
   PN is unlikely to benefit patients with advanced cancer whose malignancy is unresponsive to chemotherapy or radiation therapy.

3. Moderate to severe pancreatitis when adequate enteral intake is not expected for 5–7 days.
   PN should be used when enteral feeding exacerbates abdominal pain, ascites, or fistula output in patients with pancreatitis and limited oral intake.

4. Severe malnutrition[a] with a temporary (5–7 days) nonfunctional gastrointestinal tract.

5. Critical care
   Moderate to severe catabolism with or without malnutrition when the gastrointestinal tract is nonfunctional for 5–7 days (e.g., major surgery, trauma, sepsis).

6. Organ failures—liver, renal, respiratory
   Moderate to severe catabolism with or without malnutrition when enteral feeding is contraindicated.

7. Preoperative malnutrition[a] when the gastrointestinal tract is not functional and surgery is not expected for at least 7 days.

8. Hyperemesis gravidarum

9. Eating disorders
   PN should be considered for patients with anorexia nervosa who require nonvolitional feeding but who cannot tolerate enteral support for physical or emotional reasons.

---

[a]Malnutrition (upon initial assessment): 0–5% weight loss over past 6 months and serum albumin <3.0 g/% or 10–15% weight loss over past 6 months and serum albumin <3.5 g/%.

X

▶ TREATMENT

PARENTERAL NUTRITION COMPONENTS

- Both macronutrients (i.e., water, protein, dextrose, and intravenous lipid emulsion [IVLE]) and micronutrients (i.e., vitamins, trace elements, and electrolytes) are necessary for maintenance of normal metabolism.

Macronutrients

- Macronutrients are generally utilized for energy (dextrose, fat) and as structural substrates (protein, fats).

Amino Acids

- Protein is provided as crystalline amino acids (CAAs). Currently available standard products, which differ in amino acid, total nitrogen, and electrolyte content, are designed for patients with "normal" organ function (Table 58.2). Although optimal proportions of different amino acids have not been defined, these standard CAA products yield similar effects on protein markers.
- Nitrogen balance can be readily calculated based on the assumption that each gram of nitrogen is derived from 6.25 g of protein intake (Figure 58.1).
- Higher concentrated CAA solutions (i.e., 10% and 15%) can be useful for critically ill patients who typically require fluid restriction but have large protein needs.
- Modified amino acid solutions are designed for patients who have altered protein requirements owing to hepatic encephalopathy, renal failure, metabolic stress/trauma, or young age (i.e., neonates and children) (Table 58.3), however, these solutions tend to be expensive and their clinical role in disease-specific PN regimens is controversial.   X
- Although dipeptide amino acids have been investigated as a potential parenteral source for conditionally essential amino acids (CEAAs), further study is required to assess their long-term safety and effectiveness (Table 58.2).

Dextrose

- Carbohydrate, usually in the form of dextrose monohydrate, is available in concentrations ranging from 5–70%. When oxidized, each gram of hydrated dextrose provides 3.4 kcal.
- Recommended doses for routine clinical care rarely exceed 5 mg/kg/min; higher infusion rates may contribute to metabolic complications.
- Noninsulin-dependent sources of carbohydrate (e.g., xylitol, sorbitol, fructose, and glycerol) are currently being investigated for use in critically ill patients.

Lipid Emulsion

- Lipid emulsion may be used as a concentrated source of calories in a PN regimen as well as a source of essential fatty acids (EFAs).

TABLE 58.2. Macronutrient Components of Parenteral Nutrition Solutions

Nutritional Substrate	Intravenous Source	Commercial Product (Manufacturer)		Concentrations Available (%)
Fluid	Sterile water for injection USP			
Nitrogen	Crystalline amino acids	Various manufacturers		
		Aminosyn	(Abbott)	3.5, 5, 7, 8.5, 10
		Aminosyn II	(Abbott)	3.5, 5, 7, 8.5, 10, 15
		FreAmine III	(McGaw)	3, 8.5, 10
		Travasol	(Travenol)	5.5, 8.5, 10
		Novamine	(KabiVitrum)	15
		Investigational		
	Intravenous dipeptides			
	L-alanyl-L-glutamine			
	Glycyl-L-tyrosine	Used in Trophamine	(McGaw)	
	L-alanyl-L-tyrosine			
	N-acetyl-L-tyrosine			
Energy				
Carbohydrate	Dextrose	Various manufacturers		5, 10, 20, 25, 30, 50, 60, 70
	Glycerol	Used in Procalamine	(McGaw)	3% amino acids/3% glycerol
	Xylitol	Investigational		
Fat	Intravenous fat emulsion			
	LCT emulsions (oil source)			
		Intralipid	(Clintec)	10, 20, 30ᵃ
		(soybean)		
		Liposyn II	(Abbott)	10, 20
		(soybean/safflower)		
		Liposyn III	(Abbott)	10, 20
		(soybean)		
		Neutrilipid	(McGaw)	10, 20
		(soybean)		
		Soyacal	(Alpha Therapeutic)	10, 20
		(soybean)		
	LCT/MCT combination	Investigational		
	Short-chain fatty acids	Investigational		
	Omega 3 fatty acids	Investigational		

Key: LCT, long-chain triglycerides; MCT, medium-chain triglycerides; ( ), source of triglycerides.
ᵃApproved only for use in the preparation of total nutrient admixtures and is not intended for direct administration.

Nitrogen balance $-$ nitrogen$_{in}$ $-$ nitrogen$_{out}$

Nitrogen$_{in}$ (g/d) = protein$_{in}$ (g/d) $\div$ 6.25 g protein/g nitrogen

Nitrogen$_{out}$ (g/day) = urinary nitrogen + (nonurea nitrogen + insensible losses + integumentary losses)*

*Clinically, these measurements are usually estimated to be 2–7 g/d depending on the clinical condition of the patient (see Chapter 56).

Figure 58.1. Calculation of nitrogen balance.

TABLE 58.3. Modified Crystalline Amino Acid Solutions

Clinical Condition	Amino Acid Solution (Manufacturer)	Characteristics of Amino Acid Profile
Hepatic encephalopathy	Hepatamine 8% (McGaw)	Higher concentrations of BCAA and lower concentrations of AAA and methionine.
Renal failure	Aminosyn RF 5.2% (Abbott) NephrAmine 5.4% (McGaw) RenAmine 6.5% (Clintec) Aminess 5.2% (Clintec)	Higher concentrations of EAA and histidine.
Metabolic stress/trauma	Aminosyn HBC 7% (Abbott) FreAmine 6.9% HBC (McGaw) BranchAmin 4%[a] (Clintec)	Standard essential, semiessential, and nonessential amino acids with higher concentrations of BCAA.
Pediatrics	Aminosyn PF 7%, 10% Trophamine 6%, 10%	Standard essential, semiessential, and nonessential amino acids with lower concentrations of methionine, phenylalanine, and glycine. These solutions also contain taurine, glutamate, and aspartate.

Key: BCAA, branched-chain amino acids (leucine, isoleucine, valine); AAA, aromatic amino acids (includes phenylalanine and tyrosine); EAA, essential amino acids (leucine, isoleucine, valine, phenylalanine, tryptophan, methionine, threonine, and lysine).
[a]Used as a supplement to a standard amino acid solution to increase BCAA content.

- Current IVLE products differ in source of triglycerides, fatty acid content, and concentrations of fat source (10–30%) (see Table 58.2).
- When oxidized, 1 g of fat yields 9 kcal. Because of the caloric contribution from egg phospholipid and glycerol, caloric content of IVLE is about 1 kcal/mL per 10% emulsion.
- As a caloric source, lipid emulsion is probably most useful for metabolic stress, pancreatitis or diabetes, and carbon dioxide-retaining ventilator dependency.
- Essential fatty acid deficiency (EFAD) may be prevented by giving 500 mL of 10% IVLE two to three times weekly. Patients with clinical manifestations of EFAD usually respond after a 2-week course of IVLE, which provides 25% of total daily caloric requirements.
- Provision of approximately 1–1.5 g/kg/d, not to exceed 30–40% of total calories, infused over 24 hours appears to be a reasonable compromise in view of the lack of clear data concerning effects of rapid infusion on immunocompetency (and thereby on morbidity and mortality) in humans and the clinical utility of IVLE as a noncarbohydrate source.
- Infusions over 24 hours eliminate the need for a test dose.
- Commercially available 10% and 20% IVLE products may be administered by central or peripheral vein, added directly to PN solution as a total nutrient admixture (TNA) or 3-in-1 system (lipids, protein, glucose, and additives), or piggybacked with the CAA/dextrose solution.
- IVLE use is contraindicated if patients have impaired ability to clear lipid emulsion or history of severe egg allergy.

Micronutrients: Vitamins, Trace Elements, and Electrolytes
- Micronutrients are usually required in small amounts to support a variety of metabolic activities necessary for cellular homeostasis such as enzymatic reactions, fluid balance, and regulation of electrophysiologic processes.
- Multiple vitamin products (e.g., MVI-12, MVC 9+3, and MVI-pediatric) have been formulated to comply with guidelines established by the Nutrition-Advisory Group of the American Medical Association (NAG–AMA). These products do not contain vitamin K, which may be given intramuscularly or subcutaneously or added to the PN solution; weekly dose recommendations for adults range from 2–4 mg to 5–10 mg.
- Routine use of trace elements during short-term PN is controversial. Requirements for trace elements are age specific and may change depending on the clinical condition of the patient (e.g., higher doses of supplemental zinc are probably necessary in patients with high-output ostomies or diarrhea). Because requirements for trace elements during organ failure are not clearly defined, the recommended daily dose of a multiple trace element solution may be reduced empirically and given two to three times weekly.
- Patients who have normal organ function and relatively normal serum concentrations of any electrolyte should receive normal maintenance doses of electrolytes on initiation of PN and daily thereafter. Require-

X

ments for specific electrolytes will vary according to the disease state, organ function, previous and current drug therapy, nutrition status, and extrarenal losses of the patient.

DESIGNING PN REGIMENS

- Peripheral PN (PPN) is a relatively safe and simple method of nutritional support. PPN candidates do not have large nutritional requirements, are not fluid restricted, and are expected to begin enteral intake within 7–10 days. Advantages of PPN include avoidance of the risk of infectious, metabolic, and technical complications associated with central vein catheterization. Complications include limited peripheral venous access in some patients, relatively poor tolerance of peripheral veins to hypertonic solutions, and thrombophlebitis.
- Central PN (CPN) is useful in patients who require PN for >7–10 days during hospitalization or indefinitely at home, who have large nutrient requirements and in whom fluid volume is of concern, and who have major organ failure and metabolic stress (e.g., extensive surgery, trauma, sepsis, or malignancy). Disadvantages of CPN include risks of catheter insertion, routine use of catheter, and care of the access site.
- Formulas (Figure 58.2) and computer programs are available for calculating volumes of solutions for PN regimens.
- If CAA/dextrose is infused separately from IVLE, two clinically useful and highly concentrated base solutions are 7% CAA/15% dextrose (final concentrations), which can be prepared from 10% CAA and 70% dextrose stock solutions, or 8% CAA/25% dextrose (final concentrations), compounded from 15% CAA and 70% dextrose stock solutions.

COMPOUNDING AND STORING PN SOLUTIONS

- The two major PN solutions are traditional CAA/dextrose combination with or without IVLE piggybacked into the PN line, and TNAs.
- Advantages of TNA solutions include reduced inventory (infusion pumps, tubing, and other related supplies), decreased time for compounding and administration, potential decrease in infusion-line manipulations and decreased risk of catheter contamination, and ease of delivery and storage for home PN. Disadvantages include infectious, stability, and compatibility concerns. For example, the opaque solution that results after adding IVLE makes detection of particulate matter difficult, and TNA solutions cannot be filtered with a bacterial retentive 0.22-μm filter.
- Bacterial growth is least likely with CAA/dextrose, greatest with IVLE, and intermediate with TNA. CAA/dextrose solutions that are not administered within 1 hour after admixing should be refrigerated and used within 24 hours of compounding. Many institutions allow expiration times up to 24 hours for IVLE infusions. TNA can be safely administered over 24 hours without greater risk of contamination than with CAA/dextrose solutions.
- Because of their complex compositions, PN solutions are prone to problems with stability and compatibility. CAA/dextrose solutions are

The total daily volume of a PN solution may be determined based upon a patient's maintenance fluid requirements or an approximation of the minimum volume may be determined by calculating the volumes of stock solutions required to provide the daily nutrients desired as illustrated below.

Pt. Case: A patient's estimated nutritional requirements have been assessed at approximately 95–105 g protein/day and 1800–2100 nonprotein kcal/day. The patient has no history of hyperlipidemia or allergy to eggs and is not fluid restricted. The PN solution will be compounded as an individualized regimen utilizing a single bag, 24-hour infusion of a crystalline amino acid (CAA)/dextrose combination with intravenous lipid emulsion (IVLE) piggy-backed into the PN infusion line. The stock solutions used to compound this regimen are 10% CAA and 70% Dextrose.

- Step 1: Determine the volume of IVLE required

    2000 kcal/day × 30–40% of total as fat = 600–800 kcal*

The most clinically reasonable choice of IVLE product for this regimen is IVLE 20% 250 mL/day or IVLE 10% 500 mLs/day.

IVLE 20% 250 mL/day × 2 kcal/mL= 500 kcal/day; IVLE 10% 500 mL/day × 1.1 kcal/mL = 550 kcal/day

X

2000 kcal/day	Estimated daily nonprotein calorie requirements
−500 kcal/day	IVLE calories
1500	kcal needed from dextrose

- Step 2: Calculate the volume of 10% CAA stock solution required to provide 100 g protein

$$\frac{100 \text{ g protein}}{X \text{ mL}} = \frac{10 \text{ g protein}}{100 \text{ mL}} \qquad X = 1000 \text{ mL } 10\% \text{ CAA}$$

Figure 58.2. Calculations for compounding a parenteral nutrition regimen.

- Step 3: Calculate the volume of 70% dextrose required to provide 1500 calories

$$\begin{array}{l} 1500 \text{ kcal/day} \\ \div\ 3.4 \text{ kcal/g dextrose} \\ \overline{441 \text{ g dextrose}} \end{array} \qquad \dfrac{441 \text{ g dextrose}}{X \text{ mL}} = \dfrac{70 \text{ g dextrose}}{100 \text{ mL}}$$

$$X = 630 \text{ mL } 70\% \text{ dextrose}$$

- Step 4: Determine the infusion rate

Total base volume:

$$\begin{array}{ll} & 1000 \text{ mL} \quad 10\% \text{ CAA} \\ + & 630 \text{ mL} \quad 70\% \text{ dextrose} \\ \hline & 1630 \text{ mL base solution} \end{array}$$

$$+\ 50\text{--}100 \text{ mL/L for additives}$$

Total PN volume = 1700–1800 mL/day or 70–75 mL/h

- Step 5: Calculate the PN order

Choose 75 mL/hr or 1800 mL/day for PN volume

$$\dfrac{100 \text{ g Protein}}{1800 \text{ mL}} = \dfrac{X \text{ g protein}}{100 \text{ mL}} \qquad \begin{array}{l} X = 5.6\% \text{ CAA} \\ \text{(round down to 5.5\%)} \end{array} \qquad X$$

$$\dfrac{441 \text{ g Dextrose}}{1800 \text{ mL}} = \dfrac{X \text{ g Dextrose}}{100 \text{ mL}} \qquad \begin{array}{l} X = 24.5\% \\ \text{(round up to 25\%)} \end{array}$$

Final PN order (base solution): 5.5% CAA/25% dextrose at 75 mL/h + IVLE 20% 250 mL/day

This regimen provides approximately 99 g protein/day and 2030 nonprotein calories/day

---

* See text for IVLE dosing guidelines.

Figure 58.2. continued

generally stable for 1–2 months if refrigerated at 4°C and protected from light.

- Factors affecting TNA solution stability include pH, electrolyte charges, temperature, and time after compounding. In general, electrolytes (except phosphorus) and trace elements should be added to the dextrose solution, phosphate should be added to the CAA solution, and, finally, the amino acid solution should be added to the IVLE before or with the dextrose solution. TNA solutions should be infused within 24–48 hours after compounding, but certain TNA solutions have acceptable stability for 10–28 days when refrigerated at 4–5°C.
- Risk factors for precipitation of calcium and phosphorus include high concentrations of calcium and phosphorus salts, use of chloride salt of calcium, decreased amino acid concentrations, increased solution temperature, increased solution pH, use of improper sequence when mixing calcium and phosphorus salts, and presence of other additives including IVLE.
- Sodium bicarbonate should not be added to PN solutions. Use of a bicarbonate precursor salt (e.g., acetate) is usually preferred.
- Vitamins may be adversely affected by changes in solution pH, presence of other additives, storage time, solution temperature, and exposure to light. Vitamins should be added to PN solution near the time of administration and should not be in the PN solution >24 hours.
- Advantages of using PN admixtures as drug vehicles include consolidation of dosage units, improved pharmacotherapy for certain drugs, conservation of fluid in volume-restricted patients, fewer venous catheter violations, and decreased compounding and administration time. However, a major disadvantage is lack of compatibility and stability data in the PN solutions. Medications frequently added to PN solutions include albumin, aminophylline, hydrochloric acid, regular insulin, and histamine-2 antagonists.

ADMINISTERING PN SOLUTIONS

- PN solutions should be administered with an infusion pump.
- A 0.22-μm filter is recommended for CAA/dextrose solutions to remove particulate matter, air, and microorganisms.
- Because IVLE particles measure approximately 0.5 μm, IVLE should be administered separately and piggybacked into the PN line beyond the in-line filter.
- Routine use of in-line filters (>0.22 μm) with TNA solutions is controversial. A 1.2-μm filter may prevent catheter occlusion due to precipitates or lipid aggregates, and may also remove *C. albicans.* Alternatively, a 5-μm filter can be used to minimize occlusion alarms from infusion pumps and to remove particles that may obstruct pulmonary capillaries.
- Although protocols for initiating PN differ, many institutions gradually increase the rate during a period of 24–48 hours to prevent development of hyperglycemia.

- Cyclic PN (e.g., for 12- to 18-hours each day) is useful in hospitalized patients who have limited venous access and who require other medications necessitating interruption of PN infusion, to prevent or treat hepatotoxicities associated with continuous PN therapy, and to allow home patients to resume normal lifestyles. Cyclic PN may be poorly tolerated by patients with severe glucose intolerance or unstable fluid balance.

COMPLICATIONS

- Mechanical or technical complications include malfunctions in the delivery system (e.g., infusion pump, administration sets or tubing, and catheter). Catheter-related complications are potentially life-threatening and include pneumothorax, catheter misdirection into the wrong vein or ill-positioned within the cardiac chambers, arterial puncture, bleeding, hematoma formation, venous thrombosis, and air embolism.
- Infectious complications can be a major hazard in patients receiving central PN. Infections commonly occur when the catheter becomes colonized by direct microbial invasion of the skin at the insertion site or at the infusion site of the catheter.
- Metabolic complications are numerous, potentially fatal if not treated, and related to substrate intolerance (Table 58.4) and fluid, electrolyte, and acid–base disorders (Table 58.5).

▶ EVALUATION OF THERAPEUTIC OUTCOMES

- Routine evaluation should include the assessment of the clinical condition of the patient, with a focus on nutritional and metabolic effects of the PN regimen.
- A variety of biochemical and clinical measurements are necessary for effective monitoring of patients receiving PN (Table 58.6).
- Patients receiving their first dose of IVLE should be monitored for acute adverse reactions such as dyspnea, tightness of chest, palpitations, and chills. Headache, nausea, and fever have also been reported and may be associated with a rapid infusion rate. Hepatic abnormalities such as elevated transaminases, hepatomegaly, and intrahepatic cholestasis have been reported with multiple infusions, although these alterations are transient and are usually associated with excessive doses.

See Chapter 133, Parenteral Nutrition, authored by Todd W. Mattox, PharmD, BCNSP, for a more detailed discussion of this topic.

TABLE 58.4. Substrate Intolerance in Parenteral Nutrition

Complication	Possible Causes	Intervention
Hyperglycemia	Stress, infection, corticosteroids, pancreatitis, diabetes mellitus, peritoneal dialysis, excessive dextrose administration	Decrease dextrose load by decreasing infusion rate or dextrose concentration (may substitute fat calories); administer insulin
Hypoglycemia (rare)	Abrupt withdrawal of dextrose, insulin overdose	Increase dextrose intake; decrease exogenous insulin
Excess of carbon dioxide production	Excess dextrose intake	Decrease dextrose intake; balance calories from fat and dextrose
Hyperlipidemia (elevated cholesterol and triglyceride)	Stress, familial hyperlipidemia, pancreatitis	Decrease intake of fat or discontinue if indicated
Serum amino acid imbalance	Stress, hepatic failure	Modify amino acid intake if possible or decrease intake of amino acids
Abnormal liver function tests (elevated AST, alkaline phosphatase, and bilirubin)	Stress, infection, cancer, excess carbohydrate intake, excess caloric intake, essential fatty acid deficiency	Decrease dextrose load (substitute fat); decrease total calories; provide essential fatty acids

Key: AST, aspartate aminotransferase (SGOT).
Adapted from Teasley-Strausburg KM, Shronts EP. Metabolic and gastrointestinal complications, in Teasley-Strausburg KM (ed): Nutrition Support Handbook: A Compendium of Products with Guidelines for Usage. Cincinnati, OH, Harvey Whitney Books Company, 1992, pp 298–299, with permission.

X

TABLE 58.5. Fluid, Electrolyte, and Acid–Base Abnormalities

Problem	Possible Causes	Intervention
Hypovolemia	Gastrointestinal fluid losses, osmotic diuresis	Increase fluid intake
Hypervolemia	Renal failure, excess fluid intake	Decrease fluid intake and diuretics
Hyponatremia	Gastrointestinal losses, fluid overload, diuretics	Varies with cause
Hypernatremia	Dehydration	Increase fluid intake
Hypokalemia	Gastrointestinal losses, diuretics, anabolism	Increase potassium intake
Hyperkalemia	Renal failure	Decrease potassium intake
Hypophosphatemia	Phosphate-binding antacids, anabolism, phosphate-free dialysate	Discontinue phosphate binders, increase phosphorus intake
Hyperphosphatemia	Renal failure	Decrease phosphorus intake
Hypomagnesemia	Diarrhea, malabsorption, anabolism	Increase magnesium intake
Hypermagnesemia	Renal failure	Decrease magnesium intake
Hypocalcemia	Hypoalbuminemia, chronic renal failure	Increase calcium intake (with chronic renal failure only)
Hypercalcemia	Rare	Decrease calcium intake
Metabolic acidosis	Diarrhea, high-output fistulae, renal failure, excess amino acid intake	Treat underlying causes; increase acetate and decrease Cl in TPN solution; decrease amino acid intake
Metabolic alkalosis	Gastric losses	Treat underlying cause; increase Cl and decrease acetate in TPN solution

X

Adapted from Teasley-Strausburg KM, Shronts EP. In Teasley-Strausburg KM (ed):. Nutrition Support Handbook: A Compendium of Products with Guidelines for Usage. Cincinnati, OH, Harvey Whitney Books Company, 1992:298–299, with permission.

TABLE 58.6. Routine Monitoring Data for Parenteral Nutrition

Every Day	2–3 Times/Wk	Every Week
Weight	Complete blood count	Nitrogen balance
Vital signs (temperature, pulse, respirations)	Clotting studies (PT/PTT, platelets)	Total protein
	Creatinine	Albumin
Fluid	Calcium	Transferrin or prealbumin
Nutritional intake	Phosphorus	Liver biochemical tests
kcal, protein, fat	Magnesium	Alkaline phosphatase
Electrolytes, vitamins		AST
Trace elements		ALT
Serum electrolytes		LDH
Sodium		Bilirubin
Potassium		Other tests as warranted
Chloride		
Bicarbonate		
Glucose		
BUN		
Urine glucose, acetone (every 6 h)		
Output		
Urine		
Gastrointestinal		
Other losses		

Key: PT, prothrombin time; PTT, partial thromboplastin time; AST, aspartate aminotransferase (SGOT); ALT, alanine aminotransferase (SGPT); LDH, lactate dehydrogenase; BUN, blood urea nitrogen.

X

Oncologic Disorders
Edited by Terry L. Schwinghammer, PharmD, FCCP, BCPS

Chapter 59

▶ BREAST CANCER

▶ DEFINITION

Breast cancer is the most common cancer and the second leading cause of cancer death in women. It is potentially curable in the early stages, but metastatic breast cancer is usually incurable.

▶ PATHOPHYSIOLOGY

- The two strongest risk factors are female gender and increasing age. Additional risk factors include endocrine factors (e.g., early menarche, nulliparity, late age at first birth, estrogen therapy), environment (e.g., diet, alcohol consumption, radiation exposure), and genetics (personal and family history).
- A tumor suppresser gene known as the BRCA1 gene may be important in the development of inherited and perhaps sporadic breast and ovarian cancer.
- Spread of breast cancer via the bloodstream occurs early in the course of the disease. This results in relapse with systemic metastatic disease after local curative therapy. Tissues most commonly involved with metastases are lymph nodes, skin, bone, liver, lungs, and brain.
- The likelihood of later development of metastatic disease is related to size of the primary tumor, presence or absence of lymph node involvement, and the presence of additional prognostic factors as described below.

▶ CLINICAL PRESENTATION

- The initial sign in >90% of women with breast cancer is a painless lump that is typically solitary, unilateral, solid, hard, irregular, and non-mobile. In approximately 10% of cases, stabbing or aching pain is the first symptom. Less commonly, nipple discharge, retraction, or dimpling may be noted. In more advanced cases, prominent skin edema, redness, warmth, and induration may be observed.
- 90% of women first detect some breast abnormalities themselves, underscoring the importance of breast self-examination.
- It is increasingly common for breast cancer to be detected during routine screening mammography in asymptomatic women.
- Symptoms of bone pain, difficulty breathing, abdominal enlargement, jaundice, and mental status changes may occur in metastatic breast cancer.

▶ DIAGNOSIS

- Initial work-up for a woman presenting with a localized lesion or other suggestive symptoms should include a careful history and physical examination of the breast and three-dimensional mammography. Other breast imaging techniques such as ultrasound may also provide useful information.
- Breast biopsy is indicated for a mammographic abnormality that suggests malignancy or for a mass that is palpable on physical examination.

▶ STAGING

- Stage is defined on the basis of the size of the primary tumor (T1–4), presence and extent of lymph node involvement (N1–3), and presence or absence of distant metastases (M) (Figure 59.1 and Table 59.1). Simplistically stated, these stages may be represented as:

  Early Breast Cancer
  Stage 0: Carcinoma in situ or disease that has not invaded the basement membrane.
  Stage I: Small primary tumor without lymph node involvement.
  Stage II: Metastasis to ipsilateral axillary lymph nodes.

  Advanced Breast Cancer
  Stage III: Usually a large tumor with extensive nodal involvement in which either node or tumor is fixed to the chest wall *(locally advanced disease)*.
  Stage IV: Metastases to organs distant from the primary tumor.

- The approximate percent of patients presenting with each stage of breast cancer and an estimate of their 5-year disease-free survival (DFS) is shown in Table 59.2.

▶ PATHOLOGIC EVALUATION

- The pathologic evaluation of breast lesions serves to establish the histologic diagnosis and to confirm the presence or absence of prognostic factors.

INVASIVE CARCINOMA

- Most breast carcinomas are adenocarcinomas and are classified on the basis of their microscopic appearance as either ductal or lobular. The five most common types of invasive breast cancer include:
  - *infiltrating ductal carcinoma* (75% of cases)
  - *infiltrating lobular carcinoma* (5–10%)
  - *tubular carcinoma* (2%)

XI

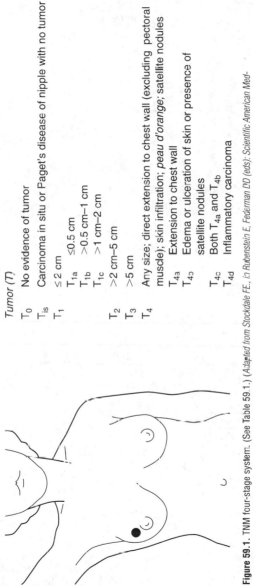

Tumor (T)

T_0 No evidence of tumor

T_{is} Carcinoma in situ or Paget's disease of nipple with no tumor

T_1 ≤2 cm

    T_{1a} ≤0.5 cm

    T_{1b} >0.5 cm–1 cm

    T_{1c} >1 cm–2 cm

T_2 >2 cm–5 cm

T_3 >5 cm

T_4 Any size; direct extension to chest wall (excluding pectoral muscle); skin infiltration; *peau d'orange*; satellite nodules

    T_{4a} Extension to chest wall

    T_{4b} Edema or ulceration of skin or presence of satellite nodules

    T_{4c} Both T_{4a} and T_{4b}

    T_{4d} Inflammatory carcinoma

Figure 59.1. TNM four-stage system. (See Table 59.1.) (*Adapted from Stockdale FE., in Rubenstein E, Federman DD (eds): Scientific American Medicine. New York, Scientific American, 1991:1–17, with permission.*)

XI

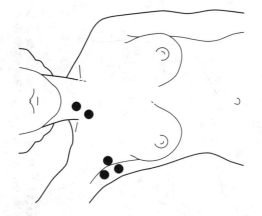

Nodes (N)

N_0 No regional lymph node metastasis

N_1 Metastasis to movable ipsilateral axillary lymph node or nodes

N_2 Metastasis to ipsilateral axillary node or nodes fixed to one another or other structures

N_3 Metastasis to ipsilateral internal mammary node or nodes

Figure 59.1. continued

Metastasis (M)

M₀   No distant metastases

M₁   Distant metastasis, including metastasis to ipsilateral
       supraclavicular lymph node or nodes

Figure 59.1. continued

XI

TABLE 59.1. Stages of Primary Breast Cancer

	T	N	M
Stage 0	T_{is}	N_0	M_0
Stage I	T_1	N_0	M_0
Stage IIA	T_0	N_1	M_0
	T_1	N_1	
	T_2	N_0	
Stage IIB	T_2	N_1	M_0
	T_3	N_0	
Stage IIIA	T_0	N_2	M_0
	T_1	N_2	
	T_2	N_2	
	T_3	N_1, N_2	
Stage IIIB	T_4	Any N	M_0
	Any T	N_3	
Stage IV	Any T	Any N	M_1

[a]See Fig. 59.1.
Adapted from Stockdale FE. Breast cancer, in Rubenstein E, Federman DD (eds): Scientific American Medicine. New York, Scientific American, 1991, pp 1–17, with permission.

- *medullary carcinoma* (5–7%)
- *mucinous* (or *colloid*) *carcinoma* (about 3%)
- Paget's disease of the breast (1–4% of all breast cancer cases) is manifested by a relatively long history of eczematous changes in the nipple with itching, burning, oozing, and/or bleeding that is associated with a palpable lesion.
- Inflammatory breast cancer is characterized clinically by prominent skin edema, redness and warmth, visible erysipeloid margin, and induration of the underlying tissue. Biopsies of the involved skin reveal cancer cells in the dermal lymphatics.

XI

TABLE 59.2. Estimated Stage at Presentation and 5-Year Disease-Free Survival: Breast Cancer 1994

	Percent of Total Cases	5-Year DFS[a] (%)
Stage I	40	70–90
Stage II	40	50–70
Stage III	15	20–30
Stage IV	5	0–10[b]

[a] With current conventional local and systemic therapy.
[b] Patients in stage IV are rarely free of disease, however, 10–20% of these patients may survive with minimal disease for 5–10 years.

NONINVASIVE CARCINOMA

- Noninvasive lesions may also be divided into ductal and lobular categories. In situ carcinoma (ductal and lobular) has also been referred to as intraductal carcinoma.
- These lesions histologically appear as their invasive counterparts, however invasion through the basement membrane is absent.

PATHOLOGIC PROGNOSTIC FACTORS

- Tumor size and the presence and number of involved axillary lymph nodes are primary factors in assessing the risk for breast cancer recurrence and subsequent metastatic disease.
- Response to hormonal manipulation and duration of disease-free survival (DFS) are highly correlated with the presence of both positive estrogen receptor (ER) protein and positive progesterone receptor (PR) protein. Approximately 70–80% of patients who are ER positive and PR positive will respond to hormonal manipulation. PR negative patients rarely respond, and patients who are ER negative and PR positive lie somewhere in between.
- The rate of tumor cell proliferation can be determined by either the tritiated-thymidine labeling index (TLI) or DNA flow cytometry, which determines the percentage of tumor cells actively dividing (S-phase fraction). Patients with rapidly proliferating tumors have a decreased DFS compared to patients with slowly proliferating tumors. Flow cytometry can also detect abnormal DNA content, or aneuploidy, in breast cancer cells, which may be associated with shorter relapse-free survival times than for patients with diploid tumors.
- Additional potential prognostic factors include nuclear grade and tumor (histologic) differentiation, overexpression of the HER-2/*neu* oncogene and the c-ERB-B2 protein, the epidermal growth factor receptor (EGFR), cathepsin-D, angiogenic growth factors, and mutations in the tumor suppressor *p53* gene.

▶ DESIRED OUTCOME

XI

The goal of therapy with early and locally advanced breast cancer is to cure the patient of the disease. However, once breast cancer has advanced beyond a local-regional disease, it is currently incurable. The goals of treatment of metastatic breast cancer are to improve symptoms and quality of life and prolong survival.

▶ TREATMENT

TREATMENT OF EARLY BREAST CANCER

Local-Regional Therapy

- Surgery alone can cure most, if not all, patients with in situ cancers and approximately half of all patients with stage II cancers.

- *Breast conservation* is an appropriate primary therapy for the majority of women with stages I and II disease; it is preferable to modified radical mastectomy because it produces equivalent survival rates with cosmetically superior results. Breast conservation consists of lumpectomy (also referred to as segmental mastectomy or partial mastectomy) and is defined as excision of the primary tumor and adjacent breast tissue followed by radiation therapy to reduce the risk of local recurrence. Sampling of axillary lymph nodes is recommended for completeness of staging and prognostic information.
- *Simple* or *total mastectomy* involves removal of the entire breast without resection of the underlying muscle or axillary nodes. This procedure is used in patients with carcinoma in situ where there is a 1% incidence of axillary node involvement, or in cases of local recurrence following breast conservation therapy. Simple mastectomy may be a reasonable alternative for women who wish to avoid the inconvenience of radiation therapy and preserve their option for breast reconstruction in the future.

Systemic Adjuvant Therapy

- Systemic adjuvant therapy is the administration of systemic therapy following definitive therapy (surgery, radiation, or both) when there is no evidence of metastatic disease but a high likelihood of recurrence owing to the presence of undetectable micrometastases. The goal of such therapy is cure of disease.
- According to a large overview analysis, in women <50 years of age, adjuvant chemotherapy alone reduces the annual odds of recurrence by 37% and the annual odds of death by 27%. In contrast, tamoxifen alone reduces the annual odds of recurrence by 27% and the annual odds of death by 17%. Ovarian ablation (oophorectomy) has approximately the same magnitude of benefit as chemotherapy in this age group.
- In women ≥50 years old, adjuvant tamoxifen reduces the annual odds of recurrence by 30% and the annual odds of death by 19%. Chemotherapy offers smaller benefits in this group reducing the annual odds of recurrence and death by 22% and 14%, respectively.
- Between the ages of 50 and 69, chemotherapy plus tamoxifen is superior to chemotherapy alone for both recurrence and mortality and better than tamoxifen alone for recurrence.
- The overview also demonstrated that the proportional benefits of chemotherapy in node negative and node positive patients are comparable, combination chemotherapy is superior to single agents, and adjuvant treatment duration of 12–24 months is no more effective than 6 months of treatment. Indirect comparisons showed that long-term tamoxifen (2–5 years) is significantly more effective than tamoxifen treatment programs of shorter duration and that tamoxifen doses >20 mg are not associated with better responses than 20-mg daily doses.
- Recommendations on the treatment of early stage breast cancer that resulted from a 1990 NIH consensus conference and from an interna-

XI

tional group of researchers who met at St. Gallen in 1992 are found in Table 59.3. The recommendations put forward at St. Gallen differ from the NIH conference in that they are also more aggressive in use of combined chemohormonal therapy in hormone receptor–negative patients as well as in postmenopausal patients in general.

- The risks of metastases and cancer death are of a sufficient magnitude to justify the use of adjuvant chemotherapy for all node positive, premenopausal women and adjuvant tamoxifen for all node positive, ER positive, postmenopausal women.
- The options are less certain for node positive, ER negative postmenopausal women. Chemotherapy is strongly favored by the St. Gallen recommendations; tamoxifen may also represent a possible treatment.
- Node negative patients with primary breast tumors of <1 cm have an excellent prognosis, and the benefits of adjuvant therapy may be too small to justify its use. Decisions regarding adjuvant therapy in node-

TABLE 59.3. Comparison of the Treatment Guidelines for Premenopausal and Postmenopausal Women

Node Status	1990 NIH	1992 St. Gallen
Premenopausal Women		
Node negative		
Low/minimal[a]	No treatment	No treatment or tamoxifen
Good risk[b]	No treatment	Tamoxifen
High risk[c]		
ER+	CT or tamoxifen	CT $\pm$ Tamoxifen
ER−	CT or tamoxifen	CT
Node positive		
ER+	CT	CT $\pm$ Tamoxifen
ER−	CT	CT
Postmenopausal Women		
Node negative		
Low/minimal risk[a]	No treatment	No treatment or tamoxifen
Good risk[b]	No treatment	Tamoxifen
High risk[c]		
ER+	CT or tamoxifen	Tamoxifen $\pm$ CT
ER−	CT or tamoxifen	CT $\pm$ Tamoxifen
Node positive		
ER+	Tamoxifen or CT	Tamoxifen $\pm$ CT
ER−	Tamoxifen or CT	CT $\pm$ Tamoxifen

Key: CT, chemotherapy.
[a] Small (≤1 cm) invasive carcinoma, *in situ,* or good histopathology (colloid, tubular, papillary).
[b] ER+, low nuclear grade, or tumor size 1–2 cm.
[c] ER−, cancers of ≥1 cm; ER+, cancers ≥2 cm, and all cancers with nuclear grade III.
Adapted from Clin Oncol Alert 1993;2:15, with permission.

negative patients should be individualized based on the estimated risk of relapse and death, the expected benefits of treatment, the toxicity of treatment, and the impact of therapy on quality of life.

Adjuvant Chemotherapy

- The most common combination chemotherapy regimens employed in the adjuvant setting are listed in Table 59.4.
- Chemotherapy should be initiated within 3 weeks of surgical removal of the primary tumor. The optimal duration of treatment appears to be about 4–6 months.
- The short-term toxic effects of chemotherapy used in the adjuvant setting are generally well tolerated, especially with the availability of serotonin-antagonist antiemetics and colony-stimulating factors for preventing febrile neutropenia. Other common side effects include alopecia, weight gain, and fatigue. Patients who are menstruating will expe-

TABLE 59.4. Combination Chemotherapy of Breast Cancer

Abbreviation	Regimen
FAC	5-Fluorouracil, 400–500 mg/m^2 IV, days 1 and 8 Adriamycin, 40–50 mg/m^2 IV, day 1 Cyclophosphamide, 400–500 mg/m^2 IV, day 1 Repeat every 28 days as tolerated
CMFVP (Cooper)	Cyclophosphamide, 80–100 mg PO per day Methotrexate, 20–25 mg IV per week 5-Fluorouracil, 500 mg IV per week Vincristine, 1 mg IV per week Prednisone, 45 mg PO per day × 14 days, then 30 mg PO per day × 14 days, then 15 mg PO per day
CAF	Cyclophosphamide, 500 mg/m^2 IV, day 1 Adriamycin, 50 mg/m^2 IV, day 1 5-Fluorouracil, 500 mg/m^2 IV, day 1 Repeat every 21 days as tolerated
CMF (original)	Cyclophosphamide, 100 mg/m^2 PO, per day × 14 days Methotexate, 40 mg/m^2 IV days 1 and 8 5-Fluorouracil, 600 mg/m^2 IV days 1 and 8 Repeat every 28 days as tolerated
CMF (revised)	Cyclophosphamide, 600 mg/m^2 IV, day 1 Methotrexate, 40 mg/m^2 IV, day 1 5-Fluorouracil, 600 mg/m^2 IV, day 1 Repeat every 21 days as tolerated
AC	Adriamycin, 30–40 mg/m^2 IV, day 1 Cyclophosphamide, 150–200 mg/m^2 PO, days 3–6 Repeat every 21 days as tolerated

Note: Doses are modified for leukopenia, thrombocytopenia, impaired renal and liver function, etc. Maximum tolerated doses should be used.

XI

rience a cessation of menses that may or may not return; signs and symptoms of menopause accompany cessation of menses. Rare effects include deep vein thrombosis, secondary leukemia from cyclophosphamide-based regimens, and cardiomyopathy induced by doxorubicin (incidence <1% if total dose <320 mg/m^2 body surface area).

Adjuvant Hormonal Therapy

- Tamoxifen is the adjuvant hormonal therapy of choice. It blocks hormone receptors and may stimulate the production of transforming growth factor beta, an inhibitory growth factor that could inhibit not only estrogen receptor positive cancer cells, but also estrogen receptor negative cancer cells. Tamoxifen reduces the incidence of contralateral breast cancer and has beneficial estrogenic effects on the cardiovascular system and bone density.
- The optimal dose of tamoxifen appears to be 20 mg/d, which can be given as a single daily dose. Therapy is usually initiated shortly after surgery or as soon as pathology results are known and the decision to administer tamoxifen as adjuvant therapy is made. The optimal duration of therapy has not been defined; most recommendations suggest 2–5 years, and even longer courses have been advocated.
- Tamoxifen is usually well tolerated. Symptoms of estrogen withdrawal (hot flashes and vaginal bleeding) may occur but decrease in frequency and intensity over time. A dose- and duration-dependent proliferation of the endometrium has been linked to a two-fold increase in endometrial cancer in women receiving 20 mg/d continuously for 5 years.

TREATMENT OF LOCALLY ADVANCED BREAST CANCER (STAGE III)

- The term *locally advanced disease* refers to breast carcinomas with significant primary tumor and nodal disease but where distant metastases cannot be documented. This stage is poorly controlled by radical surgery alone and has a poor prognosis.
- Local regional therapy of locally advanced disease consists of surgery, radiation, or both. There is apparently no advantage to mastectomy over primary radiation therapy in patients with stage III disease. The benefit of combining mastectomy and postoperative radiation is controversial.
- Neoadjuvant (or primary) chemotherapy is the administration of systemic chemotherapy prior to a definitive local-regional procedure. It should be the initial choice of treatment because systemic relapse and death occur in the majority of patients even when local-regional control is accomplished. Neoadjuvant chemotherapy has been used to control micrometastases, reduce tumor bulk, and allow for more limited procedures for local control. It is then followed by surgery or radiation therapy (or both), and then adjuvant systemic therapy. Most tumors respond with >50% decrease in tumor size, about 70% of patients experience downstaging, breast conservation is possible for many patients, and almost all patients initially are rendered disease free.

XI

TREATMENT OF METASTATIC BREAST CANCER (STAGE IV)

The choice of therapy for metastatic disease is based on the site of disease involvement and presence or absence of certain characteristics, as described below.

Endocrine Therapy

- The presence of estrogen and progesterone receptors in the primary tumor tissue is the most important factor in predicting response to endocrine therapy. Fifty to 60% of ER positive patients and 75–80% of ER and PR positive patients respond to hormonal therapy; those with ER and PR negative tumors have <10% response rate.
- Patients who experience a long disease-free survival following local-regional therapy or are late premenopausal or postmenopausal will likely respond to endocrine therapy.
- Endocrine therapy is more likely to be effective in patients with bone and soft tissue metastases. Visceral involvement (i.e., liver) and central nervous system involvement are generally nonresponsive to hormonal therapy and seldom respond to chemotherapy.
- Endocrine therapy is the treatment of choice for patients who are hormone receptor positive and exhibit the first sign of metastatic disease in soft tissue, bone, or pleura, owing to the equal probability of response to hormonal compared to chemotherapy and the lower toxicity profile of endocrine therapy. Patients are sequentially treated with endocrine therapy until they have progressive symptoms resulting from rapidly growing metastatic disease, at which time cytotoxic chemotherapy can be given.
- Women with hormone receptor–negative tumors, with rapidly progressive lung, liver, or bone marrow involvement, or those having failed initial endocrine therapy are not likely to benefit from endocrine therapy and are usually treated initially with cytotoxic chemotherapy.
- Because most endocrine therapies are equally effective, the choice of a particular one is based primarily on toxicity (Table 59.5).
  - Tamoxifen (10 mg twice daily or 20 mg once daily) is usually the agent of choice in both premenopausal and postmenopausal women who are also hormone receptor positive. It remains the preferred initial agent in women who received the drug as adjuvant therapy. The maximum beneficial effects are not observed for at least 2 months. In addition to the side effects described previously, in the setting of metastatic breast cancer a tumor flare or hypercalcemia occurs in approximately 5% of patients after the initiation of therapy. This may be a positive indication that the patient will respond to endocrine therapy.
  - Ovarian ablation (oophorectomy) is considered by some specialists to be the endocrine therapy of choice in premenopausal women and produces similar overall response rates to tamoxifen.
  - In premenopausal women, medical castration with luteinizing hormone-releasing hormone (LHRH) analogues (leuprolide or goserelin)

XI

TABLE 59.5. Endocrine Therapies Used For Metastatic Breast Cancer

Class	Drug	Dose	Side Effects
Antiestrogen	Tamoxifen	10–20 mg PO bid	Disease flare, hot flashes, nausea, vomiting, edema
LHRH analogs	Leuprolide	7.5 mg sq q28d	Amenorrhea, hot flashes, occasional nausea
	Goserelin	3.6 mg sq q28d	
Progestins	Medroxyprogesterone acetate	400–1000 mg IM qwk	Weight gain, hot flashes, vaginal bleeding
	Megestrol acetate	40 mg PO qid	
Aromatase inhibitors	Aminoglutethimide	250 mg PO bid × 2 weeks then qid with hydrocortisone 40 mg/d	Lethargy, rash, postural dizziness, ataxia, nystagmus
Estrogens	Diethylstilbestrol	5 mg PO tid	Nausea/vomiting, fluid retention, hot flashes, anorexia, thromboembolism, hepatic dysfunction
	Ethinylestradiol	1 mg PO tid	
	Conjugated estrogens	2.5 mg PO tid	
Androgens	Fluoxymesterone	10 mg PO bid	Deepening voice, alopecia, hirsutism, facial/truncal acne, fluid retention, menstrual irregularities, cholestatic jaundice

induces remissions in about one-third of unselected cases. Down-regulation of LHRH receptors in the pituitary and decreased levels of lutcinizing-hormone subsequently lead to a decrease in estrogen to castration levels, thereby simulating oophorectomy.

- Studies using tamoxifen, oophorectomy, or LHRH analogues as first-line therapy in premenopausal patients with metastatic breast cancer are necessary to determine the definitive choice for initial therapy.
- Progestins such as megesterol acetate (Megace) and medroxyprogesterone acetate (Provera) may be an alternative to first-line therapy with tamoxifen.
- Aminoglutethimide and hydrocortisone are generally considered third-line hormonal therapy in the treatment of metastatic breast cancer. Aminoglutethimide decreases peripheral estrogen concentrations by inhibiting cytochrome P-450–dependent conversion of androstenedione to estrone in target tissues. Hydrocortisone, 40 mg/d, is usually administered concomitantly in doses of 10 mg at 3:00 PM and 6:00 PM and 20 mg at 10:00 PM to mimic the natural cortisol production.
- Estrogens and androgens are used rarely today because they are more toxic than other alternatives. It is generally accepted that estrogens are not effective in premenopausal patients. Estrogen initiation is sometimes associated with a disease flare manifested by the appearance of flu-like symptoms or an exacerbation of disease symptoms

XI

(e.g., achiness or pain at sites of metastases); this subsides spontaneously within a month. Hypercalcemia is the most serious side effect
associated with the tumor flare and is seen most commonly in women
with metastatic bone disease.

- Androgens are less effective than estrogens and have masculinizing
  side effects. They are occasionally useful in older women with congestive heart failure because androgen use is not accompanied by
  fluid retention that can exacerbate congestive heart failure.

Cytotoxic Therapy

- Chemotherapy is eventually required in most patients with metastatic
  breast cancer, and patients with hormone receptor–negative tumors usually require chemotherapy at the first sign of symptomatic metastases.
- Although combination chemotherapy results in an objective response in
  approximately two-thirds of patients previously unexposed to chemotherapy, the majority have only partial responses and complete remissions occur in <20% of patients. The median duration of response is
  5–12 months and median survival is 14–33 months. In general, once a
  chemotherapy regimen has been initiated, it is continued until there is
  unequivocal evidence of progressive disease.
- Agents with demonstrated activity in the treatment of breast cancer
  include doxorubicin, cyclophosphamide, fluorouracil, methotrexate,
  mitoxantrone, vinblastine, mitomycin-C, thiotepa, and melphalan. The
  objective response rates to single-agent therapy range from 20–40%.
- Paclitaxel, docetaxel, and vinorelbine have been associated with
  response rates of up to 40–50%. Paclitaxel (175 mg/m^2 infused intravenously over 3 hours every 3 weeks) and docetaxel (60–100 mg/m^2
  infused intravenously over 1 hour every 3 weeks) are FDA-approved
  for single-agent treatment of metastatic breast cancer in patients who
  relapse after therapy with an anthracycline-containing regimen.
- Combination regimens have been associated with higher response rates
  than single-agent therapy; the first-line regimens in the metastatic setting are similar, if not identical, to the ones used in the adjuvant setting.
  If doxorubicin was included in the first-line regimen, second-line combinations in common use include:
  - Mitomycin-C (10 mg/m^2) on day 1 and vinblastine (5 mg/m^2) on days
    1 and 15 repeated every 4 weeks.
  - VATH (vinblastine 4.5 mg/m^2 IV day 1, doxorubicin 45 mg/m^2 IV
    day 1, thiotepa 12 mg/m^2 IV day 1, fluoxymesterone [Halotestin] 10
    mg PO TID).
  - Single-agent treatment with paclitaxel, docetaxel, vinorelbine,
    nitrosourea derivatives, platinum derivatives, or mitoxantrone. Com-
    bination regimens that include vinorelbine or paclitaxel are currently
    being investigated.
- Very high doses of single agents or combinations have been used with
  autologous bone marrow transplant to circumvent dose-limiting myelosuppression. Patients with refractory metastatic disease have a high

XI

response rate, but the duration of response is brief. However, it appears that 10–20% of patients who receive high-dose chemotherapy with autologous marrow transplantation after obtaining a complete (or near complete) response to conventional chemotherapy may be cured of their disease or at least achieve a prolonged disease-free interval.

PREVENTION AND EARLY DETECTION OF BREAST CANCER

- The American Cancer Society recommends that all women over the age of 20 perform monthly breast self-examinations.
- Most guidelines recommend annual mammography for women 50 years old and older.
- The American Cancer Society recommends that a baseline mammography be performed between 35 and 40 years of age, and that screening mammography occur every 1–2 years in the 40- to 50-year-old age group. However, in December 1993, the National Cancer Institute withdrew its support of screening mammography in women less than 50 years of age. This controversy remains unresolved.

▶ EVALUATION OF THERAPEUTIC OUTCOMES

EARLY BREAST CANCER

- The overall goal of adjuvant therapy in early stage disease is to cure the patient; this goal cannot be fully evaluated for years after initial diagnosis and treatment. Since there is no clinical evidence of disease at the time adjuvant therapy is administered, assessment of disease response is not possible.
- Adjuvant chemotherapy is often associated with substantial toxicity. Maintaining dose intensity is important in cure of disease and, therefore, optimizing supportive care measures such as antiemetics and growth factors is highly recommended.

METASTATIC BREAST CANCER

- Optimizing quality of life is the therapeutic endpoint in the treatment of patients with metastatic breast cancer. A number of valid and reliable tools are available for objective assessment of quality of life.
- The least toxic therapies are used initially with increasingly aggressive therapies applied in a sequential fashion and in a manner that does not significantly compromise the quality of the patient's life.
- Tumor response is measured by clinical chemistry (e.g., liver enzyme elevation in patients with hepatic metastases) or imaging techniques such as bone scans or chest x-rays.
- Assessment of the clinical status and symptom control of the patient is often adequate to evaluate response to the therapy.

See Chapter 120, Breast Cancer, authored by Celeste Lindley, PharmD, MS, FCCP, FASHP, for a more detailed discussion of this topic.

Chapter 60

▶ COLORECTAL CANCER

▶ DEFINITION

Colorectal cancer involves the colon, rectum, and anal canal. It is one of the three most common cancers in adults and the third leading cause of cancer-related deaths in the United States.

▶ PATHOPHYSIOLOGY

- Risk increases with increasing age. Multiple factors are associated with development of colorectal cancer, including acquired and inherited genetic susceptibility, environmental elements, and lifestyle. Etiologic and clinical risk factors include high dietary fat intake, low dietary fiber intake, no postmenopausal hormone replacement therapy, chronic ulcerative colitis, Crohn's disease, familial adenomatosis polyposis, and hereditary nonpolyposis colorectal cancer.
- Development of a colorectal neoplasm is a multistep process of genetic and phenotypic alterations of normal bowel epithelium structure and function. Sequential mutations within colonic epithelium result in cellular replication or enhanced invasiveness. Genetic changes include mutational activation of oncogenes and inactivation of tumor suppressor genes.
- Adenocarcinomas account for >90% of tumors of the large intestine. Other histologic types (e.g., mucinous adenocarcinoma, signet ring adenocarcinoma, carcinoid simplex, and carcinoid tumors) occur less frequently.
- The most differentiated adenocarcinomas (i.e., grade I) generally resemble adenomas, whereas the most undifferentiated tumors (i.e., grade III) are considered "high-grade" and have frequently lost characteristics of mature normal cells.

▶ CLINICAL MANIFESTATIONS

- Signs and symptoms of colorectal cancer can be extremely varied, subtle, and nonspecific. Patients with early stage colorectal cancer are often asymptomatic.
- Although rectal bleeding and abdominal pain are the most common signs, any change in bowel habits, vague abdominal discomfort, or distention may be warning signs.
- Nausea, vomiting, and abdominal discomfort are often secondary signs of a larger underlying problem such as obstruction, perforation, and/or bleeding.
- Approximately 20–25% of patients with colorectal cancer present with metastatic disease. The most common site of metastasis is the liver, followed by the lungs and then bones.

▶ DIAGNOSIS

- When a patient is suspected of having colorectal carcinoma, a careful history and physical examination should be performed to detect risk factors and clinical manifestations.
- Evaluation of the entire large bowel is undertaken with colonoscopy, or sigmoidoscopy and air-contrast barium enema.
- Baseline laboratory tests should include complete blood cell count, platelet count, prothrombin time (PT), activated partial thromboplastin time (aPTT), liver function tests, and serum carcinoembryonic antigen (CEA). Red blood cell indices and workup of iron status may be useful to confirm acute or chronic blood loss and/or iron-deficiency anemia. Serum CEA can serve as a "marker" for colorectal cancer and for monitoring response to treatment, but it is too insensitive and nonspecific to be used as a screening test for early-stage colorectal cancer.
- Radiographic imaging studies help evaluate extent of disease involvement and may include chest x-ray, bone scan, abdominal computed tomography (CT) scan or ultrasound, intrarectal or transrectal ultrasonography, and intraluminal and hepatic magnetic resonance imaging (MRI) studies.
- Immunodetection of tumors using tumor-directed antibodies is being recognized as an imaging technique for early detection of colorectal cancers. OncoScint CR/OV, an indium-111-labeled monoclonal antibody targeted to the TAG-72 antigen, is an FDA-approved diagnostic imaging agent.

STAGING

- Dukes' classification, originally published in 1932, has traditionally been used to stage colorectal cancers.
- To standardize the staging system, the American Joint Committee on Cancer and the International Union Against Cancer agreed to use the TNM classification. This system considers three aspects of cancer growth—T = *t*umor size, N = lymph *n*ode involvement, and M = presence or absence of *m*etastases (Figure 60.1).
- Stage of colorectal cancer upon diagnosis is the most important independent prognostic factor for survival and disease recurrence. For example, 5-year survival rates for colorectal cancer drop from 70–95% for stage I disease to ≤12% for stage IV disease. Stage of disease is also useful for determining initial treatment.

PREVENTION AND SCREENING

- Cancer prevention efforts can be primary or secondary. Primary prevention requires identification of etiologic factors followed by eradication or alteration of their effects on carcinogenesis. Promising strategies include dietary supplementation (e.g., fiber, calcium, and antioxidants such as vitamin A) and chemoprevention (e.g., α-difluoromethylornithine [DFMO] and nonsteroidal anti-inflammatory agents).

XI

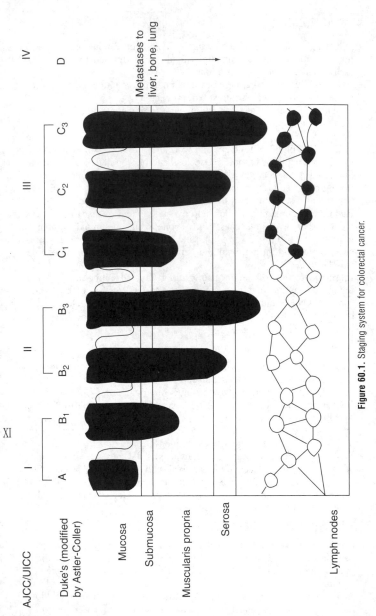

Figure 60.1. Staging system for colorectal cancer.

AJCC/UICC

XI

I   II   III   IV

Duke's (modified by Astler-Coller)

A B_1 B_2 B_3 C_1 C_2 C_3 D

Mucosa

Submucosa

Muscularis propria

Serosa

Lymph nodes

Metastases to liver, bone, lung

- Secondary prevention includes procedures that range from colono-scopic removal of precancerous polyps to total colectomy for high-risk individuals.
- American Cancer Society guidelines for average-risk individuals include annual digital rectal examination starting at age 40 years, annual occult fecal blood testing starting at age 50 years, and sigmoid-oscopic examination starting at age 50 years.

► DESIRED OUTCOME

The goal of treatment depends on the stage of disease at diagnosis. If colorectal cancer is resectable, the goal is to remove the tumor and pre-vent recurrence. Because metastatic colorectal cancer is incurable, the goal is to alleviate symptoms and preserve quality of life. In either case, treatment decisions require careful assessment of relative risks and ben-efits.

► TREATMENT

GENERAL PRINCIPLES

- Treatment modalities are surgery, radiation therapy, chemotherapy, and immunotherapy. These modalities can be used as primary treatment for resectable disease, adjuvant therapy to be combined with primary treat-ment, and options for metastatic disease. Each of these therapeutic strategies is addressed separately, later in this chapter.
- Adjuvant therapy is administered after complete tumor resection to eliminate residual local or metastatic microscopic disease.
- Adjuvant therapy is different for colon and rectal cancer because nat-ural history and recurrence patterns are different. Rectal tumors are more difficult to resect with wide margins, so local recurrences are more frequent than with colon cancers. Adjuvant radiation therapy plus chemotherapy is considered standard for stage II/III rectal cancer, and adjuvant chemotherapy is standard for stage III colon cancer. Because most patients with stage I colorectal cancer are cured by surgical resec-tion alone, adjuvant therapy is not indicated. By definition, adjuvant therapy is not indicated for metastatic disease.
- For the best results, chemotherapeutic agents with proven activity should be administered at maximally tolerated doses when the tumor burden is minimal and tumor growth kinetics is optimal.

TREATMENT MODALITIES

Surgery

- Surgical removal of the primary tumor is the treatment of choice for most patients.
- Surgery generally involves complete tumor resection with an appropri-ate margin of tumor-free bowel and a regional lymphadenectomy.

XI ·

- Only about 1 in 7 patients require permanent colostomy for rectal cancer. Other surgical complications can include infection, adhesion formation, and malabsorption syndromes.

Radiation Therapy

- Radiation therapy (XRT) can be administered with curative surgical resection to reduce local tumor recurrence, or in advanced or metastatic disease to reduce symptoms.
- Acute adverse effects associated with XRT include hematologic depression, dysuria, diarrhea, abdominal cramping, and proctitis. Chronic symptoms may persist for months following discontinuation of XRT and may involve diarrhea, proctitis, enteritis, small bowel obstruction, perineal tenderness, and impaired wound healing.

Chemotherapy

- 5-Fluorouracil (5-FU) is the most active and widely used chemotherapeutic agent for colorectal cancer. Biochemical modulating agents can be added to 5-FU to modify its activity and improve its response rates.

5-Fluorouracil and 5-Fluoro-2'-Deoxyuridine

- As a prodrug, 5-fluorouracil (5-FU) undergoes anabolism to two active metabolites, 5-fluorouridine-5'-triphosphate (FUTP) and 5-fluoro-deoxyuridine-5'-monophosphate (FdUMP). FUTP is incorporated into RNA, thereby impairing protein synthesis. FdUMP bonds with thymidylate synthase (TS), the key enzyme for de novo synthesis of thymidylate, which is a major constituent for DNA synthesis, replication, and repair.
- 5-FU is typically administered by intravenous (IV) bolus, generally once weekly or daily for 5 days each month, or by continuous IV infusion usually over 5 days. Continuous infusion appears to have more favorable clinical activity, which is consistent with evidence that duration of infusion may be an important determinant of the biologic activity.
- 5-Fluoro-2'-Deoxyuridine (FUDR; floxuridine) produces the same cytotoxic effect as 5-FU through conversion to FdUMP. FUDR can be administered IV, but intrahepatic use is more common.
- Toxicity patterns depend on dose, route, and schedule of administration. Leukopenia is the primary dose-limiting toxicity of IV bolus 5-FU, although diarrhea, stomatitis, nausea, and vomiting can also occur. Stomatitis can be reduced with oral cryotherapy, which involves chewing ice chips and holding them in the mouth for 5 minutes prior to until 30 minutes following bolus injection of 5-FU.
- Continuous IV infusion 5-FU is generally well tolerated, but dose-limiting toxicities can be substantial. The most common toxicities are stomatitis and a distinct toxicity, palmar-plantar erythrodysesthesia (hand-foot syndrome), which is characterized by painful swelling and erythroderma of the soles of the feet, palms of the hands, and distal fingers. Although reversible and not life threatening, this skin toxicity can be acutely disabling.

XI

- Complications of hepatic infusion of 5-FU are generally mild and include nausea, vomiting, hematologic depression, hepatotoxicity, and infection.
- Common toxicities of hepatic artery infusion of FUDR include gastric ulceration and hepatobiliary toxicity, which usually require transient interruption of therapy, decreased dosage, or discontinuation of therapy. Rest periods between therapy have also been recommended to prevent or minimize toxicity.
- Combined 5-FU and XRT therapy results in severe hematologic toxicity, enteritis, and diarrhea compared with either chemotherapy or XRT alone.

Levamisole (Ergamisol)

- Levamisole is a synthetic, oral anthelmintic drug with immunomodulatory properties (e.g., T cell activation, augmentation of macrophage activity, and enhancement of chemotaxis by polymorphonuclear cells and monocytes).
- Although the mechanism of its synergistic effect with 5-FU is unknown, proposed mechanisms include immunomodulatory activity, biochemical modulation, or possibly inhibition of cellular phosphatases.
- Toxicities are generally mild, infrequent, and clinically tolerable. Levamisole is associated with taste abnormalities, arthralgias, myalgias, and rare (<5% of patients) central nervous system (CNS) toxicities (e.g., anxiety, irritability, somnolence, depression, insomnia, agitation, confusion, or cerebellar ataxia). Up to 40% of patients treated with levamisole plus 5-FU show laboratory abnormalities consistent with hepatic toxicity, which are mild, rarely symptomatic, and reversible on discontinuation of therapy.

Leucovorin Calcium (Folinic Acid, Citrovorum Factor)

- Leucovorin enhances 5-FU cytotoxicity by increasing intracellular concentrations of reduced folate.
- Leucovorin is generally nontoxic in therapeutic doses, although hypersensitivity reactions (e.g., anaphylaxis and urticaria) have been reported. Combining 5-FU with leucovorin, however, produces greater toxicity to the gastrointestinal epithelium. Dose-limiting toxicities are characterized by stomatitis for low-dose leucovorin and diarrhea for high-dose regimens.
- Diarrhea should initially be treated with bowel rest, IV fluids, and interruption of chemotherapy until symptoms are resolved. Loperamide and diphenoxylate can be used for symptomatic treatment. Octreotide acetate can be administered subcutaneously at a dosage of 100 μg two or three times daily or 50–150 μg/h via continuous IV infusion for refractory 5-FU-induced diarrhea.

Interferon

- Interferon (IFN) may enhance the cytotoxic activity of 5-FU by pharmacodynamic mechanisms (e.g., augmenting binding of active 5-FU metabolite to its target site) or pharmacokinetic mechanisms (e.g., decreasing 5-FU clearance).

- Toxicities of combination therapy include flu-like symptoms, lethargy, stomatitis, and leukopenia. Most toxicities resolve spontaneously or upon dose reduction or discontinuation of IFN or 5-FU.

ADJUVANT THERAPY FOR COLON CANCER

- There is currently no definitive role for adjuvant XRT in extrapelvic colon cancer.
- Single-agent 5-FU or FUDR increased overall survival rates 5–10% in four large randomized trials, but this improvement was not statistically significant.
- In 1990, the NIH Consensus Development Conference recommended that the use of 5-FU and levamisole be considered standard therapy for patients with surgically treated stage III colon cancer (Table 60.1). This combination has been shown to reduce the recurrence rate by 40% and death rate by 33%.
- 5-FU plus high- or low-dose leucovorin has been shown to improve rates of recurrence and survival. Optimal doses, administration schedule, and duration of therapy have yet to be determined (Table 60.1). Although efficacy and toxicity of different regimens are similar, costs of leucovorin doses ranging from 20–500 mg/m^2 are substantially different.
- Direct hepatic infusion of 5-FU provides high local concentrations of the drug at the most common site of recurrence and minimizes systemic toxicity. The value of portal vein infusion of 5-FU, however, remains unproven and controversial because of inconsistent effects on disease recurrence or survival in clinical studies.
- Immunomodulating agents continue to be evaluated. Early results from some studies of autologous tumor cell vaccines and monoclonal anti-

XI

TABLE 60.1. Adjuvant Chemotherapy Regimens for Stages II and III Colon Cancer

Standard Regimen for Stage III:
5-FU + levamisole (begin simultaneously 3–5 weeks after surgery)
  5-FU 450 mg/m^2 rapid IV injection (IVP) for 5 days, then weekly starting at day 28 for 1 year
  Levamisole 50 mg orally (PO) three times daily for 3 days, repeated every 2 weeks for 1 year

Regimens with Potential Value:
Intensive course of 5-FU + low-dose leucovorin
  5-FU 425 mg/m^2 IVP + leucovorin 20 mg/m^2 IVP on days 1–5, repeated every 4–5 weeks for 6 months
Intensive course of 5-FU + high-dose leucovorin
  5-FU 370–400 mg/m^2 IVP + leucovorin 200 mg/m^2 IVP on days 1–5, repeated every 5 weeks for 6 months
Weekly 5-FU + high-dose leucovorin (begin within 6 weeks after surgery)
  5-FU 500 mg/m^2 IVP + leucovorin 500 mg/m^2 IVP weekly during 6 of every 8 weeks for 1 year

bodies suggest that they may help reduce tumor recurrence rates and, perhaps, influence survival.

ADJUVANT THERAPY FOR RECTAL CANCER

- The goal of adjuvant radiation therapy for rectal cancer is to decrease local tumor recurrence after surgery, not to improve survival.
- 5-FU may sensitize rectal tumor cells to cytotoxic effects of XRT. Compared with XRT alone, the combination reduces local tumor recurrence and improves patient survival in high-risk patients.
- Several combinations have been evaluated in clinical studies (Table 60.2), but no single regimen is clearly superior to the others. Continuous infusions of 5-FU, which may provide more effective radiosensitization, significantly improved disease-free and overall survival compared with IV bolus injections. The incidence of leukopenia was greater with 5-FU bolus, whereas the incidence of diarrhea was greater with continuous infusion.
- More research is needed to establish the best combination of surgery, XRT, and chemotherapy, because no single modality satisfactorily prevents recurrence and improves survival. Interest in preoperative adjuvant therapy has resurfaced because of advances in imaging techniques and preoperative staging.

TREATMENT OF METASTATIC COLORECTAL CANCER

- Site(s) of tumor involvement and symptoms help to define appropriate initial management strategy (Figure 60.2). In general, treatment options are similar for metastatic cancer of the colon and rectum.
- Surgical resection of isolated hepatic and pulmonary metastases may offer selected patients an opportunity to experience extended disease-free survival.
- Chemotherapy is the primary treatment modality for unresectable metastatic colorectal cancer.
- 5-FU can be administered by IV bolus, continuous infusion, or hepatic artery infusion. IV bolus schedules are favored because of low cost, ease of administration, and documented efficacy. Typical regimens con-

XI

TABLE 60.2. Adjuvant Chemotherapy Regimen for Stages II and III Rectal Cancer

5-FU 500 mg/m^2 IVP for 5 days, starting on days 1 and 28, begin 22–70 days after surgery

XRT 5040 cGy in 180-cGy fractions for 5 days each week for 6 weeks, begin on day 56 after initiation of therapy

5-FU 500 mg/m^2 IVP for 3 days, begin simultaneously with XRT and repeated on the first 3 days of the last week of XRT

5-FU 400 mg/m^2 IVP for 5 days, beginning 1 month after XRT and followed in 4 weeks by 5-FU 500 mg/m^2 IVP for 5 days

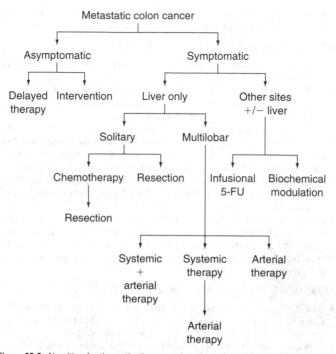

Figure 60.2. Algorithm for the methodic approach to the patient with metastatic colorectal cancer. *(From Kemeny N, Lokich JJ, Anderson N, et al. Cancer 1993;71:16, with permission.)*

sist of 5-FU 450–500 mg/m²/d for 5 days every 4–5 weeks, or doses ranging up to 600 mg/m² weekly for 6 of 8 weeks. Although no significant improvement in survival has been gained with IV bolus, patients receiving weekly IV bolus injections who achieve objective responses have a small survival benefit (12–18 versus 6–8 months).

- The relatively low response rates achieved with bolus 5-FU administration are consistent with tumor cell and drug kinetics. Since 5-FU primarily kills actively dividing tumor cells and has a short plasma half-life, susceptible tumor cells may not be exposed to 5-FU for an adequate period of time.

- Continuous IV infusion regimens (e.g., 8- to 24-hour, 4- to 5-day) have been developed to increase the duration of drug exposure. Even protracted continuous infusions (e.g., 250–300 mg/m²/d IV over 24 hours for up to 10 weeks) are not associated with substantial toxicity. Comparative studies have shown that continuous infusion significantly improved response rates compared with IV bolus (30–44% versus

TABLE 60.3. 5-FU/Leucovorin Therapy for Metastatic Colorectal Cancer

Standard Regimen:
5-FU + low-dose leucovorin
   5-FU 425 mg/m^2 IVP + leucovorin 20 mg/m^2 IVP on days 1–5, repeated at 4 and 8 weeks and
   every 5 weeks thereafter.

Other Regimens:
5-FU + high-dose leucovorin
   5-FU 500 mg/m^2 IVP + leucovorin 500 mg/m^2 IV weekly for 6 weeks, followed by a 2-week rest
   period prior to repeating the cycle
5-FU + high-dose leucovorin
   5-FU 370 mg/m^2 IVP + leucovorin 200 mg/m^2 IVP on days 1–5, repeated at 4 and 8 weeks, and
   every 5 weeks thereafter

7–22%), but only a small number of patients were studied and the benefit did not translate into survival advantages.
- 5-FU plus low-dose leucovorin (Table 60.3) is currently recommended as standard systemic treatment for metastatic colorectal cancer based on response rates, toxicity, lower estimated drug costs, and quality of life indices.
- Promising activity has been reported in a phase II study evaluating 5-FU, leucovorin, and IFN-α in previously untreated patients with good performance status and measurable metastatic disease.
- Options for patients who no longer respond to standard treatments for metastatic colorectal cancer are limited.
- Pharmacokinetic properties of FUDR provide for rapid systemic clearance and high liver drug extraction. Delivery of FUDR 0.3 mg/kg/d via the hepatic artery as a continuous 24-hour infusion for 14 days results in increased local drug concentrations. Heparin 10,000–17,500 units/50 mL of solution is often added to prevent arterial thromboses. Prospective randomized studies have consistently demonstrated significantly higher response rates compared with IV therapy (50–60% versus 20%) and slightly higher median survival rates (17–20 versus 11–12 months). Because of significant costs and toxicities, hepatic artery infusions should be reserved for palliative treatment of isolated liver metastases in patients who have failed systemic therapy.
- Investigational treatments include monoclonal antibodies directed against tumor-associated antigens, biologic modifier therapy, gene therapy techniques, and new chemotherapeutic agents.

▶ EVALUATION OF THERAPEUTIC OUTCOMES

- Patients who undergo curative surgical resection, with or without adjuvant therapy, require close follow-up (Table 60.4).

TABLE 60.4. General Guidelines for Follow-up After Curative Resection

Procedure or Test	Frequency
History and physical exam Fecal occult blood testing CEA Sigmoidoscopy	Every 3–4 months for 3 years, then every 6 months for 2 years, then annually
Colonoscopy or sigmoidoscopy + barium enema	Annually for several years, then every 2–3 years
Chest x-ray	Annually
Liver function tests	As indicated by above findings
Chest, abdominal, or pelvic CT scan	
Liver ultrasound	
Liver–spleen scan	
Bone scan	
Laparotomy	

Adapted from Cohen AM, Minsky BD, Schilsky RL, in DeVita VT, Hellmann S, Rosenberg SA, (eds): Cancer: Principles and Practice of Oncology, 4E, Philadelphia, PA. JB Lippincott. 1993:939–945, with permission.

- The goal of monitoring is to evaluate whether the patient is receiving any benefit from the management of their disease or to detect recurrence.
- Symptoms of recurrence such as pain syndromes, changes in bowel habits, rectal or vaginal bleeding, pelvic masses, anorexia, and weight loss develop in <50% of patients. More recurrences are detected in asymptomatic patients due to increased serum CEA levels that lead to further examination.

XI *See Chapter 122, Colorectal Cancer, authored by Lisa E. Davis, PharmD, and Motria M. Krawczeniuk, PharmD, for a more detailed discussion of this topic.*

Chapter 61

► LEUKEMIAS, ACUTE

► DEFINITION

Acute lymphocytic leukemia (ALL) and acute nonlymphocytic leukemia (ANLL) are hematologic malignancies characterized by unregulated proliferation of the blood-forming cells of the bone marrow. They differ from each other and from chronic leukemias with respect to differences in cell of origin and cell line maturation, patient life expectancy, clinical presentation, rapidity of progression of the untreated disease, and response to therapy. Untreated, the acute leukemias are rapidly progressive, resulting in death in 2–3 months.

► PATHOPHYSIOLOGY

- Both ANLL and ALL arise from a single leukemic cell that proliferates. There is a failure to maintain a relative balance between proliferation and differentiation, so that the cells do not differentiate past a particular stage of hematopoiesis but then proliferate uncontrollably.
- These immature proliferating cells (blasts) physically crowd out or inhibit normal cellular maturation in bone marrow, resulting in anemia, granulocytopenia, and thrombocytopenia. Leukemic blasts may also leave the bone marrow and infiltrate a variety of tissues such as lymph nodes, skin, liver, spleen, kidney, and the central nervous system (CNS).
- ANLL affects the immature precursors of the myeloid blood-forming cells. The French–American–British (FAB) classification system outlined in Table 61.1 identifies eight different morphologic subtypes of ANLL.
- ALL is characterized by proliferation of immature lymphoblasts. Markers on the cell surface or membrane of the lymphoblast can be used to classify ALL (Table 61.2).
- The genetic defect that leads to leukemia may be activation of a normally suppressed gene to create an oncogene that signals unregulated proliferation, differentiation, or survival. A second genetic cause is the loss or disturbance of genes such as $p53$ (tumor suppressor genes) that suppress the development of cancer.

► CLINICAL PRESENTATION

- The symptoms of acute leukemia are nonspecific.
  - Anemia often manifests as fatigue, lassitude, malaise, and pallor; palpitations or dyspnea on exertion may also be noted.
  - Granulocytopenia may present as fever with or without frank infection.

TABLE 61.1. Morphologic (FAB) Classification of Acute Nonlymphocytic Leukemia

Subtype	Morphologic Features
M_1 Acute myeloblastic leukemia with minimal differentiation	Myeoblasts with scant granules
M_2 Acute myeloblastic leukemia with maturation	Myeloblasts with granules, promyelocytes, few myelocytes
M_3 Acute promyelocytic leukemia	Promyelocytes with prominent granules
M_4 Acute myelomonocytic leukemia	Myeloblasts, promyelocytes, monoblasts, promonoblasts
M_{5a} Acute monoblastic leukemia without differentiation	Large monoblasts with lacy nuclear chromatin and abundant cytoplasm
M_{5b} Acute monoblastic leukemia with differentiation	Monoblasts, promonocytes, monocytes, blood monocytosis
M_6 Acute erythroleukemia	Megaloblastic erythroid precursors, myeloblasts
M_7 Megakaryocytic leukemia	Megakaryocytes, lymphoid morphology, cytoplasmic budding

Adapted from Lukens JN. In Lee GR, Bithell TC, Foerster J, et al (eds): Wintrobe's Clinical Hematology, 9th ed. Philadelphia, Lea and Febiger, 1993, pp. 1873–1891, with permission.

TABLE 61.2. Morphologic (FAB) Classification of Acute Lymphocytic Leukemia

Subtype	Cells of Origin	Morphologic Features
L_1	Early pre-B cell Pre-B cell B cell T cell	Small cell with indistinct nucleoli, scant cytoplasm, regular nucleus shape
L_2	Early pre-B cell Pre-B cell B cell T cell	Large cell with prominent nucleoli, abundant cytoplasm, irregular nucleus shape
L_3	B cell	Large cell with prominent nucleoli, abundant cytoplasm, regular nucleus shape

Adapted from Lukens JN. In Lee GR, Bithell TC, Foerster J, et al (eds): Wintrobe's Clinical Hematology, 9th ed. Philadelphia, Lea and Febiger, 1993, pp 1873–1891, with permission.

XI

- Thrombocytopenia may manifest as simple petechiae or frank bleeding or bruising, often involving the gums, skin, or GI tract. Menorrhagia may be seen in premenopausal women.
- Seizures, gum hypertrophy, loss of vision, the presence of an abnormal mass, or bone pain may result from leukemic infiltrates. Headache, diplopia, nausea, or vomiting may indicate leukemic meningitis.
- Physical findings are compatible with anemia (pallor, tachycardia, cardiac murmurs), granulocytopenia (infection, fever), thrombocytopenia (bruising, frank bleeding, petechiae, ecchymoses, purpura, menorrhagia), and leukemic infiltration (lymphadenopathy, splenomegaly, hepatomegaly, sternal tenderness, gingival hypertrophy, cranial palsies, and skin infiltration).
- On laboratory testing, the anemia is usually normocytic and normochromic with decreased reticulocytes. The platelet count is reduced in nearly all patients (median 40,000–50,000/μL.) The WBC count is normal or elevated in about 85% of patients with ALL; in some patients, it exceeds 50,000/μL. In adults with ANLL, the WBC count at the time of diagnosis may be elevated, normal, or low. The peripheral blood smear usually demonstrates a decrease in normal granulocytes, with an increase in blasts. Other laboratory findings include hyperuricemia, serum calcium imbalances, hyperkalemia, hypoalbuminemia, and hypogammaglobulinemia.

▶ DIAGNOSIS

- In patients with signs, symptoms, and laboratory findings suggestive of leukemia, marrow biopsy and aspirate are necessary to establish a diagnosis and follow disease progression and response to therapy.
- The marrow is usually hypercellular with a predominance of blasts. Leukemia is diagnosed if >30% of the marrow cells are blasts. If the percentage is <5%, then the marrow is considered normal. If the marrow has 5–30% leukemic blasts, the term "myelodysplasia" is used, which is a preleukemic state that will eventually evolve into ANLL.
- Identification of clinical and laboratory risk factors at diagnosis may allow the clinician to better understand the disease and to tailor treatment according to the predicted response.

XI

▶ DESIRED OUTCOME

- The short-term treatment goal for acute leukemia is to rapidly achieve a complete clinical and hematologic remission (defined as the disappearance of all clinical and bone marrow evidence of leukemia, with restoration of normal hematopoiesis).
- After a complete remission is achieved, the goal is to maintain the patient in continuous complete remission, as relapse may ultimately lead to a fatal outcome.

▶ TREATMENT

GENERAL MANAGEMENT PRINCIPLES

- Acute leukemia patients, particularly those with an initial elevated WBC count, should receive allopurinol prior to and during chemotherapy to prevent the development of urate nephropathy from rapid destruction of white cells. In adults, 300 mg of allopurinol once daily, started 1–2 days prior to chemotherapy, is usually adequate.
- Platelet transfusions are often given for peripheral counts <5000/µL or clinical signs of bleeding.
- Transfusions of packed red cells may be indicated for a hematocrit <20%, profound fatigue, or chest pain.
- Because of the GI toxicity of chemotherapy, parenteral nutrition should be used liberally.
- Patients frequently receive infusions of antibiotics, fluids, hyperalimentation, and blood products simultaneously; a triple lumen central venous access device (e.g., Hickman catheter) is placed at the start of therapy to provide the total support needed.

ACUTE LYMPHOCYTIC LEUKEMIA

Remission Induction Therapy

- In adult ALL, prednisone, vincristine, daunorubicin, and asparaginase are a common combination for remission induction therapy (Table 61.3). Other agents that are sometimes included in remission induction regimens are cyclophosphamide, cytarabine (high dose or standard dose), mercaptopurine, methotrexate (standard dose or high dose), and mitoxantrone. The value of adding more drugs to the basic three- or four-drug regimen is unclear.
- In pediatric ALL, low-risk patients commonly receive only a glucocorticoid, vincristine, and asparaginase for remission induction, and the complete remission rate is near 99%. In high-risk patients, the induction regimen includes the same three drugs plus two or three others (e.g., daunorubicin and cyclophosphamide or etoposide, cytarabine, and high-dose methotrexate).

Central Nervous System Prophylaxis

- After patients achieve complete remission, they usually receive CNS prophylaxis because the CNS is a potential sanctuary for leukemic cells from chemotherapeutic agents and because undetectable leukemic cells are present in the CNS in many patients.
- In adults with ALL, CNS prophylaxis usually includes cranial irradiation (2-Gy fractions to a total dose of 18–24 Gy) and intrathecal methotrexate (10–15 mg intrathecally once or twice weekly for four to six doses) to eradicate undetectable leukemia in the cranial region and spinal column, respectively. Intrathecal cytarabine (20–100 mg), hydrocortisone (10–35 mg), and methotrexate (12–15 mg) have also been given together.

XI

TABLE 61.3. Representative Chemotherapy Regimens for Adult Acute Lymphocytic Leukemia

Remission Induction Drug & Dose	Days	CNS Prophylaxis Drug & Dose	Days	Consolidation Drug & Dose	Days	Maintenance (Drug, Dose, & Schedule)
German Regimen						
PRED (PO) 60 mg/m²	1–28	Cranial irradiation & MTX (IT) 10 mg/m²[2b]	31,38,45,52	DEX (PO) 10 mg/m²	1–28	MP (PO) 60 mg/m² QD and MTX (PO/IV) 20 mg/m² weekly Weeks 10–18 and 29–130
VCR (IV) 1.5 mg/m²[2a]	1,8,15,22			VCR (IV) 1.5 mg/m²[2a]	1,8,15,22	
DNR (IV) 25 mg/m²	1,8,15,22			DOX (IV) 25 mg/m²	1,8,15,22	
ASP (IV) 5000 U/m²	1–14			CTX (IV) 650 mg/m²[2c]	29	
CTX (IV) 650 mg/m²[2c]	29,43,57			ARA-C (IV) 75 mg/m²	31–34,38–41	
ARA-C (IV) 75 mg/m²	31–34,38–41, 45–48,52–55			TG (PO) 60 mg/m²	29–42	
MP (PO) 60 mg/m²	29–57					
University of California–San Francisco, Stanford University, and City of Hope Medical Center						
DNR (IV) 50 mg/m²	1–3	Cranial irradiation & MTX (IT) 12 mg	Weekly × 6	*Cycles 1,3,5,7*		MTX (PO) 20 mg/m² weekly
VCR (IV) 2 mg	1,8,15,22			DNR (IV) 50 mg/m²	1,2	MP (PO) 75 mg/m² daily until 30 months in continuous complete remission
				VCR (IV) 2 mg	1,8	
				PRED (PO) 50 mg/m²	1–14	
				ASP (IM) 12,000 U/m²	2,4,7,9,11,14	
If day 14 bone marrow has leukemia						
DNR (IV) 50 mg/m²	15			*Cycles 2,4,6,8*		
				TEN (IV) 165 mg/m²	1,4,8,11	
				ARA-C (IV) 300 mg/m²	1,4,8,11	
If day 28 bone marrow has leukemia						
DNR (IV) 50 mg/m²	29,30			*Cycle 9*		
VCR (IV) 2 mg	29,36			MTX (IV) 690 mg/m² over 42 h		
PRED (PO) 60 mg/m²	29–42			LEUC (IV) 15 mg/m² Q6h × 12 doses, beginning at 42 h		
ASP (IM) 6000 U/m²	29–35					

TABLE 61.3. continued

Remission Induction		CNS Prophylaxis		Consolidation		Maintenance (Drug, Dose, & Schedule)
Drug & Dose	Days	Drug & Dose	Days	Drug & Dose	Days	
CALGB 8811						
Course I				*Course II: Early Intensification*		*Course V*
CTX (IV) 1200 mg/m²	1			MTX (IT) 15 mg	1	VCR (IV) 2 mg day 1 monthly
DNR (IV) 45 mg/m²	1,2,3			CTX (IV) 1000 mg/m²	1	PRED (PO) 60 mg/m² days 1–5 monthly
VCR (IV) 2 mg	1,8,15,22			MP (PO) 60 mg/m²	1–14	MTX (PO) 20 mg/m² days 1,8,15,22 monthly
PRED (PO) 60 mg/m²	1–21			ARA-C (SC) 75 mg/m²	1–4,8–11	MP (PO) 60 mg/m² days 1–28 monthly
ASP (SC) 6000 U/m²	5,8,11,15,18,22			VCR (IV) 2 mg	15,22	
				ASP (SC) 6000 U/m²	15,18,22,25	
For patients ≥ 60 yr old, use:		*Course III*				
CTX 800 mg/m²	1	Cranial irradiation	1,8,15,22,29			
DNR 30 mg/m²	1,2,3	MTX (IT) 15 mg	1–70	*Course IV: Late Intensification*		
PRED 60 mg/m²	1–7	MP (PO) 60 mg/m²	36,43,50,57,64	DOX (IV) 30 mg/m²	1,8,15	
		MTX (PO) 20 mg/m²		VCR (IV) 2 mg	1,8,15	
				DEX (PO) 10 mg/m²	1–14	
				CTX (IV) 1000 mg/m²	29	
				TG (PO) 60 mg/m²	29–42	
				ARA-C (SC) 75 mg/m²	29–32,36–39	

XI

Key: ARA-C, cytarabine; ASP, asparaginase; CTX, cyclophosphamide; DEX, dexamethasone; DNR, daunorubicin; DOX, doxorubicin; MP, mercaptopurine; MTX, methotrexate; PRED, prednisone; TEN, teniposide; TG, thioguanine; VCR, vincristine.
[a]Maximum single dose, 2 mg.
[b]Maximum single dose, 15 mg.
[c]Maximum single dose, 100 mg.

- In children, low-risk ALL patients can be treated with a combination of intrathecal cytarabine, methotrexate, and hydrocortisone, with doses individualized by age. High-risk patients require both intrathecal chemotherapy and radiation or a combination of intrathecal and systemic chemotherapy.

Consolidation Therapy

- In adult ALL, consolidation therapy is started after a complete remission has been achieved and involves continued intensive chemotherapy in an attempt to eradicate clinically undetectable disease. The three regimens listed in Table 61.3 offer three different approaches to consolidation with similar results.
- In pediatric ALL, a phase of dose-intensified chemotherapy usually follows induction, especially in patients with recognized poor risk factors. The drugs chosen are similar to those used in adults.

Maintenance Therapy

- The goal of maintenance therapy is to further eradicate residual leukemic cells and prolong remission duration.
- In adult and childhood ALL, maintenance therapy usually consists of mercaptopurine and methotrexate, at doses that produce minimal myelosuppression, with or without intermittent pulses of vincristine and prednisone (see Table 61.3). Most treatment programs continue maintenance therapy for at least 30 months.

ACUTE NONLYMPHOCYTIC LEUKEMIA

Remission Induction Therapy

- The most active single agents in ANLL are the anthracycline antibiotics (daunorubicin, doxorubicin, and idarubicin) and the antimetabolite cytarabine (Table 61.4)
- Daunorubicin has historically been the preferred anthracycline because it has similar antileukemic activity but causes less gastrointestinal toxicity (necrotizing colitis) than doxorubicin. Recent studies of idarubicin in adult ANLL have shown a significant improvement in complete remission rate over daunorubicin (69% vs. 55%) in patients also receiving cytarabine. Idarubicin has not been as well tested in pediatric ANLL patients.
- In one study, addition of high-dose cytarabine to conventional "7 & 3" resulted in a remission rate of 89% after induction therapy.
- Most patients achieve a complete remission after one or two courses of chemotherapy. Patients who require additional chemotherapy to achieve a complete remission have been reported to have a poor prognosis, even if remission is ultimately achieved.

Central Nervous System Prophylaxis

- CNS prophylaxis is not routinely given for ANLL because the risk of CNS relapse is lower than in patients with ALL.

TABLE 61.4. Representative Chemotherapy Regimens for Adult Acute Nonlymphocytic Leukemia

Remission Induction	Intensive Postremission Therapy	Maintenance Therapy
Southeastern Cancer Study Group		
Cytarabine 100 mg/m^2/d continuous infusion days 1–7	Cytarabine 100 mg/m^2 every 12 h × 10 doses	
	Thioguanine 100 mg/m^2 PO every 12 h for 10 doses	None
Idarubicin 12 mg/m^2/d days 1–3	Idarubicin 15 mg/m^2/d on day 1 (3 courses)	
CALGB		
Cytarabine 200 mg/m^2/d continuous infusion days 1–7	Cytarabine 3 g/m^2 every 12 h days 1,3,5 (4 courses) every 12 h	Cytarabine 100 mg/m^2 SC
Daunorubicin 45 mg/m^2/d days 1–3	days 1–5	Daunorubicin 45 mg/m^2 day 1 (4 courses)
Boston Group		
Daunorubicin 45 mg/m^2/d days 1–3	*Cycle 1,3*	
Cytarabine 100 mg/m^2/d continuous infusion days 1–7	Daunorubicin 60 mg/m^2/d days 1–2	
Cytarabine 2 g/m^2/d every 12 h days 8–10	Cytarabine 200 mg/m^2/d continuous infusion days 1–5	
	Cycle 2	
	Cytarabine 2 g/m^2 every 12 h days 1–3	
	Etoposide 100 mg/m^2/d days 4–5	

Intensive Postremission Therapy

- Although most adults with ANLL achieve a complete remission, the duration of remission is short (4–8 months), and relapse is presumably due to the presence of clinically undetectable leukemic cells. The goal of intensive postremission therapy (IPRT) is to eradicate these residual leukemic cells and to prevent the emergence of drug-resistant disease.
- IPRT may consist of *consolidation,* which involves the administration of drugs that the patient has not previously received, or *intensification,* which is administration of one or two courses of high doses of the same drugs used for remission induction, immediately after a complete remission is achieved.
- The three regimens in Table 61.4 offer three distinctly different approaches to postremission therapy.

Maintenance Therapy

- Most patients receive no further treatment after induction followed by IPRT, although selected patients may go on to marrow transplantation.
- Occasionally, a maintenance phase is included and usually employs low-dose subcutaneous cytarabine as illustrated in the CALGB trial (see Table 61.4).

XI

TREATMENT OF RELAPSED ALL AND ANLL

- Most adult patients with acute leukemia who achieve complete remission eventually experience a leukemic relapse. In children, the relapse rate in ANLL is approximately the same as adults, but relapse is less frequent in pediatric ALL. After the first relapse the median survival is 6–8 months with only 7% of patients alive at 3 years.
- Salvage therapy for ALL has involved similar drugs used during initial induction administered on different schedules. The VAD regimen employs a 4–day continuous infusion of vincristine and doxorubicin with intensive dexamethasone therapy; IPRT follows for 24–30 months. Another regimen uses prednisone, intermediate-dose cytarabine, mitoxantrone, and etoposide in relapsed or refractory ALL. Combinations with high-dose cytarabine or methotrexate are also commonly employed.
- In relapsed or resistant ANLL, high dose cytarabine, etoposide, intermediate-dose or high-dose methotrexate, L-asparaginase, carboplatin, mitoxantrone, and idarubicin have been useful. If the relapse occurs 6 months or more beyond the initial remission, then induction with the original chemotherapy may be successful.

MARROW TRANSPLANTATION

For both ALL and ANLL, allogeneic or autologous marrow transplantation (BMT) is another viable treatment option once remission is induced, especially for high-risk patients and patients in relapse.

ANLL

- In the treatment of ANLL, allogeneic BMT given as IPRT (immediately after initial remission) has been shown to improve disease-free survival over chemotherapy alone. Overall survival may also have been improved.
- Patients who relapse after an initial remission should be offered allogeneic BMT if a donor is available. Long-term survival after autologous BMT appears to be similar to allogeneic BMT. Use of various techniques to purge autologous marrow of residual leukemic cells remains an unresolved issue. Patients in second or later remission who do not qualify for an allogeneic BMT should be considered for autologous BMT as soon as possible after achieving remission.

ALL

- Because the initial remission is usually easily achieved in ALL and no benefit to BMT has been demonstrated in immediate postremission BMT, allogeneic BMT is not recommended in first remission for most patients.
- Once a relapse has occurred, an allogeneic BMT should be performed if a donor is available. Autologous BMT remains an option for patients after relapse when a suitable donor is not available. Autologous BMT leads to longer disease-free survival than could be gained from conven-

XI

tional chemotherapy. Compared to allogeneic BMT for patients in second remission or later, overall survival is similar, but the relapse rate is greater with autologous BMT (79 vs. 56%).

▶ EVALUATION OF THERAPEUTIC OUTCOMES

- With the exception of prednisone, L-asparaginase, and vincristine, antineoplastic agents used to treat acute leukemias cause a rapid fall in peripheral platelet and WBC counts. During ANLL remission induction therapy, daily monitoring of the complete blood count and the absolute neutrophil count is necessary to determine when red cell and platelet transfusions are needed and when neutropenia is achieved. Less frequent monitoring than daily may be sufficient during ALL induction.
- During the period of hypoplasia, infectious complications are major causes of death. Intense monitoring of chemistry laboratory values, microbiology reports, and the patient's physical condition are necessary to identify infections early. As typical signs and symptoms of infection may be absent in the neutropenic host, frequent monitoring of vital signs and daily physical examinations are important.
- Frequent culturing and early institution of antibiotics will prevent infectious deaths.
- Close monitoring of the patient's condition and laboratory values also allows appropriate institution of nutritional support.
- The primary outcome desired initially is the establishment of remission (return of hematologic values to normal and a repeat bone marrow biopsy that demonstrates no evidence of disease).
- After the appropriate postremission therapy has been completed, the patient may return on a regular basis to check hematologic values.

See Chapter 126, Acute Leukemias, authored by Steven P. Smith, PharmD, BCPS, and Mary E. Teresi, Pharm D, for a more detailed discussion of this topic.

XI

Chapter 62

▶ LEUKEMIAS, CHRONIC

▶ DEFINITION

Chronic leukemia includes four recognized hematologic malignancies: chronic myelogenous leukemia (CML), chronic lymphocytic leukemia (CLL), prolymphocytic leukemia, and hairy cell leukemia. They differ from each other and from acute leukemias with respect to differences in cell of origin, patient life expectancy, clinical presentation, rapidity of progression of the untreated disease, and response to therapy. This chapter deals with the two most common types, CML and CLL.

▶ CML

PATHOPHYSIOLOGY

- CML is myeloproliferative disorder that results from the malignant transformation of a pluripotent stem cell leading to the clonal proliferation and accumulation of both progenitor and mature myeloid and lymphoid cells. The hematologic and cytogenetic abnormalities involve the myeloid and B-lymphoid elements of bone marrow.
- The Philadelphia chromosome (Ph[1]) abnormality, present in 90–95% of patients, is identified as a shortened long arm of chromosome 22, and is found in granulocyte and erythrocyte progenitors, macrophages, megakaryocytes, and some lymphocytes. It is the consequence of breaks in chromosomes 9 and 22, resulting in a transposition that relocates the 3′ end of the c-*abl* protooncogene from its normal site on chromosome 9 at band 34 to the 3′ end of the breakpoint cluster region *(bcr)* on chromosome 22 at band 11, which is symbolized as t(9;22)(q34;q11). This results in the formation of the hybrid *bcr-abl* fusion gene. Through this chromosomal translocation, the c-*abl* protooncogene is able to escape the normal genetic controls on its expression and is activated into a functional oncogene, directing the transcription of an 8.5-kilobase mRNA molecule that is translated into a 210-kDa protein known as p210[BCR-ABL]. The protein has a higher tyrosine phosphokinase activity than the protein translated by the mRNA of the normal c-*abl* gene, which may be essential in the development of CML.
- Carcinogenesis begins with the transformation of a single cell with an inheritable selective growth advantage, leading to the proliferation of a neoplastic, monoclonal population of pluripotent stem cells. The disease soon evolves into a Ph[1]-positive chronic phase.
- Granulocytosis results from the increased growth rate of the transformed clone and disruption of normal hematopoietic cell maturation.
- The silent monoclonal growth phase of CML evolves into the clinically recognized *chronic phase* when the malignant cells acquire Ph[1] and the

immature myeloid cells begin to lose the ability to differentiate into mature functioning cells. At this stage, therapeutic intervention can effectively control the expansion of these clonal cells and normalize the WBC count.

- An *accelerated phase* begins to emerge later as the patient's WBC count becomes increasingly difficult to manage.
- The final *acute phase* or blastic phase (blast crisis) is marked by the presence of rapidly proliferating blast cells that have lost the ability to differentiate into nonproliferating cells. CML in blastic phase is resistant to treatment owing to drug resistance and the high proliferative rate of malignant cells.

CLINICAL PRESENTATION

- CML is commonly diagnosed after the patient presents with symptoms such as weight loss, fatigue, malaise, night sweats, and fever.
- On physical examination, splenomegaly and hepatomegaly are found in 30–40% of patients.

DIAGNOSIS

- The diagnosis of CML is usually made during the chronic phase following an abnormal peripheral blood smear that may have been obtained because of the patient's presenting symptoms or during a routine physical examination.
- Laboratory findings of the peripheral blood during the chronic phase include leukocytosis (WBC often >100,000/µL), thrombocytosis, basophilia, and abnormal leukocyte alkaline phosphatase levels.
- Physical symptoms of acceleration include a resurgence of splenic enlargement, unexplained fever, and persistent bone pain. WBC counts and other signs and symptoms begin to be increasingly difficult to control with conventional oral chemotherapeutic agents.
- The presence of blastic phase is confirmed by >20% blasts in the bone marrow or peripheral blood.

XI DESIRED OUTCOME

The primary goals of therapy for CML are to control the patient's signs and symptoms, delay the onset of blastic phase, and achieve cure by eradicating the Ph[1]-positive cells.

TREATMENT

Conventional Chemotherapy

- Conventional cytotoxic chemotherapy can be used in chronic phase CML to attain hematologic remission (normalization of WBC count), but has no significant cytogenetic effects and has only marginally improved median survival in CML. Table 62.1 illustrates the effect of various treatment modalities on median survival in CML.
- Busulfan and hydroxyurea can be taken orally, are inexpensive, have a reasonable side-effect profile, and are able to rapidly normalize elevated

TABLE 62.1. Effect of Various Treatment Modalities on Survival in CML

Therapy	Median Survival (months)
No treatment	37 (mean)
Splenic irradiation	42 (mean), 28 (median)
Busulfan	35–47
Hydroxyurea	48–69
Combination chemotherapy	45–55
Bone marrow transplantation	40–70% alive at 5 years[a]
IFN-α	50–60% alive at 5 years

[a]Only therapy to eliminate Ph[1] clone.

WBC counts in chronic phase. A comparison of hydroxyurea and busulfan can be seen in Table 62.2.

- Hydroxyurea treatment has been shown to provide a significant survival advantage of >1 year over busulfan therapy. Hydroxyurea inhibits the enzyme ribonucleotide reductase, leading to suppression of DNA synthesis. It is administered either daily or intermittently. In the daily schedule, hydroxyurea is initiated at 50 mg/kg/d in divided doses until the WBC count falls below 10,000/μL; the dose can then be decreased to a maintenance level of 20 mg/kg/d or temporarily discontinued and reinitiated at the daily maintenance dose when the WBC count begins to climb. The WBC count rarely continues to fall after the drug is discontinued. Because prolonged daily administration of hydroxyurea has been associated with adverse dermatologic effects, an intermittent maintenance dose of 20 mg/kg twice daily (40 mg/kg/d) 2 days each week has been proven effective in controlling the WBC count while minimizing cutaneous toxicity.
- Busulfan may be the second-line agent because of its toxicity. Initial doses are 4–8 mg/d, continued until the WBC count approaches

XI

TABLE 62.2. Comparison of Hydroxyurea and Busulfan in Chronic Phase CML

Effect of Therapy	Hydroxyurea	Busulfan
Rate of WBC decline	Rapid	Slower
Myelosuppression	Uncommon at usual dose	Common
Side-effect profile	Mild—skin	Severe—lung
Effect on platelet count	No effect	Decreased
Effect on splenomegaly	Significant reversal	Significant reversal
Effect on Ph[1]-positive marrow	None	After prolonged myelosuppression
BMT eligible patients	Recommended	Not recommended

BMT, bone marrow transplant.

20,000/μL, and then discontinued. The WBC count will continue to fall after the drug is discontinued and appropriate WBC counts can be maintained for several weeks. Toxicities include prolonged myelosuppression, pulmonary fibrosis, and skin hyperpigmentation. Patients who have received busulfan have more complications if they undergo allogeneic bone marrow transplant (BMT) later. For this reason, and because of the possibility of inducing drug resistance, busulfan is not considered first-line therapy in patients who are candidates for BMT.

Interferons

- Two recombinant forms of alpha interferon (IFN-α) are presently marketed: IFN-α-2a (Roferon) and IFN-α-2b (Intron A).
- One proposed mechanism in the treatment of CML is the binding of IFN-α to its cell surface receptor on target cells, initiating a cascade of biochemical processes that can result in direct cytotoxicity to leukemic cells. Other mechanisms may also be operative.
- Some patients achieve cytogenetic response (a decrease or loss of Ph^1-positive cells), and up to 70–80% achieve complete hematologic remission.
- The optimal dose schedule appears to be 5×10^6 U/m^2/d with doses above that being unlikely to improve response rates while increasing the incidence of toxicities.
- Adverse effects consist of short-term constitutional effects and potentially dose-limiting long-term effects. The most predictable early toxicity is a flu-like syndrome involving fever, chills, myalgias, headache, and anorexia which can be ameliorated by starting dosing at 50% of the final dose during the first week, by giving the drug at bedtime, and by coadministering acetaminophen or indomethacin. Reduction of initial WBC counts to around 10,000/μL with hydroxyurea may also reduce these symptoms. Tachycardia and hypotension are seen in about 15% of patients in the first 1–2 weeks. Long-term adverse effects include weight loss, alopecia, neurologic effects (paresthesias, cognitive impairment, depression), and immune-mediated complications (hemolysis, thrombocytopenia, nephrotic syndrome, systemic lupus erythematosus, hypothyroidism).
- The combination of hydroxyurea and IFN-α has demonstrated promise, with hydroxyurea started first at 50 mg/kg/d and titrated to keep WBC counts at a normal level; IFN-α is then initiated at a dose of 5×10^6 U/m^2/d. The advantage of this combination is the rapid normalization of blood counts and differentials, lower incidence of IFN-α-induced symptoms associated with leukocytosis, and higher complete hematologic remission rates. However, the incidence of cytogenetic response is not significantly different from IFN-α therapy alone.

Treatment in Blastic Phase

- The more common myeloid form has been most responsive to high-dose cytarabine. The usual protocol is 3000 mg/m^2 every 12 hours for up to 12 doses, resulting in complete responses of 25–40%.

XI

- The most effective treatment of the lymphoid form is a combination vincristine–prednisone regimen; the dose of vincristine is usually 2 mg IV each week and prednisone 60 mg/m^2/d PO. The addition of doxorubicin to this protocol may enhance complete response to around 50%.

Bone Marrow Transplantation

- Allogeneic BMT is the only therapeutic option that can result in cure, which can be achieved only through eradication of the Ph^1-positive clone.
- For patients with an HLA-matched sibling donor, BMT is the treatment of choice and should be performed shortly after diagnosis. Approximately 60% of CML patients in chronic phase undergoing BMT from an HLA-identical sibling donor can be cured. When transplanted within the first year of diagnosis, 5-year survival rates approach 80%.
- Less than 30% of patients have an ideal donor, but related one-antigen-mismatch transplants have survival rates which approach HLA-matched transplants.
- Of those patients receiving marrow from an HLA-matched unrelated donor, about 40% are alive and in remission at 2 years. T cell depletion of the donor marrow reduces the morbidity and mortality associated with acute graft-versus-host disease but increases relapse rates owing to loss of the graft-versus-leukemia effect.
- Autologous BMT harvested in chronic phase and stored prior to transplantation has resulted in transient loss of the Ph^1 positive clone for several years in a few patients. Relapse rates remain very high and methods for successfully purging CML marrow have been elusive because of the similarity between CML cells and normal stem cells.

EVALUATION OF THERAPEUTIC OUTCOMES

- Chemotherapy in chronic phase CML is used to maintain a normal WBC count.
- While chemotherapy can produce hematologic remissions, it is unable to produce permanent cytogenetic responses.
- Endpoints for chemotherapy are reduction in tumor bulk and relief of symptoms.

▶ CLL

PATHOPHYSIOLOGY

- CLL is a lymphoproliferative disorder resulting in a progressive accumulation of functionally incompetent lymphocytes which usually results from malignant transformation of a B lymphocyte with subsequent clonal proliferation.

CLINICAL PRESENTATION

- The diagnosis is often made after the patient complains of constitutional symptoms (e.g., fatigue, fever).

DIAGNOSIS

- On physical examination, about 60% of patients have lymphadenopathy in the cervical, axillary, or inguinal areas. Intra-abdominal nodes may also be palpable and about 50% of patients have spleen and liver enlargement.
- An abnormal CBC is characterized by high numbers of mature-looking small lymphocytes (lymphocytosis).
- Bone marrow aspirate usually shows infiltration with mature-appearing lymphocytes making up 30% of nucleated cells.
- Diagnosis can be confirmed by analyzing phenotypic characteristics of the peripheral blood lymphocytes. Presence of a monoclonal B lymphocytosis may confirm the diagnosis.
- Anemia, thrombocytopenia, neutropenia, and hypogammaglobulinemia are frequently evident either at the time of diagnosis or sometime during the course of the disease.
- The Rai staging system has helped to design appropriate management strategies. Table 62.3 gives the staging system and median survival time for each stage.

DESIRED OUTCOME

There are no curative treatments for CLL; therapy is designed to improve quality of life.

TREATMENT

General Management Principles

- Treatment is instituted if there are signs and symptoms of progressive disease, worsening of blood dyscrasias, autoimmune complications, symptomatic splenomegaly, bulky lymph nodes, severe lymphocytosis (>100–$200,000/\mu L$), and increased infectious complications.

TABLE 62.3. Rai Staging System and 10-Year Survival

	Lymph[a]	Lymphadenopathy	Organomegaly[b]	Hgb[c]	Platelets[d]
Low Risk (Median Survival, 7–10 Years)					
Stage 0	+	−	−	−	−
Intermediate Risk (Median Survival, 5–6 Years)					
Stage I	+	+	−	−	−
Stage II	+	+/−	+	−	−
High Risk (Median Survival, 2–3 Years)					
Stage III	+	+/−	+/−	+	−
Stage IV	+	+/−	+/−	+/−	+

[a]$>15 \times 10^9$/L blood lymphocytes.
[b]Enlarged liver and spleen.
[c]Hemoglobin <11 g/dL.
[d]Platelets $<100,000 \times 10^9$/L.

- Most stage 0 patients do not require treatment and are usually managed with close observation.
- In patients with stage I or II disease, a consistent survival benefit has not been demonstrated for drug therapy.
- In stage III and IV disease, treatment is required with the intention of achieving a partial or complete remission. Drug therapy is usually begun with chlorambucil and corticosteroids; chlorambucil can be replaced with cyclophosphamide without compromising response rates. Splenic radiation or splenectomy is often recommended in patients with stage III and IV disease to reduce symptoms and to improve autoimmune blood dyscrasia.

Corticosteroid Therapy

- Response rates are low when prednisone is used alone, rarely resulting in complete remission.
- Prednisone may be helpful in treating autoimmune thrombocytopenia and anemia, both relatively frequent complications of CLL. Splenomegaly, anemia, and thrombocytopenia often improve under corticosteroid therapy.

Cytotoxic Chemotherapy

- The combination of chlorambucil and prednisone remains the standard treatment of CLL; response rates approach 70% with about 40% complete responses. Chlorambucil is dosed either on a daily basis or intermittently every 2–4 weeks.
- Cyclophosphamide gives a similar response to chlorambucil and can be used in patients who have difficulty tolerating chlorambucil or where response is not optimal.
- The purine nucleoside analogues fludarabine, 2-chlorodeoxyadenosine (2-Cda), and 2-deoxycoformycin (pentostatin) may have an important role in the management of patients who have become resistant to chlorambucil plus prednisone.

Other Treatments

- Experience regarding allogeneic BMT in CLL is limited. The available data suggest that although there may be a high complete remission rate, few patients remain free from disease after transplant as measured by molecular studies. XI
- The current role of IFN-α is limited; the response in advanced CLL is well under 20%.
- Intravenous immunoglobulin (IVIG) has been employed in an attempt to reduce infections resulting from hypogammaglobulinemia that are a major cause of morbidity and mortality in patients with CLL. Doses of 400 mg/kg every 3 weeks for 1 year have been shown to produce a significant reduction in bacterial infections. However, routine use of IVIG may be difficult to justify on a quality of life or economic basis.

See Chapter 127, Chronic Leukemias, authored by Timothy R. McGuire, PharmD and Peter W. Kazakoff, PharmD, for a more detailed discussion of this topic.

Chapter 63

▶ LUNG CANCER

▶ DEFINITION

Lung cancers are solid tumors that have been classified into four major cell types: (1) squamous cell carcinoma; (2) adenocarcinoma; (3) large cell carcinoma; and (4) small cell carcinoma. Histologic confirmation of cell type is essential in treatment planning because they differ in natural history, clinical features, and response to therapy.

▶ PATHOPHYSIOLOGY

- Lung carcinomas arise from pluripotent epithelial cells after exposure to carcinogens (especially tobacco smoke), which cause chronic inflammation and eventually lead to genetic and cytologic changes that progress to carcinoma.
- Activation of protooncogenes and uncontrolled secretion of growth factors also contribute to cellular proliferation and this malignant transformation.
- Although cigarette smoking has been estimated to be responsible for about 83% of lung cancer cases, occupational or environmental exposure to asbestos, chloromethyl ethers, various heavy metals, polycyclic aromatic hydrocarbons, and radon has also been implicated.
- The World Health Organization has classified lung cancer into four major carcinoma cell types that can be identified by light microscopy:
  - *Squamous cell* carcinoma (<30% of all lung cancers) is distinguished histologically by evidence of squamous differentiation. It (along with small cell lung cancers) has a much higher incidence among smokers and males. Most squamous cell carcinomas tend to be slow growing and confined to the lungs but may eventually metastasize to the hilar and mediastinal lymph nodes, liver, adrenal glands, kidneys, bone, and gastrointestinal tract.
  - *Adenocarcinoma* (40% of lung cancers) are distinguished pathologically by a glandular or papillary pattern and mucin production. They are likely to metastasize at an early stage (often before the diagnosis of the primary tumor) and spread widely to distant sites including the contralateral lung, liver, bone, adrenal glands, kidneys, and central nervous system.
  - *Large cell* carcinomas (15%) are anaplastic tumors that show no evidence of differentiation. They have a propensity to metastasize in a pattern similar to that of adenocarcinomas.
  - *Small cell* lung carcinomas (SCLC or "oat cell" carcinomas) account for about 25% of all lung tumors. They are distinguished by a proliferation of neoplastic cells with round to oval nuclei. SCLC is a very aggressive and rapidly growing tumor with about 60–70% of patients

initially presenting with disseminated disease. It tends to metastasize to the lymph nodes, opposite lung, liver, adrenal glands and other endocrine organs, bone, bone marrow, and central nervous system.

- In terms of management strategy and overall prognosis, adenocarcinoma squamous cell, and large cell carcinomas are frequently grouped together and referred to as non-small cell lung cancers (NSCLC).

▶ CLINICAL PRESENTATION

- The most common initial signs and symptoms include cough, dyspnea, chest pain, sputum production, and hemoptysis. Many patients also exhibit systemic symptoms such as anorexia, weight loss, and fatigue that are suggestive of a malignancy.
- Disseminated disease also may cause neurologic deficits from CNS metastases, bone pain or pathologic fractures secondary to bone metastases, or liver dysfunction from hepatic involvement.
- Paraneoplastic syndromes that commonly occur in association with lung cancers include cachexia, hypercalcemia, syndrome of inappropriate hormone secretion, and Cushing's syndrome.

▶ DIAGNOSIS

- In a patient with signs and symptoms of lung cancer, chest x-ray is the primary method of lung cancer detection. It may also be useful in measuring tumor size, establishing gross lymph node enlargement, and aiding in detection of other tumor-related findings such as pleural effusion, lobar collapse, and metastatic bone involvement of ribs, spine, and shoulders.
- Computed tomography (CT) scans are helpful in all of the above as well as in evaluation of parenchymal lung abnormalities, detection of masses only suspected on the chest x ray, and assessment of mediastinal and hilar lymph nodes.
- Pathologic confirmation of lung cancer must be established by examination of sputum cytology and/or tumor biopsy by fiber optic bronchoscopy, percutaneous needle biopsy, or open-lung biopsy.
- All patients must also have a thorough history and physical examination with emphasis on detecting signs and symptoms of the primary tumor, regional spread of the tumor, distant metastases, and paraneoplastic syndromes. The physical examination also aids in determining whether or not a patient may be able to withstand aggressive surgery or chemotherapy.

▶ STAGING

- The American Joint Committee has established a TNM staging classification for lung cancer based on the primary tumor size and extent (T),

TABLE 63.1. Tumor (T), Node (N), and Metastasis (M) Staging for Lung Cancer

T_x	Positive malignant cell; no lesion seen
T_1	≤3 cm surrounded by lung or visceral pleura
T_2	>3 cm or involvement of main bronchus 2 cm or more distal to the carina, or invasion of visceral pleura, or associated atelectasis or obstructive pneumonitis extending to hilar region
T_3	Direct invasion of chest wall, diaphragm, mediastinal pleura, or parietal pericardium; or tumor in main bronchus less than 2 cm distal to the carina; or associated atelectasis or obstructive pneumonitis of the entire lung
T_4	Invasion of mediastinum, heart, great vessel, trachea, esophagus, vertebral body, carina; or tumor with a malignant pleural effusion
N_0	No regional lymph node involvement
N_1	Metastasis in ipsilateral peribronchial and/or ipsilateral hilar lymph nodes, including direct extension
N_2	Metastasis in ipsilateral mediastinal and/or subcarinal lymph node(s)
N_3	Metastasis in contralateral mediastinal, contralateral hilar, ipsilateral or contralateral scalene, or supraclavicular lymph node(s)
M_0	No distant metastases
M_1	Distant metastases

Stage Groupings

Stage			
Stage I	T_1	N_0	M_0
	T_2	N_0	M_0
Stage II	T_1	N_1	M_0
	T_2	N_1	M_0
Stage III$_A$	T_1	N_2	M_0
	T_2	N_2	M_0
	T_3	N_0,N_1,N_2	M_0
Stage III$_B$	Any T	N_3	M_0
	T_4	Any N	M_0
Stage IV	Any T	Any N	M_1

XI

regional lymph node involvement (N), and the presence or absence of distant metastases (M) (Table 63.1).

- For comparison of treatments, a more simple stage grouping system is also used:
  - Stage I refers to tumors confined to the lung without lymphatic spread;
  - Stage II refers to large tumors with ipsilateral peribronchial or hilar lymph node involvement;
  - Stage III includes other lymph node and regional involvement; and
  - Stage IV includes any tumor with distant metastases.

- The primary tumor is assessed using chest roentgenographs and fiber optic bronchoscopy, while lymphatic spread is usually assessed by mediastinoscopy, gallium-67 citrate scanning, or CT.
- If there is evidence of metastatic disease, then special scans (e.g., bone, brain, or liver) or biopsies (e.g., bone marrow or liver) may be necessary for staging.
- A two-stage classification is widely used to stage SCLC. *Limited disease* is disease confined to one hemithorax and to the regional lymph nodes. All other disease is classified as *extensive disease*.

▶ TREATMENT

NON–SMALL CELL LUNG CANCER

- Surgical resection is the treatment of choice for patients with clinical stage I and II disease. The single most important prognostic factor in patients undergoing curative resection is the presence or absence of lymph node involvement. The size of the tumor in stage I and II disease also has prognostic importance.
- Radiation therapy is an alternative in patients with stage I or II disease who decline surgery or are considered high surgical risks because of concomitant illness or restrictive pulmonary reserve. Radiation therapy may also be utilized when the tumor is not resectable because of fixation to a major blood vessel, the trachea, or esophagus.
- The response rates for chemotherapy in NSCLC have been disappointingly low and overall survival benefits have not been clearly demonstrated. Thus, there is no standard chemotherapy regimen for NSCLC. However, it does appear that patients who respond to chemotherapy are likely to have a survival benefit over nonresponders.
  - Single-agent chemotherapy has generally demonstrated objective response rates of 5–15% with no significant effect on overall survival.
  - Response rates for combination therapy generally have been better than those for single agent therapy; consistent improvement in overall survival rates has been more difficult to demonstrate. Therefore, the use of combination chemotherapy in advanced NSCLC remains controversial.
  - Cisplatin is included in the most widely studied and recommended regimens (Table 63.2). In general, response rates have been in the range of 20–40%, with responders surviving longer than nonresponders and complete responses occurring only rarely.
  - Because of the questionable benefits of chemotherapy in terms of overall survival advantage and its toxic effects, it is common practice to reserve chemotherapy for patients with a good performance status and otherwise favorable prognosis. In patients receiving chemotherapy, a minimum of two courses of therapy is usually given before evaluating the patient for response. If no objective response is seen, the regimen should be discontinued. Patients responding to chemotherapy should continue therapy until disease progression has been documented.

XI

TABLE 63.2. Combination Chemotherapy in Non–Small Cell Lung Cancer

Combination	Dosages	Schedule	Overall Response Rate (%)
CAP			
CTX	400 mg/m^2 IV day 1		
ADR	40 mg/m^2 IV day 1	Repeat course every 4 weeks	6–39
DDP	40 mg/m^2 IV day 1		
CE			
DDP	60–100 mg/m^2 IV day 1		
ETOP	80–120 mg/m^2 IV × 3 days	Repeat course every 3–4 weeks	19–41
CAVP (or PACE)			
CTX	400 mg/m^2 IV day 3		
ADR	40 mg/m^2 IV day 2		
ETOP	50 mg/m^2 IV days 1–3	Repeat course every 4 weeks	46
DDP	20 mg/m^2 IV days 1–3		
or			
CTX	800 mg/m^2 IV day 1	Repeat course every 3 weeks	28
ADR	45 mg/m^2 IV day 1		
ETOP	100 mg/m^2 IV days 1, 3, and 5		
DDP	40 mg/m^2 IV day 1		
PEV			
DDP	60 mg/m^2 IV day 1	Repeat course every 3 weeks	40
ETOP	120 mg/m^2 IV days 3, 5, and 7		
VCR	1.5 mg/m^2 IV days 1 and 7		
DDP/VIN			
DDP	120 mg/m^2 IV days 1 and 29	Then repeat every 6 weeks	40
VIN	3 mg/m^2 IV Q week × 6	Then repeat course every 2 week	
or			
DDP	60 mg/m^2 IV days 1 and 29	Then repeat every 6 weeks	46
VIN	3 mg/m^2 IV Q week × 6	Then repeat every 2 weeks	
or			
DDP	100 mg/m^2 IV day 1	Repeat course every 4 weeks	33
VIN	3 mg/m^2 IV days 1, 8, and 15		
MV			
MIT	15–20 mg/m^2 IV day 1	Repeat dose every 6 weeks	
VIN	3 mg/m^2 IV Q week × 6	Repeat dose every 2 weeks	36
MVP			
MIT	8 mg/m^2 IV days 1 and 29		
VIN	3 mg/m^2 IV days 1, 8, 29, and 36		43
DDP	80 mg/m^2 IV days 1 and 29, then every 6 weeks		

Key: CTX, cyclophosphamide; ADR, doxorubicin or Adriamycin; MTX, methotrexate; PRO, procarbazine; BLE, bleomycin; CCNU, lomustine; VCR or ONC, vincristine or Oncovin; HN$_2$, mechlorethamine; DDP, cisplatin; ETOP, etoposide; VIN, vindesine; MIT, mitomycin.

- Patients with an unfavorable prognosis (weight loss, poor performance status) and/or significant concomitant diseases should be given supportive care and palliative radiation when necessary.
- In locally advanced disease, neoadjuvant chemotherapy (given prior to surgery) using combination regimens that include cisplatin 100

mg/m^2 plus radiation may confer a survival advantage over radiation therapy alone.

SMALL CELL LUNG CANCER

- Surgery is almost never indicated because SCLC has the propensity to disseminate early in the disease. A possible exception is the rare patient who presents with a small, isolated lesion.
- In contrast to NSCLC, the use of aggressive combination chemotherapy regimens in SCLC has demonstrated a four-fold to five-fold increase in median survival.
  - Patients who initially present with limited disease, a better performance status, and no weight loss appear to have an improved prognosis.
  - Combination chemotherapy is clearly superior to single-agent therapy, and the best results are generally observed when three or more active agents are combined. Some frequently used regimens are described in Table 63.3.
  - Restaging to determine the effects of chemotherapy is usually done after three courses of treatment. Therapy is then continued in patients

TABLE 63.3. Combination Chemotherapy in Small Cell Lung Cancer

Combination	Dosages	Schedule	Overall Response Rate (%)
CAV			
CTX	750–1500 mg/m^2 IV day 1		
ADR	45–50 mg/m^2 IV day 1	Repeat course every 3 weeks	63–100
VCR	2 mg IV day 1		
CAE			
CTX	1000 mg/m^2 IV day 1		
ADR	45 mg/m^2 IV day 1	Repeat course every 3 weeks	63–100
ETOP	50 mg/m^2 IV days 1–5		
	or		
	80 mg/m^2 IV days 1–3		
CEV			
CTX	1000 mg/m^2 IV day 1		
ETOP	50 mg/m^2 IV day 1, then 100 mg/m^2 PO days 2–5	Repeat course every 3 weeks	80
VCR	1.4 mg/m^2 IV day 1		
CE			
DDP	80 mg/m^2 IV day 1	Repeat course every 3 weeks	65
ETOP	150 mg/m^2 IV days 3–5		
CBDCA/ETOP			
CBDCA	100 mg/m^2 IV days 1–3	Repeat course every 4 weeks	77
ETOP	120 mg/m^2 IV days 1–3		

Key: CTX, cyclophosphamide; ADR, doxorubicin or Adriamycin; VCR, vincristine; ETOP, etoposide; CBDCA, carboplatin.

XI

responding to therapy and discontinued or changed in patients demonstrating evidence of disease progression.

- In patients achieving a complete response, the optimal duration to continue therapy remains unknown with recommendations ranging from 6–24 months.
  - Unfortunately, when the disease recurs, it is usually less sensitive to chemotherapy; only about 8–10% of patients survive >3 years.
- Radiotherapy has been used in combination with chemotherapy to treat tumors limited to the thoracic cavity. This combined-modality therapy may decrease the incidence and delay the onset of local tumor recurrences but has only modestly improved the overall duration of survival (e.g., 1–4 months) over chemotherapy alone.
- Because central nervous system (CNS) metastases often occur, prophylactic cranial irradiation (PCI) has been advocated in patients achieving a complete response to chemotherapy. However, neurologic and cognitive impairment and abnormalities on brain CT scans have been reported in long-term survivors, leading some experts to recommend that cranial radiation be withheld until brain metastases manifest. Others recommend PCI, but only in lower dose fractions (200–300 cGy vs. 400 cGy) after chemotherapy has been completed.

► EVALUATION OF THERAPEUTIC OUTCOMES

- Many of the chemotherapy regimens used are very intense and are associated with a wide variety of toxic effects.
  - Nausea and vomiting may be severe (especially in the cisplatin-containing regimens) and require aggressive antiemetic regimens.
  - Myelosuppression is often the dose-limiting toxic effect associated with these combinations and granulocytopenia following many of the more aggressive regimens places patients at high risk of serious infections.
  - Other toxic effects associated with these regimens include mucositis, peripheral neuropathies, nephrotoxicity, and ototoxicity.
- Patients receiving radiation therapy may experience fatigue, esophagitis, radiation pneumonitis, and cardiac toxicity.
- Patients with lung cancer frequently suffer from concomitant medical problems including chronic obstructive pulmonary diseases and cardiovascular disorders (often related to smoking), which require pharmacologic intervention and monitoring.
- Many patients receive complex pharmacologic regimens that may include chemotherapeutic agents, antiemetics, antibiotics, analgesics, bronchodilators, corticosteroids, anticonvulsants, and cardiovascular agents. Such regimens necessitate intensive therapeutic monitoring in order to avoid drug-related toxic effects and to optimize patient management.

See Chapter 121, Lung Cancer, authored by Rebecca S. Finley, PharmD, MS, for a more detailed discussion of this topic.

XI

Chapter 64

▶ MALIGNANT LYMPHOMAS

▶ DEFINITION

Malignant lymphomas are malignant neoplasms of lymphoid and reticuloendothelial tissues, which present as solid tumors consisting of cells that appear primitive or that resemble lymphocytes, plasma cells, or histiocytes. Lymphomas are classified by cell type, degree of differentiation, and nodular or diffuse pattern. This chapter begins with Hodgkin's lymphoma and then addresses non-Hodgkin's lymphomas.

▶ HODGKIN'S DISEASE

PATHOPHYSIOLOGY

- Etiology has not been fully elucidated. Viruses, especially Epstein-Barr virus (EBV) that causes mononucleosis, have emerged as leading candidates for an infectious etiology.
- Hodgkin's disease is unique among lymphomas because only a very small percent of cells from involved tissue actually contains malignant cells.
- The exact cellular origin of the malignant cell has yet to be determined and may not be the familiar Reed-Sternberg cell. In fact, this malignant cell appears to be of multilineage origin possibly because it represents an in vivo clonal population that occurs in response to viral stimuli (EBV) that promotes fusion of the interdigitating reticular cell, B cells, T cells, or both lymphocytes.
- The Rye classification system divides Hodgkin's disease into histologic subtypes based on the characteristics of the Reed-Sternberg cell and surrounding connective tissue. The subtypes (and incidence) are lymphocyte-predominant (46%), nodular sclerosis (60%), mixed cellularity (24%), lymphocyte-depleted (4%), and unclassified (6%).
- Hodgkin's disease appears to follow a predictable pattern of nodal spread that is not seen with non-Hodgkin's lymphomas.

CLINICAL PRESENTATION

- Most patients with lymphomas present with some form of adenopathy. In Hodgkin's disease, adenopathy is usually localized to the cervical region and is painless and rubbery. Other common sites of nodal involvement include the mediastinal, hilar, and retroperitoneal regions.
- Up to 40% of patients with Hodgkin's disease also present with constitutional or "B" symptoms (e.g., fever, night sweats, weight loss, and pruritus).

DIAGNOSIS AND STAGING

- The diagnosis and pathologic classification of Hodgkin's disease can only be made by biopsy of the enlarged node and histopathologic examination under a microscope.
- Staging is performed to provide prognostic information and to guide therapy.
- The Cotswald staging classification (Table 64.1) represents modifications of previous classifications (e.g., Ann Arbor and Rye). After careful staging, roughly half the patients have localized disease (stages I, II, and IIE) and the remainder have advanced disease, of which 10–15% are stage IV.
- Clinical staging begins with a thorough history to evaluate possible symptoms. Complete physical examination is done to determine nodal and extranodal involvement. Laboratory tests assess bone marrow, renal, and hepatic function. Chest roentgenogram and thoracic computerized tomography (CT) are necessary to evaluate mediastinal involvement. Abdominal involvement is evaluated using lower extremity lymphogram and abdominal CT. Skeletal films are used to evaluate thoracic and lumbar vertebrae, pelvis, and proximal extremities.
- Pathologic staging is based on biopsy findings of strategic sites (e.g., muscle, bone, skin, spleen, abdominal nodes) using an invasive procedure (e.g., laparoscopy or laparotomy).

TABLE 64.1. Ann Arbor Staging Classification for Hodgkin's Disease

Stage I	Involvement of single lymph node region or structure (e.g., spleen, thymus).
Stage II	Involvement of two or more lymph node regions on the same side of the diaphragm (i.e., the mediastinum is a single site, hilar nodes are laterized). The number of anatomic sites should be indicated by a subscript (e.g., II_2).
Stage III	Involvement of lymph node regions on both sides of the diaphragm:
	III_1: with or without splenic hilar, celiac, or portal nodes
	III_2: with paraortic, iliac, or mesenteric nodes.
Stage IV	Involvement of one or more extranodal site(s) beyond that designated E.

A: No symptoms
B: Fever (>38°C for 3 consecutive days), sweats, weight loss (>10%)
X: Bulky disease
   $>\frac{1}{3}$ the width of the mediastinum
   >10 cm maximal dimension of nodal mass
E: Involvement of a single extranodal site, contiguous or proximal to a known nodal site
CS: Clinical stage
PS: Pathological stage.

From Lister TA, Crowther D, Sutcliffe SB, et al. J Clin Oncol 1989;7:1630–1636.

XI

DESIRED OUTCOME

The current goal in the treatment of Hodgkin's disease is to maximize curability while minimizing short- and long-term treatment-related complications.

TREATMENT

Radiation Therapy (Alone)

Indications

- Radiation therapy alone is the cornerstone of treatment for localized Hodgkin's disease (stages I and II). Mantle irradiation may be followed with extended-field radiotherapy or subtotal nodal irradiation, which involves treatment of uninvolved areas (e.g., area below aortic bifurcation).
- Patients with $IIIA_1$ disease (i.e., limited spleen, celiac, splenic, or portal nodes) are candidates for radiation therapy alone, but not the subset with bulky mediastinal and stage $IIIA_2$ disease.

Complications

- Most side effects are transient and seldom produce significant morbidity. Anorexia, xerostomia, odynophagia, skin burns, and changes in taste perception are common. Myelosuppression can also be seen.
- Serious toxic effects include paramediastinal pulmonary densities, radiation pneumonitis and fibrosis, pericardial complications, and abnormal ventricular function.
- The most common neurologic complication is Lhermitte's syndrome (i.e., numbness and tingling caused by head flexion), which occurs in up to 15% of patients.

Chemotherapy

Combination Regimens as Initial Therapy

- MOPP has been the mainstay of treatment for stage IIIB and IV advanced Hodgkin's disease because it produces complete remissions in 80% of patients and has a 10-year cure rate of 54%. MOPP consists of 28-day cycles of mechlorethamine 6 mg/m^2 IV on days 1 and 8, vincristine 1.4 mg/m^2 IV on days 1 and 8, procarbazine 100 mg/m^2 orally on days 1–14, and prednisone 40 mg/m^2 orally on days 1–14.
- Studies indicate that combination regimens produce more rapid and durable remissions than single-agent therapy. Patients should receive a minimum of six cycles of MOPP and two cycles beyond that required to produce a complete response. Maintenance therapy does not increase survival and may contribute to long-term complications. Delivering full or nearly full doses of chemotherapy is extremely important.
- MVPP, CVPP, BVCPP, and ChlVPP (Table 64.2) are attractive alternatives to MOPP because they offer equal efficacy and differing or less severe toxicities.

XI

TABLE 64.2. Results of Treatment with MOPP Variations and Other Regimens

Regimen	N	Prior Therapy	Complete Response (%)	Disease-Free Survival (%/yr)	Overall Survival (%/yr)
MVPP	133	PR	82	60/5	76/5
MVPP	114	None	74	86/5	70/5
BVCPP	188	RT	68	55/4	—
ChlVPP	59	None	73	63/5	66/5
ChlVPP	44	None/RT	76	97/3	—
ABVD	35	RT	72	80/5	73/5
MOPP-ABV	76	None	97	91/4	94/4

Key: MVPP, mechlorethamine, vinblastine, procarbazine, prednisone; BVCPP, BCNU, vinblastine, procarbazine, prednisone; ChlVPP, chlorambucil, vinblastine, procarbazine, prednisone; ABVD, doxorubicin, bleomycin, vinblastine, dacarbazine; MOPP-ABV, mechlorethamine, vincristine, procarbazine, prednisone, doxorubicin, bleomycin, vinblastine; RT, radiation therapy.

- Alternating non-cross–resistant combinations do not provide clear advantages over fully dosed four-drug regimens possibly because they are not truly non-cross–resistant with MOPP.

Salvage Chemotherapy
- For patients who relapse after an initial complete response to MOPP, reinduction is possible. However, it is doubtful that a regimen should be used for salvage if it was unable to cure when used as first-line therapy, especially when other effective regimens with less chance of cross-resistance are available.
- Choice of salvage treatment should be guided by estimation of the patient's tolerance for a particular set of agents (Table 64.3).
- Patients who relapse following salvage chemotherapy are candidates for bone marrow transplantation.

XI

Complications
- Myelosuppression is the major dose-limiting toxic effect of most combination regimens. With the advent of colony-stimulating factors (e.g., G-CSF, GM-CSF), myelosuppression can be lessened, and dose-intensification may be possible.
- Nausea and vomiting are frequently seen with dacarbazine, doxorubicin, and mechlorethamine, although this may become much less of a factor with the availability of the $5HT_3$ antagonists.
- Many patients experience neurotoxicity secondary to vincristine in MOPP therapy.
- Other acute toxic effects include alopecia, dermatitis, mucositis, phlebitis, malaise and fatigue, pulmonary reactions, cardiomyopathy, and renal dysfunction.

TABLE 64.3. Salvage Therapy for MOPP Failures

Regimen	N	Complete Response (%)	Median Duration (mo)
ABVD	54	59	17
ABDIC	34	35	47
B-CAVe	48	44	21
CEP	58	40	15
CABS	17	35	>8
VABCD	18	44	>30

Key: ABVD, doxorubicin, bleomycin, vinblastine, dacarbazine; ABDIC, doxorubicin, bleomycin, dacarbazine, CCNU, prednisone; B-CAVe, bleomycin, CCNU, doxorubicin, vinblastine; CEP, CCNU, etoposide, prednimustine; CABS, CCNU, doxorubicin, bleomycin, steptozotocin; VABCD, vinblastine, doxorubicin, bleomycin, CCNU, dacarbazine.

- Gonadal dysfunction is a major long-term complication of combination chemotherapy. Nitrogen mustard or chlorambucil consistently produces sterilization in men.
- Secondary malignancies are also major long-term complications. Solid tumors are the most common type of malignancy, and radiation therapy is most often implicated as the causative agent. The risk of developing acute leukemia is highest in patients receiving both radiation therapy and chemotherapy. Cumulative amount of chemotherapy, especially alkylating agents (e.g., mechlorethamine, procarbazine, and BCNU), is also important.
- Differences in toxicity patterns can be used to guide selection of combination chemotherapy. Fears of nausea, vomiting, and neurotoxicity generally lead to larger dose reductions of MOPP than ABVD. If fertility is an issue, ABVD may be a reasonable initial regimen. If not, the MOPP alternative, ChlVPP, may be the best choice because it is very well tolerated, does not generally cause alopecia or neuropathy, and has leukemogenic effects that are intermediate between those of MOPP and ABVD.

XI

Combined Modality Treatment
- Controversy remains regarding the true role radiotherapy plays when added to chemotherapy in the treatment of Hodgkin's disease. Combined modality therapy is beneficial only in selected patients with early disease (e.g., large mediastinal involvement).
- Radiation therapy plus ABVD is associated with an increased risk of cardiac and pulmonary complications.

▶ NON-HODGKIN'S LYMPHOMA

PATHOPHYSIOLOGY
- Etiology of non-Hodgkin's lymphoma is unknown. A relationship between certain viral infections and development of lymphoma has

been seen, especially EBV infections and Burkitt's lymphoma in Africa. Other possible etiologic factors include immune dysregulation, chromosomal rearrangements, and exposure to ionizing radiation and environmental factors (e.g., pesticide or herbicide).

- Non-Hodgkin's lymphomas are a heterogeneous group of lymphoproliferative disorders involving the lymphatic and immune systems. These neoplasms are derived from monoclonal proliferation of B or, less commonly, T lymphocytes and their precursors.

CLINICAL PRESENTATION

- Patients may present with a variety of symptoms, which depend on the site of involvement, type of non-Hodgkin's lymphoma, and stage of disease at presentation, described later in this chapter.
- Low-grade lymphomas usually arise in middle-aged or older individuals (median age, 55 years), and are uncommon before 40 years of age. Most patients present with advanced stages of disease, often the result of bone marrow involvement. Low-grade lymphomas usually have an indolent clinical course with waxing and waning adenopathy for months to years prior to diagnosis.
- Intermediate- and high-grade lymphomas occur over a broader age range. Patients present at various stages of disease. Lymphoma tends to disseminate rapidly and often involves extranodal and privileged sites.
- Patients may have localized or generalized adenopathy. Involved nodes are painless, rubbery, and discrete, and usually located in the cervical and supraclavicular regions. Mesenteric or gastrointestinal involvement may cause nausea, vomiting, obstruction, abdominal pain, palpable abdominal mass, or gastrointestinal bleeding. Bone marrow involvement may cause symptoms related to anemia, neutropenia, or thrombocytopenia.
- Only 20% of patients with non-Hodgkin's lymphoma have constitutional or "B" symptoms.

DIAGNOSIS AND STAGING

XI

- Diagnosis must be established by an appropriate biopsy of an involved lymph node.
- Diagnosis of non-Hodgkin's lymphoma is similar to that of Hodgkin's disease except as noted later in this chapter. Extent of investigative workup required prior to therapy is determined by histopathology and available treatment for the subtype of non-Hodgkin's lymphoma.
- Chest CT is usually unnecessary if chest roentgenograms are normal.
- Staging is less important in non-Hodgkin's lymphoma than in Hodgkin's disease because treatment is the same for stages II, III, and IV within a specific subtype of non-Hodgkin's lymphoma. Instead, prognosis of non-Hodgkin's lymphoma is more dependent on histologic subtype (e.g., lymphoblastic or Burkitt's lymphoma) and clinical prognostic features (e.g., "B" symptoms, advanced age, elevated lactic dehydrogenase, large tumor burden, stage II disease or greater, bone

TABLE 64.4. Comparison of Systems of Classification of Non-Hodgkin's Lymphomas: The Working Formulation and the Rappaport Scheme

Working Formulation	Rappaport Classification	Incidence (%)
Low Grade		
A. Small lymphocytic (SL)	Diffuse well-differentiated lymphocytic (DWDL)	5
B. Follicular, small cleaved cell (FSC)	Nodular poorly differentiated lymphocytic (NPDL)	25
C. Follicular mixed, small cleaved and large cell (FM)	Nodular mixed, lymphocytic-histiocytic (NM)	10
Intermediate Grade		
D. Follicular large cell (FL)	Nodular histiocytic (NH)	4
E. Diffuse small cleaved cell (DSC)	Diffuse poorly differentiated lymphocytic (DPDL)	8
F. Diffuse mixed, small cleaved and large cell (DM)	Diffuse mixed lymphocytic-histiocytic (DM)	8
G. Diffuse large cell (DL)	Diffuse histiocytic (DH)	20
High Grade		
H. Immunoblastic, large cell	Diffuse histiocytic (DH)	10
I. Lymphoblastic	Diffuse lymphoblastic (DL)	5
J. Small noncleaved cell (SNC)	Diffuse undifferentiated (DU) (Burkitt's and non-Burkitt's)	5

marrow and gastrointestinal involvement, and conversion from low- to high-grade lymphoma).

- There are many systems for classifying non-Hodgkin's lymphomas (Table 64.4).
  - The Rappaport classification is based on the architecture of the lymph node and cytologic differentiation of the predominant cell. Lymphomas are characterized as nodular or diffuse (depending on presence or absence of malignant cell clusters), and as lymphocytic (small cells) or histiocytic (large cells).
  - The Working Formulation is based not only on morphologic features of malignant cells, but also on tumor aggressiveness and survival. Lymphomas are divided into three major groups: low, intermediate, and high grade.
  - Low-grade lymphomas are termed *good risk, favorable,* and *indolent* because patients have a relatively long disease-free survival, with or without chemotherapy. In contrast, intermediate- and high-grade lymphomas are termed *unfavorable* owing to their aggressive behavior. This traditional classification is paradoxical in view of potential for cure. While low-grade lymphomas may respond to many therapeutic approaches, response is often transient, and patients are rarely cured. In contrast, aggressive lymphomas can be

cured with intensive combination chemotherapy because of their high growth fractions and rapid tumor doubling times. (Of course, intermediate- and high-grade lymphomas are rapidly fatal if not treated.)

DESIRED OUTCOME

The primary treatment goals for non-Hodgkin's lymphoma are to relieve symptoms and cure the patient of disease whenever possible, and to do this with acceptable toxicity.

TREATMENT

General Principles

- The role of radiation therapy differs for non-Hodgkin's lymphoma versus Hodgkin's disease. Only a small percentage of patients with non-Hodgkin's lymphoma are amenable to remission induction with regional irradiation because localized disease at diagnosis is rare. Radiation therapy is used more commonly in advanced disease, but mainly as a palliative measure to control local bulky disease.
- Effective chemotherapy ranges from single-agent therapy for low-grade lymphomas to aggressive, complex combination chemotherapy regimens for intermediate- and high-grade lymphomas.
- Therapeutic approach depends on whether disease is limited (i.e., Ann Arbor stages I and II) or advanced (i.e., Ann Arbor stage III or IV, and frequently, stage II with poor prognostic features), and on histologic subtype. For the purpose of treatment, immunoblastic lymphoma will be grouped with intermediate-grade lymphomas.

Limited Disease: Low-Grade Lymphoma

- Radiation therapy is the standard treatment for early-stage low-grade lymphoma. There are no data to support the use of extended-field irradiation to clinically uninvolved contiguous lymph node chains, which is not surprising because spread of disease is frequently noncontiguous and less certain than with Hodgkin's disease.
- The role of adjuvant chemotherapy is unclear in localized stage I or II disease. Combining CHOP, but not CVP (cyclophosphamide, vincristine, and prednisone), with radiation therapy was superior to radiation alone in separate trials. CHOP consists of 21-day cycles of cyclophosphamide 750 mg/m^2 IV on day 1, doxorubicin 50 mg/m^2 IV on day 1, vincristine 1.4 mg/m^2 IV on day 1, and prednisone 100 mg/m^2 orally on days 1–5.

Limited Disease: Intermediate-Grade Lymphoma

- Radiation therapy alone appears most effective in patients with less bulky disease who have undergone staging laparotomy; however, laparotomy is associated with surgical complications and may delay initiation of therapy. Therefore, patients with early-stage aggressive lymphoma without poor prognostic features should not undergo exploratory

XI

laparotomy, but rather receive four to six cycles of combination chemotherapy followed by involved-field radiation therapy.
- If poor prognostic features are present, patients should receive treatment for advanced disease (see section on Advanced Disease).

Limited Disease: High-Grade Lymphoma
- Acute leukemia-like protocols (e.g., high-dose induction, consolidation, maintenance, and CNS prophylaxis; see Chapter 61) are used in the treatment of lymphoblastic lymphoma and small noncleaved cell lymphoma.

Advanced Disease: Low-Grade Lymphoma
- Management of stage III and IV low-grade lymphoma is controversial because standard therapeutic approaches are not curative, despite high complete-remission rates.
- Therapeutic options are diverse. Complete response can be achieved in 60–80% of patients with single-agent, combination chemotherapy, or combined modality therapy. Median remission durations range from 12–26 months. Five-year survival rates exceed 80% but fall to 30–50% by 10 years.
- Because treatment regimens have not convincingly improved survival, it has been suggested that initial therapy be withheld from asymptomatic patients (i.e., "watchful waiting"). When initial therapy was delayed, the 10-year survival was 73%, which does not differ from that of immediate therapy. However, watchful waiting may not be appropriate for follicular mixed histologies.

Advanced Disease: Intermediate-Grade Lymphoma

General Principles
- Intermediate- and high-grade non-Hodgkin's lymphomas are potentially curable diseases with intensive chemotherapy, even when they are widely metastatic.
- Intensive combination chemotherapy should be used because single-agent therapy does not consistently induce complete remission, and long-term survival is not possible without induction of a complete remission.
- Long-term maintenance therapy following a complete response has not been shown to improve survival (excluding lymphoblastic and small noncleaved cell lymphomas).
- Two cycles of chemotherapy following attainment of a complete response are usually recommended. Most current regimens last 6–9 months, except for MACOP-B, which requires only 12 weeks of therapy.
- Rapid response to chemotherapy (i.e., complete response in first three treatment cycles) is associated with a more durable remission compared with responses requiring more prolonged treatment.

XI

- Full doses of effective cytotoxic agents on schedule provides the best responses. Colony-stimulating factors (e.g., G-CSF, GM-CSF) may facilitate this goal and allow for the safer use of even more dose-intensified regimens, which may result in a new superior regimen.

Combination Regimens
- Of the first-generation regimens (Table 64.5), CHOP has gained widespread popularity. Adding agents such as bleomycin (CHOP-Bleo, BACOP) or methotrexate (COMLA) does not significantly affect treatment outcome.
- Second-generation chemotherapy consists of six or more antineoplastic agents, with more frequent cycling of myelosuppressive agents (e.g., every 3 weeks) and administration of nonmyelosuppressive, generally non-cross–resistant agents during weeks of cytopenias. Response and survival rates appear to be superior to those of first-generation regimens based on results of separate trials, but there were no differences in randomized trials.
- Third-generation treatment regimens focus on alterations in schedules (i.e., use of more drugs and early exposure to non-cross–resistant agents) and doses (i.e., increasing dose intensity). Third-generation treatment regimens appear to be superior to the first- and second-generation regimens, but there were no significant differences in a randomized trial, and third-generation regimens are more toxic.
- CHOP appears to be the therapy of choice based on response and survival rates, toxicity, and cost.

TABLE 64.5. First-Generation Chemotherapy Regimens for Advanced Intermediate- and High-Grade Lymphomas

Regimen[a]	N	Complete Response (%)	Long-Term Survival (B)[b]
C-MOPP	27	41	37
CHOP	115	67	50% (22 mo)
	418	53	30
CHOP-Bleo	26	69	—
	28	75	53
BACOP	32	48	37
COMLA	42	55	—
	72	40	30

[a]C-MOPP = cyclophosphamide, vincristine, procarbazine, prednisone; CHOP = cyclophasphamide, doxorubicin, vincristine, prednisone; CHOP-Bleo = cyclophosphamide, doxorubicin, vincristine, prednisone, bleomycin; BACOP = bleomycin, doxorubicin, cyclophosphamide, vincristine, prednisone; COMLA = cyclophosphamide, vincristine, methotrexate, leucovorin, cytarabine.
[b]Greater than 3 years.

Advanced Disease: High-Grade Lymphoma

- Treatment of advanced-stage lymphoblastic and small noncleaved cell lymphoma is essentially the same as limited disease.

Salvage Chemotherapy

- Unfortunately, second-line salvage therapies are not capable of consistently inducing remission in relapsed or refractory non-Hodgkin's lymphoma, in contrast with effective salvage regimens available for Hodgkin's disease. A possible reason for failure of salvage regimens might be the use of nearly all effective agents in primary regimens.
- A wide variety of salvage chemotherapy regimens have been used in patients with relapsed or refractory non-Hodgkin's lymphoma (Table 64.6).
- Preliminary experience suggests that high-dose chemotherapy and/or radiation with bone marrow transplantation (BMT) may improve the outlook for patients failing primary treatment.

Biologic Response Modifiers

- Biologic response modifiers (e.g., interferons [IFNs], interleukin-2 [IL-2] with or without lymphokine activated killer [LAK] cells, and monoclonal antibodies) are emerging as important investigational agents in the treatment of non-Hodgkin's lymphoma.
- The most promising results have been seen with low-grade lymphomas (i.e., follicular lymphomas).
- Recombinant IFN-α, the most extensively studied biologic agent, yields objective response rates of approximately 40% in low-grade lymphoma, with median durations of 6–12 months. The most effective dose

TABLE 64.6. Salvage Chemotherapy in Non-Hodgkin's Lymphoma

Regimen	N	Complete Response (%)	Median Duration of CR (mo)
MINE	123	32	15
DHAP	74	32	24
IMVP-16	38	37	12
CAMP	30	27	35
NOAC	66	26	7
EPOCH	70	27	6.8
IMEVC Ara C	30	53	15
DICEP	23	52	7.7

Key: MINE, mitoguazone, ifosfamide, methotrexate, etoposide; DHAP, cisplatin, high-dose cytarabine, dexamethasone; IMVP-16, ifosfamide, methotrexate, etoposide; CAMP, lomustine, cytarabine, mitoxantrone, prednisone; NOAC, mitoxantrone, high-dose cytarabine; EPOCH, etoposide, vincristine, doxorubicin, cyclophosphamide, prednisone; IMEVC Ara C, ifosfamide, mitoxantrone, etoposide, vindesine, cisplatin, cytarabine; DICEP, cyclophosphamide, etoposide, cisplatin.

XI

and schedule have not been determined, although lower doses appear to achieve similar results compared with higher doses.
- More studies are needed to confirm these preliminary results and the role of other biologic response modifiers alone or combined with chemotherapy.

AIDS-Associated Non-Hodgkin's Lymphoma
- Treatment of AIDS-associated lymphoma presents a therapeutic challenge. Standard chemotherapy regimens have been disappointing.

▶ EVALUATION OF THERAPEUTIC OUTCOMES

- The primary patient outcome to be identified is tumor response. Complete response is the desired outcome because only complete response will yield a chance for cure.
- Patients are are generally monitored at 3- to 6-month intervals for the first year or two following treatment, with longer intervals instituted when appropriate.
- The most important predictor of a positive outcome for treatment of Hodgkin's disease is dose intensity. Patients who receive full doses of chemotherapy on time do significantly better than those who do not.
- To optimize chemotherapy administration, toxicity management is key. The clinician must identify, monitor, treat, and prevent or minimize treatment-related toxicity. A review of pertinent laboratory data and other procedures will help establish a baseline for monitoring purposes. Major organ and system toxicities to be followed include hematologic, neurologic, skin, pulmonary, gastrointestinal, renal, and cardiac.
- Myelosuppression and neutropenic fever with infection are constant concerns with aggressive chemotherapy. Appropriate patient education and monitoring are critical.
- Nutritional assessment should also be undertaken.

XI *See Chapter 124, Malignant Lymphomas, authored by Jim Koeller, MS, and Val Adams, PharmD, for a more detailed discussion of this topic.*

Chapter 65

▶ PROSTATE CANCER

▶ DEFINITION

Prostate cancers are usually adenocarcinomas that are curable when local disease is present. Metastatic spread occurs most commonly to bone, but the lung, liver, brain, and adrenal glands may be involved later. There are many treatment options for advanced prostate cancer.

▶ NORMAL PROSTATE PHYSIOLOGY (Figure 65.1)

- Normal growth and differentiation of the prostate depend on the presence of androgens, specifically dihydrotestosterone (DHT), released primarily from the testes and the adrenal glands.
- Luteinizing hormone-releasing hormone (LHRH) released from the hypothalamus stimulates the release of luteinizing hormone (LH) and follicle-stimulating hormone (FSH) from the anterior pituitary gland.
  - LH complexes with receptors on the Leydig cell testicular membrane and stimulates the production of testosterone and small amounts of estrogen.
  - FSH acts on the Sertoli cells within the testes to promote the maturation of LH receptors and to produce an androgen-binding protein.
- Circulating testosterone and estradiol influence the synthesis of LHRH, LH, and FSH by a negative feedback loop operating at the hypothalamic and pituitary level.
- Testosterone accounts for 95% of the androgen concentration, and the primary source is the testes; 3–5% is derived from adrenal cortical secretion of testosterone or C19 steroids.
- Only 2% of total plasma testosterone is present in the physiologically active unbound state that penetrates the prostatic cell by passive diffusion, where it is converted to DHT by 5-α-reductase. DHT subsequently binds with a specific cytoplasmic receptor and is transported to the nucleus of the cell where transcription and ultimately, translation of stored genetic material occurs.

▶ PATHOPHYSIOLOGY

- The only widely accepted risk factors are increased age, race-ethnicity (e.g., African-American), and family history of prostate cancer. Other factors thought to be implicated include occupational exposure, diet, benign prostatic hyperplasia, and vasectomy.
- The initial step in cancer progression involves early mutations in stability genes (e.g., *p53, Rb,* E-cahedrin), resulting in unregulated cell growth.

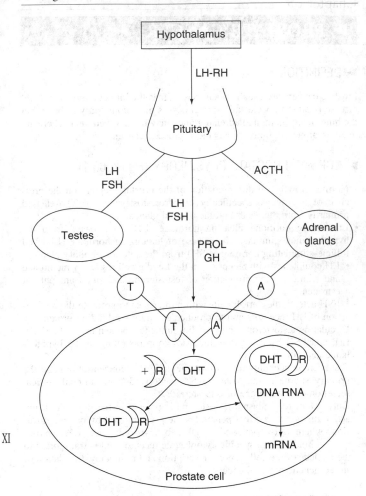

Figure 65.1. Hormonal regulation of the prostate gland. LH-RH, luteinizing hormone-releasing hormone; LH, luteinizing hormone; FSH, follicle-stimulating hormone; PROL, prolactin; ACTH, adrenocorticotropic hormone; GH, growth hormone; A, androgens; T, testosterone; R, receptor; DHT, dihydrotestosterone.

- The normal prostate is composed of acinar secretory cells that are almost always altered in size, shape, or number when invaded by carcinoma; the major pathologic cell type is adenocarcinoma (>95% of cases).
- Prostate cancer can be graded and then grouped into highly, moderately, or poorly differentiated grades. Well-differentiated tumors grow slowly, whereas poorly differentiated tumors grow rapidly and are associated with a poorer prognosis.
- Metastatic spread can occur by local extension, lymphatic drainage, or hematogenous dissemination. Skeletal metastases from hematogenous spread are the most common sites of distant spread. The lung, liver, brain, and adrenal glands are the most common sites of visceral involvement, but these organs are not usually involved initially.

▶ CLINICAL PRESENTATION

- Localized prostatic carcinoma may be asymptomatic, and most patients with signs and symptoms have advanced disease at presentation. Patients with locally invasive disease commonly have complaints arising from ureteral dysfunction or impingement, such as alterations in micturition (urinary frequency, hesitancy, and dribbling).
- Patients with advanced disease commonly present with back pain and stiffness due to osseous metastases. Untreated spinal cord lesions may ultimately lead to cord compression; rarely do pathologic fractures occur. Lower extremity edema can occur as a result of lymphatic obstruction. Anemia and weight loss are nonspecific signs of advanced disease.

▶ DIAGNOSIS

- Digital rectal exam (DRE) is commonly employed for detection of prostate cancer; it has a sensitivity of 55–69%, specificity of 89–97%, positive predictive value of 11–26%, and a negative predictive value of 85–96%.
- Prostate-specific antigen (PSA), a prostate-specific glycoprotein produced only in the cytoplasm of benign and malignant prostate cells, is the most sensitive biochemical marker available for the diagnosis, staging, and monitoring of prostate cancer. Estimated sensitivity, specificity, and positive predictive values are 67%, 97%, and 43%, respectively.
  - PSA screening is able to identify nonpalpable cancers, and it increases the detection rate of prostate cancer in asymptomatic men older than 50 years of age by 50%, compared to DRE alone.
  - Unfortunately, only 38–48% of men with clinically significant prostate cancer have a serum PSA above the reference range.
  - Although PSA is prostate specific, an elevated PSA does not always indicate prostate cancer. Benign conditions, including acute urinary

XI

795

retention, acute prostatitis, prostatic ischemia or infarction, and benign prostatic hypertrophy (BPH), will cause an elevation of PSA.
- The age-specific PSA reference ranges are included in Table 65.1.
- The American Cancer Society currently recommends that all men older than 50 years of age should have an annual PSA and DRE. If both tests are normal, no further diagnostic action is required; however, if either is abnormal, further workup by transrectal ultrasonography (TRUS) is indicated (Table 65.1).
- The actual diagnosis and histologic grading can only be established by biopsy (e.g., transperianal or transrectal needle biopsy).
- The diagnostic staging workup should include a thorough history and physical examination with careful digital inspection of the rectum and palpation of regional lymph nodes, abdomen, and spine. The posterior lobe of the prostate is palpated for size, configuration, and consistency. Prostatic carcinoma is characterized by a rock-hard nodule or mass, whereas in BPH the gland is smooth and rubbery. The lower extremities should be tested for strength and reflex symmetry.
- Initial laboratory tests should include a complete blood chemistry, liver function tests, serum creatinine, serum acid phosphatase, serum alkaline phosphatase, and urinalysis. Alkaline phosphatase is frequently increased in prostate cancer owing to the metabolic activity of the bone surrounding the bone metastases.
- A bone scan may be indicated in certain circumstances to detect early disease. Pelvic lymph node dissection has high morbidity but may be necessary for patients in whom the information obtained will directly affect treatment decisions.

TABLE 65.1. Diagnostic Algorithm for Prostate Cancer

PSA[a]	DRE[b]	Diagnostic Action
≤Age-specific range[c]	Neg	Annual PSA and DRE
>Age-specific range[c]	Neg	TRUS: Biopsy visible lesions. Sextant biopsy of remaining prostate, with 2 cores containing transition zone tissue
Any value	Pos	TRUS: Biopsy palpable and visible lesions; sextant biopsy of remaining prostate

[a] Tandem-R or IM_x PSA.
[b] Digital rectal exam.
[c] 40–49: 0–2.5 ng/mL
50–59: 0–3.5 ng/mL
60–69: 0–4.5 ng/mL
70–79: 0–6.5 ng/mL
From Oesterling JE, Cooner WH, Jacobsen SJ, et al. Influence of patient age on the serum PSA concentration. An important clinical observation. Urol Clin North Am 1993;20:671–680.

- The results of diagnostic testing are used to stage the patient. The Whitmore classification is most commonly used; patients are assigned to stages A through D based on size of the tumor, local or regional extension, presence of involved lymph node groups, and presence of metastases (Table 65.2). Stage D accounts for the majority of cases. An additional subclassification system further divides the stages into subcategories. The international classification system (TNM) may also be used for staging.

▶ DESIRED OUTCOME

- The goals of treatment for localized prostate cancer are to cure the patient and prevent postprocedure complications (e.g., impotence, stricture, and incontinence). Advanced prostate cancer (stage D) is not currently curable, and treatment is intended to provide symptom relief, maintain quality of life, and prolong survival. With treatment, the 5-year survival rates for patients with stages A, B, C, and D are 77%, 65%, 48%, and 21%, respectively.

▶ TREATMENT

GENERAL MANAGEMENT PRINCIPLES

- The treatment for prostate cancer depends on the stage of the disease (Table 65.3).
- Patients with incidental carcinoma found at the time of a transurethral resection for BPH (stage A_1) require only careful observation owing to the slow progression of the disease.
- For select patients with either stage A_2 or B disease, radical prostatectomy with staging pelvic lymphadenectomy or interstitial irradiation therapy may be used.
- For stage A_2 or B patients who are not surgical candidates, external beam irradiation is the more common treatment.
- Ongoing studies are attempting to define the best treatment for patients with stage C disease, because some stage C patients may, in fact, have occult disease dissemination at presentation. Although external beam radiotherapy has been the primary treatment option, some investigators feel there is also a role for androgen deprivation.
- There is controversy about the best approach to stage D because most therapy is palliative and cure is not possible. Patients with stage D_0 prostate cancer may be carefully watched and appropriate local therapy (surgery or radiation) instituted when symptoms appear; most of these patients will have metastatic disease requiring systemic therapy. Stage D_1 patients may be treated similarly, but early hormonal intervention may be beneficial because it is known that stage D_2 patients with minimal disease have better overall survival with hormonal therapy than those patients with a large tumor burden.

XI

TABLE 65.2. Staging and Classification Systems for Prostate Cancer

AUS[a] Stage (A–D)	AJC–UICC[b] Classification (TNM)
A (occult, nonpalpable)	$T_xN_xM_x$ (cannot be assessed)
	$T_0N_0M_0$ (nonpalpable)
A_1: Focal	T_0: Focal or diffuse
A_2: Diffuse	
B (confined to prostate)	$T_1N_0M_0$, $T_2N_0M_0$
B_1: single nodule in 1 lobe, <1.5 cm	T_1 (Clinically inapparent tumor not palpable or visible by imaging)
	T_{1a}: Tumor incidental histologic finding in 5% or less of tissue resected
	T_{1b}: Tumor incidental histologic finding in 5% or more of tissue resected
	T_{1c}: Tumor identified by needle biopsy (e.g., because of elevated PSA)
B_2: Diffuse involvement of whole gland, >1.5 cm	T_2: (Tumor confined within the prostate[c])
	T_{2a}: Tumor involves half of a lobe or less
	T_{2b}: Tumor involves more than half a lobe, but not both lobes
	T_{2c}: Tumor involves both lobes
C (localized to periprostatic area)	$T_3N_0M_0$, $T_4N_0M_0$
C_1: No seminal vesicle involvement, <70 grams	T_3: (Tumor extends through the prostatic capsule[d])
	T_{3a}: Unilateral extracapsular extension
	T_{3b}: Bilateral extracapsular extension
	T_{3c}: Tumor invades the seminal vesicle(s)
C_2: Seminal vesicle involvement, >70 grams	T_4: (Tumor is fixed or invades adjacent structures other than the seminal vesicles)
	T_{4a}: Tumor invades any of bladder neck, external sphincter, or rectum
	T_{4b}: Tumor invades levator muscles and/or is fixed to the pelvic wall
D (metastatic disease)	Any T, N_{1-4}, M_0, or N_{0-4}, M_1
D_1: Pelvic lymph nodes or ureteral obstruction	N_1: Metastasis in a single lymph node, 2 cm or less in greatest dimension
D_2: Bone, distant lymph node, organ, or soft tissue metastases	N_2: Metastasis in single lymph node more than 2 cm but not more than 5 cm in greatest dimension; or multiple lymph node metastases, none more than 5 cm in greatest dimension
	N_3: Metastasis in lymph node more than 5 cm in greatest dimension
	M_{1a}: Nonregional lymph node(s)
	M_{1b}: Bone(s)
	M_{1c}: Other site(s)

[a]American Urologic System or Whitmore classification.
[b]American Joint Committee—International Union Against Cancer.
[c]Tumor found in one or both lobes by needle biopsy, but not palpable or visible by imaging, is classified as T_{1c}.
[d]Invasion into the prostatic apex or into (but not beyond) the prostatic capsule is not classified as T_3 but as T_2.
From Beahrs OH, D.E. H, Hutter RVP, et al. Manual for Staging Cancer, 4th ed. Philadelphia, JB Lippincott, 1992, with permission.

XI

TABLE 65.3. Treatment of Prostate Cancer by Stage of Disease

Stage	Treatment
A_1	Transurethral resection followed by close observation
A_2	Radical prostatectomy or radiation therapy
B	Radical prostatectomy Radiation therapy
C	Radiation therapy Hormonal manipulation[a]
D_0	Treat local symptoms if necessary If urinary obstruction present Transurethral prostatectomy or radiation therapy
D_1	Systemic treatment[a] Close observation alone or early endocrine therapy Radical prostatectomy, lymph node dissection, and orchiectomy
D_2	Pharmacotherapy Hormonal manipulation Combination hormonal therapy Cytotoxic chemotherapy Combination hormonal/chemotherapy Palliative radiation therapy for symptomatic areas

[a]Under investigation.

From Garnick, M. Urologic cancer. In Rubenstein E, Federman DD, eds. Scientific American Medicine, Sec. 12, Vol. IX. New York: Scientific American, 1993.

- The major treatment modality for advanced prostate cancer (stage D_2) is pharmacotherapy in the form of hormonal manipulation or cytotoxic chemotherapy. Local radiation therapy also is commonly used to palliate painful skeletal metastases in patients relapsing after endocrine therapy.

THERAPY OF ADVANCED PROSTATE CANCER

Hormonal Manipulation

- Hormonal manipulation is used in the treatment and palliation of advanced prostate cancer because prostatic epithelium undergoes atrophy when the normal physiologic effect of androgens is reduced.
- Hormonal manipulations to ablate or reduce circulating androgens can occur through several mechanisms, as discussed below.

Androgen Source Ablation

- Orchiectomy is the preferred surgical procedure; adrenalectomy and hypophysectomy can remove the extratesticular sources of androgens, but these procedures are not commonly performed owing to high mortality and the availability of medical alternatives.

XI

- Many patients are not surgical candidates because of their advanced age, and other patients find orchiectomy psychologically unacceptable; these patients are candidates for pharmacotherapy.

LHRH or LH Inhibition

- Estrogens, LHRH agonists, progestogens, and cyproterone acetate suppress the release of LH from the pituitary gland resulting in reduced testosterone production.
- Estrogens (e.g., diethylstilbestrol or DES) may directly inhibit LH release, interfere with hormone synthesis, act directly on the prostate cell and/or increase the steroid-binding globulin level, thereby reducing the amount of free circulating androgens.
  - Estrogen therapy provides symptomatic relief in 60–80% of previously untreated patients. The onset of response is usually 1–2 weeks after initiation of therapy and is manifested by decreased bone pain and relief of urinary symptoms. The usual duration of response is 1–2 years, and almost all patients progress to metastatic disease. There is no benefit to using orchiectomy and estrogens simultaneously.
  - In studies of patients with advanced disease, deaths from cardiovascular complications were more common in patients >75 years of age, those with a prior history of cardiovascular disease, and those receiving the highest DES dose of 5 mg/d. For this reason, young patients with good performance status should be considered for early hormonal intervention.
  - There is no standard initial DES dose. DES 3 mg/d in three divided doses may be given to uniformly suppress testosterone production and hopefully reduce the incidence of cardiovascular complications. An initial dose of 1 mg/d may be used, but incomplete testosterone suppression may occur in up to 70% of patients; testosterone concentrations and PSA should be carefully monitored in those patients to ensure that castration levels have been achieved.
  - Other complications from DES therapy include fluid retention, nausea, vomiting, impotence, and painful gynecomastia.
  - Ethinyl estradiol, conjugated estrogens, chlorotrianisene, and polyestradiol phosphate offer no therapeutic advantage and are more expensive but can be used if patients cannot tolerate DES.
- LHRH agonists (leuprolide, goserelin) cause release of both LH and FSH, and new products with long durations of action inhibit gonadotropin release owing to a decrease both in number and sensitivity *(down-regulation)* of pituitary receptors and a decrease in testosterone production.
  - As initial therapy, LHRH agonists produce similar response rates to orchiectomy and estrogen administration and have a lower incidence of cardiovascular toxicity than estrogens.
  - Usual doses are leuprolide acetate 1 mg SC daily, leuprolide depot 7.5 mg IM once monthly, and goserelin acetate 3.6 mg SC every 28 days. Products for every-3-months administration are also available.

The long-acting preparations have similar efficacy and toxicity to the regular leuprolide formulation and are preferred because of extended duration of action.

- During the first week of treatment, a flare in disease may occur, usually manifested by increased bone pain; this corresponds with the initial increase in both LH and FSH and resolves by the second week of continued therapy. Other adverse effects may include hot flashes/sweats, sexual dysfunction manifested by erectile impotence and decreased libido, and minor irritation at the injection site.
- Both megestrol acetate (a progestational agent) and cyproterone acetate (a progestogenic antiandrogen) inhibit the release of LH from the pituitary in addition to their antiandrogen action at the target tissue level.

Androgen Synthesis Inhibition

- Aminoglutethimide, ketoconazole, and progestational agents interfere with the synthesis of androgens by the testes or adrenal gland.
- Aminoglutethimide inhibits the desmolase enzyme complex in the adrenal gland, thereby preventing the conversion of cholesterol to pregnenolone, the precursor substrate for all adrenal-derived steroids (androgens, glucocorticoids, and mineralocorticoids).
  - Medical adrenalectomy using aminoglutethimide is the preferred alternative to surgical adrenalectomy in order to reduce extratesticular sources of androgens in patients with advanced disease who progress after initial hormonal therapy. Although response rates with surgical adrenalectomy are 20–40%, the operative morbidity and mortality are high.
  - Aminoglutethimide can delay disease progression and produce symptomatic relief for a short time in up to 50% of patients with progressive disease, despite previous estrogen administration or orchiectomy.
  - Therapy is usually initiated with aminoglutethimide 250 mg PO twice daily and increased gradually to 250 mg PO 3 or 4 times daily depending on patient tolerance. Supplementation with physiologic doses of hydrocortisone or cortisone acetate is begun concomitantly to prevent negative feedback increases in ACTH production, which could competitively overcome the adrenal blockade. Mineralocorticoid replacement may be necessary in select patients. If the patient is taking an estrogen, it is continued to suppress the testicular source of androgen production. The duration of therapy should be at least 4–6 weeks to properly assess efficacy.
  - The major adverse effects that occur in about 50% of patients include lethargy, ataxia, and dizziness. A transient pruritic rash has been reported in up to 30% of patients that usually resolves within 5–8 days with continued therapy.
- Ketoconazole (400 mg given PO every 8 hours) results in a dose-related, reversible reduction in serum cortisol and testosterone concentration by inhibiting both adrenal and testicular steroidogenesis.

XI

- In uncontrolled trials, ketoconazole relieved symptoms in previously untreated patients with stage D prostate cancer. Responses were manifested by rapid pain relief and discontinuation of narcotic analgesics, decrease in prostatic acid phosphatase, and decrease in prostate size.
- Adverse effects included gastrointestinal intolerance, transient rises in liver and renal function tests, and hypoadrenalism.
- Megestrol acetate inhibits the synthesis of androgens, primarily at the adrenal level.

Antiandrogens

- Flutamide, bicalutamide, and nilutamide inhibit the formation of the DHT-receptor complex and thereby interfere with androgen-mediated action at the cellular level.
  - In patients with advanced prostate cancer, monotherapy with flutamide (250 mg PO three times daily) produces a favorable response (improvement in bone pain, decrease in prostate size, or improvement in performance status) in the majority of patients.
  - Gynecomastia is a common adverse reaction; liver function test abnormalities and methemoglobinemia may also occur.
  - Flutamide and bicalutamide are currently FDA approved only for combination with an LHRH agonist (see below). Nilutamide is approved for use in combination with orchiectomy.
- Megestrol acetate (120–160 mg PO per day) is a progestational agent that also blocks both androgen production and androgen action. Possible mechanisms include weak competition with DHT, inhibition of nuclear and cytosol androgen receptor formation, and moderate inhibition of 5-α-reductase.

5-α-Reductase Inhibition

- Compounds that inhibit 5-α-reductase action can block the formation of the DHT-receptor complex and prevent receptor activation. Clinical trials of finasteride in patients with advanced prostate cancer are ongoing.
  - 5-α-reductase inhibitors may ultimately prove useful in combination with other agents such as flutamide or as part of a chemoprevention program.

Combined Hormonal Blockade

- The intent of combination hormonal therapy (sometimes referred to as maximal androgen deprivation or total androgen blockade) is to interfere with multiple hormonal pathways to completely eliminate androgen action.
- This therapy includes an agent that suppresses testosterone synthesis (e.g., an LHRH agonist) and an agent that either interferes with androgen synthesis or blocks androgen action (e.g., flutamide or low-dose estrogen with megestrol).
- In a controlled trial of newly diagnosed patients with stage D disease, the combination of leuprolide plus flutamide was associated with longer

XI

survival in patients with minimal disease than those treated with leuprolide alone (61 vs. 41 months). Flutamide also reduced the symptoms
from the flare phenomenon associated with LHRH agonist therapy.
Diarrhea occurred more frequently in patients treated with flutamide.

- In contrast, a meta-analysis of 22 randomized trials comparing maximal
  androgen blockade to conventional medical or surgical castration
  showed no survival benefit for maximal androgen blockade. Consider-
  ing these conflicting results, the potential benefits must be weighed
  against the costs of combined therapy.

Hormone Withdrawal Syndromes

- Objective responses (PSA declines of approximately 50% for an average of 6 months) and improved clinical symptoms have been noted
  after the discontinuation of flutamide or bicalutamide in patients receiving these agents as part of combined androgen blockade.
- Mutations in the androgen receptor may result in antagonist compounds
  (e.g., flutamide, bicalutamide) or their metabolites becoming agonists.
- Antiandrogen withdrawal might be useful in patients progressing on
  combined androgen blockade.

Chemotherapy

- No currently approved antineoplastic agents or combinations prolong
  survival in patients with advanced prostate cancer. Although no clear
  benefit has been established, androgen ablation is usually continued
  when chemotherapy is initiated.
- Single agents with modest activity include cyclophosphamide, estra-
  mustine, 5-fluorouracil, methotrexate, DTIC, doxorubicin, and cisplatin. Combination therapy apparently does not improve response
  rates.
- Because studies using currently available cytotoxic chemotherapy for
  advanced disease have produced marginal clinical benefits and no survival advantage, its use should be limited to the investigational setting.

APPROACH TO THE PATIENT WITH ADVANCED PROSTATE CANCER

XI

- Orchiectomy is the preferred initial manipulation, especially in the
  patient with cardiovascular disease or in the emergent setting of
  impending spinal cord compression or ureteral obstruction. Addition of
  an antiandrogen (e.g., flutamide, nilutamide) to orchiectomy has produced improvements in bone pain and longer median survival than
  orchiectomy plus placebo, in some controlled studies.
- If the patient refuses orchiectomy or is not a surgical candidate, other
  forms of androgen ablation may be tried, which vary considerably in
  cost (Table 65.4). DES (1 mg 3 times/d) is least expensive; DES 1 mg/d
  requires monitoring of serum testosterone and PSA to ensure that castration levels are achieved. LHRH agonists are suitable alternatives to
  DES owing to low cardiovascular toxicity, but they are considerably
  more expensive.

TABLE 65.4. Comparative Costs of Hormonal Therapy for Advanced Prostate Cancer

Drug	Dose	Average Wholesale Price per Month of Therapy ($)
Diethylstilbestrol	3 mg/d	8.22
Leuprolide	1 mg/d	535.00
Leuprolide depot	7.5 mg/mo	472.50
Goserelin implant	3.6 mg every 28 days	358.55
Flutamide	750 mg/d	268.64
Biclutamide	50 mg/d	307.50

From Drug Topics: Annual Pharmacists' Reference (Redbook). Oradell, NJ, Medical Economics, 1995, with permission.

- Combined androgen blockade (antiandrogen plus LHRH agonist) is quite costly but may benefit patients with minimal disease and good performance status.
- When disease progression occurs despite compliance with hormonal manipulation that produced adequate testosterone suppression, a second hormonal manipulation can be attempted. If the patient is receiving an antiandrogen, it should first be discontinued and PSA monitored to assess the possible benefit of the hormonal withdrawal syndrome. Chemotherapy can be instituted, preferably as part of a research protocol. Adjunctive therapy for bone pain palliation is often the major therapeutic goal and includes reassessment of current therapy, radiation therapy, and analgesics.

▶ EVALUATION OF THERAPEUTIC OUTCOMES

- The objective measures of response to therapy include assessment of the primary tumor size, evaluation of involved lymph nodes, the response of tumor markers to treatment (e.g., PSA reduction), and survival duration.
- Subjective parameters include a scale for activity grading, an assessment of weight change, alterations in analgesic requirement, and general patient symptoms. Quality of life evaluations are important considerations in assessing the impact of prostate cancer treatments.

See Chapter 123, Prostate Cancer, authored by Barry R. Goldspiel, PharmD, Jill M. Kolesar, PharmD, and John G. Kuhn, PharmD, FCCP, for a more detailed discussion of this topic.

XI

Ophthalmic Disorders

Edited by Cindy W. Hamilton, PharmD

Chapter 66

▶ GLAUCOMA

▶ DEFINITION

The glaucomas are a group of ocular diseases characterized by changes in the optic nerve head (optic disk) and loss of visual sensitivity and field.

▶ PATHOPHYSIOLOGY

- The balance between the inflow and outflow of aqueous humor in the eye determines the intraocular pressure (IOP). The mean normal population IOP is 15.5 ± 2.5 mm Hg, with frequency distribution skewed toward higher pressures.
- The specific cause of glaucomatous optic disk changes, retinal nerve fiber damage, and visual loss is unknown. Previously, increased IOP was considered to be the sole cause of the visual damage; however, IOP is only one of many factors associated with the development and progression of glaucoma.
- Retinal ischemia, caused by either increased IOP or a reduced or dysregulated retinal and choroidal blood flow (or both), is likely to be a primary factor.
- Although IOP is a poor predictor of which patients will have visual field loss, the risk of visual field loss clearly increases with increasing IOP.
- Two major types of glaucoma have been identified. Open-angle glaucoma accounts for most cases; angle-closure glaucoma accounts for only 5%. Either type may be a primary, inherited disorder; secondary to disease, trauma, or drugs; or congenital (Table 66.1).
- The basic, underlying disorder producing the retinal nerve damage of primary open-angle glaucoma (POAG) is unknown. The increased IOP seen in most patients with POAG is caused by a decreased aqueous outflow facility, resulting in an imbalance between aqueous production and aqueous outflow.
- Angle-closure glaucoma results from mechanical blockage of the trabecular meshwork by the iris.
- A number of medications (Table 66.2) have been associated with increased IOP. The potential for a medication to produce or worsen glaucoma depends on the type of glaucoma and whether or not the patient is adequately controlled.

TABLE 66.1. Classification of Glaucoma

I. Primary glaucoma
   A. Open angle
   B. Angle closure
      1. With pupillary block
      2. Without pupillary block
II. Secondary glaucoma
   A. Open angle
      1. Pretrabecular
      2. Trabecular
      3. Post-trabecular
   B. Angle closure
      1. With pupillary block
      2. Without pupillary block
III. Congenital glaucoma

TABLE 66.2. Drugs That May Induce or Potentiate Glaucoma

Open-Angle Glaucoma	Angle-Closure Glaucoma
Corticosteroids (high risk)	Topical anticholinergics (high risk)
Topical anticholinergics	Topical sympathomimetics (high risk)
Systematic anticholinergics (low risk)	Antihistamines
Heterocyclic antidepressants (low risk)	Systemic anticholinergics
Phenothiazines (low risk)	Heterocyclic antidepressants
Vasodilators (low risk)	Phenothiazines
Cimetidine (low risk)	Ipratropium
	Benzodiazepines
	Theophylline (low risk)
	Vasodilators (low risk)
	Systemic sympathomimetics (low risk)
	CNS stimulants (low risk)
	Tetracyclines (low risk)
	Carbonic anhydrase inhibitors (low risk)
	Monoamine oxidase inhibitors (low risk)
	Topical cholinergics (low risk)

XII

▶ CLINICAL PRESENTATION

- Characteristic visual field loss occurs in glaucoma, but loss of central visual acuity does not occur until late in the disease. Visual field defects may include general peripheral visual field constriction, isolated scotomas or blind spots, nasal visual field depression or nasal step, enlargement of the blind spot, and large arclike scotomas.
- Patients with untreated angle-closure glaucoma typically experience intermittent prodromal symptoms brought on by precipitating events. The symptoms include blurred or hazy vision with halos around lights and, occasionally, headache.

▶ DIAGNOSIS

- IOP, optic disk changes, and perimetry are the primary diagnostic (and monitoring) parameters; however, increased IOP is not necessary for the diagnosis of glaucoma.
- Optic disk findings associated with glaucoma include cup:disk ratio >0.5, progressive increase in cup size, cup:disk ratio asymmetry >0.2, vertical elongation of the cup, excavation or deepening of the cup, increased exposure of lamina cribrosa, pallor of the cup, splinter hemorrhages, cupping to the edge of the disk, and notching of the cup.

▶ DESIRED OUTCOME

The ultimate goal of drug therapy in patients with glaucoma is to preserve visual function by reducing the IOP to a level at which no further optic nerve damage occurs.

▶ TREATMENT OF OPEN-ANGLE GLAUCOMA

- All patients with characteristic optic disk changes or visual field defects should be treated. Treatment of the patient with ocular hypertension remains controversial.
- Controversy exists as to whether the initial therapy of glaucoma should be surgical trabeculectomy, argon laser trabeculectomy, or medical therapy.
- Drug therapy of patients with documented glaucomatous change is initiated in a graduated manner, starting with lower concentrations of a single well-tolerated topical agent (e.g., β blocker, pilocarpine, carbonic anhydrase inhibitor, dipivefrin, or epinephrine) (Table 66.3).
- Systemic carbonic anhydrase inhibitors (CAIs) are indicated in patients failing to respond to or tolerate maximum topical therapy. The available systemic CAIs (Table 66.4) produce equivalent IOP reduction but differ in potency, side effects, dosage forms, and duration of action.

XII

XII

TABLE 66.3. Topical Agents Used in the Treatment of Glaucoma

Drug	Form	Strength%[a]	Brand Name	Dose Frequency[a]	Mechanism of IOP Reduction
β-Adrenergic Blockers					
Betaxolol	Solution	0.5	Betoptic	q 12 h	Decreased aqueous flow
	Suspension	0.25	Betoptic S	q 12 h	
Carteolol	Solution	1	Ocupress	q 12 h	
Levobunolol	Solution	0.25, 0.5	Betagan	q 12–24 h	
Metipranolol	Solution	0.3	OptiPranolol	q 12 h	
Timolol	Solution	0.25, 0.5	Timoptic	q 12–24 h	
	Gelling soln.	0.25	Timoptic XE	q 24 h	
Adrenergic Agonists					
α/β agonist					
Epinephrine HCl	Solution	0.25, 0.5, 1, 2	Epifrin, Glaucon	q 12 h	Increased aqueous outflow
Epinephrine bitartrate	Solution	2	Epinal	q 12 h	
Epinephrine borate	Solution	0.5, 1, 2		q 12 h	
Dipivefrin	Solution	0.1	Propine	q 12 h	Increased aqueous outflow
α₁ agonist					Decreased aqueous inflow
Apraclonidine	Solution	1	Iopidine	pre- and post-op	
	Solution	0.5	Iopidine	q 8–12 h	

TABLE 66.3. continued

Parasympathomimetics				
Direct acting				Increased aqueous outflow
Pilocarpine	Solution	0.25–10	Numerous	q 4–12 h	
Pilocarpine	Gel	4	Pilopine HS	q 24 h	
Carbachol	Solution	0.75, 1.5, 2.25	IsoptoCarbachol	q 8–12 h	
Cholinesterase inhibitors					Increased aqueous outflow
Physostigmine	Solution	0.25 0.5	Isopto Eserine	q 8–12 h	
Demecarium	Solution	0.125	Humorsol	q 8–72 h	
Echothiophate	Solution	0.03–0.25	Phospholine Iodide	q 12–24 h	
Isoflurophate	Ointment	0.25	Floropryl	q 8–72 h	
Carbonic Anhydrase Inhibitors					Decreased aqueous inflow
Dorzolamide	Solution	2	Trusopt	q 8–12 h	
Prostaglandin Analogues					Increased uveoscular outflow
Latanoprost	Solution	0.005	Xalatan	q 24 h	

aUse of nasolacrimal occlusion (NLO) may allow use of lower concentrations at longer intervals.

XII

809

TABLE 66.4. Carbonic Anhydrase Inhibitors

Drug	Form	Strength (mg)	Brand Name	Dose	IOP Reduction (h)		
					Onset	Peak	Duration
Acetazolamide	Injection	500	Diamox	500 mg IV or IM	2 min	0.25–0.5	2–5
	Tablets	125, 250	Diamox	125–250 mg bid-qid	1–1.5	2–4	8–12
	Capsules	500	Diamox Sequels[a]	500 mg bid	2	8–12	12–24
Dichlorphenamide	Tablets	50	Daranide	25–50 mg bid-qid	0.5–1	2–4	6–12
Methazolamide	Tablets	50	Neptazane	25–100 mg bid-tid	2–4	6–8	10–12

[a]Sustained-release capsule.

XII

▶ TREATMENT OF ANGLE-CLOSURE GLAUCOMA

- Iridectomy is the definitive treatment of angle-closure glaucoma; it produces a hole in the iris that permits aqueous flow to move directly from the posterior chamber to the anterior chamber.
- IOP in acute angle-closure glaucoma can be effectively reduced by decreasing aqueous humor production with application of a topical β blocker and a systemic CAI agent.
- An osmotic agent is often used because it rapidly decreases IOP (Table 66.5).
- Once the IOP is controlled, pilocarpine should be given every 6 hours until iridectomy is performed.

▶ EVALUATION OF THERAPEUTIC OUTCOMES

- Monitoring of therapy should be individualized: IOP should be measured initially every 1–2 weeks, then every 1–3 months after stabilization; the disk should be visualized and the visual field measured every 6–12 months (more frequently after any change in drug therapy).
- Because of the poor relationship between IOP and optic nerve damage, no specific target IOP exists. Typically, a 25–30% reduction is desired.
- The target IOP also depends on disease severity and is <21 mm Hg for early visual field loss or optic disk changes; 15–19 mm Hg for advanced disease, or even lower for very advanced disease, progressive damage at higher IOP, or low-tension glaucoma.
- Compliance with glaucoma therapy is commonly inadequate, and should always be considered a possible cause of drug therapy failure.

See Chapter 88, Glaucoma, authored by Timothy S. Lesar, PharmD, for a more detailed discussion of this topic.

XII ◀

XII

TABLE 66.5. Osmotic Agents Used in Glaucoma

Drug	Molecular Weight	Strength (%)	Dose	Route	Distribution[a]	Ocular Penetration[b]	IOP Reduction (h) Onset	IOP Reduction (h) Peak	IOP Reduction (h) Duration
Mannitol	182	5, 10, 15, 20, 25	1–2 g/kg	IV	Extracellular	Poor	0.25	0.5–1	6–9
Urea	60	30	1–1.5 g/kg	IV	Total	Good	0.25	1–2	5–6
Sodium ascorbate	198	20	0.5–1 g/kg	IV	Total	Good	0.5	1–2	8–12
Glycerin	92	50, 75	1–1.5 g/kg	PO	Extracellular	Moderate	0.25	0.5–1.5	4–6
Isosorbide	146	45	1–2 g/kg	PO	Total	Good	0.25	0.5–1.5	4–6
Ethanol	46	40–50	2–3 mL/kg	PO	Total	Good	0.5	1–2	8

[a]Distribution in body water.
[b]Prefer poor intraocular penetration for IOP reduction.

Chapter 67

▶ ALZHEIMER'S DISEASE

▶ DEFINITION

Alzheimer's Disease (AD) is a progressive dementia for which no cause is known and no cure exists. Disability progresses until AD sufferers become totally dependent. AD is the most common cause of dementia, accounting for 60% of all cases of late-life cognitive dysfunction.

▶ PATHOPHYSIOLOGY

NEUROFIBRILLARY TANGLES AND NEURITIC PLAQUES

- AD affects the brain structures associated with memory, higher learning, reasoning, behavior, and emotional control (cortex and limbic areas).
- The brains of AD patients have a drastically increased number of neurofibrillary tangles (NFTs) and neuritic plaques (NPs) in comparison to normal brains. These lesions occur particularly in the hippocampus, amygdala, and cerebral cortex in areas where cholinergic and other brain neuronal pathways have been destroyed.
- NFTs are intracellular and are comprised of paired neurofilaments with a helical shape that aggregate in dense bundles. The paired helical filaments are comprised of an abnormally phosphorylated form of tau protein. Affected cells function improperly and eventually die.
- NPs (also called *amyloid* or *senile plaques*) are extracellular and are comprised of a core of beta amyloid protein (βAP) surrounded by a snarled mass of broken neurites. Plaque formation seems to precede accumulation of NFTs. The number of NPs parallels disease severity.

BETA AMYLOID PROTEIN

- βAP deposition may initiate the process of plaque formation. Proteases cleave the amyloid precursor protein (APP) to form the βAP.
- Genetic abnormalities of the APP gene on chromosome 21 can lead to overproduction of βAP. Other early onset cases may be attributed to an Alzheimer's gene located on chromosome 14 that may play a role in the production and cleavage of APP.

APOLIPOPROTEIN E

- A subtype of apolipoprotein E (apo E) is a genetic marker for late-onset AD. The gene responsible for the production of apo E is located on chromosome 19. Ninety percent of persons inheriting two copies of apo E4 develop AD by age 80 years, and the onset of symptoms is relatively earlier. Apo E2 appears to be protective, conferring a relative resistance to AD. However, AD does occur in persons with no copies of apo E4.

INFLAMMATORY MEDIATORS

- Inflammatory mediators and other immune system constituents are present near areas of plaque formation, suggesting that the immune system plays a role in pathogenesis of AD. This could foster disease progression.

NEUROTRANSMITTER ABNORMALITIES

- The neuronal pathways most profoundly damaged are the cholinergic pathways. Logically, much research has focused on augmentation of cholinergic transmission at remaining synapses.
- Serotonergic neurons of the raphe nuclei and noradrenergic cells of the locus ceruleus are lost, whereas monoamine oxidase type-B (MAO-B) activity is increased. MAO-B is responsible for metabolizing norepinephrine (NE), serotonin (5-HT), and dopamine (DA).
- Glutamate and other excitatory amino acid neurotransmitters have been implicated as potential neurotoxins in AD.

EXOGENOUS FACTORS

- Evidence is building suggesting a role for estrogen in the prevention of AD.
- Repeated or severe head trauma has also been implicated as predisposing to AD.
- Preliminary in vitro evidence suggests that zinc may accelerate plaque formation from soluble βAP. Although the use of zinc supplements should be discouraged in patients with AD, at this time zinc should not be considered a cause of the disease.

CLINICAL PRESENTATION

- Cognitive and noncognitive symptoms of AD are shown in Table 67.1.
- Onset can be as early as age 40, but most cases occur after age 65.
- Loss of memory is typically the presenting complaint. Initially, memory complaints refer to disorientation for time or inability to recall recent events. Recall for remote events is spared until later in the disease process. Anomia is difficulty recalling names of familiar objects or people. Patients may resort to confabulation or circumlocution to compensate for their deficits.
- As speech, recall, and comprehension become impaired, there is decreased socialization and a withdrawal from casual conversation.
- At the moderate stages of severity, patients may be unable to use objects properly and unable to draw complex figures or conceptualize their orientation in space (constructional apraxia). They become unable to plan, to do household chores, and have trouble initiating activities.

XIII

TABLE 67.1. Fundamental Symptom Categories in Alzheimer's Disease

Cognitive Deficits[a]

- Memory loss: *poor recall; agnosia; losing items*
- Dysphasia: *anomia; circumlocution; aphasia*
- Dyspraxia
- Disorientation: *impaired perception of time; poor sense of direction; cannot recognize acquaintances, family, or self*
- Impaired calculation
- Impaired judgment and problem-solving skills

Noncognitive Psychiatric Symptoms and Disruptive Behaviors[b]

- Depression
- Psychotic symptoms: *hallucinations; delusions; suspiciousness*
- Nonpsychotic disruptive behaviors: *physical and verbal aggression; motoric hyperactivity; uncooperativeness; wandering; repetitive mannerisms/activities; combativeness*

[a]Cognitive deficits: symptoms occurring in all patients as disease progresses.
[b]Noncognitive symptoms: symptoms that are variably present, consisting mainly of psychiatric and behavioral problems.

- In the severe stages, patients may become lost in their homes, unable to recognize family, and unable to speak (aphasia). Judgment and reasoning are extremely impaired, and they may wander, become combative, incontinent, and require placement in a long-term care facility.
- Noncognitive symptoms are shown in Table 67.1. Depression, frustration, and irritability may occur early. Anxiety, hostility, and delusions are common in moderate stages. Disruptive behaviors and psychosis are seen in moderate to severe stages.
- Choking, aspiration, or infection generally results in death within 3 to 20 years of disease onset.

▶ DIAGNOSIS

- Early diagnosis is critical because cognition-enhancing drugs are more beneficial early in the course of the illness.
- Definitive diagnosis of AD is made by direct examination of brain tissue at autopsy or biopsy.
- In 1984, the Neurological and Communicative Disorders and Stroke and the Alzheimer's Disease and Related Disorders Association (NINCDS–ADRDA) developed criteria for AD (Table 67.2). These criteria establish a diagnosis of probable AD and are used to identify patients for research trials. These criteria reduce erroneous diagnosis to less than 10%.
- All patients should have a thorough history (from patient and caregiver) and physical exam. The history should include review of drug use, his-

TABLE 67.2. NINCDS–ADRDA Criteria and Diagnostic Workup for Probable Alzheimer's Disease

1. History of progressive cognitive decline of insidious onset
   - In-depth interview of patient and caregivers
2. Deficits in at least two or more areas of functioning
   - Confirmation with use of dementia rating scale (i.e., Mini-Mental Status Exam [MMSE[a]] or Blessed Dementia Scale)
3. No disturbance of consciousness
4. Age between 40 and 90 (usually >65)
5. No other explainable cause of symptoms
   - Normal laboratory tests including hematology, full chemistries, B_{12} and folate, thyroid function tests, VDRL (to rule out venereal disease or syphilis)
   - Normal electrocardiogram and electroencephalogram
   - Nominal physical exam, including thorough neurologic exam
   - Neuroimaging: CT or MRI scanning; no focal lesions signifying other possible causes of dementia are allowed. Abnormalities that are common, but not diagnostic for Alzheimer's disease include general cerebral wasting, widening of sulci, widening of the ventricles, and lesions of white matter surrounding the ventricle deep in the brain.

---

[a]The Folstein Mini-Mental Status Exam (MMSE) is a commonly used scale that measures orientation, recall, short-term memory, concentration, constructional praxis, and language. The MMSE is scored from 0 to 30, with a score of 10 to ~28 typical of moderate to very early Alzheimer's disease.

---

tory of alcohol or other substance use, family medical history, and history of trauma, depression, or head injury.

- Medication use (anticholinergics, sedatives) must be ruled out as contributing to the symptoms.
- The Folstein Mini-Mental Status Exam (MMSE) can be used to establish history of deficits in two or more areas of cognition.
- Other causes of dementia must be excluded (e.g., cerebral vascular disease, subcortical stroke, alcoholism, vitamin B_{12} deficiency, head trauma, Parkinson's disease, Huntington's disease, Pick's disease, Creutzfeldt-Jakob disease, hypothyroidism).
- Routine laboratory tests, physical and neurologic exams, and brain imaging tools help establish the diagnosis.
- Following diagnosis, AD is staged using a scale such as the Global Deterioration Scale (GDS) (Table 67.3), which is useful in monitoring cognitive decline.

XIII
- Two potential methods of early diagnosis are undergoing research.
  - It may be possible to identify patients in the early stages of AD by ophthalmic application of 0.01% tropicamide solution followed by measurement of pupil size.
  - Another strategy under investigation combines two less specific tests, genetic testing for the apo E4 gene and position emission tomography (PET) scan measures for decreased parietal glucose metabolism and left–right asymmetry.

TABLE 67.3. Stages of Cognitive Decline: the Global Deterioration Scale (GDS)

Stage 1	Normal	No subjective or objective change in intellectual functioning.
Stage 2	Forgetfulness	Complaints of losing things or forgetting names of acquaintances. Does not interfere with job or social functioning. Generally a component of normal aging.
Stage 3	Early confusion	Cognitive decline causes interference with work and social functioning. Anomia, difficulty remembering right word in conversation, and recall difficulties are present and noticed by family members. Memory loss may cause anxiety for patient.
Stage 4	Late confusion (early Alzheimer's)	Patient can no longer manage finances or homemaking activities. Difficulty remembering recent events. Begins to withdraw from difficult tasks and give up hobbies. May deny memory problems.
Stage 5	Early dementia (moderate Alzheimer's)	Patient can no longer survive without assistance. Frequently disoriented with regard to time (date, year, season). Difficulty selecting clothing. Recall for recent events is severely impaired; may forget some details of past life (i.e., school attended or occupation). Functioning may fluctuate from day to day. Patient generally denies problems. May become suspicious or tearful. Loses ability to drive safely.
Stage 6	Middle dementia (moderately severe Alzheimer's)	Patients need assistance with activities of daily living (i.e., bathing, dressing, and toileting). Patients experience difficulty interpreting their surroundings; may forget names of family and caregivers; forgets most details of past life; difficulty counting backward from 10. Agitation, paranoia, and delusions are common.
Stage 7	Late dementia	Patient loses ability to speak (may only grunt or scream), walk, and feed self. Incontinent of urine and feces. Consciousness reduced to stupor or coma.

▶ DESIRED OUTCOME

XIII

• The goals of therapy of AD are to improve cognitive functioning and/or slow the cognitive decline and to eliminate or minimize noncognitive symptoms such that social functioning and self-care are enhanced. Additional goals are to allow the patient to be maintained at home as long as possible. Although the needs of the patient are paramount, all therapeutic plans must consider the effect of treatment on the caregiver.

► TREATMENT

PHARMACOTHERAPY OF COGNITIVE SYMPTOMS

Tacrine

- Tacrine is a competitive, reversible inhibitor of both acetylcholinesterase and butyrylcholinesterase. This results in increases in the amount of acetylcholine available for binding to muscarinic receptors. The synthesis, turnover, and release of 5-HT, NE, and DA are also increased by tacrine in animal studies.
- Efficacy of tacrine has been documented in two large multicenter trials.
- As a result of adverse effects (elevated hepatic enzymes and peripheral cholinergic side effects), after 6 months of treatment, only 11–12% of patients started on tacrine were still taking it and demonstrating clinical improvement, and an additional 11–12% tolerated the drug and showed no cognitive decline.
- A positive dose-response relationship and serum concentration–response relationship exists for efficacy as well as for side effects. However, the rise in alanine aminotransferase (ALT) does not appear to be dose related.
- Elevated transaminases (i.e., ALT or aspartate aminotransferase [AST] greater than 3 times the upper limits of normal) occurred in 23.5% of patients receiving tacrine. These tend to occur during the first 8 weeks of therapy and are more common in females.
- Liver enzymes return to normal within 4–6 weeks following dosage decrease or discontinuation.
- Other common adverse effects include nausea, vomiting, diarrhea, and abdominal pain.
- Bioavailability is low (17%) and nonlinear. The rate and extent of absorption is decreased when tacrine is taken within 2 hours after a meal.
- Tacrine is metabolized primarily by cytochrome P-450IA2 to an active metabolite. The multiple dose half-life of elimination is short (3.5 hours), thus requiring multiple doses daily.
- Tacrine decreases theophylline clearance by approximately 50%, and cimetidine decreases tacrine clearance by approximately 30%.

Therapeutic Principles for Use of Tacrine

- Tacrine should be used only in patients with mild to moderate dementia. The MMSE can be used as a screening tool, with patients scoring a ≥10 being placed on the drug.
- The initial dosage should be 10 mg PO four times daily with the dose titrated, if tolerated, in 40 mg/d increments every 4–6 weeks up to a maximum of 40 mg four times daily.
- ALT should be monitored weekly for the first 18 weeks, and weekly for 6 weeks after any increase in dose. The dose should be decreased if the ALT exceeds three times the upper limit of normal and discontinued if the ALT exceeds five times the upper limit of normal.

► XIII

- Three months of treatment is considered minimal to assess therapeutic response.
- Tacrine should be continued as long as the patient is tolerating it and showing no rapid cognitive decline. If tacrine is discontinued, tapering is recommended.

Donepezil

- Donepezil is a second generation reversible cholinesterase inhibitor that is specific to brain acetylcholinesterase with minimal effect on peripheral butyrylcholinesterase.
- Unlike tacrine, donepezil's pharmacokinetics are linear at therapeutic doses. Its long elimination half-life (70 hours) enables once daily administration.
- Donepezil demonstrates dose-related efficacy within a range of 3–10 mg/d, and appears to cause fewer gastrointestinal and other peripheral cholinergic effects than tacrine.
- Significant improvement compared to placebo has been demonstrated in memory, reasoning, orientation, language, general functioning, behavior, and activities of daily living.
- Doses of 5 mg once daily and doses of 10 mg once daily have been shown to be effective. Treatment with a dose of 10 mg daily should not be contemplated until patients have been on a daily dose of 5 mg for 4–6 weeks. Donepezil should be taken in the evening, just prior to retiring, and may be taken with or without food.
- Liver function monitoring is not required. The most common reasons for drug discontinuation are nausea, vomiting, and diarrhea.

Other Drugs

- Evidence continues to accumulate supporting the role of low-dose ibuprofen in preventing or delaying the onset of AD symptoms.
- In a small study, patients taking nimodipine, 90 mg daily, but not 180 mg daily, showed significant improvement on selected memory tests.

PHARMACOTHERAPY OF NONCOGNITIVE SYMPTOMS

- General guidelines for management include starting with small doses, monitoring closely, and carefully documenting response and side effects. Most psychotropic medications have anticholinergic effects that may worsen cognition. Suggested doses of commonly used medications are provided in Table 67.4.

XIII

Depression

- Patients with AD respond to antidepressant medications, but response is not as dramatic as in depressed nondemented patients.
- Secondary amine tricyclic antidepressants (TCAs) (e.g., nortriptyline, desipramine) or selective 5-HT reuptake inhibitors (SSRIs) (e.g., fluoxetine, paroxetine, sertraline) are usually preferred. For a more complete discussion refer to Chapter 70, Depressive Disorders.

Psychiatric Disorders

TABLE 67.4. Medications Used in Treating Noncognitive Symptoms of Dementia

Drugs	Suggested Dosage in Dementia (mg/d)	Indications
Antipsychotics		Psychosis: hallucinations, delusions, suspiciousness
Haloperidol	0.5–5 mg	Disruptive behaviors: agitation, aggression
Thioridazine	30–150 mg	
Antidepressants[b]		Depression: poor appetite, insomnia, hopelessness,
Desipramine	50–100[a] mg	anhedonia, withdrawal, suicidal thoughts, agitation
Nortriptyline	25–100[a] mg	
Fluoxetine	5–20 mg	
Sertraline	50–200 mg	
Paroxetine	10–40 mg	
Trazodone	150–400[a] mg	
Anticonvulsants		
Carbamazepine	100–1000[a] mg	
Valproic acid	1000–2500[a] mg	
Others		
L-Deprenyl	10 mg	Disruptive behaviors, agitation, anxiety, depression
Buspirone	10–45 mg[a]	Disruptive behaviors
Oxazepam	10–60 mg[a]	Disruptive behaviors

[a] Administer in divided doses.
[b] Newer antidepressants such as venlafaxine and nefazodone theoretically could be used but have not been reported. Concurrent use of fluvoxamine with tacrine should be avoided due to fluvoxamine's capacity to inhibit cytochrome P=450–IA2.

Antipsychotics

- Antipsychotics are used to treat disruptive behaviors and psychosis in AD patients, but they are moderately effective at best. Symptoms responding include assaultiveness, extreme agitation and hyperexcitability, hallucinations, delusions, suspiciousness, hostility, and uncooperativeness. Symptoms not responding include withdrawal, apathy, cognitive deficits, and incontinence.
- Patients with AD are more sensitive to antipsychotic side effects than are other patient groups. Especially problematic are extrapyramidal side effects, orthostatic hypotension, anticholinergic effects, and worsening cognition.
- The most widely used antipsychotic in AD is haloperidol, likely due to its relatively low incidence of anticholinergic effects, sedation, and orthostatic hypotension. However, if extrapyramidal effects are bothersome, thioridazine in low doses is an acceptable substitute.
- The suggested therapeutic range for haloperidol (5–12 ng/mL) should not be used as a guide for dosing in AD because efficacy and adverse effects occur well below this range in many patients.
- If delusions and problem behaviors are not particularly disturbing to the patient or caregiver, they may not require treatment.

XIII

- Attempts to taper and discontinue antipsychotic medication should be made at least every 3 months.

Miscellaneous Therapies
- Doses of selected medication are listed in Table 67.4.
- Benzodiazepines, particularly oxazepam, have been used to treat anxiety, agitation, and aggression, but generally show inferior efficacy when compared to antipsychotics. Their routine use is not advised because they may impair cognition and increase the risk of falls.
- Buspirone has shown benefit in treating agitation and aggression in a limited number of patients.
- L-deprenyl has been shown to decrease anxiety, depression, and agitation.
- There is less documentation to support use of carbamazepine or valproate, and lithium thus far has shown no benefit.

▶ EVALUATION OF THERAPEUTIC OUTCOMES

- A thorough assessment at baseline should define goals and document cognitive status, physical status, functional performance, mood, thought processes, and behavior. Both the patient and caregiver should be interviewed.
- The MMSE (or a variation) can be used to objectively assess multiple spheres of cognition.
- A list of symptoms to be treated and potential side effects should be documented.
- Periodic assessment for efficacy, compliance, side effects, need for dosage adjustment, or change in treatment should occur at least monthly.
- A treatment period of 6 months to 1 year may be necessary before it can be determined whether therapy is beneficial.

See Chapter 64, Alzheimer's Disease, authored by Andrea Eggert, PharmD, M. Lynn Crimson, PharmD, FCCP, and Larry Ereshefsky, PharmD, FCCP, for a more detailed discussion of this topic.

XIII

Chapter 68

► ANXIETY DISORDERS

► DEFINITION

Anxiety disorders include a constellation of disorders in which anxiety and associated symptoms are irrational or experienced at a level of severity that impairs normal daily functioning. The characteristic features are anxiety and avoidance behavior.

► PATHOPHYSIOLOGY

- Noradrenergic Model: This model suggests that the autonomic nervous system of anxious patients is hypersensitive and overreacts to various stimuli. The locus coeruleus may have a role in regulating anxiety, as it activates norepinephrine (NE) release and stimulates the sympathetic nervous system. Chronic noradrenergic overactivity down-regulates alpha$_2$ adrenoreceptors in patients with generalized anxiety disorder (GAD).
- Benzodiazepine Receptor Model: Benzodiazepine receptors are linked to γ-aminobutyric acid, type A (GABA$_A$) receptors and chloride ion channels. GABA is the major inhibitory neurotransmitter in the central nervous system (CNS). Anxiety symptoms may be related to underactivity of GABA systems.
- Serotonin Model: GAD symptoms may reflect excessive serotonin (5-HT) transmission or overactivity of the stimulatory 5-HT pathways.

► CLINICAL PRESENTATION

- The *Diagnostic and Statistical Manual of Mental Disorders,* fourth edition (DSM-IV) classifies anxiety disorders into several categories (Table 68.1).

GENERALIZED ANXIETY DISORDER

- The DSM-IV diagnostic criteria for GAD are shown in Table 68.2. The illness has a gradual onset, usually in the early twenties. The course of the illness is chronic, with multiple spontaneous exacerbations and remissions.

SOCIAL PHOBIA

- The essential feature is a marked and persistent fear of social or performance situations in which embarrassment may occur. The fear and avoidance of the situation must interfere with daily routine or social or occupational functioning.

SPECIFIC PHOBIA

- The primary characteristic is a marked and persistent fear of a specific object or situation such as thunderstorms, snakes, insects, or heights.

TABLE 68.1. DSM-IV Classification of Anxiety Disorders

A. Generalized anxiety disorder

B. Panic disorder
   With agoraphobia
   Without agoraphobia

C. Agoraphobia without a history of panic disorder

D. Phobic disorders
   Social phobia
   Special phobia

E. Obsessive–compulsive disorder

F. Post-traumatic stress disorder

G. Acute stress disorder

These patients are not seriously impaired in their daily functioning, as they simply avoid the feared object.

PANIC DISORDER

• Symptoms begin as a series of unexpected panic attacks. These are followed by at least 1 month of persistent concern about having another

TABLE 68.2. DSM-IV Diagnostic Criteria for Generalized Anxiety Disorder

A. Excessive anxiety and worry (apprehensive expectation), occurring more days than not for at least 6 months, about a number of events or activities (such as work or school performance),

B. The person finds it difficult to control the worry.

C. The anxiety and worry are associated with three (or more) of the following six symptoms (with at least some symptoms present for more days than not for the past 6 months):
   1. Restlessness or feeling keyed up or on edge
   2. Being easily fatigued
   3. Difficulty concentrating or mind going blank
   4. Irritability
   5. Muscle tension
   6. Sleep disturbance

D. The anxiety and worry is not confined to features of another psychiatric illness (e.g., having a panic attack, being embarrassed in public).

E. The constant worry causes significant distress, and significant impairment in social, occupational, or other important areas of functioning.

F. The excessive anxiety and worry are not caused by a drug substance (e.g., drugs of abuse or medications), or a general medical disorder, and do not occur exclusively as part of another psychiatric disorder (e.g., an affective disorder).

XIII

Adapted from the Diagnostic and Statistical Manual of Mental Disorders, 4th ed. Washington, DC: American Psychiatric Association, 1994; 435–436.

panic attack, worry about the consequences of the panic attack, or behavior change related to the panic attack.

- During an attack there must be four or more of the following symptoms: palpitations or an accelerated heart rate; sweating, trembling or shaking; sensations of shortness of breath; feeling of choking; chest pain or discomfort; nausea; dizziness; derealization or depersonalization; fear of losing control; fear of dying; numbness or tingling; and chills or hot flushes. The attacks reach a peak within 10 minutes and usually last no more than 20 minutes.
- Many patients eventually develop agoraphobia, which is avoidance of specific situations (e.g., crowded places, bridges, leaving home) where they fear a panic attack might occur.
- Patients may become homebound, and complications may include suicide attempts, depression, and alcohol abuse.
- The illness usually begins between late adolescence and the mid-thirties.

▶ DIAGNOSIS

- Evaluation of the anxious patient requires a complete physical and mental status exam, appropriate laboratory tests, and a medical, psychiatric, and drug history.
- Anxiety symptoms may be associated with medical illnesses (Table 68.3) or drug therapy (Table 68.4).
- Anxiety symptoms may be a concomitant symptom of several major psychiatric illnesses (e.g., mood disorders, schizophrenia, organic mental syndromes, substance withdrawal).
- Patients with panic disorder may be hypersensitive to even small doses of caffeine and other CNS stimulants. Anxiety symptoms are common as part of the withdrawal syndrome associated with abrupt discontinuation of CNS depressants.

TABLE 68.3. Common Medical Disorders Associated with Anxiety Symptoms

Cardiovascular/Respiratory System
Arrhythmias, chronic obstructive lung disease, hyperdynamic beta-adrenergic state, hypertension, hyperventilation, mitral valve prolapse, myocardial infarction, angina, pulmonary embolus

Endocrine System
Cushing's disease, hyperthyroidism, hypothyroidism, hypoglycemia, pheochromocytoma

Gastrointestinal System
Colitis, irritable bowel syndrome, peptic ulcer, ulcerative colitis

Miscellaneous
Epilepsy, migraine, pain, pernicious anemia, porphyria

XIII

TABLE 68.4. Drugs Associated with Anxiety Symptoms

CNS Depressants

Anxiolytics/sedatives, ethanol, narcotic agonists (withdrawal)

CNS Stimulants

Prescription products

Albuterol (Proventil, Ventolin), amphetamine sulfate, cocaine, diethylpropion (Tenuate), fenfluramine (Pondimin), isoproterenol (Isuprel, Medihaler-Iso), methylphenidate (Ritalin)

Nonprescription products

Caffeine (NoDoz, Vivarin), ephedrine (Efedron Nasal), naphazoline (Privine, Allerest Eye Drops), oxymetazoline (Afrin, Dristan), phenylephrine (Neo-Synephrine, Sinex), phenylpropanolamine (Dexatrim, Acutrim), pseudoephedrine (Sudafed, Novafed)

Miscellaneous

Anticholinergic toxicity, baclofen (Lioresal), digitalis toxicity, dapsone (Avlosulfon), cycloserine (Seromycin)

► DESIRED OUTCOMES

- The desired outcomes of treatment for patients with anxiety disorders are to minimize anxiety symptoms (including panic attacks), minimize impairment of social and occupational functioning, minimize side effects and other drug-related problems, ensure compliance with the drug regimen, and, in most cases, ultimately to discontinue medication.
- The goals of therapy of panic disorder include a complete resolution of panic attacks (not always achievable), marked reduction in anticipatory anxiety and phobic fears, and resumption of normal activities.

► TREATMENT

NONDRUG TREATMENT

- For patients with GAD, nonpharmacologic modalities include short-term counseling, stress management, psychotherapy, meditation, and exercise. Cognitive therapy is the most effective psychological therapy for GAD patients. Supportive therapy can benefit most patients.
- For panic disorder patients, it is critical that patients be educated to avoid substances that may precipitate panic attacks. These substances include caffeine, drugs of abuse, and nonprescription stimulants. In addition to drug therapy, patients often require behavioral therapy (e.g., exposure therapy, cognitive therapy, cognitive–behavioral therapy) to alleviate their avoidance behavior. XIII

GENERALIZED ANXIETY DISORDER

General Therapeutic Principles

- For patients experiencing functional disability, antianxiety medication is indicated.

- Benzodiazepines (BZs) are the most effective and widely prescribed medication for GAD.
- Buspirone, autonomic blocking agents, and antidepressants are additional anxiolytic options (Table 68.5).
- An algorithm for management of GAD is shown in Figure 68.1.

Benzodiazepine Therapy
- The BZs are drugs of choice for treating GAD (Table 68.6).
- It is theorized that BZs ameliorate anxiety through potentiation of the inhibitory activity of GABA. Serotonergic involvement may also contribute to anxiolytic effects.

Pharmacokinetics
- BZ pharmacokinetic properties are shown in Table 68.7.
- Diazepam and clorazepate have high lipophilicity and are rapidly absorbed and quickly distributed into the CNS (this may be associated with a "rush"). However, they have a shorter duration of effect after a single dose than would be predicted based on half-life because they are rapidly distributed to the periphery.
- Lorazepam, oxazepam, and prazepam are less lipophilic and have a slower onset but a longer duration of action. They are not recommended for immediate relief of anxiety.
- Many BZs are converted to desmethyldiazepam (DMDZ), an active metabolite with a long-elimination half-life and long-lasting antianxiety effect.
- Prazepam and clorazepate are prodrugs. Prazepam is converted to DMDZ in the liver, and clorazepate is converted to DMDZ in the stom-

TABLE 68.5. Nonbenzodiazepine Antianxiety Agents

Class/Generic Name	Approved for Anxiety	Usual Dosage Range (mg/d)[a]
Diphenylmethanes	No	25–200
Diphenhydramine	Yes	50–400
Hydroxyzine		
β-Blockers		
Propranolol	No	80–160
Azapirones		
Buspirone	Yes	15–60[b]

[a]Elderly patients are usually treated with approximately one-half of the dose listed.
[b]The dosage range in elderly patients appears to be the same, but is not established.

XIII

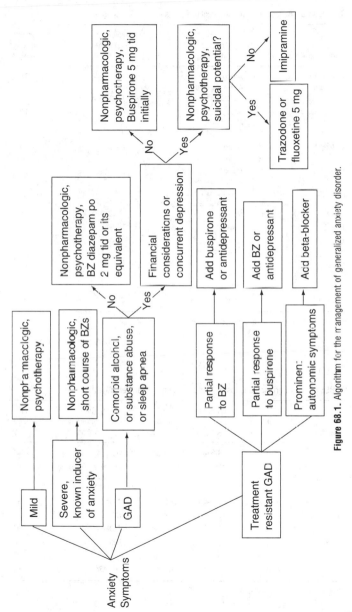

Figure 68.1. Algorithm for the management of generalized anxiety disorder.

XIII

TABLE 68.6. Benzodiazepine Antianxiety Agents

Generic Name	Approved Indications	Approved Dosage Range (mg/d[a])	Approximate Equivalent Dose (mg)
Alprazolam	Anxiety Anxiety-depression Panic disorder	0.75–4 1.5–10	0.5
Chlordiazepoxide	Anxiety Alcohol withdrawal Pre-op sedation	25–200	10
Clorazepate	Anxiety Seizure disorders	7.5–90	7.5
Diazepam	Anxiety Alcohol withdrawal Muscle spasm Pre-op sedation Status epilepticus	2–40	5
Halazepam	Anxiety	20–160	20
Lorazepam	Anxiety Pre-op sedation	0.5–10	1
Oxazepam	Anxiety Anxiety-depression Alcohol withdrawal	30–120	15
Prazepam	Anxiety	20–60	10

[a]Elderly patients are usually treated with approximately one-half of the dose listed.

TABLE 68.7. Pharmacokinetics of Benzodiazepine Antianxiety Agents

Generic Name	Peak Plasma Level (h)	Elimination Half-Life Parent (h)	Metabolic Pathway	Clinically Significant Metabolites	Protein Binding (%)
Alprazolam	1–2	12–15	Oxidation	None	80
Chlordiazepoxide	1–4	5–30	N-Dealkylation Oxidation	Desmethylchlordiazepoxide Demoxepam N-DMDZ[a]	96
Clorazepate	1–2	Prodrug	Oxidation	N-DMDZ	97
Diazepam	0.5–2	20–80	Oxidation	N-DMDZ	98
Halazepam	1–3	14	Oxidation	N-DMDZ	97
Lorazepam	2–4	10–20	Conjugation	None	85
Oxazepam	2–4	5–20	Conjugation	None	97
Prazepam	6	Prodrug	Oxidation	N-DMDZ	97

[a]N-desmethyldiazepam half-life 36–200 h.

ach. The later is a pH-dependent process that may be impaired by concurrent antacid use.

- Immediate- or short-acting BZs are preferred for chronic use in the elderly and those with liver disorders because of minimal accumulation and achievement of steady state within 1–3 days.
- BZs with long-elimination half-lives may be dosed once daily at bedtime and may provide both hypnotic and daytime anxiolytic activity.

Drug Interactions

- Drug interactions with the BZs are summarized in Table 68.8.
- The combination of BZs with alcohol or other CNS depressant agents is potentially fatal.
- Cimetidine inhibits the metabolism of the BZs metabolized by oxidation. This appears to have minimal clinical importance for healthy patients on chronic BZ therapy. However, when chronic therapy is indicated in elderly or debilitated patients receiving cimetidine, oxazepam or lorazepam is the BZ of choice.
- The alprazolam dose should be reduced by 50% if nefazodone or fluvoxamine is added.

TABLE 68.8. Drug Interactions with the Benzodiazepines

Drug	Effect
Alochol	Decreased clearance of chlordiazepoxide and diazepam; additive psychomotor impairment
Antacids	Decreased rate and extent of clorazepate absorption; decreased rate of diazepam and chlordiazepoxide absorption
Cimetidine	Decreased clearance of alprazolam, diazepam, chlordiazepoxide, and clorazepate and increased elimination half-life
Clozapine	Respiratory suppression, possibly death
Disulfiram	Decreased clearance of chlordiazepoxide and diazepam by 40–50%, and probably alprazolam, clorazepate, halazepam, prazepam
Fluoxetine	Decreased clearance of diazepam
Fluvoxamine	Decreased clearance of alprazolam and prolonged half-life
Isoniazid	Decreased metabolism of diazepam
Nefazodone	Decreased clearance of alprazolam, AUC doubled and half-life prolonged
Omeprazole	Decreased clearance of diazepam
Oral contraceptives	Increased free concentration of chlordiazepoxide and slightly decreased clearance; decreased clearance and increased half-life of diazepam and alprazolam
Rifampin	Increased metabolism of diazepam
Theophylline	Decreased alprazolam concentrations

XIII

Adverse Drug Effects
- The most common adverse event associated with BZ therapy is CNS depression. Tolerance usually develops to this effect. Other side effects include disorientation, confusion, aggression, and impaired memory (anterograde amnesia).

Abuse, Dependence, Withdrawal, and Tolerance
- Individuals with a history of drug abuse are at the greatest risk for becoming BZ abusers.
- With abrupt discontinuation of BZs, a mild withdrawal syndrome may occur in up to 44% of patients ingesting therapeutic doses of BZs for only 4–6 weeks.

Benzodiazepine Discontinuation
- After BZ therapy is abruptly discontinued, several events can occur:
  - Rebound symptoms represent an immediate, but transient, return of original symptoms with an increased intensity compared with baseline.
  - Recurrence or relapse is the return of original symptoms at the same intensity as before treatment (occurs in 50–65% of GAD patients treated with BZs for more than 1 year).
  - Withdrawal is the emergence of new symptoms and a worsening of preexisting symptoms. Withdrawal symptoms include anxiety, insomnia, restlessness, muscle tension, nausea, diaphoresis, nightmares, hallucinations, and seizures.
- The onset of withdrawal symptoms is 24–48 hours after discontinuation of the short-elimination half-life drugs and 3–8 days after discontinuation of the long-elimination half-life drugs.
- Discontinuation strategies include:
  - Twenty-five percent per week reduction in dosage until 50% of the dose is reached, then dosage reduction by one-eighth every 4–7 days.
- A BZ with a long elimination half-life (e.g., diazepam) may be substituted for a drug with a short elimination half-life (e.g., lorazepam, oxazepam, alprazolam). The substituted drug should be given for several weeks before gradual tapering begins.

General Prescribing Guidelines
- When dosage adjustments are made, all agents share similar anxiolytic and hypnotic activity.
- The dose must be individualized to avoid adverse effects.
- Duration of BZ therapy should be monitored and usually should not exceed 4 months. However, some patients require longer treatment.
- Abuse of BZs is unusual except in patients with a history of alcohol or sedative– hypnotic dependence.
- The elderly have an enhanced sensitivity to BZs.

Buspirone Therapy
- Buspirone is an azapirone and lacks anticonvulsant, muscle relaxant, hypnotic, motor impairment, and dependence properties. It is as efficacious as BZs after 4 weeks of therapy.

XIII

- Buspirone is a 5-HT$_{1A}$ partial agonist, binding presynaptically in the dorsal raphe and postsynaptically in the hippocampus and cortical brain areas.
- It is 95% protein bound, and the mean elimination half-life is 2.5 hours. It is metabolized oxidatively to active and inactive metabolites. Although unaffected by age, its clearance is decreased in patients with cirrhosis and in patients with renal impairment.
- Side effects include dizziness, nausea, headaches, and nervousness. Gynecomastia, galactorrhea, and extrapyramidal symptoms are rare.
- It has a low potential for abuse.

Drug Interactions
- Buspirone increases the area under the concentration-versus-time curve of haloperidol.
- It lacks a pharmacokinetic interaction with alcohol and does not potentiate performance impairment induced by alcohol.
- Concurrent monoamine oxidase inhibitor (MAOI) use with buspirone may cause elevated blood pressure, and this combination should be avoided.
- Fluoxetine is reported to antagonize buspirone's anxiolytic activity.

General Prescribing Guidelines
- The usual therapeutic dose of buspirone is 20–30 mg/d, with a maximum of 60 mg/d.
- The onset of antianxiety effects may require 4 weeks or more, and maximum therapeutic benefit may not be evident for 4–6 weeks.
- It is not useful in situations requiring immediate antianxiety effects or as-needed therapy.
- When a patient is switched from a BZ to buspirone, the BZ should be tapered slowly.

Adrenergic Blocking Agents
- The usefulness of propranolol and other beta-blocking agents may be restricted to patients whose physical symptoms, especially cardiovascular complaints, have not responded adequately to BZ therapy.
- Dosing should begin at 10 mg twice daily. Doses of propranolol ranging from 40–360 mg/d are used in managing GAD, and it should be dosed at least twice daily.
- To avoid rebound anxiety and cardiovascular effects, propranolol should be tapered prior to discontinuation.

XIII ◀

Antidepressants
- Although not first-line agents, imipramine and trazodone are effective after 3–8 weeks for treatment of GAD. Low doses of selective serotonin reuptake inhibitors (SSRIs) are also effective.
- They are useful adjuncts in patients with partial response to BZs or buspirone and as monotherapy for patients with contraindications to BZ therapy.

Evaluation of Therapeutic Outcomes
- Initially, anxious patients should be monitored twice weekly for a reduction in the frequency, duration, and severity of anxiety symptoms and improvement in occupational, social, and interpersonal functioning.
- Patients should be monitored for the occurrence of side effects.
- A Visual Analogue Scale, the State–Trait Anxiety Inventory, or the Zung Self-Rating Anxiety Scale may assist in the evaluation of drug response.

PANIC DISORDER

General Therapeutic Principles
- Panic disorder is treated effectively with several drugs including imipramine, alprazolam, phenelzine, and SSRIs (Table 68.9).
- Most patients without agoraphobia improve with pharmacotherapy alone, but if agoraphobia is present, cognitive–behavioral therapy typically is initiated concurrently.

Antidepressants
- Imipramine is effective in 75% of patients within 3–5 weeks. Maximal improvement may require 6–10 weeks. Other tricyclic antidepressants (TCAs) (e.g., desipramine, clomipramine) may be effective.
- With imipramine, 20–30% of patients experience stimulatory side effects including insomnia, jitteriness, and unusual energy. These side effects often affect patient compliance negatively and prevent increases in medication dosage. Reducing the dose may eliminate these effects.
- Approximately 40–50% of panic disorder patients respond to fluoxetine.
- With phenelzine, the antipanic effect is delayed for 3–5 weeks, and the antiphobic effect does not occur for 6–10 weeks. Side effects and dietary restrictions adversely affect patient acceptance.
- High dose alprazolam is effective and is well tolerated except for sedation. Diazepam, lorazepam, and clonazepam are possibly effective when taken in sufficient doses.
- Onset of therapeutic response to BZs is 1–2 weeks, but improvement continues for 4–6 weeks.

Clinical Guidelines
- Antidepressants are considered first-line therapy for patients with panic disorder who are clinically depressed or have a history of depression.
- BZs should be avoided in patients with panic disorder who have a history of alcohol or drug abuse.
- Some clinicians view SSRIs as first-line agents because of their tolerability.
- Phenelzine is a last-line medication, and is reserved for the most reliable patients.

Acute Phase
- The acute phase is 2–3 months for antidepressants and 1–3 weeks for BZs. Medication should be started in low doses but increased to adequate doses.

XIII

TABLE 68.9. Drugs Used in the Treatment of Panic Disorder

Class/Generic Name	Antipanic Dosage[a] Range (mg)	Comments
Benzodiazepines		
Alprazolam	1–10[b]	Effective in high doses, rapid response
		Problems: side effects, withdrawal
Diazepam	30–40	Possibly effective, needs more study
Clonazepam	3–6	Possibly effective, needs more study
Lorazepam	3–4	Possibly effective, needs more study
Tricyclic antidepressants		
Imipramine	~50–300	Effective
		Problems: lag time, side effects
Monoamine oxidase inhibitors		
Phenelzine	45–90	Effective
		Problems: patient acceptance, dietary restrictions, side effects
Serotonin reuptake inhibitors		
Fluoxetine	2.5–20	Effective
		Problems: lag time, expensive
Fluvoxamine	~50–300	Effective
		Problems: lag time, expensive
Paroxetine	~0–60	Effective
		Problems: lag time, expensive
Sertraline	25–100	Effective
		Problems: lag time, expensive
Miscellaneous agents		
Clonidine	0.2–0.5	Reserved as last-line agent; tolerance develops to antipanic effects
Valproic acid	500–2000	Reserved as last-line agent

[a]Dosage used in clinical trials but not FDA approved. [b]Dosage is FDA approved.

XIII

- Imipramine should be initiated with 10 mg/d at bedtime and slowly increased by 10 mg every 2–4 days as tolerated to 100–200 mg/d over a 2- to 4-week period. Most patients require 150 mg/d of imipramine or a combined imipramine–desipramine plasma concentration of 100–150 ng/mL.
- Similarly, low initial doses of SSRIs (2.5–5 mg/d of fluoxetine) are recommended.
- Phenelzine should be started at 15 mg/d and titrated upward. A dose of less than 45 mg/d is rarely effective. Consult Chapter 70 (Depressive Disorders) for precautions guiding the use of MAOIs.
- Although a few patients respond to alprazolam doses as low as 2–3 mg/d, many require 3–6 mg/d, and some need 6–10 mg/d. Because of its long half-life, clonazepam is an alternative if breakthrough panic attacks occur at the end of a dosing interval.

Continuation Phase
- The continuation phase lasts 2–4 months, and the goals are to extend the treatment response, especially with regard to phobic avoidance.

Maintenance Phase and Discontinuation
- The duration of the maintenance phase is 3–12 months, and the goals of treatment are to maintain response and to allow the patient to resume normal functioning.
- Usually patients are treated for 8–12 months before discontinuation is attempted, but many require longer treatment. Many patients may be tapered off medication during the second year of therapy. Approximately 20–40% of patients require chronic therapy.
- In patients taking alprazolam doses greater than 3 mg/d, dosage reduction should proceed by 0.5 mg every 2 weeks until 3 mg/d is reached, then 0.25 mg every 2 weeks until 1 mg is reached, then 0.125 mg every 2 weeks. The taper phase is most successful when it is accomplished over a 3- to 6-month period.
- TCAs should be reduced by 25 mg every 2–4 weeks. Phenelzine should be reduced by 15 mg every 2–4 weeks.

Treatment Resistance
- All standard treatments should be tried before using augmentation strategies. The most common strategy used in patients with a partial response to one agent is to augment with low doses of another agent. Limited data support the use of valproate.

XIII Evaluation of Therapeutic Outcomes
- Patients with panic disorder should be seen twice weekly for 2 weeks to adjust medication doses based on improvement in panic symptoms and to monitor for adverse events. Once stabilized, the patients can be seen weekly until antipanic response is achieved, then monthly.
- Patients should be encouraged to maintain a diary to document panic and avoidance symptoms.

- During discontinuation, patients should be monitored closely for withdrawal symptoms and relapse.

OTHER ANXIETY DISORDERS

Specific Phobias
- Specific phobia is considered unresponsive to drug therapy.

Social Phobia
- Generalized social phobia may respond to MAOIs, BZs, or SSRIs.
- Patients responded to phenelzine (doses similar to those in panic disorder) after 8–12 weeks.
- Clonazepam 1.5–2 mg/d or alprazolam 3 mg/d have shown effectiveness after 2 weeks.
- Propranolol is not effective for generalized social phobia, but may be used to manage performance anxiety in doses of 40 mg 1 hour before the performance.
- Fluoxetine (10–80 mg/d) and sertraline (50–200 mg/d) reduce avoidance and social anxiety. Fluvoxamine 150 mg/d improves social and general anxiety symptoms.

See Chapter 69, Anxiety Disorders, authored by Cynthia K. Kirkwood, PharmD, FASHP, FCCP, and Peggy E. Hayes, PharmD, for a more detailed discussion of this topic.

XIII

▶ BIPOLAR DISORDERS

Bipolar disorder, previously known as manic–depressive illness, is a cyclical disorder with recurrent fluctuations in mood, energy, and behavior. Diagnosis requires the occurrence of a manic, hypomanic, or mixed episode during the course of the illness.

▶ PATHOPHYSIOLOGY

- From 80–90% of bipolar patients have a parent, sibling, or child with a mood disorder.
- Theories involve neurotransmitter alterations in the central nervous system (CNS).
  - This may include a functional deficit of norepinephrine (NE) and/or serotonin (5-HT) in depression and an excess of NE in mania.
  - The permissive hypothesis posits that there is low central 5-HT in both mania and depression.
  - Mood disorders may be caused by a dysregulation between neurotransmitter systems.
  - Hyperdopaminergic activity may cause hyperactivity and psychosis in the severe stages of mania.
  - A deficiency of γ-aminobutyric acid (GABA) may cause mood disorders. GABA is the main inhibitory neurotransmitter in the CNS.
- Recurrences of the illness may result in behavioral sensitivity and electrophysiologic kindling. Initially, psychosocial or physical stressors may trigger episodes, but later, the episodes may occur spontaneously due to the increased CNS sensitivity and kindling.
- Electrolyte theories have been proposed. High serum and cerebrospinal fluid (CSF) calcium concentrations were found in patients with depression, whereas low CSF levels were reported in manic patients.
- Circadian rhythm desynchronization or seasonal rhythms may cause diurnal variations in mood and seasonal recurrences of episodes. Incidence of depression peaks in the spring and incidence of mania during the summer months.

▶ CLASSIFICATION AND CLINICAL PRESENTATION

The *Diagnostic and Statistical Manual of Mental Disorders,* 4th ed. (DSM-IV) divides bipolar disorders into four subtypes: (1) bipolar I, (2) bipolar II, (3) cyclothymic disorder, and (4) bipolar disorder not otherwise specified (NOS).
- Bipolar I is characterized by one or more manic or mixed episodes and is usually accompanied by major depressive episodes.
- Bipolar II disorder is characterized by one or more major depressive episodes and at least one hypomanic episode (Table 69.1).

TABLE 69.1. Comparison of Bipolar I and Bipolar II Disorders

	Bipolar I	Bipolar II
Episodes	Manic Hypomanic Mixed Major depression	Hypomanic Major depression
Lifetime prevalence	0.4–1.6%	0.5%

Sex differences	Female = male
	First episode in males more
	  likely manic episode
	First episode in females more
	  likely depressive episode
		Female > male

Clinical course	60–70% of manic episodes occur
	  just before/after a depressive
	  episode; interval between
	  episodes decreases with age
		60–70% of hypomanic
		  episodes occur just before/
		  after a depressive episode

Lifetime episodes	More episodes than major
	  depressive disorder
		More episodes than major
		  depressive disorder

Rapid cycling	5–15% of patients	5–15% of patients
% of patients that do not recover between episodes	20–30%	15%
Precipitants of episodes	Changes in sleep-wake cycle Sleep deprivation	Postpartum period

Familial pattern	First-degree biological relatives
	  with mood disorder:
	    Bipolar I (4–24%)
	    Bipolar II (1–5%)
	    Major depression (4–24%)
		Higher rates of mood disorder
		  than general population

- Cyclothymic disorder is characterized by at least 2 years of numerous episodes of both hypomanic and depressive symptoms, but they do not meet the criteria for a manic or major depressive episode.

MAJOR DEPRESSIVE EPISODE

XIII

- The clinical presentation and diagnostic criteria for bipolar depression are the same as those for major depressive episode, as discussed in Chapter 70 (Depressive Disorders).
- Bipolar depression is characterized by hypersomnia, fatigue, psychomotor retardation, decreased sexual activity, slowed speech, carbohydrate craving, and weight gain.

MANIC EPISODE

- DSM-IV diagnostic criteria include at least a 1-week period of abnormal and persistently elevated mood (expansive or irritable) and at least three of the following symptoms (four if the mood was only irritable): inflated self-esteem, decreased need for sleep, pressured speech, racing thoughts (flight of ideas), distractibility, increased activity, and excessive involvement in activities that are pleasurable but have a high risk for serious consequences. In addition, there must be marked impairment in functioning or the need for hospitalization.
- Seasonal changes, stressors, antidepressants, bright light, or electroconvulsive therapy (ECT) can precipitate a manic episode.
- Approximately two-thirds of bipolar patients have psychotic symptoms at some point, primarily paranoid or grandiose delusions.

MIXED EPISODE

- Mixed episodes are characterized by symptoms of a manic episode and a major depressive episode occurring nearly every day for at least a 1-week period.
- Symptoms are severe enough to cause impairment in social or occupational functioning or to require hospitalization.

HYPOMANIC EPISODE

- Hypomanic episodes are characterized by elevated, expansive, or irritable mood and associated symptoms, such as increased psychomotor activity, decreased need for sleep, pressure of speech, flight of ideas, and distractibility, but no marked impairment in social or occupational functioning, no delusions, and no hallucinations.
- During a hypomanic episode, some patients may be more productive and creative.
- Five percent to 15% of hypomanic patients may rapidly "switch" to a manic episode.

▶ COURSE OF ILLNESS

- Average age of onset of a first manic episode is in the early twenties.
- Recurrences may become more frequent as the disease progresses.
- Rapid cyclers are defined as individuals having four or more episodes per year (major depressive, manic, mixed, or hypomanic).
  - Rapid-cycling and mixed states are associated with a poorer prognosis and nonresponse to antimanic agents.
  - Tricyclic antidepressants (TCAs) and monoamine oxidase inhibitors (MAOIs) or subclinical hypothyroidism may exacerbate rapid cycling.

▶ DIFFERENTIAL DIAGNOSIS

- The diagnostic workup includes longitudinal psychiatric data; family history; a thorough medical, drug, and alcohol history; a complete physical examination; and appropriate laboratory tests.

XIII

- The majority of bipolar patients with depression or mixed episodes are nonsuppressors to the dexamethasone suppression test (DST). A blunted thyroid-stimulating hormone (TSH) response to the thyrotropin-releasing hormone (TRH) stimulation test has been reported in mania.
- Although these tests are rarely used for diagnosis, they may predict recovery, because patients have an increased risk for relapse if both tests do not return to normal.
- Several medical conditions, medications, and drug withdrawal syndromes can induce or present as mania (Table 69.2).

TABLE 69.2. Nonpsychiatric Causes of Manic and Hypomanic Symptoms

Medical Conditions
AIDS (HIV)
Addison's disease
Carcinoid tumors
Cushing's disease
Epilepsy (temporal lobe)
Hemodialysis
Huntington's disease
Hyperthyroidism
Multiple sclerosis
Neoplasm
Neurosyphilis
Postconcussion
Postinfection (viral, encephalitis, influenza)
Postcerebrovascular accident
Subarachnoid hemorrhage
Surgical trauma

Medications
Alcohol
Amantadine
Amphetamines
Anabolic steroids
Anticholinergics
Anticonvulsants
Antidepressants (TCAs, MAOIs, SSRIs)
Baclofen
Benzodiazepines
Bronchodilators
Caffeine
Calcium replacement
Captopril

Cimetidine
Cocaine
Corticosteroids (ACTH)
Disulfiram
Ephedrine
Hallucinogens
Indomethacin
Isoniazid
Levodopa
Methylphenidate
Phenylpropanolamine
Procainamide
Procarbazine
Quinacrine
Sympathomimetics (decongestants)
Theophylline
Thyroid supplements
Tolmetin
Yohimbine

Drug Withdrawal Syndromes
Antidepressants (TCAs, MAOIs)
Baclofen
Benzodiazepines
Clonidine
Corticosteroids
Guanabenz
Guanfacine
Methyldopa

Somatic Treatments
Electroconvulsant therapy
Bright light therapy

▶ DESIRED OUTCOMES

- The goal of treatment is to minimize target symptoms, toxicity, and adverse effects of medications while optimizing social and occupational functioning.
- Ideally, the patient and family should be involved in treatment to ensure compliance and adequate monitoring.

▶ TREATMENT

NONPHARMACOLOGIC THERAPY

- Bipolar disorder is most effectively treated with a combination of medications and adjunctive psychotherapy (individual, group, or family).
- ECT has approximately an 80% response rate. Preliminary data suggest that, in mania, bilateral ECT may be more effective than unilateral ECT.

GENERAL THERAPEUTIC PRINCIPLES

- Manic episodes are often treated first with lithium (plus short-term adjunctive agents, such as benzodiazepines for sleep). Recurrent manic episodes can be treated with either lithium, carbamazepine (CBZ), or valproic acid (VPA) along with adjunctive benzodiazepines.
- Severe manic episodes, with psychosis or agitation, often require longer term adjunctive benzodiazepines and/or antipsychotics along with lithium, CBZ, or VPA until the mania subsides. If the patient has not responded within 2–3 weeks, a second mood stabilizer can be added to the regimen.
- Maintenance therapy is recommended for any patient with at least two major episodes.
- In spite of adequate maintenance treatment, some patients may have "breakthrough" episodes of hypomania or depression that require short-term adjunctive medication (benzodiazepines or antipsychotics for mania and antidepressants for depression).
- Depressed patients on lithium should always be evaluated for lithium-induced hypothyroidism, because thyroid supplementation may reverse the depression.
- Monotherapy is preferred for long-term maintenance, but combinations of drugs may be necessary for patients with mixed episodes or rapid cyclers (e.g., lithium plus CBZ, lithium plus VPA, CBZ plus VPA).

XIII LITHIUM

- Lithium is generally 70–80% effective in aborting an acute manic or hypomanic episode within 7–14 days after starting therapy. Prophylactic lithium therapy is approximately 70–80% effective in preventing or attenuating recurrences of mania, hypomania, and depression.
- Maintenance lithium therapy may be more effective in patients with fewer prior episodes, a history of euthymia between episodes, a family

history of good response to lithium, and plasma concentrations between 0.8–1.0 mEq/L (vs 0.4–0.6 mEq/L).
- Lithium may be less effective in severe mania with psychotic features, mixed episodes, rapid/continuous cycling, and in organic-induced mood states.

Pharmacokinetics
Absorption
- Regular-release tablets or capsules are 95–100% absorbed, and peak plasma concentrations occur within 1–3 hours. Absorption is complete within 6–8 hours.
- Slow- or controlled-release tablets are 80–97% absorbed and have a slower absorption with lower and delayed peak plasma concentrations (within 2–6 hours) and complete absorption in 6–10 hours.
- Oral solutions of lithium citrate are rapidly and completely absorbed, with peak concentrations occurring within 15–60 minutes.

Distribution
- Lithium is widely distributed into most body tissues and follows a biphasic model.
- Distribution is usually complete within 6–10 hours after oral adminis-tration of regular-release tablets or capsules.
- Lithium is not bound to plasma proteins.

Elimination
- Lithium is primarily excreted renally and is not metabolized. Less than 5% of a lithium dose is excreted through the feces, sweat, and saliva.
- The average half-life of elimination is approximately 24 hours in adults, 36 hours in the elderly, and 40–50 hours in patients with impaired renal function.
- Approximately 80% of the lithium filtered through the glomeruli is reabsorbed in the proximal renal tubules.

Initiation of Therapy
- The recommended guidelines for baseline and routine laboratory testing are listed in Table 69.3.

Dosing
- Therapy is usually initiated with moderate doses (900–1200 mg/d) for prophylaxis and higher doses (1200–1800 mg/d) for acute mania, dosed two to four times daily. The dose should be adjusted based on the steady-state plasma concentrations drawn 12 hours ± 30 minutes after the last dose.
- When mania begins to resolve, the dose should be adjusted downward to decrease the risk of toxicity.
- A therapeutic trial should last a minimum of 4–6 weeks and maintain lithium plasma concentrations in the therapeutic range.
- Lithium therapy should not be discontinued abruptly.

XIII

TABLE 69.3. Recommendations for Baseline and Routine Laboratory Testing for Lithium Therapy

	Baseline	12 Months
Cardiac		
ECG[a]	•	
Pulse and blood pressure	•	
Hematologic		
CBC with differential	•	•
Metabolic/endocrine		
Weight	•	•
Serum electrolytes (sodium, potassium, calcium, phosphate)	•	•
T₃, T₄, free thyroxine index, TSH[b]	•	•
Renal function		
Serum creatinine[c]	•	•
24-hour creatinine clearance[d]	•	•
Urinalysis/osmolality/specific gravity	•	•
Pregnancy test		
In women of childbearing age	•	
Plasma lithium concentrations[e]		

[a] Patients older than 50 or those with preexisting cardiovascular disease; measure at baseline and every 6–12 months as indicated.

[b] TSH is a better indicator of hypothyroidism and should be obtained every 3–6 months during maintenance therapy if thyroid function tests change, if TSH >4 mIU/mL, or if symptoms of hypothyroidism occur.

[c] Measure every 3 months in patients with impaired renal functioning.

[d] Indicated at baseline for patients with a history of renal disease or abnormally high serum creatinine or significant increases in serum creatinine.

[e] Measure every 1–3 months during maintenance therapy; every 5–7 days after any dosage change or possible drug interactions; less frequent monitoring in stable patients (every 6–12 months).

Special Considerations for Dosing

- Lower initial doses are prescribed for elderly patients and when lithium excretion is impaired (low salt diet, diuretic therapy, renal disease, decreased cardiac output).
- In patients with polyuria, single-daily dosing at bedtime with extended-release products may be used to reduce urine output.
- When therapy is initiated in children, the dose should be low (e.g., 300–900 mg/d, or 30 mg/kg/d in divided doses) with gradual increases after laboratory monitoring.

XIII

Blood Level Monitoring

- The usual therapeutic range is 0.6–1.2 mEq/L. Acutely manic patients require a plasma concentration of at least 0.8 mEq/L, and some patients may require 1.2–1.5 mEq/L.

TABLE 69.4. Factors that Can Affect the Accuracy and Reliability of Plasma Lithium Concentrations or Alter Dose/Blood Relationship

Compliance before the blood test
Timing of blood sampling after last dose
Inadequate time to reach steady state
Product formulation and bioequivalency differences
Accuracy and reliability of the laboratory
Changes in sodium intake or excretion
Caffeine and alcohol intake
Concomitant drugs that alter lithium clearance
Medical illnesses (renal disease, dehydration, diarrhea, vomiting, anorexia, etc.)
Alterations in diet or physical activity
Pregnancy and delivery

- Onset of the acute antimanic effect usually requires 5–7 days, and the full antimanic effect may require 10–21 days and up to 28 days for a full antidepressant effect.
- When lithium is started, a nonsteady-state plasma concentration is recommended every 2–3 days in patients prone to toxicity. When the desired plasma concentration is achieved, blood levels should be monitored weekly for 3–4 weeks or until stabilized.
- Several variables can influence plasma lithium concentrations (Table 69.4).

Maintenance Therapy

- Standard therapeutic plasma concentrations (0.8–1.0 mEq/L) may decrease the risk of relapses, but lower concentrations (0.4–0.6 mEq/L) are better tolerated and are effective for some patients. The National Institutes of Mental Health/National Institutes of Health (NIMH/NIH) Consensus Development Conference on Mood Disorders recommended a maintenance range of 0.6–0.8 mEq/L for most patients. Elderly patients can be maintained on 0.6 mEq/L or less to avoid neurotoxicity.
- Breakthrough episodes during maintenance therapy should be treated by increasing the dose of lithium to achieve higher plasma concentrations (1.0–1.2 mEq/L). XIII
- During maintenance therapy, plasma concentrations should be obtained every 1–3 months. If a patient has been stable for 1 year, lithium concentrations may be checked less frequently (every 6–12 months).
- Plasma concentrations should be obtained 5–7 days after any change in the dose, whenever there is suspected toxicity, a possible drug interaction, a major change in diet, or significant weight fluctuations.

Duration of Treatment
- Patients with only one manic episode should be continued on a mood stabilizer for 9–12 months. Lifetime antimanic therapy should be given to patients with two or three prior episodes, frequent episodes (greater than one per year), or rapid onset of manic episodes.

Adverse Effects
- Side effects of lithium are summarized in Table 69.5.

Early Side Effects
- Gastrointestinal disturbances occur in 10–30% of patients, but are usually mild and transient. If nausea is significant, patients should take lithium after food, take a smaller dose more frequently, or switch to an extended-release product.
- Polydipsia, polyuria, and nocturia occur in up to 70% of patients initially but usually diminish with time.
- A fine hand tremor may occur in up to 50% of patients initially, and may persist in up to 4% of patients. The tremor is seen at rest and increases with voluntary movement. Propranolol in divided doses, 20–80 mg daily,

TABLE 69.5. Adverse Effects Associated with Lithium Therapy

Early Onset	Long Term	Toxicity
GI upset	Weight gain	Severe drowsiness
Nausea	Altered taste	Coarse hand tremor
Polydipsia	Decreased libido	Muscle twitching
Polyuria	Hypothyroidism	Myoclonus
Nocturia	Rash	Choreoathetosis
Dry mouth	Acne	Cogwheel rigidity
Fine hand tremor	Psoriasis	Vomiting
Leukocytosis	Alopecia	Loss of appetite
Muscle weakness	Nonspecific	Confusion
Difficulty concentrating	T-wave changes	Ataxia
Impaired memory	Premature ventricular beats (rare)	Hyperreflexia
	Nephrogenic diabetes insipidus	Nystagmus
	Nephrotoxicity (rare)	Seizures
	Fine hand tremor	Coma

XIII

is commonly used to treat lithium-induced tremor. Atenolol, 50 mg/d, and metoprolol, 20–80 mg/d, have also been used.

Long-Term Side Effects

- Lithium blocks the action of antidiuretic hormone (ADH) by interfering with cAMP production in the distal tubule and, in some patients, produces a nephrogenic diabetes insipidus (NDI) manifested as urinary output >3 L/day. Reduction in lithium dose, changing to single-daily dosing with an extended-release product, adding a potassium supplement (10–20 mEq/d), or discontinuation of therapy may alleviate polyuria or NDI. Lithium-induced NDI has also been treated with loop diuretics, thiazide diuretics, or triamterene that paradoxically decreases water excretion. Amiloride has been used to treat lithium-induced polyuria in doses of 10–20 mg/d. Frequent monitoring of serum electrolytes and lithium concentrations are required for patients with NDI, and fluid restriction is not recommended.
- In general, lithium causes minimal nephrotoxicity if patients are maintained on the lowest effective dose, if adequate hydration is maintained, and if toxicity is avoided.
- Up to 30% of patients on maintenance lithium therapy develop transiently elevated TSH concentrations and 5–15% develop a goiter and/or hypothyroidism. Hypothyroidism is not dose-related, occurs 10 times more frequently in women, and is almost always reversible with drug discontinuation. Subclinical hypothyroidism (normal total and free T_4 with TSH >6 mIU/mL) is indicative of insufficient thyroid functioning. If the TSH is >5.0 mIU/mL, levothyroxine 0.05 mg/day can be added (followed by a TSH level in 1 month) and increased up to 0.2 mg or higher (to achieve TSH >0.1 and <5.0).
- Lithium may cause T-wave flattening or inversion in up to 30% of patients and may aggravate ventricular arrhythmias and atrial premature contractions.
- In patients with preexisting cardiac disease, consultation with a cardiologist is recommended before lithium is initiated.

Toxicity

- Several situations predispose patients to the risk of elevated lithium concentrations and potential toxicity (Table 69.6).
- Mild toxicity (gastrointestinal upset, fatigue, impaired memory) may occur at plasma concentrations of 1.2–1.5 mEq/L. Moderate toxicity (agitation, confusion, ataxia, dysarthria, nystagmus, course tremors) may occur at plasma concentrations >1.5 mEq/L. In concentrations >3.0 mEq/L, the syndrome may progress with clonic–tonic twitching, seizures, irreversible brain damage, coma, and death.

Special Considerations for Pregnancy and Lactation

- Lithium use during the first trimester of pregnancy has been associated with Epstein's anomaly.

XIII

TABLE 69.6. Situations that May Increase Plasma Lithium Concentrations

Decreased sodium intake or increased sodium excretion
Low-sodium diet
Diuretics
Excessive exercise/sweating
Protracted diarrhea/vomiting
Salt deficiency

Decreased water intake or increased water excretion
Dehydration
Diuretics (thiazide and potassium sparing)
Fever
Physical illness (flu, surgery, diarrhea, vomiting)
Postpartum fluid changes
Slimming diets

Renal disease or decreased renal blood flow
Renal dysfunction
Nonsteroidal anti-inflammatory agents

- During pregnancy, glomerular filtration rate (GFR) and plasma volume increase, and lithium dosage should be adjusted based on regular monitoring of plasma concentration. Lithium dosage should be reduced by one-half 1 week before or discontinued 2–3 days before the delivery date. It is restarted a few days after delivery at the regular dosage.
- Lithium may impair thyroid function in the fetus.
- Plasma concentrations in the nursing infant are 10–50% of the mother's, and breast-feeding is discouraged.

Drug Combinations and Drug Interactions
- Several drug–drug interactions have been reported and are summarized in Table 69.7.

Antipsychotics
- Lithium and antipsychotics may be coadministered safely if lower doses are used and if lithium plasma concentrations are maintained below 1.0 mEq/L.

XIII Benzodiazepines
- Benzodiazepines may be used instead of antipsychotics to calm agitated manic patients.
- The oral dose of lorazepam is 1–4 mg three times daily, with gradual increments to achieve maximum effects (approximately 0.5–1.0 mg clonazepam is equivalent to 2.0 mg lorazepam). Lower lorazepam doses are required if administered intramuscularly or intravenously.

TABLE 69.7. Drug Interactions with Lithium

Class/Generic Name	Effect on Plasma Lithium Concentration	Significance
Antibiotics		
Erythromycin	Unclear	Case report of possible increase in lithium
Metronidazole		concentrations (from nephrotoxic effect of antibi-
Spectinomycin		otics); tetracycline may be safe, as drug interaction
Tetracycline		not substantiated
Antidepressants		
Fluoxetine	Increase	Case reports of increased lithium concentrations and neurotoxicity
Tricyclic	Unknown	May cause switch to mania; increase in tremors
Monoamine oxidase inhibitors		May cause switch to mania
Anti-inflammatory drugs		
Diclofenac	Increase	All nonsteroidals (except sulindac) interfere with
Ibuprofen		clearance and increase lithium concentrations
Indomethacin		
Mefenamic acid		
Naproxen		
Phenylbutazone		
Piroxicam		
Sulindac	No effect	May be used with lithium
Antipsychotics		
Chlorpromazine	Unclear	All antipsychotics may increase lithium's neurotoxicity;
Fluphenazine		may increase RBC lithium concentrations; haloperi-
Haloperidol		dol may increase plasma lithium concentrations
Perphenazine		
Thioridazine		
Cardiovascular drugs		
ACE inhibitors		
Lisinopril	Increase	Case reports of increased lithium concentrations due
Catopril		to decreased renal elimination
Enalapril		
Calcium channel blockers		
Verapamil	Unclear	Case reports of neurotoxicity and bradycardia; case
Diltiazem		reports of decreased lithium concentrations
Digoxin	Unknown	Case report of CNS confusion and bradycardia
Methyldopa	Unclear	Case reports of neurotoxicity at low lithium
Diuretics		concentrations
Carbonic anhydrase inhibitors	Decrease	Increase lithium excretion
Acetazolamide		
Loop diuretics		
Ethacrynic acid	Possible increase	May increase lithium concentrations; less likely than
Furosemide		distal tubule diuretics
Distal tubule diuretics		
Chlorthalidone	Increase	Well-documented interaction with increase in lithium
Metolazone		concentrations
Thiazides		
Osmotic diuretics		
Mannitol	Decrease	Increase lithium excretion
Urea		

XIII

(continued) **847**

TABLE 69.7. continued

Class/Generic Name	Effect on Plasma Lithium Concentration	Significance
Potassium-sparing diuretics		
Amiloride	No effect	May be used to treat lithium-induced polyuria
Spironolactone	Increase	May increase lithium concentrations
Triamterene		
Xanthines		
Caffeine	Decrease	Increase lithium excretion
Theophylline		
Neuromuscular blocking drugs		
Pancuronium bromide	Unknown	May prolong neuromuscular blockade
Succinylcholine		
Miscellaneous		
Alcohol	Unknown	Increased lithium toxicity in animals; acute alcohol ingestion may increase peak lithium concentration
Carbamazepine	Unknown	May have synergistic effect in treating mania and depression; case reports of neurotoxicity
Clonazepam	Unknown	May potentiate lithium toxicity and neurotoxicity
Insulin and oral hypoglycemics	Unclear	Careful monitoring of glucose is needed as lithium can alter glucose tolerance
Metoclopramide	Unknown	Case report of extrapyramidal symptoms
Metronidazole	Unknown	May increase lithium concentrations
Phenytoin	Unknown	Case reports of lithium toxicity even at therapeutic concentrations and changes in phenytoin concentrations
Sodium bicarbonate	Decrease	Alkalinization of urine increases lithium excretion
Sodium chloride	Decrease	Increase lithium excretion

Diuretics
- Before starting a patient on a thiazide diuretic, the plasma lithium concentration should be within the therapeutic range (0.6–1.2 mEq/L), and the lithium dose should be reduced by about 50%. Plasma lithium concentrations should be ordered biweekly until the concentration restabilizes. Loop diuretics have less effect on lithium clearance. Restricted sodium intake also significantly increases plasma lithium concentrations.

XIII

▶ ALTERNATIVE TREATMENTS FOR BIPOLAR DISORDER

- CBZ and VPA are now being used as first-line mood stabilizers. Twenty percent to 40% of patients cannot tolerate the adverse effects or do not respond to lithium. Rapid cycling, mixed episodes, and severe manic stages are often resistant to monotherapy with lithium.

CARBAMAZEPINE

- CBZ has acute antimanic (60% response), antidepressant (50–60% response), and prophylactic effects (60–75% response) comparable with lithium in bipolar disorders.
- It may be more effective than lithium in severe mania, rapid–continuous cycling, and in mixed episodes.
- The antimanic response may be faster than that of lithium.
- CBZ is preferred over lithium for patients with dementia and organic causes of mania.
- Predictors of CBZ response include severe manic episodes, anxiety, dysphoria, schizoaffective–psychotic features, brain damage, patients with early onset manic episodes, and negative family history for mood disorders.

Proposed Mechanism of Action

- CBZ blocks reuptake and decreases the release of NE, increases acetylcholine (ACh) in the striatum, decreases dopamine and GABA turnover, decreases the activity of adenylate cyclase, and inhibits amygdala kindling.

Dosing

- CBZ should be administered with meals to minimize gastrointestinal side effects.
- During an acute manic episode, CBZ should be started at 200–400 mg/d and increased by 200 mg every 3–5 days up to 600–1200 mg/d in divided doses (two to four times daily). If there is no response after 2 weeks, then the dose can be increased gradually to obtain plasma concentrations between 6 and 12 μg/mL. When patients are symptom free, CBZ can be initiated at lower doses (e.g., 100–200 mg/d, and increased by 100–200 mg/d every 3–5 days to 600–1200 mg/d).
- When CBZ is combined with lithium, VPA, or antipsychotics, lower doses and blood levels of CBZ are recommended.

Plasma Concentrations

- During the first month of therapy, plasma concentrations of CBZ may decrease due to autoinduction of hepatic oxidative enzymes, and the dose may need to be increased.
- Plasma concentrations should be ordered twice monthly during the first 2 months of therapy. Once steady-state concentrations are stabilized, plasma CBZ concentrations can be monitored every 2–4 months.

Baseline and Routine Laboratory Monitoring

- Baseline laboratory testing should include a complete blood count (CBC) with differential and platelet count, liver enzymes, thyroid function (T_3, T_4, and TSH), serum electrolytes, blood urea nitrogen, urine specific gravity, serum creatinine, neurologic assessment, and electrocardiogram (ECG) if the patient is older than 40 years or has cardiac disease.

XIII ◄

- Patients with low-normal or below-normal pretreatment white blood cell (WBC) and neutrophil counts should be monitored more closely due to increased risks of developing leukopenia (e.g., every 2 weeks for the first 1–3 months of treatment). A transient decrease in WBC and platelets can occur during the first few months of treatment and does not require discontinuation of drug.
- If symptoms of bone marrow suppression occur (e.g., sores, infections, fever, fatigue, petechiae, easy bruising), a CBC with differential, platelet count, and liver enzymes should be ordered to rule out aplastic anemia, agranulocytosis, or thrombocytopenia.
- If leukopenia occurs (WBC <3000/mm^3 or neutrophil counts <1000/mm^3), then the dose of CBZ should be decreased or discontinued. CBZ may be restarted at lower doses when WBC and neutrophils return to normal.

Adverse Effects

- Neurologic side effects (e.g., dizziness, fatigue, ataxia, blurred vision, nystagmus, dysarthria, confusion) may be minimized by low initial doses with gradual increments. Dosage reduction or giving a larger bedtime dose may also reduce side effects.
- Gastrointestinal side effects occur frequently early in therapy and may be minimized by giving the drug with food or by reducing the daily dose.
- Mild to moderate rashes may be treated with 20–30 mg of prednisone and/or antihistamines for a few weeks. However, more serious and life-threatening reactions include erythema multiforme, Stevens–Johnson syndrome, exfoliative dermatitis, and toxic epidermal necrolysis.
- Agranulocytosis and aplastic anemia occur in approximately 1 in 125,000 patients, and fatal toxicity is uncommon. Patients with a history of bone marrow suppression and concomitant use of medications that have an increased incidence of causing agranulocytosis (such as clozapine) should not receive CBZ.
- CBZ may cause syndrome of inappropriate antidiuretic hormone (SIADH) or water intoxication secondary to its antidiuretic activity.
- Mild transient elevation of liver enzymes occurs commonly but does not necessitate drug discontinuation. Yearly monitoring of liver function tests is recommended.

Pregnancy and Lactation

XIII

- CBZ may cause craniofacial defects, fingernail hypoplasia, and developmental delays. Maternal plasma concentrations and umbilical cord concentrations are identical. CBZ concentrations in breastmilk are about 60% of the mother's plasma concentration.

Drug Combinations

- Lithium and CBZ may be synergistic in refractory patients. Neurotoxicity and thyroid suppression may be additive when these two drugs are coadministered.

- Neurotoxicity has also been reported with the combination of CBZ and haloperidol.
- Concomitant drug therapies that may result in CBZ toxicity include cimetidine, erythromycin, isoniazid, verapamil, diltiazem, propoxyphene, and fluoxetine.

DIVALPROEX SODIUM, SODIUM VALPROATE, OR VALPROIC ACID

- VPA, a branched-chain fatty acid is available as sodium valproate, valproic acid, and divalproex sodium. Valproate sodium is rapidly converted to VPA in the stomach; divalproex sodium delayed-release tablets is converted to VPA in the small intestine.
- Divalproex sodium is approved by the US Food and Drug Administration (FDA) as a mood stabilizer for the treatment of bipolar mania. It is as effective as lithium for mania and may be more effective for rapid cycling, mixed mania, secondary bipolar disorder, and comorbid substance abuse.
- Predictors of response include rapid cycling, a high level of dysphoria or depression during the manic episode (mixed episode), concomitant panic attacks, mania with organic features, history of head trauma, and mental retardation.
- Antimanic effects of VPA may be augmented by lithium, CBZ, antipsychotics, or benzodiazepines.

Proposed Mechanism of Action
- The mechanism of action may be related to the inhibition of GABA metabolism, stimulation of GABA synthesis and release, and augmentation of the postsynaptic inhibitory effect of GABA.

Dosing
- The initial dose of VPA is 250–750 mg/d (5–10 mg/kg/d) divided into three doses, and the dose is adjusted up by 250 mg every 2–3 days to 750–3000 mg/d (maximum of 60 mg/kg/d). Higher initial doses (20 mg/kg/d or 1200–1500 mg/d in divided doses) have been used as a loading dose in acutely agitated manic patients.
- Most clinicians use the anticonvulsant therapeutic range of 50–150 µg/mL (12 hours after the last dose) as the desired plasma concentration range.

Adverse Effects
- The most common side effects are gastrointestinal upset and sedation. Gastrointestinal complaints can be minimized by giving the drug with food, using lower initial doses, or switching to the delayed-release product (divalproex sodium).
- Additional side effects are ataxia, lethargy, fine tremor, alopecia, pruritus, prolonged bleeding (inhibition of platelet aggregation), transient increases in liver enzymes, and weight gain. Liver function tests should be obtained at baseline and at 6- to 12-month intervals. VPA should not be administered to patients with hepatic disease or significant hepatic

XIII

dysfunction. Rare cases of hepatitis have been reported; most cases were in children on multiple-drug regimens.

- Thrombocytopenia may be dose related.
- VPA is not recommended during the first trimester of pregnancy (1–2% incidence of neural tube defects), and it is excreted into breast milk in low concentrations.

Drug Interactions

- VPA may cause additive CNS depression when given with other CNS depressants.
- VPA may displace CBZ from plasma proteins and thereby cause CBZ toxicity.
- CBZ may decrease VPA plasma concentrations due to induction of hepatic metabolism.
- VPA may potentiate the anticoagulant effects of warfarin and aspirin.

▶ EVALUATION OF THERAPEUTIC OUTCOMES

- Patients with bipolar disorder should be seen regularly and monitored for response of target symptoms and presence of side effects.
- Patients should receive regular laboratory monitoring and be monitored for compliance with drug regimen. Ideally, they should be actively involved in their own treatment.

See Chapter 68, Bipolar Disorders, authored by Martha P. Fankhauser, MS, and William H. Benefield, Jr., PharmD, FASCP, for a more detailed discussion of this topic.

XIII

Chapter 70

► DEPRESSIVE DISORDERS

► DEFINITION

Depressive disorders include major depressive disorder and dysthymic disorder. The essential feature of major depressive disorder is a clinical course that is characterized by one or more major depressive episodes without a history of manic, mixed, or hypomanic episodes. Dysthymic disorder is a chronic disturbance of mood involving depressed mood and at least two other symptoms, and it is generally less severe than major depressive disorder.

► PATHOPHYSIOLOGY

- Biogenic Amine Hypothesis: Depression may be caused by inadequate monoamine neurotransmission, most notably norepinephrine (NE).
- Permissive Hypothesis: Low serotonin (5-HT) activity may permit the expression of the affective state, but the type is governed by the level of NE. Low NE levels cause depression, and high NE levels cause mania.
- Postsynaptic Changes in Receptor Sensitivity: Changes in sensitivity of NE or $5-HT_2$ receptors may relate to onset of depression.
- Dysregulation Hypothesis: This theory emphasizes a failure of homeostatic regulation of neurotransmitter systems, rather than absolute increases or decreases in their activities.
- The Role of Dopamine (DA): Recent reviews suggest that increased DA neurotransmission in the nucleus accumbens may be related to the mechanism of action of antidepressants.

► CLINICAL PRESENTATION

- Emotional symptoms of a major depressive episode may include diminished ability to experience pleasure, loss of interest in usual activities, sadness, pessimistic outlook, crying spells, hopelessness, anxiety, and feelings of guilt. These symptoms may be accompanied by psychotic features (e.g., auditory hallucinations, delusions).
- Physical symptoms may include fatigue, pain (especially headache), sleep disturbance, appetite disturbance (decreased or increased), loss of sexual interest, gastrointestinal or cardiovascular complaints (especially palpitations).
- Intellectual or cognitive symptoms may include decreased ability to concentrate or slowed thinking, poor memory for recent events, confusion, and indecisiveness.
- Psychomotor disturbances may include psychomotor retardation (slowed physical movements, thought processes, and speech) or psychomotor agitation.

▶ DIAGNOSIS

- Major depression is characterized by one or more episodes of major depression as defined by the *Diagnostic and Statistical Manual of Mental Disorders,* Fourth Edition (DSM-IV; Table 70.1).
- When a patient presents with depressive symptoms, it is necessary to investigate the possibility of a medical, psychiatric, and/or drug-induced cause (Table 70.2).
- Depressed patients should have a medication review, physical examination, mental status examination, a complete blood count with differential, thyroid functions tests, and electrolyte determinations.

▶ DESIRED OUTCOMES

- The goals of treatment of the acute depressive episode are to eliminate or reduce the symptoms of depression, minimize adverse effects, ensure compliance with the therapeutic regimen, and facilitate a return to a premorbid level of functioning.
- Seventy percent of patients with a single depressive episode experience a relapse. For about 20–35% of patients, depression is chronic with considerable residual symptoms. Older persons are less likely to fully recover.

TABLE 70.1. DSM-IV Criteria for Major Depressive Episode

A. Five (or more) of the following symptoms have been present during the same 2-week period and represent a change from previous functioning; at least one of the symptoms is either (1) depressed mood or (2) loss of interest or pleasure.

  1. Depressed mood most of the day, nearly every day

  2. Markedly diminished interest or pleasure in all, or almost all, activities

  3. Significant weight loss (not dieting) or weight gain, or decrease or increase in appetite nearly every day

  4. Insomnia or hypersomnia nearly every day

  5. Psychomotor agitation or retardation nearly every day (observable)

  6. Fatigue or loss of energy nearly every day

  7. Feelings of worthlessness or excessive or inappropriate guilt (may be delusional) nearly every day

  8. Diminished ability to think or concentrate, or indecisiveness

  9. Recurrent thoughts of death, recurrent suicidal ideation without a specific plan, or a suicide attempt or a specific suicide plan

B. The symptoms cause clinically significant distress or impairment in social, occupational, or other important areas of functioning.

C. The symptoms are not due to the direct physiologic effects of a substance or a general medical condition (e.g., hypothyroidism).

Modified from American Psychiatric Association, Diagnostic and Statistical Manual of Mental Disorders, Fourth Edition. Washington, DC, American Psychiatric Association, 1994, p 327.

TABLE 70.2. Common Medical Disorders, Psychiatric Disorders, and Drug Therapy Associated with Depression

Medical Disorders		**Psychiatric Disorders**
Endocrine diseases	Systemic lupus erythematosus	Alcoholism
Hyperthyroidism	Metabolic disorders	Anxiety disorders
Hypothyroidism	Electrolyte imbalance	Eating disorders
Addison's disease	Hypokalemia	Schizophrenia
Cushing's disease	Hyponatremia	**Drug Therapy**
Deficiency states	Hepatic encephalopathy	Alcohol
Pernicious anemia	Cardiovascular disease	Antihypertensives
Wernicke's encephalopathy	Cerebral arteriosclerosis	Reserpine
Severe anemia	Congestive heart failure	Methyldopa
Infections	Myocardial infarction	Propranolol hydrochloride
Encephalitis	Neurologic disorders	Guanethidine sulfate
Influenza	Alzheimer's disease	Hydralazine hydrochloride
Mononucleosis	Huntington's disease	Clonidine hydrochloride
Tuberculosis	Multiple sclerosis	Diuretics
AIDS	Parkinson's disease	Oral contraceptives
Collagen disorders	Poststroke	Steroids/ACTH
	Malignant disease	

▶ TREATMENT

NONDRUG TREATMENT

- Electroconvulsive therapy (ECT) is a safe and effective treatment for all subtypes of major depressive disorder. It is considered when a rapid response is needed, risks of other treatments outweigh potential benefits, there has been a poor response to drugs, and the patient expresses a preference for ECT. A rapid therapeutic response (10–14 days) has been reported. Relative contraindications include increased intracranial pressure, cerebral lesions, recent myocardial infarction, recent intracerebral hemorrhage, bleeding, or otherwise unstable vascular condition. Adverse effects of ECT include cognitive dysfunction (e.g., confusion, memory impairment), prolonged apnea, treatment emergent mania, headache, nausea, and muscle aches. Relapse rates during the year following ECT are high unless maintenance antidepressant medications are prescribed.   XIII
- The efficacy of psychotherapy and antidepressant medication is considered to be additive. Psychotherapy alone is not recommended for the acute treatment of patients with severe and/or psychotic major depressive disorders. For uncomplicated nonchronic major depressive disorder, combined treatment may provide no unique advantage. Cognitive therapy, behavioral therapy, and interpersonal psychotherapy appear to be equal in efficacy.

GENERAL THERAPEUTIC PRINCIPLES

- In general, antidepressants are equal in efficacy when administered in comparable doses.
- Factors that influence the choice of antidepressant include the patient's past history of response, history of familial response, subtype of depression, concurrent medical history, potential for drug–drug interactions, side effect profile of various drugs, and drug cost.
- Sixty percent to 70% of patients with varying types of depression improve with drug therapy.
- Melancholic depression appears to respond well to tricyclic antidepressants (TCAs) and selective 5-HT reuptake inhibitors (SSRIs).
- A preferential response to monoamine oxidase inhibitors (MAOIs) has been reported in patients with atypical depression.
- Patients who fail to respond to a TCA may well respond to an SSRI and vice versa.
- Psychotically depressed individuals generally require either ECT or combination therapy with an antidepressant plus an antipsychotic agent.

DRUG CLASSIFICATION

- Table 70.3 shows the commonly accepted classification of available antidepressant drugs and their suggested therapeutic plasma concentration ranges, initial doses, and usual dosage ranges.
- TCAs are effective in treating all depressive subtypes, especially the severe melancholic subtype.
- The potency and selectivity of the antidepressants for the inhibition of NE and 5-HT reuptake vary greatly among these agents. Table 70.4 shows these affinities as well as the relative propensity for side effects of the various antidepressants.
- The MAOIs increase the concentrations of NE, 5-HT, and DA within the neuronal synapse through inhibition of the monoamine oxidase enzyme system.
- The triazolopyradines, trazodone and nefazodone, are antagonists at the 5-HT$_2$ receptor and inhibit the reuptake of 5-HT. They have negligible affinity for cholinergic and histaminergic receptors.
- Bupropion's most potent neurochemical action is blockade of DA reuptake.
- Mirtazapine, a piperazinoazepine, is an antagonist of α_2-adrenergic autoreceptors and heteroreceptors on both NE and 5-HT presynaptic axons, and an antagonist of postsynaptic 5-HT$_2$ and 5-HT$_3$ receptors. The net effect is increased noradrenergic activity and increased serotonergic activity, especially at 5-HT$_{1A}$ receptors.

XIII

ADVERSE EFFECTS

- Adverse effect profiles of the various antidepressants are summarized in Table 70.4.

TABLE 70.3. Adult Dosages for Currently Available Antidepressant Medications

Generic Name	Suggested Therapeutic Plasma Concentration Range (ng/mL)	Initial Dose[a] (mg/d)	Usual Dosage Range[a] (mg/d)
Tricyclic antidepressants			
Tertiary amines			
Amitriptyline	120–250[b]	50–75	100–300
Clomipramine		25	100–250
Doxepin	110–250[b]	50–75	100–300
Imipramine	200–300[b]	50–75	100–300
Trimipramine		50–75	100–300
Secondary amines			
Desipramine	125–300	50–75	100–300
Nortriptyline	50–150	25–50	50–150
Protriptyline	70–240	10–20	15–60
Dibenzoxazepine			
Amoxapine	200–400[c]	50–150	100–400

XIII

XIII

TABLE 70.3. continued

Generic Name	Suggested Therapeutic Plasma Concentration Range (ng/mL)	Initial Dose[a] (mg/d)	Usual Dosage Range[a] (mg/d)
Tetracyclic			
Maprotiline	200–300[b]	50–75	100–225
Triazolopyridines			
Nefazodone		200	300–600
Trazodone		50–150	150–400
Aminoketone			
Bupropion	50–100	200	300–450
Piperazinoazepine			
Mirtazepine		15	15–45
Monoamine oxidase inhibitors			
Phenelzine		15	15–90
Tranlycypromine	20	20–60	
Selective serotonin reuptake inhibitors			
Fluoxetine		10–20	10–80
Fluvoxamine		50	50–300
Paroxetine		20	20–50
Sertraline		50	100–200
Serotonin/norepinephrine reuptake inhibitor			
Venlafaxine		75	75–375

[a]Doses listed are total daily doses; elderly patients are usually treated with approximately one-half of the dose listed.
[b]Parent drug plus demethylated metabolite.
[c]Parent drug plus hydroxymetabolite.

TABLE 70.4. Relative Potencies of Norepinephrine and Serotonin Reuptake Blockade and Side-Effects Profile of Antidepressant Drugs

	Reuptake Antagonism		Anticholinergic Effects	Sedation	Orthostatic Hypotension	Seizures	Conduction Abnormalities
	Norepinephrine	Serotonin					
Tertiary amines							
Amitriptyline	++	+++	++++	++++	+++	+++	+++
Clomipramine	++	+++	++++	++++	+++	++++	+++
Doxepin	++	++	+++	++++	++	+++	++
Imipramine	+++	+++	+++	+++	++++	+++	+++
Trimipramine	++	+-	++++	++++	+++	+++	+++
Secondary amines							
Desipramine	++++	+	++	++	++	++	++
Nortriptyline	+++	++	++	++	+	++	++
Protriptyline	+++	++	++	+	++	++	+++
Dibenzoxazepine							
Amoxapine[a]	+++	+	+++	++	++	+++	++
Tetracyclic							
Maprotiline	+++	+	+++	+++	++	++++	++
Triazolopyridines							
Nefazodone	0	++	0	+++	+++	++	+
Trazodone	0	++	0	++++	+++	++	++
Aminoketone							
Bupropion	+	+	+	0	0	++++	+
Piperazinoazepine							
Mirtazapine	+		+	+++	+	+	
Monoamine oxidase inhibitors							
Phenelzine			++	++	++	++	+
Tranylcypromine			++	+	++	++	+
Selective serotonin reuptake inhibitors							
Fluoxetine	0	+++	0	0	0	++	0
Fluvoxamine	0	+++	0	0	0	++	0
Paroxetine	0	+++	+	+	0	++	0
Sertraline	0	+++	0	0	0	++	0
Serotonin/norepinephrine reuptake inhibitor							
Venlafaxine	++++	+++	+	+	0	++	+

Key: ++++, high; +++, moderate; ++, low; +, very low; 0, none. aAlso blocks dopamine receptors.

XIII

Tricyclic Antidepressants and Other Heterocyclics

- Anticholinergic side effects (e.g., dry mouth, blurred vision, constipation, urinary retention, tachycardia, and memory impairment) and sedation are more likely to occur with the tertiary amine TCAs than with the secondary amine TCAs.
- A common and potentially serious adverse effect of the TCAs is orthostatic hypotension with resultant syncope. This occurs as a result of α_1-adrenergic antagonism.
- Additional side effects include cardiac conduction delays and heart block, especially in patients with preexisting conduction disease.
- Other side effects that may lead to noncompliance include weight gain, excessive perspiration, and sexual dysfunction.
- Abrupt withdrawal of TCAs (especially high doses) may result in symptoms of cholinergic rebound (e.g., dizziness, nausea, diarrhea, insomnia, restlessness).
- Amoxapine is a demethylated metabolite of loxapine, and as a result of its postsynaptic receptor DA-blocking effects, may be associated with extrapyramidal side effects (EPS).
- Maprotiline, a tetracyclic drug, causes seizures at a higher incidence than do standard TCAs and is contraindicated in patients with a history of seizure disorder. The ceiling dose is considered to be 225 mg/d.

Venlafaxine

- Venlafaxine may cause a dose-related increase in diastolic blood pressure, and baseline blood pressure is not a useful predictor of this phenomenon. Dosage reduction or discontinuation may be necessary if sustained hypertension occurs.

Selective Serotonin Reuptake Inhibitors

- The SSRIs produce fewer sedative, anticholinergic, and cardiovascular adverse effects than the TCAs and are not associated with weight gain. The primary adverse effects include nausea, vomiting, diarrhea, and sexual dysfunction. Headache, insomnia, and fatigue also are reported commonly with SSRIs.

Triazolopyradines

- Trazodone and nefazodone cause minimal anticholinergic and gastrointestinal effects. Sedation and orthostatic hypotension are the most frequent dose-limiting side effects.
- Priapism occurs rarely with trazodone use (1 in 6000 male patients).

Aminoketone

- The occurrence of seizures with bupropion is dose-related and may be increased by predisposing factors (e.g., history of head trauma or central nervous system [CNS] tumor). At the ceiling dose (450 mg/d), the incidence of seizures is 0.4%.

Monoamine Oxidase Inhibitors

- The most common adverse effect of MAOIs is postural hypotension, and this is more likely to occur with phenelzine than with tranylcypromine. Anticholinergic side effects are common but less severe than with the TCAs. Phenelzine causes mild to moderate sedating effects, but tranylcypromine is often stimulating, and the last dose of the day is administered in early afternoon. Sexual dysfunction in both genders is common. Phenelzine has been associated with hepatocellular damage and weight gain.

- Hypertensive crisis is a potentially fatal adverse reaction that can occur when MAOIs are taken concurrently with certain foods, especially those high in tyramine (Table 70.5) and with certain drugs (Table 70.6). Ten milligrams of tyramine can cause a marked pressor response, and 25 mg can result in serious hypertensive crisis. Symptoms of hypertensive crisis include occipital headache, stiff neck, nausea, vomiting, sweating, and sharply elevated blood pressure. The hypertensive crisis can be treated with 10–20 mg of nifedipine sublingually or swallowed or 5 mg of phentolamine intravenously. Education of patients taking MAOIs regarding dietary and medication restrictions is critical.

PHARMACOKINETICS

- The pharmacokinetics of the antidepressants are summarized in Table 70.7.

TABLE 70.5. Dietary Restrictions for Patients Taking Monoamine Oxidase Inhibitors

Aged cheeses[a]	Liver (chicken or beef, more than 2 days old)
Sour cream[b]	Fermented foods
Yogurt[b]	Canned figs
Cottage cheese[b]	Raisins
American cheese[b]	Pods of broad beans[a] (fava beans)
Mild Swiss cheese[b]	Yeast extract[a] and other yeast products
Wine[c] (especially Chianti and sherry)	Meat extract (Marmite)
Beer	Soy sauce
Herring[a] (pickled, salted, dry)	Chocolate[b]
Sardines	Coffee[d]
Snails	Ripe avocado
Anchovies	Sauerkraut
Canned, aged, or processed meats	Licorice
Monosodium glutamate	

[a]Clearly warrants absolute prohibition (e.g., English Stilton, blue, Camembert, cheddar).
[b]Up to 2 oz. daily is acceptable.
[c]3 oz. white wine or a single cocktail is acceptable.
[d]Up to 2 oz. daily is acceptable; larger amounts of decaffeinated coffee are acceptable.

XIII ◄

TABLE 70.6. Medication Restrictions for Patients Taking Monoamine Oxidase Inhibitors

Amphetamines	Levodopa
Appetite suppressants	Local anesthetics containing sympathomimetic
Asthma inhalants	vasoconstrictors
Buspirone	Meperidine
Carbamazepine	Methyldopa
Cocaine	Methylphenidate
Cyclobenzaprine	Other antidepressants
Decongestants (topical and systemic)	Other MAOIs
Dextromethorphan	Reserpine
Dopamine	Stimulants
Ephedrine	Sympathomimetics
Epinephrine	Tryptophan
Guanethidine	

- Substantial amounts of TCAs pass into breast milk; breast-feeding is not advised.
- The major metabolic pathways of the TCAs are demethylation, hydroxylation, and glucuronide conjugation. Metabolism of the TCAs appears to be linear within the usual dosage range, but dose-related kinetics cannot be ruled out in elderly patients.
- All four SSRIs may have a nonlinear pattern of drug accumulation with chronic dosing.
- Factors reported to influence TCA plasma concentrations include: disease states (e.g., renal or hepatic dysfunction), genetics, age, cigarette smoking, and concurrent drug administration. Similarly, hepatic impairment, renal impairment, and age have been reported to influence pharmacokinetics of SSRIs.
- Studies in acutely depressed patients have demonstrated a correlation between antidepressant effect and plasma concentrations for some TCAs. Table 70.3 shows suggested therapeutic plasma concentration ranges. The best established therapeutic range is for nortriptyline, and these data suggest a therapeutic window.
- Some indications for plasma level monitoring include inadequate response, relapse, serious or persistent adverse effects, use of higher than standard doses, suspected toxicity, elderly patients, children and adolescents, pregnant patients, patients of African or Asian descent (because of slower metabolism), cardiac disease, suspected noncompliance, suspected pharmacokinetic drug interactions, and changing brands.
- Plasma concentrations should be obtained at steady state, usually after a minimum of 1 week at constant dosage. Sampling should be done

XIII

TABLE 70.7. Pharmacokinetic Properties of Antidepressants

Generic Name	Elimination Half-Life (h)[a]	Time of Peak Plasma Concentration (h)	Plasma Protein Binding (%)	% Bioavailable	Clinically Important Metabolites
Tricyclic antidepressants					
Tertiary amines					
Amitriptyline	9–46	1–5	90–97	30–60	Nortriptyline
Clomipramine	20–24	2–6	97	36–62	10-Hydroxynortriptyline
Doxepin	8–36	1–4	68–82	13–45	Desmethyldoxepin
Imipramine	6–34	1.5–3	63–96	22–77	2-Hydroxyimipramine; desipramine; 2-hydroxydesipramine
Trimipramine	7–40	3	94–96	18–63	None
Secondary amines					
Desipramine	11–46	3–6	75–92	33–51	2-Hydroxydesipramine
Nortriptyline	16–38	3–12	87–95	46–70	10-Hydroxynortriptyline
Protriptyline	54–198	6–12	90–94	75–90	None
Dibenzoxazapine					
Amoxapine	8–30[b]	1–2	90	—[c]	8-Hydroxyamoxapine
Tetracyclic					
Maprotiline	28–105	4–24	88	79–87	Desmethylmaprotiline
Triazolopyridines					
Nefazodone	2–4	1	99	20	*meta*-Chlorophenylpiperazine; hydroxynefazodone; triazole-dione
Trazodone	6–11	1–2	92	—[c]	*meta*-Chlorophenylpiperazine
Aminoketone					
Bupropion	10–21	3	82–88	—[c]	Bupropion threo-amino alcohol; bupropion morpholinol

(continued)

XIII

863

TABLE 70.7. continued

Generic Name	Elimination Half-Life (h)[a]	Time of Peak Plasma Concentration (h)	Plasma Protein Binding (%)	% Bioavailable	Clinically Important Metabolities
Piperazinoazepine					
Mirtazapine	13–34	2	85	50	N-Demethylmirtazapine
Monoamine oxidase inhibitors					
Phenelzine	1.5–4	—[c]	—[c]	—[c]	
Tranylcypromine	1.5–3	—[c]	—[c]	—[c]	
Selective serotonin reuptake inhibitors					
Fluoxetine	24–120	4–8	94	95	Norfluoxetine
Fluvoxamine	15–26	2–8	77	53	None
Paroxetine	24–31	5–7	95	None
Sertraline	27	6–8	99	36[d]	N-Desmethylsertraline
Serotonin/norepinephrine reuptake inhibitor					
Venlafaxine	5	2	27–30		O-Desmethylvenlafaxine

[a] Biologic half-life in slowest phase of elimination.
[b] Amoxapine, 8 hours; 8-hydroxyamoxapine, 30 hours.
[c] No data available.
[d] Increases 30–40% when taken with food.

during the elimination phase, usually in the morning, 12 hours after the last dose. Samples collected in this manner are comparable for patients on once daily, twice daily, or three times daily regimens.

DRUG INTERACTIONS

- As TCAs are hepatically metabolized by the cytochrome P-450 system and they are highly protein bound, many drugs can interact when given concurrently. Drug interactions are summarized in Tables 70.8 and 70.9.
- Table 70.10 summarizes the drug interactions of non-TCA antidepressants.
- The very slow elimination of fluoxetine and norfluoxetine makes it critical to ensure a 5-week washout after fluoxetine discontinuation before starting an MAOI. Potentially fatal reactions may occur when any SSRI or TCA is coadministered with an MAOI.
- Potential exists for an interaction between venlafaxine and drugs that inhibit the P-450IID6 system. Dosage reduction of alprazolam and triazolam is required if either drug is coadministered with nefazodone.
- As nefazodone is an in vitro inhibitor of cytochrome P-450IIIA4, it should not be coadministered with astemizole or terfenadine.

TABLE 70.8. Pharmacokinetic Drug Interactions Involving Tricyclic Antidepressants

Elevates plasma concentrations of TCAs
  Cimetidine
  Diltiazem
  Ethanol, acute ingestion
  SSRIs
  Haloperidol
  Labetalol
  Methylphenidate
  Phenothiazines
  Propoxyphene
  Quinidine
  Verapamil

Lowers plasma concentrations of TCAs
  Barbiturates
  Carbamazepine
  Ethanol, chronic ingestion
  Phenytoin

Elevates plasma concentrations of interacting drug
  Hydantoins
  Oral anticoagulants
  Phenytoin

Lowers plasma concentrations of interacting drug
  Levodopa

XIII

TABLE 70.9. Pharmacodynamic Drug Interactions Involving Tricyclic Antidepressants

Interacting Drug	Effect
Alcohol	Increased CNS depressant effects
Amphetamines	Increased effect of amphetamines
Androgens	Delusions, hostility
Anticholinergic agents	Excessive anticholinergic effects
Bethanidine	Decreased antihypertensive efficacy
Clonidine	Decreased antihypertensive efficacy
Disulfiram	Acute organic brain syndrome
Estrogens	Increased or decreased antidepressant response; increased toxicity
Guanadrel	Decreased antihypertensive efficacy
Guanethidine	Decreased antihypertensive efficacy
Insulin	Increased hypoglycemic effects
Lithium	Possible additive lowering of seizure threshold
Methyldopa	Decreased antihypertensive efficacy; tachycardia; CNS stimulation
Monoamine oxidase inhibitors	Increased therapeutic and possibly toxic effects of both drugs; hypertensive crisis; delirium; seizures; hyperpyrexia; serotonin syndrome
Oral hypoglycemics	Increased hypoglycemic effects
Phenytoin	Possible lowering of seizure threshold and reduced antidepressant response
Sedatives	Increased CNS depressant effects
Sympathomimetics	Increased pharmacologic effects of direct-acting sympathomimetics; decreased effects of indirect acting sympathomimetics
Thyroid hormones	Increased therapeutic and possibly toxic effects of both drugs; CNS stimulation; tachycardia

SPECIAL POPULATIONS

Elderly Patients

- The SSRIs are often selected as first-choice antidepressants in elderly patients, and they may enable one to avoid adverse effects commonly associated with the TCAs.
- In healthy elderly patients, cautious use of a secondary amine TCA (desipramine or nortriptyline) may be appropriate because of their defined therapeutic plasma concentration ranges, well-established efficacy, and well-known adverse effect profiles.
- Trazodone, nefazodone, and bupropion are also often chosen because of their milder anticholinergic and less frequent cardiovascular side effects.

XIII

TABLE 70.10. Drug Interactions of Non-TCA Antidepressants

Non-TCA	Interacting Drug/Drug Class	Effect
Dibenzoxazepine Amoxapine	Many of the drugs that interact with the TCAs	Similar response to that seen with TCA interaction
Tetracyclic Maprotiline	Many of the drugs that interact with the TCAs	Similar response to that seen with TCA interaction
Triazolopyridine Nefazodone	Alprazolam	Increased plasma concentrations of alprazolam
	Astemizole	Theoretically increased plasma concentrations of astemizole with potentially serious cardiovascular adverse effects
	Digoxin	Increased C_{max}, C_{min}, and AUC of digoxin by 29, 27, and 15%, respectively
	Haloperidol	Decreased clearance of haloperidol by 35%
	MAOIs	Hypertensive crisis; serotonin syndrome; delirium; coma; seizures; hyperpyrexia
	Propranolol	Decreased C_{max} and AUC of propranolol; increased C_{max}, C_{min}, and AUC of m-CPP metabolite of nefazodone
	Terfenadine	Theoretically increased plasma concentrations of terfenadine with potentially serious cardiovascular adverse effects
	Triazolam	Increased plasma concentrations of triazolam, increased psychomotor impairment
Trazodone	CNS depressants	Increased CNS depression
	Digoxin	Increased serum concentrations of digoxin
	Ethanol	Additive impairment in motor skills
	Fluoxetine	Increased plasma concentrations of trazodone
	MAOIs	Theoretically, central serotonin syndrome could occur
	Neuroleptics	Increased hypotension
	Phenytoin	Increased serum concentrations of phenytoin
	Tryptophan	Agitation, restlessness, poor concentration, nausea
	Warfarin	Decreased hypoprothrombinemic response
Aminoketone Bupropion	MAOIs	Increased toxicity of bupropion
	Medications that lower seizure threshold	Increased incidence of seizures
	Levodopa	Increased incidence of adverse experiences
Selective serotonin reuptake inhibitors Fluoxetine	Alprazolam	Increased plasma concentrations and half-life of alprazolam; increased psychomotor impairment
	Anticoagulants	Possible increased risk of bleeding
	β-Adrenergic blockers	Increased metoprolol serum concentrations and bradycardia; possible heart block
	Buspirone	Decreased therapeutic response to buspirone
	Carbamazepine	Increased plasma concentrations of carbamazepine with symptoms of carbamazepine toxicity
	Dextromethorphan	Visual hallucinations (one patient only)

(continued)

TABLE 70.10. continued

Non-TCA	Interacting Drug/Drug Class	Effect
	Haloperidol	Increased haloperidol concentrations and increased extrapyramidal side effects
	Lithium	Neurotoxicity—confusion, ataxia, dizziness, tremor, absence seizures
	MAOIs	Severe or fatal reactions—confusion, nausea, double vision, hypomania, hypertension, tremor, serotonin syndrome
	Phenytoin	Increased plasma concentrations of phenytoin and symptoms of phenytoin toxicity
	TCAs	Markedly increased TCA plasma concentration with symptoms of TCA toxicity
	Terfenadine	Arrhythmias, shortness of breath and orthostasis
	Trazodone	Headaches, dizziness, sedation
	Tryptophan	Agitation, restlessness, poor concentration, nausea
	Valproate	Increased valproate serum concentrations
Fluvoxamine	Alprazolam	Increased AUC of alprazolam by 96%, increased alprazolam half-life by 71%, and increased psychomotor impairment
	Astemizole	Theoretically, increased plasma concentrations of astemizole with potentially serious cardiovascular effects
	β-Adrenergic blockers	Fivefold increase in propranolol serum concentrations; bradycardia and hypotension with combined fluvoxamine and metoprolol
	Carbamazepine	Possible carbamazepine toxicity, although a controlled study did not support this
	Clozapine	Increased clozapine serum concentrations and increased risk for seizures and orthostatic hypotension
	Diazepam	Decreased clearance of diazepam and its active metabolite
	Diltiazem	Bradycardia
	Haloperidol	Increased haloperidol plasma concentrations
	Lithium	Increased serotonergic effects; seizures, nausea, tremor
	MAOIs	Potential for hypertensive crisis, serotonin syndrome, seizures, delirium
	Methodone	Increased methodone plasma concentrations with symptoms of methodone toxicity
	TCAs	Increased TCA plasma concentration
	Terfenadine	Theoretically, increased plasma concentrations of terfenadine with potentially serious cardiovascular effects
	Theophylline	Increased serum concentrations of theophylline with symptoms of theophylline toxicity
	Tryptophan	Increased serotonergic effects and severe vomiting
	Warfarin	Increased hypoprothrombinemic response to warfarin
Paroxetine	Cimetidine	Increased paroxetine serum concentrations
	Desipramine	Increased plasma concentrations and half-life of desipramine

TABLE 70.10. continued

Non-TCA	Interacting Drug/Drug Class	Effect
	MAOIs	Potential for hypertensive crisis, serotonin syndrome, seizures, delirium
	Warfarin	Possible increased risk for bleeding
Sertraline	Carbamazepine	Increased plasma concentrations of carbamazepine
	Diazepam	Small decrease in clearance of diazepam
	MAOIs	Serotonin syndrome, myoclonus, violent shaking
	TCAs	Increased plasma concentrations of secondary amine TCAs (desipramine, nortriptyline)
	Tolbutamide	Decreased clearance of tolbutamide (16%)
	Warfarin	Increased protime
Serotonin/norepinephrine reuptake inhibitor		
Venlafaxine	Cimetidine	Reduced clearance of venlafaxine by 43%: AUC and peak serum concentration of venlafaxine increased by 60%
	MAOIs	Potential for hypertensive crisis, serotonin syndrome, seizures, delirium

Children and Adolescents

- Data supporting efficacy of antidepressants in children and adolescents are sparse. The SSRIs are better tolerated than the TCAs and are relatively safer on overdose (suicide is the second leading cause of death in adolescents).
- Several cases of sudden death have been reported in children and adolescents taking desipramine. A baseline electrocardiogram (ECG) is recommended before initiating a TCA in children and adolescents, and an additional ECG is advised when steady-state plasma concentrations are achieved. Plasma concentration monitoring is critical.

Pregnancy

- As a general rule, nondrug approaches to the treatment of depression in the pregnant patient are preferred.
- The TCAs are usually given preference, and nortriptyline or desipramine may be the treatment of choice because of the experience that has been gained with these agents in pregnant patients and because therapeutic plasma concentration ranges have been established. When TCAs are withdrawn during pregnancy, they should be tapered gradually to avoid withdrawal symptoms. If possible, drug tapering is usually begun 5–10 days before the estimated day of confinement.

DOSING

- Dosing recommendations are shown in Table 70.3. The usual initial adult dose of most TCAs is 50 mg at bedtime, and the dose may be increased by 25–50 mg every third day.

XIII

- Bupropion is usually initiated at 100 mg twice daily, and this dose may be increased to 100 mg three times daily after 3 days. An increase to 450 mg/d (the ceiling dose), given as 150 mg three times daily, may be considered in patients with no clinical response after several weeks of treatment at 300 mg/d.
- A 6-week trial at a maximum dosage is considered an adequate trial. Patients must be told about the expected lag time of 2–4 weeks before the onset of antidepressant effect.
- Elderly patients should receive half the initial dose given to younger adults, and the dose is increased at a slower rate. They may require 6–12 weeks of treatment to achieve the desired antidepressant response.
- Some investigators recommend life-long maintenance therapy for persons at greatest risk for recurrence (e.g., persons >50 years of age at onset of the first episode, persons >40 years of age and with 2 or more prior episodes, and persons of any age with 3 or more prior episodes).

REFRACTORY PATIENTS

- Most "treatment-resistant" depressed patients have received inadequate therapy. Issues to be considered in patients who have not responded to treatment include: (1) Is the diagnosis correct? (2) Does the patient have a psychotic depression? (3) Has the patient received an adequate dose and duration of treatment? (4) Do adverse effects preclude adequate dosing? (5) Has the patient been compliant with the prescribed regimen? (6) Was treatment outcome measured adequately? (7) Is there a coexisting or preexisting medical or psychiatric disorder?
- The current antidepressant may be stopped and a trial with an unrelated agent initiated. Alternatively, the current antidepressant may be augmented (potentiated) by the addition of lithium, liothyronine, or an anticonvulsant such as carbamazepine or valproic acid.
- Switching medications is often preferred over augmentation as an initial strategy.
- A third approach is to use two different classes of antidepressants concurrently (e.g., TCA plus an MAOI). Concurrent use of a TCA and an MAOI should be undertaken only by a clinician experienced in the use of such combinations. When this is undertaken, the MAOI is slowly added to the TCA. Desipramine is not recommended to be used in combination with an MAOI. When the combination is discontinued, the MAOI should be stopped first. The combination of an SSRI and MAOI should never be used. An algorithm for treatment of depression including refractory patients is shown in Fig 70.1.

EVALUATION OF THERAPEUTIC OUTCOMES

- Several monitoring parameters, in addition to plasma concentrations, are useful in managing patients. Patients must be monitored for adverse effects, remission of previously documented target symptoms, and changes in social or occupational functioning. Regular monitoring

XIII

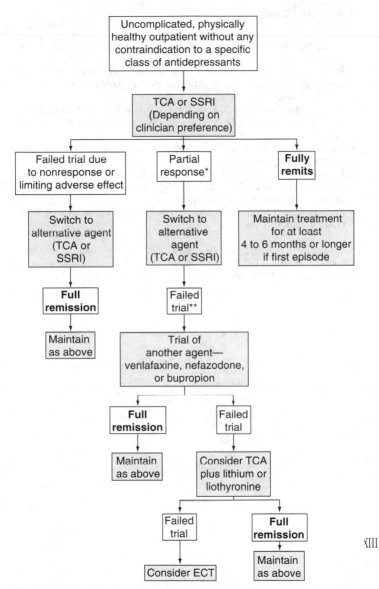

Figure 70.1. Algorithm for treatment of uncomplicated major depression. *Be certain patient is receiving an adequate dose and treatment duration has been at least 3–4 weeks; **some clinicians attempt augmentation (with lithium or liothyronine) at this point. *(Modified from Preskorn SH, Burke MJ, J Clin Psychiatry 1992; 53 (suppl 9): 5–18.)*

should be assured for several months after antidepressant therapy is discontinued.
- Patients given venlafaxine and those given TCAs concurrently with adrenergic neuronal blocking antihypertensives should have blood pressure monitored regularly.
- Patients older than age 40 should receive a pretreatment ECG before starting TCA therapy, and follow-up ECGs should be performed periodically.
- Patients should be monitored for emergence of suicidal ideation after initiation of any antidepressant.
- In addition to the clinical interview, psychometric rating instruments allow for rapid and reliable measurement of the nature and severity of depressive and associated symptoms.
- Patients should be monitored closely for relapse or recurrence if the brand of antidepressant is changed.

See Chapter 67, Depressive Disorders, authored by Barbara G. Wells, PharmD, FASHP, FCCP, Laura A. Mandos, PharmD, and Peggy E. Hayes, PharmD, for a more detailed discussion of this topic.

XIII

Chapter 71

▶ SCHIZOPHRENIA

▶ DEFINITION

Schizophrenia is a heterogeneous syndrome of disorganized and bizarre thoughts, delusions, hallucinations, inappropriate affect, and impaired psychosocial functioning.

▶ PATHOPHYSIOLOGY

- Dopaminergic Hypothesis: Psychosis may result from hyper- or hypoactivity of dopaminergic processes in specific brain regions.
- Phospholipid Abnormalities: Phosphoinositide serves as a second messenger system for the dopamine$_2$ (D$_2$) receptor.
- Dysregulation Hypothesis: Aberrant homeostatic control mechanisms cause erratic neurotransmission.
- Serotonin (5-HT) Abnormalities: Increased peripheral serotonin concentrations have been found in schizophrenics in some studies.
- Norepinephrine Abnormalities: Increased concentrations of norepinephrine have been observed in the limbic structures of patients with chronic paranoid schizophrenia, but not in patients with other subtypes.
- Imbalance in activity between dopaminergic and glutamatergic neurons with relative deficiency of glutamatergic activity is proposed as being at least partially responsible for psychotic symptomatology.
- Increased ventricular size, small decrease in brain size, and brain asymmetry has been reported.

▶ CLINICAL PRESENTATION

- Symptoms of the acute episode may include: out of touch with reality; hallucinations (especially hearing voices); delusions (fixed false beliefs); ideas of influence (actions controlled by external influences); disconnected thought processes (loose associations); ambivalence (contradictory thoughts); flat (no emotional expression), inappropriate, or labile affect; autism (withdrawn and inwardly directed thinking and approach to life); uncooperativeness, hostility, and verbal or physical aggression; impaired self-care skills; and disturbed sleep and appetite.
- When the acute psychotic episode remits, the patient typically has residual features (e.g., anxiety; suspiciousness; lack of volition; lack of motivation; poor insight; impaired judgment; social withdrawal; difficulty in learning from experience).

► DIAGNOSIS

- The *Diagnostic and Statistical Manual of Mental Disorders,* 4th ed. (DSM-IV) specifies the following criteria for the diagnosis of schizophrenia.
  - Persistent dysfunction lasting longer than 6 months.
  - Two or more symptoms including: hallucinations, delusions, disorganized speech, grossly disorganized or catatonic behavior, and negative symptoms. These symptoms must have been present for at least one month.
  - Significantly impaired functioning (work, interpersonal, or self-care).
- DSM-IV classifies symptoms as positive or negative.
  - Positive symptoms include delusions, disorganized speech (association disturbance), hallucinations, behavior disturbance (disorganized or catatonic), and illusions.
  - Negative symptoms include alogia (poverty of speech), avolition, affective flattening, anhedonia, and social isolation.
- Positive and negative symptoms may provide a framework for subtypes of schizophrenia that may correlate with prognosis, cognitive functioning, structural abnormalities in the brain, and response to typical antipsychotic (AP) drugs (Table 71.1). Typical APs include all available APs except clozapine, risperidone, and olanzapine.

► TREATMENT

- A thorough mental status examination (MSE), physical and neurologic examination, a complete family and social history, and laboratory workup (vital signs, complete blood count, electrolytes, hepatic function, renal function, cardiac function, thyroid function, and toxicology) must be performed prior to treatment.

GENERAL THERAPEUTIC PRINCIPLES

- All typical APs are equal in efficacy in groups of patients when used in equipotent doses.
- Selection of medication should be based on the need to avoid certain side effects and in view of concurrent medical or psychiatric disorders. Patient or family history of response is also helpful in the selection of an AP.
- Traditional dosage equivalents [expressed as "chlorpromazine (CPZ) equivalent dosages"—the equipotent dosage of any AP compared with 100 mg of CPZ] may assist in determining the range of effective dosage when switching to another AP drug (Table 71.2).

MECHANISMS OF ACTION

- AP medications are putative dopaminergic antagonists. Multiple dopamine (DA) receptor subtypes exist, with D_1 and D_2 being the best studied. D_1 receptors are at least partially responsible for AP activity.

XIII

TABLE 71.1. Features of Schizophrenic Subtypes Based on the Positive and Negative Models

Characteristic	Syndrome Type I (Good Prognosis)	Syndrome Type II (Poor Prognosis)
Premorbid adjustment	Good	Poor
Precipitating factors	Present	Not obvious
Onset	Abrupt (<6 months)	Insidious
Family history of schizophrenia	Less frequent	More frequent
Family history of affective disorder	More frequent	Less frequent
Sensorium	Dreamlike or "spacy"	Clear
Symptoms	Predominance of positive symptoms	Predominance of negative symptoms
Outcome of treatment	Potentially reversible	More chronic course
Intellectual impairment dysfunction	Absent	Neurocognitive
Postulated pathophysiology	D_2 overactivity	D_2 hypoactivity (?), cell loss in prefrontal cortex and temporal lobes
Ventricle:brain ratio	Normal	Increased
Response to antipsychotics	Marked to moderate	Variable response
Response to clozapine	Marked to moderate	Marked to moderate
Response to dopamine agonists and stimulants	Exacerbation common	Little effect or symptoms are improved
Importance of dopamine dysfunction	Highly important	Possibly implicated

The D_2 receptor is also associated with AP efficacy, and appears to be the primary receptor involved in the pathogenesis of extrapyramidal side effects (EPS). However, some D_1 blockade appears to be necessary to produce EPS.
- Therapeutic effects of APs are thought to occur in the limbic system, including the ventral striatum, whereas the EPS are thought to be related to DA blockade in the dorsal striatum.
- Atypical is the term applied to APs that produce little or no EPS, and potentially have clinical response patterns different than traditional APs. The mechanism of action of atypical APs is unknown. It may be related to one or more of the following pharmacodynamic effects: relative D_1, D_4, or D_5 specificity; relative selectivity for limbic dopaminergic receptors; 5-HT_2, 5-HT_6, and 5-HT_7 antagonism; or α_1-adrenergic antagonism.

XIII

875

TABLE 71.2. Available Antipsychotics: Doses and Dosage Forms

Generic Name	Traditional Equivalent Dose (mg)	Dosage Range (mg/d)	Geriatric Maximum Dose (mg/d)	Dosage Forms[a]
Aliphatic Phenothiazines				
Chlorpromazine	100	60–2000	800	T,L,LC,I,C-ER,S
Piperazine Phenothiazines				
Fluphenazine	2	2–40	20	T,L,LC,I
Perphenazine	10	8–64	32	T,LC,I
Trifluoperazine	5	2–80	40	T,LC,I
Piperidine Phenothiazines				
Mesoridazine	50	50–500	250	T,LC,I
Thioridazine	100	50–800	400	T,LC
Thioxanthenes				
Chlorprothixene	100	100–1600	800	T,LC,I
Thiothixene	4	5–60	30	C,LC,I
Butyrophenone				
Haloperidol	2	1–100	50	T,LC,I
Dibenzoxapine				
Clozapine	50	75–900	NL[b]	T
Loxapine	10	20–250	125	C,LC,I
Dihydroindolone				
Molindone	10	15–225	112	T,LC
Benzisoxazole				
Risperidone	ND[c]	2–16	8	T
Thienobenzodiazepine				
Olanzapine	1	5–20		T

[a]T, tablet; C, capsule; ER or SR, extended- or sustained-release; I, injection; L, liquid solution, elixir, or suspension; LC, liquid concentrate; R, rectal suppositories; S, syrup.
[b]NL, not listed.
[c]ND, no data available.

PHARMACOKINETICS

- Absorption of AP drugs can be variable. Low-potency APs are prone to a large first-pass effect. The systemic bioavailability is significantly higher with the concentrate than with tablet formulations.
- Among the APs, mean relative bioavailability between oral and intramuscular administration ranges from 25% with CPZ to 65% with haloperidol (HPD).
- The APs are highly lipophilic and have large volumes of distribution.
- APs are metabolized primarily through oxidative microsomal enzyme processes in the liver, and metabolites may be active or inactive.
- APs have fairly long elimination half-lives, most in the range of 20–40 hours. Thus after dosage stabilization, most APs can be dosed once daily.

- The approximate therapeutic peak plasma concentration (Cp) range of HPD is between 5 and 12 ng/mL, and this may represent a therapeutic window. Daily dosage of HPD HCl 10 mg results in a HPD Cp in this range in about 50% of patients.
- Although the research with fluphenazine (FPZ) is less extensive, preliminary results suggest that the therapeutic range is approximately 0.5–3.0 ng/mL.
- In patients refractory to the typical APs, a clozapine (CLZ) plasma concentration greater than approximately 350 ng/mL was associated with a significantly greater probability of efficacy.
- Cp monitoring may be considered in patients who do not respond to reasonable AP doses within a 6-week period; in patients who develop unusual or severe adverse experiences; in patients who are taking concomitant medications that may cause drug interactions; in patients who have age or pathophysiologic changes suggesting a change in pharmacokinetics; and in occasional patients to assess compliance.
- The depot APs are useful in the outpatient treatment of schizophrenia, where noncompliance with medications is a significant problem. The first dose of depot AP may be administered in the outpatient setting or just prior to hospital discharge.
  - Patients may be dosed with FPZ decanoate on a 1- to 3-week interval, and with HPD decanoate usually once a month. The elimination half-life of FPZ decanoate is 14 days and the elimination half-life of HPD decanoate is 21 days.
  - There is a lower incidence of psychotic exacerbation after 6 and 12 months of treatment if the patient's predose FPZ Cps is greater than 1 ng/mL.

INITIAL TREATMENT

- The goals during the first 7 days are decreased agitation, hostility, combativeness, anxiety, tension, aggression, and normalization of sleep and eating patterns.
- The usual recommendation is to initiate therapy with the equivalent of 400–600 mg CPZ unless the patient's physiologic status or history suggests otherwise.
- Fixed-dose studies of low versus high daily doses do not reveal any differences in time to AP response or length of hospitalization.
- Rapid neuroleptization is the administration of repeated doses of a high-potency AP (e.g., HPD 5 mg IM) every 30–60 minutes over a period of less than 24 hours. The goal is to obtain a rapid calming effect (not sedation) in severely agitated patients.
- Intramuscular administration of lorazepam is equivalent to intramuscular APs in the management of acute agitation or aggression.

STABILIZATION OF THERAPY

- During weeks two and three, the goals should be to increase socialization and improve self-care habits and mood.

XIII

- Most patients receive a dosage of 500–800 CPZ equivalents daily for the acute stabilization phase. Typically, the patient should remain at this dosage as long as symptoms continue to improve. If necessary, dose titration may continue every 1–2 weeks, and most patients can also be switched to once-daily dosing.
- An adequate trial to evaluate response is at least 6 weeks at an AP dose equivalent to 800 mg CPZ. However, a fixed-dose study indicated that 50% of patients nonresponsive after 6 weeks responded by 12 weeks when continued on the same dose of FPZ.

MAINTENANCE THERAPY

- Medication should be continued for at least 12 months after remission of the first psychotic episode. Patients who have had multiple acute psychotic episodes and who respond well to medication should be treated for at least 5 years. Then low-dose strategies or complete drug withdrawal may be attempted.
- APs should be tapered slowly before discontinuation to avoid rebound cholinergic withdrawal symptoms.

Depot Antipsychotics

- The principles for conversion from oral APs to depot formulations are as follows:
  - Stabilization on an oral dosage form of the same agent (or at least a short trial of 3–7 days) to determine that the medication is tolerated adequately.
  - Use of an appropriate conversion factor, taking into account whether the patient is still acutely ill or relatively stable.
  - Overlap with the oral agent until adequate Cps can be achieved with the depot agent alone.
  - For FPZ, the simplest conversion is the Stimmel method, which uses 1.2 times the oral daily dose for stabilized patients, rounding up to the nearest 12.5-mg interval, administered in weekly doses for the first 4–6 weeks (1.6 times the oral daily dose for patients who are more acutely ill). Subsequently, FPZ decanoate may be administered once every 2–3 weeks. Oral FPZ may be overlapped for 1 week.
  - For HPD, a factor of 10–15 times the oral daily dose is commonly recommended, rounding up to the nearest 50-mg interval, administered in a once-monthly dose with oral HPD overlap for the first month.
  - Depot APs should be administered by a deep, "Z-tract" intramuscular method, although there is some evidence that FPZ decanoate can be administered subcutaneously with similar results.

MANAGEMENT OF THE REFRACTORY PATIENT

Atypical Antipsychotics

- Common to all definitions of "atypical AP" is the ability of the drug to produce AP response with little or no EPS. Other attributes that have

XIII

been ascribed to atypical APs include enhanced efficacy (particularly on negative symptoms), absence of propensity to cause tardive dyskinesia (TD), and lack of effect on serum prolactin (PRL).

- Clozapine
  - CLZ was effective in approximately 32% of refractory schizophrenic patients compared with only 2% treated with a combination of CPZ and benztropine.
  - CLZ may be more effective against negative symptoms than typical APs.
  - To minimize orthostasis and sedation, a CLZ test dose of 12.5–25 mg should be given, followed by slow titration until a daily dose of 300–450 mg is reached. If inadequate response is obtained after 6 weeks, then further titration may occur. However, patients receiving greater than 600 mg daily must be monitored carefully for side effects.
  - Individual patient trials of at least 6 months have been recommended.
  - CLZ use has been associated with a decrease in total patient care costs of nearly $10,000 per patient annually.
- Risperidone
  - Risperidone may be superior to HPD in treatment of negative symptoms.
  - The mean optimal dose in fixed-dose studies was 4–6 mg daily. At doses greater than 10 mg daily, risperidone's side effect profile is more similar to that of a typical AP.
  - Risperidone has not been evaluated systematically in treatment of refractory patients; however, because of drug acquisition cost differences and the agranulocytosis associated with CLZ, clinicians often use risperidone before proceeding on to CLZ.
- Olanzapine
  - Olanzapine is superior to HPD in treatment of negative symptoms.
  - Olanzapine appears less likely to cause EPS and TD than HPD.
  - Olanzapine is usually dosed 5–20 mg/day.

ANTIPSYCHOTIC ADVERSE EFFECTS

Table 71.3 presents the relative incidence of common categories of AP side effects.

Autonomic Nervous System

- Anticholinergic (ACh) side effects include impaired memory, dry mouth, constipation, tachycardia, blurred vision, inhibition of ejaculation, and urinary retention. Elderly patients are especially sensitive to these effects.
  - Dry mouth can be managed with increased intake of fluids, oral lubricants (Xerolube), ice chips, or use of sugarless chewing gum or hard candy.
  - Constipation can be treated with increases in fluid and dietary fiber intake, and also with exercise.

XIII

TABLE 71.3. Relative Side Effects Incidence of Commonly Used Antipsychotics

	Sedation	EPS	Anticholinergic	Cardiovascular
Chlorpromazine	+ + + +	+ + +	+ + +	+ + + +
Clozapine	+ + + + +	+	+ + + + +	+ + + +
Fluphenazine	+ +	+ + + + +	+ +	+ +
Haloperidol	+	+ + + + +	+	+
Loxapine	+ + +	+ + + +	+ +	+ + +
Molindone	+	+ + +	+ +	+ +
Olanzapine	+ +	+	+ +	+ +
Perphenazine	+ +	+ + + +	+ +	+ +
Risperidone	+	+ +	+	+ +
Thioridazine	+ + + +	+ +	+ + + +	+ + + +
Trifluoperazine	+ +	+ + + +	+ +	+ +
Thiothixene	+ +	+ + + +	+ +	+ +

Key: +, very low; + +, low; + + +, moderate; + + + +, high; + + + + +, very high.

Central Nervous System
Extrapyramidal System
- Dystonia is defined as a state of abnormal muscle tonicity, sometimes described simplistically as a severe "muscle spasm."
  - Dystonias usually occur within 24–96 hours of dosage initiation or dosage increase and may be life threatening, as in the case of pharyngeal–laryngeal dystonias.
  - Treatment includes intramuscular or intravenous AChs (Table 71.4) or benzodiazepines. Benztropine mesylate 2 mg or diphenhydramine 50 mg may be given intramuscularly or intravenously, or diazepam 5–10 mg slow intravenous push or lorazepam 1–2 mg intramuscularly may be given. Relief usually occurs within 15–20 minutes of an intramuscular injection and within 5 minutes of intravenous administration. This dose should be repeated if no response is seen within 15 minutes of intravenous injection or 30 minutes of intramuscular injection.
  - A five- to eightfold reduction in dystonia is seen when ACh prophylaxis is used, especially in young males on high-potency APs; a 1.9-fold reduction is seen when taking all APs into account, and no benefit occurs in patients older than 45 years or in patients treated with low-potency agents.
  - Dystonias may also be minimized by the use of lower initial doses of APs.
- Akathisia
  - Diagnosis is made by combining subjective complaints (feeling of inner restlessness) with objective symptoms (pacing, shuffling, or tapping feet).

XIII

TABLE 71.4. Anti-Parkinsonian Agents

Generic Name	Equivalent Dose (mg)	Dosage Range (mg)	Dosage Forms[a]
Antimuscarinics			
Benztropine	1	1–8[b]	T,I
Biperiden	2	2–8	T,I
Orphenadrine	50	50–250	T
Procyclidine	2	7.5–20	T
Trihexyphenidyl	2	2–15	T,C-ER,L
Antihistaminic			
Diphenhydramine	50	50–400	C,T,L,I
Dopamine agonist			
Amantadine	N/A	100–400	C,L

[a]Abbreviations as per Table 71.2.
[b]Dosage may be titrated to 12 mg with care; nonlinear pharmacokinetics have been demonstrated.

- Treatment with ACh agents is disappointing, and reduction in AP dosage is perhaps the best intervention. Another alternative is to switch to a lower potency agent.
- Efficacy of diazepam 5 mg three times per day has been reported, but some researchers failed to demonstrate efficacy.
- Propranolol (up to 160 mg daily), nadolol (up to 80 mg daily), and metoprolol (100 mg daily or less) were reported to be effective.
- Pseudoparkinsonism has four cardinal symptoms: (1) Akinesia, bradykinesia, or decreased motor activity, including masklike facial expression, micrographia, slowed speech, and decreased arm swing; (2) tremor, predominantly at rest, decreases with movement, and usually involves the fingers and hands; (3) rigidity, which may present as stiffness. Cogwheel rigidity is seen as the patient's limbs yield in jerky, rachet-like fashion when moved passively by the examiner; and (4) stooped, unstable posture and a gait that ranges from slow and shuffling to festinating.
- Accessory symptoms include seborrhea, sialorrhea, hyperhidrosis, fatigue, dysphagia, and dysarthria. A variant of pseudoparkinsonism is rabbit syndrome, a perioral tremor.
- The onset of symptoms is usually 1–2 weeks after initiation of AP therapy or dose increase.
- Benztropine has a longer half-life, which allows once- to twice-daily dosing. Dosage increases higher than 6 mg daily must be slow, as benztropine displays nonlinear pharmacokinetics. Trihexyphenidyl, diphenhydramine, and biperiden usually require three-times daily dosing.
- Symptoms usually begin to resolve within 3–4 days of initiation of treatment, but at least 2 weeks is normally required for full response.
- Amantadine is generally as efficacious as AChs, but has less effect on memory.

XIII

- An attempt should be made to taper and discontinue these agents 6 weeks to 3 months after symptoms resolve.
- Tardive dyskinesia is sometimes irreversible and is characterized by abnormal involuntary movements (AIMs) occurring with chronic AP therapy.
  - The classic presentation of TD is bucco-lingual-masticatory (BLM) movements, the onset of which is usually insidious. Symptoms may become severe enough to interfere with chewing, speech, respiration, or swallowing. Facial movements include frequent blinking, brow arching, grimacing, upward deviation of the eyes, and lip smacking. Involvement of the extremities occurs in later stages (restless choreiform and athetotic movements of limbs). The final area of involvement is the truncal movements. Movements may worsen with stress, and may decrease with sedation.
  - The Abnormal Involuntary Movement Scale (AIMS) may be used for general screening, but is not diagnostic by itself.
  - The Dyskinesia Identification System: Condensed User Scale (DISCUS) is the first involuntary movement scale to be valid psychometrically.
  - Dosage reduction alone may have a significant effect on outcome, with a complete disappearance of symptoms in some patients.
- Prevention of TD is best accomplished by: (1) using APs only when there is a clear indication and at the minimum effective dose for the shortest duration possible; (2) using the DISCUS or other scales to assess for early signs of TD, at least quarterly; (3) discontinuing APs at the earliest symptoms of TD, if possible; and (5) using APs only short-term to abort aggressive behavior in nonpsychotic patients.
  - Lecithin (phosphatidylcholine), in doses up to 24 g daily, demonstrated a statistically significant treatment effect, but the clinical significance was questionable.
  - Baclofen (60–75 mg/d) has been partially effective, but muscular hypotonia and sedation are common.
  - Although there are successful reports of benzodiazepines improving symptoms of TD, recent analyses have shown no efficacy.
  - CLZ does not appear to cause TD, and reduced AIMs by 50% or greater in 43% of patients with TD.
- Sedation
  - Administration of most or all of the daily dosage at bedtime can decrease daytime sedation and may eliminate the need for hypnotics.
- Seizures
  - There is an increased risk of drug-induced seizures in all patients treated with APs. The highest risk for AP-induced seizures is with the use of CPZ or CLZ, followed by trifluoperazine and perphenazine. Seizures are more likely with initiation of treatment and with the use of higher doses and rapid dosage increases.
  - When an isolated seizure occurs, a dosage decrease is first recommended, and anticonvulsant therapy is usually not recommended.

XIII

- If a change in AP therapy is required in the management of AP-induced seizures, molindone, thiordiazine (TRD), HPD, or FPZ are recommended.
- Thermoregulation
  - Hyperpyrexia can lead to heat stroke. Hypothermia is also a risk, particularly in elderly patients. These problems are more common with the use of low-potency APs.
- Neuroleptic Malignant Syndrome
  - Neuroleptic malignant syndrome (NMS) occurs in 0.5–1% of patients receiving APs. NMS may occur more frequently in patients receiving high-potency, injectable, or depot APs, and in patients who are dehydrated or who have organic mental disorders.
  - The onset of symptoms varies from early in treatment to months later. It develops rapidly, over the course of 24–72 hours.
  - Cardinal signs and symptoms of NMS are body temperature exceeding 38°C, altered level of consciousness, autonomic dysfunction (tachycardia, labile blood pressure, diaphoresis, tachypnea, urinary or fecal incontinence), and ridgidty.
  - Laboratory evaluation frequently shows leukocytosis, increases in creatine kinase (CK), aspartate aminotransferase (AST), alanine aminotransferase (ALT), lactate dehydrogenase (LDH), and myoglobinuria.
  - Treatment should begin with AP discontinuation and supportive care.
  - The DA agonist bromocriptine, used in theory to reverse DA blockade, reduces rigidity, fever, or CK in up to 94% of patients.
  - Amantadine has been used successfully in up to 63% of patients.
  - Dantrolene has been used as a skeletal muscle relaxant, with effects on temperature, respiratory rate, and CK in up to 81% of patients.
  - Rechallenge may be considered only for those patients in greatest need of reinstitution of APs, but careful monitoring is required. The patient must be observed for at least 2 weeks without APs, and the lowest effective AP dose must be used.
- Psychiatric Side Effects
  - Akathisia has resulted in impulsivity and, in extreme cases, violence and suicide.
  - Delirium and psychosis are reported with large doses of APs or combinations of AChs with APs.

Endocrine System

- Galactorrhea and menstrual irregularities are common. These effects may be dose related and are more common with the use of high-potency APs.
- Possible management strategies for galactorrhea include switching AP agents, bromocriptine in doses up to 15 mg daily, or amantadine in doses up to 300 mg daily.
- Weight gain is frequently reported in patients receiving APs.
- APs may affect glucose levels.

XIII

Cardiovascular System

- Orthostatic hypotension, defined as a greater than 20 mm Hg drop in systolic pressure, is caused by α-adrenergic blockade. Incidence is greatest with lower potency APs (especially with intramuscular or intravenous administration).
  - Tolerance to this effect usually occurs within 2–3 months. Reducing the dose or changing a higher potency AP may be attempted.
  - For severe hypotensive episodes, volume expansion through the use of intravenous fluids should be attempted before the use of pressor agents.
  - Pure α-adrenergic pressor agents, such as phenylephrine or metaraminol, can be used, as well as norepinephrine, which has β_1-adrenergic properites. Epinephrine, with α- and β-adrenergic effects, should never be used because unopposed β-adrenergic stimulation lowers blood pressure further. Isoproterenol should also be avoided.
- Electrocardiogram (ECG) Changes
  - APs have direct myocardial depression and quinidine-like effects on cardiac conduction, and they also antagonize sympathetic nervous system activity in the hypothalamus and stabilize cardiac tissue through local anesthetic properties. Low-potency agents, such as TRD and CLZ, are more likely to have cardiac effects.
  - ECG changes include increased heart rate, flattened T waves, ST segment depression, prolongation of QT and PR intervals, and torsades de pointes.
  - In patients older than 40 years, a pretreatment ECG is recommended.

Ophthalmic

- Impairment in visual accommodation results from paresis of ciliary muscles. Photophobia may also result. If severe, pilocarpine ophthalmic solution may be necessary.
- Exacerbation of narrow-angle glaucoma can occur.
- Opaque deposits in the cornea and lens may occur with chronic phenothiazine treatment, especially with CPZ. Although visual acuity is not usually affected, periodic slit-lamp examinations are recommended in patients receiving phenothiazines long term.
- Retinitis pigmentosis can result from use of TRD doses greater than 800 mg daily (the manufacturer's recommended maximum dose). It is caused by melanin deposits, and can result in permanent visual impairment or blindness.

XIII Hepatic System

- Liver function test (LFT) abnormalities are common. If aminotransferases are greater than three times the upper limit of normal, the AP should be changed to a chemically unrelated AP.
- Cholestatic hepatocanalicular jaundice can occur in up to 2% of patients receiving phenothiazines, and the onset is usually within the first 2 weeks of therapy. Symptoms resolve within 2–8 weeks of discontinuation of the AP.

Genitourinary System

- Urinary hesitancy and retention is commonly reported, especially with low-potency APs, and men with benign prostatic hypertrophy are especially prone. Urinary incontinence is reported more frequently in older patients, especially women.
- Erectile dysfunction, considered an ACh effect, occurs in 25–60% of patients, most frequently with TRD.
- Anorgasmia and decreased libido in women have also been proposed to be ACh effects.
- α-Adrenergic bloackade is proposed to be the mechanism behind priapism and retarded and retrograde ejaculation.
- Using lower AP doses, changing to high-potency APs, or discontinuation of ACh medications are potential interventions.

Hematologic System

- Transient leukopenia may occur with AP therapy, but it typically does not progress to clinically significant parameters.
- If the white blood cell (WBC) count is less than $3000/mm^3$ or the absolute neutrophil count (ANC) is $<1000/mm^3$, the AP should be discontinued, and the WBC monitored closely until it returns to normal.
- Agranulocytosis reportedly occurs in 0.01% of patients receiving typical APs, and of the typical APs, it may occur most frequently with CPZ and piperazine phenothiazines. The onset is usually within the first 8 weeks of therapy. Agranulocytosis may initially manifest as a local infection (e.g., sore throat, leukoplakia, and erythema and ulcerations of the pharynx). If these symptoms occur, an immediate WBC should be ordered.
- The 18-month treatment risk of developing agranulocytosis with CLZ appears to be approximately 0.91%. Increasing age and female gender are associated with greater risk. The greatest risk appears to be between months 1 and 6 of treatment. Weekly WBC monitoring is mandated. If the total WBC drops to less than $2000/mm^3$, or the ANC is less than $1000/mm^3$, CLZ should be discontinued.
- In cases of mild to moderate neutropenia (granulocytes between 2000 and $3000/mm^3$, or ANC $1000–1500/mm^3$), which occurs in up to 2% of patients, CLZ should be discontinued with daily monitoring of complete blood counts until values return to normal.

Dermatologic System

- Allergic reactions are rare and usually occur within 8 weeks of initiating therapy, manifesting as maculopapular, erythematous, pruritic rashes. Drug discontinuation and topical steroids are recommended.
- Contact dermatitis, including the oral mucosa, may occur. In susceptible patients, mixing the concentrate in a sufficient quantity of a nonacidic liquid and swallowing it quickly decreases problems.
- Phenothiazines can absorb ultraviolet light and energy. Erythema and severe sunburns can occur. Patients should be educated to use maximally blocking sunscreens, hats, protective clothing, and sunglasses when in the sun.

XIII

- Blue-gray or purplish discoloration of skin exposed to sunlight may occur in patients receiving higher doses of low-potency phenothiazines (especially CPZ) long term.

Sudden Death Syndromes

- The cause of death may be ventricular arrhythmias; laryngeal–pharyngeal dystonia leading to aspiration and hypoxia; hyperpyrexia; NMS; seizures; and toxic megacolon.

DRUG INTERACTIONS

- Most AP drug interactions are relatively minor and often involve additive CNS effects. The most common drug interactions seen in schizophrenia involve AChs and drugs causing sedation.
- AP pharmacokinetics can be significantly affected by concomitant enzyme inducers or inhibitors. Smoking is a potent inducer of hepatic enzymes and may increase AP clearance by as much as 50%. Consult the published literature for a listing of drug interactions.

USE IN PREGNANCY AND LACTATION

- Case reports implicating limb malformations are rare, but should be considered in deciding whether to use APs during the first trimester of pregnancy. During pregnancy, HPD and other high-potency agents appear to be the preferred APs (primarily due to a lack of published reports over decades of use).
- Other potential but largely unknown risks of APs throughout pregnancy are behavioral teratogenicity on the neonate, receptor changes, perinatal effects (e.g., tonicity, strength, sucking), EPS, jaundice, respiratory depression, and intestinal obstruction.
- APs appear in breast milk with milk to plasma ratios of 0.5 to 1.

▶ EVALUATION OF THERAPEUTIC OUTCOMES

- Clinicians should use standardized psychiatric rating scales to rate response objectively.
- The Brief Psychiatric Rating Scale (BPRS) is recognized as the primary instrument to determine AP efficacy in phase II and III clinical trials. Other scales [e.g., Comprehensive Psychiatric Rating Scale (CPRS), Positive and Negative Syndrome Scale (PANSS)] are also available, but are less commonly used.

XIII *See Chapter 66, Schizophrenia, authored by M. Lynn Crimson, PharmD, FCCP, and Peter G. Dorson, PharmD, for a more detailed discussion of this topic.*

Chapter 72

▶ SLEEP DISORDERS

▶ DEFINITION

Abnormalities in the normal physiology of sleep often cause patients to complain of three types of sleep problems: (1) insomnia, (2) excessive daytime sleepiness, and (3) abnormal sleep behaviors.

▶ NEUROCHEMISTRY AND SLEEP PHYSIOLOGY

- The reticular activating system (RAS) is responsible for maintaining wakefulness. Neurochemically, norepinephrine (NE) and acetylcholine in the cortex and histamine and neuropeptides (e.g., substance P, corticotropin-releasing factor) in the hypothalamus modulate neuronal activity during wakefulness.
- As the RAS decelerates, information transfer to the cortex ceases and serotonin (5-HT) neurotransmission in the raphe nuclei reduces sensory input to inhibit motor activity. NE is involved in dreaming, whereas 5-HT is active during nondreaming sleep.
- Polysomnography (PSG) is a procedure that measures multiple electrophysiologic parameters simultaneously during sleep, such as an electroencephalogram (EEG), electrooculogram (EOG), and electromyogram (EMG). Two EOGs, one EEG, and one EMG are the minimal recordings used in scoring sleep stages.
- The two types of sleep are nonrapid eye movement (NREM; stages 1–4) and rapid eye movement (REM). During NREM sleep, skeletal muscle tone and eye movements are low in comparison with wakefulness, and respiratory activity occurs at a slow, regular pace.
  - Stage 1 sleep represents a transition between wakefulness and sleep that lasts between 0.5 and 7 minutes. The EEG reveals low-voltage (3–7 Hz), desynchronized activity.
  - Stage 2 sleep is characterized by a low-voltage EEG, frequent "sleep spindles" (10–16 Hz spindle-shaped waves), and "K-complexes" (high-voltage spikes).
  - Stages 3 and 4 are called delta sleep and consist of high-amplitude, slow waves.
- REM sleep is marked by the onset of a low-voltage, mixed frequency EEG and bursts of bilaterally conjugate REMs. During REM sleep, muscle tone is low, but autonomic functions (e.g., heart rate, perspiration, penile erection) are active. Dream reports occur in 80–90% of subjects if awakened during or at the end of a REM period.
- Within 90 minutes of falling asleep, the first REM period commences and lasts only 5–7 minutes. The cycle lasts approximately 70–120 minutes and is repeated four to six times during the night. Most delta sleep occurs during the first half of the night. REM periods lengthen progres-

sively throughout the night. A sleep histogram for a normal young adult is depicted in Figure 72.1.

- In elderly individuals the sleep pattern is altered, with a considerable decrease in delta sleep, REM sleep, and total sleep time. Correspondingly, there is an increase in the number of awakenings and total time spent awake at night. In elderly persons, the incidence of sleep pathology may be as high as 40%.

► CLASSIFICATION

- The *Diagnostic and Statistical Manual of Mental Disorders,* Fourth Edition (DSM-IV) classifies sleep disorders into three categories:
  - Primary sleep disorders result from endogenous abnormalities in the sleep–wake timing or generating processes and are further classified as dyssomnias (abnormalities in the amount, timing, or quality of sleep) or parasomnias (abnormal behaviors associated with sleep, such as somnambulism, sleep terrors, and nightmares). Primary sleep disorders include primary insomnia, primary hypersomnia, narcolepsy, breathing-related sleep disorder, and circadian rhythm sleep disorder.
  - Sleep disorders related to another mental disorder.
  - Other sleep disorders include sleep disorders due to a medical condition and substance-induced sleep disorders.

► INSOMNIA

CLINICAL PRESENTATION

- Patients complain of difficulty falling asleep, maintaining sleep, or of not feeling rested in spite of a sufficient opportunity to sleep.
- Transient (2–3 night) and short-term (less than 3 weeks) insomnia are typical of individuals without a history of sleep problems. Long-term or chronic insomnia (exceeding 3 weeks) may be related to medical or psychiatric disorders, or may be psychophysiologic.

DIAGNOSIS

- Common identifiable causes of insomnia are situational (e.g., stress, jet lag, shift work), medical (e.g., cardiovascular, respiratory, pain, endocrine, gastrointestinal, neurologic), psychiatric (e.g., mood disorders, anxiety disorders, substance abuse), and medications (e.g., central adrenergic blockers, diuretics, selective 5-HT reuptake inhibitors, steroids, stimulants). Evaluation of the patient with transient insomnia should focus on possible acute stresses, environmental disruptions, and drug-related causes. In patients with chronic disturbances, a complete diagnostic evaluation should include physical and mental status examinations and routine laboratory tests, as well as medication and substance abuse histories to rule out medical and psychiatric etiologies.

XIII

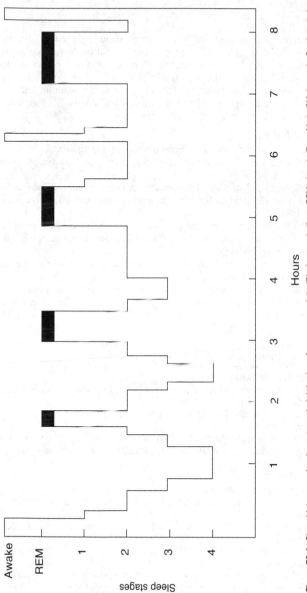

Figure 72.1. Sleep histogram showing a typical night's sleep for a young adult. (Black areas indicate REM sleep.) *(From Morin CM. Insomnia: Psychological Assessment and Management. New York: Guilford Press, 1993, p. 16.)*

XIII

TREATMENT

Nonpharmacologic

- Behavioral and educational interventions include cognitive therapy, relaxation therapy, stimulus control therapy, light therapy, sleep deprivation, and sleep hygiene education. Nonpharmacologic recommendations for insomnia are shown in Table 72.1.
- Individuals with insomnia should avoid all products containing caffeine and chocolate for at least 8 hours before bedtime. Alcoholics frequently have insomnia for months to years after recovery.

Hypnotic Agents

- Table 72.2 lists the commonly prescribed hypnotic agents.
- Benzodiazepines (BZs) are the class of choice for the symptomatic relief of insomnia.
- Excluding zolpidem, the nonbarbiturate, non-BZ hypnotics have associated risks identical to those of the barbiturates and offer no advantages over the BZs.
- The antidepressants (e.g., amitriptyline, doxepin, trazodone) are alternatives in patients who complain of nonrestorative sleep and those who should not receive BZs.
- Antihistamines are less effective than the BZs, and their use may be complicated by anticholinergic effects.
- Zolpidem acts selectively at the BZ_1 receptor and has minimal anxiolytic and no muscle relaxant or anticonvulsant effects. It increases stages 2, 3, and 4 sleep and decreases REM. Its half-life is approxi-

---

TABLE 72.1. Nonpharmacologic Recommendations for Insomnia

Stimulus Control Procedures
1. Establish a regular time to wake up and to go to sleep (including weekends).
2. Sleep only as much as necessary to feel rested.
3. Avoid long periods of wakefulness in bed. Use the bed only for sleep or intimacy; do not read or watch television in bed.
4. Avoid trying to force sleep. If you do not fall asleep within 20–30 minutes, leave the bed and perform a relaxing activity (e.g., read, listen to music, watch television) until drowsy. Repeat this as often as necessary.
5. Avoid daytime naps.

Sleep Hygiene Recommendations
1. Exercise routinely (e.g., three to four times weekly), but not close to bedtime because this may cause arousal.
2. Create a comfortable sleep environment by avoiding temperature extremes, loud noises, and illuminated clocks.
3. Discontinue or reduce the use of alcohol, caffeine, and nicotine.
4. Avoid excessive fulllness or hunger at bedtime.
5. Avoid drinking large quantities of liquids in the evening to prevent nighttime trips to the restroom.

Adapted from Hartmann PM, Am Fam Physician 1995;51:191–194, with permission.

XIII

TABLE 72.2. Classification and Dosages of Hypnotics

Generic Name	Trade Name (Manufacturer)	Daily Dosage Range (mg)
Benzodiazepines		
Estazolam	ProSom (Abbott)	1–2
Flurazepam	Dalmane (Roche)	15–30
	Generics (various)	
Quazepam	Doral (Baker Cummins)	7.5–15
Temazepam	Restoril (Sandoz)	15–30
	Generics (various)	
	Halcion (Upjohn)	0.125–0.25
Triazolam	Generics (various)	
Nonbarbiturate, Nonbenzodiazepines		
Chloral hydrate	Noctec (Squibb Mark)	500–2000
	Generics (various)	
Zolpidem	Ambien (Searle)	5–10
Antidepressants[a]		
Trazodone	Desyrel (Mead Johnson)	50–100
	Generics (various)	
Antihistamines		
Diphenhydramine	Benadryl (Parke–Davis)	25–100
	Generics (various)	
Doxylamine	Unisom (Leeming)	25–100

[a]Non–FDA-approved for insomnia.

mately 2.5 hours, and duration of effect is 6–8 hours. Lower doses should be used in elderly patients and in patients with hepatic impairment.

Benzodiazepines

- BZs decrease the duration of stages 1 and 4 sleep, and increase stage 2 sleep. They do not decrease REM sleep.
- Triazolam maintained its hypnotic efficacy for only 2 weeks whereas flurazepam, quazepam, and temazepam maintained their efficacy for 1 month, and estazolam may maintain its efficacy for up to 12 weeks. Long-term use of low doses of BZs is associated with loss of efficacy and worsened sleep in chronic insomniacs.

XIII ◄

Pharmacokinetics

- The pharmacokinetic properties of BZ hypnotics are summarized in Table 72.3.
- Flurazepam and triazolam are rapidly absorbed. Temazepam is less lipophilic and has a slower onset of effect. Estazolam and quazepam are similar to flurazepam in their onset of effect.

TABLE 72.3. Pharmacokinetics of Benzodiazepine Hypnotic Agents

Generic Name	Time to Peak Plasma Concentration (h)	Elimination Half-Life Parent (h)	Metabolic Pathway	Clinically Significant Metabolites
Estazolam	2	12–15	Oxidation	—
Flurazepam	1	8	Oxidation	Hydroxyethylflurazepam Flurazepam aldehyde
			N-Dealkylation	N-DAF[a]
Quazepam	2	39	Oxidation	2-Oxo-quazepam
			N-Dealkylation	N-DAF[a]
Temazepam	1.5	10–15	Conjugation	—
Triazolam	1	2	Oxidation	—

[a]N-desalkylflurazepam, mean half-life 47–100 hours.

- The duration of effect of triazolam is short, whereas that of temazepam and estazolam is intermediate, and flurazepam and quazepam have a long duration of effect.
- Drugs that inhibit cytochrome P450IIIA4 (e.g., erythromycin, nefazodone, ketaconazole) reduce the clearance of triazolam.
- Desalkylflurazepam (DAF) is a long half-life metabolite of flurazepam, and it accounts for most of flurazepam's pharmacologic effects.
- DAF helps alleviate daytime anxiety or early morning awakening, but daytime drowsiness and impaired psychomotor performance may be a problem.

Adverse Effects
- Tolerance to the carryover central nervous system (CNS) effects (e.g., drowsiness, psychomotor incoordination, decreased concentration, cognitive deficits) may develop in some individuals.
- Anterograde amnesia occurs more frequently with triazolam than temazepam; however, flurazepam demonstrated more anterograde amnestic effects than triazolam in one study. Using the lowest dose possible minimizes amnestic effects.
- Triazolam is associated with a higher reported rate of confusion, bizarre behavior, agitation, and hallucinations than the other BZ hypnotics.
- Daytime anxiety and rebound insomnia are associated with the use of triazolam.
- Rebound insomnia can be minimized by using the lowest effective dose and tapering the dose on discontinuation.
- The rapidly eliminated BZs are associated with less daytime sedation and fewer performance deficits; however, they may increase the chance of daytime anxiety.

XIII

- There is an association between falls and hip fractures and the use of long-elimination half-life BZs, thus use of flurazepam and quazepam should be avoided in elderly patients.

General Therapeutic Principles
- Patients with difficulty initiating sleep and patients who require daytime alertness should receive the short-acting BZ hypnotics. Patients who have difficulty maintaining sleep may benefit from intermediate elimination half-life agents. Long-elimination half-life BZs should be considered if management of daytime anxiety is required.
- BZs should not be given to persons with sleep apnea, a history of substance abuse, or to pregnant individuals.
- Patients taking BZs should be instructed to avoid alcohol, as even alcohol on the day after ingestion of a long-elimination half-life BZ can result in additive CNS impairment.

► SLEEP APNEA

- Apnea is the cessation of airflow at the nose and mouth lasting at least 10 seconds.

OBSTRUCTIVE SLEEP APNEA
Clinical Presentation
- Obstructive sleep apnea (OSA) is potentially life-threatening and is characterized by repeated episodes of nocturnal breathing cessation with loud snoring and gasping. It is caused by an occlusion of the upper airway.
- The apneic episode is terminated by a reflex action to the fall in O_2 saturation that causes a brief arousal during which breathing resumes.
- OSA patients usually present with complaints of excessive daytime sleepiness. Additional symptoms include morning headache, poor memory, and irritability.
- Most individuals with OSA are overweight.

Treatment
- Patients with severe apnea (greater than 20 apneas/hour on PSG) and moderate apnea (5–20 apneas/hour on PSG) have shown significant improvement and reduction in mortality with treatment.
- Nonpharmacologic approaches are the treatment of choice [e.g., weight loss, tonsillectomy, nasal septal repair, nasal continuous positive airway pressure (CPAP), uvulopalatopharyngoplasty, upper airway resection]. XIII
- The most important pharmacologic intervention is avoidance of all CNS depressants. Other pharmacologic interventions should be reserved for patients with mild forms of OSA and in patients who have failed other treatments.
- Protriptyline 10–30 mg/d reduces the frequency of apneas and increases O_2 saturation.
- Fluoxetine 20 mg/d was effective in reducing apneas in some patients.

CENTRAL SLEEP APNEA

Clinical Presentation

- Central sleep apnea (CSA) accounts for <10% of all apneas. It is characterized by repeated episodes of apnea caused by temporary loss of respiratory effort during somnolence.
- Patients present with morning headache, daytime somnolence, insomnia, and nocturnal awakenings with shortness of breath or gasping.

Treatment

- The primary treatment is ventilatory support with O_2 and CPAP; acetazolamide, theophylline, and medroxyprogesterone have shown mixed results.
- In refractory cases, diaphragmatic pacing, tracheostomy, or positive pressure ventilation are helpful. In nonhypercapneic patients, treatment may consist of BZs to reduce arousals, and acetazolamide, CPAP, and O_2 to stabilize breathing patterns.

▶ NARCOLEPSY

CLINICAL PRESENTATION

- The essential feature is excessive daytime sleepiness with sleep attacks that may last up to 30 minutes. Other features are hypersomnia, fatigue, impaired performance, disturbed nighttime sleep, cataplexy, hypnagogic hallucinations, hypnopompic hallucinations, and sleep paralysis.

TREATMENT

- Good sleep habits should be encouraged, and the patient should be encouraged to take at least two naps during the day if possible.
- The psychostimulants (Table 72.4) can be used for excessive daytime sleepiness and antidepressants for cataplexy.
- Amphetamines and methylphenidate have a fast onset of effect and durations of 3–4 hours and 6–10 hours, respectively. Divided daily doses are recommended. Amphetamines are associated with more likelihood of abuse and tolerance.
- Pemoline has a delayed onset of effect, but its duration is 8–10 hours. Liver function must be monitored at 1 month, then yearly.
- The tricyclic antidepressants (TCAs) are effective in reducing cataplexy and sleep paralysis. Imipramine (50–250 mg/d), protriptyline (5–30 mg/d), and nortriptyline (50–200 mg/d) are effective in 80% of patients.
- Selegiline in daily doses of 20–40 mg improves hypersomnolence and cataplexy.
- Hydroxybutyrate, 60 mg/kg/night, is a therapeutic option without anticholinergic side effects.
- The goal of therapy is to maximize alertness during waking hours or at selected times. Cataplexy can be treated on an as-needed basis in some patients.

XIII

TABLE 72.4. Stimulant Drugs Used to Treat Narcolepsy

Generic Name	Trade Name (Manufacturer)	Daily Dosage Range (mg)
Dextroamphetamine	Dexedrine (SmithKline Beecham) Generics (various)	5–60
Dextroamphetamine/ amphetamine salts[a]	Adderall (Richwood)	5–60
Methamphetamine[b]	Desoxyn (Abbott)	5–15
Methylphenidate	Ritalin (Ciba) Generics (various)	38–80
Pemoline	Cylert (Abbott)	37.5–112.5

[a]Dextroamphetamine sulfate, dextroamphetamine saccharate, amphetamine aspartate, amphetamine sulfate.
[b]Not available in some states.

▶ EVALUATION OF THERAPEUTIC OUTCOMES

- Patients with short-term or chronic insomnia should be evaluated after 1 week of therapy to assess for drug effectiveness, adverse events, and compliance with nonpharmacologic recommendations. Patients should be instructed to maintain a sleep diary, including a daily recording of bedtime, arising time, sleep onset latency, number and duration of awakenings, medication ingestions, naps, and an index of sleep quality.
- Patients with sleep apnea should be evaluated after 2–4 weeks of treatment for improvement in alertness, daytime symptoms, and weight reduction. The bed partner can be consulted regarding snoring and gasping. The goals of therapy are to reduce apneic episodes and to improve O_2 saturation.
- Monitoring parameters for pharmacotherapy of narcolepsy include reduction in daytime sleepiness, cataplexy, hypnagogic and hypnopompic hallucinations, and sleep paralysis. Patients should be evaluated monthly until an optimal dose is achieved, then every 6–12 months to assess for the development of adverse drug events (e.g., mood changes, sleep disturbances, cardiovascular abnormalities). If symptoms increase during therapy, PSG should be performed.

See Chapter 71, Sleep Disorders, authored by Cynthia K. Kirkwood, XIII *PharmD, and Rakesh K. Sood, MD, for a more detailed discussion of this topic.*

Chapter 73

▶ DEFINITIONS

The substance-related disorders include disorders related to the taking of a drug of abuse (including alcohol), to the side effects of a medication, and to toxin exposure.

- Drug abuse: Use of a drug in a manner inconsistent with social norms with the intent of altering mood or feeling.
- Addiction or drug dependence: Behavioral patterns of compulsive drug use in which obtaining and using a drug constitute the principal focus of the user's life.
- Physical dependence: State of physiologic adaptation to chronic use of a drug such that abrupt dosage reduction or discontinuation results in an abstinence syndrome.
- Tolerance: State of physiologic adaptation to a drug such that higher-than-usual dosages are required to achieve the usual effect.
- Withdrawal or abstinence syndrome: Characteristic physical and emotional signs and symptoms precipitated by the abrupt reduction or discontinuation of a drug.
- Cross-tolerance and cross-dependence: Ability of one drug to suppress the manifestations of physical withdrawal produced by another drug and to maintain the physically dependent state.

▶ PATHOPHYSIOLOGY

MECHANISMS OF TOLERANCE, DEPENDENCE, AND WITHDRAWAL

- The euphoriant or other pleasant properties of a drug initially act as reinforcers of continued drug use. As tolerance develops, pleasant effects diminish, and higher doses are required to produce the same feelings. Also, the user continues drug use to avoid the abstinence syndrome.
- There are two types of physiologic tolerance: (1) dispositional tolerance (metabolic or pharmacokinetic tolerance), which results from changes in pharmacokinetic handling, and (2) pharmacodynamic tolerance (cellular or functional tolerance), which results from adaptive changes at the site of action.

CENTRAL NERVOUS SYSTEM DEPRESSANTS

- Alcohol: Alcohol disrupts neuronal membrane function and membrane-mounted proteins. It potentiates γ-aminobutyric acid type A ($GABA_A$) receptor function and inhibits the function of the N-methyl-D-aspartate (NMDA) receptors. The principal mechanism of tolerance appears to

be pharmacodynamic, such as cell membrane changes and changes in cell function mediated by neurotransmitters and ion transport. Withdrawal appears to be mediated by sympathetic nervous system overactivity.
- Barbiturates: The primary mechanism of barbiturate tolerance appears to be dispositional, as they induce their own metabolism.
- Benzodiazepines (BZs): Tolerance appears to be primarily pharmacodynamic, possibly a decrease in the number or sensitivity of BZ receptors.
- Opiates: Tolerance to opiates appears to be pharmacodynamic. With chronic use there is a decrease in production of the endogenous substance enkephalin and a decrease in the binding sensitivity of the opiate receptor system (down-regulation). Thus larger doses are required to achieve the same degree of inhibition of noradrenergic activity. Opiate withdrawal can be conceptualized as a syndrome of noradrenergic hyperactivity.

CENTRAL NERVOUS SYSTEM STIMULANTS

- Cocaine: Tolerance to cocaine is pharmacodynamic. Withdrawal effects (e.g., depression, fatigue, increased sleep and appetite) are the opposite of the usual effect of the drug. Chronic cocaine use may cause a catecholamine depletion in the brain.
- Phencyclidine (PCP): Tolerance to PCP may be dispositional in nature.
- Marijuana: Tolerance to marijuana appears to be more pharmacodynamic than dispositional.

▶ CLINICAL PRESENTATION, PATTERNS OF USE, AND DIAGNOSIS

- The *Diagnostic and Statistical Manual of Mental Disorders,* Fourth Edition (DSM-IV) categorizes substance-related disorders as substance use disorders and substance-induced disorders.
- Substance use disorders include dependence and abuse; substance-induced disorders include intoxication, withdrawal, dementia, psychosis, mood disorders, and anxiety.
- The essential feature of substance dependence is the continued use of the substance despite adverse consequences. To meet the criteria for diagnosis, at least three of the following must be present at any time in a 12-month period: (1) tolerance; (2) withdrawal, (3) the substance is taken in larger amounts or over a longer period of time than was intended; (4) persistent desire or unsuccessful efforts to cut down or control use; (5) time spent in activities necessary to obtain the substance, use it, or recover from its effects; (6) effects on social, occupational, or recreational activities; and (7) substance use continues despite knowledge of resultant physical or psychological problems.
- The essential feature of substance abuse is a maladaptive pattern of substance use with repeated adverse consequences related to repeated use.

XIII

897

- Intoxication refers to the development of a substance-specific syndrome after recent ingestion and presence in the body of a substance and is associated with maladaptive behavior during the waking state caused by the effect of the substance.

ALCOHOL

- Signs and symptoms of alcohol intoxication and withdrawal are shown in Table 73.1.
- Medical complications of alcoholism include liver disease, cardiomyopathy, pancreatitis, gastrointestinal (GI) disease, anemia, central nervous system (CNS) disturbances, and fetal alcohol syndrome.
- Mild intoxication can cause an apparent stimulation that is a disinhibition effect.
- Alcohol withdrawal.
  - Phase I. Begins within hours of cessation, lasts for 3–5 days, and consists of tremor, tachycardia, diaphoresis, labile blood pressure, anxiety, nausea, and vomiting. Most patients do not progress beyond phase I even if untreated.
  - Phase II. Includes perceptual disturbances, most commonly auditory or visual.
  - Phase III. Includes seizures (usually tonic–clonic) lasting 30 seconds to 4 minutes and progressing to status epilepticus in about 3% of cases. Seizures occur in 10–15% of untreated withdrawal patients.
  - Phase IV *(delirium tremens)*. Occurs in <1% of patients. It manifests as acute autonomic hyperactivity and delirium including severe hyperthermia. The mortality rate for patients who progress to phase IV is 20%.

CHAPTER 73.1. Signs and Symptoms of Alcohol Intoxication and Withdrawal

Intoxication	Withdrawal
Slurred speech	Tremor
Ataxia	Tachycardia
Nystagmus	Diaphoresis
Sedation	Labile blood pressure
Flushed face	Anxiety
Mood change	Nausea and vomiting
Irritability	Hallucinations
Euphoria	Seizures
Loquacity	Hyperthermia
Impaired attention	Delirium

XIII

BENZODIAZEPINES AND OTHER SEDATIVE-HYPNOTICS

- Abusers usually prefer the shorter acting barbiturates (e.g., secobarbital, pentobarbital). Short-acting nonbarbiturates (e.g., meprobamate, methyprylon, ethchlorvynol, glutethimide) are also abused. Among the BZs, faster onset drugs, especially diazepam, are often preferred. Alprazolam may be particularly dependence-producing.
- Although infrequent, tolerance and withdrawal have been reported with zolpidem use.
- Withdrawal from shorter-acting drugs (e.g., lorazepam, alprazolam) has an onset within 12–24 hours of the last dose. Withdrawal from longer-acting drugs (e.g., diazepam, chlordiazepoxide, clorazepate, phenobarbital, amobarbital) may be delayed for several days after discontinuation.
- Dependence on sedative-hypnotics and BZs is summarized in Table 73.2. The likelihood and severity of withdrawal is a function of both dose and duration of exposure.

OPIATES

- IV injection of an opiate causes a flushing of the skin and a lower abdominal sensation described as similar to orgasm. Following the

TABLE 73.2. Dependence on Sedative–Hypnotics[a]

Generic Name	Oral Sedating Dose (mg)	Physical Dependence Dose and Time Needed to Produce Dependence	Time Before Onset of Withdrawal (h)	Peak Withdrawal Symptoms (d)
Benzodiazepines				
Diazepam	5–10	40–120 mg × 42–120 d	12–24	5–8
Chlordiazepoxide	10–25	75–600 mg × 42–120 d	12–24	5–8
Clorazepate	7.5–15	45–180 mg × 42–120 d (est.)	12–24	5–8
Alprazolam	0.25–8	8–16 mg × 42 d (est.)	8–24	2–3
Barbiturates				
Secobarbital	100	800–2200 mg × 35–37 d	6–12	2–3
Pentobarbital	100	Same	6–12	2–3
Equal parts of seco- and amobarbital	100	Same	6–12	2–3
Amobarbital	65–100	Same	8–12	2–5
Nonbarbiturate Sedative—Hypnotics				
Ethchlorvynol	200	1–1.5 g × 30 d	6–12	2–3
Chloral hydrate	250	Exact dose unknown: 12 g/d chronically has led to delirium upon sudden withdrawal	6–12	2–3
Meprobamate	400	1.6–3.2 g × 270 d	8–12	3–8

[a] Withdrawal symptoms are tremor, tachycardia, diaphoresis, nausea, vomiting, blood pressure lability, delirium, seizures, and hallucinations.

XIII

rush, there is a period of detachment for a few hours, then the drug effects wear off. Tolerance may develop rapidly.

- Drug combinations involving opiates are quite popular [e.g., pentazocine with tripelennamine, opiates with cocaine (speedball), opiates with alcohol].

- Complications of opiate use include overdoses, anaphylactic reactions to impurities, nephrotic syndrome, septicemia, endocarditis, and acquired immune deficiency syndrome (AIDS).

- Some opiate-dependent persons use methadone as part of their treatment. A more recent development is the availability of levo-alpha-acetylmethadol (LAAM) in some treatment programs. LAAM is a pro-drug related to methadone that has a long half-life.

- Signs and symptoms of opioid intoxication and withdrawal are shown in Table 73.3. Onset of withdrawal ranges from a few hours after stopping heroin to 3–5 days after stopping methadone, and duration is 3–14 days. Withdrawal is not fatal unless there is a concurrent medical problem. Delirium is not characteristic of opioid withdrawal.

COCAINE

- Cocaine is perhaps the most behaviorally reinforcing of all drugs of abuse. Common slang terms are "coke," "snow," "girl," and "nose candy."

- Cocaine blocks reuptake of norepinephrine (NE) and dopamine (DA).

- The most characteristic systemic effect of cocaine is stimulation of the CNS. The most common clinical manifestations are euphoria, decreased fatigue, and increased alertness.

- In the presence of alcohol, cocaine is metabolized to cocaethylene, a longer acting, but more lethal psychoactive compound compared to the parent drug.

TABLE 73.3. Signs and Symptoms of Opioid Intoxication and Withdrawal

Intoxication	Withdrawal
Euphoria	Lacrimation
Dysphoria	Rhinorrhea
Apathy	Mydriasis
Motor retardation	Piloerection
Sedation	Diaphoresis
Slurred speech	Diarrhea
Attention impairment	Yawning
Miosis	Fever
	Insomnia
	Muscle aching

XIII

- Many users convert the cocaine hydrochloride to cocaine base, also known as "crack" or "rock," which is absorbed immediately by inhalation and produces intense euphoria.
- Complications: At toxic doses, it causes cardiac failure due to a direct effect on myocardial contractility. Cocaine also causes a toxic psychosis characterized by hallucinations, paranoid thinking, and looseness of associations.
- Signs and symptoms of cocaine intoxication are summarized in Table 73.4.
- Withdrawal is characterized by fatigue, sleep disturbance, nightmares, and depression, beginning within hours of discontinuing the drug and lasting up to several days.

AMPHETAMINES AND OTHER STIMULANTS

- Physiologic and psychologic effects are qualitatively similar to those of cocaine.
- Amphetamines block the reuptake and inhibit degradation of NE and DA. Amphetamines are psychotomimetic. The onset of effects of amphetamines is not as abrupt, and the duration of action is longer than that of cocaine.
- The IV use of methamphetamine is known as speed. Methamphetamine base ("ice") can be smoked, and the duration of effect is much longer than that of cocaine.

PHENCYCLIDINE

- Phencyclidine, also known as "PCP," "angel dust," and "crystal," is most often used as a substitute for or contaminant of other drugs.
- When used intentionally, PCP is commonly smoked with marijuana, but may also be taken orally or IV.

TABLE 73.4. Signs and Symptoms of Cocaine Intoxication and Withdrawal

Intoxication	Withdrawal
Motor agitation	Fatigue
Elation/euphoria	Sleep disturbance
Grandiosity	Nightmares
Loquacity	Depression
Hypervigilance	Increased appetite
Tachycardia	
Mydriasis	
Elevated or lowered blood pressure	
Sweating or chills	
Nausea and vomiting	

XIII

- PCP blocks the reuptake of serotonin (5-HT), NE, and DA, blocks activity of the NMDA receptor, and binds at an opiate receptor associated with psychotomimetic properties.
- Signs and symptoms of PCP intoxication include very unpredictable behavior, increased blood pressure, tachycardia, ataxia, slurred speech, euphoria, agitation, anxiety, hostility, delusions, and hallucinations. Psychosis may last for weeks.

HALLUCINOGENS

- Hallucinogens cause a heightened awareness of sensation and a diminished ability to differentiate boundaries of objects or self from the environment.
- Lysergic acid diethylamide (LSD) and similar drugs stimulate presynaptic 5-HT_{1A} and postsynaptic 5-HT_2 receptors in brain.
- Signs and symptoms of intoxication include intensified perceptions, depersonalization, derealization, hallucinations, mydriasis, tachycardia, diaphoresis, palpitations, blurred vision, tremor, incoordination, dizziness, drowsiness, and paresthesias.
- LSD is the most potent and long acting of the hallucinogens. DMT is inactive when ingested orally, but can be smoked, inhaled, or injected. There is a cross-tolerance among LSD, psilocybin, and mescaline.
- There is no physical withdrawal syndrome associated with hallucinogens.
- Complications include prolonged episodes of panic (the "bad trip") and flashbacks. Flashbacks can occur spontaneously up to several years after the last drug exposure.

MARIJUANA

- Marijuana, referred to as "reefer," "pot," "grass," or "weed," is the most commonly used illicit drug. The principal psychoactive component is tetrahydrocannabinol (THC). Hashish, the dried resin of the top of the plant, is more potent than the rest of the plant.
- Chronic exposure is not associated with a significant withdrawal syndrome on discontinuation, but many users exhibit compulsive drug-seeking behavior.
- Physiologic effects include sedation, difficulty in performing complex tasks, and disinhibition. Endocrine effects include amenorrhea, decreased testosterone production, and inhibition of spermatogenesis. Signs and symptoms of marijuana intoxication are shown in Table 73.5.
- Although duration of effect may be only several hours, THC is detectable on toxicologic screening for up to 4–5 weeks in chronic users.

XIII

INHALANTS

- Organic solvents inhaled by abusers include gasoline, glue, aerosols, amyl nitrite, typewriter correction fluid, and nitrous oxide. Toluene is a component of several inhaled solvents.

TABLE 73.5. Signs and Symptoms of Marijuana Intoxication

Tachycardia	Euphoria
Conjunctival congestion	Sensory intensification
Increased appetite	Apathy
Dry mouth	Hallucinations

- Physiologic effects include CNS depression, headache, nausea, hallucinations, and delusions. With chronic use the drugs are toxic to virtually all organ systems.

▶ DESIRED OUTCOMES

- The goals of treatment are cessation of use of the drug in question and termination of associated drug-seeking behaviors. The goals of treatment of the withdrawal syndrome are prevention of progression of withdrawal to life-threatening severity, thus enabling the patient to be sufficiently comfortable and functional in order to participate in a behavioral treatment program and supportive therapy. The ultimate goal of treatment is to allow the patient to return to normal social and occupational functioning.

▶ TREATMENT

INTOXICATION

- Whenever possible, drug therapy should be avoided. However, drug therapy may be indicated when patients are agitated, combative, assaultive, hallucinatory, or delusional (Table 73.6).
- Toxicology screens are useful in evaluating patients. When they are desired, blood or urine should be collected immediately on the patient's arrival.
- Flumazenil is not indicated in all cases of suspected BZ overdose, and it is specifically contraindicated in cases in which cyclic antidepressant involvement is known or suspected because of the risk of seizures. It should be used with caution when BZ physical dependence is suspected, as it may precipitate BZ withdrawal.
- In opiate intoxication, naloxone may be used to revive unconscious patients with respiratory depression. However, it may also precipitate physical withdrawal in dependent patients.
- Cocaine intoxication is treated pharmacologically only if the patient is agitated and psychotic.
- Many patients with hallucinogen intoxication respond to simple reassurance. When necessary, short-term antianxiety and/or antipsychotic therapy can be used. The same approach applies to marijuana and inhalant intoxication.

XIII

TABLE 73.6. Treatment of Substance Intoxication

Drug Class	Pharmacologic Therapy	Nonpharmacologic Therapy
Benzodiazepines	Flumazenil 0.1–0.2 mg/min IV up to 1 mg	Support vital functions
Alcohol, barbiturates, and sedative–hypnotics (nonbenzodiazepines)	None	Support vital functions
Opiates	Naloxone 0.4–2.0 mg IV every 3 min	Support vital functions
Cocaine and other CNS stimulants	Lorazepam 2–4 mg IM every 30 min to 6 h prn agitation Haloperidol 2–5 mg IM (or other antipsychotic agent) every 30 min to 6 h prn psychotic behavior	Monitor cardiac function
Hallucinogens, marijuana, and inhalants	Lorazepam and/or haloperidol as above	Reassurance; "talk-down therapy"; support vital functions
Phencyclidine	Lorazepam and/or haloperidol as above	Minimize sensory input

WITHDRAWAL

- Treatment of drug withdrawal is summarized in Table 73.7.

Alcohol

- Most clinicians agree that the BZs are the drugs of choice in treatment of alcohol withdrawal.
- The long-acting drugs (e.g., chlordiazepoxide, diazepam) control withdrawal effectively with few rebound effects after discontinuation. A dosage regimen for detoxification with chlordiazepoxide is 50 mg tid × 1 d, then 50 mg bid × 1 d, then 25 mg tid × 1 d, then 25 mg bid × 1 day, then 25 mg daily × 1 d, then discontinue.
- The short- to intermediate-acting BZs (e.g., oxazepam, lorazepam) are also used for alcohol detoxification. An example regimen is lorazepam, 2 mg tid × 2 d, then 2 mg bid × 2 d, then 2 mg daily × 1 d, then discontinue.
- More aggressive treatment with a BZ, often by injection (e.g., lorazepam 2–4 mg IM or IV, or diazepam 10 mg IV), may be required to bring alcohol withdrawal under better control.
- Patients with severe withdrawal symptoms may require higher doses and longer tapering periods. Monitoring parameters should include vital signs, tremor, sweating, and other withdrawal symptoms.
- Antipsychotic therapy is not generally indicated and may lower seizure threshold.

XIII

TABLE 73.7. Treatment of Withdrawal From Common Drugs of Abuse

Drug or Drug Class	Pharmacologic Therapy
Alochol	
Detoxification	Chlordiazepoxide 50 mg tid-qid or lorazepam 2 mg tid-qid; taper over 5–7 d
Withdrawal hallucinations	Lorazepam 2 mg IM, may be repeated; higher detoxification dosage and slower taper may be needed
Withdrawal seizures	Supportive treatment only during seizure unless condition progresses to status epilepticus; lorazepam 2 mg IM after seizure ends; use higher detoxification dosage and slower taper
Supportive drug therapy	Thiamine 100 mg IM, then 100 mg PO daily; multivitamin, one daily; magnesium sulfate 1 g IM × 1–3 d
Benzodiazepines	
Short- to intermediate acting	Chlordiazepoxide 50 mg tid-qid or lorazepam 2 mg tid-qid; taper over 5–7 d
Long-acting	Chlordiazepoxide 50 mg tid-qid or lorazepam 2 mg tid-qid; taper over additional 5–7 d
Barbiturates and other sedative–hypnotics	Pentobarbital tolerance test; initial detoxification at upper limit of tolerance test; decrease dosage by 100 mg every 2–3 d
Opiates	Methadone 20–80 mg PO daily; taper by 5–10 mg daily or clonidine 2 μg/kg tid × 7 d; taper over additional 3 d
Mixed-substance withdrawal	
Drugs are cross-tolerant	Detoxify according to treatment for longer acting drug used
Drugs are not cross-tolerant	Detoxify from one drug while maintaining second drug (cross-tolerant drugs), then detoxify from second drug
CNS stimulants	Supportive treatment only; pharmacotherapy often not used; bromocriptine 2.5 mg tid or higher may be used for severe craving associated with cocaine withdrawal

- Alcohol withdrawal seizures do not require anticonvulsant treatment unless they progress to status epilepticus. Phenytoin does not prevent or treat withdrawal seizures.
- Patients with seizures should be treated supportively, and an increase in the dosage and lengthening of the tapering schedule of the BZ used in detoxification or a single injection of a BZ may be necessary to prevent further seizures. Patients with a history of withdrawal seizures can be given a higher initial dose of a BZ and a slower tapering period of 7–10 days.

XIII

Benzodiazepines

- Detoxification is approached by initiating treatment at usual doses (e.g., chlordiazepoxide 50 mg three times daily, or lorazepam 2 mg three times daily) and maintaining on this dose for 5 days. Then gradually

taper the dose over an additional 5 days. A more gradual taper may be required for patients in alprazolam withdrawal.
• In patients with a history of long exposure to BZs, protracted minor abstinence symptoms (e.g., anxiety, insomnia, irritability, muscle spasms) may remain for several weeks.

Barbiturates and Other Sedative-Hypnotic Drugs

• Determine the level of tolerance by giving 200 mg of pentobarbital orally and observing for 2–3 hours for signs of a mild intoxication, including sedation, slurred speech, and ataxia. Repeat one or more times if necessary until one or more signs of intoxication are seen. The total dose required can be used as an approximate initial daily starting dose for detoxification. This dose is then reduced in decrements of 100 mg every third day at first, then every other day if the patient tolerates initial dosage reductions.

Opiates

• Unnecessary detoxification with drugs should be avoided if possible (e.g., if symptoms are tolerable).
• Detoxification of heroin users usually requires a starting dose of methadone of no more than 20 mg daily. If LAAM is used instead of methadone, dosing is three times weekly.
• Clonidine can attenuate the noradrenergic hyperactivity of opiate withdrawal without interfering significantly with activity at the opiate receptors. Monitoring should include blood pressure checks, supine and standing, at least daily.

Withdrawal from Other Substances

• Treatment of cocaine withdrawal is mostly supportive, but bromocriptine has been used usually short term to reduce craving.

Mixed Substance Withdrawal

• If the drugs used are cross-tolerant (e.g., alcohol and diazepam), treatment for withdrawal from diazepam, the longer acting of the two drugs, also concurrently treats alcohol withdrawal. If the drugs are not cross-tolerant (e.g., alcohol and opiates), withdrawal from each drug must be treated separately. In a young healthy individual, withdrawal from both drugs can be treated concurrently. Otherwise, when detoxification from one drug is completed, the second drug can be tapered and discontinued.

SUBSTANCE DEPENDENCE

XIII • The treatment of drug dependence, or addiction, is primarily behavioral. The goal of treatment is complete abstinence, and treatment is a lifelong process. Most drug-dependence treatment programs embrace a treatment approach based on Alcoholics Anonymous (AA).

Drug Therapy

• Disulfiram is an inhibitor of aldehyde dehydrogenase that serves as a disincentive to drink alcohol. It is an adjunct to behavioral treatment. In the presence of alcohol, it inhibits the metabolism of acetaldehyde, causing flushing, nausea, vomiting, headache, palpitations, fever, and hypotension. Severe reactions may include respiratory depression, arrhythmias, myocardial infarction, and cardiovascular collapse. Inhibition of the enzyme continues for as long as 2 weeks after discontinuing disulfiram. Disulfiram reactions have occurred with the use of alcohol-containing mouthwashes and aftershaves. The usual dosage is 250–500 mg/d.

- Naltrexone has been approved as an adjunctive treatment for alcoholism. Doses of 50 mg daily have been associated with reduced craving and fewer drinking days. Naltrexone-treated patients should be monitored for hepatic toxicity.
- Naltrexone is also useful in blocking the euphoric effects of opiates, thus interrupting the reinforcement process. It is especially useful during the first several months after initial withdrawal from opiates. Usual dosage is 50 mg daily or 350 mg per week in three divided doses.
- Tricyclic antidepressants, primarily desipramine, have been used to decrease cocaine craving. It may treat the depression associated with cocaine withdrawal and block cocaine-induced euphoria.

COEXISTENT DRUG DEPENDENCE AND PSYCHIATRIC DISORDERS: THE DUAL DIAGNOSIS PATIENT

- The prevalence of substance dependence in clinical psychiatric settings is about 50%, but the prevalence of psychiatric disorders in addiction treatment populations is much lower.
- Treatment of the dual diagnosis patient involves initial treatment of the substance use disorder, especially when the patient is in physical withdrawal. If symptoms of psychiatric disorder continue after the patient has been drug free for 2 weeks, then treatment of the psychiatric disorder must be considered.

See Chapter 65, Substance-Related Disorders, authored by Brian L. Crabtree, PharmD, and Alexis Polles, MD, for a more detailed discussion of this topic.

XIII

Chapter 74 _____

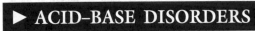

▶ ACID–BASE DISORDERS

▶ DEFINITION

Acid–base disorders are caused by disturbances in hydrogen ion homeostasis, which is ordinarily maintained by extracellular buffering, renal regulation of hydrogen ion and bicarbonate, and ventilatory regulation of carbon dioxide elimination.

▶ GENERAL PRINCIPLES

PATHOPHYSIOLOGY

- Buffering refers to the ability of a solution to resist change in pH with the addition of a strong acid or base. The principal buffer system utilized by the body is the carbonic acid/bicarbonate (H_2CO_3/HCO_3^-) system. Noncarbonate buffers (e.g., phosphate and protein) act primarily intracellularly.
- There are four primary types of acid–base disturbances. Disturbances in hydrogen ion (H^+) homeostasis initially caused by a gain or loss of H^+ or HCO_3^- are of metabolic origin (i.e., metabolic acidosis and metabolic alkalosis). Disturbances initially caused by a rise or fall in arterial carbon dioxide tension ($Paco_2$) are of respiratory origin (i.e., respiratory acidosis and respiratory alkalosis). These processes may occur independently or together as a compensatory response.
- General principles that are common to all types of acid–base disturbances are addressed first, followed by separate discussions of each type of acid–base disturbance.

DIAGNOSIS

- Arterial blood gases, along with serum electrolytes, medical history, medication history, and clinical condition, are the primary tools for determining cause of acid–base disorders and for designing therapy.
- Arterial blood gases are measured to determine oxygenation and acid–base status (Figure 74.1). Low pH values (<7.35) indicate acidemia, while high values (>7.45) indicate alkalemia. $Paco_2$ value helps to determine if there is a primary respiratory abnormality, while HCO_3^- concentration enables assessment of metabolic component.
- Current methods of arterial blood gas analysis are similar and measure pH, Pco_2, and Po_2 directly. Bicarbonate values and O_2 saturation (Sao_2) are calculated.

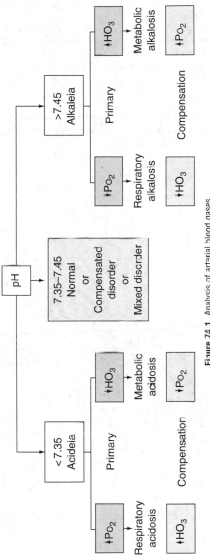

Figure 74.1. Analysis of arterial blood gases.

XIV

- If a given set of blood gases does not fall within the range of expected responses for a single acid–base disorder (Figure 74.2), a mixed disorder should be suspected.
- Ratio of change in anion gap (AG) to change in bicarbonate ($\Delta AG/\Delta HCO_3$) is a helpful diagnostic parameter, particularly for mixed acid–base disorders. The ratio is usually 1.0 for common organic acidoses (e.g., diabetic ketoacidosis or lactic acidosis); however, mixed acid–base disorder is probably present if the ratio is >1.2 or <0.8.

DESIRED OUTCOME

Initial treatment is usually aimed at immediately stabilizing the acute condition, followed by identifying and correcting underlying cause(s) of

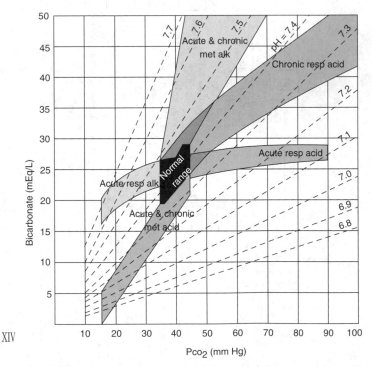

Figure 74.2. Acid–base nomogram. met, metabolic; alk, alkalosis; resp, respiratory; acid, acidosis. *(From CMAJ 1973;109:291–293, with permission.)*

XIV

acid–base disturbances. Additional treatment may be required depending on the severity of symptoms and to prevent recurrence, especially in patients with ongoing initiating events.

▶ RESPIRATORY ALKALOSIS

PATHOPHYSIOLOGY

- Respiratory alkalosis, one of the most common acid–base disturbances, is characterized by an initial decrease in $Paco_2$, hypocapnia, which raises pH and results in a secondary decrease in plasma bicarbonate concentration.
- $Paco_2$ decreases when ventilatory excretion exceeds metabolic production because of hyperventilation.
- Potential causes of respiratory alkalosis include increases in neurochemical stimulation via central (e.g., anxiety, pain, fever, brain tumor, vascular accident, salicylates), or peripheral (e.g., pulmonary emboli, congestive heart failure, altitude, asthma) mechanisms, or physical increases in ventilation via voluntary or artificial means (e.g., mechanical ventilation).
- The earliest compensatory response is to chemically buffer excess bicarbonate by moving hydrogen ions extracellularly from intracellular proteins, phosphates, and hemoglobin. If respiratory alkalosis is prolonged beyond >6 hours, the kidneys attempt to further compensate by increasing bicarbonate elimination (i.e., decreasing reabsorption of filtered bicarbonate and net acid excretion).

CLINICAL PRESENTATION

- Light-headedness, confusion, decreased intellectual functioning, syncope, and seizures may be caused by decreased cerebral blood flow
- Nausea and vomiting may occur, probably as a result of cerebral hypoxia.
- Cardiac arrhythmias may occur in severe respiratory alkalosis.
- Serum chloride concentration is usually slightly increased and serum potassium concentration may be slightly decreased. Serum phosphorus concentration may decrease by as much as 1.5–2.0 mg/dL. Ionized calcium is reduced, which may be partially responsible for muscle cramps and tetany.

TREATMENT

- Direct measures (e.g., treatment of pain, hypovolemia, fever, infection, or salicylate overdose) may prove effective. A rebreathing device (e.g., paper bag) may help control hyperventilation.
- If the patient is receiving mechanical ventilation, respiratory alkalosis may often be corrected by decreasing minute ventilation (i.e., number of mechanical breaths per minute), using a capnograph and spirometer to more precisely adjust ventilator settings, or increasing dead space in the ventilator circuit.

XIV

▶ RESPIRATORY ACIDOSIS

PATHOPHYSIOLOGY

- Respiratory acidosis is initially caused by primary retention of carbon dioxide that lowers blood pH and results in a compensatory increase in plasma bicarbonate concentration.
- Respiratory acidosis results from a disorder that restricts ventilation or increases CO_2 production, such as perfusion abnormalities (e.g., massive pulmonary embolism, cardiac arrest), airway and pulmonary abnormalities (e.g., airway obstruction, severe pulmonary edema, severe pneumonia), neuromuscular abnormalities (e.g., trauma, stroke, brainstem or cervical cord injury, myasthenia gravis, narcotic or sedative overdose), or mechanical ventilator problems (e.g, malfunction).
- The early compensatory response to acute respiratory acidosis is buffering by noncarbonate systems. If respiratory acidosis is prolonged >12–24 hours, renal excretion of hydrogen ion also increases, which generates new bicarbonate.

CLINICAL PRESENTATION

- Neuromuscular symptoms include altered mental status, abnormal behavior, seizures, stupor, and coma. Hypercapnia may mimic stroke or central nervous system (CNS) tumor by producing headache, papilledema, focal paresis, and abnormal reflexes. CNS symptoms are caused by increased cerebral blood flow and are variable depending in part on acuity of onset.
- The degree of altered cardiac contractility and heart rate depends on severity of acidosis, whether it is metabolic or respiratory, and rapidity of onset.
- Serum sodium and chloride concentrations remain normal or increase slightly. Serum potassium concentration increases secondary to intracellular movement.

TREATMENT

- If carbon dioxide excretion is acutely and severely impaired, and life-threatening hypoxia is present (PO_2 <40 mm Hg), adequate ventilation should be provided, which may involve maintaining a patent airway (e.g., emergency tracheotomy, bronchoscopy, or intubation), clearing excessive secretions, administering oxygen, and mechanical ventilation.
- Underlying cause of acute acidosis should be treated aggressively (e.g, bronchodilators, stopping respiratory depressants such as narcotics and benzodiazepines).
- Bicarbonate administration is rarely necessary and potentially harmful.
- Treatment is essentially similar for acute respiratory acidosis in a patient with chronic respiratory acidosis (e.g., chronic obstructive pulmonary disease), with a few important exceptions. Because the drive to breathe depends on hypoxemia rather than hypercarbia, oxygen therapy

should be initiated carefully and only if Pao_2 is <50 mm Hg. Measures should be taken to treat underlying causes of acute exacerbation (e.g., antibiotics).

- Chronic respiratory acidosis is discussed in Chapter 82.

► METABOLIC ACIDOSIS

PATHOPHYSIOLOGY

- Metabolic acidosis is characterized by decreased pH and low serum bicarbonate concentrations, which can result from adding organic acid to extracellular fluid (ECF) (e.g., lactic acid, ketoacids), loss of bicarbonate stores (e.g., in diarrhea), or accumulation of endogenous acids due to impaired renal function (e.g., phosphates, sulfates).
- Patients with metabolic acidosis may have an elevated or normal anion gap. The normal anion gap is approximately 12 mEq/L with a range of 8–16 mEq/L.
- Normal anion gap metabolic acidosis occurs when bicarbonate losses from ECF are replaced by chloride, which may be caused by diarrhea, pancreatic fistula, other gastrointestinal disorders, acid ingestion, carbonic anhydrase inhibitors, dilutional acidosis, renal acidification defects, ureterosigmoidostomy, and ileostomy.
- Metabolic acidosis with an increased anion gap is most often present when bicarbonate losses are replaced by an anion other than chloride, which may result from accumulation of endogenous organic acids (e.g., lactic acid, acetoacetic acid, or β-hydroxybutyric acid), toxin ingestion (e.g., methanol or ethylene glycol), salicylate overdose, starvation, or chronic renal failure.
- Lactic acidosis is one of the most common causes of metabolic acidosis. Lactic acidosis is caused by tissue hypoxia (i.e., type A) or systemic disorders (i.e., type B). Type A, the more frequent form, is most likely to be caused by cardiovascular collapse (e.g., shock, congestive heart failure). Type B may result from systemic diseases (e.g., diabetes mellitus, neoplastic disease, liver or renal failure), drugs (e.g., phenformin), toxins (e.g., methanol, ethylene glycol), or congenital enzyme deficiency.
- The primary compensatory mechanism is increased carbon dioxide excretion due to increasing respiratory rate, which decreases $Paco_2$. Ventilatory compensation begins rapidly and does not reach steady state until 12–24 hours after onset of metabolic acidosis.

CLINICAL PRESENTATION

- Hyperventilation is often the first sign of metabolic acidosis. In extremely severe acidosis (pH <6.8), CNS function may be disrupted to such a degree that the respiratory center is depressed. Respiratory compensation may occur as Kussmaul's respirations (i.e., deep, rapid respirations characteristic of diabetic ketoacidosis). XIV

- Peripheral vasodilation is characterized by flushing, a rapid heart rate, and wide pulse pressure. Cardiac output may be initially increased, but it falls as hypotension worsens.
- Gastrointestinal symptoms include loss of appetite, nausea, and vomiting. These symptoms occur commonly in patients with renal insufficiency who experience mild acidosis. Severe acidosis (pH <7.1) interferes with carbohydrate metabolism and insulin use, resulting in hyperglycemia.
- Effect on serum potassium concentrations depends on type of acidosis, ranging from consistent increases with mineral acids to smaller increments with organic acids (e.g., lactic acidosis).

DIAGNOSIS

- Definitive diagnosis of lactic acidosis is made by measuring serum lactate concentrations. Although the diagnostic threshold has not been defined, lactate concentrations of ≥ 4.0–5.0 mEq/L with simultaneous decreases in bicarbonate and arterial pH are highly suggestive of lactic acidosis.

TREATMENT

- Administration of sodium bicarbonate has been recommended to raise arterial pH to 7.15–7.20, but no controlled clinical trials demonstrate reduced morbidity and mortality compared with general supportive care. Although excessive sodium bicarbonate is potentially detrimental, sodium bicarbonate administration may be necessary for acute situations (e.g., cardiac arrest; see Chapter 6) after more proven interventions have been employed.
- Other alkalinizing agents (e.g., lactate, acetate, and citrate ions) may have an advantage over bicarbonate because of their compatibility and stability in parenteral solutions.
- Investigational agents include Carbicarb, an equimolar mixture of sodium carbonate (Na_2CO_3) and sodium bicarbonate ($NaHCO_3$), and dichloroacetate (DCA).
- Treatment of renal tubular acidosis depends on whether it is type I (i.e., classic, distal, or gradient limited), type II (i.e., proximal or quantity limited), or another type. Alkali administration ranges from 1–3 mEq/kg/day for type I to 10–25 mEq/kg/day for type II. Potassium supplementation may also be necessary (e.g., potassium citrate, which would provide both potassium and alkali).
- Treatment of diabetic ketoacidosis is covered in Chapter 17.

XIV ▶ **METABOLIC ALKALOSIS**

PATHOPHYSIOLOGY

- Metabolic alkalosis, a common condition in hospitalized patients, is characterized by a primary increase in plasma bicarbonate concentration.

- Bicarbonate concentration elevation can be generated by net loss of hydrogen ion from ECF space, net addition of bicarbonate or its precursors (i.e., carbonate, citrate, acetate) to ECF space, or loss of chloride-rich bicarbonate-poor fluid (i.e., gastric HCl).
- Initiating events can be categorized as sodium chloride responsive or resistant, depending on response to saline volume expansion. Sodium chloride-responsive disorders are associated with urinary chloride concentrations of <10 mEq/mL, while sodium chloride-resistant disorders are associated with concentrations of >20 mEq/mL.
  - The most common initiating event is loss of chloride-rich, bicarbonate-poor fluid (e.g., diuretic use, nasogastric suctioning, or vomiting); these are sodium chloride-responsive disorders.
  - Many sodium chloride-resistant disorders are associated with excess mineralocorticoid activity, which may result from primary adrenal overproduction (e.g., hyperaldosteronism) or oversupply of endogenous mineralocorticoids (e.g., licorice ingestion), and oversecretion of mineralocorticoid secondary to increased renin activity. These disorders are also caused by persistent hypokalemia.
  - Miscellaneous causes include large doses of penicillins (e.g., ticarcillin).
- The immediate compensatory response is chemical buffering, which involves movement of intracellular hydrogen ions to the ECF in exchange for potassium and sodium. The second phase is respiratory compensation (i.e., hypoventilation to raise the $PaCO_2$).

CLINICAL PRESENTATION

- No unique signs or symptoms are associated with metabolic alkalosis.
- Patients may complain of symptoms related to the underlying disorder (e.g., muscle weakness with hypokalemia or postural dizziness with volume depletion).

DIAGNOSIS

- Patient history (e.g., vomiting, gastric drainage, or diuretic use) is especially useful in the diagnosis of metabolic alkalosis because of the lack of unique signs and symptoms.

TREATMENT

- Treatment of underlying cause(s) may not correct metabolic alkalosis.
- Therapy depends on whether the disorder is sodium chloride responsive or resistant (Figure 74.3).
- Initial therapy of sodium chloride–responsive disorders is directed at expanding intravascular volume and replenishing chloride stores by administering sodium chloride and potassium solutions. If patients are volume expanded or intolerant to sodium volume loads (e.g., congestive heart failure), a carbonic anhydrase inhibitor may be beneficial. One or two doses of acetazolamide 250 or 500 mg may be administered.

XIV

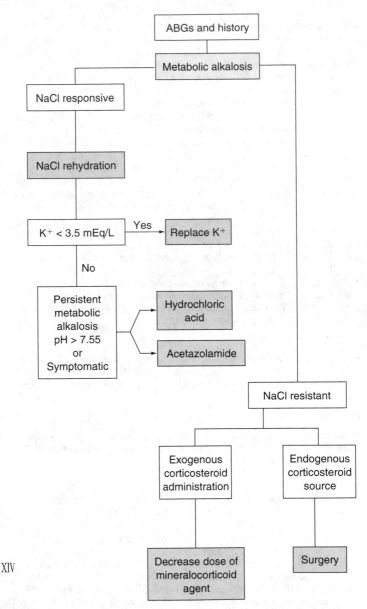

Figure 74.3. Treatment algorithm for patients with primary metabolic alkalosis.

XIV

- Other agents sometimes used to treat sodium chloride–responsive metabolic alkalosis include hydrochloric acid, ammonium chloride, and arginine monohydrochloride.
- Standard doses of histamine H_2-receptor antagonists and omeprazole have been used to decrease the volume and hydrogen ion content in gastric fluids in patients with metabolic alkalosis caused by nasogastric suction.
- Treatment of sodium chloride-resistant disorders involves removal of excess mineralocorticoid activity (e.g., decreasing the corticosteroid dose, surgical correction of excess endogenous mineralocorticoid activity).

▶ MIXED ACID–BASE DISORDERS

PATHOPHYSIOLOGY

- Failure of compensation is responsible for mixed acid–base disorders such as respiratory acidosis and metabolic acidosis, or respiratory alkalosis and metabolic alkalosis. In contrast, excess compensation is responsible for metabolic acidosis and respiratory alkalosis, or metabolic alkalosis and respiratory acidosis.
- Mixed respiratory and metabolic acidosis may develop in patients with cardiorespiratory arrest, in chronic lung disease patients who are in shock, and in metabolic acidosis patients who develop respiratory failure.
- The most common mixed acid–base disorder is respiratory and metabolic alkalosis, which occurs in critically ill surgical patients with respiratory alkalosis caused by mechanical ventilation, hypoxia, sepsis, hypotension, neurologic damage, pain, or drugs, and with metabolic alkalosis caused by vomiting or nasogastric suctioning and massive blood transfusions. It may also occur in patients with hepatic cirrhosis, hyperventilation, diuretic use, or vomiting, and in patients with chronic respiratory acidosis and an elevated plasma bicarbonate concentration who are placed on mechanical ventilation and undergo a rapid fall in $Paco_2$ to hypocapnic levels.
- Metabolic acidosis and respiratory alkalosis may be seen in patients with advanced liver disease, salicylate intoxication, and pulmonary-renal syndromes.
- Mixed metabolic alkalosis and respiratory acidosis may occur in patients with chronic obstructive pulmonary disease and respiratory acidosis who are treated with salt restriction, diuretics, and possibly, glucocorticoids.

DIAGNOSIS

XIV ◀

- Because it is often difficult to correctly identify mixed metabolic alkalosis and respiratory acidosis, it is helpful to observe the patient's response to discontinuation of diuretics and administration of sodium and potassium chloride. This treatment will correct the metabolic alkalosis component if it is a simple metabolic alkalosis, but will only minimally affect $PaCO_2$ if it is a mixed disorder.

TREATMENT

- Mixed respiratory and metabolic acidosis should be treated by responding to both the respiratory and metabolic acidosis. Improved oxygen delivery must be initiated to improve hypercarbia and hypoxia. Mechanical ventilation may be needed to reduce $PaCO_2$. During the initial stage of therapy, appropriate amounts of $NaHCO_3$ should be given to reverse the metabolic acidosis.
- The metabolic component of mixed respiratory and metabolic alkalosis should be corrected by administering sodium chloride and potassium chloride solutions. The respiratory component should be treated by readjusting the ventilator or by treating the underlying disorder causing hyperventilation.
- Treatment of mixed metabolic acidosis and respiratory alkalosis should be directed at the underlying cause. Because of the enhanced compensation, pH is usually closer to normal than in either of the two individual disorders.
- In metabolic alkalosis and respiratory acidosis, pH may not deviate significantly from normal, but treatment may be required to maintain PaO_2 and $PaCO_2$ at acceptable levels. Treatment should be aimed at decreasing plasma bicarbonate with sodium and potassium chloride therapy, allowing the renal excretion of retained bicarbonate from the diuretic-induced metabolic alkalosis.

▶ EVALUATION OF THERAPEUTIC OUTCOMES

- Patients should be monitored closely because acid–base disorders can be serious and even life-threatening.
- Arterial blood gases are the primary tools for evaluation of therapeutic outcome. They should be monitored closely to ensure resolution of simple acid–base disorders without deterioration to mixed disorders due to compensatory mechanisms. For example, arterial blood gases should be obtained every 2–4 hours during the acute phase of respiratory acidosis and less frequently (every 12–24 hours) as the acidosis improves.

See Chapter 52, Acid–Base Disorders, authored by Robert A. Kilroy, PharmD, BCPS, for a more detailed discussion of this topic.

XIV

Chapter 75

▶ DIALYSIS

▶ DEFINITION

Dialysis is one of the primary treatment modalities for patients with renal failure. Two of the principle functions of the kidney (i.e., removal of endogenous waste products and maintenance of water [fluid] balance) can be accomplished by a well-designed dialysis prescription based on the diffusion of solutes (movement from an area of high to low concentration, or from blood to dialysate) and ultrafiltration of water (movement from an area of high to low pressure, or from blood to dialysate) across a semipermeable membrane (dialysis filter).

▶ PATHOPHYSIOLOGY, CLINICAL PRESENTATION, AND DIAGNOSIS

- The delivery of chronic renal replacement therapy is evolving. New methodologic approaches introduced in the last 5–10 years continue to be evaluated. The definition of optimal dose of dialysis remains in question. Recommendations for the management of acute complications of dialysis, particularly peritonitis, are evolving. Therefore, this chapter incorporates new observations and recommendations that were not available when the third edition of *Pharmacotherapy: A Pathophysiologic Approach* was published.
- The number of patients receiving chronic renal replacement therapy has steadily increased by nearly 10% per year since the early 1970s. It is estimated that more than 325,000 patients will receive some type of maintenance dialysis by the year 2000.
- Hemodialysis (Table 75.1) and peritoneal dialysis (Table 75.2) are the predominant treatment options for acute and chronic renal failure (see Chapters 78 and 79). Each type of dialysis has unique advantages and disadvantages that facilitate individualization of therapy. Therefore, the two types are discussed separately in this chapter.
- In patients with chronic renal failure, dialysis should be initiated electively rather than urgently to allow time to educate the patient, create a suitable access, and prevent complications. Because of the progressive nature of chronic renal failure, the need should be anticipated when serum creatinine or blood urea nitrogen (BUN) rises above 8–10 or 100 mg/dL, respectively.

▶ DESIRED OUTCOME

The ultimate goal of dialysis is to provide the optimal dose of dialysis for each individual patient; that is, the amount of therapy above which there is no cost-effective increment in the patient's quality-adjusted life expectancy.

TABLE 75.1. Advantages and Disadvantages of Hemodialysis (HD)

Advantages

1. Higher solute clearance allows intermittent treatment.
2. Parameters of adequacy of dialysis better defined and therefore underdialysis can be detected early.
3. Technique failure rate is low.
4. Even though intermittent heparinization is required, hemostasis parameters are better corrected with hemodialysis than peritoneal dialysis.
5. In-center hemodialysis enables closer monitoring of the patient.

Disadvantages

1. Requires multiple visits each week to the hemodialysis center, which translates into loss of control by the patient.
2. Disequilibrium, dialysis hypotension, and muscle cramps are common. May require months before the patient adjusts to hemodialysis.
3. Bioincompatibility causes activation of complement and cytokines, and, perhaps, predisposes to dialysis-related amyloidosis.
4. Infections in hemodialysis patients may be related to the choice of membranes, the complement activating membranes being more deleterious.
5. Vascular access frequently associated with infection and thrombosis.
6. Decline of residual renal function more rapid compared to peritoneal dialysis.

TABLE 75.2. Advantages and Disadvantages of Peritoneal Dialysis (PD)

Advantages

1. Little risk of disequilibrium due to slow solute removal rate.
2. CAPD becomes more effective than HD as the solute size increases, which may explain good clinical state of the patient in spite of lower urea clearance.
3. Hypotension less frequent.
4. Better control of blood pressure.
5. Better preservation of residual renal function.
6. Convenient intraperitoneal route of administration of drugs such as antibiotics and insulin.
7. Can be done in elderly and the very young—age groups who may not tolerate HD well.
8. Freedom from the "machine" gives the patient a sense of independence.

Disadvantages

1. Protein losses through peritoneum and reduced appetite due to continuous glucose load and sense of abdominal fullness predispose to malnutrition.
2. Risk of peritonitis.
3. Catheter malfunction, exit site, and tunnel infection.
4. Inadequate ultrafiltration.
5. Patient burnout and high rate of technique failure.
6. Risk of obesity with excessive glucose absorption.
7. Mechanical problems such as hernias, dialysate leaks, hemorrhoids, or back pain.
8. Extensive abdominal surgery may preclude peritoneal dialysis.

CAPD, continuous ambulatory peritoneal dialysis.

► TREATMENT: HEMODIALYSIS

GENERAL PRINCIPLES

- Hemodialysis consists of perfusion of heparinized blood and physiologic salt solution on opposite sides of a semipermeable membrane. Waste products (e.g., urea and creatinine) move from blood into the dialysate by passive diffusion along concentration gradients.
- Diffusion rate depends on the difference between solute concentrations in blood and dialysate, solute characteristics, dialysis filter composition, and blood and dialysate flow rates.
- Ultrafiltration or convection, the primary mode for removal of excess body fluids, also occurs during hemodialysis. If the filter pore size is large enough, drugs and endogenous waste products in plasma water are also removed.
- Hemodialysis consists of an external vascular circuit through which blood is transferred in sterile polyethylene tubing to the dialysis filter via a mechanical pump (Figure 75.1). The patient's blood then passes through the dialyzer on one side of the semipermeable membrane material and is returned to the patient. The dialysate solution, which consists of purified water and electrolytes, is pumped through the dialyzer countercurrent to the flow of blood on the other side of the semipermeable membrane. The dialysate circuit is not sterile and is a potential source of infection, particularly if the membrane ruptures.
- Permanent access to the bloodstream for hemodialysis may be accomplished by several techniques. Native arteriovenous fistula (AV fistula) has the longest survival of all blood access devices and is associated with the lowest complication rate. Synthetic vascular grafts are the access of choice for most patients, especially those who have poor peripheral vasculature, and are found in more than 60% of all patients. Vascular access for acute dialysis is usually achieved by inserting a dual lumen catheter into a large vein (e.g., internal jugular). The primary complications of vascular accesses are infection, thrombosis, and stenosis.
- In conventional or standard hemodialysis, low-permeability (low-flux) membranes are made of natural products (i.e., cellulose). Each session usually lasts 4 to 5 hours.
- Rapid high efficiency dialysis (RHED) has the advantages of increased clearance of low molecular weight solutes (e.g., urea) and shorter procedure times due to the use of larger filters (some with increased water permeability), and increased blood and dialysate flow rates. However, clearance of middle and high molecular weight solutes, including many drugs, is not increased because the membrane pore size is still small.
- High-flux dialysis (HFD) combines diffusion and convection. The membrane pores are more open than those found in RHED filters and therefore have higher clearance rates for middle molecules. HFD filters are more expensive than low- or medium-flux filters, and require more precise ultrafiltration controllers to avoid large rapid fluid shifts.

XIV

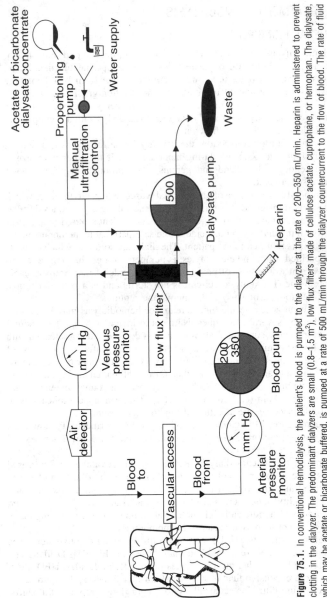

Figure 75.1. In conventional hemodialysis, the patient's blood is pumped to the dialyzer at the rate of 200–350 mL/min. Heparin is administered to prevent clotting in the dialyzer. The predominant dialyzers are small (0.8–1.5 m²), low flux filters made of cellulose acetate, cuprophane, or hemophan. The dialysate, which may be acetate or bicarbonate buffered, is pumped at a rate of 500 mL/min through the dialyzer countercurrent to the flow of blood. The rate of fluid removal from the patient is manually controlled by adjusting the pressure in the dialysate compartment.

Despite these drawbacks, use of HFD is increasing. HFD is used by more than 35% of hemodialysis patients in the United States.

HEMODIALYSIS PRESCRIPTION

- Although there is no clear agreement on the optimal dose of dialysis that should be prescribed, several clinical trials are in progress that will likely clarify this issue.
- In centers where the dose of dialysis has been proactively increased, mortality rates and duration of hospitalization have decreased.
- Many nephrologists recommend a target urea reduction ratio (URR) of 65 or a *Kt/V* of >1.2 for nondiabetic patients receiving standard dialysis, and a URR of >70 or a *Kt/V* of ≥1.4–1.5 for diabetics and/or patients receiving RHED or HFD therapy. *Kt/V* is a unitless parameter that represents the fraction of the patient's urea distribution volume that is cleared of urea during a dialysis session.
- URR can be calculated as follows:

$$URR = BUN_{pre} - BUN_{post}/BUN_{pre}$$

where BUN_{pre} is predialysis BUN and BUN_{post} is postdialysis BUN.
- The most accurate way to determine the delivered *Kt/V* requires collection of BUN concentrations prior to, during, or after the dialysis session and application of a nomographic or computerized urea kinetic modeling approach.
- The delivered *Kt/V* can be estimated as follows:

$$Kt/V = -\ln[(BUN_{post}/BUN_{pre}) - 0.008t] + [(4 - 3.5BUN_{post}/BUN_{pre})UF/Wt]$$

where K is dialyzer clearance of urea (in L/h), V is patient's distribution volume (in L), t is duration of dialysis (in h), and UF is ultrafiltration volume removed (in L).
- Post-treatment BUN samples should be obtained 15–30 minutes after the end of the treatment to assure re-equilibration of urea. In most dialysis facilities, however, samples are collected within 2 minutes of the end of treatment, which overestimates the true delivered dose of dialysis.

COMPLICATIONS OF HEMODIALYSIS

- Intradialytic complications are frequent in patients receiving hemodialysis (Table 75.3). Despite use of higher blood flow rates and dialyzers with increased K_{uf}, the incidence of almost all of these complications is 30–40% lower in patients receiving RHED or HFD compared with standard hemodialysis.

Acute Complications

- Type A dialyzer reactions are similar to drug-induced anaphylactic reactions and may be due to hypersensitivity to ethylene oxide (a common dialyzer sterilant), heparin, formaldehyde, or glutaraldehyde

XIV

TABLE 75.3. Common Complications During Hemodialysis

	Incidence	Etiology/Predisposing Factors	Management
Hypotension	20–30%	Excessive ultrafiltration	Place in Trendelenburg position
		Target weight too low	100–200 mL bolus of normal saline
		Acetate dialysate→vasodilation	Decrease ultrafiltration rate
		Autonomic neuropathy	10–20 ml of 23.4% hypertonic saline
		Patient unable to compensatorily increase cardiac output	over 5 minutes
Cramps	5–20%	Hypotension	100–200 mL bolus of normal saline
		Dehydration	10–20 ml of 23.4% hypertonic saline over 5 minutes
		Sodium level in dialysate too low	Give oxazepam 5–10 mg 2 h before dialysis
			Prophylaxis with carnitine 20 mg/kg IV TIW
Nausea and vomiting	5–15%	Hypotension	Treat hypotension
		May be an early sign of disequilibrium syndrome	Prochlorperazine 10 mg po or 2.5 mg IV
Headache	5%	For most, mechanism unknown	Acetaminophen 650 mg po (PRN)
		Acute caffeine withdrawal due to dialytic removal	
		Vasodilatation secondary to acetate dialysate solution	
Chest or back pain	2.5%	Type B dialyzer reaction	Change dialyzer or start reuse program
		Underlying cardiac disease	Nasal oxygen
Itching	5%	Uremic toxins	Activated charcoal 6 g daily
		Elevated calcium-phosphorus produce	Reduce hyperphosphatemia
		Dry skin	Topical emollients
		Allergy to heparin, plasticizers in dialysis tubing, sterilizer used or any other medication	Topical capsaicum cream 0.025%
			Diphenhydramine 25–50 mg po
			Switch from ethylene oxide to gamma-ray-sterilized dialyzer

(common reuse sterilants). This type of reaction has also been associated with bradykinin system activation by some dialyzer membranes (predominantly AN69), particularly in patients receiving angiotensin-converting enzyme (ACE) inhibitors. These reactions can be managed by immediately stopping the dialysis procedure. Resuscitative therapy (e.g., epinephrine, antihistamines, and steroids) will likely be required.

- Type B dialyzer reactions are more common than Type A but less severe. Chest and back pain, the most frequently reported symptoms, may be noted within minutes or up to 1–2 hours into the session. Although patients can continue dialysis, they should be switched to a more biocompatible dialyzer and/or placed on a reprocessing program to minimize future reactions.

XIV

Chronic Complications

- Patients with end-stage renal disease (ESRD) demonstrate several immune abnormalities, some of which may be aggravated if bio-incompatible filters (e.g., cellulose and cuprophane) are utilized.
- Disequilibrium syndrome is characterized by systemic and neurologic symptoms and EEG changes that may occur during, but generally soon (hours) after, the end of dialysis. In mild cases, symptoms are nonspecific (e.g., nausea, vomiting, headache, or restlessness). Severe disequilibrium is characterized by the development of seizures, obtundation, or coma. The risk can be minimized by adjusting dialysate sodium (at least 140 mEq/L) and glucose (at least 200 mg/dL) levels, and by reducing ultrafiltration rate and target urea reduction ratio.
- Dialysis-related amyloidosis is common in patients who receive dialysis for >8–10 years secondary to accumulation of β_2 microglobulin. The first and most prominent clinical manifestation is carpal tunnel syndrome. Other clinical manifestations include pain and stiffness of other major joints, and soft-tissue swelling.

▶ TREATMENT: PERITONEAL DIALYSIS

GENERAL PRINCIPLES

- In peritoneal dialysis (PD), the dialysate-filled compartment is the peritoneal cavity, into which dialysate is instilled via a permanent peritoneal catheter that traverses the abdominal wall. The peritoneal membrane functions as the semipermeable membrane.
- Access to the peritoneal cavity is via placement of an indwelling catheter, which is manufactured from a silastic material that is soft, flexible, and biocompatible.
- PD dialysate solutions contain dextrose 1.5–4.25%. The osmolarity of the solutions, which ranges from 350–480 mOsm/L and exceeds that of serum (280 mOsm/L), provides the drawing force for water and solute movement across the peritoneal membrane. Dextrose is not an ideal osmotic agent, in part because it alters peritoneal mesothelial cells and leukocyte function.
- Commercial PD solutions also contain electrolytes to minimize their removal by reducing the diffusion gradient. Electrolytes in PD solutions include sodium 132 mEq/L (132 mmol/L), chloride 102 mEq/L (102 mmol/L), lactate 35 mEq/L, magnesium 1.5 mEq/L (0.75 mmol/L), and calcium 3.5 mEq/L (1.75 mmol/L) or 2.5 mEq/L (1.25 mmol/L).
- PD is much less efficient per unit time than hemodialysis, and must therefore be a more frequent or virtually continuous procedure. Quantity of dialysis delivered may be regulated by altering the number of daily exchanges, volume of each exchange, or dextrose concentration. Additional disadvantages (and advantages) of PD can be found in Table 75.3.

XIV

- Continuous ambulatory PD (CAPD) is the most common of the available PD procedures. Others include continuous cycling (CCPD), daily ambulatory (DAPD), and nightly intermittent (NIPD).
- In a basic CAPD prescription, dialysate flows into the peritoneal cavity under gravity over about 15 minutes, dwells within the peritoneal cavity, and then is drained out of the peritoneal cavity into the original container for about 30 minutes. Typically a patient instills a 2-liter exchange of dialysate about every 4 hours during the day and then a single 2-liter exchange, often using a higher dextrose concentration, for an overnight, 12-hour dwell.

DESIGN AND ASSESSMENT

- The peritoneal equilibration test (PET) is a diagnostic test that determines the peritoneal membrane clearance and ultrafiltration characteristics. PET quantitates the ability with which solutes and water transfer across the membrane.
  - PET test results determine which, if any, variant of PD is appropriate for an individual. Table 75.4 illustrates the prognostic interpretation where APD is nightly automated PD; DAPD is daily ambulatory PD; standard dose PD is CAPD or standard CCPD; and high dose is CAPD with >9 L dialysate/d, or CCPD with >8 L dialysate overnight and >2 L dialysate during the day.
  - PET also provides quantitative guidance regarding the design of the PD prescription (e.g., volume of PD in each exchange, number per day).
- Assessment of adequacy of dialysis requires more than a simple examination of BUN profile. The most common assessment methods are Kt/V and creatinine clearance.
- To calculate Kt/V for PD, a dialysate-to-plasma (D/P) urea concentration is determined, and Kt is estimated as:

$$Kt = D/P \times \text{volume drained (L/day)}$$

TABLE 75.4. Prognostic Value of PET Results

Creatinine or Dextrose Transport	Ultrafiltration Rate	Predicted Solute Clearance	Preferred Type[a]
High	Poor	Adequate	APD, DAPD
High average	Adequate	Adequate	Standard dose PD
Low average	Good	Adequate/inadequate	Standard to high dose PD
Low	Excellent	Inadequate	High dose PD, hemodialysis

[a] See text for discussion of terms.

From Twardowski ZJ. Blood Purif 1989;7:95–108, p 102, with permission.

XIV

The urea volume of distribution can be approximated as 0.6 L/kg in men and as 0.55 L/kg in women. Alternatively, V can be estimated as follows:

V in men = [2.447 + 0.3362 × weight (kg)] + [0.1074 × height (cm)] − [0.09516 × age (y)]

V in women = [−2.097 + 0.2466 × weight (kg)] + [0.1069 × height (cm)]

- The resultant dialytic Kt/V must be multiplied by 7 and divided by 3 to produce a value that can be compared with that of intermittent, thrice-weekly hemodialysis. Consequently, appropriate Kt/Vs for PD should be ≥0.5–0.6.
- Determination of weekly creatinine clearance can also be used to assess adequacy of peritoneal dialysis; however, this method may overestimate the amount of dialysis delivered. A minimum weekly dialytic clearance of 40 liters has been recommended, which is in addition to the patient's residual renal creatinine clearance.

COMPLICATIONS OF PERITONEAL DIALYSIS

- Mechanical complications include those effected by technical issues (e.g., kinking of catheter, inflow and outflow obstruction), which are solved by manipulation of the catheter, or prevented by careful initial placement of the catheter. Other mechanical problems include excessive catheter motion at the exit site, pain from catheter-tip impingement on viscera, or inflow pain.
- PD patients have numerous metabolic and nutritional abnormalities (e.g., exacerbation of diabetes mellitus due to absorption of dextrose from the peritoneal cavity, electrolyte abnormalities especially hypercalcemia or hypocalcemia, sustained uremia, accumulation of "middle molecule" toxins, amino acid and albumin loss into the dialysate, loss of muscle mass and increased adipose tissue, and poor appetite and malnutrition). Other medical complications include fluid overload, chemical peritonitis, and fibrin formation in dialysate.

Infectious Complications

- Infectious complications (e.g., peritonitis and catheter related) are a major cause of morbidity and mortality, and the leading cause of technique failure and transfer from PD to hemodialysis.
- Peritonitis is a common clinical problem. Approximately 1.1 to 1.3 episodes/patient/year were reported in the 1980s and 1990s.
- Most infections (40–65%) are caused by gram-positive bacteria (Table 75.5), of which *Staphylococcus epidermidis* and *S. aureus* predominate. The relative probability of gram-negative infection is increased in patients using the disconnect systems because of the reduced incidence of gram-positive infections.

XIV

927

TABLE 75.5. Organisms Causing Peritonitis

Organisms	% Episodes
Gram positive	40–65
S. epidermidis	30–45
S. aureus	10–20
Streptococci	10–15
Enterococci	3–5
Diphtheroids	<5
Gram negative	20–35
E. coli	5–12
P. aeruginosa	5–8
Enterobacter	2–3
Acinetobacter	2–3
Klebsiella	2–3
Proteus	2–3
Mixed gram positive and negative	10–15
Fungi	5–10
Sterile culture, presumed bacterial	5–20
Other	5

- Although available literature suggests ambivalent results using antibiotics or vaccines to prevent peritonitis, reductions in catheter-related infections may be possible with appropriate prophylaxis.
- The emergence of vancomycin resistance has created a therapeutic dilemma of international proportions. While the resistance gene was initially confined to enterococci, the rapidly escalating prevalence of vancomycin-resistant enterococci raises the concern that the gene may be transmitted to staphylococci. Vancomycin resistance has been associated with resistance to penicillins and aminoglycosides, which could preclude the use of many second-line agents. Consequently, the Advisory Committee on Peritonitis Management recommended major modifications in therapeutic options in 1996, as summarized in Table 75.5.

Initial Therapy of Peritonitis
- Patients with cloudy fluid and symptoms (i.e., abdominal pain or fever) require prompt initiation of empiric therapy (Figure 75.2). In asymptomatic patients with only cloudy fluid, it is reasonable to delay initiation of therapy until cell count, differential, and gram stain results are available.
- Initial empiric therapy should consist of a first-generation cephalosporin and an aminoglycoside (Table 75.6).

XIV

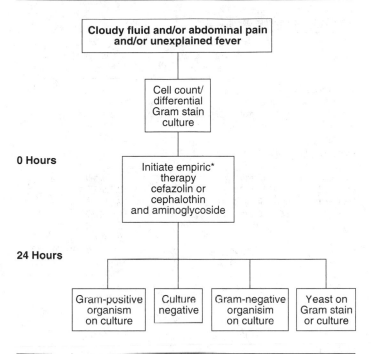

Figure 75.2. Assessment and therapy of peritonitis. *(From Keane WF, Alexander SR, Bailie GR, et al. Perit Dial Int 1996; 16[6]:557–573, with permission.)*

TABLE 75.6. Antimicrobial Dosing for Patients with Peritonitis[a]

Drug	Intermittent Dosing (dose in 1 bag/day unless otherwise specified)	Continuous Dosing (mg/L unless otherwise specified)
Aminoglycosides		
Amikacin	2 mg/kg	LD 25, MD 12
Gentamicin	0.6 mg/kg	LD 8, MD 4
Netilmicin	0.6 mg/kg	LD 8, MD 4
Tobramycin	0.6 mg/kg	LD 8, MD 4
Cephalosporins		
Cefazolin	15 mg/kg	LD 500, MD 125
Cephalothin	15 mg/kg	LD 500, MD 125
Cephradine	15 mg/kg	LD 500, MD 125
Cephalexin	500 mg po QID	NA
Cefamandole	1000 mg	LD 500, MD 250
Cefmenoxime	1000 mg	LD 100, MD 50
Cefoxitin	ND	LD 200, MD 100
Cefuroxime	400 mg po/IV QD	LD 200, MD 100–200
Cefixime	400 mg po QD	NA
Cefoperazone	ND	LD 500, MD 250
Cefotaxime	2000 mg	LD 500, MD 250
Cefsulodin	500 mg	LD 50, MD 25
Ceftazidime	1000 mg	LD 250, MD 125
Ceftizoxime	1000 mg	LD 250, MD 125
Ceftriaxone	1000 mg	LD 250, MD 125
Penicillins		
Azlocillin	ND	LD 500, MD 250
Mezlocillin	3000 mg IV BID	LD 3 g IV, MD 250
Piperacillin	4000 mg IV BID	LD 4 g IV, MD 250
Ticarcillin	2000 mg IV BID	LD 1–2 g IV, MD 125
Ampicillin	ND	MD 125; or 250–500 mg po BID
Dicloxacillin	ND	MD 125
Oxacillin	ND	MD 125
Nafcillin	ND	250–500 mg po Q12h
Quinolones		
Ciprofloxacin	500 mg po BID	Not recommended
Fleroxacin	800 mg po, then 400 mg po QD	Not recommended
Ofloxacin	400 mg po, then 200 mg po QD	Not recommended
Others		
Vancomycin	15–30 mg/kg Q5–7d	LD 1000, MD 25
Aztreonam	1000 mg	LD 1000, MD 250
Clindamycin	ND	LD 300, MD 150
Erythromycin	500 mg po QID	LD ND, MD 150
Metronidazole	500 mg po/IV TID	ND

XIV

TABLE 75.6. continued

Drug	Intermittent Dosing (dose in 1 bag/day unless otherwise specified)	Continuous dosing (mg/L unless otherwise specified)
Minocycline	100 mg po BID	NA
Rifampin	450–600 mg po QD or 150 mg ip TID-QID	NA
Antifungals		
Amphotericin	NA	1.5
Flucytosine	1 g QD po or 100 mg/L ip each exch x 3d, then 50 mg/L/exch 200–800 mg po QD	50 QD
Fluconzaole	ND	ND
Ketoconazole		NA
Miconazole		LD 200, MD 100–200
Combinations		
Ampicillin/sulbact	2 g Q12h	LD 1000, MD 100
Imipenem/cilistat	1 g BID	LD 500, MD 200
Trimeth/sulfameth	320/1600 Q1–2d po	LD 320/1600, MD 80/400

ᵃThe route of administration is intraperitoneal unless otherwise specified. These pharmacokinetic data and proposed dosage regimens presented here are based on published literature reviewed through January 1996. There is no evidence that mixing different antibiotics in dialysis fluid (except for aminoglycosides and penicillins) is deleterious for the drugs or patients. Do not use the same syringe to mix antibiotics.

LD = Loading dose; MD = Maintenance dose; NA = Not applicable; ND = No data; IV = Intravenous; IP = Intraperitoneally; po = Oral; QD = Once a day; BID = Twice a day; TID = Three times a day; QID = Four times a day.

Note: CAPD patients with residual renal function may require increased doses or more frequent dosing, especially when using intermittent regimens.

From Keane WF, Alexander SR, Bailie WR, et al. Perit Dial Int 1996; 16(6):557–573, with permission.

Modification of Treatment for Peritonitis Based on Culture and Sensitivity

- Within 24–48 hours after culture of dialysate fluid, 70–90% of samples yield a specific microorganism, which is usually gram positive. Antimicrobial therapy is modified accordingly (Figure 75.3).
- If the culture reveals gram-negative organisms, it is imperative to modify the therapeutic plan (Figure 75.4). Surgical intervention may be necessary if multiple types of gram-negative organisms are seen.
- If gram stain reveals yeast, antifungal therapy should be initiated promptly (Figure 75.5).
- If the culture is negative and not suggestive of gram-negative organisms, and the patient is clinically improving after 4–5 days, only the cephalosporin should be continued (Figure 75.6).

XIV

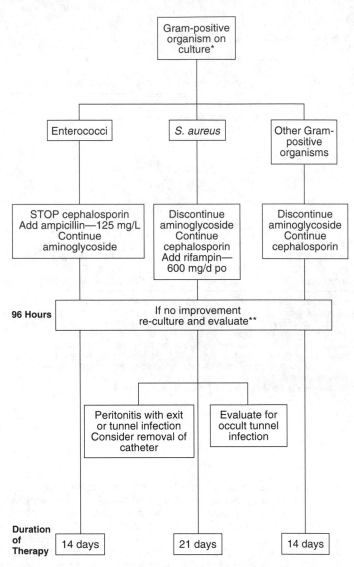

Gram-positive organism on culture*

Enterococci | S. aureus | Other Gram-positive organisms

Enterococci:
STOP cephalosporin
Add ampicillin—125 mg/L
Continue aminoglycoside

S. aureus:
Discontinue aminoglycoside
Continue cephalosporin
Add rifampin—600 mg/d po

Other Gram-positive organisms:
Discontinue aminoglycoside
Continue cephalosporin

96 Hours — If no improvement re-culture and evaluate**

Peritonitis with exit or tunnel infection Consider removal of catheter

Evaluate for occult tunnel infection

Duration of Therapy — 14 days | 21 days | 14 days

* Choice of therapy should always be guided by sensitivity patterns.

XIV ** If MRSA is cultured and the patient is not clinically responding, clindamycin or vancomycin should be used.

Figure 75.3. Management of gram-positive peritonitis. *(From Keane WF, Alexander SR, Bailie GR, et al. Perit Dial Int 1996; 16[6]:557–573, with permission.)*

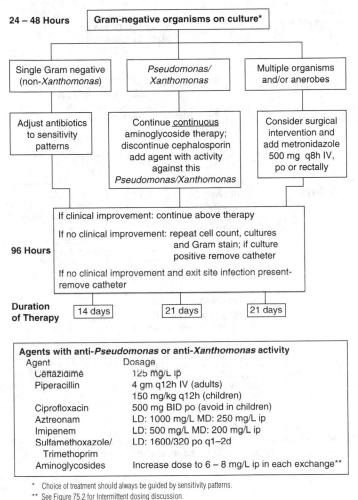

Figure 75.4. Management of gram-negative peritonitis. *(From Keane WF, Alexander SR, Bailie GR, et al. Perit Dial Int 1996; 16[6]:557–573, with permission.)*

XIV ◀

24–48 Hours

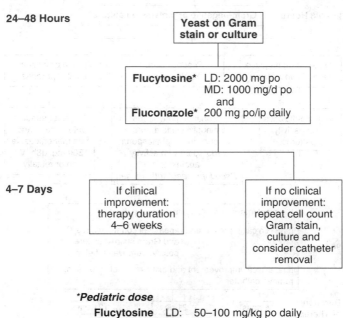

Yeast on Gram stain or culture

Flucytosine* LD: 2000 mg po
MD: 1000 mg/d po
and
Fluconazole* 200 mg po/ip daily

4–7 Days

If clinical improvement: therapy duration 4–6 weeks

If no clinical improvement: repeat cell count Gram stain, culture and consider catheter removal

*Pediatric dose

Flucytosine LD: 50–100 mg/kg po daily
MD: 25–50 mg/kg po daily

Fluconazole 1–3 mg/kg ip q2

Figure 75.5. Management of peritonitis caused by yeast. *(From Keane WF, Alexander SR, Bailie GR, et al. Perit Dial Int 1996; 16[6]:557–573, with permission.)*

Assessment of Patients with Peritonitis

- Within 48 hours after initiating therapy, most patients with PD-related peritonitis show considerable improvement. In this setting, therapy is continued for at least 14 days.
- If symptoms persist, the presence of the following is considered: intra-abdominal or gynecologic pathology requiring surgical intervention, or unusual organisms (e.g., mycobacteria, fungi, or fastidious organisms).

Prophylaxis and Treatment of Exit-Site Infections

- Exit-site infection is defined by the presence of purulent drainage with or without erythema of the skin at the catheter-epidermal interface. Empiric antibiotic therapy may be initiated immediately if the clinical appearance warrants early intervention, or delayed until culture results are available.

XIV

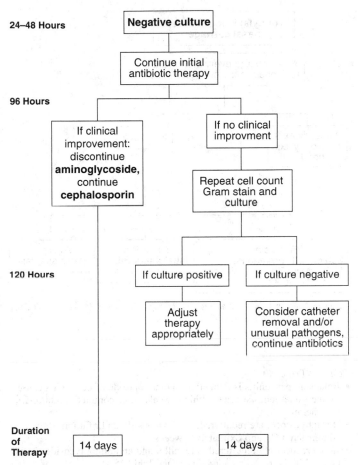

Figure 75.6. Management of culture-negative peritonitis. *(From Keane WF, Alexander SR, Bailie GR, et al. Perit Dial Int 1996; 16[6]:557–573, with permission.)*

- Nasal carriage of *S. aureus* is associated with exit-site/tunnel infections or peritonitis. Because of the efficacy shown in clinical trials, prophylaxis (e.g., intranasal mupirocin, exit-site mupirocin, or oral rifampin) is recommended for adults with positive nasal cultures (Figure 75.7).

XIV

935

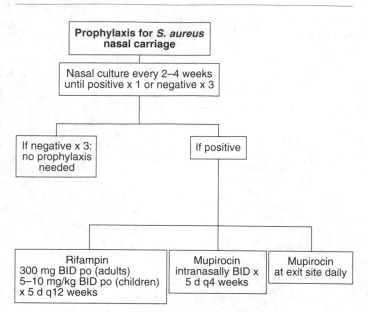

Figure 75.7. Prophylaxis for *S. aureus* nasal carriage. *(From Keane WF, Alexander SR, Bailie GR, et al. Perit Dial Int 1996; 16[6]:557–573, with permission.)*

Relapsing Peritonitis
- Relapsing peritonitis is defined as another episode of peritonitis caused by the same genus/species within 4 weeks after completing antimicrobial therapy.
- If staphylococci are recultured, a cephalosporin and rifampin should be administered for approximately 4 weeks.
- If enterococci are recultured, ampicillin and an aminoglycoside should be used in the recommended doses (see Table 75.1).
- If gram-negative organisms are recultured, intra-abdominal abscess, catheter removal, and surgical exploration should be considered. After culture results are available, ceftazidime or aminoglycoside monotherapy can be used.

INTRAPERITONEAL DRUG THERAPY

XIV
- Drug-dosing in renal insufficiency is covered in Chapter 76.
- For management of systemic infections, potential benefits of the IP method include use of an established access, ability to treat infections in outpatient settings and associated cost savings, possible avoidance of IV drug-related toxicities, and improved patient acceptance.

- For insulin, possible advantages of the IP method include avoidance of erratic absorption, convenience, avoidance of subcutaneous injection-site complications, and prevention of peripheral hyperinsulinemia.
- Instillation of heparin 500 U/L to each exchange may prevent fibrin formation.
- Pilot data suggest that amino acids are absorbed from the IP method (IPAA) and may positively influence nutritional parameters. In addition, higher concentrations of IPAAs may produce adequate ultrafiltration. Before use of IPAA is generally accepted, however, results of long-term studies on patient outcome should be awaited.
- Other drugs that have been administered by the IP method include calcitriol for secondary hyperparathyroidism, deferoxamine for aluminum bone disease and hyperaluminumism, erythromycin for diabetic gastroparesis, lithium for bipolar affective disorder, streptokinase and urokinase for recurrent peritonitis, and erythropoietin for anemia.

See Chapter 46, Principles and Practice of Chronic Renal Replacement Therapy, authored by Gary R. Matzke, PharmD, FCP, FCCP, and George R. Bailie, MSc, PharmD, PhD, FCCP, for a more detailed discussion of this topic.

XIV

Chapter 76

▶ DRUG DOSING IN RENAL INSUFFICIENCY

▶ DEFINITION

The primary reason to individualize drug therapy for patients with renal insufficiency is to minimize the toxicities associated with drug accumulation, which may occur owing to reduced renal clearance. Drug therapy may also need to be altered in patients with renal insufficiency because of changes in bioavailability, protein binding, distribution volume, and metabolic activity.

▶ PATHOPHYSIOLOGY, CLINICAL PRESENTATION, DIAGNOSIS, AND TREATMENT

- The pathophysiology, clinical manifestations, diagnosis, and treatment of acute and chronic renal failure are discussed in Chapters 78 and 79, respectively.

▶ GENERAL PRINCIPLES

- Drug therapy individualization for patients with renal insufficiency may require only a simple proportional dose adjustment based on the fractional reduction in creatinine clearance. Alternatively, complex adjustments may be required for medications that are extensively metabolized or for which dramatic changes in protein binding and/or distribution volume have been reported.
- Furthermore, patients may demonstrate an altered pharmacodynamic response to a given medication because of the physiologic and biochemical changes associated with progressive renal insufficiency.

BIOAVAILABILITY

- There is little quantitative information regarding influence of impaired renal function on drug absorption and bioavailability.
- Factors that may theoretically affect bioavailability include alterations in gastrointestinal (GI) emptying time, gastric pH, complications of severe renal insufficiency (e.g., edema of the GI tract, vomiting, and diarrhea), and concomitant drug therapy, especially antacid or H_2 antagonist administration.
- Increased bioavailability has been reported for propranolol, tolamolol, bufuralol, oxprenolol, dextropropoxyphene, and dihydrocodeine in patients with renal insufficiency. However, clinical consequences have been demonstrated only with dextropropoxyphene and dihydrocodeine.

DISTRIBUTION

- Volume of distribution of many drugs is significantly increased in patients with end-stage renal disease (ESRD) (Table 76.1). Changes may result from altered protein or tissue binding, or pathophysiologic alterations in body composition (e.g., fractional contribution of total body water to total body weight).
- Generally, plasma protein binding of acidic drugs (warfarin, phenytoin) is decreased in uremia (Table 76.2), whereas binding of basic drugs (quinidine, lidocaine) is usually normal or slightly decreased.
- In patients with renal insufficiency, particularly those with ESRD, "normal" total drug concentration may be associated with adverse reactions secondary to elevated unbound drug concentrations or subtherapeutic responses because of an altered plasma/tissue drug concentration ratio. Unbound (versus total) drug concentrations should be monitored for drugs that have a narrow therapeutic range, are highly protein bound

TABLE 76.1. Effect of ESRD on the Volume of Distribution of Selected Drugs[a]

	Normal	ESRD
Amikacin	0.20	0.29
Azlocillin	0.21	0.28
Bretylium	3.58	4.48
Cefazolin	0.13	0.16
Cefonicid	0.11	0.14
Cefoxitin	0.16	0.26
Cefuroxime	0.20	0.26
Clofibrate	0.14	0.24
Cloxacillin	0.14	0.26
Dicloxacillin	0.08	0.18
Erythromycin	0.57	1.09
Furosemide	0.11	0.18
Gentamicin	0.20	0.32
Isoniazid	0.6	0.8
Minoxidil	2.6	4.9
Nalmefene	7.9	14.7
Phenytoin	0.64	1.4
Sisomicin	0.19	0.25
Sulfamethopyrazine	0.21	0.38
Trimethoprim	1.36	1.83
Vancomycin	0.64	0.85

[a]All data are in liters per kilogram unless otherwise stated.

XIV ◄

TABLE 76.2. Protein Binding of Acidic Drugs in Patients with Normal Renal Function and ESRD

	Normal	ESRD
Abecarnil	94–98	85
Azlocillin	35–40	25
Cefazolin	84	71
Cefoxitin	73	41
Ceftriaxone	90	80
Clofibrate	97	91
Cloxacillin	95	80
Diazoxide	94	84
Dicloxacillin	97	91
Diflunisal	88	56
Doxycycline	88	72
Furosemide	96	94
Methotrexate	42.8	36.2
Metolazone	95	90
Moxalactam	52	36
Naproxen	99.8	99.2
Pentobarbital	66	59
Phenylbutazone	93–96	82–86
Phenytoin	90	74–85
Piretanide	94	88
Salicylate	92	80
Sulfamethoxazole	66	42
Valproic acid	92	77
Warfarin	99	98
Zomepirac	98.7	96.2

(free fraction of <20%), and have marked variability in the free fraction (e.g., phenytoin and disopyramide).

- Methods for calculating volume of distribution may be influenced by renal disease. Of the most commonly used terms (i.e., volume of central compartment [V_c], volume of terminal phase [V_β, V_{area}], and volume of distribution at steady state [V_{SS}]), V_{SS} may be the most appropriate for comparing patients with renal insufficiency versus those with normal renal function because V_{SS} has the advantage of being independent of drug elimination.

XIV

TABLE 76.3. Effect of ESRD on Nonrenal (Hepatic) Clearance

		Decreased	
Acyclovir	Aztreonam	Bufuralol	Captopril
Cefmenoxime	Cefmetazole	Cefonicid	Cefotaxime
Cefotiam	Cefsulodin	Ceftizoxime	Cilastatin
Cimetidine	Cortisol	Encainide	Erythromycin
Erythromycin	Imipenem	Isoniazid	Methylprednisolone
Metoclopramide	Moxalactam	Nicardipine	Nimodipine
Nitrendipine	Procainamide	Quinapril	Verapamil
Zidovudine			
		Unchanged	
Acetaminophen	Chloramphenicol	Clonidine	Codeine
Diflunisal	Indomethacin	Insulin[a]	Isradipine
Lidocaine	Morphine	Metoprolol	Nisoldipine
Nortriptyline	Pentobarbital	Propafenone	Quinidine
Theophylline	Tocainide	Tolbutamide	
		Increased	
Antipyrine	Bumetanide	Cefpiramide	Fosinopril
Nifedipine	Phenytoin	Sulfadimidine	

[a]May be unchanged or decreased.

METABOLISM

- The kidney contributes to the biotransformation of many drugs. Several cytochrome P-450 enzymes are present in the kidney that contribute to the metabolism of endogenous substances (e.g., vitamin D) and drugs. Furthermore, chronic renal impairment may also have a detrimental effect on drug metabolism within the liver.
- Drug metabolism may be increased, decreased, or unaffected by renal failure (Table 76.3).
- Patients with severe renal insufficiency may experience accumulation of metabolite(s) as well as parent compound (Table 76.4).

RENAL EXCRETION

- Differences in pharmacokinetic parameters among patients with similar reductions in glomerular filtration rate may be due to differences in their types of renal disease. Therefore, dosage-adjustment methodologies may need to be developed to take into consideration the impact of altered tubular as well as glomerular function.
- Clinical measurement or estimation of creatinine clearance remains the guiding factor for drug dosage regimen design because there are no clinically useful techniques to quantitate tubular function.

XIV

TABLE 76.4. Pharmacologic Activity of Selected Drug Metabolites

Parent Drug	Metabolite	Pharmacologic Activity of Metabolites
Acetaminophen	*N*-acetyl-*p*-benzo-quinoneimine	Responsible for hepatotoxicity
Allopurinol	Oxipurinol	Metabolite primarily responsible for suppression of xanthine oxidase
Azathioprine	Mercaptopurine	All of the immunosuppressive activity resides in the metabolite
Cefotaxime	Desacetyl cefotaxime	Similar antimicrobial spectrum, but one-fourth to one-tenth as potent
Chlorpropamide	2-Hydroxychlorpropamide	Similar in vitro insulin-releasing activity
Clofibrate	Chlorophenoxyisobutyric acid	Primarily responsible for hypolipidemic effect and direct muscle toxicity
Codeine	Morphine-6-glucuronide	Possibly more active than parent compound, which may prolong narcotic effect
Imipramine	Desmethylimipramine	Similar antidepressant activity
Meperidine	Normeperidine	Less analgesic activity than parent, but more CNS-stimulatory effects
Morphine	Morphine-6-glucuronide	Possibly more active than parent compound, which may prolong narcotic effect
Procainamide	*N*-acetyl procainamide	Distinct antiarrhythmic activity, with different mechanism compared with parent compound
Sulfonamides	Acetylated metabolites	Devoid of antibacterial activity, but elevated concentrations are associated with increased toxicity
Theophylline	1,3-Dimethyl uric acid	Cardiotoxicity has been demonstrated
Zidovudine	Zidovudine triphosphate	Primarily responsible for antiretroviral activity

▶ CALCULATION OF DRUG DOSAGE

- Most dosage adjustment guidelines propose the use of a fixed dose or interval for patients with broad ranges of renal function. These categories encompass up to a ten-fold range in renal function and, thus, the drug regimen may not be optimal for all patients.
- Design of the optimal dosage regimen for patients with renal insufficiency requires an individualized assessment and depends on the availability of an accurate characterization of the relationship between the

TABLE 76.5. Relationship Between Renal Function and Pharmacokinetic Parameters of Selected Drugs

Drug	Total Body Clearance	Elimination Rate Constant
Acyclovir	$CL = 3.37 \, (CL_{cr}) + 0.41$	
Amikacin	$CL = 0.6 \, (CL_{cr}) + 9.6$	$k_{el} = 0.0026 \, (CL_{cr}) + 0.02$
Cefazolin		$k_{el} = 0.003 \, (CL_{cr}) + 0.02$
Cefmetazole	$CL = 1.18 \, (CL_{cr}) - 0.29$	
Ceftazidime	$CL = 1.15 \, (CL_{cr}) + 10.6$	$k_{el} = 0.004 \, (CL_{cr}) + 0.004$
Ciprofloxacin	$CL = 2.83 \, (CL_{cr}) + 363$	
Digoxin	$CL = 0.88 \, (CL_{cr}) + 23$	
Gentamicin	$CL = 0.983 \, (CL_{cr})$	$k_{el} = 0.00315 \, (CL_{cr})$
Netilmicin	$CL = 0.65 \, (CL_{cr}) + 3.72$	$k_{el} = 0.003 \, (CL_{cr}) + 0.013$
Ofloxacin	$CL = 1.04 \, (CL_{cr}) + 38.7$	
Piperacillin	$CL = 1.36 \, (CL_{cr}) + 1.50$	
Procainamide	$CL = 3 \, (CL_{cr}) + 0.23 \, (ABW)$	
Teicoplanin	$CL = 7.09 \, (CL_{cr}) - 16.2$	
Tobramycin	$CL = 0.801 \, (CL_{cr})$	$k_{el} = 0.00382 \, (CL_{cr})$
Vancomycin	$CL = 0.69 \, (CL_{cr}) + 3.7$	$k_{el} = 0.00083 \, (CL_{cr}) + 0.0044$

pharmacokinetic parameters of the drug and renal function, and an accurate assessment of the patient's renal function (i.e., creatinine clearance).
- Consideration must be given to stability of renal function and type of dialysis.

STABLE RENAL INSUFFICIENCY

- If the relationship between creatinine clearance and the kinetic parameters of a drug (i.e., total body clearance [CL], elimination rate constant [K_{el}], and V_{SS}) have been characterized, these data should be used to individualize drug therapy (Table 76.5). The kinetic parameter/dosage adjustment factor (Q) is the ratio of the patient's predicted CL or K_{el} to the value derived from the relationship for individuals with normal creatinine clearance of 120 mL/min/1.73 m².

Estimation of Kinetic Parameters

- If relevant data are not available for patients with renal insufficiency, kinetic parameters must be estimated. Kinetic parameters are based on fraction of the drug that is eliminated renally unchanged (f_e) in subjects with normal renal function. These approaches assume that the decrease in CL and k are proportional to CL_{cr}, renal disease does not alter drug metabolism, any metabolites are inactive and nontoxic, and the drug obeys first-order (linear) kinetic principles and is adequately described by a one-compartment model.

XIV

- The Q factor for dosage adjustment can be calculated as:

$$Q = 1 - [f_e(1 - KF)]$$

where KF is the ratio of the patient's CL_{cr} to the assumed normal value of 120 mL/min/1.73 m^2. Estimated total body clearance can be calculated as:

$$CL_{PT} = CL_{norm} \times Q$$

where CL_{norm} is the mean value in patients with normal renal function from the literature.
- The best method for dosage regimen adjustment depends on whether the desired goal is maintenance of a similar peak, trough, or average steady-state drug concentration.
- The principal choices are to decrease the dose, prolong the dosing interval, or both. Prolonging the interval is generally preferred because it is likely to yield cost savings by reducing nursing and pharmacy time as well as associated supplies.
- The prolonged dosing interval (τ_f) may be calculated from the following relationships, where τ_n is the normal dosing interval:

$$\tau_f = \tau_n Q$$

This approach assumes that similar peak and trough concentrations will be attained.
- The reduced maintenance dose (DF) to be administered at τ_n may be calculated from the following relationship:

$$D_f = D_n \times Q$$

where D_n is the normal dose.

Estimation of Kinetic Parameters for Altered Volume of Distribution (V_d) or to Achieve Target V_d

- If V_{SS} is significantly altered or a specific maximum or minimum concentration is desired, estimation of a dosage regimen becomes more complex.
- The dosing interval (τ_f) is calculated as:

$$t_f = -1/k_f [\ln C_{trough}/C_{peak}] + t'$$

where t' is the infusion duration.
- The dose to be administered by intravenous infusion is calculated as:

$$\text{Dose}_{IV} = (k_f)(V_f)(C_{peak})t' [(1 - e^{-k}f'f/(1 - e^{-k}f'))]e^{-k}f'z$$

where t_z is the time after the end of the infusion.

- For orally administered drugs, τ_f can be calculated as:

$$\tau_f = [(-1/k_f)(\ln[C_{min}/C_{max}])] + t_{peak}$$

Dose can be approximated as, where C_p^t equals the desired plasma concentration at time t and k_a is the absorption rate constant:

$$\text{Dose}_{PO} = [SFC_p^t V_d \, (k_a - k)]/[k_a((e^{-kt}/1 - e^{-k\tau}) - (e^{-k}a^t/1 - e^{-ka\tau}))].$$

If the drug is absorbed extremely rapidly ($t_{peak} < 1$ hour), τ_f can be approximated as:

$$\tau_f = (-1/k_f)(\ln [C_{min}/C_{max}])$$

and the dose as:

$$\text{Dose} = V_d \times (C_{max} - C_{min})$$

CONTINUOUS RENAL REPLACEMENT THERAPY

- Drug therapy individualization for patients receiving continuous renal replacement therapy (CRRT) is simple because the procedure results in a consistent increment in the residual total body clearance of the patient. However, individualization is complicated by higher residual nonrenal clearance of some drugs in patients with acute versus chronic renal insufficiency. Furthermore, there are marked differences in drug removal between intermittent hemodialysis and the three primary types of CRRT (i.e., continuous arteriovenous ultrafiltration [CAVU] or slow continuous ultrafiltration [SCUF], continuous arteriovenous or venovenous hemofiltration [CAVH or CVVH], and continuous arteriovenous or venovenous hemodialysis [CAVHD/CVVHD]).
- During CAVU/SCUF and CAVH/CVVH, drug clearance is a function of membrane permeability for the drug, which is called the sieving coefficient (SC) and the rate of ultrafiltrate formation (UFR). SC can be calculated as:

$$SC = C_{UF}/C_a$$

where C_a and C_{UF} are the concentration in plasma going into the filter and ultrafiltrate, respectively. SC is often approximated by the fraction unbound (f_{ub}) because this information may be more readily available (Table 76.6). Thus, clearance by these two modes of CRRT can be calculated as:

$$CL_{CVVH} = UFR \times SC$$

- Clearance by CVVHD (CL_{CVVHD}) can be calculated as the product of the combined ultrafiltrate and dialysate volume (V_{df}) and drug concentration in this fluid (C_{df}) divided by the plasma concentration going into the filter (C_a^{mid}) at the midpoint of the V_{df} collection period:

$$CL_{CVVHD} = (V_{df} \times C_{df})/C_a^{mid}$$

XIV

945

TABLE 76.6. Predicted and Measured Sieving Coefficients of Selected Drugs

Drug	Predicted	Measured
Amikacin	0.95	0.88
Amphotericin	0.01	0.32–0.4
Ampicillin	0.8	0.6–0.69
Cefoperazone	0.10	0.27–0.69
Cefotaxime	0.62	0.55–1.1
Cefoxitin	0.30	0.32
Ceftazidine	0.90	0.38–0.78
Ceftriaxone	0.10	0.71–0.82
Clindamycin	0.25	0.49–0.98
Digoxin	0.75	0.96
Erythromycin	0.25	0.37
5-Flurocytosine	0.96	0.98
Gentamicin	0.95	0.81–0.75
Imipenem	0.80	0.78
Metronidazole	0.80	0.80
Mezlocillin	0.68	0.68
Nafcillin	0.20	0.47
N-acetyl procainamide	0.80	0.92
Netilmicin	—	0.85
Oxacillin	0.05	0.02
Phenobarbital	0.60	0.86
Phenytoin	0.10	0.45
Procainamide	0.80	0.86
Theophylline	0.47	0.85
Tobramycin	0.95	0.78–0.86
Vancomycin	0.90	0.5–0.8

Clearance by CVVHD for a given drug and filter is primarily affected by the dialysate flow rates (Table 76.7).

- After the total clearance has been calculated, the optimal dosage regimen can be calculated using the same approach described for patients with stable renal function.

PERITONEAL DIALYSIS

- Peritoneal dialysis has the potential to affect drug disposition; however, drug therapy individualization is often less complicated in these patients owing to the continuous nature of chronic ambulatory peritoneal dialysis (CAPD).

TABLE 76.7. Clearance of Selected Drugs by CAVHD/CVVHD

	Dialysate Flow Rate (mL/min)				
	5	*10*	*16.7*	*33.3*	*50–60*
Ceftazidime	—	—	13–17	15.2	24
Cefuroxime	—	—	14–19	16.2	35
Ciprofloxacin	—	—	16.3	19.9	—
Digoxin	2.6	4.2	6.4–10.0	11	—
Gentamicin	—	—	20.5	26.0	—
Phenytoin	1.4	3.0	6.5	—	—
Theophylline	4.0	7.8	14.8	—	—
Tobramycin	—	—	11.1–29	14.9	16–37
Urea	—	—	13–28	18–36	27–40
Vancomycin	3.3	6.7	8.1–11.7	23–28	—

- Factors that influence drug dialyzability include drug-specific characteristics (e.g., molecular weight, solubility, degree of ionization, protein binding, and volume of distribution) and intrinsic properties of the peritoneal membrane (e.g., blood flow, pore size, and peritoneal membrane surface area).
- In general, hemodialysis is more effective in removing drug substances, especially small molecules, than peritoneal dialysis. If a drug is not removed by hemodialysis, it is not likely to be removed by peritoneal dialysis.
- The ratio of the half-life of drugs in CAPD patients to that of patients with normal renal function (Table 76.8) can be used to calculate the dosage adjustment factor as:

$$Q = t_{1/2norm}/t_{1/2CAPD}$$

CHRONIC HEMODIALYSIS

- Impact of hemodialysis on drug therapy depends on drug characteristics, dialysis conditions (e.g., dialysis membrane composition, filter surface area, blood and dialysate flow rates, and whether or not the dialysis unit reuses the dialysis filter), and clinical indication for dialysis.
- In the mid 1980s, rapid high-efficiency hemodialysis (RHED) and high-flux dialysis (HFD) began to be used in the United States (see Chapter 75). HFD allows free passage of most solutes with molecular weights of ≤20,000, and therefore is more likely to remove high molecular weight drugs (e.g., vancomycin) as well as drugs with low molecular to midmolecular weights (i.e., 100–1000) (Table 76.9).
- RHED differs from conventional hemodialysis because the size of RHED filters is larger, and blood and dialysate flow rates are increased. These changes result in up to 50% increased clearance of small mole-

XIV

TABLE 76.8. Half-lives of Antibiotics in Patients with Normal Renal Function and Renal Insufficiency

	Half-Life (h)		
	Normal	*ESRD*	*CAPD*
Aminoglycosides			
Amikacin	1.6	39	40
Gentamicin	2.2	53	32
Netilmicin	2.1	42	18
Tobramycin	2.5	58	36
Cephalosporins			
First Generation			
Cefazolin	2.2	28	30
Cefonicid	4.0	68	50
Cephalothin	0.2	3.7	ND
Cephradine	0.9	12	ND
Cephalexin	0.8	19	9
Second Generation			
Cefamandole	1.0	10	8.0
Cefmenoxime	1.3	11.3	6.0
Cefoxitin	0.8	20	15
Cefuroxime	1.3	18	15
Third Generation			
Cefixime	3.2	11.5	15
Cefoperazone	1.8	2.3	2.2
Cefotaxime	0.9	2.5	2.4
Cefsulodin	1.8	11	11
Ceftazidime	1.8	26	13
Ceftizoxime	1.6	28	11
Ceftriaxone	8.0	15	12
Moxalactam	2.2	20	16
Penicillins			
Azlocillin	0.9	5.1	ND
Mezlocillin	1.0	4.3	ND
Piperacillin	1.2	3.9	2.4
Ticarcillin	1.2	15	ND
Quinolones			
Ciprofloxacin	4.0	8.0	11
Fleroxacin	13.0	27	27
Ofloxacin	7.0	30	25
Vancomycin and Others			
Vancomycin	6.9	161	92
Teicoplanin	50	260	260
Aztreonam	2.0	7.0	9.3
Clindamycin	2.8	2.8	ND
Erythromycin	2.1	4.0	ND
Metronidazole	7.9	7.7	11
Rifampin	4.0	8.0	ND
Antifungal Agents			
Amphotericin	360	360	ND
Flucytosine	4.2	115	ND
Fluconazole	22	125	72

XIV

TABLE 76.8. continued

	Half-Life (h)		
	Normal	*ESRD*	*CAPD*
Antifungal Agents (continued)			
Ketoconazole	2.0	1.8	2.4
Miconazole	24	25	ND
Combinations			
Ampicillin	1.3	15	9.5
Sulbactam	1.0	19	9.7
Imipenem	0.9	3.0	6.4
Cilistatin	0.8	15	19
Sulfamethoxazole	10	13	14
Trimethoprim	14	33	34

Key: ESRD, creatinine clearance <10 mL/min, patient not on dialysis; ND, no data.

cules (e.g., gentamicin) primarily because of increased blood flow. The clearance of midmolecular weight substances may also be increased due to the larger surface area for diffusion.

- The dialysate recovery clearance approach has become the benchmark for determination of dialyzer clearance. It can be calculated as:

$$CL_D^r = R/AUC_{0-t}$$

where R is total amount of drug recovered unchanged in dialysate and AUC_{0-t} is area under the prefilter plasma concentration–time curve during hemodialysis. To determine AUC_{0-t}, at least two and preferably three to four plasma concentrations should be obtained during dialysis.

- Total clearance during dialysis can be calculated as the sum of the total body clearance of the patient during the interdialytic period (CL_{PT}) and dialyzer clearance (CL_D):

$$CL_T = CL_{PT} + CL_D$$

Half-life during the period between dialysis treatments and during dialysis can then be calculated from the following relationships using an estimate of the drug's distribution volume (V), which can be obtained from the literature:

$$t_{1/2, \text{ offHD}} = 0.693 \ [V/CL_{PT}] \text{ and}$$

$$t_{1/2, \text{ onHD}} = 0.693 \ [V/(CL_{Pt} + CL_D)]$$

- After key pharmacokinetic parameters (CL, CL_D, and V) have been XIV estimated or calculated, they may be used to simulate the plasma concentration–time profile of the drug for the individual patient and ascertain how much drug to administer and when.

TABLE 76.9. Drug Disposition During Dialysis Depends on Filter Characteristics

Drug	Hemodialysis Clearance (mL/min)		Half-Life During Dialysis (h)	
	Conventional	*High-Flux*	*Conventional*	*High-Flux*
Ceftazidime	55–60	155[a]	3.30	1.2[a]
Cefuroxime	NR	103[b]	3.75	1.6[b]
Gentamicin	58.2	41.7[b]	3.0	4.3[b]
Netilmicin	46	87–109	5.0–5.2	2.9–3.4
Vancomycin	9–21	31–60[c]	35–38	12.0[c]
		40–150[b]		4.5–11.8[b]
		72–116[d]		NR

Key: NR, not reported.
[a]Polyamide filter.
[b]Polysulfone filter.
[c]Polyacrylonitrile filter.
[d]Polymethylmethacrylate.

- The first step is to estimate the pharmacokinetic parameters for the drug based on published population data.
- Plasma concentrations of the drug over the interdialytic interval of 24–48 hours can be predicted. The concentration at the end of the 30-minute infusion (C_{max}) would be:

$$C_{max} = (dose/t')1 - e^{-kt'}/CL$$

The plasma concentration prior to the next dialysis session (C_{bD}) can be calculated as:

$$C_{bD} = C_{max} \times e^{-(CL/V) \times t}$$

- The hemodialysis clearance of most drugs is dialysis filter dependent, and a value can be extrapolated from the literature. The concentration after dialysis can be calculated as:

$$C_{aD} = C_{bD} \times e^{-(CL + CL_D)/Vt}$$

- The postdialysis dose can be calculated as follows because the elimination half-life is extremely prolonged relative to the infusion time and thus minimal drug is eliminated during the infusion period:

$$Dose = V_d \times (C_{max} - C_{min})$$

See Chapter 50, Drug Therapy Individualization for Patients with Renal Insufficiency, authored by Gary R. Matzke, PharmD, FCP, FCCP, and Reginald F. Frye, PharmD, PhD.

Chapter 77

▶ ELECTROLYTE HOMEOSTASIS

▶ DEFINITION

An electrolyte is any salt that dissociates in water; however, the term usually refers to sodium, potassium, chloride, carbon dioxide, calcium, magnesium, and phosphorus. Electrolytes are involved in movement of body water, acid–base balance, muscle contractility, enzyme systems, blood coagulation, energy production, and other life-sustaining functions. Homeostatic mechanisms exist to preserve serum concentrations within relatively narrow ranges. Electrolyte imbalances may result from numerous causes and can be associated with substantial morbidity and mortality. This chapter reviews disorders of sodium, potassium, calcium, magnesium, and phosphorus homeostasis.

▶ DESIRED OUTCOME

The goals of therapy for disorders of electrolyte homeostasis are to promptly identify and correct reversible underlying causes; institute corrective treatment, if indicated, to relieve symptoms and prevent serious complications; and to normalize the serum electrolyte concentration.

▶ DISORDERS OF SODIUM HOMEOSTASIS

HYPONATREMIA (SERUM SODIUM <135 mEq/L)

Etiology

Isotonic Hyponatremia

- Hyponatremia associated with normal serum osmolality may be observed in patients with hyperlipidemia or hyperproteinemia (pseudohyponatremia) and during IV infusion of isotonic, sodium-free solutions.

Hypertonic Hyponatremia

- Hyponatremia in the presence of elevated serum osmolality is most frequently encountered in the settings of hyperglycemia or the administration of hyperosmolar glycerin or mannitol solutions.

Hypotonic Hyponatremia

- Hypotonic hyponatremia may be classified as hypovolemic, hypervolemic, or isovolemic hyponatremia (Figure 77.1).
  - Hypovolemic hyponatremia is associated with a deficit of extracellular fluid (ECF) volume and sodium, with a proportionally greater deficit of sodium than water (e.g., from diuretic use).

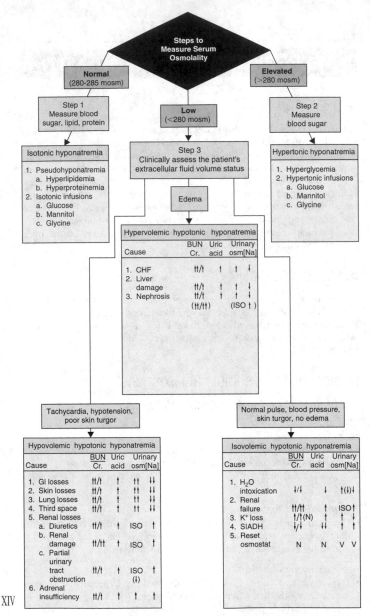

Figure 77.1. Diagnostic approach to hyponatremia. Arrows indicate direction of change. Single and double arrows define the magnitude of change. ISO, isotonic; N, normal; V, variable. *(From Narins RG, Jones RE, Stom MC, et al. Am J Med 1982;72(3):498, reprinted with permission.)*

- Isovolemic hyponatremia is associated with a normal total body sodium content and small increases in ECF volume. Altered thirst, antidiuretic hormone (ADH) secretion, and defective renal diluting mechanisms cause water retention and hyponatremia in patients who appear clinically euvolemic (e.g., the syndrome of inappropriate ADH secretion [SIADH]).
- Hypervolemic hyponatremia (also referred to as dilutional hyponatremia) is associated with an elevated total body sodium content and an expanded ECF volume and is manifested clinically as edema and weight gain (e.g., congestive heart failure and hypoalbuminemic syndromes such as cirrhosis or nephrotic syndrome).

Clinical Presentation

- In hypovolemic hyponatremia, most of the clinical manifestations are due to hypovolemia (poor skin turgor, tachycardia, orthostatic hypotension, oliguria, and azotemia) and not hypotonicity.
- In contrast, the hypotonicity associated with isovolemic and hypervolemic hyponatremia may result in symptoms related to cellular swelling; cerebral edema with increased intracranial pressure is the most severe.
- A decrease in serum sodium from 140 to 130 mEq/L over minutes to hours may be accompanied by moderate symptoms such as bloating, headache, anorexia, muscle cramps, nausea, and vomiting. A decrease of >10 mEq/L over a similar period may be associated with more severe syndromes such as headache, lethargy, and disorientation, which may progress to seizures and coma. However, patients with serum sodium concentrations of 115–120 mEq/L may be free of symptoms, particularly in chronic cases where hyponatremia developed slowly.

Treatment

- Hypovolemic hyponatremia is rarely associated with hypotonic symptoms, so therapy is directed toward replacing the sodium and volume losses with normal saline over a period of 6–12 hours. Infusion of hypertonic saline (3 or 5% NaCl) is rarely necessary, because isotonic saline corrects the pathophysiologic factors that led to impaired free water excretion. Ongoing sodium losses must be accounted for by appropriate maintenance fluid adjustments.
- Isovolemic hyponatremia associated with a nonacute reduction of serum sodium concentrations to values not less than 115 mEq/L and an absence of symptoms may be treated conservatively by water restriction. Fluids are provided to allow for mandatory urinary solute excretion, allowing insensible water loss to correct the hyponatremia. Fluid restrictions of 500 mL/d or less may be necessary to correct hyponatremia over 3 to 5 days. Chronic SIADH due to an underlying cause that cannot be corrected may require pharmacologic intervention (e.g., demeclocycline 600–1200 mg/d) in addition to water restriction. Because its onset of action ranges from 5–8 days, demeclocycline has no role in the acute treatment of severe hyponatremia.

XIV

- Hypervolemic hyponatremia is treated by correcting the underlying disease and restricting both water and salt. Loop diuretics may be necessary to elicit a loss of free water.
- Slow correction of serum sodium concentration (an increase of <12 mEq/L/d) is recommended for most cases of nonemergent symptomatic hyponatremia to prevent the *osmotic demyelinization syndrome* (quadriparesis, mutism, pseudobulbar palsy) that sometimes follows rapid treatment of symptomatic hyponatremia. Rapid correction of hyponatremia should be reserved for true emergencies (seizures or coma in any hyponatremic patient) or in cases of known rapid onset of severe hyponatremia (water intoxication).

HYPERNATREMIA (SERUM SODIUM >150 mEq/L)

Etiology
- Hypernatremia is always associated with hypertonicity and results from a state of relative water deficit. Patients who cannot express their thirst (infants, unconscious patients) or who are unable to ambulate (elderly and disabled patients) to obtain fluids are at the highest risk for developing hypernatremia.
- Hypernatremia may be classified according to the status of the ECF volume (Figure 77.2).
  - Hypovolemic hypernatremia occurs in the setting of ECF volume depletion and is caused by water losses exceeding sodium losses (e.g., profound diarrhea, excessive sweating). Important drug-induced causes include osmotic diuresis with mannitol, diuretics, and laxative-induced diarrhea.
  - Isovolemic hypernatremia is associated with an isolated pure water loss, and total body sodium content is normal. Iatrogenic causes include failure to replace insensible water loss or the replacement of insensible water losses with relatively hypertonic solutions. Excessive insensible water loss may occur with fever or high ambient temperatures. Insufficient fluid intake may result from lack of access to water (e.g., elderly patients with decreased levels of consciousness). Diabetes insipidus (DI) is associated with the production of large amounts of hypotonic urine.
  - Hypervolemic hypernatremia results from an increase in total body sodium and water, with the gain of sodium exceeding that of water (e.g., excessive sodium administration).

Clinical Presentation
- Cellular dehydration may lead to symptoms of thirst, restlessness, irritability, tremulousness, spasticity, hyperreflexia, ataxia, seizures, coma, and death.
- The shrinking effect of hypernatremia may result in the tearing of cerebral blood vessels, leading to intracranial bleeding.

XIV

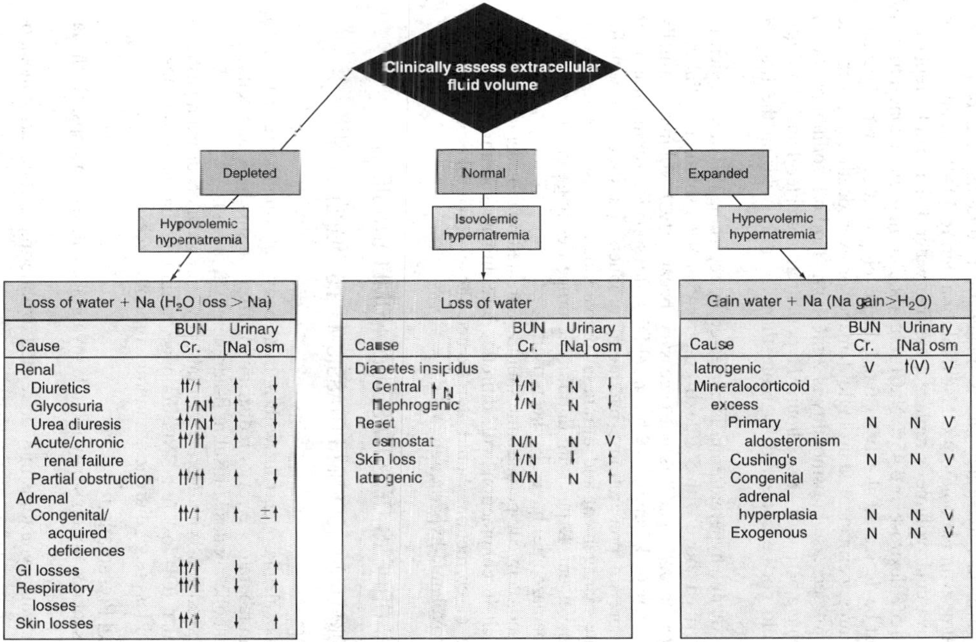

Loss of water + Na (H_2O loss > Na)

Cause	BUN Cr.	Urinary [Na]	Urinary osm
Renal			
Diuretics	↑↑/↑	↑	↓
Glycosuria	↑/N↑	↑	↓
Urea diuresis	↑↑/N↑	↑	↓
Acute/chronic renal failure	↑↑/↑↑	↑	↓
Partial obstruction	↑↑/↑↑	↑	↓
Adrenal			
Congenital/acquired deficiences	↑↑/↑	↑	±↑
GI losses	↑↑/↑	↓	↑
Respiratory losses	↑↑/↑	↓	↑
Skin losses	↑↑/↑	↓	↑

Loss of water

Cause	BUN Cr.	Urinary [Na]	Urinary osm
Diabetes insipidus			
Central	↑/N	N	↓
Nephrogenic	↑/N	N	↓
Reset osmostat	N/N	N	V
Skin loss	↑/N	↓	↑
Iatrogenic	N/N	N	↑

Gain water + Na (Na gain > H_2O)

Cause	BUN Cr.	Urinary [Na]	Urinary osm
Iatrogenic	V	↑(V)	V
Mineralocorticoid excess			
Primary aldosteronism	N	N	V
Cushing's	N	N	V
Congenital adrenal hyperplasia	N	N	V
Exogenous	N	N	V

Figure 77.2. Diagnostic approach to hypernatremia. Arrows indicate direction of change. Single and double arrows define the magnitude of change. N, normal; V, variable. *(From Narins RG, Jones RE, Stom MC et al. Am J Med 1982;72(3):501, reprinted with permission.)*

Treatment

- The goal of therapy is normalization of serum tonicity by correcting reversible causes, treating underlying disorders, and normalizing ECF volume status.
- Hypovolemic hypernatremia is treated by restoration of intravascular volume with isotonic 0.9% NaCl solution during 30–45 minutes. Once intravascular volume is replaced, the free-water deficit can be replaced with 5% dextrose or 0.45% NaCl solution. Serum sodium concentration must be decreased slowly to avoid the development of cerebral edema, seizures, permanent neurologic damage, or even death. An acceptable rate of decrease in osmolality is 2 mOsm/h (1 mEq/L sodium per hour) during a period of 48–72 hours. Hypernatremia greater than 175 mEq/L should not be corrected by more than 15 mEq/L during the first 24 hours.
- Isovolemic hypernatremia is corrected by replacing the water deficit as described above with 5% dextrose or 0.45% NaCl solution. Initial therapy with 0.9% NaCl is not necessary, because ECF volume is usually not decreased. Patients with central DI will respond to administration of vasopressin preparations; parenteral products are usually given for acute management and intranasal preparations are used for long-term management. Drugs with antidiuretic properties (e.g., chlorpropamide, carbamazepine) have also been used.
- Hypervolemic hypernatremia should be treated by replacement of water deficit in conjunction with diuretics to eliminate sodium excess. The rate of correction should not exceed those previously proposed for hypovolemic hypernatremia.

▶ DISORDERS OF POTASSIUM HOMEOSTASIS

HYPOKALEMIA (SERUM POTASSIUM <3.5 mEq/L)

Etiology

- Hypokalemia occurring with normal body potassium stores can result from laboratory error or redistribution from plasma back into cells (e.g., metabolic alkalosis, insulin, β-adrenergic agonists).
- Hypokalemia with decreased total body stores can occur from gastrointestinal (GI) loss (e.g., NG drainage, vomiting, diarrhea), skin loss, or renal loss (e.g., diuretics, mineralocorticoid excess).

Clinical Presentation

- Muscular symptoms may include myalgia, weakness, cramps, akathisia, and paralysis.
- Metabolic symptoms may be related to abnormal carbohydrate metabolism (e.g., glucose intolerance).
- ECG effects are characterized by ST segment lowering or flattening, inversion of the T wave, and elevation of the U wave. A widening of the PR interval, an increase in P wave amplitude, and widening of the QRS complex may also occur.

XIV

- Cardiac arrhythmias include bradyarrhythmias, heart block, atrial flutter, paroxysmal atrial tachycardia with block, atrioventricular dissociation, premature ventricular contractions, and ventricular fibrillation. Hypokalemia lowers the threshold for digitalis cardiotoxic arrhythmias.

Treatment

- Potassium replacement therapy is indicated for: (1) symptomatic hypokalemia; (2) starvation and debilitation; (3) potassium loss associated with vomiting or diarrhea; (4) acidosis leading to increased renal potassium excretion; (5) digitalis intoxication leading to cardiac arrhythmias; (6) myocardial infarction with low serum potassium; (7) diabetic ketoacidosis treated with insulin; and (8) adrenocortical hyperactivity.
- Sustained-release potassium products are good choices for oral administration because they disperse potassium in the gut gradually, thereby minimizing gastric irritation and ulceration associated with enteric-coated products. Liquid potassium preparations are inexpensive but are often poorly tolerated because of unpleasant taste, aftertaste, nausea, heartburn, and diarrhea. Salt substitutes are an effective, inexpensive alternative; potassium-rich food sources (i.e., bananas, orange juice) are generally not recommended for chronic supplementation because they often contain less chloride than other potassium sources and may add unwanted calories.
- When metabolic alkalosis accompanies hypokalemia, the administration of the chloride salt is essential for correction of both the alkalosis and the potassium deficit. Nonchloride salts (e.g., phosphate, gluconate) are indicated only for hypokalemia associated with metabolic acidosis.
- IV potassium (usually 10–20 mEq/h) is indicated when the oral route is not feasible and/or in the presence of life-threatening hypokalemia (paralysis, arrhythmias). Rates of administration >10–20 mEq/h should be accompanied by ECG monitoring. The maximally tolerated concentration for peripheral-vein administration is 40–60 mEq/L.
- For patients on diuretic therapy with serum potassium <3.0 mEq/L (or symptoms) 50–60 mEq/d KCl oral solution or wax matrix can be used. Potassium-sparing diuretics (spironolactone, triamterene, amiloride) are an alternative to exogenous potassium during diuretic therapy. Combined use of potassium chloride supplements and potassium-sparing diuretics is generally contraindicated.
- For edematous patients (i.e., congestive heart failure, cirrhosis with ascites, severe aldosteronism), oral therapy with 40–80 mEq/d should be used for mild deficits and up to 100–120 mEq/d with careful monitoring for more severe deficits.

HYPERKALEMIA (SERUM POTASSIUM >5.5 mEq/L)   XIV

Etiology

- Hyperkalemia associated with normal total body stores may result from redistribution of potassium from the intracellular to the extracellular space in vivo (e.g., acidosis, insulin deficiency, cellular injury), and pseudohyperkalemia, an in vitro phenomenon in which the measured serum potassium level is falsely elevated because of potassium release from red blood cells, white blood cells, or platelets.

- Hyperkalemia associated with elevated total body potassium stores is due to excessive potassium ingestion, reduced potassium excretion (e.g., renal impairment, use of ACE inhibitors), or both.

Clinical Presentation

- Hyperkalemia may be manifested clinically as paresthesias, muscle weakness, and paralysis. Weakness often begins in the lower extremities, ascending to the trunk and upper extremities. At concentrations ≥6.5 mEq/L muscle twitching, weakness, nausea, and cramping can occur.

- The earliest ECG changes (serum potassium 5.5–6 mEq/L) are peaked T waves and shortening of the QT interval. Between 6 and 7 mEq/L, the PR interval and QRS duration are prolonged. When the concentration exceeds 7–8 mEq/L, there is widening of the QRS complex and decreased amplitude, widening, and eventual loss of the P wave. When concentrations exceed 9–10 mEq/L, the QRS complex merges with the T wave, resulting in a sine-wave pattern, which may deteriorate to ventricular fibrillation or asystole at concentrations from 10–12 mEq/L.

Treatment (Table 77.1)

- Severe hyperkalemia (>8 mEq/L) or moderate hyperkalemia (6.5–8 mEq/L) with symptoms or ECG changes requires immediate treatment. Exogenous potassium must be withheld, and potentially reversible causes of hyperkalemia must be reversed.

- Calcium administration rapidly reverses ECG manifestations and arrhythmias. Calcium does not lower serum potassium concentrations and, because it is short acting, it must be repeated if signs or symptoms recur, until serum potassium can be lowered.

- Promoting intracellular movement of potassium effectively lowers extracellular serum levels (e.g., IV glucose and insulin infusion, inhaled or IV β-adrenergic agonist therapy, or sodium bicarbonate).

- Sodium polystyrene sulfonate is a cation-exchange resin that removes potassium from the body. It has a slow onset of action and should not be used as monotherapy for patients who already exhibit EKG changes. Each gram of resin may bind as much as 1 mEq of potassium and release 1–2 mEq of sodium. Doses of 40 g given orally in four divided doses may decrease serum potassium concentrations by 1.0 mEq/L in 24 hours in patients with renal failure. It should be administered with sorbitol to prevent constipation and retention of the resin. Prepackaged suspensions in sorbitol are commercially available.

- If hyperkalemia persists, especially if the patient is in renal failure (acute or chronic), hemodialysis is indicated.

XIV

TABLE 77.1. Treatment of Hyperkalemia

Medication	Dose	Route of Administration	Mechanism of Action	Expected Result	Onset/Duration
Albuterol	10–20 mg	Nebulized over 10 min	Stimulates Na$^+$/K$^+$-ATPase pump	Redistribution of K$^+$ into the cell	30 min/1–2 h
Calcium chloride	1 g (13.5 mEq)	IV over 5–10 min	Raises threshold potential and reestablishes cardiac excitability	Reverses ECG effects	1–2 min/10–30 min
Dextrose 50%	50 mL (25 g)	IV over 5 min	Increases insulin release	Redistribution of K$^+$ into cell	30 min/2–6 h
Dextrose 10%	1000 mL (100 g)	IV over 1–2 h	Increases insulin release	Redistribution of K$^+$ into cell	30 min/2–6 h
Sodium bicarbonate	50–100 mEq	IV over 2–5 min	Increases serum pH	Redistribution of K$^+$ into cell	30 min/2–6 h
Insulin (regular)	1 unit per 3–5 g dextrose	IV with 10% dextrose SC	Stimulates potassium intracellular uptake	Redistribution of K$^+$ into cell	30 min/2–6 h
Sodium polystyrene sulfonate	15–60 g	Orally or rectally	Exchanges resin Na$^-$ for K$^+$	Increase in K$^+$ elimination	1 h/variable
Hemodialysis	2–4 h	—	Removes from plasma	Increase in K$^+$ elimination	Immediate/variable

XIV

► DISORDERS OF CALCIUM HOMEOSTASIS

HYPERCALCEMIA (TOTAL SERUM CALCIUM >10.5 mg/dL)

Etiology

- Hypercalcemia of malignancy is most commonly observed in squamous cell carcinomas of the lung, head, and neck; hematologic malignancies such as multiple myeloma and T cell lymphomas; and carcinomas of breast, ovary, kidney, and bladder.
- Hyperparathyroidism is the most common cause of hypercalcemia in the general population. Benign parathyroid adenomas account for 70–85% of cases of hyperparathyroidism, with parathyroid hyperplasia accounting for the remaining 15%.

Clinical Presentation

- Mild to moderate hypercalcemia (<13 mg/dL) may be asymptomatic, as is often the case in drug-induced hypercalcemia and in most patients with hyperparathyroidism.
- Symptoms of hypercalcemia associated with malignancy may have an acute presentation because the onset of hypercalcemia is rapid. A symptom complex characterized by anorexia, nausea and vomiting, constipation, polyuria, polydipsia, and nocturia is common.
- Patients infrequently present in hypercalcemic crisis, manifested by the acute onset of severe hypercalcemia, acute renal failure, and obtundation. If untreated, hypercalcemic crisis may progress to oliguric renal failure, coma, and malignant ventricular arrhythmias, which may result in death.
- Disorders associated with long-standing hypercalcemia (i.e., hyperparathyroidism) are more likely to present with metastatic calcification, nephrolithiasis, and chronic renal insufficiency caused by deposition of calcium phosphate in soft tissue.
- ECG changes associated with hypercalcemia include shortening of the QT interval, and coving of the ST-T wave; very high serum calcium concentrations may cause T wave widening.

Treatment (Figure 77.3)

- Patients with hypercalcemic crisis or symptomatic hypercalcemia should be treated immediately. Asymptomatic patients with mild hypercalcemia may be carefully observed, especially if treatment for the underlying condition (i.e., malignancy, hyperparathyroidism) is initiated.
- In patients with functioning kidneys, treatment involves rehydration by infusion of normal saline at rates of 200–300 mL/h. Fluid status should be assessed by intake/output or by central venous pressure monitoring.
- Once rehydration has been accomplished, loop diuretics such as furosemide (40–80 mg IV every 1–4 hours) may be instituted to increase urine output to a goal of 200–250 mL/h.

XIV

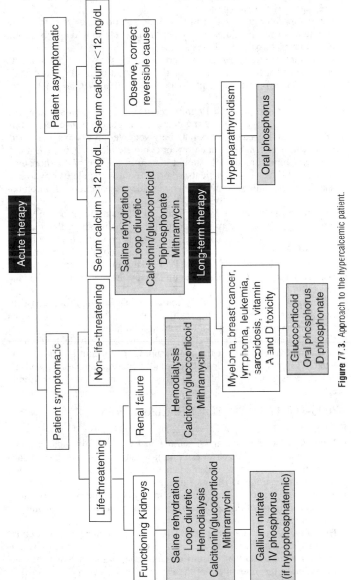

Figure 77.3. Approach to the hypercalcemic patient.

Acute therapy

Patient asymptomatic

Serum calcium <12 mg/dL
Observe, correct reversible cause

Serum calcium >12 mg/dL
Saline rehydration
Loop diuretic
Calcitonin/glucocorticoid
Diphosphonate
Mithramycin

Patient symptomatic

Non–life-threatening

Life-threatening

Renal failure
Hemodialysis
Calcitonin/glucocorticoid
Mithramycin

Functioning Kidneys
Saline rehydration
Loop diuretic
Hemodialysis
Calcitonin/glucocorticoid
Mithramycin
Gallium nitrate
IV phosphorus
(if hypophosphatemic)

Long-term therapy

Hyperparathyroidism
Oral phosphorus

Myeloma, breast cancer, lymphoma, leukemia, sarcoidosis, vitamin A and D toxicity
Glucocorticoid
Oral phosphorus
D phosphonate

- Saline rehydration and furosemide often decrease serum calcium by 2–3 mg/dL within 24–48 hours.
- Potassium chloride is added to the saline solution after rehydration to maintain normokalemia; serum magnesium levels should also be monitored during furosemide diuresis.
- In life-threatening hypercalcemic crisis, acute, short-term therapy with calcitonin (4 MRC units/kg SQ or IM every 12 hours, or constant IV infusion of 10–12 MRC units/h) rapidly (within 1–2 hours) reduces serum calcium levels.
- Mithramycin (25 µ/kg via IV infusion over 1–3 hours in saline or 5% dextrose solution) has an onset within 12 hours and a peak effect within 48–96 hours. Repeated doses may be given every 3–4 days as needed, along with frequent determinations of complete blood count, liver function, and renal function. It should generally be limited to short-term therapy (2–3 weeks) in patients who have not responded to hydration and diuretics; mithramycin should be avoided in patients with thrombocytopenia, liver disease, or renal disease.
- The bisphosphonates etidronate and pamidronate are effective in the treatment of hypercalcemia associated with malignancy. Pamidronate (60–90 mg by IV infusion during 24 hours) is preferred because it may be more effective and requires only a single dose. Treatment with etidronate (7.5 mg/kg/d by slow IV infusion during 3 hours) may be necessary for 4–5 days, so calcitonin therapy may be necessary if rapid reduction is required.
- Gallium nitrate (200 mg/m^2/d by continuous IV infusion for 5 consecutive days) is indicated for the treatment of symptomatic hypercalcemia of malignancy not responsive to hydration therapy.
- Glucocorticoids (40–60 mg/d of prednisone or equivalent) are usually effective for hypercalcemia resulting from multiple myeloma, leukemia, lymphoma, sarcoidosis, and hypervitaminoses A and D, but there is a lag time of 5–10 days before onset of hypocalcemic effect.

HYPOCALCEMIA (TOTAL SERUM CALCIUM <8.5 mg/dL)

Etiology

- Vitamin D–deficiency states resulting in hypocalcemia include nutritional deficiency, GI disease resulting in vitamin D and calcium malabsorption, gastric surgery, chronic pancreatitis, small-bowel disease, and intestinal resection and bypass surgery.
- Symptomatic hypocalcemia most commonly occurs because of parathyroid gland dysfunction secondary to surgical procedures involving the thyroid, parathyroid, and neck.
- Hypoalbuminemia is a common cause of laboratory hypocalcemia. Patients remain asymptomatic because the ionized fraction of serum calcium remains normal. Serum albumin concentration is a vital consideration in the assessment of the cause of hypocalcemia.

XIV

- Hypomagnesemia of any cause may be associated with severe symptomatic hypocalcemia that is unresponsive to calcium replacement therapy.

Clinical Presentation

- The hallmark sign of acute hypocalcemia is tetany, which manifests as paresthesias around the mouth and in the extremities, muscle spasms and cramps, carpopedal spasms, and rarely, laryngospasm and bronchospasm.
- Cardiovascular manifestations result in ECG changes characterized by a prolonged QT interval and symptoms of decreased myocardial contractility often associated with congestive heart failure.

Treatment

- Hypocalcemia associated with hypoalbuminemia requires no treatment because ionized plasma calcium concentrations are normal.
- Acute, symptomatic hypocalcemia requires parenteral administration of soluble calcium salts (Table 77.2).
  - The initial goal is to administer 200–300 mg of elemental calcium IV (at a rate ≤30–60 mg/min) and repeat until symptoms are fully controlled.
  - Calcium gluconate (2–3 g) is preferred over calcium chloride (1 g) for peripheral venous administration because extravasation of calcium chloride may result in tissue necrosis.

TABLE 77.2. Calcium Preparations

Calcium salt	Elemental Calcium per Gram of Salt		Route
	(mg)	(mEq)	
Calcium carbonate	400	20.0	PO
Calcium chloride	270	13.5	IV
Calcium citrate	211	10.6	PO
Calcium glubionate	64	3.2	PO
Calcium gluceptate	82	4.1	IV
Calcium gluconate	90	4.5	IV/PO
Calcium glycerophosphate	191	9.6	IV
Calcium lactate	130	6.5	PO
Calcium phosphate (dibasic anhydrous)	290	14.5	PO
Calcium phosphate (dibasic dihydrate)	230	11.5	PO
Calcium phosphate (tribasic)	400	20.0	PO

XIV

- If symptoms recur after initial IV calcium replacement, a slow IV infusion of 15 mg/kg of elemental calcium during 4–6 hours may be administered.
- If hypomagnesemia is present, magnesium supplementation is indicated.
- Chronic hypocalcemia from hypoparathyroidism and vitamin D-deficient states may be managed by oral calcium supplementation (e.g., 2–4 g/d of elemental calcium). If serum calcium does not normalize, a vitamin D preparation should be added.
- Treatment of hypocalcemia due to vitamin D-deficient states should be individualized depending upon the underlying cause.

▶ DISORDERS OF MAGNESIUM HOMEOSTASIS

HYPERMAGNESEMIA (SERUM MAGNESIUM >2 mEq/L OR >2.4 mg/dL)

Etiology
- Hypermagnesemia most commonly occurs in the setting of renal insufficiency, when glomerular filtration rates are <30 mL/min.
- Use of magnesium-containing laxatives or antacids can lead to hypermagnesemia in renal failure patients.
- Patients with multiple-system organ failure receiving magnesium-containing antacids for stress ulcer prophylaxis or magnesium-containing parenteral fluids are at high risk.
- Parenteral treatment of eclampsia with magnesium sulfate or its use in the therapy of preterm labor can potentially cause hypermagnesemia.

Clinical Presentation
- Hypermagnesemia may cause hypotonic, diminished, or absent deep tendon reflexes, varying degrees of muscle weakness, and complete flaccid paralysis with resultant respiratory depression, depending on the serum concentration of magnesium attained.
- CNS depression may result in varying degrees of lethargy and sedation, which may progress to stupor and coma, especially at high (≥6 mEq/L) serum concentrations.
- Hypotension and cutaneous vasodilation may occur above serum levels of 3 mEq/L. Sinus bradycardia, first-degree heart block, nodal rhythms, or bundle branch block may occur at concentrations ≥5–10 mEq/L. Complete heart block progressing to asystole and cardiac arrest may occur at concentrations ≥14–15 mEq/L.

Treatment
- Treatment is indicated in symptomatic patients with serum magnesium levels of 5–8 mEq/L and in all patients whose serum level is >8 mEq/L.
- Administration of IV calcium (100–200 mg of elemental calcium) is indicated to directly antagonize the neuromuscular and cardiovascular

XIV

effects of magnesium. Repeated doses may be necessary in life-threatening situations.

- Hemodialysis is the treatment of choice in all patients with renal dysfunction. Supportive care with mechanical ventilation, pressors, and cardiac pacemakers may be necessary until serum magnesium concentrations are lowered.
- In patients with adequate renal function and non-life–threatening hypermagnesemia, promotion of renal magnesium excretion may be accomplished by administering IV saline and furosemide.

HYPOMAGNESEMIA (SERUM MAGNESIUM <1.5 mEq/L OR <1.8 mg/dL)

Etiology

- Dietary magnesium deprivation rarely leads to significant magnesium depletion unless it is prolonged.
- Generalized malabsorption syndromes associated with hypomagnesemia occur in various intestinal mucosal diseases (e.g., celiac sprue, Whipple's disease, radiation enteritis), massive intestinal resection, and pancreatic insufficiency.
- Magnesium losses exceeding intake may occur in GI disorders secondary to loss of intestinal fluids (which have a magnesium concentration of 14 mEq/L) or biliary, gastric, and pancreatic fluids (magnesium concentration 0.4–1.1 mEq/L).
- Renal magnesium wasting may be due to intrinsic tubular disorders and drug-induced, hormone-induced, and ion- or nutrient-induced renal tubular magnesium losses.
- Patients at highest risk for development of hypomagnesemia from chronic diuretic therapy include elderly patients, alcohol abusers, and patients consuming diets low in magnesium
- Other agents associated with magnesium wasting include aminoglycosides, amphotericin B, foscarnet, pentamidine, cisplatin, and cyclosporine.

Clinical Presentation

- Manifestations of hypomagnesemia include neuromuscular hyperactivity (muscle twitching and tremor, muscle weakness, hyperreflexia, paresthesias), psychiatric effects (depression, delirium, agitation, confusion, hallucinations), and cardiac effects (premature ventricular beats, ventricular fibrillation or tachycardia, torsades de pointes).
- ECG changes are nonspecific and include wide QRS complexes and tall, peaked T waves in moderate deficiency, and prolonged PR, QRS, and QT intervals, ST-segment depression, and flat, broad T waves with prominent U waves in severe deficiency.
- Hypocalcemia is a prominent manifestation of magnesium deficiency, and serum calcium concentration should be assessed if hypomagnesemia is discovered.

XIV

Treatment (Table 77.3)

- Patients with asymptomatic hypomagnesemia and levels >1 mEq/L (1.2 mg/dL) are treated with oral magnesium supplements.
- Patients who are symptomatic or have serum magnesium levels <1 mEq/L (1.2 mg/dL) should receive parenteral magnesium therapy.
- Patients with renal insufficiency are treated with lower doses and must have serum levels monitored frequently.
- Because 50% of the dose is excreted in the urine, magnesium replacement must be continued during the course of 3–5 days or longer.
- Rapid IV bolus injection is avoided because of flushing, sweating, and a sensation of warmth.
- Direct IV administration of 50% magnesium sulfate may produce pain and venosclerosis; therefore, it should be diluted to 20% before administration. Intramuscular injections are reserved for situations in which peripheral venous access is not readily available.

TABLE 77.3. Guidelines for Treatment of Magnesium Deficiency in Adults

1. Serum magnesium <1 mEq/L (1.2 mg/dL) with life-threatening symptoms (seizure, arrhythmia)

   Day 1

   a. 2 g $MgSO_4$[a] mixed with 6 mL 0.9% NaCl in 10-mL syringe and administer IV push over 1 min

   b. Follow with 0.5 mEq Mg^{2+}/kg lean body weight IV infusion over 5–6 h, then 0.5 mEq Mg^{2+}/kg lean body weight IV infusion over 17–18 h

   Days 2–5

   0.5 mEq Mg^{2+}/kg lean body weight per day divided in maintenance IV fluids

2. Serum magnesium <1 mEq/L (1.2 mg/dL) without life-threatening symptoms

   Day 1

   Total of 1 mEq Mg^{2+}/kg lean body weight per day as continuous IV infusion, or divided and given IM every 4 h for five doses

   Days 2–5

   Total of 0.5 mEq Mg^{2+}/kg lean body weight IV infusion per day as continuous IV infusion or divided and given IM every 6–8 h

3. Serum magnesium >1 mEq/L (1.2 mg/dL) and <1.5 mEq/L (1.8 mg/dL) without symptoms

   As in No. 2, or

   a. Milk of Magnesia 5 mL four times daily as tolerated

   b. Magnesium-containing antacid 15 mL three times daily as tolerated

   c. Magnesium oxide tablets 300 mg four times daily, increase to two tablets four times daily as tolerated

XIV

[a]1 g $MgSO_4$ = 8.1 mEq Mg^{2+}.

▶ DISORDERS OF PHOSPHORUS HOMEOSTASIS

HYPERPHOSPHATEMIA (SERUM PHOSPHORUS CONCENTRATION >4.5 mg/dL)

Etiology
- The most common cause of hyperphosphatemia is a decrease in urinary phosphorus excretion secondary to decreased glomerular filtration rate (GFR).
- Patients with excessive exogenous phosphorus administration or endogenous intracellular phosphorus release in the setting of acute renal failure may develop profound hyperphosphatemia.
- In chronic renal insufficiency, severe hyperphosphatemia is usually encountered in advanced disease (GFR <25 mL/min).
- Hypoparathyroidism results in increased renal tubular reabsorption of phosphorus and may result in hyperphosphatemia.
- Iatrogenic causes include sodium phosphate enemas, laxatives containing phosphate salts, and IV phosphorus given for treatment of hypercalcemia.
- Rhabdomyolysis and chemotherapy treatment of acute leukemia and lymphoma may result in the release of large amounts of phosphorus from intracellular stores.

Clinical Presentation
- The major effect of hyperphosphatemia is related to the development of hypocalcemia and damage resulting from the deposition of calcium phosphate crystals.
- Metastatic calcification leading to band keratopathy, "red eye," pruritus, vascular calcification, and periarticular calcification is most common in renal failure.
- Soft-tissue calcifications in the conjunctiva, skin, heart, cornea, lung, gastric mucosa, and kidney have also been observed in chronic renal failure patients.
- Hyperphosphatemia associated with chronic renal disease may result in azotemic osteodystrophy (osteitis fibrosis cystica and osteomalacia).

Treatment
- In general, the most effective way to treat hyperphosphatemia itself is to decrease phosphate absorption in the lumen of the GI tract by the use of phosphate binders (e.g., antacids containing divalent cations). Because of concerns over aluminum toxicity, calcium salts are now the preferred phosphate binders in chronic renal failure patients.
- Severe symptomatic hyperphosphatemia manifesting as hypocalcemia and tetany is treated by the IV administration of calcium salts.

XIV

HYPOPHOSPHATEMIA (SERUM PHOSPHORUS CONCENTRATION <2.5 mg/dL)

Etiology

- Phosphate depletion may occur from dietary deficiency or chronic ingestion of phosphate-binding substances such as sucralfate, calcium carbonate, and aluminum/magnesium-containing antacids.
- Excess renal excretion can occur with the marked diuretic phase that accompanies recovery from extensive third-degree burns.
- Rapid refeeding of malnourished patients with high-carbohydrate, high-calorie nutritional diets with inadequate amounts of supplemental phosphorus may result in severe symptomatic hypophosphatemia.
- Severe and prolonged respiratory alkalosis may cause profound hypophosphatemia from intracellular shifts of phosphorus.
- Patients with diabetic ketoacidosis (DKA) may present with hyperphosphatemia, but DKA treatment may ultimately result in hypophosphatemia.
- Malnutrition, poor dietary intake, diarrhea, vomiting, and the use of phosphate-binding antacids may contribute to the hypophosphatemia of alcoholism.

Clinical Presentation

- CNS manifestations of severe hypophosphatemia include a progressive syndrome of irritability, apprehension, weakness, numbness, paresthesias, dysarthria, confusion, obtundation, seizures, and coma.
- Skeletal muscle dysfunction in severe hypophosphatemia may result in myalgia, weakness, and potentially fatal rhabdomyolysis. Acute respiratory failure due to respiratory muscle weakness and diaphragmatic contractile dysfunction has been observed.
- Congestive cardiomyopathy, hemolysis, increased risk of infection, and platelet defects may also occur.

Treatment

- The routine addition of phosphorus in concentrations of 12–15 mmol/L in IV hyperalimentation solution is of utmost importance for prevention of the severe hypophosphatemia associated with phosphorus-free hyperalimentation solutions.
- Mild to moderate asymptomatic hypophosphatemia are treated by oral administration of phosphorus salts (Table 77.4). Patients with moderate hypophosphatemia and concomitant renal dysfunction receive reduced daily oral doses (i.e., 1 g or approximately 30 mmol of phosphorus) with careful monitoring of serum phosphorus concentration.
- Severe symptomatic hypophosphatemia is treated with parenteral phosphorus replacement. Infusion of 9–15 mmol of phosphorus (0.15–0.25 mmol/kg) over 4–12 hours has been shown to be safe and effective. Patients should be closely monitored with frequent serum phosphorus determinations and assessment of serum calcium concentration. Therapy with parenteral phosphorus should be undertaken with great caution

TABLE 77.4. Phosphorus Replacement Therapy

Moderate hypophosphatemia (serum phosphorus 1.0–2.5 mg/dL)
  Oral therapy
    1.5–2 g (50–60 mmol) phosphorus per day, divided into three or four doses
  Parenteral therapy
    0.15 mmol/kg lean body weight infused in 250–1,000 mL D_5W over 12 h; repeat until serum
    phosphorus >2 mg/dL
Severe hypophosphatemia (serum phosphorus <1 mg/dL)
  Parenteral therapy
    0.25 mmol/kg lean body weight infused in 250–500 mL D_5W by infusion pump over 4–6 h;
    repeat until serum phosphorus >2 mg/dL

and at reduced dosage for patients with baseline hypercalcemia, renal dysfunction, or evidence of tissue injury.

See Chapter 51, Body Electrolyte Homeostasis, authored by Nathan J. Schultz, PharmD, BCPS, and Kerri K. Chitwood-Dagner, PharmD, BCPS, for a more detailed discussion of this topic.

XIV

Chapter 78

▶ RENAL FAILURE: ACUTE

▶ DEFINITIONS

- *Acute renal failure* is an abrupt decline in renal function characterized by the inability of the kidneys to excrete metabolic waste products (nitrogenous wastes and water) and maintain acid–base balance.
- *Azotemia* is an elevation in nitrogenous waste products (e.g., creatinine and urea nitrogen).
- *Uremia* is the clinical syndrome resulting from azotemia characterized by anorexia, nausea, vomiting, and mental status changes.
- The most commonly used definition of acute renal failure is an increase in the serum creatinine concentration of 0.5 mg/dL when the baseline creatinine is <3.0 mg/dL, or an increase of 1.0 mg/dL when the baseline is ≥3.0 mg/dL.

▶ PATHOPHYSIOLOGY

CLASSIFICATION

The classification of acute renal failure into broad categories based on precipitating factors facilitates diagnosis and patient management.

Prerenal Azotemia

- Prerenal acute renal failure results from hypoperfusion of the renal parenchyma, with or without systemic arterial hypotension.
  - Renal hypoperfusion with hypotension may be caused by a decline in intravascular volume (e.g., hemorrhage, dehydration) or a decline in effective blood volume (e.g., congestive heart failure, liver failure).
  - Renal hypoperfusion without hypotension most commonly results from bilateral renal artery occlusion or unilateral occlusion in a patient with a single functioning kidney.

Functional Acute Renal Failure

- Functional acute renal failure is a reversible decline in glomerular ultra-filtrate production secondary to a reduced glomerular hydrostatic pressure without damage to the kidney itself.
- The decline in glomerular hydrostatic pressure is a consequence of changes in glomerular afferent (vasoconstriction) and efferent (vasodilation) arteriolar circumference.
- This condition occurs in individuals who have reduced effective blood volume (e.g., congestive heart failure, cirrhosis, severe pulmonary disease, hypoalbuminemia) or renovascular disease (e.g., renal artery stenosis) and cannot compensate for changes in afferent or efferent arteriolar tone.

- Disorders that result in afferent arteriolar vasoconstriction include hypercalcemia and the administration of cyclosporine and NSAIDs. Decreases in efferent arteriolar resistance usually result from administration of ACE inhibitors.

Acute Intrinsic Renal Failure
- Acute intrinsic renal failure results from damage to the kidney itself and may result from:
  - Small vessel vasculitis (e.g., polyarteritis nodosa, hemolytic uremic syndrome, malignant hypertension) or cholesterol emboli to small vessels.
  - Acute glomerular inflammation (acute glomerulonephritis) from a variety of precipitating causes (e.g., systemic lupus erythematosus, antiglomerular basement membrane disease).
  - Renal tubular injury secondary to ischemia (e.g., from severe hypotension or vasoconstricting drugs) or exogenous toxins (e.g., contrast agents, heavy metals, aminoglycosides, amphotericin B, foscarnet) and endogenous toxins (e.g., myoglobin, hemoglobin, uric acid). Acute intrinsic renal failure secondary to tubular injury is referred to as acute tubular necrosis (ATN).
  - Acute interstitial nephritis (e.g., from medications or infections).

Postrenal Obstruction
- Bladder outlet obstruction (e.g., from benign prostatic hyperplasia or cervical cancer) is the most common cause of obstructive uropathy.
- Crystal deposition within the tubules (e.g., secondary to uric acid, sulfonamide, or oxalate) and ureteral obstruction (e.g., secondary to shed renal papilla or calculi) are infrequent causes.

CLINICAL COURSE
- Pathophysiologic processes can affect the four basic components of the kidney: the vasculature, the glomeruli, the tubules, and the interstitium surrounding the other three parts. The clinical manifestations of acute renal failure differ depending upon which of the component parts are involved.
- Many texts divide the clinical course of ATN into an initial, oliguric, and recovery phase, but the utility of this approach is questionable because recovery from acute tubular necrosis does not begin at a defined time from onset of renal failure. Rather, recovery from ATN occurs 10–14 days after the last insult to the kidney. Treatment with nephrotoxins may delay the recovery process, and renal vasoconstriction results in continued reduced blood flow to the nephron even after the insult to the kidneys is removed and the tubules begin recovering. Actual improvements in glomerular filtration rate will not be manifested until tubular cell necrosis is repaired and renal blood flow is normalized.

XIV ◄

▶ CLINICAL PRESENTATION

- A change in voiding habits (increased urinary frequency or nocturia) suggests a urinary concentrating defect.
- A decrease in the force of the urinary stream may suggest an obstructive process.
- The presence of cola-colored urine, indicating the presence of blood in the urine, is common in acute glomerulonephritis. If the accompanying proteinuria is heavy, the patient may note excessive foaming of the urine in the toilet.
- The onset of bilateral flank pain may suggest swelling of the kidneys secondary to either acute glomerulonephritis or acute interstitial nephritis.
- Recent onset of severe headaches may suggest the development of hypertension as a result of acute renal failure.
- A recent increase in weight secondary to salt and water retention also may be helpful in defining the onset of renal failure.

▶ DIAGNOSIS

- Rapid determination of the etiology of acute renal failure is essential; a delay may result in a more severe nephrologic injury.

MEDICAL HISTORY AND PHYSICAL EXAMINATION (Table 78.1)

- The medical history, previous laboratory data, and recent medication use of the patient may suggest whether the renal failure is acute or chronic.
- Significant renal injury can occur prior to an increase in the serum creatinine, so clinicians must pay careful attention to subtle changes in weight, blood pressure, and urine output to diagnose the onset of acute renal failure.
- Acute anuria (<50 mL urine production/24 hours) is either secondary to complete urinary obstruction or a catastrophic event (e.g., shock). Oliguria (≤400 mL urine production/24 hours) suggests prerenal azotemia, functional acute renal failure, or acute intrinsic renal failure. Nonoliguric renal failure (>400 mL urine production/24 hours) usually results from acute intrinsic renal failure or incomplete urinary obstruction.
- Common physical findings in patients with acute renal failure are listed in Table 78.1.

LABORATORY EVALUATION

- Urinalysis revealing a high urinary specific gravity, in the absence of glucosuria or mannitol administration, suggests an intact urinary concentrating mechanism and prerenal azotemia or functional acute renal failure. The presence of proteinuria and hematuria indicates a glomerular injury. Glucosuria, aminoaciduria, and phosphaturia are associated with acute proximal tubular dysfunction. A benign urine sediment sug-

TABLE 78.1. Physical Examination Findings in Acute Renal Failure

Physical Examination Finding	Clinical Implication If Present	Possible Diagnoses	Category of Acute Renal Failure	Possible Confounding Factors
Vital Signs				
Orthostatic hypotension	Intravascular volume status	Volume depletion	Prerenal azotemia	Antihypertensive therapy Neuropathies (diabetes mellitus)
Skin				
Tenting	Volume status	Volume depletion	Prerenal azotemia	Advanced age
Rash	Allergic reaction	Hypersensitivity reaction	Acute interstitial nephritis	Contact dermatitis
Petechiae	Platelet dysfunction	Thrombotic thrombocytopenic purpura Hemolytic uremic syndrome Sepsis	Acute intrinsic renal failure— vasculitis	Bone marrow suppression Antiplatelet drugs
Splinter hemorrhages Janeway lesions Osler's nodes	Embolic phenomenon	Endocarditis	Acute intrinsic renal failure—acute Glomerulonephritis	Small vessel vasculitis
Edema	Volume status	Total body volume overload	Suggests prerenal azotemia unlikely	Right heart failure, deep venous thrombosis
HEENT				
Hollenhorst plaque	Embolic phenomenon	Cholesterol emboli	Acute intrinsic renal failure—vascular	Plaque must be in aorta to affect kidney
Roth spots	Embolic phenomenon	Endocarditis	Acute intrinsic renal failure— Glomerulonephritis	Other systemic infection

(continued)

XIV

973

TABLE 78.1. continued

Physical Examination Finding	Clinical Implication If Present	Possible Diagnoses	Category of Acute Renal Failure	Possible Confounding Factors
Heart				
S₃ heart sound	Left ventricular dysfunction	Congestive heart failure	Prerenal azotemia	Preexisting compensated congestive heart failure (CHF)
New murmur (particularly diastolic murmurs)	Valvular dysfunction	Endocarditis	Acute intrinsic renal failure—acute Glomerulonephritis	Preexisting valvular disease Hyperdynamic state
Lung				
Rales	Pulmonary congestion	Pulmonary edema with volume overload or left ventricular dysfunction	Prerenal azotemia	Compensated CHF
Abdomen				
Renal artery bruit	Arterial integrity	Renal artery stenosis	Prerenal azotemia	Generalized atherosclerosis
Ascites	Elevated venous pressure	Liver failure or right heart failure	Prerenal azotemia Hepatorenal syndrome	Peritoneal membrane disorder (tumor)
Bladder distention	Bladder capacity	Bladder outlet obstruction	Postobstruction renal failure	
GU				
Prostatic enlargement	Prostate enlargement	Prostatic hypertrophy or cancer	Postobstruction renal failure	Nonenlarged prostate does not exclude obstruction
GYN				
Abnormal bimanual exam	Uterine size Cervical status	Bilateral ureteral obstruction or cervical cancer	Postobstruction renal failure	

gests prerasal azotemia, functional acute renal failure, or urinary obstruction. The presence of red blood cells and red blood cell casts indicates a glomerular injury. The finding of white blood cells and white blood cell casts results from interstitial inflammation (i.e., interstitial nephritis), which can be secondary to an allergic, granulomatous, or infectious process.

- Simultaneous measurement of serum and urinary chemistries is often helpful in determining the etiology (Table 78.2). The equation for the calculation of the fractional excretion of sodium is:

$$FE_{Na} = (U_{Na} \times P_{Cr} \times 100)/(U_{Cr} \times P_{Na})$$

where U_{Na} = urine sodium, P_{Cr} = plasma creatinine, U_{Cr} = urine creatinine, and P_{Na} = plasma sodium.

- A low urinary sodium concentration and low FE_{Na} (<1%) in a patient with oliguria is characteristic of prerenal azotemia or functional acute renal failure; a FE_{Na} >1–2% suggests acute intrinsic renal failure.

- A highly concentrated urine (>500 mOsm/L) suggests stimulation of antidiuretic hormone, indicating prerenal azotemia secondary to either hypovolemia or a decrease in effective blood volume; the urine creatinine to serum creatinine ratio usually exceeds 40.

- Estimation of glomerular filtration rate is difficult because this patient population is usually not in a steady-state situation. Methods of estimating the glomerular filtration rate and creatinine clearance from serum creatinine determinations (e.g., Cockcroft–Gault, Jelliffe equa-

TABLE 78.2. Diagnostic Parameters for Differentiating Causes of Acute Renal Failure[a]

Lab Test	Prerenal Azotemia	Acute Intrinsic Renal Failure	Postrenal Obstruction
Urine sediment	Normal	Casts, cellular debris	Cellular debris
Urinary RBC	None	2–4+	Variable
Urinary WBC	None	2–4+	1+
Urine sodium	<20	>40	>40
FE_{Na} (%)	<1	>1–2	Variable
Urine osmolality/ Serum osmolality	>1.5	<1.3	<1.5
Urine creatinine/ Plasma creatinine	>40:1	<20:1	<20:1
BUN/S_{Cr}	>20	15	15

[a]Common laboratory tests are listed that are used to classify the cause of acute renal failure. Functional acute renal failure, which is not included in this table, would have laboratory values similar to those seen in prerenal azotemia. However, the urine osmolality to plasma osmolality ratios may not exceed 1.5 depending on the circulating levels of antidiuretic hormone. The laboratory results listed under acute intrinsic renal failure are those seen in acute tubular necrosis, the most common cause of acute intrinsic renal failure.

XIV

tions) assume the patient has stable renal function. Creatinine clearance can be estimated in patients with acute renal failure using equations specially designed for nonsteady-state conditions.

DIAGNOSTIC PROCEDURES

- In hospitalized patients with previously normal renal function, insertion of a urinary catheter into the bladder is usually adequate to exclude postrenal obstruction as the cause.
- For outpatients presenting with acute renal failure, renal ultrasound is instrumental in determining whether the renal failure is acute or chronic and whether obstruction is present.
- A plain film radiograph of the abdomen will document the presence of two kidneys and also provide a check for renal stones.
- If the possibility of renal artery obstruction exists, a radioisotope scan or renal angiography may be required.
- Cystoscopy with retrograde pyelography may be helpful if the possibility of obstruction exists.
- Intravenous pyelography is rarely used in the diagnostic work-up of acute renal failure.
- A percutaneous renal biopsy may be indicated if the etiology of the acute renal failure is unclear despite a careful history, physical examination, and the above diagnostic tests.

▶ DESIRED OUTCOME

The goals of therapy are to identify and remove the underlying cause, if possible, to prevent progression to irreversible renal injury, and provide adequate metabolic, electrolyte, and fluid control until recovery.

▶ TREATMENT

PREVENTION OF ACUTE RENAL FAILURE

- Preventive therapy should be instituted in patients who are at risk for developing acute renal failure and are about to receive known nephrotoxins or procedures likely to induce nephrotoxicity.
- The simplest and most effective method of acute renal failure prevention is to ensure that the patient is adequately hydrated (e.g., with 0.45% or 0.9% NaCl) prior to nephrotoxic events. Adequate hydration improves renal perfusion, lowers tubular workload by reducing the need for urinary concentration, and dilutes the nephrotoxin concentration within the tubule.
- Sodium loading prior to the scheduled nephrotoxic event (e.g., amphotericin therapy) enhances the tubular glomerular reflex. The increased delivery of sodium chloride reduces renal blood flow, glomerular filtration rate, and tubular flow, decreasing the amount of the nephrotoxin delivered to the distal nephron.

XIV

- Diuretics increase tubule fluid flow and may prevent tubular obstruction from cellular debris, which is often associated with vasoconstriction and a reduced glomerular filtration rate. Loop diuretics increase renal blood flow via their vasodilating effects, which may be beneficial in the prevention of acute renal failure. Mannitol, an osmotic diuretic, may reduce tubular cell damage by acting as an impermeable solute that reduces cell swelling. Although diuretic therapy has potential benefits, most controlled trials found no benefit to these treatments, and some studies have found that preventive diuretic therapy may increase the incidence of acute renal failure. Overaggressive preventive diuresis can result in hypovolemia and may induce or worsen acute renal failure. Adequate hydration and tissue perfusion is probably of more value than diuretic use in this setting.
- Low-dose dopamine (1–3 µg/kg/min) selectively increases renal blood flow, but pretreatment has been shown to be ineffective in preventing radiocontrast-induced nephropathy in patients with chronic renal insufficiency.
- Calcium channel blocker administration prior to the nephrotoxic insult may be a promising prophylactic therapy. These drugs inhibit the vasoconstrictive response of the afferent arterioles of the kidney to vasoconstrictive agonists, and a subsequent increase in glomerular filtration occurs because the efferent arterioles are relatively resistant to the vasodilating effects of the drug.

PHARMACOLOGIC TREATMENT OF ACUTE RENAL FAILURE

- The initial treatment of acute renal failure should be to alleviate the underlying cause, when possible.
- Because the most common cause of acute renal failure in the hospital setting is ATN from renal hypoxia, immediate attention should be given to improving renal oxygenation and perfusion through the use of oxygen and hydration. Once fluid repletion has been accomplished, sodium and fluid restriction may be necessary to avoid fluid overload in oliguric patients. Identifiable nephrotoxins such as amphotericin B and the aminoglycosides should be avoided if possible. Other important supportive therapies include adequate nutrition and renal replacement therapy.
- Diuretics are the most common therapy used to change the status from oliguria to nonoliguria, but most studies have shown that diuretics do not improve patient outcome in established acute renal failure. However, secondary considerations such as increased urine output and reduced need for renal replacement therapy have been documented with diuretic use. Use of mannitol or loop diuretics in the early reversible phase of acute renal failure may improve survival.
  - When given in equipotent doses, the parenteral loop diuretics furosemide, bumetanide, and torsemide have similar efficacy in acute renal failure. The equipotency ratio of parenteral bumetanide:

XIV

TABLE 78.3. Agents Used in the Treatment of Acute Renal Failure

Agent	Adult Dosage	Special Considerations
Furosemide	100 mg IV; if no response within 1 hour, give 240 mg IV; if urine output follows, give 5–50 mg/h continuous infusion or 500–1500 mg/d in divided doses to maintain urine output	Other IV loop diuretics probably offer no additional benefit. Monitor urine output and serum electrolytes. Infuse ≤4 mg/min to avoid ototoxicity.
Metolazone	10 mg PO Q12h can be given along with loop diuretic therapy to increase urine output	If patient cannot take oral meds, IV chlorothiazide 500 mg Q12h can be used. Same monitoring as for furosemide.
Mannitol (20%)	12.5–25 g IV over 3–5 min, may repeat in 1 hour if no response; if urine output follows, give 20 mL/h mannitol 20% along with furosemide	Monitor patient's fluid status, urine output, and serum electrolytes. Serum osmolality >310 mOsm/L is contraindication for mannitol therapy.
Dopamine	1–5 µg/kg/min IV	Monitor urine output, blood pressure, IV site for extravasation.

torsemide:furosemide in patients with normal renal function is 1:20:40, but in renal failure this ratio changes to 1:11:11.

- Nearly all studies in acute renal failure were conducted with furosemide, and it is commonly used for reasons of familiarity and cost. Adult dosage is contained in Table 78.3. Response to an initial dose of furosemide should be followed with subsequent intermittent dosing or the institution of a continuous infusion. Continuous infusion may result in an improved, titratable, diuretic response.
- Combination therapy with a loop diuretic and a diuretic from a different pharmacologic class and with a different mechanism of action can be effective in overcoming diuretic resistance. Diuretics that work at the distal convoluted tubule (thiazides) or the collecting duct (amiloride, triamterene, spironolactone) may have a synergistic effect when administered with loop diuretics by blocking compensatory increases in sodium and chloride reabsorption. Metolazone is commonly used because, unlike other thiazides, it produces effective diuresis at glomerular filtration rates below 20 mL/min.
- Low-dose dopamine infusions combined with diuretics may increase urine output in poor responders to diuretics alone, but the combination has not been documented to improve survival.
- Administration of calcium channel blockers early in the course of acute renal failure in an attempt to prevent mitochondrial changes and cell death may ultimately be shown to be beneficial.

XIV

COMPLICATIONS OF ACUTE RENAL FAILURE

Hyperkalemia

- The clinical presentation, diagnosis, and treatment of hyperkalemia are included in Chapter 77.

Infection

- Infection is the most common cause of death in patients with acute renal failure.
- Acute renal failure contributes to the high infection rate by altering leukocyte function and cell-mediated immunity.
- Indwelling vascular or peritoneal access devices and indwelling urinary catheters also predispose patients to infection.
- Critically ill patients with acute renal failure often have failures of other organ systems that predispose them to infection.
- Concomitant cardiopulmonary failure necessitating mechanical ventilation increases the risk of pneumonia.
- High-dose vasopressor therapy results in reduced blood flow to the gastrointestinal (GI) tract, which may cause ischemia and introduction of gut flora to the bloodstream.
- Management of infection requires aggressive antibiotic therapy that has been adjusted appropriately for renal disease and renal replacement therapy.

Cardiovascular

- Hypertension, hypotension, heart failure, pericarditis, arrhythmias, and pulmonary edema all may be associated with acute renal failure.
- Causes include electrolyte disturbances, impaired acid base balance, uremia, and volume overload.
- Volume overload may be best treated with diuretics and renal replacement therapy.
- Aggressive renal replacement therapy can also alleviate uremic pericarditis and electrolyte and acid–base disorders.

Gastrointestinal

- Hypotension, vasoconstrictive agents, and a high catabolic state can contribute to stress ulceration and GI bleeding. The uremic state also may induce bleeding by causing a defect in platelet function.
- Other common GI complaints in patients with acute renal failure include nausea and vomiting associated with uremia and electrolyte imbalances.

Neurologic

- The neurologic sequelae associated with uremia may include altered mentation, myoclonus, and lethargy.
- Other causes of neurologic symptoms include electrolyte (calcium, phosphate, and sodium) disturbances.
- Adverse effects from improperly dosed, renally eliminated drugs can also manifest as seizures or somnolence.

XIV

RENAL REPLACEMENT THERAPIES

- The most common reasons to begin renal replacement therapy in acute renal failure are for control of azotemia, hyperkalemia, and fluid overload. The advantages and disadvantages of intermittent and continuous renal replacement therapies are listed in Table 78.4. (Also see Chapter 75.)
- Hemodialysis is effective for azotemic control, but it must be performed 5–6 times per week to achieve control similar to that achieved by some continuous therapies.
- Peritoneal dialysis is relatively easy to perform once the dialysis catheter is placed into the peritoneum, but it is not very efficient for volume and solute removal and can provide a large glucose load to the patient.
- Continuous hemofiltration and hemodiafiltration are more technically difficult and require more nursing time to perform but provide improved fluid and metabolic control, especially in patients unable to tolerate hemodialysis. Continuous therapies are generally better tolerated because the fluid and electrolyte shifts are more gradual than with the intermittent therapies.
- Hemofiltration is more effective than dialytic therapies in the removal of large molecular weight substances.
  - With continuous arteriovenous hemofiltration (CAVH), ultrafiltrate production is dependent on cardiovascular status, which frequently yields adequate volume control but inadequate solute removal in critically ill patients. However, no special machinery is needed to conduct CAVH, making it a widely used renal replacement modality.
  - Continuous venovenous hemofiltration (CVVH) does not require arterial access but uses pumps to move blood through the circuit and to regulate ultrafiltrate production. This increase in complexity, compared to CAVH, is balanced by more effective volume and solute control in patients with acute renal failure.
  - The most common method of hemodiafiltration, continuous venovenous hemodiafiltration (CVVHD), provides the most solute removal of any of the continuous therapies but requires more complex machinery and increased training for intensive care unit personnel.

▶ EVALUATION OF THERAPEUTIC OUTCOMES

- Close monitoring of the patient's status is essential during the recovery period, which may occur quickly, within a few months, or never.
- Azotemic control can be assessed in the physical examination by looking for signs of uremia. The sound of a friction rub on chest examination can be a sign of a pericardial effusion caused by uremia. Fluid status should be assessed by checking lung sounds and inspecting for edema. Rales can be indicative of pulmonary edema secondary to fluid overload.

XIV

TABLE 78.4. Advantages and Disadvantages of Common Renal Replacement Therapies for Acute Renal Failure

	Intermittent Hemodialysis	Intermittent Hemofiltration	Peritoneal Dialysis	Slow Continuous Ultrafiltration (SCUF)	Continuous Arteriovenous Hemofiltration (CAVH)	Continuous Venovenous Hemofiltration (CVVH)	Continuous Arteriovenous Hemodiafiltration (CAVHD)	Continuous Venovenous Hemodiafiltration (CVVHD)
Solute control	Usually adequate	Inadequate	Inadequate	Inadequate	Inadequate	Adequate	Adequate	Adequate
Volume control	Variable	Adequate	Adequate	Adequate	Adequate	Adequate	Adequate	Adequate
Hemodynamic stability	Variable	Well tolerated	Well tolerated	Well tolerated	Well tolerated	Well tolerated	Well tolerated	Well tolerated
Access	Venous	Venous	Peritoneal	Arterial and venous	Arterial and venous	Venous	Arterial and venous	Venous
Anticoagulation	Short duration	Short duration	None	Continuous high dose	Continuous low dose	Continuous high dose	Continuous low dose	Continuous
Technical complexity	High	High	Low	Low	Low	Moderate	Moderate	High
Workload	Intermittent	Intermittent	Low	Low	Low	Moderate	Moderate	High
Drug dosing ease	Many published recommendations	Difficult	Difficult	Negligible drug removal	Difficult	Many published recommendations	Difficult	Difficult
Convective clearance (small and middle molecules)	Mixed	Minimal	Moderate	Moderate	Large	Large	Large	Large
Dialytic clearance (small molecules)	Large	None	Large	None	None	None	Large	Large
Common complications	Hypotension	Hypotension	Hyperglycemia, atelectasis, peritonitis	Arterial bleeding, hypotension	Arterial bleeding, filter clotting	Hypotension	Arterial bleeding, ↑ serum lactate	↑ Serum lactate, hypotension

- Measurements of daily weight and fluid intake/output help gauge day-to-day recovery, especially in patients receiving continuous hemofiltration or hemodiafiltration. Urine output may be the best single test to assess recovery from acute renal failure.
- Critically ill patients with acute renal failure frequently receive continuous hemodynamic monitoring via a Swan–Ganz catheter to assess fluid status and determine fluid replacement needs.
- Urine collection and measurement of urinary creatinine may be beneficial to assess changes in renal function. Urinalysis also can help discern the cause of acute renal failure, so attention should be given to the presence of urinary sediment, specific gravity, and sodium concentration in order to decide on a therapy to treat the cause of the acute renal failure. Blood urea nitrogen and creatinine measurements are useful, but creatinine clearance calculations may be unreliable in patients with changing serum creatinine values.
- Therapeutic drug monitoring should be performed frequently, not only because these patients are not at steady state, but also because of the paucity of data regarding drug disposition in acute renal failure.
- Serum electrolytes should be monitored daily with particular attention given to potassium, phosphorus, and calcium in early acute renal failure.
- Arterial blood gas determinations can help determine the respiratory status of critically ill patients and assess whether the kidney is able to compensate for any acid–base disturbances.
- Monitoring parameters for agents used in the treatment of acute renal failure are listed in Table 78.3.
- Peritoneal and vascular access sites should be monitored routinely for signs of infection (erythema or purulent drainage). Frequent evaluation of urine for signs of infection is warranted.

See Chapter 43, Acute Renal Failure, authored by Bruce A. Mueller, PharmD, BCPS, and William L. Macias, MD, PhD, for a more detailed discussion of this topic.

XIV

Chapter 79

► RENAL FAILURE: CHRONIC

► DEFINITION

Chronic renal failure is a progressive process that may occur even when the primary renal insult has been corrected or treated, or become inactive. Adaptive mechanisms may play a major role as evidenced by the common histologic appearance of kidneys from patients with end-stage renal disease (ESRD). Although progression is a continuous process, categoric classifications of patients are often utilized to guide decision making.

► OVERVIEW

PATHOPHYSIOLOGY

- Many diseases of the kidney, either idiopathic or secondary to systemic illness, ultimately result in ESRD. Overall, the incidence of patients starting ESRD therapy has increased 8.8% annually with the largest increase in the 65- to 74-year old population.
- Diabetes and hypertension are the most common causes of ESRD in the United States (Figure 79.1). Hyperlipidemia is also a major risk factor associated with progression of renal disease.
- As renal disease progresses, adaptations take place in functioning (remnant) nephrons that blunt the drop in total glomerular filtration rate (GFR). Changes in other renal functions, (e.g., hydroxylation of vitamin D), however, are not preserved.
- Although there are multiple primary causes of renal injury, adaptive hyperfiltration ultimately contributes to glomerular hypertension, which plays a significant role in progressive loss of renal function. When serum creatinine rises above 2 mg/dL or creatinine clearance (Cr Cl) falls to approximately 60 mL/min, injury usually progresses to end-stage renal disease (ESRD) regardless of the primary etiology of kidney disease.
- Although exact pathogenic mechanisms have not been identified, hemodynamic changes at the glomerulus influence and/or regulate progression of renal disease. Increased glomerular capillary plasma flow and glomerular capillary hydraulic pressure lead to glomerular hyperfiltration. Glomerular hyperfiltration and hypertension lead to progressive glomerular sclerosis and development of overt proteinuria. Systemic hypertension is not required for development of glomerular hyperfiltration and hypertension but, when present, may amplify the pathologic effects of intrarenal changes.

CLINICAL MANIFESTATIONS

- Clinical course of progressive renal disease can be divided into four stages. Accompanying signs and symptoms and laboratory parameters are described in Figure 79.2.

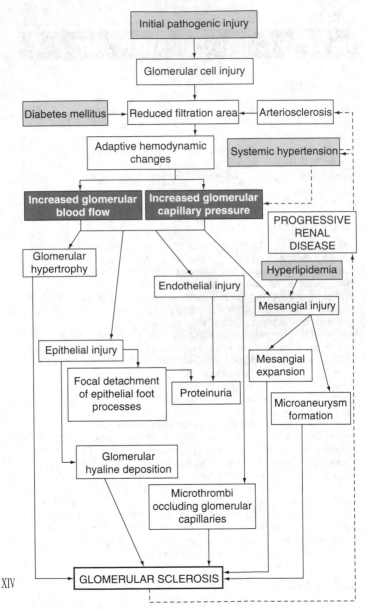

Figure 79.1. Proposed mechanisms of progressive glomerular sclerosis in chronic renal failure.

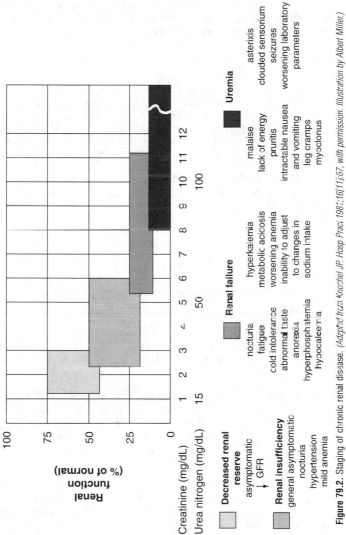

Figure 79.2. Staging of chronic renal disease. (Adapted from Knochel JP. Hosp Pract 1981;16(11):67, with permission. Illustration by Albert Miller.)

Renal function (% of normal)

100 — 75 — 50 — 25 — 0

Creatinine (mg/dL): 1 2 3 4 5 6 7 8 9 10 11 12

Urea nitrogen (mg/dL): 15 — 50 — 100

Decreased renal reserve
asymptomatic
↓ GFR

Renal insufficiency
general asymptomatic
nocturia
hypertension
mild anemia

Renal failure
nocturia
fatigue
cold intolerance
abnormal taste
anorexia
hyperphosphatemia
hypocalcemia

hyperkalemia
metabolic acicosis
worsening anemia
inability to adjust
to changes in
sodium intake

Uremia
malaise
lack of energy
pruritis
intractable nausea
and vomiting
leg cramps
myoclonus

asterixis
clouded sensorium
seizures
worsening laboratory
parameters

XIV

DESIRED OUTCOME

The ultimate goal of therapy is to prevent progression of renal disease. Additional goals include the prevention and management of complications such as anemia, secondary hyperparathyroidism, hyperlipidemia, hypertension, and renal osteodystrophy.

TREATMENT

Diabetics

- Early detection of microalbuminuria in the diabetic patient facilitates therapeutic intervention that can slow progression of renal disease and other vascular complications (Figure 79.3).
- Adequate blood pressure control can reduce the rate of decline in GFR and albuminuria in hypertensive patients with either insulin-dependent or noninsulin-dependent diabetes mellitus (IDDM or NIDDM).
- Angiotensin-converting enzyme inhibitors (ACEI) have been shown to decrease proteinuria and preserve GFR independent of blood pressure control. ACEI should be started in patients with IDDM who have persistent microalbuminuria.
- Intensive blood glucose control in IDDM patients has been reported to reduce the frequency, decrease severity, and delay development or progression of diabetic complications, including nephropathy, in several randomized clinical trials (see Chapter 17).
- Correction of lipid abnormalities in patients with renal damage may be important in retarding the progression of renal disease (see section on Hyperlipidemia).

Non-diabetics

- Non-diabetic renal disease is often considered collectively, but these disease states (e.g., hypertensive nephrosclerosis, glomerular and tubulointerstitial disease, and polycystic kidney disease) may respond differently to treatment.
- A low-protein diet is of questionable benefit in patients with moderate renal impairment (GFR = 25–55 mL/min/1.73 m^2), so a standard protein diet (>0.8 g/kg/d) should be followed unless there is rapid progression of renal failure or uremia. For severe renal impairment (GFR = 13–24 mL/min/1.73 m^2), a low-protein diet of 0.6 g/kg/d may reduce the rate of decline in renal function, time to reach ESRD, and onset of uremic symptoms.
- Pharmacologic treatment of hypertension in non-diabetic patients delays the progression of renal disease. In most studies, renal function remained stable, or the rate of decline was reduced, but more follow-up is needed to confirm that short-term benefits persist.

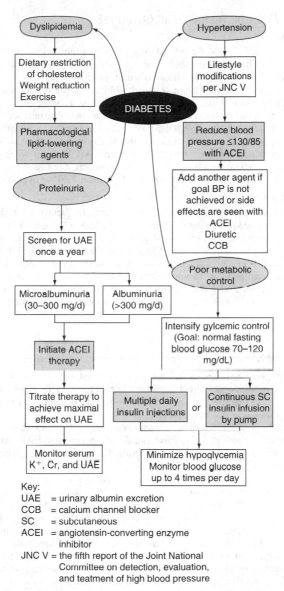

Key:
UAE = urinary albumin excretion
CCB = calcium channel blocker
SC = subcutaneous
ACEI = angiotensin-converting enzyme inhibitor
JNC V = the fifth report of the Joint National Committee on detection, evaluation, and teatment of high blood pressure

XIV

Figure 79.3. Therapeutic strategies to prevent progression of renal disease in diabetic individuals.

EVALUATION OF THERAPEUTIC OUTCOMES

Diabetics

- Patients with IDDM for >5–10 years, and/or a family history of renal disease or hypertension should be screened every year for microalbuminuria (annual UAE or urinary albumin-to-creatinine ratio).
- Blood glucose should be maintained within, or close to, normal range either by frequent insulin injections or use of an insulin pump.
- If there are no contraindications, ACEI therapy should be initiated in normotensive or hypertensive IDDM patients with persistent microalbuminuria or overt albuminuria (>300 mg/d). ACEI should be titrated every 1 to 3 months to achieve a maximal effect on UAE. Within 1 week of initiating or increasing a dose of an ACEI, serum creatinine and potassium should be evaluated to detect abrupt reductions in GFR or hyperkalemia.

Non-diabetics

- Nutritional management should be monitored frequently, regardless of the prescribed protein intake, to avoid malnutrition (Figure 79.4). Nutrition goals are serum albumin >4 g/dL and transferrin >200 mg/dL.
- Blood pressure control should target normotensive levels (130/80–85 mm Hg). If proteinuria >1 g/d is present and there are no contraindications, blood pressure should be reduced to 125/75 mm Hg. If a patient has proteinuria >3 g/d and chronic renal failure, ACEI and perhaps calcium channel blockers should be considered as first-line therapy.

▶ HYPERTENSION

TREATMENT

- All hypertensive agents do not preserve renal function to the same degree despite equal blood pressure control (Table 79.1). Antihypertensive agents that maintain renal blood flow, reduce glomerular pressure, and proteinuria are preferred.
- Regardless of the regimen, hypertension should be controlled. If proteinuria is present, ACEI and nondihydropyridine calcium channel blockers may be superior to conventional treatment in decreasing proteinuria and glomerular hypertension.
- Hyperkalemia can complicate ACEI use, especially in diabetics or those using nonsteroidal anti-inflammatory agents. Except for fosinopril, the half-lives of ACEI (or active metabolites) are prolonged in renal failure and lower doses may suffice. In patients with renal insufficiency, dosage alterations are unnecessary with most calcium channel blocking agents.
- Other antihypertensive drugs may also be required to lower blood pressure in patients with ESRD, but they have not been shown to retard progression of renal failure. Drugs that interfere with renin release may be useful (e.g., β blockers or the combined α- and β-blocker, labetolol); effects of ESRD and dialysis on drug pharmacokinetics impact on choice of β blocker (see Chapter 76). Sympathetic nervous system

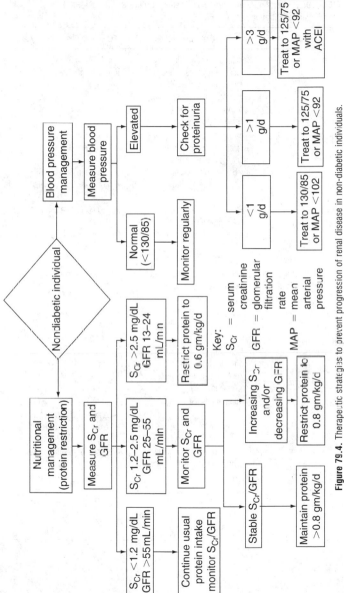

Key:
S_{Cr} = serum creatinine
GFR = glomerular filtration rate
MAP = mean arterial pressure

Figure 79.4. Therapeutic strategies to prevent progression of renal disease in non-diabetic individuals.

XIV

TABLE 79.1. Effects of Antihypertensive Agents on Renal Blood Flow (RBF) and Glomerular Filtration Rate (GRF)

Antihypertensive Agent	Mechanism of Action	Effects on Renal Hemodynamics
Diuretics	Sodium and volume depletion	⇓ in GFR and RBF
	⇑ vasodilatory prostaglandin levels [intravenous (IV) loop diuretics]	⇑ in RBF
	Renal vasoconstriction (IV thiazide)	⇓ in GFR and RBF
β-Adrenergic blockers	⇓ cardiac output	⇓ in GFR and RBF
	⇑ renal vascular resistance (nonselective agents)	⇓ in GFR and RBF
	⇓ renal vascular resistance (β₁-selective agents)	No change in GFR and RBF
		⇓ or no change in microalbuminuria
Centrally acting antiadrenergic drugs	⇓ renal vascular resistance (α-methyldopa)	No change in GFR and RBF
	⇓ renal perfusion pressure (clonidine, α₂-adrenergic agonist)	GFR and RBF are preserved
Peripherally acting antiadrenergic drugs	Direct vasodilation (postsynaptic α₁-adrenoreceptor blocking agents)	No adverse effect on GFR and RBF
Direct vasodilator agents	⇓ renal vascular resistance (hydralazine, minoxidil)	⇑ in RBF and no effect on GFR
Direct vasodilator agents	Arterial vasodilation plus dilatation of venous capacitance vessels (nitroprusside) (diazoxide-less venous dilatation)	⇓ in GFR and RBF (acute effect)
ACEI	Dilation of efferent arteriole	⇑ in RBF and GFR (only in patients with hypertension, renal insufficiency, and ⇑ renin states)
	Dilatation of efferent arteriole plus inhibition of angiotensin II	⇓ glomerular capillary pressure
Calcium channel blockers	⇓ renal vascular resistance by vasodilation of afferent arterioles (hypertensive patients)	⇑ in RBF ⇑/no change in GFR
	⇓ renal vasoconstriction (isolated perfused kidney)	⇑ in RBF and GFR

XIV

active agents (e.g., prazosin, terazosin, doxazosin, clonidine, guanabenz, or guanfacine) may be required in patients unresponsive to dialytic therapy plus ACEI, calcium channel blocker, or β-blocker therapy. Adding vasodilators (e.g., minoxidil or hydralazine) may be useful in patients resistant to previously mentioned agents; most patients require a β blocker or a central α adenoreceptor agonist to suppress minoxidil-induced reflex tachycardia.

EVALUATION OF THERAPEUTIC OUTCOMES

- Achievement of an individual's "dry weight" should be attempted (Figure 79.5). Control of total body sodium via dialysis normalizes blood pressure in 50–60% of patients with ESRD.
- Precipitous falls in blood pressure to normotensive levels may be acutely deleterious to renal function in patients with impaired renal function. Target blood pressure should be achieved reasonably slowly to allow adaptation to reduced perfusion pressures.

▶ END-STAGE RENAL DISEASE

PATHOPHYSIOLOGY

- No single toxin is responsible for all of the abnormalities associated with ESRD. The clinical picture likely results from an interplay of multiple factors.
- Organic compounds known to accumulate in uremia include metabolic by-products of protein metabolism, and biologically and endogenous active substances (e.g., parathyroid hormone and atrial natriuretic peptide, gastrin, growth hormone, glucagon, somatostatin, prolactin, calcitonin, and insulin).
- Uremic syndrome is most likely caused by retention of by-products of protein metabolism because many manifestations can be improved with protein restriction.

CLINICAL PRESENTATION

- Renal osteodystrophy (bone disease) is a common manifestation of chronic renal disease (discussed later in this chapter)
- Hematologic complications of chronic renal failure include nor mochromic, normocytic anemia secondary to decreased erythropoietin production (discussed later in this chapter), and prolonged bleeding time and a bleeding diathesis due to platelet dysfunction.
- Sodium retention leads to volume expansion, which can result in volume overload and cardiovascular (e.g., pulmonary edema) and pulmonary complications (e.g., noncardiogenic pulmonary edema).
- Common gastrointestinal (GI) complications of chronic renal failure include anorexia, hiccups, and a metallic taste in the mouth. Nausea, vomiting, diarrhea, abdominal distention, and GI bleeding may also occur.

XIV

991

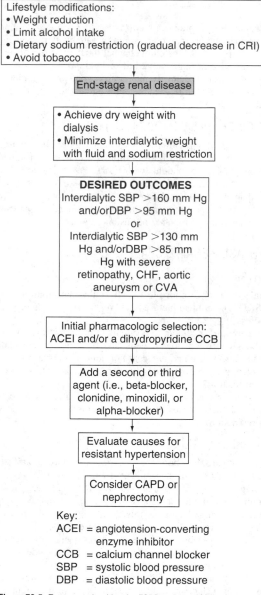

Key:
ACEI = angiotension-converting
enzyme inhibitor
CCB = calcium channel blocker
SBP = systolic blood pressure
DBP = diastolic blood pressure

Figure 79.5. Treatment algorithm for ESRD patients with hypertension.

- Uremic toxins may increase neuromuscular irritability and result in leg cramps, restless leg syndrome, and reversal of the sleep–wake cycle. Uremic toxins can induce peripheral neuropathy. Uremic encephalopathy is manifested by clouded sensorium, coma, seizures, myoclonic jerks, and asterixis.
- Endocrine and metabolic abnormalities are common in ESRD. Most patients are clinically hypothyroid (i.e., low energy, cold intolerance, constipation). Hyperglycemia secondary to peripheral resistance to insulin can occur. Primary hypogonadism and hypothalamic abnormalities contribute to sexual dysfunction and sterility.
- Common dermatologic manifestations of uremia include dry, flaking skin and generalized pruritus, which is not consistently alleviated by any single therapeutic modality.
- Infectious diseases are common and result in significant morbidity and mortality in patients with chronic renal failure/ESRD.

TREATMENT

- Dialysis, discussed in Chapter 75.

▶ RENAL OSTEODYSTROPHY AND SECONDARY HYPERPARATHYROIDISM

PATHOPHYSIOLOGY

- Calcium and phosphorus balance is mediated through a complex interplay of hormones and their effects on bone, GI tract, kidney, and parathyroid gland. Phosphate retention inhibits renal activation (C_1-α hydroxylation) of vitamin D, which in turn reduces gut absorption of calcium. Low blood calcium concentration stimulates parathyroid hormone (PTH) secretion. As functional renal mass declines, serum calcium balance can only be maintained at the expense of increased bone resorption (Figure 79.6).
- Secondary hyperparathyroidism can result in osteitis fibrosa cystica, which is characterized by high bone-formation rate.
- Two additional types of metabolic bone disease are frequently associated with ESRD. Osteomalacia is characterized by a high volume of osteoid tissue and impaired calcification of new bone. A dynamic bone disease is characterized by low bone-formation rates, which results from aluminum toxicity, peritoneal dialysis with high dialysate calcium concentrations along with high doses of calcium-containing phosphate binders, aggressive vitamin D therapy, diabetes, and advanced age.
- Although once a major problem, aluminum toxicity occurs less frequently due to use of deionizers and reverse osmosis filters for dialysate water purification and decreased use of aluminum phosphate binders.

XIV ◀

993

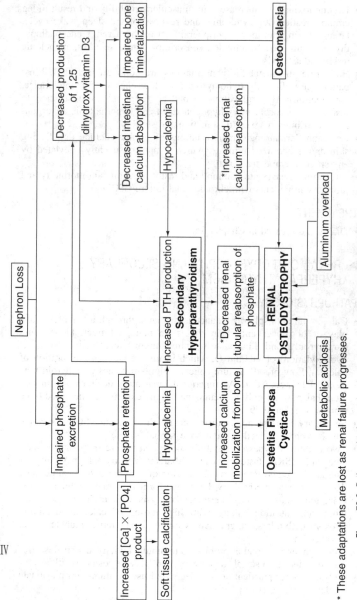

* These adaptations are lost as renal failure progresses.

Figure 79.6. Pathogenesis of secondary hyperparathyroidism and renal osteodystrophy in patients with chronic renal failure.

XIV

CLINICAL MANIFESTATIONS

- Excess PTH promotes progression of osteitis fibrosa cystica and may adversely affect lipid metabolism, myocardial and skeletal muscle, and neurologic function. Common signs and symptoms include fatigue and musculoskeletal and GI complaints.
- Hyperphosphatemia can lead to metastatic calcification of joints, vessels, and soft tissue.
- Although bone symptoms are rare in mild to moderate renal impairment, bone pain and skeletal fractures are characteristic of advanced renal osteodystrophy.

DIAGNOSIS

- Although transiliac bone biopsy is the gold standard for evaluation of renal osteodystrophy, this biopsy is infrequently performed because it is invasive.
- Bone mineral densitometry studies are used to monitor therapeutic intervention.
- Serum calcium, phosphorous, PTH, alkaline phosphatase, and osteocalcin are useful biochemical markers and the primary markers of renal osteodystrophy.

TREATMENT

- Dietary phosphorus restriction (6.5–12.0 mg/kg/d) should be initiated in patients with Cr Cl <50 mL/min.
- By the time ESRD develops, most patients require a combination of phosphate-binding medication and/or vitamin D therapy to prevent development of secondary hyperparathyroidism, renal osteodystrophy, and metastatic calcification.

Phosphate-Binding Agents

- Phosphate-binding agents decrease phosphorus absorption from the intestine and should be administered with meals to maximize this effect.
- Despite availability of many phosphate-binding medications (Table 79.2), none is ideal.
- Oral calcium compounds have emerged as first-line agents for controlling both serum phosphorus and calcium concentrations. Calcium salts have the potential advantage of partially correcting metabolic acidosis and increasing ionized calcium concentrations, thereby decreasing PTH secretion. Calcium carbonate can normalize phosphate concentrations, but large doses (average 6–14 g/d) may be required. Calcium acetate binds approximately twice as much phosphorus as calcium carbonate, but it is more expensive and causes more nausea and diarrhea. The chloride salt is very astringent and unpalatable, and absorbed chloride may contribute to systemic acidosis. The citrate salt binds phosphate poorly in vitro and markedly increases intestinal aluminum absorption owing to the formation of soluble aluminum citrate complexes.

XIV

XIV

TABLE 79.2. Phosphate-Binding Agents Used in the Treatment of Hyperphosphatemia of Renal Failure

Agents	Calcium, Aluminum, or Magnesium Content	Dosage Form	Starting Doses	Comments
Calcium Carbonate (40% calcium)			0.5–1 g (elemental calcium) tid with meals	Dissolution characteristics and phosphate binding effect may vary from product to product. Usual maintenance dosage ranges from 2.4–5.6 g (elemental calcium) or 6–14 g (calcium carbonate) per day.
Os-Cal 500	500 mg[a]	Tablet		
Caltrate 600	600 mg	Tablet		
Nephro-Calci	600 mg	Tablet		
CalCarb HD	2400 mg/packet	Powder		
Calci-Mix	500 mg	Capsule		To be mixed with food.
Calci-Chew	500 mg	Tablet		To be mixed with food.
Tums	200, 300, 400 mg	Tablet		Chewable.
Calcium carbonate[b]	500 mg/5 mL	Suspension		Chewable.
Calcium Acetate (25% calcium)			2 tablets tid with meals	Comparable efficacy to calcium carbonate with half the dose of elemental calcium.
Phos-Lo	169 mg[a]	Tablet		
Calcium Citrate (21% calcium)			0.5–1 g (elemental calcium) tid with meals	Citrate enhances absorption of aluminum. Should not be administered concurrently with aluminum binders, antacids, or sucralfate.
Citracal	200 mg[c]	Tablet		
	500 mg	Effervescent tablet		Contains aspartame.

TABLE 79.2. continued

Aluminum Carbonate		400–500 mg tid with meals	Second line agent after calcium binders. Do not use concurrently with citrate-containing products.
Basaljel	500 mg[a]	Tablet, capsule	
	400 mg/5 mL	Suspension	
Aluminum Hydroxide		300–600 mg tid with meals	Second line agent after calcium binders. Do not use concurrently with citrate-containing products
Amphogel	300, 600 mg[c]	Tablet	
AlternaGel[b]	320 mg/5 mL	Suspension	
	600 mg/5 mL	Suspension	
Magnesium Hydroxide		300–400 mg tid with meals	Magnesium concentration in dialysate needs to be reduced to avoid hypermagnesemia. Serum magnesium concentration should be routinely monitored and kept within the normal range. Diarrhea is a common side effect.
Milk of Magnesia	300, 600 mg[a]	Tablet	
	400 mg/5 mL	Suspension	
	800 mg/5 mL	Suspension	

[a]Content represents amount of elemental calcium in product.
[b]Many other trade names and generic brands available.
[c]Content represents amount of aluminum carbonate in product.
[d]Content represents amount of aluminum hydroxide in product.
[e]Content represents amount of magnesium hydroxide in product.

XIV

997

- If necessary, magnesium- or aluminum-containing phosphate binders can be added to calcium-containing phosphate binders to optimize phosphorus control. Magnesium-containing antacids are fairly effective phosphate binders, but they may cause diarrhea and hyperkalemia. Aluminum binders are quite effective; however, they may cause constipation and require periodic monitoring of serum aluminum concentrations.

Vitamin D Therapy

- Vitamin D therapy should be added in patients who do not achieve normocalcemia or those with biochemical features of progressive bone disease despite the use of calcium-containing binders.
- Only dihydrotachysterol and 1,25-dihydroxyvitamin D_3 (calcitriol) do not require hydroxylation in the kidney to become optimally physiologically active. Calcitriol has largely replaced dihydrotachysterol because it inhibits PTH secretion directly and stimulates intestinal absorption of calcium.
- Controversy exists regarding the most effective method of administration, optimal dose, and dosage interval of calcitriol.

EVALUATION OF THERAPEUTIC OUTCOMES

- Intact or N-terminal PTH concentrations of 2.0–3.0 times normal, total calcium concentrations (corrected for albumin) of 9–11 mg/dL ([4–Albumin] • 0.8] + Serum Calcium), and serum phosphorus concentrations of 4.5–6.0 mg/dL are the goals.
- A calcium (mg/dL)-phosphorus product (mg/dL) of >70 should be avoided to lessen the risk of metastatic calcification.

▶ ANEMIA OF CHRONIC RENAL FAILURE

PATHOPHYSIOLOGY

- The primary cause of anemia in patients with chronic renal failure and ESRD is erythropoietin (EPO) deficiency (see Chapter 31). Other contributing factors include blood loss, iron, folic acid, or vitamin B_{12} deficiency, severe osteitis fibrosa, systemic infection or inflammatory illness, aluminum toxicity, or hypersplenism.

CLINICAL MANIFESTATIONS

- Signs and symptoms of fatigue, exertional dyspnea, dizziness, headache, and pallor are commonly seen even though some adaptation to a decreased hematocrit (HCT) occurs during the progression of ESRD anemia.

TREATMENT

- Epoetin is the therapy of choice for long-term correction and maintenance of HCT levels in predialysis and dialysis patients. It is reasonable to begin epoetin therapy in patients with hematocrits of <30%.
- Epoetin can be administered IV, subcutaneously, or intraperitoneally. The subcutaneous method is preferable in chronic ambulatory peri-

XIV

toneal dialysis and prehemodialysis patients because they usually do not have permanent IV access.

- The major side effect of epoetin is elevated blood pressure, which occurs in 20–33% of patients.
- Although iron management may be initiated with oral agents that have relatively high bioavailability and low cost, many centers use parenteral iron exclusively.

EVALUATION OF THERAPEUTIC OUTCOMES

- Iron balance (ferritin, >100 ng/mL; transferrin saturation, >20%) should be monitored monthly for 3 months and quarterly thereafter to maximize erythropoietic response. Recommended initial dosages of epoetin are: *Predialysis,* 90–120 U/kg subcutaneously once per week; *Hemodialysis,* 30–60 U/kg IV three times per week or 30–45 U/kg subcutaneously three times per week; *Chronic ambulatory peritoneal dialysis,* 30–45 U/kg subcutaneously three times per week, 45–60 U/kg twice per week, or 90–120 U/kg once per week.
- Once epoetin is initiated, hematocrit/hemoglobin response may be delayed for approximately 2 weeks. Following initiation of epoetin or dose change, steady-state hematocrit levels will not be attained until one red blood cell (RBC) life span has occurred (approximately 2–3 months), so epoetin doses should not be adjusted more often than every 3–4 weeks.
- The rate of rise in hematocrit should not exceed four points in any 2-week period.
- Goal hematocrit is 30–36%. Hematocrit levels should be drawn weekly on the same day each week prior to hemodialysis, or anytime during the first 3 months of peritoneal dialysis then monthly thereafter.
- Patients should be monitored for potential complications. Antihypertensive agents should be added as necessary to stabilize blood pressure. Blood pressure control (goal DBP <90 mm Hg) should be attained before starting epoetin.

▶ METABOLIC ACIDOSIS

PATHOPHYSIOLOGY

- Clinically significant metabolic acidosis is uncommonly seen before the glomerular filtration rate drops below 20 mL/min.
- Ability of the kidneys to synthesize ammonia is impaired. This decrease in urinary buffer results in decreased net acid excretion, continuous positive hydrogen ion balance, and ultimately metabolic acidosis (see Chapter 74).

CLINICAL MANIFESTATIONS

- Metabolic acidosis contributes to renal bone disease, hyperkalemia, and fatigue.

XIV

TREATMENT

- Generally, treatment should be instituted when plasma bicarbonate is <20 mEq/L.
- Alkalinizing salts such as sodium bicarbonate or citrate/citric acid preparations (e.g., Shohl's Solution and Bicitra) are useful to replenish depleted body bicarbonate stores. Alkali therapy should be initiated at 0.5 mEq/kg/d in divided doses.

► HYPERLIPIDEMIA

- Chronic renal failure with or without nephrotic syndrome is frequently accompanied by abnormalities in lipoprotein metabolism.
- It has not been proven that patients with renal disease, including nephrotic syndrome, are more or less prone to the atherogenic effects of abnormal lipoprotein patterns. In the absence of solid data in this population, it seems prudent to follow guidelines set forth by the National Cholesterol Education Program Expert Panel (see Chapter 8).

See Chapter 44, Chronic Renal Failure and End-Stage Renal Disease, authored by Wendy L. St. Peter, PharmD, BCPS, Scott W. Mihalovic, PharmD, BCPS, Marigel Vargas-Ruiz, RPh, MS, and Lawrence J. Lambrecht, PharmD, BCPS, for a more detailed discussion of this topic.

Respiratory Disorders

Edited by Terry L. Schwinghammer, PharmD, FCCP, BCPS

Chapter 80

► ALLERGIC RHINITIS

► DEFINITION

Allergic rhinitis is inflammation of the nasal mucous membrane caused by exposure to inhaled allergenic materials that elicit a specific immunologic response. There are two types:

- Seasonal: occurs in response to specific allergens present seasonally (e.g., pollens).
- Perennial: occurs year-round in response to nonseasonal allergens (e.g., dust mites, animal dander, molds); usually results in more subtle chronic symptoms.

► PATHOPHYSIOLOGY

- The initial reaction occurs when airborne allergens enter the nose and are processed by lymphocytes, which produce antigen-specific IgE, thereby sensitizing genetically predisposed hosts. On reexposure, IgE bound to mast cells interacts with the airborne allergen and triggers the release of inflammatory mediators [preformed mediators and newly generated mediators from the arachidonic acid cascade (Table 80.1)]. These mediators cause vasodilatation, increased vascular permeability, and production of nasal secretions. Histamine is probably the most important mediator.
- Several hours after the initial reaction a late-phase reaction may occur, which involves an influx of inflammatory cells (e.g., eosinophils, monocytes, macrophages, basophils) and activation of the lymphocyte population. Late-phase symptoms (nasal congestion) begin 3–5 hours after antigen exposure and peak at 12–24 hours.

► CLINICAL PRESENTATION

- Symptoms include rhinorrhea, sneezing, nasal congestion, postnasal drip, allergic conjunctivitis, and pruritic eyes, ears, or nose.
- Rhinitis symptoms may lead to insomnia, malaise, fatigue, and poor work efficiency.
- Structural facial and dental problems can result from chronic allergic rhinitis.
- Allergic rhinitis is a risk factor for asthma.
- Acute and chronic sinusitis and epistaxis are complications of allergic rhinitis.

TABLE 80.1. Mast Cell Mediators

Mediator	Effect
Preformed and Rapidly Released	
Histamine	Stimulates irritant receptors
	Pruritis
	Vascular permeability
	Mucosal permeability
	Smooth muscle contraction
Neutrophil chemotactic factor	Influx of inflammatory cells
Eosinophil chemotactic factor	Influx of inflammatory cells
Kinins	Vascular permeability
N-α-tosyl L-arginine methylesterase	Vascular permeability
Newly Generated	
Leukotrienes	Smooth muscle contraction
	Vascular permeability
	Mucus secretion
Prostaglandins	Pruritis
	Vascular permeability
	Chemotaxis
	Mucus secretion
	Neutrophil chemotaxis
Thromboxanes	Smooth muscle spasm
Platelet-activating factor	Mucus secretion
	Airway permeability
	Chemotaxis
	Vascular permeability
Granule Matrix Contents	
Heparin	Anti-inflammatory
Tryptase	Protein hydrolysis
Kallekrein	Protein hydrolysis

▶ DIAGNOSIS

- Physical exam may reveal dark circles under the eyes, a transverse nasal crease, adenoidal breathing, edematous nasal turbinates, clear nasal secretions, tearing, conjunctival injection, and periorbital swelling.
- Microscopic exam of nasal scrapings reveals numerous eosinophils.
- Further support for the diagnosis is provided by presence of specific IgE by allergen skin testing or in vitro assays such as the radioallergosorbent test (RAST). RAST is rarely justified in clinical practice because it is more expensive and less sensitive than skin tests. Total IgE levels are elevated in only 30–40% of allergic rhinitis patients, and it is also elevated in some nonallergic conditions, thus limiting usefulness.

► DESIRED OUTCOME

- The goal of treatment is to prevent or minimize target symptoms while side effects are minimized and cost-effectiveness of therapy is assured.
- Patients should be knowledgeable about proper timing and monitoring of their illness.
- Allergic rhinitis should have minimal effect on social and occupational functioning.

► TREATMENT

AVOIDANCE

- Avoidance of offending allergens is difficult. Mold growth can be reduced by keeping humidity below 50% and removing obvious growth with bleach or disinfectant.
- High-efficiency particulate air (HEPA) filters may reduce allergic respiratory symptoms.
- Windows should be kept closed and time spent outdoors during pollen season should be minimized. Filter masks can be helpful when gardening or mowing the lawn.

ANTIHISTAMINES

- Antihistamines prevent the histamine response in sensory nerve endings and blood vessels. They are more effective in preventing histamine response than in reversing it.
- Antihistamines are well absorbed and are metabolized hepatically. Therapeutic effect is more prolonged than predicted by half life.
- Drowsiness is the most frequent side effect (Table 80.2), and some tolerance to sedation occurs within 24 hours of the first dose. Sedative effects can be beneficial.
- Development of peripheral-acting antihistamines (terfenadine, astemizole, loratadine, fexofenadine) is a major advance, as minimal sedation is associated with these agents.
- Terfenadine is contraindicated in patients taking ketoconazole, itraconazole, erythromycin, clarithromycin, or troleandomycin. Coadministration of any of these drugs results in increased plasma concentrations of terfenadine and astemizole, which has quinidine-like actions, and may lead to torsades de pointes and death. Torsades de pointes has also been reported with overdoses of astemizole.
- The half-life of loratadine is 7.8–15 hours, that of terfenadine is 16–23 hours, that of astemizole is 20–60 hours, and that of fexofenadine is 14 hours.
- Cetirizine, a metabolite of hydroxyzine, is associated with increased sedation at higher doses. It has a half-life of 8 hours. It is free of cardiac effects in usual doses.

XV ◄

TABLE 80.2. Relative Side Effect Profile of Antihistamines

Agent	Relative Sedative Effect	Relative Anticholinergic Effect
Alkylamine class		
Brompheniramine maleate	Low	Moderate
Chlorpheniramine maleate	Low	Moderate
Dexchlorpheniramine maleate	Low	Moderate
Ethanolamine class		
Carbinoxamine maleate	High	High
Clemastine fumarate	Moderate	High
Diphenhydramine hydrochloride	Low	High
Ethylenediamine class		
Pyrilamine maleate	Low	Low to none
Tripelennamine hydrochloride	Moderate	Low to none
Phenothiazine class		
Methdilazine hydrochloride	Low	High
Promethazine hydrochloride	High	High
Trimeprazine	Moderate	High
Piperadine class		
Azatadine maleate	Moderate	Moderate
Cyproheptadine hydrochloride	Low	Moderate
Diphenylpyraline hydrochloride	Low	Moderate
Phenindamine tartrate	Low to none	Moderate
Miscellaneous		
Astemizole	Low to none	Low to none
Terfenadine	Low to none	Low to none
Loratadine	Low to none	Low to none
Cetirizine	Low to moderate	Moderate
Fexofenadine	Low	Low

- Many patients respond to and tolerate the older agents well, and because some are available generically, they may be less expensive than the newer agents.
- Anticholinergic symptoms can be troublesome, especially for elderly men and those on concurrent anticholinergic therapy (Table 80.2). Caution should also be used in patients with increased intraocular pressure, hyperthyroidism, and cardiovascular disease.
- Other side effects include nausea, epigastric distress, constipation, and diarrhea. Taking medication with meals or a full glass of water may prevent gastrointestinal side effects.
- Antihistamines are more effective when taken approximately 1–2 hours before the anticipated exposure to the offending allergen.
- Table 80.3 lists recommended doses of commonly prescribed agents.

TABLE 80.3. Oral Dosages of Commonly Prescribed Antihistamines and Decongestants

Drug	Dosage and Interval	
	Adults	*Children*
Antihistamines		
Chlorpheniramine maleate, plain	4 mg every 6 h	6–12 yr: 2 mg every 6 h 2–6 yr: 1 mg every 6 h
Chlorpheniramine maleate, sustained release	8–12 mg at bedtime or 8–12 mg every 8 h	6–12 yr: 8 mg at bedtime <6 yr: not recommended
Cetirizine	5–10 mg daily	Not recommended
Diphenhydramine hydrochloride	25–50 mg every 8 h	5 mg/kg/d divided every 8 h (up to 25 mg per dose)
Clemastine fumarate	1.34 mg twice daily to 2.68 mg three times daily	Not recommended
Astemizole	30 mg on day 1; 20 mg on day 2; then 10 mg daily	Not recommended
Loratadine	10 mg daily	Not recommended
Terfenadine	60 mg twice daily	6–12 yr: 30–60 mg twice daily 3–6 yr: 15 mg twice daily
Fexofenadine	60 mg every 12 h	Not recommended
Decongestants		
Pseudoephedrine	60 mg every 4–6 h 120 mg every 12 h for sustained release	6–12 yr: 30 mg every 4–6 h 2–5 yr: 15 mg every 4–6 h
Ephedrine sulfate	25–50 mg every 4 h	2–3 mg/kg/d divided every 4 h (up to 25 mg every 4 h)
Phenylpropanolamine	25 mg every 4 h or 50 mg every 8 h for sustained release	6–12 yr: 12.5 mg every 4 h 2–5 yr: 6.25 mg every 4 h

DECONGESTANTS

- Topical and systemic decongestants are sympathomimetic agents that act on adrenergic receptors in the nasal mucosa to produce vasoconstriction and shrink swollen mucosa.
- Use of topical decongestants results in little or no systemic absorption (Table 80.4).
- Prolonged use of topical agents results in rhinitis medicamentosa, which is caused by severe nasal edema and reduced receptor sensitivity. Treatment options are:
  - Abrupt cessation: This option works, but rebound congestion lasts several days or weeks.
  - Nasal steroids: These require several days to work.

XV

TABLE 80.4. Duration of Action of Topical Decongestants

Drug	Duration (h)
Short-acting	Up to 4
Phenylephrine hydrochloride	
Intermediate-acting	4–6
Naphazoline hydrochloride	
Tetrahydrozoline hydrochloride	
Long-acting	Up to 12
Oxymetazoline hydrochloride	
Xylometazoline hydrochloride	

- Gradual increases in dosage interval or decreases in concentration: This method works, but it takes several weeks. Use of nasal steroids may aid this process.
- Other side effects of topical decongestants include burning, stinging, and sneezing.
- Duration of therapy with topical decongestants should be limited to 3–5 days.
- With the oral route, onset of action is delayed, but duration of action is longer. Rhinitis medicamentosa is not a problem with oral therapy. Pharmacokinetic parameters are summarized in Table 80.5.
- The therapeutic index for phenylpropanolamine and ephedrine is low. Both can cause hypertension at near-therapeutic doses. Pseudoephedrine appears to be the safest of the three—doses up to 180 mg produce no measurable change in blood pressure or heart rate, although higher doses can. Hypertensive patients should avoid these drugs, especially phenylpropanolamine and ephedrine.
- Monoamine oxidase inhibitors should be avoided in any patient taking decongestants.

TABLE 80.5. Pharmacokinetic Variables of Systemic Decongestants

Drug	Half-Life (h)	Mechanism of Metabolism or Elimination
Pseudoephedrine	3–8	Partially metabolized; majority excreted unchanged in urine
Ephedrine	3–6	Majority excreted unchanged in urine
Phenylpropanolamine	3–4	Majority excreted unchanged in urine

XV

TOPICAL CORTICOSTEROIDS

- Topical steroids are effective, have minimal side effects, and may inhibit early as well as late-phase response (Table 80.6).
- Local effects on the mucosa include decrease in the number of epithelial mediator cells, reduction in epithelial permeability, reduction in secretory response, and partial inhibition of the immediate allergen-induced nasal symptoms.
- Side effects include sneezing, stinging, epistaxis, and infections with *Candida albicans* (rare).
- Some patients improve within a few days, but peak response may require 2–3 weeks.
- Blocked nasal passages should be cleared with a decongestant before administration of corticosteroids.

CROMOLYN SODIUM

- Cromolyn sodium, a mast cell stabilizer, is available as a nasal solution.
- It prevents mast cell degranulation and release of mediators, including histamine.
- The most common side effect is local irritation.
- The dose in individuals older than 6 years is one spray in each nostril 3–4 times daily.
- For seasonal rhinitis, initiate treatment just before the start of the allergen's season, and continue throughout the season.
- Nasal passages should be cleared before administration, and inhaling during administration of cromolyn aids distribution to the entire nasal lining.

TABLE 80.6. Dosages of Topical Steroids

Drug	Dosage and Interval
Beclomethasone diproprionate	>12 yr: 1 inhalation (42 µg) per nostril 2–4 times per day (maximum, 336 µg/d) 6–12 yr: 1 inhalation per nostril 3 times per day
Budesonide	>6 yr: 2 sprays (64 µg) per nostril in AM and PM or 4 sprays per nostril in the AM (maximum, 256 µg)
Flunisolide	Adults: 2 sprays (50 µg) per nostril twice daily (maximum, 400 µg) Children: 1 spray per nostril 3 times per day
Fluticasone propionate	>12 yr: 200 µg once daily Children ≥4 yr: 100 µg once daily
Triamcinolone acetonide	>12 yr: 2 sprays (110 µg) per nostril once daily (maximum, 440 µg/d)

XV

IMMUNOTHERAPY

- Efficacy is documented for seasonal and perennial allergic rhinitis.
- Immunotherapy suppresses seasonal rises of IgE antibodies, decreases basophil reactivity and sensitivity to allergens, generates antigen-specific suppressor cells, and produces IgG antibodies that block the allergen-IgE interaction.
- Adverse reactions include swelling at the site of injection. Other reactions occurring rarely are urticaria, bronchospasm, laryngospasm, and vascular collapse.
- Patients receiving oral or topical β-adrenergic blocking agents are at risk for severe and life-threatening anaphylaxis from immunotherapy injections.
- When conducted by experienced personnel, immunotherapy with inhalant allergens is a safe mode of therapy for resistant rhinitis symptoms.
- Severe reactions are treated with epinephrine, antihistamines, and systemic corticosteroids.
- Candidates for immunotherapy are patients whose symptoms are uncontrolled by medication and who are unable to avoid the offending allergen and those with intolerable side effects or who become resistant to medication.
- Injections are given once or twice weekly, and the concentration is increased until the maximum tolerated dose is achieved. This maintenance dose is continued every 2–6 weeks.

▶ EVALUATION OF THERAPEUTIC OUTCOMES

- Patients should be monitored regularly for reduction in severity of identified target symptoms and presence of side effects.
- Patients must be educated about timing and administration of prophylactic regimens.
- Compliance must be monitored and alternative regimens explored when necessary.

See Chapter 89, Allergic Rhinitis, authored by J. Russell May, PharmD, Timothy A. Feger, MD, and Margaret F. Guill, MD, for a more detailed discussion of this topic.

Chapter 81

▶ ASTHMA

▶ DEFINITION

An Expert Panel of the National Institutes of Health National Asthma Education and Prevention Program (NAEPP) has defined asthma as a chronic inflammatory disorder of the airways in which many cells and cellular elements play a role. In susceptible individuals, inflammation causes recurrent episodes of wheezing, breathlessness, chest tightness, and coughing. These episodes are usually associated with airflow obstruction that is often reversible either spontaneously or with treatment. The inflammation also causes an increase in bronchial hyperresponsiveness to a variety of stimuli.

▶ PATHOPHYSIOLOGY

- Hyperreactivity of the airways to physical, chemical, and pharmacologic stimuli is the hallmark of asthma.
- The increased bronchial responsiveness is at least in part due to an inflammatory response within the airway. The histologic examination at autopsy is characterized by marked hypertrophy and hyperplasia of the airway smooth muscle, increased airway wall thickness caused by an exudative inflammatory reaction and edema, and mucous gland hypertrophy and mucus hypersecretion.
- Inflammation of the airways and the release of mediators of inflammation appear to be necessary for the development and maintenance of bronchial hyperreactivity. Airway inflammation is associated with epithelial cell damage and increased mucosal permeability. This facilitates access of noxious stimuli from the lumen to the airway smooth muscle, submucosal mast cells, and the cholinergic irritant receptors located in the junction between cells. Inflammation can also account for mucus hypersecretion.
- Involvement of leukocytes within the airways and surrounding tissues is important in the pathogenesis of asthma.
  - Mast cell degranulation in response to allergens results in release of mediators such as histamine; eosinophil and neutrophil chemotactic factors; leukotrienes C_4, D_4, and E_4; prostaglandins; and platelet-activating factor. Histamine is capable of inducing smooth muscle constriction and bronchospasm and is thought to play a role in mucosal edema and mucus secretion.
  - The granules within eosinophils contain major basic protein (MBP), which is responsible for damage to airway epithelium and has been found in very high quantities in the sputum of patients with asthma.
  - Neutrophils can also be a source for a variety of mediators (platelet-activating factors, prostaglandins, thromboxanes, and leukotrienes)

that contribute to bronchial hyperresponsiveness and airway inflammation.

- Alveolar macrophages produce and release a number of inflammatory mediators, including platelet-activating factor, leukotriene B_4, leukotriene C_4, and leukotriene D_4. Production of neutrophil chemotactic factor and eosinophil chemotactic factor attract neutrophils and eosinophils, which in turn further facilitate the inflammatory process.
- The presence of T lymphocytes has been correlated to bronchial hyperresponsiveness. The T_{H2} subset of T lymphocytes produces and releases interleukin (IL)-4, IL-5, IL-6, and IL-10. Conversely, T_{H1} cells secrete IL-2, IFN-γ, and tumor necrosis factor beta (TNF-β), with both T_{H1} and T_{H2} cells producing IL-3, granulocyte-macrophage colony-stimulating factor (GM-CSF), and IFN-α.
- Chemical substances known as phospholipids are found in rich supply in the membranes of most cells involved with inflammation. Several classes of inflammatory mediators, including arachidonic acid and its metabolites, prostaglandins, leukotrienes, and platelet-activating factor, are derived from these membrane phospholipids.
- The lipoxygenase pathway of arachidonic acid breakdown is responsible for production of leukotrienes. Leukotrienes C_4, D_4, and E_4 (sulfidopeptide leukotrienes) constitute the slow-reacting substance of anaphylaxis (SRS-A). These leukotrienes are liberated during inflammatory processes in the lung and have significant effects on airway smooth muscle (bronchoconstriction), mucociliary function, microvascular permeability, and airways edema.
- The exudative inflammatory process and sloughing of epithelial cells into the airway lumen impairs mucociliary transport. The bronchial glands are increased in size and the goblet cells are increased in size and number, suggesting an increased production of mucus. Expectorated mucus from patients with asthma tends to have a high viscosity.
- The airway is innervated by parasympathetic, sympathetic, and nonadrenergic inhibitory nerves. The normal resting tone of human airway smooth muscle is maintained by vagal efferent activity, and bronchoconstriction can be mediated by vagal stimulation in the small bronchi. All airway smooth muscle contains noninnervated β_2-adrenergic receptors that produce bronchodilation. The importance of α-adrenergic receptors in asthma is unknown.

▶ CLINICAL PRESENTATION

CHRONIC ASTHMA

- Classic asthma is characterized by episodic dyspnea associated with wheezing, but the clinical presentation of asthma is diverse. Patients may complain of a feeling of tightness in the chest or occasionally a burning sensation. A chronic persistent cough may be the only symptom.

- Asthma has a widely variable presentation from chronic daily symptoms to only intermittent symptoms. The interval between symptoms may be weeks, months, or years. It is a disease characterized by recurrent exacerbations and remissions.
- The severity is primarily determined by the number of medications required to adequately control symptoms. Patients can present with mild intermittent symptoms that require no medications or only occasional use of inhaled bronchodilators to severe chronic asthma symptoms despite receiving multiple medications.
- Chronic severe asthma is defined by the requirement of continuous or frequent intermittent glucocorticoids and chronic bronchodilator therapy for control of symptoms.

ACUTE SEVERE ASTHMA

- Uncontrolled asthma can progress to an acute state where inflammation, airways edema, excessive accumulation of mucus, and severe bronchospasm result in a profound airways narrowing, which is poorly responsive to usual bronchodilator therapy.
- Patients present with severe dyspnea, inspiratory as well as expiratory wheezing, anxiety, tachypnea, tachycardia, and in severe cases, cyanosis.
- They exhibit supraclavicular and intercostal retractions, a hyperinflated chest, and coughing. In severe obstruction, air movement in and out of the lungs is substantially decreased, so that wheezing may actually decrease.
- Emergency department visits for acute severe asthma often represent the failure of an adequate therapeutic regimen for chronic asthma.

▶ DIAGNOSIS

- The diagnosis of asthma is based primarily on a good history of recurrent episodes of dyspnea and/or wheezing.
- The patient may have a family history of allergy or asthma or have symptoms of allergic rhinitis. A history of exercise or cold air precipitating the dyspnea or an association of increased symptoms during specific allergen seasons would also point to asthma.
- In the older child and adult patient in whom spirometric evaluations can be performed, abnormal pulmonary functions that improve 15% or more following bronchodilator administration help confirm the diagnosis. Failure of pulmonary functions to improve acutely does not necessarily rule out asthma. If baseline spirometry is normal, challenge testing with exercise, histamine, or methacholine can be used to elicit bronchial hyperreactivity.
- Studies for atopy such as serum IgE and sputum and blood eosinophils are not necessary to make the diagnosis of asthma, but they may help differentiate asthma from chronic bronchitis in adults.

XV

▶ DESIRED OUTCOME

- The NAEP has provided the following goals for asthma management: prevent chronic and troublesome symptoms (e.g., coughing or breathlessness in the night, in the early morning, or after exertion); maintain near "normal" pulmonary function rates; maintain normal activity levels (including exercise); prevent recurrent exacerbations of asthma; minimize adverse effects from asthma medication; meet patients' and families' expectations of care.
- In patients with an acute severe asthma exacerbation, the goals of therapy are to relieve airway obstruction as quickly as possible (within minutes), relieve hypoxemia, restore lung function to normal as soon as possible (within hours), plan avoidance of future relapses, and develop a written action plan in case of further exacerbations.

▶ TREATMENT

Treatment algorithms published by the National Heart, Lung, and Blood Institute are contained in Table 81.1 and Figure 81.1.

NONPHARMACOLOGIC MANAGEMENT

- Patient education and the teaching of patient self-management skills should be the cornerstone of the treatment program; self-management programs have been shown to improve patient adherence to medication regimens, improve self-management skills, and improve utilization of health care services.
- Use of objective measurements of airflow obstruction with a home peak flow meter is integral to many of the programs. The NAEP Expert Panel has advocated the use of objective pulmonary-function monitoring at home with portable peak expiratory flow meters as a means of improving the care of asthmatics.
- Avoidance of known allergenic triggers can result in an improvement in symptoms, a reduction in medications, and a decrease in bronchial hyperreactivity. Obvious environmental triggers (e.g., animals) should be avoided, and patients who smoke should be encouraged to stop.
- Oxygen therapy is indicated in patients requiring emergency therapy for acute severe asthma. Patients hospitalized with acute severe asthma should be given adequate maintenance hydration in order to mobilize secretions, but excessive hydration should be avoided to prevent excessive lung fluid in patients with inflammation and bronchial edema.

PHARMACOLOGIC MANAGEMENT

β_2 Agonists (Table 81.2)

- The β_2 agonists are the most effective bronchodilators available. β_2-adrenergic receptor stimulation activates adenyl cyclase, which produces an increase in intracellular cyclic AMP. This increase results in a decrease in unbound intracellular calcium, producing smooth muscle

TABLE 81.1. Stepwise Approach for Managing Asthma in Adults and Children Older Than 5 Years of Age: Treatment (Preferred Treatments are in Bold Print)

	Long-Term Control	Quick Relief	Education
Step 4 Severe Persistent	Daily medications: • **Anti-inflammatory: inhaled corticosteroid (high dose) AND** • **Long-acting bronchodilator: either long-acting inhaled β₂-agonist,** sustained-release theophylline, or long-acting β₂-agonist tablets AND • Corticosteroid tablets or syrup long term (2 mg/kg/day, generally do not exceed 60 mg per day).	• Short-acting bronchodilator: **inhaled β₂-agonists** as needed for symptoms. • Intensity of treatment will depend on severity of exacerbation. • Use of short-acting inhaled β₂-agonists on a daily basis, or increasing use, indicates the need for additional long-term control therapy.	Steps 2 and 3 actions plus: • Refer to individual education/counseling

Step 3 Moderate Persistent	Daily medication:
	• Either
	  • **Anti-inflammatory: inhaled corticosteroid (medium dose)**
	  OR
	  • **Inhaled corticosteroid (low-medium dose)** and add a long-acting bronchodilator, especially for nighttime symptoms: either **long-acting inhaled β₂-agonist,** sustained-release theophylline, or long-acting β₂-agonist tablets.
	• If needed
	  • Anti-inflammatory: **inhaled corticosteroids (medium-high dose) AND**
		• Short-acting bronchodilator: **inhaled β₂-agonists** as needed for symptoms.
		• Intensity of treatment will depend on severity of exacerbation.
		• Use of short-acting inhaled β₂-agonists or a daily basis, or increasing use, indicates the need for additional long-term control therapy.	

TABLE 81.1. continued

	Long-Term Control	Quick Relief	Education
	Long-acting bronchodilator, especially for nighttime symptoms: either **long-acting inhaled β₂-agonist,** sustained-release theophylline, or long-acting β₂-agonist tablets.		
Step 2 Mild Persistent	One daily medication: • **Anti-inflammatory:** either **inhaled corticosteroid** (low doses) or **cromolyn or nedocromil** (children usually begin with a trial of cromolyn or nedocromil). • Sustained-release theophylline to serum concentration of 5–15 μg/mL is an alternative, but not preferred, therapy. Zafirlukast or zileuton may also be considered for patients ≥12 years of age, although their position in therapy is not fully established.	• Short-acting bronchodilator: **inhaled β₂-agonists** as needed for symptoms. • Intensity of treatment will depend on severity of exacerbation. • Use of short-acting inhaled β₂-agonists on a daily basis, or increasing use, indicates the need for additional long-term-control therapy.	Step 1 actions plus: • Teach self-monitoring • Refer to group education if available • Review and update self-management plan
Step 1 Mild Intermittent	• No daily medication needed.	• Short-acting bronchodilator: **inhaled β₂-agonists** as needed for symptoms. • Intensity of treatment will depend on severity of exacerbation.	• Teach basic facts about asthma • Teach inhaler/spacer/holding chamber technique • Discuss roles of medications • Develop self-management plan

TABLE 81.1. continued

Long-Term Control	Quick Relief	Education
	• Use of short-acting inhaled β₂-agonists more than 2 times a week may indicate the need to initiate long-term-control therapy.	• Develop action plan for when and how to take rescue actions, especially for patients with a history of severe exacerbations • Discuss appropriate environmental control measures to avoid exposure to known allergens and irritants

⇓ **Step down**

Review treatment every 1 to 6 months; a gradual stepwise reduction in treatment may be possible.

⇑ **Step up**

If control is not maintained, consider step up. First, review patient medication technique, adherence, and environmental control (avoidance of allergens or other factors that contribute to asthma severity).

Note: • **The stepwise approach presents general guidelines to assist clinical decision making; it is not intended to be a specific prescription. Asthma is highly variable; clinicians should tailor specific medication plans to the needs and circumstances of individual patients.**

• Gain control as quickly as possible; then decrease treatment to the least medication necessary to maintain control. Gaining control may be accomplished by either starting treatment at the step most appropriate to the initial severity of the condition or starting at a higher level of therapy (e.g., a course of systemic corticosteroids or higher dose of inhaled corticosteroids).

• A rescue course of systemic corticosteroids may be needed at any time and at any step.

• Some patients with intermittent asthma experience severe and life-threatening exacerbations separated by long periods of normal lung function and no symptoms. This may be especially common with exacerbations provoked by respiratory infections. A short course of systemic corticosteroids is recommended.

• At each step, patients should control their environment to avoid or control factors that make their asthma worse (e.g., allergens, irritants); this requires specific diagnosis and education.

From NAEPP Expert Panel Report II: Guidelines for the Diagnosis and Management of Asthma.

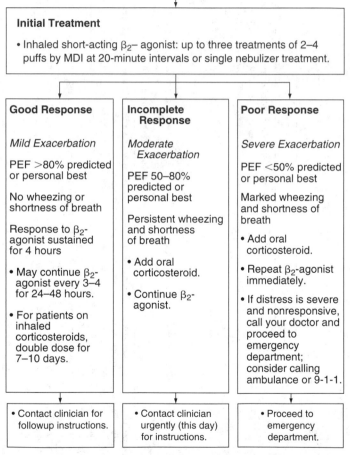

Figure 81.1. Management of asthma exacerbations: home treatment. (*Patients at high risk of asthma-related death should receive immediate clinical attention after initial treatment. Additional therapy may be required. From NAEPP Expert Panel Report II: Guidelines for the Diagnosis and Management of Asthma.*)

TABLE 81.2. Relative Selectivity, Potency, and Duration of Action of the β-Adrenergic Agonists

Agent	Selectivity			Duration of Action		
	β₁	β₂	β₂ Potency[a]	Bronchodilation (h)	Protection[b] (h)	Oral Activity
Isoproterenol	++++	++++	1	0.5–2	0.5–1.0	No
Metaproterenol	+++	+++	15	3–4	1–2	Yes
Isoetharine	++	+++	6	0.5–2	0.5–1.0	No
Albuterol	+	++++	2	4–8	2–4	Yes
Bitolterol	+	++++	5	4–8	2–4	No
Pirbuterol	+	++++	5	4–8	2–4	Yes
Terbutaline	+	++++	4	4–8	2–4	Yes
Salmeterol	+	++++	0.50	>12	>12	UK[c]

[a]Relative molar potency; 1 = most potent.
[b]Protection refers to the duration of time that bronchoconstriction may be prevented.
[c]UK, unknown.

relaxation, mast cell membrane stabilization, and skeletal muscle stimulation.

- Aerosol administration enhances bronchoselectivity and provides a more rapid response and a greater degree of protection against provocations that induce bronchospasm (e.g., exercise and allergen challenges) than does systemic administration.
- Inhaled short-acting selective β₂ agonists are indicated for the treatment of intermittent episodes of bronchospasm and are the first treatment of choice for acute severe asthma.
- In acute severe asthma, β₂ agonists should be given in high doses by jet nebulization in frequent intervals or alternatively, via metered dose inhaler (MDI) plus a spacer device by trained personnel; dosing guidelines are presented in Table 81.3. Initially, the patient should receive dosages every 20 minutes for the first 1 or 2 hours, and then the dosage should be adjusted based on response (see Table 81.1 and Figure 81.1). During the recovery phase, the dose is generally lowered first and then the dosing interval is extended.
- These agents are the treatment of choice for exercise-induced asthma (EIA). They provide complete protection for at least 2 hour after inhalation; the new long-acting agents provide significant protection for 8–12 hours.
- Their short duration limits usefulness in patients who require chronic maintenance bronchodilators to prevent and control symptoms, particularly those with nocturnal asthma.
- In chronic asthma, they may be used for chronic maintenance in patients with symptoms who are already on standard doses of anti-inflammatories prior to advancing to high-dose inhaled corticosteroids. Twice daily inhaled salmeterol is indicated for the chronic maintenance XV

TABLE 81.3. Dosages of Medications for Acute Severe Asthma

Medication	Dosage		Comment
	Pediatric	Adult	
Sympathomimetics			
Isoetharine	0.1–1.0% 0.1–0.2 mg/kg every 20 min for 3 doses, then every 1–2 h as needed	3–10 mg every 20 min for 3 doses then every 1–2 h as needed	For optimal delivery, dilute aerosols to minimum of 4 mL, maximum 6 mL; gas flow at 6–12 L/min
Metaproterenol 5% (50 mg/mL), 15-µg unit dose	0.25–0.5 mg/kg every 2–4 h as needed, maximum 15 mg	15 mg every 20 min for 3 doses, then 15–30 mg every 2–4 h as needed	Not recommended due to low potency and short duration Do not exceed maximum; not recommended in high dose due to lack of β₂ selectivity
Terbutaline Injection (1 mg/mL) Nebulizer solution (10 mg/mL)	0.1–0.3 mg/kg every 20 min or 3 doses, then every 2–4 h as needed	10 mg every 20 min then 10 mg every 2–4 h as needed	Currently not approved for this mode of administration; no advantage over albuterol so not recommended
Albuterol (5 mg/mL)	0.05–0.15 mg/kg every 20 min for 3 doses, then 0.15–0.3 mg/kg up to 10 mg every 2–4 h as needed, or 0.5 mg/kg/h by continuous nebulization	5–10 mg every 20 min for 3 doses every 2–4 h as needed, or 10–15 mg/h by continuous nebulization	May continue every 20 min for 2–4 h in severe cases
Systemic			
Epinephrine 1:1000 (1 mg/mL)	0.01 mg/kg up to 0.5 mg every 20 min for 3 doses SQ	0.3–0.5 mg every 20 min for 3 doses	No proven advantage of systemic therapy over aerosol in patients capable of moving air
Sustained-action susphrine 1:200 (5 mg/mL)	0.005–0.01 mL/kg every 6–10 h as needed SQ	0.5–0.75 mg every 6–10 h as needed	

TABLE 81.3. continued

Terbutaline (1 mg/mL)	0.01 mg/kg every 20 min for 3 doses, then every 2–6 h as needed SQ 10 μg/kg over 10 min intravenously followed by 0.4 μg/kg/min. Increase as necessary by 0.2 μg/kg/min up to 3–6 μg/kg/min	0.25–0.5 mg every 20 min for 3 doses, then every 2–6 h as needed Not recommended	Due to cardiac toxicity high dose inhaled agonists preferred

Anticholinergics

Aerosol Atropine sulfate	0.5–0.075 mg/kg every 4–6 h as needed	0.025 mg/kg or 2.5–5 mg every 4–5 h as needed	Due to excellent absorption atropine sulfate not recommended
Ipratropium bromide 0.025%	250 μg every 4–6 h as needed	250–500 μg every 4–6 h as needed	
Glycopyrrolate (Robinul) 0.2 mg/mL injection	0.025–0.05 mg/kg nebulized every 4–5 h	2 mg nebulized every 2–6 h as needed	

Glucocorticoids

Methylprednisolone	1–2 mg/kg every 6 h for 24–48 h or severe symptoms abate, then reduce to 1–2 mg/kg/c every 12 h	80–200 mg/d in 2–4 divided doses	Duration of steroid therapy is dependent on response; continue full dose until patient at least 70–75% of normal predicted FEV₁; hydrocortisone produces greater sodium retention: no advantage over parenteral therapy
Hydrocortisone	4 mg/kg every 4–6 h for 24–48 h, then reduce	200–400 mg/d 2–4 divided doses	
Prednisone	1–2 mg/kg/d in 2–3 doses for outpatient use for 3–5 days. Inpatient same as for methylprednisolone	40–160 mg/d in 2–4 divided doses	

XV

1019

therapy of asthma, but it is ineffective for acute severe asthma because it can take up to 20 minutes for onset and 1–4 hours for maximum bronchodilation. Patients should be counseled to continue to use their short-acting inhaled β_2 agonists for acute exacerbations.

Methylxanthines

- The mechanism by which theophylline produces bronchodilation is unknown but may involve inhibition of the release of intracellular calcium and/or inhibition of phosphodiesterases (PDEs). PDE inhibition may result in decreased mast cell mediator release, decreased eosinophil basic-protein release, decreased T lymphocyte proliferation, decreased T cell cytokine release, and decreased plasma exudation. Theophylline also inhibits pulmonary edema by decreasing vascular permeability, enhances mucociliary clearance, and strengthens contraction of a fatigued diaphragm.
- Methylxanthines are ineffective by aerosol and therefore must be taken systemically (orally or IV).
- Theophylline is primarily eliminated by metabolism via the hepatic cytochrome P-450 mixed-function oxidase microsomal enzymes (primarily the CYP1A2 isozyme) with 10% or less excreted unchanged in the kidney. The hepatic P-450 enzymes are susceptible to induction and inhibition by various environmental factors and drugs, as listed in Table 81.4.
- Because of a relatively large intrapatient variability in theophylline clearance, no patient should be treated with theophylline without rou-

TABLE 81.4. Factors Affecting Theophylline Clearance

Decreased Clearance	Decrease in Clearance[a] (%)	Increased Clearance	Increase in Clearance[a] (%)
Cimetidine	−35 to −60	Rifampin	+53
Troleandomycin	−25 to −50	Carbamazepine	+50
Erythromycin	−25	Phenobarbital	+34
Allopurinol	−20		
Propranolol	−30	Phenytoin	+70
Oral contraceptives	−10 to −30	Smoking	+40
Enoxacin	−65	High-protein diet	+25
Ciprofloxacin	−25 to −30	Charcoal broiled meat	+30
Norfloxacin	−10	Intravenous isoproterenol	
Ofloxacin	−26	Sulfinpyrazone	+22
Systemic viral illness	−50		
Thiabendazole	−65		

[a]Approximate means reported across studies.

tine monitoring of serum theophylline concentrations. A range of 5–15 μg/mL has been recommended by the NAEP and others as an effective and safe range of steady-state concentrations for most patients.

- Figures 81.2 and 81.3 give recommended dosages, monitoring schedules, and dosage adjustments for theophylline.
- Sustained-release oral preparations are favored for outpatient therapy, but each product has different release characteristics and the products are variably susceptible to altered absorption from food or gastric pH changes. In general, preparations unaffected by food that can be administered a minimum of every 12 hours in most patients are preferable.
- In hospitalized adult and child asthmatics, addition of aminophylline to optimal inhaled β_2 agonists and oral glucocorticoids has been shown to provide no further benefit.
- In the outpatient setting, chronic theophylline administration can reduce asthma symptoms, reduce the amount of as-needed inhaled β_2 agonists used, and reduce the oral steroid requirement in steroid-dependent asthmatics.
- Sustained-release theophylline once nightly is effective for nocturnal asthma.
- Significant disadvantages to chronic theophylline therapy include the lack of effect of theophylline on underlying bronchial hyperreactivity and the dangers inherent in giving a drug that can produce severe neurologic toxicity, including seizures, permanent neurologic deficit, and death at serum concentrations only two-fold greater than optimal therapeutic concentrations.
- Due to its high risk/benefit ratio, theophylline should be considered as a second- or third-line drug in the therapy of asthma. It may be an alternative to the long-acting inhaled β_2 agonists for patients still symptomatic despite standard or high-dose anti-inflammatory therapy.

Anticholinergics (Table 81.5)

- Anticholinergic bronchodilators are competitive inhibitors of muscarinic receptors; they only produce bronchodilation in cholinergic-mediated bronchoconstriction. Anticholinergics are effective bronchodilators but are not as potent as β_2 agonists. They attenuate, but do not block, allergen- or exercise-induced asthma in a dose-dependent fashion.
- Anticholinergics consistently produce bronchodilation in acute severe asthma. They can be expected to produce a further 20–25% improvement in FEV_1 over β_2 agonists alone.
- Quaternary ammonium derivatives (ipratropium bromide, atropine methonitrate, oxitropium, and glycopyrrolate) have the advantage of poor absorption across mucosae and the blood–brain barrier as compared to the tertiary ammonium compound, atropine sulfate. This results in negligible systemic effects with a prolonged local effect (i.e., bronchodilation) with no decrease in mucociliary clearance.

XV

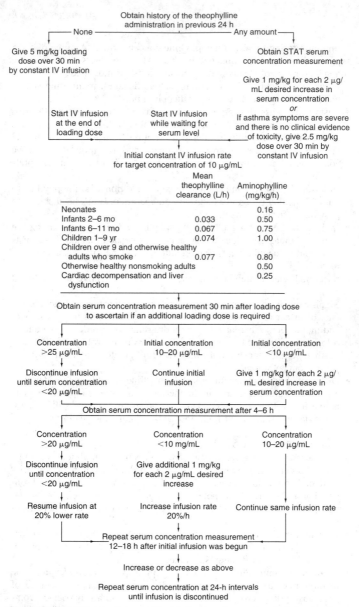

Figure 81.2. Algorithm for the use of theophylline to relieve acute symptoms of asthma. Aminophylline = 80% theophylline. *(From Jenne JW, Murphy S (eds). Drug Therapy for Asthma: Research and Clinical Practice. New York, Marcel Dekker, 1987, with permission.)*

Initial dosage
Adults and children >1 yr of age:
12–14 mg/kg per day up to a maximum of 300 mg/day

After 3 days, *if tolerated*, increase dose to:

Incremental increase
Adults and children ≥45 kg: 400 mg/day
Children <45 kg: 16 mg/kg per day up to a maximum of 400 mg/day

After 3 days, *if tolerated*, increase dose to:

Final dosage before serum concentration measurement
Adults and children ≥45 kg: 600 mg/day
Children <45 kg: 20 mg/kg per day up to a maximum of 600 mg/day

Check serum concentration ~4 hours after a morning dose of most slow-release products or 8 hours after a dose of a very slowly absorbed product given once every 24 hours, when no doses have been missed, added, or taken at unequal intervals for 3 days.

Dosage adjustment based on serum concentration

Peak serum concentration	Directions
<7.5 μg/mL	Increase dose about 25%. *Recheck serum theophylline concentration for guidance in further dosage adjustment.*
7.5 to 9.9 μg/mL	If tolerated, increase dose ~25%.
10 to 14.9 μg/mL	If tolerated, maintain dose. *Recheck serum theophylline concentration at 6- to 12-month intervals.**
15 to 19.9 μg/mL	Consider 10% decrease in dose to provide greater margin of safety.*
20 to 24.9 μg/mL	Decrease dose 10% to 25%. Recheck serum serum concentration after 3 days.
25 to 30 μg/mL	Skip next dose and decrease subsequent doses at least 25%. Recheck serum concentration after 3 days.
>30 μg/mL	Skip next 2 doses and decrease subsequent doses 50%. *Recheck serum theophylline concentration for guidance in further dosage adjustment.*[†]

*Dosage reduction or serum concentration measurement is indicated whenever adverse effects are present, physiologic abnormalities that can reduce theophylline clearance occur (e.g., persistent fever), or a drug that interacts with theophylline is added or discontinued (e.g., erythromycin, carbamazepine).
[†]Administer activated charcoal in water, 0.5 gm/kg every 2 hours until serum concentration <20 μg/mL. Consider intravenously administered phenobarbital, 20 mg/kg, to prevent seizures if excessive serum concentration has resulted from multiple doses. Consult a regional poison control center for additional advice.

Figure 81.3. Algorithm for slow titration of theophylline dosage and guide for final dosage adjustment based on serum theophylline concentration measurement. For infants <1 year of age, the initial daily dosage can be calculated by the following regression equation: Dose = (mg/kg) = (0.2)(age in weeks) + 5.0. Whenever side effects occur, dosage should be reduced to a previously tolerated lower dose.

TABLE 81.5. Comparison of Anticholinergics[a]

Agent	Availability	Relative Potency[b]	Duration (h)	Dosages Pediatrics	Dosages Adults
Atropine methonitrate	Investigational only	1	5–6	ND[c]	1.5 mg nebulized q 6 h
Ipratropium bromide (Atrovent)	MDI[d] 18 µg/actuation; 300 actuations; 0.025% (0.25 mg/mL) nebulizer solution	Unknown 0.5	5–6	2 inhalations q 6 h nebulized 250 µg nebulized q 4–6 h for acute asthma	2–4 inhalations q 6 h or 500 µg nebulized q 6 h for acute asthma
Glycopyrrolate (Robinul)	0.2 mg/mL injectable solution	1	6–12	0.025–0.05 mg/kg nebulized q 6 h	2 mg nebulized q 6 h
Oxitropium bromide	Investigational	Unknown	8	ND[c]	500 µg

[a]At the current time there are no anticholinergics approved by the FDA for use in asthma.
[b]Dose required to produce equivalent bronchodilation.
[c]ND, not determined.
[d]MDI, metered-dose inhaler.

- The time it takes to reach maximum bronchodilation from aerosolized anticholinergics is considerably longer than from aerosolized short-acting β_2 agonists (2 hours versus 30 minutes). This is of little clinical consequence because some bronchodilation is seen within 30 seconds, 50% of maximum response occurs within 3 minutes, and 80% of maximum is reached within 30 minutes.
- Anticholinergics have a limited role in the treatment of asthma, and there is no rationale for using atropine sulfate. Anticholinergics are unable to produce maximum bronchodilation in asthma and are significantly less effective than the β_2 agonists in the usual recommended doses. Both the β_2 agonists and cromolyn provide superior protection against EIA. Anticholinergics do represent a safer and more effective additional bronchodilator than theophylline in acute severe asthma and appear to be as effective as β_2 agonists for reversing the bronchospastic component of acute exacerbations of chronic bronchitis.

Cromolyn Sodium and Nedocromil Sodium

- The exact mechanism of action for these agents is unknown but is believed to result, at least in part, from mast cell membrane stabilization.
- As such, they inhibit the response to allergen challenge as well as EIA. Neither drug has a bronchodilatory effect.
- Cromolyn and nedocromil are effective only by inhalation and are available as MDIs, while cromolyn also comes as a nebulizer solution and Spinhaler.
- Both drugs are remarkably nontoxic. Cough and wheezing have been reported following inhalation of the dry powder inhaler of cromolyn and bad taste and headache after nedocromil.
- Cromolyn and nedocromil are indicated for the prophylaxis of chronic mild to moderate asthma in both children and adults regardless of etiology; approximately 60–75% of patients (adults and children) are adequately controlled.
- They are particularly effective for the allergic asthmatics on a seasonal basis or just prior to an acute exposure (i.e., animals or mowing the lawn).
- Cromolyn is the second drug of choice for the prevention of EIA and may be used in conjunction with a β_2 agonist in more severe cases not completely responding to either agent alone.
- Cromolyn and nedocromil have been advocated as the anti-inflammatories of first choice for childhood asthma due to their efficacy and safety. Nedocromil therapy may be able to produce a decrease in inhaled steroid dosage.
- Most patients will experience an improvement in 1–2 weeks. Patients should initially receive cromolyn or nedocromil four times daily and then, only after stabilization of symptoms, may the frequency be reduced to two or three times daily. It is not necessary to maintain the regular use of concomitant β_2 agonists after the patient becomes stable; they can be reduced as needed.

XV

Glucocorticoid Therapy (Table 81.6)

- The mechanisms of action of glucocorticoids in asthma include increasing the number of β_2-adrenergic receptors and improving the receptor responsiveness to β_2-adrenergic stimulation, reducing mucus production and hypersecretion, and inhibiting the inflammatory response at all levels.

- Inhaled glucocorticoids are often first-line therapy for chronic asthma because of the contribution of inflammation to the pathogenesis of asthma and because of their localized effect.

- Reversal of seasonal increased bronchial hyperreactivity requires at least 1 week of therapy. Reactivity to EIA decreases after 4 weeks of therapy.

- Acute severe asthma (status asthmaticus) is treated with high-dose systemic (parenteral or oral) glucocorticoids combined with frequent administration of inhaled β_2 agonists. From 4–12 hours may be required before any clinical response is noted. Systemic steroids should be administered in a dose approximately equivalent to methylprednisolone 0.5–1 mg/kg IV or orally every 6–8 hours. After resolution of severe obstruction (achievement of 50% of predicted normal FEV_1, which generally occurs in the first 48–72 hours), the steroid dose is reduced to 1 mg/kg/d in children or 60 mg/d in adults as one or two doses administered by the oral method. The duration of treatment is dependent on the patient's response and past history. Tapering the steroid dosage after hospitalization is unnecessary.

- Glucocorticoids are also recommended for the treatment of impending episodes of severe asthma unresponsive to bronchodilator therapy. Prednisone, approximately 1–2 mg/kg/d (up to 30–40 mg/dose), is administered orally in two divided doses for 3–7 days.

- Because short-term (1–2 weeks) high-dose steroids (1–2 mg/kg/d methylprednisolone) do not produce serious toxicities, the ideal use is to administer the glucocorticoids for a short course and then maintain the patient on bronchodilators, inhaled corticosteroids, and/or cromolyn with long periods between systemic glucocorticoid treatment.

- In patients who require chronic systemic glucocorticoids for control of asthma, the lowest possible dose required to control symptoms should be used. Toxicities of systemic glucocorticoid therapy may be decreased by alternate-day therapy or use of topical inhaled glucocorticoids.

- Patients derive increased antiasthmatic benefits from increasing the dose of inhaled glucocorticoids from 400 to 2000 µg daily. Daily aerosol glucocorticoid administration often produces greater control than alternate-day systemic glucocorticoids. Inhaled steroids may allow the systemic dose to be lowered in severe steroid-dependent asthmatics.

- The inhaled glucocorticoids produce dose-dependent suppression of the adrenal cortex, but much less than systemic glucocorticoids. Glucocorticoids can predispose adults to osteoporosis, and chronic glucocorticoid administration can result in growth retardation in prepubertal chil-

TABLE 81.6. Glucocorticoid Comparison Chart

Systemic	Relative Anti-Inflammatory Potency	Relative Sodium-Retaining Potency	Duration Biologic Activity (h)	Plasma Elimination Half-Life (h)	Equivalent Dose (mg)
Hydrocortisone	1	1	8–12	1.5–2	20
Prednisone	4	0.8	12–36	2.5–3.5	5
Prednisolone	4	0.8	12–36	2.5–3.6	5
Methylprednisolone	5	0.5	12–36	3.3	4
Triamcinolone	5	0	12–36	2.5–3.3	4
Betamethasone	25	0	36–54	5–7	0.75
Dexamethasone	25	0	36–54	3.4–4	0.75

Aerosol	Relative Topical Potency	Systemic Bioavailability (%)	Dosage per Inhalation (µg)	Plasma Elimination Half-Life (H)
Beclomethasone-16, 17-dipropionate (Forte)	0.3–0.5	<5	42(250)	15
Budesonide[a]	1.0	10	50	2–2.8
Flunisolide	0.05	20	250	1.6
Triamcinolone-16, 17-acetonide	0.2	Unknown	100	Unknown
Fluticasone dipropionate[a]	2.0	Unknown	—	3.0

[a]Investigational.

dren. Local adverse effects of inhaled steroids include oropharyngeal candidiasis and dysphonia; use of a spacer device can decrease oropharyngeal deposition and decrease the incidence and severity of local side effects. Oropharyngeal candidiasis can be reduced with less frequent administration and rinsing of the oropharynx.

Leukotriene Modifiers

- A number of compounds that either inhibit the production of leukotrienes or antagonize their receptors are undergoing clinical trials. Two agents have recently been approved for prophylaxis and chronic treatment of asthma in adults and children ≥12 years of age. Neither is indicated for reversal of acute bronchospasm.
  - Zileuton (Zyflo) is a specific inhibitor of 5-lipoxygenase, which thereby inhibits formation of leukotrienes B_4, C_4, D_4, and E_4. Adverse effects include headache (25%), unspecified pain (8%), abdominal pain (5%), and rare hepatotoxicity. Hepatic transaminases should be monitored before treatment, once a month for the first 3 months, every 2–3 months for the remainder of the first year, and then periodically thereafter. Because zileuton may increase theophylline levels approximately two-fold, theophylline dosage should be reduced by about one-half when zileuton therapy is initiated. The recommended dose is 600 mg four times daily, taken with meals and at bedtime.
  - Zafirlukast (Accolate) is a selective and competitive antagonist of the receptors for leukotrienes D_4 and E_4. Adverse effects include headache (13%), infection (3.5%), and nausea (3%). Although zafirlukast does not affect theophylline levels, theophylline may reduce plasma levels of zafirlukast by 30%. The recommended dose is 20 mg twice daily, taken at least one hour before or two hours after meals.

Methotrexate

- Low-dose methotrexate (5–25 mg/week) may act as an anti-inflammatory agent when used for the treatment of asthma. It may also have immunomodulatory effects by inhibiting chemotaxis of neutrophils, inhibiting leukotriene B_4-induced adherence to endothelium, and inhibiting the proinflammatory activity of IL-1.
- At best, methotrexate therapy results in a moderate reduction in systemic steroid dosage (14–35%) in patients with severe steroid-dependent asthma and does not induce a remission in the disease.
- Methotrexate should be considered experimental and reserved for only severe steroid-dependent asthmatics. Patients require careful monitoring, including periodic liver biopsies to detect hepatotoxicity.

▶ EVALUATION OF THERAPEUTIC OUTCOMES

CHRONIC ASTHMA

- Control of asthma is defined as achieving a minimal need for as-needed short-acting β_2 agonists (ideally none), no acute episodes, no limitation of activity, no emergency visits, no nocturnal symptoms, normal peak expiratory flow (PEF) rates, a peak flow diurnal variation of <20%, and minimal or no adverse effects from medicine.

- Monitoring consists of quantitating the use of as-needed short-acting β_2 agonists, days of limited activity, and number of symptoms.
- In moderate to severe asthmatics, daily peak flow monitoring may be warranted, particularly at times of increased symptoms.
- Patients should also be asked about exercise tolerance and nocturnal symptoms.
- All patients on inhaled drugs should have their inhalation technique evaluated periodically, every 3–6 months once optimal technique is established.
- Frequency of monitoring depends on the clinical condition, with severe patients or patients who present as adherence problems seen monthly, and mild to moderate patients evaluated every 3–6 months.
- After initiation of anti-inflammatory therapy or a change in dosage, most patients should begin experiencing a decrease in symptoms within 1–2 weeks and achieve maximum symptomatic improvement within 4–8 weeks. Improvement in baseline FEV_1 or PEF should follow a similar time frame, however a decrease in bronchial hyperreactivity as measured by diurnal variation in PEF and exercise tolerance may take longer and slowly improve over 1–3 months and continue to improve from 6 months to 1 year.

ACUTE SEVERE ASTHMA

- Patients at risk for acute severe exacerbations should monitor peak flows twice daily at home during periods of increased symptoms or acute exacerbations and continue to monitor peak flows until both the evening and morning PEFs are in the green zone (80% of normal or personal best). If in the yellow zone (50–80% of normal), patients should intensify bronchodilator and possibly anti-inflammatory therapy until they improve into the green zone, or contact their physician, or begin their home action plan if not improved in 1–2 days. Patients who fall below 50% of normal PEF should contact their physician as soon as possible and seek urgent medical care.
- In children unable to perform PEFs, supraclavicular retractions and increased respiratory rate and heart rates correlate with severe obstruction.

See Chapter 25, Asthma, authored by H. William Kelly, PharmD, and Alan K. Kamada, PharmD, for a more detailed discussion of this topic.

Chapter 82

► CHRONIC OBSTRUCTIVE LUNG DISEASE

► DEFINITIONS

- Chronic obstructive lung disease (COLD) is a term used to describe a pulmonary disorder characterized by abnormal results of tests of expiratory flow that do not change markedly over several-months of observation. The terms chronic obstructive airway disease (COAD) and chronic obstructive pulmonary disease (COPD) are synonymous with COLD.
- COLD has conventionally included the subsets of chronic bronchitis and emphysema. Chronic bronchitis is a condition with chronic or recurrent excess mucus secretion into the bronchial tree that occurs on most days during a period of at least 3 months of the year for at least 2 consecutive years. Emphysema is a condition of the lung characterized by abnormal, permanent enlargement of the airspaces distal to the terminal bronchiole, accompanied by destruction of their walls, yet without obvious fibrosis.

► PATHOPHYSIOLOGY

CHRONIC BRONCHITIS

- Excessive tracheobronchial mucous secretion results from hyperplasia and hypertrophy of mucus-producing glands and goblet cells due to continued bronchial irritation.
- Inflammation exists with mucus production and narrowing of the lumen in the more distal noncartilagenous or membranous bronchioles. In addition, there is fibrosis, tortuosity, and irregularity of these smaller airways.
- As chronic bronchitis progresses during several years, the changes in small airways begin to impair ventilation (V), while perfusion (Q) remains fairly adequate, resulting in a V/Q imbalance and hypoxemia. The hypoxemia leads to pulmonary hypertension with subsequent right ventricular failure (cor pulmonale).
- Persistent hypoxemia stimulates erythropoiesis with resultant secondary polycythemia and increased blood viscosity, with its attendant complications of mental confusion and thrombotic stroke.
- Patients are predisposed to repeated infections owing to mucus stagnation and plugging as well as lack of cilia or ciliary movement to clear mucus. The respiratory syncytial virus is considered the most common overall pathogen, while *Streptococcus pneumoniae* and *Haemophilus influenzae* are the most common bacterial pathogens.

EMPHYSEMA

- In emphysema, there is destruction of walls within the acinus such that the surface area for gas exchange is diminished.
- Centrilobular emphysema is the most common type and is characteristically seen in cigarette smokers and simple pneumoconiosis of coal workers. This type is confined largely to the proximal portion of the acinus; the respiratory bronchioles are particularly affected. Damage occurs because cigarette smoke causes a macrophage alveolitis and a respiratory bronchiolitis. These macrophages are chemotactic for neutrophils. Both the macrophages and neutrophils release a greater amount of elastase (which breaks down elastin, a protein integral to the structural integrity of alveolar walls) in smokers. The respiratory bronchiolitis leads to narrowing of the terminal bronchioles.
- As its name implies, the entire acinus is involved in panacinar emphysema. It is found in those genetically susceptible individuals who have a deficiency of protease inhibitors (α_1-antitrypsin deficiency) such that proteases are allowed to destroy the alveolar walls of the acinus.
- The destruction of the surface area for gas exchange within the acinus results in a loss of elastic recoil, which permits compression of distal airways during expiration.
- Loss of alveolar walls results in a loss of the capillary network essential to adequate perfusion. This results in a decrease in ventilation and a loss in perfusion, so the V/Q ratio is maintained better than in chronic bronchitis. Therefore, while emphysematous patients experience greater dyspnea than chronic bronchitis patients, the former are better able to preserve gas exchange because their respiratory centers are more responsive to hypoxia. The net result of this on other physiologic systems is less cor pulmonale and less polycythemia than in chronic bronchitis.

▶ CLINICAL PRESENTATION (Table 82.1)

CHRONIC BRONCHITIS

- The patient presenting with predominant chronic bronchitis is often overweight and has a history of productive cough that has been increasing in frequency and duration and has increasing dyspnea on exertion.
- Patients are often referred to as "blue bloaters" (type B) as they tend to retain carbon dioxide because of a decreased responsiveness of the respiratory center to hypoxemia and ultimately hypercarbia.
- They commonly have peripheral edema from cor pulmonale and usually have a normal or only slightly increased respiratory rate at rest.
- With advanced disease, the anteroposterior diameter of the chest is often increased, resulting in a "barrel chest" appearance.
- On physical examination, percussion of the chest is resonant, and the breath sounds are distant on auscultation. Rhonchi and wheezes are fre-

TABLE 82.1. Clinical Features of COLD

	Predominant Emphysema	Predominant Chronic Bronchitis
Age (yr)	60±	50±
Dyspnea	Severe	Mild
Cough	After dyspnea starts	Before dyspnea starts
Sputum	Scanty, mucoid	Copious, purulent
Bronchial infection	Less frequent	More frequent
Respiratory insufficiency episode	Often terminal	Repeated
Chest film	Increased diameter Flattened diaphragms	Increased bronchovascular markings, large heart
$Paco_2$ (mm Hg)	35–40	50–60
Pao_2 (mm Hg)	65–75	45–60
Hematocrit (%)	35–45	50–60
Pulmonary hypertension		
Rest	None to mild	Moderate to severe
Exercise	Moderate	Worsens
Cor pulmonale	Rare	Common
Diffusion capacity	Decreased	None to slightly decreased

Adapted from Anthonisen NR. Am Rev Respir Dis 1989;140:595–599, with permission.

quently heard and change in location as the patient breathes deeply or coughs.

- A rapid assessment of obstruction can be done by placing the stethoscope over the trachea and instructing the patient to forcefully expire. Forced expiration lasting >4 seconds correlates with obstruction in pulmonary function tests.
- The use of the scalene or sternocleidomastoid muscles of the neck to assist respiration may not be apparent unless severe obstruction is present.
- As the degree of obstruction worsens and the arterial oxygen tension (Pao_2) continues to drop, pulmonary hypertension from vasoconstriction ensues. This leads to right ventricular strain and ultimately cor pulmonale. On physical examination this is manifested by jugular venous distention, hepatomegaly, hepatojugular reflux, and peripheral edema.
- On cardiac examination, a heave may be felt (or even seen in thin patients) upon palpation of the epigastric area. Auscultation of the area may reveal a gallop rhythm suggestive of right ventricular hypertrophy.
- In the face of chronic hypoxemia, cyanosis of the lips, mucous membranes, or extremities may be seen. Clubbing of the fingers is rarely seen in chronic bronchitis.

EMPHYSEMA

- Patients with predominant emphysema are characteristically older than those with chronic bronchitis. The chief complaint is often increasing dyspnea, even at rest, with minimal cough.
- These patients have been classically termed "pink puffers" (type A) because of their obvious tachypnea and flushed appearance, which is due to their respiratory centers being quite responsive to hypoxemia as a stimulus to breathe.
- These patients are frequently thin and will present with "pursed lip" breathing. They also are tachypneic at rest and often sit with their chests forward and hands resting on their knees; this position requires the least energy for breathing. Accessory muscles of the chest and neck are frequently used to assist in the work of breathing.
- Percussion of the chest is hyperresonant, and auscultation reveals diminished breath sounds with rhonchi and minimal wheezes. Excursion of the diaphragms is limited because of persistent hyperinflation of the lungs.
- Hypoxemia is not a significant problem in the predominant emphysema patient until late in the disease state. As a result, cor pulmonale is not common until the terminal stages.

▶ DIAGNOSIS

PULMONARY FUNCTION TESTS

- In patients with chronic bronchitis and/or emphysema, there are reductions in forced expiratory volume after 1 second (FEV_1), forced vital capacity (FVC), $FEV_1/FVC\%$, and forced expiratory flow ($FEF_{25-75\%}$).
- Measurement of diffusion capacity using carbon monoxide (DCO) can help distinguish predominant bronchitis from emphysema. In emphysema, the diffusion capacity is diminished because of loss of surface area available for gas diffusion. In bronchitis the diffusion capacity is normal or only slightly decreased.

ARTERIAL BLOOD GASES

- The predominant chronic bronchitis patient is characterized as having a low arterial oxygen tension ($PaO_2 = 45-60$ mm Hg) and an elevated arterial carbon dioxide tension ($PaCO_2 = 50-60$ mm Hg).
- The predominantly emphysematous patient has by comparison a higher PaO_2 and usually normal $PaCO_2$ with similar degrees of pulmonary dysfunction.
- Because these changes in PaO_2 and $PaCO_2$ are subtle and progress over many years, the pH is usually near normal because the kidneys compensate by retaining bicarbonate.

CHEST ROENTGENOGRAM

- Characteristic findings of severe emphysema include flattened diaphragms that move <3 cm between inspiration and expiration, loss

XV

of peripheral vascular markings, bullous lesions, and increased ret-
rosternal air space, indicating extensive air trapping.

- In the patient with predominant chronic bronchitis, the only changes are
  increased bronchovascular markings in the lower lung field and an
  increased cardiac silhouette in the presence of right ventricular failure
  with prominent pulmonary arteries.

ELECTROCARDIOGRAM

- Common findings when cor pulmonale develops are right-axis deviation, prominent R waves in V1 and V2, S wave in V5 or V6 $\geq$ 7 mm,
  and tall peaked P waves in lead II.

OTHER LABORATORY TESTS

- In the predominant chronic bronchitic patient, the hemoglobin and
  hematocrit are elevated secondary to erythropoiesis caused by hypoxemia.
- In exacerbations of chronic bronchitis, the white cell count may or may
  not rise and a left shift may or may not be present.
- Examination of sputum (e.g., Gram stain) is helpful in exacerbations of
  chronic bronchitis to identify potential bacterial pathogens that may have
  precipitated the exacerbation and aid in the selection of antimicrobial
  therapy. Sputum should also be examined for eosinophils to rule out an
  allergic component that would be consistent with asthmatic bronchitis.

DIAGNOSIS OF ACUTE RESPIRATORY FAILURE IN COLD

- The diagnosis of acute respiratory failure in COLD is made on the basis
  of an acute drop in PaO_2 of 10–15 mm Hg or any acute increase in
  $PaCO_2$ that decreases the serum pH to 7.30 or less.
- Additional acute clinical manifestations include restlessness, confusion,
  tachycardia, diaphoresis, cyanosis, hypotension, irregular breathing,
  miosis, and unconsciousness.
- The most common cause of acute respiratory failure in COLD is
  acute exacerbation of bronchitis with an increase in the volume and
  viscosity of sputum. This serves to worsen obstruction and further
  impair alveolar ventilation, resulting in worsening hypoxemia and
  hypercapnea. Additional causes are pneumonia, pulmonary embolism,
  left ventricular failure, pneumothorax, and central nervous system
  depressants.

▶ DESIRED OUTCOME

The goals of therapy are to improve the chronic obstructive state, treat
and prevent acute exacerbations, reduce the rate of progression of the disease, improve the physical and psychologic well-being of the patient so
that daily activities can be resumed or maintained, reduce the number of
days lost from work, reduce hospitalizations, and reduce mortality.

▶ TREATMENT

GENERAL PRINCIPLES

- Smoking cessation is a critical first step that will slow the rate of decline in pulmonary function tests, decrease symptoms, and improve the patient's quality of life.
- Many individuals with COLD obtain some degree of improvement in their obstruction from bronchodilators, even though tests of reversibility using an inhaled sympathomimetic followed by pulmonary function tests do not indicate a positive response.
- An algorithm to provide guidance in the choice of therapy for COLD is shown in Figure 82.1. Individualized treatment regimens are necessary in order to optimize outcome because patients differ in their compliance with medication, technique in using inhalers and equipment, and values in terms of quality of life.

ANTICHOLINERGICS

- When given by inhalation, atropine and ipratropium bromide produce bronchodilation by competitively inhibiting cholinergic receptors in bronchial smooth muscle. This activity blocks acetylcholine, with the net effect being a reduction in cyclic guanosine monophosphate (GMP), which normally acts to constrict bronchial smooth muscle.
- These drugs have emerged as first-line therapy for the stable COLD patient. Anticholinergic agents produce greater improvement in pulmonary function tests than the sympathomimetics in patients with COLD, pointing out the relative importance of the cholinergic system as a mediator of bronchial tone. These agents maintain their effectiveness during years of regular continuous use.
- Ipratropium bromide is preferred over atropine sulfate because it has fewer systemic side effects. It is available as a metered dose inhaler (MDI) and a solution for inhalation and provides a peak effect in 1.5–2 hours with a duration of 4–6 hours. Systemic absorption is minimal because of its quaternary ammonium structure.
- Although the recommended dose is two puffs 4 times a day, many clinicians prescribe two to three times that dose to produce maximal bronchodilation.
- Spacer devices improve aerosol delivery from MDIs in patients who are unable to adequately coordinate MDI actuation with inhalation (e.g., elderly COLD patients).

SYMPATHOMIMETICS

- β_2-selective sympathomimetics cause bronchodilation by stimulating the enzyme adenyl cyclase to increase the formation of adenosine $3',5'$ monophosphate ($3',5'$-cAMP). In addition, they are thought to improve mucociliary clearance.

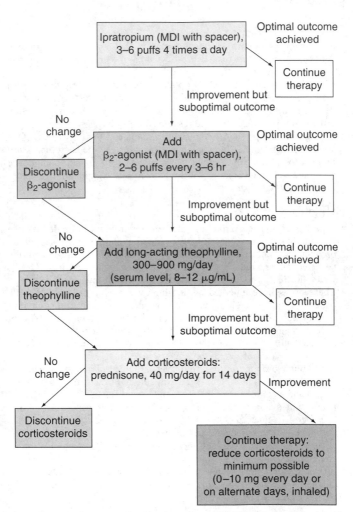

Figure 82.1. Typical treatment algorithm for patients with COLD. Outcome is measured in terms of improvement in the FEV₁:FVC and peak flow; improvement in the distance covered in a 6- or 12-minute walk; and objectively observed reduction in dyspnea, medication use, and nocturnal symptoms. MDI, metered dose inhaler. *(Reprinted by permission of The New England Journal of Medicine, vol 328, pp 1017–1022, 1993.)*

- Agents with greater β_2 selectivity and longer duration of action are preferred and include albuterol, bitolterol, salmeterol, and terbutaline. The inhalation route is preferred over the oral and parenteral route in terms of both efficacy and toxicity.
- Sympathomimetics are the bronchodilators of choice for acute exacerbations of COLD.
- All patients with COLD deserve a trial of inhaled β_2 agonist even if their FEV_1 is not changed, because mechanisms other than bronchodilation may be helpful (e.g., increase in mucociliary clearance). An individual's perceived benefit from these agents may significantly affect their usefulness.
- The dose can be increased in an acute exacerbation, although the limiting factor is an excessive increase in heart rate.

COMBINATION ANTICHOLINERGICS AND SYMPATHOMIMETICS

- The combination of inhaled anticholinergic and sympathomimetic regimens may be more effective than either one alone.
- Before the combination is used, the dose of the anticholinergic should first be titrated.
- With the products currently available, the anticholinergic should be used 2 hours prior to using the sympathomimetic.

METHYLXANTHINES

- In addition to inhibition of phosphodiesterase, numerous other mechanisms have been proposed to explain bronchodilation and other respiratory effects of methylxanthines, including inhibition of calcium ion influx into smooth muscle, prostaglandin antagonism, stimulation of endogenous catecholamines, adenosine receptor antagonism, and inhibition of release of mediators from mast cells and leukocytes.
- Because not all studies have demonstrated that theophylline improves symptoms in COLD patients, it is considered third-line therapy after anticholinergics and sympathomimetics. When methylxanthines are used, parameters other than objective measurements, such as FEV_1, should be monitored to assess efficacy. Subjective parameters, such as perceived exercise tolerance, are important in assessing the acceptability of methylxanthines for COLD patients.
- Sustained-release theophylline (1,3-dimethylxanthine) improves patient compliance and achieves more consistent serum concentrations than rapid-release theophylline and aminophylline preparations, but there are considerable variations in sustained-release characteristics.
- Administration of long-acting theophylline preparations at bedtime has been demonstrated to reduce overnight declines in FEV_1 and morning respiratory symptoms.
- Administration of IV aminophylline is indicated for severe acute decompensation or if the patient is unable to take oral medications. Recommended loading doses are 6–9 mg/kg (actual body weight) for patients who have not taken any theophylline in the previous 24 hours, XV

TABLE 82.2. Maintenance Doses of Parenteral Aminophylline in Exacerbations of COLD

Age (>50 yr)	0.6–0.7 mg/kg/h
Bacterial or viral pneumonia	0.45–0.7 mg/kg/h
Heart failure (left or right)	0.45–0.7 mg/kg/h
Liver disease (total bilirubin >1.5 mg/dL)	0.2–0.25 mg/kg/h

or 3 mg/kg if they have taken sustained-release theophylline within the past 24 hours or rapid-release theophylline within the past 12 hours. The administration rate should not exceed 25 mg/min, to avoid cardiac arrhythmias or cardiovascular collapse.

- The desired therapeutic range in older COLD patients is 10–15 μg/mL in order to minimize the likelihood of toxicity.
- Initial maintenance dose recommendations for various conditions are included in Table 82.2. Serum concentrations should be obtained 12–24 hours after the initiation of therapy and every 24 hours thereafter until the patient is stable.
- When switching to oral therapy, the oral sustained-release preparation can be initiated at the time the IV infusion is stopped. The total 24-hour IV dose may be divided in thirds or in halves depending on the desired interval and strength of preparation available. Follow-up trough serum concentrations should be obtained several days later to ensure the appropriateness of the dose and dosing interval. Once a dose is established, it is not necessary to routinely monitor serum concentrations unless the patient's disease worsens or toxicity is suspected.

CORTICOSTEROIDS

- The anti-inflammatory mechanisms whereby corticosteroids exert their beneficial effect in COLD include reduction in capillary permeability to decrease mucus, inhibition of release of proteolytic enzymes from leukocytes, and inhibition of prostaglandins.
- Corticosteroids may be initiated during an acute exacerbation when the patient is deteriorating or not improving as expected, despite adequate anticholinergic and/or sympathomimetic therapy and possibly methyl-xanthines.
- Patients taking chronic oral steroids who present in acute distress should be immediately started on parenteral steroids. Therapy is initiated with methylprednisolone or its equivalent 0.5–1.0 mg/kg IV every 6 hours. It generally requires 3–6 hours for a beneficial effect to be observed.
- As soon as symptoms have stabilized, the patient may be switched to 40–60 mg of prednisone daily. Steroids should be stopped in 7–14 days, if possible, to minimize HPA suppression.
- If prolonged therapy is needed, a low morning daily dose (e.g., prednisone, 7.5 mg/d) or alternate-day therapy should be employed.

- In patients requiring continuous steroid therapy, giving short bursts of higher doses of oral prednisone during periods of worsening clinical status may be effective in decreasing hospitalizations.
- Although inhaled corticosteroids may be of some benefit in COLD, asthmatic patients tend to gain greater benefit than COLD patients.

LONG-TERM OXYGEN

- Stable outpatients receiving optimal pharmacotherapy should have long-term oxygen therapy instituted if either of two conditions exists: (1) a resting PaO_2 of <55 mm Hg; or (2) evidence of right heart failure, polycythemia, or impaired neuropsychiatric function with a PaO_2 of <60 mm Hg.
- Oxygen therapy may also be used during exercise in those patients who show serious hypoxemia during episodes of increased activity, and during the night in individuals who have nocturnal hypoxemia.
- The most practical means of administering long-term oxygen is with the nasal cannula, which provides 24–28% oxygen. The goal is to raise the PaO_2 above 60 mm Hg. Patients known to retain carbon dioxide should be cautioned to not raise the PaO_2 so high that they depress their respiratory drive.
- The use of an oxygen concentrator may cost between $200 and $400 per month. Portable oxygen tanks may cost about $300 per month.

ANTIBIOTICS

- Antibiotics are reasonable in patients who exhibit signs suggestive of bronchial infection, such as increased sputum, increased viscosity of sputum, and/or change in sputum color. Sputum Gram stain is more helpful in determining the need for oral antibiotic therapy than sputum cultures. Patients may not have fever, chills, or a leukocytosis in the early stage of infectious exacerbations.
- Therapy should be initiated within 24 hours of symptoms to prevent unnecessary hospitalization.
- The bacterial organisms usually responsible for exacerbations are *Streptococcus pneumoniae* and *Haemophilus influenzae*.
- Oral ampicillin and amoxicillin are the agents of choice in patients not allergic to penicillins. Other acceptable oral alternatives include tetracyclines, cephalosporins, and cotrimoxazole. If bacterial resistance to the penicillins through β-lactamase is suspected, a β-lactamase inhibitor such as clavulanate may be an appropriate choice (e.g., amoxicillin/clavulanate).
- Therapy should generally be continued for at least 7–10 days. Azithromycin for 3–5 days is also effective.
- If the patient deteriorates or does not improve as anticipated, hospitalization may be necessary and more aggressive attempts should be made to identify potential pathogens responsible for the exacerbation. Parenteral antibiotics may be required.

XV

- COLD patients should receive one dose of pneumococcal vaccine and a yearly influenza vaccination. If a patient has been exposed to influenza before vaccination, a course of amantadine or rimantadine may be considered.

▶ EVALUATION OF THERAPEUTIC OUTCOMES

- The pharmacologic plan for a given patient requires weighing the risk/benefit ratio carefully and having a comprehensive plan to assess subjectively and objectively the efficacy and toxicity of the chosen therapy.
- Objective outcome measures include improvement in the FEV_1:FVC and peak flow; improvement in the distance covered in a 6- or 12-minutes walk; and objectively observed reduction in dyspnea, medication use, and nocturnal symptoms.
- Subjective parameters, such as perceived improvement in exercise tolerance should also be considered; although objective improvement may be minimal with some therapies, clinical benefit to the individual may be meaningful.

See Chapter 26, Chronic Obstructive Lung Disease, authored by Margaret A. Noyes, PharmD, BCPS, and Mark A. Stratton, PharmD, BCPS, FASHP, for a more detailed discussion of this topic.

Chapter 83

▶ CYSTIC FIBROSIS

▶ DEFINITION

Cystic fibrosis is a genetically inherited disease caused by a chloride transport channel defect at the secretory epithelial cell level. The disorder primarily involves the exocrine glands, gastrointestinal (GI) system, and pulmonary system. Most pathology is due to production of viscous secretions. Cystic fibrosis is inherited through an autosomal (Mendelian) recessive genetic mode.

▶ PATHOPHYSIOLOGY

- Cystic fibrosis is basically a disease of secretory epithelial cells or tissues. Such tissues are involved with the transport of chloride, sodium, and water in and out of the blood.
- An apical membrane chloride channel is apparently affected in cystic fibrosis, leading to a decrease in secretion of chloride, sodium, and water. In the most common genetic mutation, individuals have this abnormal chloride channel in the cells of several exocrine organs including pancreatic and hepatobiliary ducts, microvilli of the GI tract, and the lungs. These changes lead to the thick, dehydrated mucus that can block pancreatic and hepatobiliary exocrine outflow and also accumulate in and obstruct the airways.
- Involvement of the GI tract is owing to both the increased viscosity of mucus secretions and a relative deficiency of pancreatic digestive enzymes.
- A deficiency of pancreatic digestive enzymes (pancreatic achylia) is present in 85% of patients. Pancreatic lesions include fibrosis, fatty replacement, and cyst formation and are secondary to obstruction of small pancreatic ducts by thickened secretions and cellular debris. This leads to a maldigestion of ingested nutrients including fats and protein.
- Because of lipase deficiency, fat-soluble vitamin (A, D, E, and K) deficiencies sometimes occur.
- Insulin deficiency and carbohydrate intolerance has been described in many older cystic fibrosis patients; 8% of cystic fibrosis children older than 12 years of age require insulin therapy.
- Biliary cirrhosis secondary to bile duct obstruction occurs in as many as 18% of patients, while fatty infiltration may occur in about 30% of patients.
- Pulmonary obstruction of both small and large airways by thick mucus results in air trapping, bronchiectasis, and atelectasis, resulting in a COPD phenomenon not unlike emphysema. The persistence of mucus is an excellent growth medium for microorganisms, and pulmonary infections are common despite normal host defense mechanisms. The

three most common bacterial pathogens isolated from sputum are *Staphylococcus aureus, Pseudomonas aeruginosa,* and *Haemophilus influenzae,* with *P. aeruginosa* predominating throughout life. Viruses and other nonbacterial pathogens may also play a pathologic role.

- The inflammatory reaction in response to the inability to clear the lower airways of bacterial pathogens tends to be excessive. Excess amounts of inflammatory mediators can initiate a self-sustaining, vicious cycle leading to progressive and often permanent tissue damage. The major consequence of these pulmonary processes is a decrease in gas exchange by the lungs.

- The abnormally high concentrations of both sodium and chloride in the sweat, owing to defective salt reabsorption, can result in the need for supplementary dietary intake of these electrolytes, and forms the basis for the diagnosis of the disease. There is a failure of the sweat ducts to reabsorb these electrolytes in a normal fashion, apparently because of chloride impermeability in the sweat ducts and salivary glands.

- 95% of males are sterile because of abnormal development or obstruction of the epididymis, vas deferens, and seminal vesicles, with resulting aspermia. Females also have less than normal fertility owing to the production of abnormal cervical mucus.

▶ CLINICAL PRESENTATION

- Intestinal obstruction causes symptoms such as vomiting of bile-stained material, abdominal distention, and pain.

- Maldigestion of ingested food results in steatorrhea and malnutrition. Stools are characterized by their foul smell, bulky, greasy nature, and abnormally high number per day.

- Obstructive pulmonary disease and hypoxia result in cyanosis, digital clubbing, labored breathing with retractions and resultant increased anterior-posterior chest diameter (also referred to as "barrel chest"), flattened diaphragm, and overaeration observed on chest roentgenogram.

- Marked declines in pulmonary status (presumably secondary to infection) are referred to as acute respiratory exacerbations and are generally associated with fever, increased coughing, increased sputum production, change in sputum character (e.g., thicker, change in color), increased respiratory rate, dyspnea on exertion, increased oxygen requirements, and decreased exercise tolerance. Concomitantly, laboratory tests of peripheral blood reveal an increased white blood count with increased polymorphonuclear leukocytes and immature forms consistent with acute infection.

- The upper respiratory tract may also be involved; sinusitis and nasal polyposis occur in 90 and 50% of patients, respectively. Symptoms of chronic sinusitis and nasal polyposis may include rhinorrhea, nasal obstruction, pain over affected sinuses, and disturbances of smell.

- Tests of pulmonary function often demonstrate both acute and long-term changes in forced vital capacity, forced expiratory volume, and residual volume. Arterial blood gases typically reveal hypoxia and hypercapnia.

- Despite the chronic hypoxia characteristic of cystic fibrosis, erythropoietin concentrations are normal or low. The condition is characterized by decreased hematocrit and serum ferritin, increased carboxyhemoglobin, and normal or low hemoglobin.
- An arthritis can occur that may be either mono- or polyarticular but is usually nondestructive. Osteopenia and osteoporosis also occur with abnormally high frequency in adult cystic fibrosis patients.

▶ DIAGNOSIS

- Diagnosis on the basis of an abnormal sweat test involves collection of a sweat sample (usually with the use of pilocarpine iontophoresis) and determination of the concentration of chloride. A concentration of 60 mEq/L or more is generally considered to be diagnostic.
- The presence of chronic obstructive respiratory disease, exocrine pancreatic insufficiency, and/or a positive family history of the disease help to confirm the diagnosis.
- Genetic analysis is now also possible and may be used to diagnose the disease in utero or to detect heterozygotes (carriers) with obvious implications for genetic counseling

▶ DESIRED OUTCOME

The goals of treatment for cystic fibrosis are to relieve the patient's signs and symptoms, prevent and treat acute and chronic complications, provide optimal nutrition, improve quality of life, and prolong life by slowing chronic deterioration of pulmonary function.

▶ TREATMENT

PANCREATIC ENZYME SUPPLEMENTATION

- The treatment of GI involvement is usually required to correct nutritional deficits due to pancreatic enzyme deficiency and other causes.
- Microencapsulated products are preferred, because the enzymes are protected from destruction by gastric acid, and much lower doses can be used than were required with previous products susceptible to acid breakdown.
- Patients who are unable to swallow capsules may empty the contents into applesauce, jelly, or some other vehicle provided that the microencapsulated beads are not chewed. Powders may also be useful in patients unable to swallow capsules or to otherwise use the microencapsulated beads they contain.
- The most contemporary enzyme replacement products vary mainly in enzyme content per capsule, with lipase content being the chief variable (Table 83.1).

XV ◀

TABLE 83.1. Pancreatic Enzyme Products

Trade Name	Enzyme Content (units)			Form[a]
	Lipase	Protease	Amylase	
Cotazym	8000	30,000	30,000	C
Cotazym-S	5000	20,000	20,000	ECM
Creon	8000	13,000	30,000	ECM
Ilozyme	11,000	30,000	30,000	T
Pancrease	4000	25,000	20,000	ECM
Pancrease MT4	4000	12,000	12,000	ECM
Pancrease MT10	10,000	30,000	30,000	ECM
Pancrease MT16	16,000	48,000	48,000	ECM
Ultrase MT12	12,000	39,000	39,000	ECM
Ultrase MT20	20,000	65,000	66,000	ECM
Ultrase MT24	24,000	78,000	78,000	ECM
Viokase	8000	30,000	30,000	T
Viokase	16,800	70,000	70,000	P[b]
Zymase	12,000	24,000	24,000	ECM

[a]Dosage form: C, capsule; ECM, enteric coated microspheres or beads; T, tablet; P, powder.
[b]Viokase powder, units of enzymes per 700 mg.

- Histamine H_2-receptor antagonists have been used to reduce the enzyme dose when residual acid breakdown is suspected. Omeprazole has been shown to be effective in patients with steatorrhea despite high-dose enzyme supplementation.
- Side effects are unusual and may include perianal irritation resembling diaper rash in infants fed excess quantities of enzyme powders, hyper-uricosuria apparently related to high purine content, and dose-related colonic strictures (fibrosing colonopathy) in patients receiving per meal lipase doses in excess of 6000 units/kg.

VITAMIN SUPPLEMENTATION

- Clinically evident fat-soluble vitamin deficiencies are unusual in patients taking adequate pancreatic enzymes and receiving a balanced diet, but supplementation of vitamin A, vitamin E, and vitamin K has been recommended.

RESPIRATORY THERAPY

- Percussion and postural drainage aids in the clearance of pulmonary mucus and is performed as often as five times daily or more during an acute pulmonary exacerbation.
- Percussion is often preceded by nebulizer therapy during which nebulized sterile water or 0.9% sodium chloride solution is breathed to liquefy pulmonary secretions. Bronchodilators and/or mucolytic agents

(e.g., *N*-acetylcysteine) may be added to the nebulizer solution to prevent bronchospasm and further liquefy pulmonary secretions, respectively.

- Recombinant human DNase (dornase alfa) given by inhalation (2.5 mg once or twice daily) reduces the viscosity of cystic fibrosis sputum and leads to statistically significant, although modest, improvement in indices of pulmonary function. The cost of this therapy may not be justified for the majority of cystic fibrosis patients because the average improvement in pulmonary function is small.

- Alternate-day prednisone has been shown to be neither effective nor safe for inhibiting the inflammatory component of the disease, but a recent long-term trial of oral ibuprofen indicates a positive effect in slowing pulmonary deterioration.

- Systemic bronchodilators such as theophylline and β agonists may be of benefit for patients with a reactive airways component to their pulmonary disease. Responsiveness to such agents should be documented before a protracted course is begun. Theophylline clearance may be altered in cystic fibrosis, and determination of a theophylline dose should be based on the pharmacokinetic values of the individual.

- Influenza vaccine should be administered on a yearly basis because cystic fibrosis patients are at high risk to develop the complications of influenza. Amantadine prophylaxis or treatment may be indicated as well.

ANTIBIOTIC THERAPY

- Although not all acute pulmonary exacerbations are due to bacteria, and viral infection and air pollutants might contribute to such episodes, the routine presence of known bacterial pathogens dictates antibiotic use, and most clinicians regularly employ antibiotic therapy.

- Therapy is directed at proven or likely pathogens such as *P. aeruginosa* and *S. aureus,* and usually includes an aminoglycoside and an extended-spectrum penicillin. Such combinations are sometimes synergistic in vitro and may act to suppress or delay the emergence of resistance.

- Single-agent therapy (e.g., ceftazidime, aztreonam, ciprofloxacin) on an outpatient basis is employed at some centers where significant resistance to these agents has not yet emerged. However, some evidence supports the clinical superiority of two-drug combinations.

- Organism-specific drug treatment may be based on results from sputum cultures in cystic fibrosis patients because good agreement between sputum and thoracotomy cultures has been demonstrated.

- Many cystic fibrosis patients have increased total body clearance for many antibiotics, including the aminoglycosides, some of the β-lactams, and trimethoprim/sulfamethoxazole (Table 83.2). Thus, higher doses of these agents may be necessary to produce therapeutic concentrations in some patients. Aminoglycoside doses are often adjusted to desirable concentrations based on measured serum concentrations and subsequent pharmacokinetic calculations during a course of therapy. XV

TABLE 83.2. Changes in Pharmacokinetics in Cystic Fibrosis

Agent	$\beta t_{1/2}$	V_d	CL_B	CL_R
Antibiotics				
Methicillin	NC	I	I	I
Cloxacillin	D	I	I	I
Dicloxacillin	I	NR	NR	I
Azlocillin	D	I	I	NR
Piperacillin	D	I	I	NR
Ticarcillin	D	NC	I	I
Aztreonam	D	I	I	I
Ceftazidime	D	I	I	I
Imipenem	NC	I	I	NR
Trimethoprim/sulfamethoxazole	D/D	NC/NC	I/I	I/NC
Gentamicin	NC	I	I	NR
Tobramycin	NC	I	I	NC
Amikacin	NC	I	I	I
Netilmicin	NC	I	I	NR
Fleroxacin	D	D	I	D
Other				
Theophylline	D	I	I	I
Furosemide	NC	NC	I	NC
Acetaminophen	NC	NR	I	NR

Key: $\beta t_{1/2}$, elimination half-life; V_d, apparent volume of distribution; CL_B, total body clearance; CL_R, renal clearance; D, decreased; I, increased; NC, no change; NR, not reported.

- Inhalation of aerosolized solutions of antibiotics (e.g., β-lactams, aminoglycosides, polymyxins) have been administered and may produce small but significant improvements in pulmonary function tests, organism density in sputum, and peripheral white blood cell count.
- The selection of antibiotics should be based on specific culture and susceptibility results (Table 83.3). Aminoglycosides should be initially dosed at the upper end of the normal dosage range (e.g., 6–7.5 mg/kg/d for tobramycin), and serum concentrations should be determined frequently so that dosage can be appropriately adjusted to achieve peak concentrations of at least 8 but not exceeding 12 μg/mL. Efficacy of once-daily administration of aminoglycosides in cystic fibrosis patients has not yet been determined.
- β-lactam antibiotics such as extended-spectrum penicillins should be prescribed with aminoglycosides to take advantage of their frequent synergy and prevent the emergence of resistance. These agents should be prescribed in large doses to delay stepwise resistance. Ticarcillin,

TABLE 83.3. Antibiotic Doses in Cystic Fibrosis

Antibiotic	Dose (mg/kg/d)	Regimen	Adult Maximum Dose (g/d)
Parenteral Antibiotics			
Tobramycin,[a] Gentamicin,[a] or Netilmicin[a]	6–9	q 6–8 h	NA
Amikacin[a]	20–30	q 6–8 h	NA
Azlocillin	400–600	q 4–6 h	24
Aztreonam	200	q 6 h	8
Carbenicillin	400–600	q 4–6 h	40
Ceftazidime	150	q 8 h	6
Colistin	6–8	q 6–8 h	NA
Imipenem	45–100	q 6 h	4
Nafcillin	100	q 4–6 h	6
Ticarcillin	400–600	q 4–6 h	18
Ticarcillin/clavulanate	400–600	q 4–6 h	18
Piperacillin	400–600	q 4–6 h	18
Oral Antibiotics			
Ciprofloxacin[b]	1500 mg/d	q 12 h	1.5
Cephalexin	50–100	q 6–8 h	6
Dicloxacillin	80–100	q 6 h	6
Trimethoprim/sulfamethoxazole	10–15[c]	q 12 h	0.64[c]
Inhaled Antibiotics			
Colistin	150 mg/d	q 6–12 h	NA
Gentamicin or Tobramycin	60–1800 mg/d	q 6–12 h	NA
Polymyxin B	250 mg/d	q 6–12 h	NA

[a]Starting doses; adjust to desired serum concentrations based on dose/serum concentration relationship.
[b]Adult dose.
[c]Based on trimethoprim.

azlocillin, and piperacillin should be prescribed in a dose of at least 350 mg/kg/d divided into 4–6 doses. For patients with *P. aeruginosa* and *S. aureus,* the combination of an aminoglycoside and ticarcillin/clavulanate or piperacillin/tazobactam should be as effective as an aminoglycoside plus an extended-spectrum penicillin and nafcillin. Selection among these agents should be based on local susceptibility patterns and cost considerations.

- Oral antibiotics should be prescribed in symptomatic outpatients with susceptible pathogens in their sputum (e.g., first-generation cephalosporins, trimethoprim/sulfamethoxazole, and amoxicillin/clavulanic acid).

▶ EVALUATION OF THERAPEUTIC OUTCOMES

- The nutritional status of the patient should be closely monitored on both short- and long-term bases. Height and weight should be followed with time and anthropometric measures to give more precise information.

XV

- The adequacy of pancreatic enzyme replacement can be grossly assessed by following stool patterns with the goal of normal number per day and normal consistency. Any evidence of steatorrhea indicates suboptimal enzyme therapy.
- Vitamin status can be assessed though serum monitoring of fat-soluble vitamin concentrations.
- Pulmonary status can be monitored by a combination of clinical observation and examination and a variety of laboratory tests. Physical examination should focus on signs and symptoms of upper and lower respiratory tract infection.
- During acute respiratory exacerbations, bacterial eradication is desirable but other attainable endpoints that serve as useful monitoring parameters include bacterial density in sputum and sputum DNA and protein content. Plasma inflammatory markers such as C-reactive protein may also be useful.
- Pulmonary function tests correlate best with clinical observations and scoring systems. Response to IV antibiotics and aggressive chest physiotherapy, as measured by FEV_1 at the end of 1 week of treatment, has been used to predict total necessary length of therapy.
- Oral antibiotic therapy should also be limited in length with specific endpoints, such as decreased cough and/or improved pulmonary function, identified as treatment commences.

See Chapter 29, Cystic Fibrosis, authored by John A. Bosso, PharmD, FCCP, for a more detailed discussion of this topic.

Appendices

▶ DRUG-INDUCED SKIN DISORDERS

TABLE A1.1. Drugs Associated with Maculopapular Eruptions

Allopurinol	Penicillamine
Barbiturates	Penicillins
Benzodiazepines	Phenothiazines
Carbamazepine	Phenylbutazone
Chloramphenicol	Piroxicam
Erythromycin	Pyrazolon derivatives
Ethionamide	Rifampin
Gold salts	Streptomycin
Hydantoin derivatives	Sulfonamides (including sulfonylureas and thiazide diuretics)
Ibuprofen	Sulindac
Indomethacin	Tetracyclines
Isoniazid	Tolmetin
Nitrofurantoin	

TABLE A1.2. Drugs Associated with Urticaria

Acetylsalicylic acid	Opiates
Gold	Penicillins
Heparin	Sulfonamides
Ibuprofen	Sulindac
Indomethacin	Tartrazine
Iodinated radiocontrast media	Tolmetin
Naproxen	

TABLE A1.3. Drugs that Produce Fixed-Drug Eruptions

Barbiturates	Ibuprofen
Dapsone	Ipecac
Digitalis compounds	Metronidazole
Diphenhydramine	Phenolphthalein
Disulfiram	Phenothiazines
Epinephrine	Phenylbutazone
Erythromycin	Quinidine
Gold	Sulfonamides
Griseofulvin	Sulindac
Hydralazine	Tetracyclines
Hydroxyurea	Trimethoprim

TABLE A1.4. Drugs that Produce Photosensitivity Reactions

Amiodarone	Piroxicam
Carbamazepine	Protriptyline
Dacarbazine	Quinidine
Furosemide	Sulfonamides
Ketoprofen	Sulfonylureas
Naproxen	Sulindac
Oral contraceptives	Tetracyclines
Phenothiazines/chlorpromazine	Thiazides
Phenylbutazone	

TABLE A1.5. Drugs Associated with Alopecia

Carbamazepine	Hydantoin derivatives
Clofibrate	Isotretinoin
Colchicine	Propranolol
Ethionamide	Valproate sodium
Etretinate	Vitamin A (high dose)

TABLE A1.6. Drugs Associated with Vasculitis

Allopurinol	Phenylbutazone
Anticoagulants	Phenytoin
Cimetidine	Piroxicam
Fluoxetine	Propylthiouracil
Hydralazine	Quinine
Ibuprofen	Sulfonamides
Indomethacin	Thiazides
Penicillins	

TABLE A1.7. Heavy Metal–Induced Hyperpigmentation

Agent	Color	Region Involved	Special Features
Mercury	Gray brown, slate green	Skin folds (topical), gingival pigmentation (systemic)	Caused by deposition of metallic granules and increased melanin production; formerly used in bleaching agents
Silver	Slate gray, blue gray	Sun-exposed areas, mucosa, sclerae, nails	Silver granule deposition that activates melanin production; occurs months to years after ingestion
Bismuth	Blue gray	Skin, conjunctiva, oral and vaginal mucosa, black line along gingival margin	Deposition of metallic granules or interaction with bacteria in mouth; more common with parenteral use
Arsenic	Brown, bronze	Trunk, "raindrop"-shaped hyperkeratotic papulonodular lesions; palms, soles	Activates enzymes that form melanin and deposit in skin; used systemically for psoriasis and as a health tonic; pigmentation appears 1–20 years after exposure
Gold	Blue gray	Periorbital, generalized chrysiasis, sun-exposed areas	Caused by deposition of metallic particles in epidermis; occurs months to years after exposure and is permanent

TABLE A1.8. Chemotherapeutic Agents Associated with Hyperpigmentation

Agent	Color	Region Involved	Special Features
Busulfan	Brown	Face, forearms, chest, trunk, hands	Accelerates melanin formation by enzymes; incidence more frequent in dark-skinned patients; resolves on discontinuation
Bleomycin	Brown	Linear bands on chest, back	Incidence 8–20%; reversible on discontinuation
Doxorubicin	Black-brown	Tongue, palms, soles, nails	Increased incidence in dark-skinned patients; reversible on discontinuation
Mechlorethamine (topical)	Brown	Areas of contact	Toxic effect on keratinocytes; increased melanocytes; some aggregation

TABLE A1.9. Drugs Associated with Erythema Multiforme

Barbiturates	Propranolol
Carbamazepine	Quinine
Diflunisal	Salicylates
Hydantoins	Sulfonamides
Ibuprofen	Sulfonylureas
Penicillins	Sulindac
Phenolphthalein	Thiazides
Phenylbutazone	

TABLE A1.10. Drugs Associated with Toxic Epidermal Necrolysis

Allopurinol	Penicillins
Barbiturates	Phenylbutazone
Chloramphenicol	Quinine
Hydantoin derivatives	Sulfonamides
Ibuprofen	Sulindac
Indomethacin	Tolmetin

See Chapter 91, Drug-Induced Skin Disorders, authored by Phillip A. Nowakowski, PharmD, Jean A. Rumsfield, PharmD, and Dennis P. West, PhD, FCCP, for a more detailed discussion of this topic.

Appendix 2

▶ DRUG-INDUCED RENAL DISEASE

TABLE A2.1. Classification of Nephrotoxic Drugs by their Therapeutic Use

Cardiovascular
Angiotensin-converting enzyme inhibitors (H)
Calcium channel blockers (H)
Captopril (G, H,[a] I)
Hydralazine (G)
Mannitol (T, H)
Methyldopa (I)
Propranolol (H)
Thiazide and loop diuretics (I)
Triamterene (H, I, N[a])
Thromboclytics (V)
Warfarin sodium (I, V)

Antimicrobial
Acyclovir (O)
Aminoglycosides (T,[a] I)
Amphotericin B (T)
Aztreonam (I)
Cephalosporins (I,[a] T)
Ciprofloxacin (I)
Erythromycin (I)
Penicillins (I)
Pentamidine (T)
Rifampin (I,[a] G)
Sulfadiazine (O)
Sulfonamides (I,[a] O)
Tetracyclines (P, T, I)
Trimethoprim (P)
Vancomycin (I)

Rheumatologic
Acetaminophen (T, PN)
Acetylsalicylic acid (H)
Allopurinol (I,[a] N)
d-Penicillamine (G)
Nonsteroidal anti-inflammatory drugs (G, H,[a] I, T, PN)
Gold (G,[a] I)

Neuropsychiatric
Amoxapine (T)
Carbamazepine (I)

Lithium (G, I)
Phenobarbital (I)
Phenytoin (I)
Valproic acid (I)

Gastrointestinal
Cimetidine (I, P[a])
Magnesium antacids (N)
Phosphate enemas (O)
Ranitidine (I)
Vasopressin (O)

Cancer Chemotherapy
Carboplatinum (T)
Cisplatin (T,[a] V)
Interleukin 2
Methotrexate (O)
Mithramycin (T)
Mitomycin C (V)
Nitrosoureas (methyl CCNU) (I)
Streptozotocin (T)

Immunosuppressive
Corticosteroids (P)
Cyclosporine (H,[a] I,[a] T, V)
Tacrolimus (FK 506) (H, I)
Interferon alfa (G, I)
Muromonab-CD3 (OKT3) (H)

Drugs of Abuse
Amphetamine (V)
Cocaine (O)
Heroin (G, O)
Phencyclidine (O)

Miscellaneous
Ascorbic acid (O)
Glyburide (I)
Lovastatin (O)
Methoxyflurane anesthesia (T, O)
Radiographic contrast agents (H, T)

Key: I, interstitial nephritis; H, hemodynamically mediated; N, nephrolithiasis; G, glomerulopathy; T, tubular necrosis; O, intratubular obstruction; P, pseudo renal failure; V, vasculopathy; PN, papillary necrosis.
[a]Most common of multiple mechanisms.

TABLE A2.2. Drugs that Interfere with the Jaffe Measurement of Creatinine and Can Falsely Increase the Serum Creatinine Concentration

Cefoxitin
Cephalothin
Cefazolin
Cefotaxime
Flucytosine
Methyldopa

TABLE A2.3. Drugs that Cause Tubular Necrosis

Higher Incidence	Lower Incidence
Acetaminophen (overdose)	Amoxapine
Aminoglycosides	Carboplatin
Amphotericin B	Cyclosporine
Cisplatin	Low-molecular-weight dextran
Radiographic contrast agents	Mannitol
Streptozocin	Methoxyflurane anesthesia
	NSAIDs
	Tetracycline

TABLE A2.4. Potential Risk Factors for Aminoglycoside Nephrotoxicity

A. Aminoglycoside dosing:
    Large total cumulative dose
    Prolonged therapy
    High 1-hour postdose concentration
    Trough concentration >2 mg/L
    Recent previous aminoglycoside therapy

B. Synergistic nephrotoxicity. Aminoglycosides in combination with:
    Cyclosporine
    Amphotericin B
    Vancomycin
    Diuretics

C. Predisposing conditions in the patient:
    Preexisting renal insufficiency
    Increased age
    Poor nutrition
    Shock
    Gram-negative bacteremia
    Liver disease
    Hypoalbuminemia
    Obstructive jaundice
    Dehydration
    Potassium or magnesium deficiencies

TABLE A2.5. Considerations for Use of Newer, Lower Osmolar Radiocontrast Agents Compared to Older, Higher Osmolar Ionic Radiocontrast Agents

Advantages:
    Less histamine release with fewer allergic or hemodynamic adverse effects.
    Less nephrotoxicity (30–50% decreased incidence in patients with preexisting nondiabetic or diabetic renal insufficiency).

Disadvantage:
    Greater than 10-fold higher cost.

TABLE A2.6. Commonly Used Drugs that Cause Allergic Interstitial Nephritis

Antibiotics
  Acyclovir
  Aminoglycosides
  Amphotericin B
  Aztreonam
  Cephalosporins
  Ciprofloxacin
  Erythromycin
  Ethambutol
  Penicillins
  Polymyxin B
  Rifampin
  Sulfonamides
  Tetracyclines
  Trimethoprim-sulfamethoxazole
  Vancomycin

Neuropsychiatric
  Carbamazepine
  Lithium
  Phenobarbital
  Nonsteroidal anti-inflammatory drugs
  Phenytoin
  Valproic acid

Diuretics
  Acetazolamide
  Amiloride
  Chlorthalidone
  Furosemide
  Triamterene
  Thiazides

Miscellaneous
  Acetaminophen
  Allopurinol
  Interferon alfa
  Aspirin
  Captopril
  Cimetidine
  Clofibrate
  Cyclosporine
  Glyburide
  Gold
  Methyldopa
  p-Aminosalicylic acid
  Phenylpropanolamine
  Propylthiouracil
  Radiographic contrast media
  Ranitidine
  Sulfinpyrazone
  Warfarin sodium

Appendix 3

TABLE A3.1. Drugs that Induce Apnea

Central Nervous System Depression	
Narcotic analgesics	F[a]
Barbiturates	F
Benzodiazepines	F
Other sedatives and hypnotics	I
Tricyclic antidepressants	R
Phenothiazines	R
Ketamine	R
Promazine	R
Anesthetics	R
Antihistamines	R
Alcohol	I
L-Dopa	R
Oxygen	R
Respiratory Muscle Dysfunction	
Aminoglycoside antibiotics	I
Polymyxin antibiotics	I
Neuromuscular blockers	I
Quinine	R
Digitalis	R
Myopathy	
Corticosteroids	F
Diuretics	I
Aminocaproic acid	R
Clofibrate	R

[a]Relative frequency of reactions: F, frequent; I, infrequent; R, rare.

TABLE A3.2. Drugs that Induce Bronchospasm

Anaphylaxis (IgE-Meditated)		Anaphylactoid Mast Cell Degranulation	
Penicillins	F[a]	Narcotic analgesics	I
Sulfonamides	F	Ethylenediamine	R
Serum	F	Iodinated-radiocontrast media	F
Cephalosporins	F	Platinum	R
Bromelin	R	Local anesthetics	I
Cimetidine	R	Steroidal anesthetics	I
Papain	F	Iron–dextran complex	I
Pancreatic extract	I	Pancuronium bromide	R
Psyllium	I	Benzalkonium chloride	I
Subtilase	I	**Pharmacologic Effect**	
Tetracyclines	I	β-Adrenergic receptor blockers	I–F
Allergen extracts	I	Cholinergic stimulants	I
L-Asparaginase	F	Anticholinesterases	R
Pyrazolone analgesics	I	α-Adrenergic agonists	R
Direct Airway Irritation		Ethylenediamine tetraacetic acid (EDTA)	R
Acetate	R	**Unknown Mechanisms**	
Bisulfite	F	ACE inhibitors	I
Cromolyn	R	Anticholinergics	R
Smoke	F	Hydrocortisone	R
N-Acetylcysteine	F	Isoproterenol	R
Inhaled steroids	I	Monosodium glutamate	I
Precipitating IgG Antibodies		Piperazine	R
α-Methyl dopa	R	Tartrazine	R
Carbamazepine	R	Sulfinpyrazone	R
Spiramycin	R		
Cyclooxygenase Inhibition			
Aspirin/NSAIDs	F		
Phenylbutazone	I		
Acetaminophen	R		

[a]Relative frequency of reactions: F, frequent; I, infrequent; R, rare.

TABLE A3.3. Therapeutic Agents that Induce Pulmonary Edema

Cardiogenic Pulmonary Edema

Excessive intravenous fluids	F[a]
Blood and plasma transfusions	F
Corticosteroids	F
Phenylbutazone	R
Sodium diatrizoate	R
Hypertonic intrathecal saline	R
β_2-Adrenergic agonists	I

Noncardiogenic Pulmonary Edema

Heroin	F
Methadone	I
Morphine	I
Oxygen	I
Propoxyphene	R
Ethchlorvynol	R
Chlordiazepoxide	R
Salicylate	R
Hydrochlorothiazide	R
Triamterene + hydrochlorothiazide	R
Iron dextran	R
Methotrexate	R
Cytosine arabinoside	R
Nitrofurantoin	R
Dextran 40	R
Fluorescein	R
Amitriptyline	R
Colchicine	R
Nitrogen mustard	R
Epinephrine	R
Metaraminol	R
Bleomycin	R
Iodide	R
Cyclophosphamide	R
Teniposide	R

[a]Relative frequency of reactions: F, frequent; I, infrequent; R, rare.

TABLE A3.4. Drugs that Induce Pneumonitis and/or Fibrosis

Oxygen	F[a]
Radiation	F
Bleomycin	F
Busulfan	F
Carmustine	F
Hexamethonium	F
Paraquat	F
Amiodarone	F
Mecamylamine	I
Pentolinium	I
Cyclophosphamide	I
Methotrexate	I
Mitomycin	I
Nitrofurantoin	I
Methysergide	I
Azathioprine, 6-mercaptopurine	R
Chlorambucil	R
Melphalan	R
Lomustine and semustine	R
Procarbazine	R
Teniposide	R
Sulfasalazine	R
Phenytoin	R
Gold salts	R
Pindolol	R
Imipramine	R
Penicillamine	R
Phenylbutazone	R

[a]Relative frequency of reactions: F, frequent; I, infrequent; R, rare.

TABLE A3.5. Drugs that Induce Pulmonary Infiltrate with Eosinophilia (Loeffler's Syndrome)

Nitrofurantoin	F[a]	Tetracycline	R
para-Aminosalicylic acid	F	Procarbazine	R
Sulfonamides	I	Cromolyn	R
Penicillins	I	Niridazole	R
Methotrexate	I	Gold salts	R
Imipramine	I	Chlorpromazine	R
Chlorpropamide	R	Naproxen	R
Carbamazepine	R	Sulindac	R
Phenytoin	R	Ibuprofen	R
Mephenesin	R		

[a]Relative frequency of reactions: F, frequent; I, infrequent; R, rare.

TABLE A3.6. Drugs that May Induce Pleural Effusions and Fibrosis

Idiopathic	
Methysergide	F[a]
Pindolol	R
Methotrexate	R
Nitrofurantoin	R
Due to Drug-Induced Lupus Syndrome	
Procainamide	F
Hydralazine	F
Isoniazid	R
Phenytoin	R
Mephenytoin	R
Griseofulvin	R
Trimethadione	R
Sulfonamides	R
Phenylbutazone	R
Streptomycin	R
Ethosuximide	R
Tetracycline	R
Pseudolymphoma Syndrome	
Cyclosporine	R
Phenytoin	R

[a]Relative frequency of reactions: F, frequent; I, infrequent; R, rare.

INDEX

Page numbers of chapter titles are in *italicized* type. Page numbers followed by t and f refer to tables and figures.

Index

Index

Index

Index

Candidiasis (cont.)
hematogenous, 461–462
in HIV-infected patient, treatment, 488t
mucocutaneous, 460–461
Candiduria, 462
Cannabinoids, for chemotherapy-induced nausea and vomiting, 304t–305t, 308–309
CAPD. *See* Continuous peritoneal dialysis, ambulatory
Capsaicin, for osteoarthritis, 13
Captopril
hemodynamics, 73t
for hypertension, 101t, 105, 112
Carbamazepine
for bipolar disorders, 848, 849–851
adverse effects, 850
baseline and routine laboratory monitoring, 849–850
in combination therapy, 850–851
dosing, 849
plasma concentrations, 849
in pregnancy and lactation, 850
proposed mechanism of action, 849
for epileptic seizure, 628t, 629t, 631t, 632t, 633–634
thyroid preparations and, 228
Carbamide peroxide, for chronic purulent otitis media, 521
Carbenicillin, for peritonitis, 499
Carbidopa-levodopa, for Parkinson's disease, 672t, 673–675
Carbohydrate metabolism, 203–204
Carbonic anhydrase inhibitors, for open-angle glaucoma, 807, 809t, 810t
Carcinoma. *See* Oncologic disorders; *specific cancers*
Cardiac Arrhythmias Suppression Trial, 41
Cardiac catheterization, for unstable angina pectoris, 125
Cardiac conditions, endocarditis prophylaxis and, 450t
Cardiac surgery
prophylaxis prior to, 575t, 577
valve replacement, 170–171
Cardiogenic shock. *See also* Shock, hypovolemic and cardiogenic
defined, 141
hemodynamic profile, 146t
pathophysiology, 141
Cardiopulmonary resuscitation, 55–61
clinical manifestations, 55–56
defined, 55
desired outcomes, 56
diagnosis, 56
long-term strategies, 60
outcome evaluation, 60–61
pathophysiology, 55

pharmacotherapy in
for asystole and PEA, 59–60
for VF and pulseless VT, 57–59
principles, 56
Cardiovascular disease, in women
as menopause indication, 346
treatment, estrogen replacement, 350
Cardiovascular disorders
arrhythmias, *37–54*
cardiopulmonary resuscitation, *55–61*
congestive heart failure, *62–78*
hyperlipidemia, *79–94*
hypertension, *95–113*
ischemic heart disease, *114–127*
myocardial infarction, acute, *128–140*
shock, hypovolemic and cardiogenic, *141–160*
stroke, *161–171*
thromboembolic disorders, *172–187*
Cardiovascular drugs, used in sepsis, 537t
Cardiovascular system
acute renal failure effect on, 979
antipsychotics effect on, 883–884
Cardioversion, for atrial fibrillation or atrial flutter, 43, 44–45
Carnitine, status assessment, 692, 696
Carotid endarterectomy, in occlusive cerebrovascular disease, 169–170
Carteolol, for hypertension, 103t, 104
Carvedilol, for chronic CHF, 77
Casanthrol, for constipation, 248t, 249
Cascara sagrada, for constipation, 248t, 249
CAST. *See* Cardiac Arrhythmias Suppression Trial
Castor oil, for constipation, 250
Cat bites, infection from, 565–566
Catecholamines, for shock, 146–147
Cathartics, saline, for constipation, 248t, 249–250
Catheterized patients, urinary tract infection in, 604
CAVH. *See* Continuous hemofiltration, arteriovenous
CBZ. *See* Carbamazepine
CCPD. *See* Continuous peritoneal dialysis, cycling
Cefaclor
for diabetic foot infection, 568
for otitis media, 518t–520t, 521
Cefadroxil, for bacterial cellulitis, 559t, 560
Cefazolin
for bacterial cellulitis, 559t, 560
for endocarditis
staphylococcal, 443t, 444
streptococcal, 439, 442t
for osteomyelitis, 416
for surgical prophylaxis, 575t
Cefixime, for otitis media, 518t–520t, 521
Cefonicid, for osteomyelitis, 418

Index

Chemotherapy (cont.)
for chronic leukemias
lymphocytic, 773
myeloproliferative, 768–771, 769t
for colorectal cancer, 750–755, 752t, 753t,
754f, 755t
emetogenic potential of, 301t
for Hodgkin's disease, 783–785, 784t,
785t
hyperpigmentation caused by, 1052t
for lung cancer, 777–779, 778t, 779t
nausea and vomiting induced by, pharmacologic treatment, 304t–305t,
307–309
for prostate cancer, 803
Chest pain, as hemodialysis complication,
924t
Chest roentgenogram, for COLD diagnosis,
1033–1034
CHF. See Congestive heart failure
Child-Pugh classification, liver disease, 233,
233t
Children
antidepressant therapy for, 869
chlamydia treatment in, 549, 550t
constipation in, management recommendations, 251
dog bite treatment in, 565
gonorrhea treatment in, 542t, 544
hepatitis B vaccine for, 286, 287t
immunization schedules for, 608t
tuberculous treatment in, 591
upper respiratory infections in
antibiotic regimen for, 517, 520t
otitis media management, 522f
Chlamydia
clinical presentation, 548–549
diagnosis, 549
epidemiology, 548
treatment, 549, 550t
outcome evaluation, 549
Chlamydia trachomatis infection. *See*
Chlamydia
Chloramphenicol
for epiglottitis, 528
for infectious arthritis, 418
interactions, 408t
for meningococcus, 428
for osteomyelitis, 417
for salmonellosis, 472
Chlorpromazine, for schizophrenia, 874
dosage and dosage forms, 876t
initial therapy, 877
pharmacokinetics, 876
stabilization of therapy, 878
Chlorpropamide
for diabetes type 2, 207, 210t
metabolite of, pharmacologic activity,
942t

Chlorprothixene, for schizophrenia, 876t
ChlVPP, for Hodgkin's disease, 783–784,
784t, 785
Cholangitis, treatment for, 501t. *See also*
Intra-abdominal infections
Cholecystitis, acute, treatment for, 501t. *See
also* Intra-abdominal infections
Cholera, 466–467, 469
antibiotic selection for, 468t
Cholestyramine
for hyperlipidemia, 86, 88, 89t
thyroid preparations and, 228
Choloxin. *See* Dextrothyroxine
Cholybar. *See* Cholestyramine
Chronic bronchitis. *See also* Chronic
obstructive lung disease
clinical presentation, 505–506, 506t,
1031–1032, 1032t
desired outcome, 506
epidemiology and etiology, 505
pathophysiology, 505, 1030
treatment, 506–508, 507t
Chronic disease, anemia treatment in,
373–374
Chronic hypertension, in pregnancy,
357–358
Chronic leukemias. *See* Chronic lymphocytic
leukemia; Chronic myelogenous
leukemia
Chronic lymphocytic leukemia
clinical presentation, 771
defined, 767
diagnosis, 772, 772t
pathophysiology, 771
treatment
desired outcome, 772
methods, 773
principles, 772–773
Chronic myelogenous leukemia
clinical presentation, 768
defined, 767
diagnosis, 768
pathophysiology, 767–768
treatment
in blastic phase, 770–771
conventional chemotherapy, 768–770,
769t
desired outcome, 768
interferons, 770
marrow transplantation, 771
outcome evaluation, 771
Chronic obstructive lung disease, *1030–1040*
clinical presentation, 1031–1033
definitions, 1030
diagnosis, 1033–1034
pathophysiology, 1030–1033, 1032t
treatment
antibiotics, 1039–1040
anticholinergics, 1036

Index

Index

Diarrhea, *252–259*
  bacterial causes
    antibiotic selection for, 468t
    enterotoxigenic, 466–470
    invasive, 470–474
  clinical presentation, 253–254
  defined, 252
  drugs inducing, 253t
  epidemiology, 252
  pathophysiology, 252
  treatment
    for acute diarrhea, 255f
    for chronic diarrhea, 256f
    desired outcome, 254
    outcome evaluation, 259
    pharmacologic therapy, 254, 258–259
    principles, 254, 255f–256f, 257t
    rehydration therapy, 257t, 465, 467t
  viral causes, 474–475
Diazepam
  for chemotherapy-induced nausea and
    vomiting, 305t, 309
  for convulsive status epilepticus, 680,
    681t, 682t
  pharmacokinetic changes during liver fail-
    ure, 236t
Diazoxide, for hypertension, in urgencies
  and emergencies, 112
Dibenzoxapines, for schizophrenia, 876t
Dibenzoxazepines, for depressive disorders,
  857t, 860
  drug interactions, 867t
  pharmacokinetics, 863t
  side effects, 859t
DIC. *See* Disseminated intravascular coagulation
Dicloxacillin
  for bacterial cellulitis, 558, 559t
  for osteomyelitis, 417
Didanosine, for HIV-infected patient, 483,
  484t, 490, 491t
Diet, nutrition assessment. *See* Nutrition
  assessment
Dietary therapy, for hyperlipidemia, 85t,
  85–86
Diethylstilbestrol, fetal drug effects, 365
Digitalis, for chronic congestive heart failure, 75–76
  hemodynamics, 73t
  toxicity, 77t
Digoxin
  for atrial fibrillation and atrial flutter, 44, 45
  for chronic congestive heart failure
    hemodynamics, 73t
    pharmacokinetics, 76
Dihydroindolone, for schizophrenia, 876t
Diltiazem
  for acute myocardial infarction, 136
  for hypertension, 101t, 107

  for ischemic heart disease, 122
    coronary artery spasm and variant
      angina pectoris, 126
    effect on myocardial oxygen demand,
      119t, 123
    unstable angina pectoris, 124
Diphenoxylate, for diarrhea, 258t
Diphenylmethane derivatives, for constipation, 248t, 249
Diphtheria antitoxin, 609
Diphtheria toxoid adsorbed, 609
Diplococcus, 426t, 428–429
Dipyridamole, following prosthetic cardiac
  valve replacement, 170
Direct-current cardioversion, for atrial fibrillation or atrial flutter, 43, 44–45
Disease-modifying antirheumatic drugs
  azathioprine, 35
  cyclophosphamide, 35
  cyclosporine, 35D36
  gold preparations, 33
  hydroxychloroquine, 35
  methotrexate, 32
  penicillamine, 35
  sulfasalazine, 35
  treatment principles, 32, 34t
Disinfection, infected pressure ulcers, 563,
  564t
Disseminated intravascular coagulation
  clinical presentation, 378, 379t
  diagnosis, 380
  in pregnancy, 354
  treatment, 388–389
    sequential therapy, 388–389
Distribution, of drugs. *See* Volume of distribution
Disulfiram, for drug dependence reduction,
  906–907
Diuretics
  for acute renal failure, 977–978
    prevention, 977
  for ascites, 240
  for congestive heart failure
    acute or severe form, 66t, 72
    chronic form, 73t, 73–74
  for hypertension, 98–99, 100t
  and lithium interaction, 847t–848t, 849
  for osteoporosis prevention, 23
  septic shock and, 538
Divalproex sodium, for bipolar disorders,
  851–852
  adverse effects, 851–852
  dosing, 851
  drug interactions, 852
  proposed mechanism of action, 851
DKA. *See* Diabetic ketoacidosis
DMARDs. *See* Disease-modifying
  antirheumatic drugs
DMPA (depomedroxyprogesterone acetate),

Index

Index

Index

Index

Index

Ischemia, cerebral, pathophysiology, 162f, 163
Ischemic heart disease, 114–127. *See also* Angina pectoris
  clinical presentation, 115, 116t
  defined, 114
  diagnosis, 116–118
  pathophysiology, 114–115
  treatment
    for coronary artery spasm and variant angina pectoris, 126–127
    desired outcome, 118
    drug therapy, 118–122, 119t
    outcome evaluation, 127
    risk factor modification, 118
    for stable exertional angina pectoris, 122–123
    for unstable angina pectoris, 124, 125f, 126
ISDN. *See* Isosorbide dinitrate
ISMN. *See* Isosorbide mononitrate
Isolated systolic hypertension, defined, 95
Isoniazid
  interactions, 408t
  for *Mycobacterium tuberculosis,* in HIV-infected patient, 485
  for tuberculosis, 586–587
  for tuberculous meningitis, 431, 432
Isoproterenol, for shock, 151t
Isosorbide dinitrate
  for chronic CHF, 74
    hemodynamics, 73t
  for ischemic heart disease, 120
    coronary artery spasm and variant angina pectoris, 126
Isosorbide mononitrate, for ischemic heart disease, 120
Isosporiasis, treatment in HIV-infected patient, 489t
Isotonic hyponatremia
  diagnostic approach, 952f
  etiology, 951
Isotretinoin
  for acne, 191t, 193–194
  fetal drug effects, 365
Isovolemic hyponatremia
  clinical presentation, 953
  etiology, 953
  treatment, 953
Isuprel. *See* Isoproterenol
Itching. *See* Pruritus
Itraconazole
  for coccidioidomycosis, 458
  for histoplasmosis, in HIV-infected patient, 488t
  interactions, 408t
  for invasive aspergillosis, 464
IUD contraception, 334t–335t

Jaffe measurement of creatinine, drugs interfering with, 1054t
Jarisch-Herxheimer reaction, 548
Joints
  disorders. *See* Bone and joint disorders
  infections. *See* Bone and joint infections

Kabikinase. *See* Streptokinase
Kaolin-pectin mixture, for diarrhea, 258t
Karaya, infected pressure ulcer treatment and, 564
Keratolytics
  for acne, 191t, 192
  for psoriasis, 197t, 198
Ketoconazole
  for blastomycosis, 457
  for candidiasis
    in HIV-infected patient, 488t
    in non-HIV-infected patient, 460, 461
  for coccidioidomycosis, 458
  for prostate cancer, 801
Kidney. *See* Renal *entries*
Koate-HP, for von Willebrand's disease, 386
Koate-HS, for von Willebrand's disease, 386
Kytril. *See* Granisetron

Labetalol
  for hypertension, 103t
    in urgencies and emergencies, 112–113
  in liver failure, pharmacokinetic changes, 236t
Labor
  induction, 361
  preterm, treatment, 359–360
Lactation
  antipsychotics use in, 886
  carbamazepine therapy in, 850
  drug use during, 365–366
    anticonvulsants, 366
    hypoglycemic agents, 366
    insulin, 366
    selected drugs, 366
  lithium therapy and, 845
  pregnancy and, therapeutic considerations, *352–366*
Lactobacillus preparations, for diarrhea, 258, 258t
Lactulose
  for constipation, 248t, 249
  for hepatic encephalopathy, 241, 242f
Lacunar infarcts
  clinical presentation, 165
  diagnosis, 166
  pathophysiology, 162f, 163
Lamivudine, for HIV-infected patient, 483, 484t, 490, 491t

Index

Metoprolol
  for acute myocardial infarction
    early administration, 136, 137f
    late administration, 136
  for chronic CHF, 77
  for hypertension, 103t, 103–104
Metronidazole
  for hepatic encephalopathy, 243
  for inflammatory bowel disease, 295
  interactions, 408t
  for intra-abdominal infections, 498
  for peptic ulcer disease, 327, 328t
  for trichomoniasis, 554, 555t
Mevacor. *See* Lovastatin
MI. *See* Myocardial infarction, acute
Micronase. *See* Glyburide
Micronutrients, in nutrition assessment, 697, 698t
Midazolam, for status epilepticus, 682t, 683, 684
Middle ear infections. *See* Otitis media
Midrin, for migraine headache, 645
Migraine headache, *641–649*
  clinical presentation, 641–642
  diagnosis, 642–643
  pathophysiology, 641, 642t
  treatment
    abortive therapy, 643, 644t, 645
    prophylactic therapy, 645–647, 646t
Milk of magnesia, for constipation, 249
Milrinone
  for congestive heart failure, 70–71
    hemodynamic effects, 66t
  for shock, 151t
Mineral oil, for constipation, 247–248, 248t
Minoxidil, for hypertension, 101t, 106–107
Mirtazepine, for depressive disorders, 856, 858t, 859t
Mixed acid–base disorders
  diagnosis, 917–918
  pathophysiology, 917
  treatment, 918
Mixed episode, in bipolar disorder, 838
Mixed substance withdrawal, treatment, 906
Molindone, for schizophrenia, 876t
Monoamine oxidase inhibitors
  for depressive disorders, 858t, 861
    dietary restrictions, 861t
    medication restrictions, 862t
    pharmacokinetics, 864t
    side effects, 859t
  for panic disorders, 832, 833t, 834
MOPP chemotherapy regimen, for Hodgkin's disease, 783–784, 784t, 785t
Morphine
  for acute myocardial infarction, 132
  for acute pain management, 656t, 658–659, 659t
  metabolite of, pharmacologic activity, 942t

  for sickle cell anemia, 394
Mucocutaneous candidiasis, 460–461
  chronic form, 460
  esophageal, 461
  oral, 460–461
  vaginal, 461
Mucocutaneous herpes simplex infection, treatment in HIV-infected patient, 489t
Mucosal protectants
  for gastroesophageal reflux disease, 269
  thyroid preparations and, 228
Mumps vaccine, 616
Muscle function, nutrition assessment and, 692
MVPP, for Hodgkin's disease, 783–784, 784t
Mycobacterium avium complex, in HIV-infected patient
  clinical presentation, 479
  diagnosis, 480
  treatment, 486, 489t
Mycobacterium tuberculosis infection
  central nervous system, 431–432
  in HIV-infected patient, treatment, 485, 591
  pulmonary. *See* Tuberculosis
Mycoplasma pneumonia, 511–512
Mycoses, systemic. *See* Fungal infections
Myocardial infarction, acute, 128–140
  clinical presentation, 130
  defined, 128
  diagnosis, 130–131
  pathophysiology, 128–130, 129f
  treatment
    desired outcome, 131
    drug therapy, 132–139
    outcome evaluation, 139
    principles, 131–132
Myocardial oxygen demand, 128–140
Myringotomy, for recurrent acute otitis media, 520
Myxedema coma, treatment, 230

Nabilone, for chemotherapy-induced nausea and vomiting, 305t, 309
Nadolol
  for hypertension, 103t, 104
  for thyrotoxicosis, 222t, 224
Nafcillin
  for bacterial cellulitis, 558, 559t
  for infectious arthritis, 418
  for lymphangitis, 561
  for staphylococcal endocarditis, 439, 443t
Naloxone, septic shock and, 538
Naltrexone, for drug dependence reduction, 906–907
Narcolepsy
  clinical presentation, 894

Index

Index

Index

Index

Index

Index

Index